D0687661

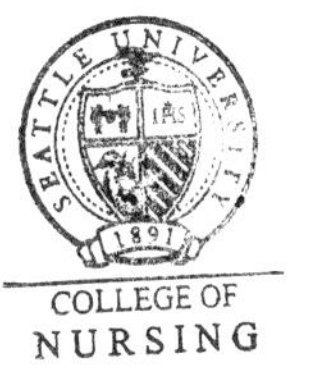
SEATTLE UNIVERSITY
1891
COLLEGE OF
NURSING

EVIDENCE-BASED GERIATRIC NURSING PROTOCOLS FOR BEST PRACTICE

Marie Boltz, PhD, RN, GNP-BC, FGSA, FAAN, is associate professor at the Boston College William F. Connell School of Nursing, where she teaches both advanced practice nursing and doctoral students. Also, she is currently a senior nurse scientist at the Munn Center for Nursing Research, Massachusetts General Hospital, and a gerontological nurse consultant at the Hospital of the University of Pennsylvania, the Office of Inspector General, and the Department of Justice. She served as director of practice at the Hartford Institute for Geriatric Nursing from 2003 to 2013. Her areas of research are the geriatric care environment including measures of quality, dementia-capable and family-centered interventions, the prevention of functional decline in hospitalized older adults, and the functional recovery of older adults during post-acute care. She has presented nationally and internationally, and authored and coauthored numerous journal publications, organizational tools, and book chapters in these areas, and has coedited five books. She is the lead editor for *Evidence-Based Geriatric Nursing Protocols for Best Practice.*

Dr. Boltz is a former John A. Hartford Foundation Claire Fagin fellow (2009–2011), recipient of the American Nurses Credentialing Center (ANCC) Margretta Madden Styles Credentialing Scholar Award, and Eastern Nursing Research Society John A. Hartford Geriatric Nursing Research Award. She is a fellow in the American Academy of Nursing and the Gerontological Society of America. Dr. Boltz received her bachelor's degree in nursing from LaSalle University, her master's degree as a geriatric nurse practitioner from the University of Pennsylvania, and her doctoral degree from New York University. She participated in postdoctoral study at the University of Maryland.

Elizabeth (Liz) Capezuti, PhD, RN, FAAN, is the William Randolph Hearst chair in gerontology and assistant dean for research at the Hunter-Bellevue School of Nursing of Hunter College of the City University of New York (CUNY). Dr. Capezuti teaches in the graduate doctor of nursing practice (DNP) program and is a professor in the Graduate Center and the PhD program in nursing science of CUNY. She is known for her work in improving the care of older adults by interventions and models that positively influence health care providers' knowledge and work environment. Dr. Capezuti's research interests include fall prevention, restraint and side-rail elimination, APN-facilitated models, palliative care, the geriatric nursing work environment, and the design of the "built environment" to facilitate function. Dr. Capezuti has disseminated the findings of 35 funded projects in five coedited books and more than 100 peer-reviewed articles and book chapters. She is the recipient of the Otsuka/American Geriatrics Society Outstanding Scientific Achievement for Clinical Investigation Award in 2001 and received the American Academy of Nursing Nurse Leader in Aging Award in 2013. Dr. Capezuti received her bachelor's degree in nursing at the Lehman College (CUNY), her master's degree as a geriatric advanced practice nurse from Hunter College, and her doctoral degree in nursing from the University of Pennsylvania.

Terry Fulmer, PhD, RN, FAAN, is president of the John A. Hartford Foundation and leads its work to improve the health of older adults in the United States. Dr. Fulmer was previously university distinguished professor and dean of the Bouvé College of Health Sciences at Northeastern University where she was also professor of Public Policy and Urban Affairs in the College of Social Sciences and Humanities. Previous to her role as dean of the Bouvé College of Health Sciences, Dr. Fulmer served as the Erline Perkins McGriff Professor of Nursing and founding dean of the New York University (NYU) College of Nursing. Dr. Fulmer is nationally and internationally recognized as a leading expert in geriatrics, and is best known for her research on elder abuse and neglect, which has been funded by the National Institute on Aging and the National Institute for Nursing Research. Dr. Fulmer is an elected member of the Institute of Medicine and serves as the chair of the National Advisory Committee for the Robert Wood Johnson Foundation Executive Nurse Fellows program. She has served as the first nurse on the board of the American Geriatrics Society and as the first nurse to serve as president of the Gerontological Society of America. For 15 years, Dr. Fulmer served as the codirector of the Hartford Institute for Geriatric Nursing at NYU, which the foundation began supporting in 1996. She has also held faculty appointments at Boston College, Columbia University, Yale University, and the Harvard Division on Aging. Dr. Fulmer received her bachelor's degree from Skidmore College, her master's and doctoral degrees from Boston College, and her geriatric nurse practitioner postmaster's certificate from NYU. She has received the status of fellow in the American Academy of Nursing, the Gerontological Society of America, and the New York Academy of Medicine.

DeAnne Zwicker, DrNP, AGNP-BC, is an American Nurses Credentialing Center (ANCC)-certified adult nurse practitioner and geriatric nurse practitioner. She is currently working as an independent geriatric consultant. She completed her doctor of nursing practice degree in 2010 with a primary focus as a clinical scientist and secondary in nursing education at Drexel University in Philadelphia. Her dissertation was a mixed-method study titled, "Preparedness, Appraisal of Behaviors, and Role Strain in Dementia Family Caregivers and the Caregiver Perspective of Preparedness." She has been a coeditor and chapter author for many versions of the *Evidence-Based Geriatric Nursing Protocols for Best Practice* book, as well as a content editor for ConsultGeriRN.org since its inception. She has been a registered nurse for 32 years with clinical practice experience as a geriatric nurse practitioner since 1992 in primary care, subacute, long-term care, and recently palliative care and a clinical expert consultant in many domains in geriatrics. She has also taught nursing at the graduate level at New York University, Drexel University, and George Mason University. Her areas of interest in geriatrics include proactive intervention in older adults to prevent adverse drug events, pain control to aid in maintaining function and quality of life, and preventing hospital iatrogenesis particularly in persons with dementia.

EVIDENCE-BASED GERIATRIC NURSING PROTOCOLS FOR BEST PRACTICE

Fifth Edition

Marie Boltz, PhD, RN, GNP-BC, FGSA, FAAN

Elizabeth Capezuti, PhD, RN, FAAN

Terry Fulmer, PhD, RN, FAAN

DeAnne Zwicker, DrNP, AGNP-BC

Editors

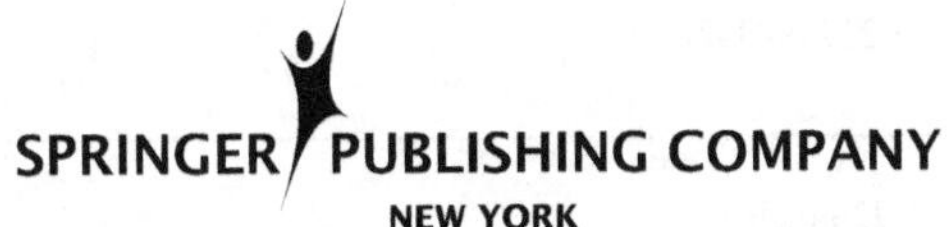

SPRINGER PUBLISHING COMPANY
NEW YORK

Springer Publishing Company, LLC
11 West 42nd Street
New York, NY10036
www.springerpub.com

Acquisitions Editor: Elizabeth Nieginski
Composition: Newgen KnowledgeWorks

ISBN: 978-0-8261-7166-5
e-book ISBN: 978-0-8261-7167-2
PowerPoint ISBN: 978-0-8261-7169-6
Test Bank ISBN: 978-0-8261-7189-4

Instructors' materials: Qualified instructors may request supplements by e-mailing textbook@springerpub.com

16 17 18 19 / 5 4 3 2 1

Library of Congress Cataloging-in-Publication Data
Names: Boltz, Marie, editor. | Capezuti, Liz, editor. | Fulmer, Terry T., editor. | Zwicker, DeAnne, editor.
Title: Evidence-based geriatric nursing protocols for best practice / Marie Boltz, Elizabeth Capezuti, Terry Fulmer, DeAnne Zwicker, editors.
Description: 5th edition. | New York, NY : Springer Publishing Company, LLC, [2016] | Preceded by Evidence-based geriatric nursing protocols for best practice / [edited by] Marie Boltz ... [et al.]. 4th ed. 2012. | Includes bibliographical references and index.
Identifiers: LCCN 2015048172| ISBN 9780826171665 | ISBN 1617181954321 (e-book)
Subjects: | MESH: Geriatric Nursing—methods | Nursing Care | Nursing Assessment | Aged | Evidence-Based Nursing
Classification: LCC RC954 | NLM WY 152 | DDC 618.97/0231—dc23
LC record available at http://lccn.loc.gov/2015048172

Printed in the United States of America by R. R. Donnelley.

Contents

PART V. MODELS OF CARE

Contributors

Elizabeth A. Ayello, PhD, RN, ACNS-BC, CWON, ETN, MAPWCA, FAAN
Faculty
Excelsior College School of Nursing
Clinical Editor
Advances in Skin and Wound Care
Senior Advisor
John A. Hartford Institute for Geriatric Nursing, New York University
Course Coordinator
International Interprofessional Wound Care Course (IIWCC), New York University
New York, New York

Michele C. Balas, PhD, RN, APRN-NP, CCRN
Associate Professor
Center of Excellence in Complex and Critical Care
The Ohio State University, College of Nursing
Columbus, Ohio

Melissa Batchelor-Murphy, PhD, RN-BC, FNP-BC
Assistant Professor
Duke University School of Nursing
Durham, North Carolina

Cheri Blevins, MSN, RN, CCRN, CCNS
Clinical Nurse Specialist
Medical Intensive Care Unit
Adjunct Faculty
University of Virginia School of Nursing
Charlottesville, Virginia

Rebecca Bolton, BSN, RN
Boston College
Chestnut Hill, Massachusetts

Marie Boltz, PhD, RN, GNP-BC, FGSA, FAAN
Associate Professor
William F. Connell School of Nursing
Boston College
Chestnut Hill, Massachusetts

Stewart M. Bond, PhD, RN, AOCN
Assistant Professor
William F. Connell School of Nursing
Boston College
Chestnut Hill, Massachusetts

Cheryl M. Bradas, PhD(c), RN, GCNS-BC, CNRN
Geriatric Clinical Nurse Specialist
Specialty Care Patient Care Unit: Acute Care Units
MetroHealth Medical Center
Cleveland, Ohio

Christine Bradway, PhD, GNP-BC, FAAN
Associate Professor of Gerontological Nursing
Biobehavioral Health Sciences Department
University of Pennsylvania School of Nursing
Philadelphia, Pennsylvania

Pamela Z. Cacchione, PhD, RN, CRNP, BC, FGSA, FAAN
Ralston House Term Chair in Gerontological Nursing
Associate Professor of Geropsychiatric Nursing-Clinician Educator
Associate Director of the Center for Integrative Science of Aging
PENN SON Liason, National Hartford Centers of Gerontological Nursing Excellence
Interim Program Director of Psychiatric Mental Health Nursing Program
University of Pennsylvania School of Nursing
Philadelphia, Pennsylvania

Billy A. Caceres, MSN, RN-BC, AGPCNP-BC
PhD Candidate
New York University College of Nursing
New York, New York

Elizabeth Capezuti, PhD, RN, FAAN
William Randolph Hearst Foundation Chair in Gerontology
Assistant Dean for Research
Hunter-Bellevue School of Nursing
Hunter College of the City University of New York (CUNY)
Professor
Nursing PhD Program
CUNY Graduate Center
New York, New York

Colleen M. Casey, PhD, ANP-BC, CNS
Assistant Professor
Division of General Internal Medicine and Geriatrics
Director of Geriatric Outpatient Initiatives
Oregon Health & Science University, School of Medicine
Assistant Professor
Oregon Health & Science University, School of Nursing
Portland, Oregon

Eileen R. Chasens, PhD, RN, FAAN
Associate Professor and Vice-Chair for Administration
Department of Health and Community Systems
School of Nursing
University of Pittsburgh
Pittsburgh, Pennsylvania

Valerie T. Cotter, DrNP, AGPCNP-BC, FAANP
Advanced Senior Lecturer
University of Pennsylvania School of Nursing
Philadelphia, Pennsylvania

Sarah Crowgey, BSN, RN
Duke University School of Nursing
Durham, North Carolina

Lauren Crozier
Undergraduate Honors
BSN Nursing Student
The Ohio State University, College of Nursing
Columbus, Ohio

Constance Dahlin, ANP-BC, ACHPN, FPCN, FAAN
Palliative Care Specialist
Director of Professional Practice
Hospice and Palliative Nurses Association
Pittsburgh, Pennsylvania
Consultant, Center to Advance Palliative Care
New York, New York
Palliative Nurse Practitioner
North Shore Medical Center
Salem, Massachusetts

Grace E. Dean, PhD, RN
Adjunct Assistant Professor
Roswell Park Cancer Institute
Associate Professor
School of Nursing
State University of New York University at Buffalo
Buffalo, New York

Rose Ann DiMaria-Ghalili, PhD, RN, CNSC, FASPEN
Associate Professor
Doctoral Nursing
College of Nursing and Health Professions
Drexel University
Philadelphia, Pennsylvania

Annemarie Dowling-Castronovo, PhD, RN, GNP-BC
Associate Professor
The Evelyn L. Spiro School of Nursing
Wagner College
Staten Island, New York

Regina M. Fink, PhD, RN, AOCN, CHPN, FAAN
Research Nurse Scientist
Associate Professor
University of Colorado, College of Nursing and School of Medicine
Anschutz Medical Campus
Aurora, Colorado

Johan Flamaing, MD, PhD
Department of Geriatric Medicine
University Hospitals Leuven
Department of Clinical and Experimental Medicine
KU Leuven
Leuven, Belgium

Kathleen Fletcher, DNP, RN, GNP-BC, FAAN
Director, Geriatric Nurse Clinical Practice Program
Research Associate in Gerontological and Population Health
Riverside Center for Excellence in Aging and Lifelong Health
Riverside Health System
Newport News, Virginia
Clinical Assistant Professor of Nursing
University of Virginia School of Nursing
Charlottesville, Virginia

Marquis D. Foreman, PhD, RN, FAAN
John L. and Helen Kellogg Dean of Nursing
Professor, Adult Health and Gerontological Nursing
College of Nursing
Rush University
Chicago, Illinois

Janice B. Foust, PhD, RN
Assistant Professor
College of Nursing, Health Science
University of Massachusetts
Boston, Massachusetts

Terry Fulmer, PhD, RN, FAAN
President
John A. Hartford Foundation
New York, New York

Elizabeth Galik, PhD, CRNP
Associate Professor
University of Maryland School of Nursing
Baltimore, Maryland

Mindy S. Grall, PhD, APRN-BC
Director
Stroke and Cerebrovascular Program
Chair
Pain Resource Team
Baptist Health
Jacksonville, Florida

Deanna Gray-Miceli, PhD, GNP-BC, FGSA, FAANP, FAAN
Assistant Professor
Rutgers, School of Nursing
Newark, New Jersey; and
Institute of Health, Health Care Policy and Aging Research
New Brunswick, New Jersey

Mary Beth Happ, PhD, RN, FGSA, FAAN
Distinguished Professor of Critical Care Research
Director
Center of Excellence in Critical and Complex Care
The Ohio State University, College of Nursing
Columbus, Ohio

Theresa A. Harvath, PhD, RN, FAAN
Clinical Professor and Director of Clinical Education
Betty Irene Moore School of Nursing
University of California—Davis
Sacramento, California

Pieter Heeren, MSc, RN
Department of Public Health and Primary Care
Academic Centre for Nursing and Midwifery
KU Leuven
Department of Geriatrics
University Hospitals Leuven
Leuven, Belgium

Karen Hertz, RGN, MSc, BSc
Advanced Nurse Practitioner
University Hospital of North Midlands
Stoke-on-Trent, United Kingdom
Chair
International Collaboration of Orthopaedic Nursing (ICON)

Ami Hommel, RN, CNS, PhD
Associate Professor
Skane University Hospital and Malmo University
Malmo, Sweden
Ambassador
International Collaboration of Orthopaedic Nursing (ICON)

Ann L. Horgas, PhD, RN, FGSA, FAAN
Associate Professor
University of Florida
College of Nursing
Gainesville, Florida

Michelle L. Klimpt, BSN, RN
Nurse II
Department of Nursing
Roswell Park Cancer Institute
Buffalo, New York

Denise M. Kresevic, PhD, RN, APN-BC
Louis Stokes Cleveland VAMC
Geriatric Research Education Clinical Center (GRECC)
Associate Director of Education/Evaluation
Clinical Nurse Specialist
University Hospitals Case Medical Center
Cleveland, Ohio

Susan Kaplan Jacobs, MLS, MA, RN, AHIP
Health Sciences Librarian/Associate Curator
Elmer Holmes Bobst Library
New York University
New York, New York

Rona F. Levin, PhD, RN
Clinical Professor and Director
Doctor of Nursing Practice Program
New York University College of Nursing
New York, New York

Fidelindo Lim, DNP, CCRN
Clinical Assistant Professor
New York University College of Nursing
New York, New York

Valerie MacDonald, RN, MSN, ONC, CNS
Fraser Health Authority
Burnaby General Hospital, British Columbia
Adjunct Professor
University of British Columbia School of Nursing
Vancouver, British Columbia
Ambassador
International Collaboration of Orthopaedic Nursing (ICON)

Ann Butler Maher, MS, RN, FNP-BC, ONC
Family Nurse Practitioner
Long Branch, New Jersey
Ambassador
International Collaboration of Orthopaedic Nursing

Mary Beth Flynn Makic, RN, PhD, CNS, CCNS, FAAN, FNAP
Associate Professor
University of Colorado
Anschutz Medical Campus
College of Nursing
Aurora, Colorado

Michael L. Malone, MD
Medical Director
Aurora Senior Services & Aurora Visiting Nurse Association of Wisconsin
Aurora Health Care
Clinical Adjunct Professor of Medicine
University of Wisconsin School of Medicine and Public Health
Milwaukee, Wisconsin

Donna McCabe, DNP, APRN-BC, GNP, CWCN
Clinical Assistant Professor
New York University College of Nursing
New York, New York

Glenise L. McKenzie, PhD, RN
Associate Professor
Program Director
Baccalaureate Completion Program for RNs
Oregon Health & Science University, School of Nursing
Portland, Oregon

Anita J. Meehan, MSN, RN-BC, ONC, FNGNA
Clinical Nurse Specialist, Gerontology
Cleveland Clinic Akron General
Akron, Ohio
Ambassador
International Collaboration of Orthopaedic Nursing (ICON)

Janet C. Mentes, PhD, APRN, BC, FGSA, FAAN
Associate Professor and Co-Director
Center for the Advancement of Gerontological Nursing Science
University of California Los Angeles, School of Nursing
Los Angeles, California

Deborah C. Messecar, PhD, MPH, AGCNS-BC, RN
Associate Professor
Oregon Health & Science University, School of Nursing
Portland, Oregon

Koen Milisen, PhD, RN
Professor
Department of Public Health and Primary Care
Academic Centre for Nursing and Midwifery
KU Leuven
Department of Geriatrics
University Hospitals Leuven
Leuven, Belgium

Lorraine C. Mion, PhD, RN, FAAN
Independence Foundation Professor of Nursing
Director
Vanderbilt Center for Gerontological Nursing Excellence
Vanderbilt School of Nursing
Nashville, Tennessee

Jonna Lee Morris, MSN, RN
Doctoral Student
School of Nursing
University of Pittsburgh
Pittsburgh, Pennsylvania

Madeline A. Naegle, PhD, CNS-PMH, BC, FAAN
Professor
New York University College of Nursing
New York, New York

Linda J. O'Connor, MSN, RNC, GCNS-BC, LNC
Assistant Administrator for Nursing
and Hospital Affairs
Mount Sinai Health System
Mount Sinai Hospital
New York, New York

Kathleen S. Oman, PhD, RN, FAEN, FAAN
Children's Hospital
Colorado Chair in Pediatric Nursing
Associate Professor
University of Colorado, College of Nursing
Aurora, Colorado

Janine Overcash, PhD, GNP-BC, FAANP
Director of the Adult/Gerontological Nurse
Practitioner Program
Clinical Associate Professor
The Ohio State University, College of Nursing
Columbus, Ohio

Robert M. Palmer, MD, MPH
Director
Glennan Center for Geriatrics and Gerontology
Professor of Internal Medicine
Eastern Virginia Medical School
Norfolk, Virginia

Lenard L. Parisi, RN, MA, CPHQ, FNAHQ
Vice President
Quality Management and Performance Improvement
Metropolitan Jewish Health System
Brooklyn, New York

Ana Julia Parks
Undergraduate Nursing Student
Boston College
Chestnut Hill, Massachusetts

Linda Farber Post, JD, MA, BSN
Director, Bioethics
Medical Affairs
Hackensack University Medical Center
Hackensack, New Jersey

Patricia A. Quigley, PhD, MPH, APRN, CRRN, FAAN, FAANP
Retired Associate Chief
Nursing Service for Research
Retired Associate Director VISN 8 Patient Safety Center of Inquiry
James A. Haley Veterans Administration Medical Center Health Services Research and Development Center of Innovation on Disability and Rehabilitation Research Veterans Integrated Services Network 8
Tampa, Florida

Barbara Resnick, PhD, CRNP, FAAN, FAANP
Professor and Sonya Ziporkin Gershowitz
Chair in Gerontology
University of Maryland School of Nursing
Baltimore, Maryland

Satinderpal K. Sandhu, MD
Primary Care
Syracuse, Virginia

Judith E. Schipper, DNP, NPC, CLS, CHFN, FNLA, FPCNA
Clinical Coordinator
Heart Failure Program
New York University Langone Medical Center
New York, New York

R. Gary Sibbald, MD, FRCPC, ABIM, DABD, Med
Director
Wound Healing Clinic
The New Women's College Hospital
Professor
Public Health Sciences and Medicine
University of Toronto, Toronto, Ontario, Canada

Larry Z. Slater, PhD, RN-BC, CNE
Clinical Assistant Professor
New York University College of Nursing
New York, New York

Constance M. Smith, PhD, RN
President
C.M. Smith Technical Writing, Inc.
Wilmington, Delaware

Amala Sooklal, BSN, RN
Boston College William F. Connell School of Nursing
Chestnut Hill, Massachusetts

Elaine E. Steinke, PhD, APRN, CNS-BC, FAHA, FAAN
Professor
School of Nursing
Coordinator, Adult-Gerontology Acute Care
Nurse Practitioner Program
Wichita State University
Wichita, Kansas

Jos Tournoy, MD, PhD
Geriatric Medicine and Memory Clinic
University Hospitals Leuven
Department of Clinical and Experimental Medicine
KU Leuven
Leuven, Belgium

Dorothy F. Tullmann, PhD, RN, CNL
Associate Professor
Director, MSN and DNP Programs
University of Virginia School of Nursing
Charlottesville, Virginia

Janet H. Van Cleave, PhD, RN
Assistant Professor
New York University College of Nursing
New York, New York

Heidi L. Wald, MD, MSPH
Associate Professor and Vice Chair
for Quality Control
Department of Medicine
University of Colorado
School of Medicine
Aurora, Colorado

Saunjoo L. Yoon, PhD, RN
Associate Professor
University of Florida, College of Nursing
Gainesville, Florida

DeAnne Zwicker, DrNP, AGNP-BC
Inova Medical Group/Geriatrics SNF Department
Reston, Virginia

Foreword

For more than 60 years, the National Institutes of Health (NIH) has supported research to improve the health of and prolong the lives of people in the United States and around the world. Over that time, mean life expectancy worldwide has doubled to more than 70 years, due in large part to medical and public health interventions developed with NIH funding (Fauci & Collins, 2015). More than 60 years of biomedical and social sciences research have yielded much of the scientific foundation on which the knowledge base of nursing has been and is being built. The editors and contributing authors of *Evidence-Based Geriatric Nursing Protocols for Best Practice* have been well supported by the NIH and other federal and nonfederal funding agencies; many are graduates of the National Hartford Center of Gerontological Nursing Excellence (NHCGNE) and the Patricia G. Archbold Predoctoral and/or Claire M. Fagin Postdoctoral Awards programs. The NHCGNE is a collaboration among the coordinating center housed at the Gerontological Society of America and schools of nursing and international institutions, that have demonstrated the highest level of commitment to the field of gerontological nursing. NHCGNE is unique in that its sole focus is gerontological nursing and because it builds on the legacy of the John A. Hartford Foundation. Their mission is to enhance and sustain the capacity and competency of nurses to provide quality care to older adults through faculty development, advancing gerontological nursing science, facilitating adoption of best practices, fostering leadership, and designing and shaping policy. Their vision is optimal health for all older adults.

The editors and contributing authors of *Evidence-Based Geriatric Nursing Protocols for Best Practice* are experts in gerontological nursing; they are scientists, educators, leaders, and clinicians dedicated to an interdisciplinary approach to clinical practice that can be defined in terms of a "three-legged stool" integrating three basic principles: (a) the best available research evidence bearing on whether and why a treatment works, (b) clinical expertise (clinical judgment and experience) to rapidly identify each patient's unique health state and diagnosis and the individual risks and benefits of potential clinical interventions, and (c) client preferences and values (Lilienfeld, Ritschel, Lynn, Cautin, & Latzman, 2013; Spring, 2007). This book is uniquely positioned to assist nurses across health care sectors, as well as students and members of an interdisciplinary health team, to improve geriatric patient care and outcomes. For me, since my day job is more research administration than practice, this book keeps me connected and grounded in research evidence, practice, and patient outcomes.

The benefits of having a competent gerontological nurse at the bedside, when needed, cannot be overstated. Nursing is critical for older adults desiring to maintain health, improve health behaviors, avoid unnecessary hospitalizations, and live full and physically functional lives. Gerontological nursing is an evidence-based nursing specialty practice committed to improving the health, outcomes, and lives of older adult patients, their families, communities, and support systems. *Evidence-Based Geriatric Nursing Protocols for Best Practice* should be a part of every gerontological clinician's toolkit. It helps to make sense of an often confusing system and educates patients, families, and friends about evidence-based best practices for older adults and how to access the valuable resources available to them.

I am most impressed by the behavioral objectives, which immediately provide information about what can be achieved by reading the chapters, the refined and complex case studies that challenge one's depth of knowledge and skill in diagnosis, and chapter summaries listing nursing standards of practice. In addition, resources are included; many link to organizations that provide relevant tools and current information. For example, in Chapter 26, "Excessive Sleepiness," the link to the basics-of-sleep guide at www.sleepresearchsociety.org/Products.aspx may prove highly valuable given the prevalence of apnea in older adults. References in each chapter are keyed to the level of quantitative evidence available for each clinical topic. If you do not understand or are unable to use the pyramid in Figure F.1, do not miss reading Chapter 1, "Developing and Evaluating Clinical Practice Guidelines: A Systematic Approach." As the authors state, "Clinical decision making that is grounded in the best available evidence is essential to promote patient safety and quality health care outcomes." They provide expert guidance on how to best evaluate the evidence.

This book does much to advance clinical decision making based on research evidence. However, there remains critical work to generate research at the highest levels of the pyramid to facilitate evidence-based practice, enhance education, and improve health care systems and patient outcomes. The nursing profession is engaging in more interventions research; however, much of this research suffers from small sample sizes and a lack of seasoned clinical trialists. This is slowly changing.

This text, now in its fifth edition, serves us well as a foundation for clinical decision making in 39 clinical topics. *Evidence-Based Geriatric Nursing Protocols for Best Practice* saves time for clinicians and educators because the evidence presented, which was exhaustively chronicled, is outstanding and addresses issues, such as the of lack of time, knowledge, experience, and skill with evidence-based practice, and is a model for establishing nursing's best practices. In this fifth edition, there are six new chapters, including "The Frail Hospitalized Older Adult," "Perioperative Care of the Older Adult," "General Surgical Care of the Older Adult," "Care of the Older Adult With Fragility Hip Fracture," "Care of the Older Adult in the Emergency Department" and "Palliative Care Models."

As evidence-based practice continues to evolve and adapt, it is time to refine our approaches and enhance the

FIGURE F.1

Level of evidence hierarchy.

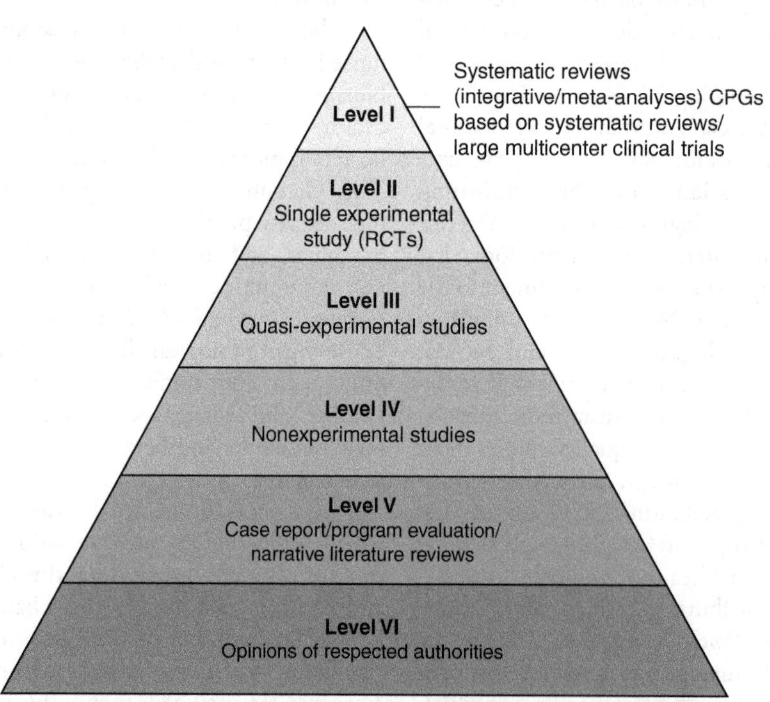

CPG, clinical practice guidelines; RCT, randomized controlled trials.
Originally published in Levin (2011). Reprinted with permission.

levels of evidence supporting gerontological nursing practice. History shows that the tools of modern science and research offer the opportunity to significantly alter major diseases that sap human health and exacerbate instability in the lives of older adults. It is imperative that gerontological nursing sustains momentum and works to deliver care founded on evidence-based protocols for best practices to older adults who need them most.

J. Taylor Harden, PhD, RN, FGSA, FAAN
Executive Director
National Hartford Center of
Gerontological Nursing Excellence
Former Assistant to the Director for
Special Populations, Retired
National Institute on Aging

REFERENCES

Fauci, A. S., & Collins, F. S. (2015). NIH research: Think globally. *Science, 348*(6231), 159. doi:10.1126/science.aab2733

Levin, R. F. (2011). Edifices of evidence: The proliferation of pyramids. *Research and Theory for Nursing Practice, 25*(1), 8–10.

Lilienfeld, S. O., Ritschel, L. A., Lynn, S. J., Cautin, R. L., & Latzman, R. D. (2013). Why many clinical psychologists are resistant to evidence-based practice: Root causes and constructive remedies. *Clinical Psychology Review, 33*(7), 883–900.

Spring, B. (2007). Evidence-based practice in clinical psychology: What it is; why it matters; what you need to know. *Journal of Clinical Psychology, 63*(7), 611–631.

Preface

The phenomenon of population aging is readily apparent to nurses who work in the acute care setting. Older adults represent the majority of hospitalized patients and also are the most clinically and socially complex patients. Acute care nurses have an enormous responsibility when providing care to older adults in this rapidly changing health care environment with its increasing regulatory requirements, shrinking reimbursement, and variable staffing levels. The nurse who is armed with information on the unique clinical presentations and response to treatment in older adults, and who has knowledge about evidence-based assessment and interventions, is situated to not only prevent complications but also to promote their functional recovery.

As in the previous editions of *Evidence-Based Geriatric Nursing Protocols for Best Practice*, we present assessment and interventions for common geriatric syndromes. Geriatric syndromes are increasingly recognized as being related to preventable iatrogenic complications, or those that occur as a direct result of medical and nursing care, causing serious adverse outcomes in older patients. We have expanded our content to include evidence-based interventions in specialty areas (e.g., surgical, perioperative, fragility hip fractures), geriatric organizational models (including palliative care and senior-friendly emergency departments), and frailty prevention and management.

In this fifth edition, we provide guidelines that are developed by experts on the topics of each chapter and are based on the best available evidence. A systematic method, the AGREE (Appraisal of Guidelines for Research and Evaluation) appraisal process (AGREE Next Steps Consortium, 2013; Levin & Vetter, 2007; Singleton & Levin, 2008), was used to evaluate the protocols and identify a process to help us improve validity of the book's content. Thus, a systematic process, described in Chapter 1, was developed to retrieve and evaluate the level of evidence of key references related to specific assessment and management strategies in each chapter. The chapter authors rated the levels of evidence based on the work of Stetler et al. (1998) and Melnyk and Fineout-Overholt (2011). The first chapter in this book, "Developing and Evaluating Clinical Practice Guidelines: A Systematic Approach," details the process of how the clinical practice guidelines were developed and how they complied with the AGREE items for rigor of development (AGREE Next Steps Consortium, 2013). Chapter 1, written by leaders in the field of evidence-based practice in the United States, is an important chapter reference for understanding the rating of the levels of evidence throughout the book.

HOW TO BEST USE THIS BOOK

Chapters provide overview and background information on the topic, evidence-based assessment and intervention strategies, and a topic-specific case study with discussion. The text of the chapter provides the context and detailed evidence for the protocol; the tabular protocol is not intended to be used in isolation of the text. We recommend that the reader take the following approach when reviewing the chapters:

1. Review the *objectives* to ascertain what is to be achieved by reviewing the chapter.
2. Review the *text*, noting the level of evidence presented in the reference section: Level I, being the highest (e.g., systematic reviews/meta-analyses), and Level VI, the lowest (e.g., expert opinions). Refer back to Chapter 1, Figure 1.1, for the definitions of the levels of evidence to understand the quantitative evidence that supports each of the recommendations. Keep in mind that it is virtually impossible to have evidence for all assessments and interventions, which does not mean they are not going to be used as an intervention. Many interventions that have been successfully used for years have

not been quantitatively researched but are well known to be effective to experts in the field of geriatrics.

3. Review the *protocols*, and remember that they reflect assessment and intervention strategies for acute care recommended by experts who have reviewed the evidence. This evidence is from all levels of care (e.g., community, primary care, long-term care, etc.) and not necessarily the hospital setting and should be applied to the unique needs of the individual patient.
4. Review the *case study* on each topic, which provides a more real-life, practical manner in which the protocol may be applied in clinical practice.

The *resources* in each chapter provide easy access to tools discussed in the chapter and link readers with organizations that provide ongoing, up-to-date information on the topic. **A PowerPoint presentation and Test Bank are available to qualified instructors from Springer Publishing by e-mailing requests to *textbook@springerpub.com.***

Although this book is titled *Evidence-Based Geriatric Nursing Protocols for Best Practice*, the text may be used by educators for geriatric nursing courses, advanced practice nurses, and by many other disciplines, including interprofessional team members, nursing home and other staff educators, social workers, dietitians, and physicians. Many interventions that are proactively identified and implemented by nurses can make a significant difference in improving outcomes, but nurses cannot provide for the complex needs of older adults in isolation. Research has shown that interprofessional teams have dramatically improved geriatric patient care and outcomes. We know that communication and collaboration are essential to improve care coordination, prevent iatrogenic complications, and improve clinical outcomes and quality of life (Institute of Medicine, 2001). Each of us must work together and be committed to provide the culture of safety that vulnerable older adults need to receive the safest, evidence-based clinical care with optimum outcomes.

Marie Boltz
Elizabeth Capezuti
Terry Fulmer
DeAnne Zwicker

REFERENCES

AGREE Next Steps Consortium. (2013). Appraisal of guidelines for research and evaluation II. Retrieved from http://www.agreetrust.org/wp-content/uploads/2013/10/AGREE-II-Users-Manual-and-23-item-Instrument_2009_UPDATE_2013.pdf

Institute of Medicine. (2001). *Crossing the quality chasm: A new health system for the 21st century*. Washington, DC: The National Academies Press.

Levin, R. F., & Vetter, M. (2007). Evidence-based practice: A guide to negotiate the clinical practice guideline maze. *Research and Theory for Nursing Practice, 21*(1), 5–9.

Melnyk, B. M., & Fineout-Overholt, E. (2011). *Evidence-based practice in nursing & healthcare: A guide to best practice* (2nd ed.). Philadelphia, PA: Lippincott Williams & Wilkins.

Singleton, J., & Levin, R. (2008). Strategies for learning evidence-based practice: Critically appraising clinical practice guidelines. *Journal of Nursing Education, 47*(8), 380–383.

Stetler, C. B., Morsi, D., Rucki, S., Broughton, S., Corrigan, B., Fitzgerald, J., . . . Sheridan, E. A. (1998). Utilization-focused integrative reviews in a nursing service. *Applied Nursing Research, 11*(4), 195–206.

Acknowledgments

We would like to thank the following for their involvement, support, and leadership during the production of this book:

- All the authors for this fifth edition
- Those nursing experts who participated in the Nurse Competence in Aging project, who contributed the first protocols to GeroNurseOnline, and led the way for the ongoing dissemination of evidence-based protocols
- Those who provided a valuable contribution in previous editions and their ongoing gerontological scholarship
- The institutions that supported faculty and geriatric clinicians who were contributors to this book
- The older adults and families who teach and inspire us to continually seek new and effective ways to improve care delivery
- Springer Publishing Company for its ongoing support of quality geriatric nursing publications

Acknowledgments

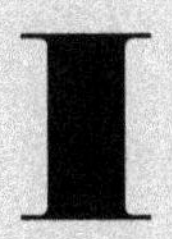

Incorporating Evidence Into Practice

1 Developing and Evaluating Clinical Practice Guidelines: A Systematic Approach

Rona F. Levin and Susan Kaplan Jacobs

EDUCATIONAL OBJECTIVES

1. Describe how to level the evidence used to develop and substantiate a practice protocol
2. Differentiate among recommendations, guidelines, and practice protocols
3. Evaluate clinical practice guidelines using AGREE II
4. Identify the five steps of the process for discovery of best evidence and integration into practice
5. Describe the best sources of evidence available to answer background/overview questions to support protocol development
6. Describe the specialized evidence sources most appropriate to support protocol development for specific patients and/or problems

OVERVIEW

Clinical decision making that is grounded in the best available evidence is essential to promoting patient safety and quality health care outcomes. With the knowledge base for geriatric nursing rapidly expanding, assessing geriatric clinical practice guidelines (CPGs) for their validity and incorporation of the best available evidence is critical to the safety and outcomes of care. In the second edition of this book, Lucas and Fulmer challenged geriatric nurses to take the lead in the assessment of CPGs, recognizing that, in the absence of best evidence, guidelines and protocols have little value for clinical decision making (Lucas & Fulmer, 2003). In the third edition of this book Levin, Singleton, and Jacobs (2008) proposed a method for ensuring that the protocols included here were based on a systematic review of the literature and synthesis of best evidence.

The purpose of this chapter is to describe the process that was used to create the fourth and current fifth edition of *Evidence-Based Geriatric Nursing Protocols for Best Practice*. Before the third edition of this book, there was no standard process or specific criteria for protocol development, nor was there any indication of the "level of evidence" of each source cited in a chapter (i.e., the evidence base for the protocol). In the third and fourth editions of this book, the process previously used to develop the geriatric nursing protocols was enhanced and described in detail. That process differed from the procedures followed in the current edition. This chapter is a guide to understanding how the protocols contained in this book were developed, and it details how to use a systematic, efficient, and evidence-based approach to discovering and evaluating evidence, which is the process needed to guide the assessment, development, and updating of practice protocols in any area of nursing practice.

DEFINITION OF TERMS

Evidence-based practice (EBP) is a framework for clinical decision making that uses (a) the best available evidence, (b) the clinician's expertise, and (c) a patient's values and circumstances to guide judgments about a patient's personal health condition (Keefer & Levin, 2013; Melnyk & Fineout-Overholt, 2011; Straus, Glasziou, Richardson, &

Haynes, 2010). Health care professionals often use the terms *recommendations*, *guidelines*, and *protocols* interchangeably but they are not synonymous.

A recommendation is a suggestion for practice, not necessarily sanctioned by a formal, expert group. A CPG is an "official recommendation" or suggested approach to diagnose and manage a broad health condition or problem (e.g., heart failure, smoking cessation, or pain management). A protocol is a more detailed guide for approaching a clinical problem or health condition and is tailored to a specific practice situation. For example, guidelines for falls prevention recommend developing a protocol for toileting elderly, sedated, or confused patients (National Guideline Clearinghouse, 2013). The specific practices or protocols that each health care organization implements, however, are agency specific. The validity of any of these practice guides can vary depending on the type and the level of evidence on which they are based. Using standard criteria to develop or refine CPGs or protocols assures reliability of their content. Standardization gives both nurses, who use the guideline/protocol, and patients, who receive care based on the guideline/protocol, assurance that the geriatric content and practice recommendations are based on the best evidence.

In contrast to these practice guides, "standards of practice" are not specific or necessarily evidence based; rather, they are a generally accepted, formal, and published framework for practice. As an example, the American Nurses Association document, *Nursing: Scope and Standards of Practice*, contains a standard regarding nurses' accountability for making an assessment of a patient's health status (American Nurses Association, 2010). The standard is a general statement. A protocol, on the other hand, may specify the measurement tool(s) to use in that assessment—for example, STRATIFY, an instrument used to measure the risk of falls (Smith, Forster, & Young, 2006).

The AGREE (Appraisal of Guidelines for Research and Evaluation) and AGREE II Instruments

The AGREE instrument, originally created and evaluated by a team of international guideline developers and researchers for use by the National Health Service (AGREE Enterprise, 2003), has been revised and updated and remains a generic tool designed primarily to help guideline developers and users assess the methodological quality of guidelines (Brouwers et al., 2010). This appraisal includes evaluation of the methods used to develop the CPG, assessment of the validity of the recommendations made in the guideline, and consideration of factors related to the use of the CPG in practice. Although the AGREE instrument was created to critically appraise CPGs, the process and criteria can also be applied to the development of clinical practice protocols. Thus, the AGREE instrument has been expanded for that purpose to standardize the creation and revision of the geriatric nursing practice protocols in this book.

The initial AGREE instrument and the one used for clinical guideline/protocol development in the third edition of this book has six quality domains: *scope and purpose, stakeholder involvement, rigor of development, clarity and presentation, application,* and *editorial independence.* A total of 23 items divided among the domains were rated on a four-point Likert-type scale from "strongly disagree" to "strongly agree." Appraisers evaluate how well the guideline they are assessing meets the criteria (i.e., items) of the six quality domains. For example, when evaluating the rigor of development, appraisers rated seven items. The reliability of the AGREE instrument is increased when each guideline is appraised by more than one appraiser. Each of the six domains receives an individual domain score and, based on these scores, the appraiser subjectively assesses the overall quality of a guideline.

Important to note, however, is that the original AGREE instrument was revised in 2009 (AGREE Next Steps Consortium, 2013), is now called AGREE II, and is the version that we used for the fourth and fifth editions of this book. The revision added one new item to the rigor of development domain. This is the current item 9, which underscores the importance of evaluating the evidence that is applied to practice. Item 9 reads: "The strengths and limitations of the body of evidence are clearly described" (Table 1.1). The remainder of the changes included a revision of the Likert-type scale used to evaluate each item in the AGREE II, a reordering of the number assigned to each item based on the addition of the new item 9, and minor editing of items for clarity. No other substantive changes were made. Table 1.1 includes the items that are in the rigor of development domain and were used for evaluation of evidence in the current edition of this book. A 2013 update of the AGREE II instrument includes a history of the project, information about language translations, and enhanced online training tools freely available to support guideline developers (AGREE Enterprise, 2014).

The rigor of development section of the AGREE instrument provides standards for literature searching and documenting the databases and terms searched. Adhering to these criteria to find and use the best available evidence on a clinical question is critical to the validity of geriatric nursing protocols and ultimately to patient safety and outcomes of care.

Published guidelines can be appraised using the AGREE II instrument, as discussed previously. In the process of guideline development, however, the clinician is faced with the added responsibility of appraising all

TABLE 1.1

Sample Domain and Items From the AGREE II Instrument for Critical Appraisal of Clinical Practice Guidelines

Domain 3: Rigor of Development
7. Systematic methods were used to search for evidence.
8. The criteria for selecting the evidence are clearly described.
9. The strengths and limitations of the body of evidence are clearly described.
10. The methods for formulating the recommendations are clearly described.
11. The health benefits, side effects, and risks have been considered in formulating the recommendations.
12. There is an explicit link between the recommendations and the supporting evidence.
13. The guideline has been externally reviewed by experts prior to its publication.
14. A procedure for updating the guideline is provided.

AGREE, Appraisal of Guidelines for Research and Evaluation.
Reprinted from the AGREE II Instrument by permission of Melissa Brouwers. www.agreetrust.org

available evidence for its quality and relevance. In other words, how well does the available evidence support recommended clinical practices? The clinician needs to be able to support or defend the inclusion of each recommendation in the protocol based on its level and quality of evidence. To do so, the guideline must reflect a systematic, structured approach to find and assess the available evidence.

Searching for the Best Evidence

Models of EBP describe the evidence-based process in five steps (Melnyk & Fineout-Overholt, 2011; Titler, 2010):

1. Develop an answerable question
2. Locate the best evidence
3. Critically appraise the evidence
4. Integrate the evidence into practice using clinical expertise with attention to patient's values and perspectives
5. Evaluate the outcome(s)

Although the evidence-based process encompasses these five steps, for the purposes of this volume of protocols and their development, this chapter focuses on the first three steps in more detail.

Step 1: Develop an Answerable Question

Developing an answerable question is critical before one can choose relevant sources to search. The information needed may be in the form of a specific "foreground" question (one that is focused on a particular clinical issue) or it may be a broad question (one that asks for overview information about a disease, condition, or aspect of health care) (Melnyk & Fineout-Overholt, 2011; Straus, Glasziou, Richardson, & Haynes, 2010) to gain some background of the practice problem and interventions, and gain insight into its significance. Background information includes both internal data from a specific agency and external data to place the health condition or problem in a broader societal context. Internal data usually include quality metrics from the health care agency in conjunction with health care providers' observations. External data might require a search for local and/or national benchmarking data and prevalence statistics as well as general literature describing the local problem as one that goes beyond a specific health care setting, population, or intervention.

An example of a background query might be one that seeks data: What is the prevalence of falls in elderly residents in a long-term care facility? Should these data demonstrate an unacceptable fall rate compared to national benchmark and safety target statistics, then the local problem can be shown to have significance beyond the specific clinical agency. A broad research query (an example of an overarching background question) related to a larger category of disease or health problem and encompassing multiple interventions might be: What is the best evidence for fall prevention in hospitalized older adults? A first place to search for evidence would be the National Guideline Clearinghouse (http://guidelines.gov) as described in Table 1.2).

A related question—What is the best evidence for falls prevention for the elderly in hospitals and long-term care facilities?—is addressed in a systematic review from the Cochrane Library, cited in Table 1.2. The Cochrane Library of Systematic Reviews contains rigorous and comprehensive narrative and statistical (meta-analyses) reviews that synthesize multiple studies of interventions (Cameron et al., 2012). The information contained in this review synthesizes multifactorial interventions and may help to further focus the inquiry into a question about the effectiveness of a specific intervention.

A similar example in Table 1.2 cites a Joanna Briggs Institute evidence summary, which answers a general background or overview question: What is the evidence regarding specific interventions to prevent falls in older adults? (Slade, 2013).

Once the overall evidence regarding a background question is uncovered, the question can be narrowed into a specific "PICO" format to specify the intervention or

TABLE 1.2

Selected Databases, Examples of Types of Questions, Sample Citations, and Level of Evidence of Citation

Database/Description/Access	Overview Question	PICO or Focused Clinical Question	Sample Citation	Level of Evidence
PubMed/MEDLINE Premier biomedical database produced by the U.S. National Library of Medicine containing more than 25 million citations for biomedical literature from MEDLINE, life science journals, and online books. http://pubmed.gov		In hospitalized elders, does the STRATIFY falls risk assessment tool predict falls in hospital and after discharge?	Smith et al. (2006)	Level IV
CINAHL Cumulative Index to Nursing and Allied Health Literature (authoritative index for more than 5,000 nursing and allied health journals) http://health.ebsco.com/products/the-cinahl-database/allied-health-nursing		Does the introduction of an educational video recording for staff decrease the rate of falls for hospitalized patients?	Cangany et al. (2015)	Level V
PsycINFO Indexes the professional and academic literature in the behavioral sciences and mental health, including medicine, psychiatry, nursing, sociology, pharmacology, physiology, and linguistics. http://www.apa.org/pubs/databases/psycinfo		Does exercise improve static and dynamic balance and dual-task ability in healthy older adults?	Gobbo, Bergamin, Sieverdes, Ermolao, and Zaccaria (2014)	Level I
Joanna Briggs Institute EBP Database Evidence summaries (short abstracts that summarize existing international evidence on common health care interventions and activities based on structured searches of the literature and selected evidence-based health care databases). http://connect.jbiconnectplus.org	What is the evidence regarding specific interventions to prevent falls in older adults?		Slade (2013)	Level VI
Cochrane Database of Systematic Reviews Produced by the Cochrane Library, one of the six databases that contain different types of high-quality, independent evidence to inform health care decision making. http://www.cochranelibrary.com	What is the best evidence for falls prevention for the older adult in hospitals and long-term care facilities?		Cameron et al. (2012)	Level I
ClinicalTrials.gov A service of the U.S. National Institutes of Health, an international registry of publicly and privately supported clinical studies of human participants. https://clinicaltrials.gov		Are high-intensity exercise programs an effective intervention for patients with Parkinson's disease, compared with the usual care (low-intensity group therapy)?	ClinicalTrials.gov (2014)	NA
National Guideline Clearinghouse Published by the AHRQ, U.S. Department of Health and Human Services, a public resource for evidence-based clinical practice guidelines. http://guideline.gov	What is the best evidence for fall prevention in hospitalized older adults?		National Guideline Clearinghouse (NGC, 2013)	Level I

AHRQ, Agency for Healthcare Research and Quality; EBP, evidence-based practice; PICO, population, intervention, comparison group or standard practice, outcomes.

assessment tool being examined (Straus et al., 2010, p. 15). PICO stands for:

- P = Population or patient problem
- I = Intervention
- C = Comparison group or standard practice
- O = Outcomes

The focused clinical or PICO question now specifies a patient problem or population and focuses on a specific intervention, for example, Does the introduction of an educational video recording for staff decrease the rate of falls for hospitalized patients?

A case study, located in the Cumulative Index to Nursing and Allied Health Literature (CINAHL) article database, provides an example of evidence in a specialized hospital setting (Cangany et al., 2015). Foreground questions are best answered by individual primary studies or syntheses of multiple studies, such as systematic reviews or meta-analyses. PICO templates work best to gather the evidence for focused clinical questions. In the question mentioned earlier, the *problem* was identified as a hospital unit with a fall rate higher than the National Database for Nursing Quality Indicators (NDNQI) benchmark, for a population of patients with heart disease in a progressive care unit. The *intervention* was the implementation of an educational video for staff, along with improved signage, improved documentation of a bed alarm, a risk assessment, and a "patient/family fall teaching contract." The *comparison* implied was the usual care, and the *outcome* measures were both a reduction in the fall rate and the costs associated with falls.

Step 2: Locate the Best Evidence

Step 2, locate the evidence, requires an evidence search based on the elements identified in the clinical question. Gathering the evidence for the protocols in this book presented the challenge of conducting literature reviews encompassing *both* the breadth of overview information as well as the depth of specificity represented in high-level systematic reviews and clinical trials to answer specific clinical questions.

Not every nurse, whether he or she is a clinical practitioner, educator, or administrator, has developed proficient database search skills to conduct a literature review to locate evidence. Beyond a basic knowledge of Boolean logic, truncation, and applying categorical limits to filter results, competency in "information literacy" requires experience with the idiosyncrasies of databases, selection of terms, and ease with controlled vocabularies and database functionality (Association of College & Research Libraries, 2013). Many nurses report that limited access to resources, gaps in information literacy skills, and, most of all, a lack of time are barriers to "readiness" for evidence-based practice (Pravikoff, Tanner, & Pierce, 2005).

The digital age presents both consumers of research evidence and researchers with an array of tools for searching, managing, and citing both the published literature and the unpublished literature. The ever-changing electronic environment provides an array of search engines, "apps," and specialized discovery tools. Such an environment can be daunting and often overwhelming to novice and experienced users alike. Research portals promoting "one-box" search tools purport comprehensiveness, yet search results are often vast and unfiltered. The apparent ease of keyword searching invites cherry picking from the first few pages of results, and can unwittingly introduce "search bias" (Wentz, 2002) into the quest for evidence, thus negating the sophisticated methodologies that were employed in primary studies to decrease experimenter bias and increase quality of evidence.

Health sciences librarians as intermediaries have been called "an essential part of the health care team by allowing knowledge consumers to focus on the wise interpretation and use of knowledge for critical decision making, rather than spending unproductive time on its access and retrieval" (Homan, 2010, p. 51). The *Cochrane Handbook* points out the complexity of conducting a systematic literature review, and highly recommends enlisting the help of a health care librarian when searching for evidence (Higgins & Green, 2011a).

Search Strategies

General or overview/background questions may be answered in textbooks, review articles, and "point of care" tools that aggregate overviews of best evidence, for example, online encyclopedias, systematic reviews, and synthesis tools. Locating systematic or narrative review articles or clinical guidelines based on systematic reviews (as pointed out earlier) may be helpful in the initial steps of gathering external evidence to support the significance of a problem before developing a narrower PICO question and investing a great deal of time in a question for which there might be limited evidence.

A search for individual studies in the published literature begins with database selection and translation of search terms into the controlled vocabulary of the database, if possible. In addition to the published literature, unpublished "grey" literature, should be considered. Unpublished evidence, though it may not be peer reviewed or evaluated, is nonetheless a part of a comprehensive gathering of evidence as a source for CPGs and protocols. One example in Table 1.2, clinical trials.gov, lists a study that proposes an exercise program for patients who have Parkinson's disease, with the status "recruiting participants" as of 2014 (ClinicalTrials.gov, 2014). Trial registries and open access repositories of clinical trials provide study criteria, outcome measures, and historical revisions to studies. They may be specialized for a particular kind of publication, for example, the Cochrane Library and the PROSPERO database, both examples of systematic review protocol repositories (Cochrane Library, 2015; University of York Centre for Reviews and Dissemination, 2015). Another of many sources of ongoing trials for nursing research is the Sigma Theta Tau International Honor Society of Nursing, 2015. The major article databases for finding the best primary evidence for most clinical nursing questions are the CINAHL database (www.ebscohost.com/academic/the-cinahl-database) and MEDLINE, the U.S. National Library of Medicine's premier biomedical article database (www.ncbi.nlm.nih.gov/pubmed). The PubMed interface to MEDLINE includes newly added citations to provide access to the most recently published literature. Another of many sources of ongoing trials for nursing research is the Virginia Henderson Global Nursing e-Repository (Sigma Theta Tau International Honor Society of Nursing, 2015). The Cochrane Library (which includes the Database of Systematic Reviews) and the Joanna Briggs publications (including evidence summaries, practice sheets, and systematic reviews) are examples of synthesized, appraised sources of evidence for broad topic areas (Cochrane Library, 2015; JBI COnNECT+ (Clinical Online Network of Evidence for Care and Therapeutics), n.d.)

The AGREE II instrument was used as a standard against which we could evaluate the process for evidence searching and use in chapter and protocol development (AGREE Next Steps Consortium, 2013). Domain 3, rigor of development, Item 7, states: "Systematic methods were used to search for evidence." And the user's manual directs: "The search strategy should be as comprehensive as possible and executed in a manner free from potential biases and sufficiently detailed to be replicated" (AGREE Next Steps Consortium, 2013, p. 23). Taking a tip from the *Cochrane Handbook*, a literature search should capture both the subject terms and the methodological aspects of studies when gathering relevant records (Higgins & Green, 2011b). The following guidelines reflect the process used to gather evidence for this book's protocols and are recommended guidelines for conducting a literature search.

- To facilitate replication and update of searches save a search strategy listing the keywords/descriptors and search string used in each database searched (e.g., MEDLINE, PsycINFO, CINAHL, trial registries)
- Specify the time period searched (e.g., 2010–2015).
- Specify categorical limits or methodological filters used (e.g., the article type: "meta-analysis" or the "systematic review subset" in PubMed; the "methodology" limit in PsycINFO for meta-analysis *or* clinical trial; the "research" limit in CINAHL).

Aggregate and organize evidence in a bibliographic management tool (e.g., Endnote [www.endnote.com], Refworks [www.refworks.com], or Zotero [www.zotero.org]). Gathering evidence to support broader topics, such as the protocols in this book, presents the searcher with a greater challenge. Limiting searches by methodology can unwittingly eliminate the best evidence for study designs that do not lend themselves to these methods. For example, a cross-sectional retrospective design may provide the highest level of evidence for a study that examines "nurses' perception" of the practice environment (Boltz et al., 2008).

A challenge to a searcher is the need to balance the comprehensiveness of recall (or "sensitivity") with precision ("specificity") to retrieve a manageable number of references. The *Cochrane Handbook* states: "Searches should seek high sensitivity, which may result in relatively low precision" (Higgins & Green, 2011a, section 6.1). Thus, retrieving a large set of articles may include many irrelevant hits. Conversely, putting too many restrictions on a database search may exclude relevant studies. The goal of retrieving the relevant studies for broad topic areas requires "sacrificing precision" and manually filtering false or irrelevant hits. Pitfalls of computerized retrieval are justification for the review by the searcher to weed false hits from the retrieved list of articles.

Repeatable search strategies were supplied to protocol developers enabling authors to revisit and rerun a database search for this fifth edition. The iterative nature of any literature search means that an initial set of relevant references for both broad or specific questions serves to point protocol authors toward best evidence as an adjunct to their own knowledge and their own pursuit of "chains of citation" (McLellan, 2001), related records, and their clinical expertise. For example, a core list of references on the topic of physical restraints might lead to exploring citations related to wandering, psychogeriatric care, or elder abuse.

Step 3: Critically Appraise the Evidence

Step 3, critically appraise the evidence, begins with identifying the methodology used in a study (often evident from reviewing the article abstract) followed by a critical reading and evaluation of the research methodology and results. The coding scheme described subsequently provides the first step in filtering retrieved studies based on research methods.

FIGURE 1.1

Level of evidence hierarchy.

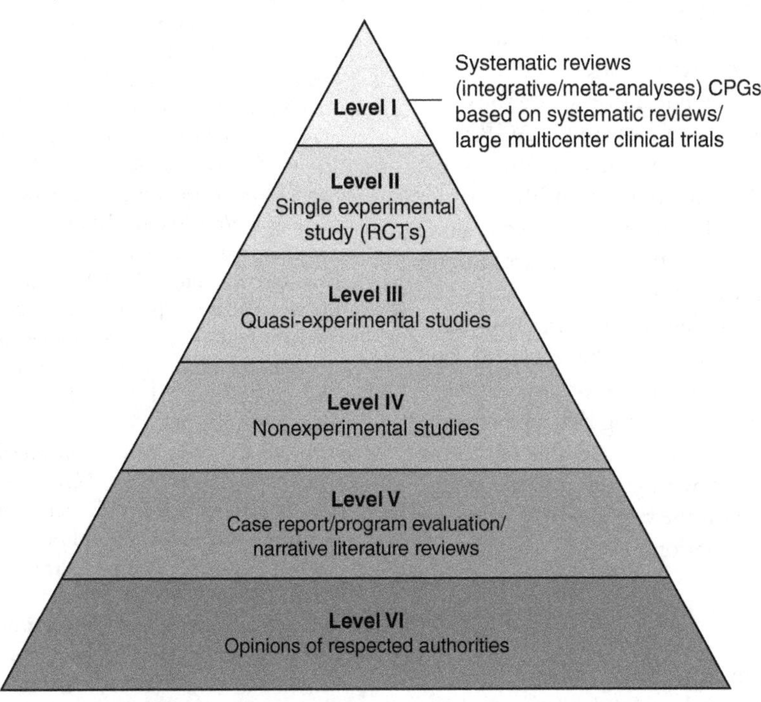

CPG, clinical practice guidelines; RCT, randomized controlled trials.
Originally published in Levin (2011). Reprinted with permission.

Levels of evidence (LOE) offer a schema that, once known, helps the reader to follow an efficient path for evidence searching as well as understand the relative value of the information presented to the clinical topic or question under review. There are many extant schemas used to identify the LOE of sources. Although multiple schemas exist, there are commonalities in their hierarchical structure, often represented by a pyramid or "publishing wedge" (DiCenso, 2009). The highest level of evidence is seen at the top of a pyramid, usually systematic reviews (meta-analyses) and CPGs based on high-level evidence. The schema used by the authors in previous editions of this book for rating the level of evidence came from the work of Stetler et al. (1998) and Melnyk and Fineout-Overholt (2011). As knowledge and thinking evolve, so do models or schemas for guiding the search for evidence. The LOE for the current edition can be seen in Figure 1.1 (Levin, 2011). Two major differences exist between the former and current pyramids that are recommended for guiding your evidence search. The first is that quantitative and qualitative research ask very different questions and thus cannot be included in the same hierarchy-of-evidence scheme. The second is that both the previously used and current LOE pyramids list individual randomized controlled trials (RCTs) as Level II. The former pyramid did not include multicenter clinical trials; thus, Levin addressed this issue and added multicenter clinical trials as Level I evidence in a quantitative pyramid (Figure 1.1).

A Level I evidence rating is given to evidence from synthesized sources: systematic reviews, which can either be meta-analyses or structured integrative reviews of evidence, and CPGs based on Level I evidence as well as multicenter clinical trials. Evidence that is judged to be at Level II comes from a single RCT. A quasi experimental study, such as a nonrandomized controlled single group pretest/posttest, time series or matched case-controlled study, is considered Level III evidence. Level IV evidence comes from a nonexperimental study, such as correlational descriptive research or case-control studies. A narrative literature review, a case report systematically obtained and of verifiable quality, or program evaluation data are rated as Level V. Level VI evidence is identified as the opinion of respected authorities (e.g., nationally known) based on their clinical experience or the opinions of an expert committee, including their interpretation of nonresearch-based information. This level also includes regulatory or legal opinions. Level I evidence is considered the strongest.

The critical appraisal of extant CPGs and research studies uses specialized tools designed to evaluate the quality of each type of evidence. Examples are the AGREE II instrument (which this volume of protocols conforms to), the Critical Appraisal Skills Programme (CASP), and the PRISMA checklist (a 27-item list of criteria for evaluation) for reporting systematic reviews and meta-analyses, among others (CASP, 2013; PRISMA, 2009).

An additional feature implemented in the third edition of this book was the inclusion of the level and type of evidence for references in chapter citations, which leads to a recommendation for practice. Using this type of standard approach ensures that this book contains protocols and recommendations for use with geriatric patients and their families that are based on the best available evidence and a similar standard of evaluation.

SUMMARY

The protocols contained in this edition, therefore, have been refined, revised, and/or developed by the authors using the best available research evidence as a foundation, with the ultimate goal of improving patient safety and outcomes. The systematic process used for finding, retrieving, and disseminating the best evidence for the fifth edition of *Evidence-Based Geriatric Nursing Protocols for Best Practice* provides a model for the use of research evidence in nursing education and in clinical practice. Translating nursing research into practice requires competency in information literacy, knowledge of the evidence-based process, and the ability to discern the context of a research study as ranked hierarchically. The following chapters and protocols present both overview (background) and foreground information in readiness for taking the next steps in the EBP process: Step 4: Integrate the evidence into practice using clinical expertise with attention to patient's values and perspectives, and Step 5: Evaluate the outcome(s).

REFERENCES

AGREE Enterprise. (2003). *The original AGREE Instrument.* Retrieved from http://www.agreetrust.org/resource-centre/the-original-agree-instrument

AGREE Enterprise. (2014). *AGREE II training tools.* Retrieved from http://www.agreetrust.org/resource-centre/agree-ii-training-tools

AGREE Next Steps Consortium. (2013). *AGREE II Instrument.* Retrieved from http://www.agreetrust.org/wp-content/uploads/2013/10/AGREE-II-Users-Manual-and-23-item-Instrument_2009_UPDATE_2013.pdf

American Nurses Association. (2010). *Nursing: Scope and standards of practice* (2nd ed.). Silver Spring, MD: Author.

Association of College & Research Libraries. (2013). *Information literacy competency standards for nursing.* Retrieved from http://www.ala.org/acrl/standards/nursing

Boltz, M., Capezuti, E., Bowar-Ferres, S., Norman, R., Secic, M., Kim, H., . . . Fulmer, T. (2008). Hospital nurses' perception of the geriatric nurse practice environment. *Journal of Nursing Scholarship: An Official Publication of Sigma Theta Tau International Honor Society of Nursing / Sigma Theta Tau, 40*(3), 282–289. Retrieved from http://doi.org/10.1111/j.1547-5069.2008.00239.x

Brouwers, M. C., Kho, M. E., Browman, G. P., Burgers, J. S., Cluzeau, F., Feder, G., . . . AGREE Next Steps Consortium. (2010). AGREE II: Advancing guideline development, reporting, and evaluation in health care. *Preventive Medicine, 51*(5), 421–424. Retrieved from http://doi.org/10.1016/j.ypmed.2010.08.005

Cameron, I. D., Gillespie, L. D., Robertson, M. C., Murray, G. R., Hill, K. D., Cumming, R. G., & Kerse, N. (2012). Interventions for preventing falls in older people in care facilities and hospitals. *Cochrane Database of Systematic Reviews, 2012*(12), CD005465. Retrieved from http://doi.org/10.1002/14651858.CD005465.pub3

Cangany, M., Back, D., Hamilton-Kelly, T., Altman, M., & Lacey, S. (2015). Bedside nurses leading the way for falls prevention: An evidence-based approach. *Critical Care Nurse, 35*(2), 82–84.

ClinicalTrials.gov. (2014). *High-intensity exercise and fall prevention boot camp for Parkinson's disease.* Retrieved from https://clinicaltrials.gov/ct2/show/study/NCT02230267?term=falls+exercise&rank=3

Cochrane Library. (2015). Retrieved from http://www.cochranelibrary.com

Critical Appraisal Skills Programme. (2013). *Critical Appraisal Skills Programme (CASP).* Retrieved from http://www.casp-uk.net

DiCenso, A. (2009). Accessing pre-appraised evidence: Fine-tuning the 5S model into a 6S model. *Evidence Based Nursing, 12*(4), 99.

Gobbo, S., Bergamin, M., Sieverdes, J. C., Ermolao, A., & Zaccaria, M. (2014). Effects of exercise on dual-task ability and balance in older adults: A systematic review. *Archives of Gerontology and Geriatrics, 58*(2), 177–187.

Higgins, J. P. T., & Green, S. (2011a). 6.3.1 Involving trials search co-ordinators and healthcare librarians in the search process. In J. P. T. Higgins & S. Green (Eds.), *Cochrane handbook for systematic reviews of interventions.* Version 5.1.0. Retrieved from http://handbook.cochrane.org

Higgins, J. P. T., & Green, S. (Eds.). (2011b). *Cochrane handbook for systematic reviews of interventions.* Version 5.1.0. The

Cochrane Collaboration. Retrieved from http://handbook.cochrane.org

Homan, J. M. (2010). Eyes on the prize: Reflections on the impact of the evolving digital ecology on the librarian as expert intermediary and knowledge coach, 1969–2009. *Journal of the Medical Library Association: JMLA, 98*(1), 49–56. Retrieved from http://doi.org/10.3163/1536–5050.98.1.016

JBI COnNECT+ (Clinical Online Network of Evidence for Care and Therapeutics). (n.d.). Retrieved from http://connect.jbiconnectplus.org

Keefer, J. M., & Levin, R. F. (2013). Integration of critical thinking and EBP. In R. F. Levin & H. R. Feldman (Eds.), *Teaching evidence-based practice in nursing* (2nd ed., pp. 85–101). New York, NY: Springer Publishing Company.

Levin, R. F. (2011). Edifices of evidence: The proliferation of pyramids. *Research and Theory for Nursing Practice, 25*(1), 8–10.

Levin, R. F., Singleton, J. K., & Jacobs, S. K. (2008). Developing and evaluating clinical practice guidelines: A systematic approach. In E. Capezuti, D. Zwicker, M. D. Mezey, T. Fulmer, D. Gray-Miceli, & M. Kluger (Eds.), *Evidence-based geriatric nursing protocols for best practice* (3rd ed.). New York, NY: Springer Publishing Company.

Lucas, J. A., & Fulmer, T. (2003). Evaluating clinical practice guidelines: A best practice. In M. D. Mezey, T. Fulmer, & A. Ivo (Eds.), *Geriatric nursing protocols for best practice* (2nd ed.). New York, NY: Springer Publishing Company.

McLellan, F. (2001). 1966 and all that—When is a literature search done? *The Lancet, 358*(9282), 646.

Melnyk, B. M., & Fineout-Overholt, E. (2011). *Evidence-based practice in nursing & healthcare: A guide to best practice* (2nd ed.). Philadelphia, PA: Lippincott, Williams, and Wilkins.

National Guideline Clearinghouse (NGC). (2013). Fall prevention. In *Evidence*-based *geriatric nursing protocols for best practice*. Retrieved from http://www.guideline.gov/content.aspx?id=43933

Pravikoff, D. S., Tanner, A. B., & Pierce, S. T. (2005). Readiness of U.S. nurses for evidence-based practice. *American Journal of Nursing, 105*(9), 40–51.

PRISMA. (2009). *PRISMA checklist.* Retrieved from http://www.prisma-statement.org

Sigma Theta Tau International Honor Society of Nursing. (2015). Virginia Henderson Global Nursing e-Repository. Retrieved from http://www.nursinglibrary.org/vhl

Slade, S. (2013). *Falls (older adults): Preventative interventions.* Retrieved from Joanna Briggs Institute EBP library database.

Smith, J., Forster, A., & Young, J. (2006). Use of the "STRATIFY" falls risk assessment in patients recovering from acute stroke. *Age and Ageing, 35*(2), 138–143. Retrieved from http://doi.org/10.1093/ageing/afj027

Stetler, C. B., Morsi, D., Rucki, S., Broughton, S., Corrigan, B., Fitzgerald, J., . . . Sheridan, E. A. (1998). Utilization-focused integrative reviews in a nursing service. *Applied Nursing Research: ANR, 11*(4), 195–206.

Straus, S. E., Glasziou, P., Richardson, W. S., & Haynes, R. B. (2010). *Evidence-based medicine: How to practice and teach it* (4th ed.). Edinburgh, UK: Churchill Livingstone.

Titler, M. (2010). Iowa model of evidence-based practice. In J. Rycroft-Malone & T. Bucknall (Eds.), *Models and frameworks for implementing evidence-based practice: Linking evidence to action.* Chichester, UK: Wiley-Blackwell.

University of York Centre for Reviews and Dissemination. (2015). *PROSPERO—International prospective register of systematic reviews.* Retrieved from http://www.crd.york.ac.uk/prospero

Wentz, R. (2002). Visibility of research: FUTON bias. *Lancet, 360*(9341), 1256. Retrieved from http://doi.org/10.1016/S0140–6736(02)11264–5

2

Measuring Performance and Improving Quality

Lenard L. Parisi

EDUCATIONAL OBJECTIVES

After completion of this chapter, the reader should be able to:

1. Discuss key components of the definition of *quality* as outlined by the Institute of Medicine
2. Describe three challenges of measuring quality of care
3. Delineate three strategies for addressing the challenges of measuring quality
4. List three characteristics of a good performance measure

OVERVIEW

Nadzam and Abraham (2003) state that "The main objective of implementing best practice protocols for geriatric nursing is to stimulate nurses to practice with greater knowledge and skill, and thus improve the quality of care to older adults" (p. 11). Although certainly improved patient care and safety are necessary goals, providers also need to be focused on the implementation of evidence-based practice and improvement of outcomes of care. The implementation of evidence-based nursing practice as a means to providing safe, quality patient care and positive outcomes is well supported in the literature. However, in order to ensure that protocols are implemented correctly, as is true with the delivery of all nursing care, it is essential to evaluate the care provided. Outcomes of care are gaining increased attention and will be of particular interest to providers as the health care industry continues to move toward "pay for performance (P4P)/value-based purchasing (VBP)," bundled payment reimbursement models and other quality incentive programs.

The improvement of care and clinical outcomes, commonly known as performance improvement, requires a defined, organized approach. Improvement efforts are typically guided by the organization's quality-assessment (measurement) and performance-improvement (process-improvement) model. Some well-known models or approaches for improving care and processes include Plan–Do–Study–Act (PDSA), Institute for Health Care Improvement (www.ihi.org/IHI/Topics/Improvement/ImprovementMethods/Tools/Plan-Do-Study-Act%20(PDSA)%20Worksheet). These methodologies are simply an organized approach to defining improvement priorities, collecting data, analyzing the data, making sound recommendations for process improvement, implementing identified changes, and then reevaluating the measures. Through performance improvement, standards of care (Nurses Improving Care for Health System Elders [NICHE] protocols, in this case) are identified, evaluated, and analyzed for variances in practice and then improved. The goal is to standardize and improve patient care and outcomes. Improvements in quality of patient care occur through restructuring, redesigning, and innovating processes. For these changes to occur, nursing professionals need to be supported by a structure that provides a vision for continuous improvement, empowers them to make changes, and delivers ongoing and reliable outcome information (Johnson, Hallsey, Meredith, & Warden, 2006).

From the very beginning of the NICHE project in the early 1990s (Capezuti et al., 2013), the NICHE team has struggled with the following questions: How can we measure whether the combination of models of care, staff education and development, and organizational change leads to improvements in patient care? How can we provide hospitals and health systems that are committed to improving their nursing care to older adults with guidance and frameworks, let alone tools for measuring the quality of geriatric care? In turn, these questions generated many other questions: Is it possible to measure quality? Can we identify direct indicators of quality? Or do we have to rely on indirect indicators (e.g., if 30-day readmissions of patients older than 65 years drop, can we reasonably state that this reflects an improvement in the quality of care?)? What factors may influence our desired quality outcomes, whether these are unrelated factors (e.g., the pressure to reduce length of stay) or related factors (e.g., the severity of illness)? How can we design evaluation programs that enable us to measure quality without adding more burden (of data collection, of taking time away from direct nursing care)? No doubt, the results from evaluation programs should be useful at the "local" level. Would it be helpful, though, to have results that are comparable across clinical settings (within the same hospital or health system) and across institutions (e.g., as quality benchmarking tools)? Many of these questions remain unanswered today, although the focus on defining practice through an evidence-based approach is becoming the standard, for it is against a standard of care that we monitor and evaluate expected care. Defining outcomes for internal and external reporting is expected, as is the improvement of processes required to deliver safe, affordable quality patient care.

This chapter provides guidance in the selection, development, and use of performance measures to monitor quality of care as a springboard to performance-improvement initiatives. Following a definition of quality of care, the chapter identifies several challenges in the measurement of quality. The concept of performance measures as the evaluation link between care delivery and quality improvement is introduced. Next, the chapter offers practical advice on what and how to measure (Capezuti et al., 2013). It also describes external comparative databases sponsored by Centers for Medicare & Medicaid Services (CMS) and other quality-improvement organizations. It concludes with a description of the challenges inherent in selecting performance measures.

It is important to reaffirm two key principles for the purposes of evaluating nursing care in this context. First, at the management level, it is indispensable to measure the quality of geriatric nursing care; however, doing so must help those who actually provide care (nurses) and must impact those who receive care (older adult patients). Second, measuring quality of care is not the end goal; rather, it is done to enable the continuous use of quality-of-care information to improve patient care.

QUALITY HEALTH CARE DEFINED

It is not uncommon to begin a discussion of quality-related topics without reflecting on one's own values and beliefs surrounding quality health care. Many have tried to define the concept, but like the old cliché "beauty is in the eye of the beholder" so is our own perception of quality. Health care consumers and providers alike are often asked: What does quality mean to you? The response typically varies and includes statements such as: a safe health care experience; receiving correct medications and receiving them in a timely manner; a pain-free procedure or postoperative experience; compliance with regulation; accessibility to services; effectiveness of treatments and medications; efficiency of services; good communication among providers (information sharing); and a caring environment. These are important attributes to remember when discussing the provision of care with clients and patients.

The Institute of Medicine (IOM) defines *quality of care* as "the degree to which health services for individuals and populations increase[s] the likelihood of desired health outcomes and are consistent with current professional knowledge" (Kohn, Corrigan, & Donaldson, 2000, p. 211). Note that this definition does not tell us what quality is, but what quality should achieve. This definition also does not say that quality exists if certain conditions are met (e.g., a ratio of *x* falls to *y* older orthopedic surgery patients, a 30-day readmission rate of *z*, etc.). Instead, it emphasizes that the likelihood of achieving desired levels of care is what matters. In other words, quality is not a matter of reaching something but, rather, the challenge, over and over, of improving the odds of reaching the desired level of outcomes. Thus, the definition implies the cyclical and longitudinal nature of quality: What we achieve today must guide us as to what to do tomorrow—better and better, over and over. The focus being on improving processes while demonstrating sustained improvement.

The IOM definition stresses the framework within which to conceptualize quality: knowledge. The best knowledge to have is research evidence—preferably from randomized clinical trials (experimental studies)—yet without ignoring the relevance of less rigorous studies (nonrandomized studies, epidemiological investigations, descriptive studies, even case studies). To be realistic, in nursing we have limited evidence to guide the care of older adults. Therefore, professional consensus among clinical and research experts is a critical factor in determining quality. Furthermore, knowledge is needed at three levels: To achieve quality, we need to know what to do (knowledge about best practice), we need to know how to do it (knowledge about behavioral skills), and we need to know what outcomes to achieve (knowledge about best outcomes).

The IOM definition of quality of care contains several other important elements. "Health services" focuses the definition on the care itself. Granted, the quality of care provided is determined by factors such as knowledgeable professionals, good technology, and efficient organizations; yet these are not typically the focus of quality measurement. Rather, the definition implies a challenge to health care organizations: The system should be organized in such a way that knowledge-based care is provided and that its effects can be measured. This brings us to the "desired health outcomes" element of the definition. Quality is not an attribute (as in, "My hospital is in the top 100 hospitals in the United States as ranked by *U.S. News & World Report*"), but an ability (as in "Only *x*% of our older adult surgical patients develop acute confusion; of those who do, *y*% return to normal cognitive function within *z* hours after onset").

In the IOM definition, *degree* implies that quality occurs on a continuum from unacceptable to excellent. The clinical consequences are on a continuum as well. If the care is of unacceptable quality, the likelihood that we will achieve the desired outcomes is nil. In fact, we probably will achieve outcomes that are the opposite of what are desired. As the care moves up the scale toward excellent, the more likely the desired outcomes will be achieved. "Degree" also implies quantification. Although it helps to be able to talk to colleagues about, say, unacceptable, poor, average, good, or excellent care, these terms should be anchored by a measurement system. Such systems enable us to interpret what, for instance, poor care is by providing us with a range of numbers that correspond to "poor." In turn, these numbers can provide us with a reference point for improving care to the level of average: We measure care again, looking at whether the numbers have improved, then checking whether these numbers fall in the range defined as "average." Likewise, if we see a worsening of scores, we will be able to conclude whether we have gone from, say, good to average. "Individuals and populations" underscores that quality of care is reflected in the outcomes of one patient and in the outcomes of a set of patients. It focuses our attention on providing quality care to individuals while aiming to raise the level of care provided to populations of patients.

In summary, the IOM definition of quality of care forces us to think about quality in relative and dynamic rather than in absolute and static terms. Quality of care is not a state of being but a process of becoming. Quality is and should be measurable, using performance measures: "a quantitative tool that provides an indication of an organization's performance in relation to a specified process or outcome" (Schyve & Nadzam, 1998, p. 222).

Quality improvement is a process of attaining ever better levels of care in parallel with advances in knowledge and technology. It strives toward increasing the likelihood that certain outcomes will be achieved. This is the professional responsibility of those who are charged with providing care (clinicians, managers, and their organizations). On the other hand, consumers of health care (patients, but also purchasers, payers, regulators, and accreditors) are much less concerned with the processes in place as with the results of those processes.

CLINICAL OUTCOMES AND PUBLICLY REPORTED QUALITY MEASURES

Although it is important to evaluate clinical practices and processes, it is equally important to evaluate and improve outcomes of care. Clinical outcome indicators are receiving unprecedented attention within the health care industry from providers, payers, and consumers alike. Regulatory and accrediting bodies review outcome indicators to evaluate the care provided by the organization before and during regulatory and accrediting surveys, and to evaluate clinical and related processes. Organizations are expected to use outcome data to identify and prioritize the processes that support clinical care, and demonstrate an attempt to improve performance. Providers may use outcome data to support best practices by benchmarking their results with similar organizations. The benchmarking process is supported through publicly reported outcome data at the national and state levels. National reporting occurs on the CMS website, where consumers and providers alike may access information and compare hospitals, home care agencies, nursing homes, and managed care plans. For example, these websites (www.hospitalcompare.hhs.gov; www.medicare.gov/NHCompare; and www.medicare.gov/HHCompare) list outcome indicators relative to the specific service or delivery model. Consumers may use those websites to select organizations and compare outcomes, one against another, to aid in their selection of a facility or service. These websites also serve as a resource for providers to benchmark their outcomes against those of another organization. Outcome data also become increasingly important to providers as the industry continues the shift toward P4P/VBP models. With these models, practitioners are reimbursed for achieving quality-of-care outcomes.

One important nationwide quality initiative, which is sure to have a positive impact on the care for older adults, is the focus on readmissions (www.cms.gov/Medicare/Medicare-Fee-for-Service-Payment/AcuteInpatientPPS/Readmissions-Reduction-Program.html). This is an important outcome measure that is sure to foster improved evaluation of clinical processes across the health care continuum.

MEASURING QUALITY OF CARE

Schyve and Nadzam (1998) identified several challenges to measuring quality. First, the suggestion that quality of care is in the eye of the beholder points to the different interests of multiple users. This issue encompasses both measurement and communication challenges. Measurement and analysis methods must generate information about the quality of care that meets the needs of different stakeholders. In addition, the results must be communicated in ways that meet these different needs. Second, we must have good and generally accepted tools for measuring quality. Thus, user groups must come together in their conceptualization of quality care so that relevant health care measures can be identified and standardized. A common language of measurement must be developed, grounded in a shared perspective on quality that is cohesive across the continuum, yet meets the needs of various user groups. Third, once the measurement systems are in place, data must be collected. This translates into resource demands and logistic issues as to who is to report, record, collect, and manage data. Fourth, data must be analyzed in statistically appropriate ways. This is not just a matter of using the right statistical methods. More important, user groups must agree on a framework for analyzing quality data to interpret the results. Fifth, health care environments are complex and dynamic in nature. There are differences across health care environments, between types of provider organizations, and within organizations. Furthermore, changes in health care occur frequently, such as the movement of care from one setting to another and the introduction of new technology. Finding common denominators is a major challenge.

ADDRESSING THE CHALLENGES

These challenges to measuring quality are not insurmountable. However, making a commitment to quality care entails a commitment to putting the processes and systems in place to measure quality through performance measures, and to report quality-of-care results. This commitment applies as much to a quality-improvement initiative on a nursing unit as it does to a corporate commitment by a large health care system. In other words, once an organization decides to pursue excellence (i.e., quality), it must accept the need to overcome the various challenges to measurement and reporting. Let us examine how this could be done in a clinical setting.

McGlynn and Asch (1998) offer several strategies for addressing the challenges to measuring quality. First, the various user groups must identify and balance competing perspectives. This is a process of giving and taking: proposing highly clinical measures (e.g., prevalence of pressure ulcers), but also providing more general data (e.g., use of restraints). It is a process of asking and responding: asking management for monthly statistics on medication errors, but also agreeing to provide management with the necessary documentation of the reasons stated for restraint use. Second, there must be an accountability framework. Committing to quality care implies that nurses assume several responsibilities and are willing to be held accountable for each of them: (a) providing the best possible care to older patients, (b) examining their own geriatric nursing knowledge and practice, (c) seeking ways to improve it, (d) agreeing to evaluation of their practice, and (e) responding to needs for improvement. Third, there must be objectivity in the evaluation of quality. This requires setting and adopting explicit criteria for judging performance, then building the evaluation process on these criteria. Nurses, their colleagues, and their managers need to reach consensus on how performance will be measured and what will be considered excellent (and good, average, etc.) performance. Fourth, once these indicators have been identified, nurses need to select a subset of indicators for routine reporting. Indicators should give a reliable snapshot of the team's care to older patients. Fifth, it is critical to separate as much as possible the use of indicators for evaluating patient care and the use of these indicators for financial or nonfinancial incentives. Should the team be cost conscious? Yes, but cost should not influence any clinical judgment as to what is best for patients. Finally, nurses in the clinical setting must plan how to collect the data. At the institutional level, this may be facilitated by information systems that allow performance measurement and reporting. Ideally, point-of-care documentation will also provide the data necessary for a systematic and goal-directed quality-improvement program, thus eliminating separate data abstraction and collection activities.

The success of a quality-improvement program in geriatric nursing care (and the ability to overcome many of the challenges) hinges on the decision as to what to measure. We know that good performance measures must be objective, that data collection must be easy and as burdenless as possible, that statistical analysis must be guided by principles and placed within a framework, and that communication of results must be targeted toward different user groups. Conceivably, we could try to measure every possible aspect of care; realistically, however, the planning for this will never reach the implementation stage. Instead, nurses need to establish priorities by asking these questions: Based on our clinical expertise, what is critical for us to know? What aspects of our care to older patients are of high risk or high volume? What parts of our elder care are problem prone, either because we have experienced difficulties in the past or because we can anticipate problems as a result of the lack of knowledge or resources? What clinical indicators would be of interest to other user groups: patients, the general public, management, payors, accreditors, and practitioners? Throughout this prioritization process, nurses should keep asking themselves: What questions are we trying to answer, and for whom?

MEASURING PERFORMANCE-SELECTING QUALITY INDICATORS

The correct selection of performance measures or quality indicators is a crucial step in evaluating nursing care and is based on two important factors: frequency and volume. Clearly high-volume practices or frequent processes require focused attention—to ensure that the care is being delivered according to protocol or processes are functioning as designed. Problem-prone or high-risk processes would also warrant a review as these are processes with inherent risk to patients or variances in implementing the process. The selection of indicators must also be conistent with organizational goals for improvement. In today's health care environment, selection of indicators may be based on external requirements such as P4P measures or reporting of publicly reported measures. This provides buy-in from practitioners as well as administration when reporting and identifying opportunities for improvement. Performance measures (indicators) must be based on a standard of care, policy, procedure, or protocol. These documents, or standards of care, define practice and expectations in the clinical setting and therefore determine the criteria for the monitoring tool. The measurement of these standards simply reflects adherence to or implementation of these standards. Once it is decided what to measure, nurses in the clinical geriatric practice setting face the task of deciding how to measure performance. There are two possibilities: either the appropriate measure (indicator) already exists, or a new performance measure must be developed. Either way, there are a number of requirements of a good performance measure that will need to be applied.

Although indicators used to monitor patient care and performance do not need to be subject to the rigors of research, it is imperative that they reflect some of the attributes necessary to make relevant statements about the care. The measure and its output need to focus on improvement, not merely the description of something. It is not helpful to have a very accurate measure that just tells the status of a given dimension of practice. Instead, the measure needs to inform us about current quality levels and relate them to previous and future quality levels. It needs to be able to compute improvements or declines in quality over time so that we can plan for the future. For example, to have a measure that only tells the number of medication errors in the past month would not be helpful. Instead, a measure that tells what types of medication errors were made, perhaps even with a severity rating indicated, compares this to medication errors made during the previous months, and shows in numbers and graphs the changes over time that will enable us to do the necessary root cause analysis to prevent more medication errors in the future.

Performance measures need to be clearly defined, including the terms used, the data elements collected, and the calculation steps employed. Establishing the definition before implementing the monitoring activity allows for precise data collection. It also facilitates benchmarking with other organizations, when the data elements are similarly defined and the data-collection methodologies consistent. Imagine that we want to monitor falls on the unit. The initial questions would be: What is considered a fall? Does the patient have to be on the floor? Does a patient slumping against the wall or onto a table while trying to prevent himself or herself from falling to the floor constitute a fall? Is a fall caused by physical weakness or orthostatic hypotension treated the same way as a fall caused by tripping over an obstacle? The next question would be: Over what time period are falls measured: a week, a fortnight, a month, a quarter, or a year? The time frame is not a matter of convenience, but of accuracy. To be able to monitor falls accurately, we need to identify a time frame that will capture enough events to be meaningful and interpretable from a quality-improvement point of view. External indicator definitions, such as those defined for use in the National Database of Nursing Quality Indicators, provide guidance for both the indicator definition as well as the data-collection methodology for "nursing-sensitive indicators." The nursing-sensitive indicators reflect the structure, process, and outcomes of nursing care. The *structure* of nursing care is indicated by the supply of nursing staff, the skill level of the nursing staff, and the education/certification of nursing staff. *Process* indicators measure aspects of nursing care such as assessment, intervention, and RN job satisfaction. Patient *outcomes* that are determined to be nursing sensitive are those that improve if there is a greater quantity or quality of nursing care (e.g., pressure ulcers, falls, IV [intravenous] infiltrations). However, frequency of primary cesarean sections and cardiac failure are not considered "nursing-sensitive" (for details, see http://pressganey.com/ourSolutions/performance-and-advanced-analytics/clinical-business-performance/nursing-quality-ndnqi). Several nursing organizations across the country participate in data collection and submission, which allows for a robust database and excellent benchmarking opportunities.

Additional indicator attributes include validity, sensitivity, and specificity. *Validity* refers to whether the measure actually measures what it says it measures. *Sensitivity* and *specificity* refer to the ability of the measure to capture all true cases of the event being measured, and only true cases. We want to make sure that a performance measure identifies true cases as true and false cases as false and does not identify a true case as false or a false case as true. Sensitivity of a performance measure determines the likelihood of a positive test when a condition is present. Lack of sensitivity is expressed as false positives: The indicator calculates a condition as present when in fact it is not. *Specificity* refers to the likelihood of a negative test when a condition is not present. False negatives reflect lack of specificity: The indicators calculate that a condition is not present when in fact it is. Consider the case of depression and the recommendation in Chapter 15 to use the Geriatric Depression Scale, in which a score of 11 or greater is indicative of depression. How robust is this cutoff score of 11? What is the likelihood that someone with a score of 9 or 10 (i.e., negative for depression) might actually be depressed (false negative)? Similarly, what is the likelihood that a patient with a score of 13 would not be depressed (false positive)?

Reliability means that results are reproducible; the indicator measures the same attribute consistently across the same patients and across time. Reliability begins with a precise definition and specification, as described earlier. A measure is reliable if different people calculate the same rate for the same patient sample. The core issue of reliability is measurement error, or the difference between the actual phenomenon and its measurement: The greater the difference, the less reliable the performance measure. For example, suppose that we want to focus on pain management in older adults with end-stage cancer. One way of measuring pain would be to ask patients to rate their pain as none, a little, some, quite a bit, or a lot. An alternative approach would be to administer a visual analog scale, a 10-point line on which patients indicate their pain levels. Yet another approach would be to ask the pharmacy to produce monthly reports of analgesic use by type and dose. Generally speaking, the more subjective the scoring or measurement, the less reliable it will be. If all these measures were of equal reliability, they would yield the same result. The concept of reliability, particularly inter-rater reliability, becomes increasingly important to consider in those situations in which data collection is assigned to several staff members (Albanese et al., 2010). It is important to review the data-collection methodology, and the instrument in detail, to avoid different approaches and interpretation by the various people collecting the data.

Several of the examples given earlier imply the criterion of interpretability. A performance measure must be interpretable; that is, it must convey a result that can be linked to the quality of clinical care. First, the quantitative output of a performance measure must be scaled in such a way that users can interpret it. For example, a scale that starts with 0 as the lowest possible level and ends with 100 is a lot easier to interpret than a scale than starts with 13.325 and has no upper boundary except infinity. Second, we should be able to place the number within a context. Suppose we are working in a hemodialysis center that serves quite a large proportion of end-stage renal disease (ESRD) patients older than 60 years—the group least likely to be fit for a kidney transplant yet with several years of life expectancy remaining. We know that virtually all ESRD patients develop anemia (hemoglobin [Hb] < 11 g/dL), which in turn impacts on their activities of daily living (ADL) and instrumental activities of daily living (IADL) performance. In collaboration with the nephrologists, we initiate a systematic program of anemia monitoring and management, relying in part on published best practice guidelines. We want to achieve the best practice guideline of 85% of all patients having hemoglobin levels equal to or greater than 11 g/dL. We should be able to succeed because the central laboratory provides us with Hb levels, which allows us to calculate the percentage of patients at Hb of 11 g/dL or greater.

The concept of risk-adjusted performance measures or outcome indicators is an important one. Some patients are sicker than others, some have more comorbidities, and some are older and frailer. No doubt, we could come up with many more risk variables that influence how patients respond to nursing care. Good performance measures take this differential risk into consideration. They create a "level playing field" by adjusting quality indicators on the basis of the risk for severity of illness of the patients. It would not be fair to the health care team if the patients on the unit are a lot sicker than those on the unit a floor above. The team is at greater risk of having lower quality outcomes, not because it provides inferior care, but because the patients are a lot sicker and are at greater risk of a compromised response to the care provided. The sicker patients are more demanding in terms of care, and ultimately are less likely to achieve the same outcomes as less-ill patients. Performance measures must be easy to collect. The many examples cited earlier also refer to the importance of using performance measures for which data are readily available, can be retrieved from existing sources, or can be collected with little burden. The goal is to gather good data quickly without running the risk of having "quick and dirty" data.

We begin the process of deciding how to measure by reviewing existing measures. There is no need to reinvent the wheel, especially if good measures are out there. Nurses should review the literature, check with national organizations, and consult with colleagues. Yet we should not adopt existing measures blindly. Instead, we need to subject them to a thorough review using the characteristics identified earlier. Also, health care organizations that have adopted these measures can offer their experience.

It may be that, after an exhaustive search, we cannot find measures that meet the various requirements outlined earlier. We decide instead to develop our own in-house measure. Here are some important guidelines.

1. Zero in on the population to be measured. If we are measuring an undesirable event, we must determine the group at risk of experiencing that event, then limit the denominator population to that group. If we are measuring a desirable event or process, we must identify the group that should experience the event or receive the process. Where do problems tend to occur? What variables of this problem are within our control? If some are not within our control, how can we zero in even more on the target population? In other words, we exclude patients from the population when good reason exists to do so (e.g., those allergic to the medication being measured).
2. Define terms. This is a painstaking but essential effort. It is better to measure 80% of an issue with 100% accuracy than 100% of an issue with 80% accuracy.
3. Identify and define the data elements and allowable values required to calculate the measure. This is another painstaking but essential effort. The 80/100 rule applies here as well.
4. Test the data-collection process. Once we have a prototype of a measure ready, we must examine how easy or difficult it is to get all the required data.

IMPLEMENTING THE QUALITY-ASSESSMENT AND PERFORMANCE-IMPROVEMENT PROGRAM

Successful performance-improvement programs require an organizational commitment to implementation of the performance-improvement processes and principles outlined in this chapter (Kliger, Lacey, Olney, Cox, & O'Neil, 2010). Consequently, this commitment requires a defined, organized approach, which most organizations embrace and define in the form of a written plan. The plan outlines the approach the organization uses to improve care and safety for its patients. There are several important elements that must be addressed in order to implement the performance-improvement program effectively. The scope of service, which addresses the types of patients and care that is rendered, provides direction on the selection of performance measures. An authority and responsibility statement in the document defines who is able to implement the quality program and make decisions that will affect its implementation. Finally, it is important to define the committee structure used to effectively analyze and communicate improvement efforts to the organization.

The success of the performance-improvement program is highly dependent on a well-defined structure and appropriate selection of performance measures. The following is a list of issues that, if not addressed, may negatively impact the success of the quality program.

1. Lack of focus: A measure that tries to track too many criteria at the same time or is too complicated to administer, interpret, or use for quality monitoring and improvement
2. Wrong type of measure: A measure that calculates indicators the wrong way (e.g., uses rates when ratios are more appropriate, uses a continuous scale rather than a discrete scale, measures a process when the outcome is measurable and of greater interest)
3. Unclear definitions: A measure that is too broad or too vague in its scope and definitions (e.g., population is too heterogeneous, no risk adjustment, unclear data elements, poorly defined values)
4. Too much work: A measure that requires too much clinician time to generate the data or too much manual chart abstraction
5. Reinventing the wheel: A measure that is a reinvention rather than an improvement of a performance measure
6. Events not under control: A measure focusing on a process or outcome that is out of the organization (or the unit's) control to improve
7. Trying to do research rather than quality improvement: Data collection and analysis are done for the sake of research rather than for improvement of nursing care and the health and well-being of the patients.
8 Poor communication of results: The format of communication does not target and enable change.
9. Uninterpretable and underused: Uninterpretable results are of little relevance to improving geriatric nursing care.

In summary, the success of the quality-assessment performance-improvement program's ability to measure, evaluate, and improve the quality of nursing care to health system elders is in the planning. First, it is important to define the scope of services provided and those to be monitored and improved. Second, identify performance measures that are reflective of the care provided. Indicators may be developed internally or obtained from external sources of outcomes and data-collection methodologies. Third, it is important to analyze the data, pulling together the right people to evaluate processes, make recommendations, and improve care. Finally, it is important to communicate findings across the organization and celebrate success.

REFERENCES

Albanese, M. P., Evans, D. A., Schantz, C. A., Bowen, M., Disbot, M., Moffa, J. S., ... Polomano, R. C. (2010). Engaging clinical nurses in quality and performance improvement activities. *Nursing Administration Quarterly, 34*(3), 226–245.

Capezuti, E., Boltz, M. P., Shuluk, J., Denysyk, L., Brouwer, J. P., Roberts, M. C., ... Secic, M. (2013). Utilization of a benchmarking database to inform NICHE implementation. *Research in Gerontological Nursing, 6*(3), 198–208.

Johnson, K., Hallsey, D., Meredith, R. L., & Warden, E. (2006). A nurse-driven system for improving patient quality outcomes. *Journal of Nursing Care Quality, 21*(2), 168–175.

Kliger, J., Lacey, S. R., Olney, A., Cox, K. S., & O'Neil, E. (2010). Nurse-driven programs to improve patient outcomes: Transforming care at the bedside, integrated nurse leadership program, and the clinical scene investigator academy. *Journal of Nursing Administration, 40*(3), 109–114.

Kohn, L. T., Corrigan, J. M., & Donaldson, M. S. (Eds.). (2000). *To err is human: Building a safer health system.* Washington, DC: The National Academies Press.

McGlynn, E. A., & Asch, S. M. (1998). Developing a clinical performance measure. *American Journal of Preventive Medicine, 14*(Suppl. 3), 14–21.

Nadzam, D. M., & Abraham, I. L. (2003) Measuring performance, improving quality. In M. Mezey, T. Fulmer, & I. Abraham (Eds.). *Geriatric nursing protocols for best practice* (2nd ed., pp. 15–30). New York, NY: Springer Publishing Company.

Schyve, P. M., & Nadzam, D. M. (1998). Performance measurement in healthcare. *Journal of Strategic Performance Measurement, 2*(4), 34–42.

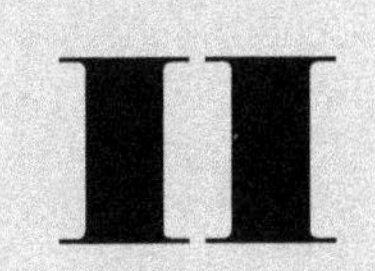

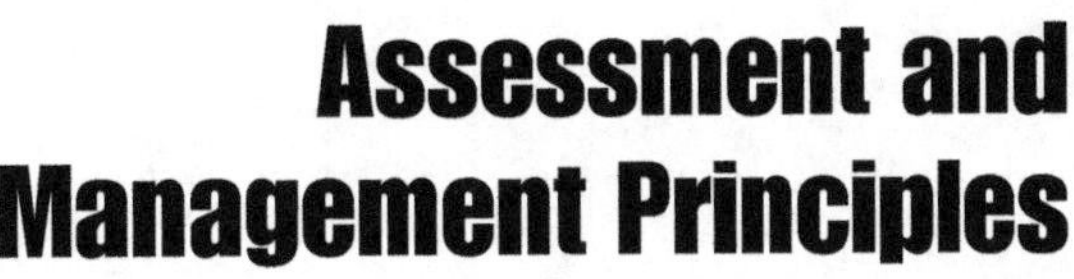

II Assessment and Management Principles

3

Age-Related Changes in Health

Constance M. Smith and Valerie T. Cotter

EDUCATIONAL OBJECTIVES

On completion of this chapter, the reader should be able to:

1. Describe the structural and functional changes in multiple body systems that occur during the normal aging process
2. Understand the clinical significance of these age-related changes regarding the health and disease risks of the older adult
3. Discuss the components of a nursing assessment for the older adult in light of the manifestations of normal aging
4. Identify care strategies to promote successful aging in older adults, with consideration of age-related changes

OVERVIEW

The process of normal aging, independent of disease, is accompanied by a myriad of changes in body systems. As evidenced by longitudinal studies, such as the Baltimore Longitudinal Study of Aging (2015), modifications occur in both structure and function of organs and are most pronounced at an advanced age of 85 years or older (Hall, 2002). Many of these alterations are characterized by a decline in physiological reserve. Although baseline function is preserved, organ systems become progressively less capable of maintaining homeostasis in the face of stresses imposed by the environment, disease, or medical therapies (Miller, 2009). Age-related changes are strongly impacted by genetics (Harada, Natelson Love, & Triebel, 2013), as well as by long-term lifestyle factors, including physical activity, diet, alcohol consumption, and tobacco use (Kitzman & Taffet, 2009). Furthermore, great heterogeneity occurs among older adults; clinical manifestations of aging can range from stability to significant decline in function of specific organ systems (Beck, 1998).

The clinical implications of these age-related alterations are important in nursing assessment and care of the older adult for several reasons (Smith & Cotter, 2012). First, changes associated with normal aging must be differentiated from pathological processes in order to develop appropriate interventions (Gallagher, O'Mahony, & Quigley, 2008). Manifestations of aging can also adversely impact the health and functional capability of older adults and require therapeutic strategies to correct (Matsumura & Ambrose, 2006). Age-associated changes predispose older persons to selected diseases (Kitzman & Taffet, 2009). Thus, nurses' understanding of these risks can serve to develop more effective approaches to assessment and care. Finally, aging and illness may interact reciprocally, resulting in altered presentation of illness, response to treatment, and outcomes (Hall, 2002).

For a description of evidence levels cited in this chapter, see Chapter 1, "Developing and Evaluating Clinical Practice Guidelines: A Systematic Approach."

This chapter describes age-dependent changes for several body systems. Clinical implications of these alterations, including associated disease risks, are then discussed, followed by nursing assessment and care strategies related to these changes.

CARDIOVASCULAR SYSTEM

Cardiac reserve declines in normal aging. This alteration does not affect cardiac function at rest and resting heart rate, ejection fraction, and cardiac output remain virtually unchanged with age. However, under physiological stress, the ability of the older adult's heart to increase both rate and cardiac output, in response to increased cardiac demand, such as physical activity or infection, is compromised (Lakatta, 2000). Such diminished functional reserve results in reduced exercise tolerance, fatigue, shortness of breath, slow recovery from tachycardia (Watters, 2002), and intolerance of volume depletion (Mick & Ackerman, 2004). Furthermore, because of the decreased maximal attainable heart rate with aging, a heart rate greater than 90 beats per minute (bpm) in an older adult indicates significant physiological stress (Kitzman & Taffet, 2009).

Age-dependent changes in both the vasculature and the heart contribute to the impairment in cardiac reserve. An increase in the wall thickness and stiffness of the aorta and carotid arteries results in diminished vessel compliance and greater systemic vascular resistance (Thomas & Rich, 2007). Elevated systolic blood pressure (BP) with constant diastolic pressure follows, increasing the risk of isolated systolic hypertension and widened pulse pressure (AlGhatrif & Lakatta, 2015). Strong arterial pulses, diminished peripheral pulses, and increased potential for inflamed varicosities commonly occur with age. Reductions in capillary density restrict blood flow in the extremities, producing cool skin (Mick & Ackerman, 2004).

As an adaptive measure to increased workload against noncompliant arteries, the left ventricle and atrium hypertrophy and become rigid. The ensuing impairment in relaxation of the left ventricle during diastole places greater dependence on atrial contractions to achieve left ventricular filling (Lakatta, 2000; Shah et al., 2008). In addition, sympathetic response in the heart is blunted because of diminished beta-adrenergic sensitivity, resulting in decreased myocardial contractility (Thomas & Rich, 2007).

Additional age-related changes include sclerosis of atrial and mitral valves, which impairs their tight closure and increases the risk of dysfunction. The ensuing leaky heart valves may result in aortic regurgitation or mitral stenosis, which present on examination as heart murmurs (Kitzman & Taffet, 2009). Loss of pacemaker and conduction cells contributes to changes in the resting electrocardiogram (EKG) of older adults. Isolated premature atrial and ventricular complexes are common arrhythmias, and the risk of atrial fibrillation is increased (Thomas & Rich, 2007). Because of atrial contractions in diastole, S_4 frequently develops as an extra heart sound, occurring immediately before the normal S_1 and S_2 (Lakatta, 2000; Shah et al., 2008).

Baroreceptor function, which regulates BP, is impaired with age, particularly with change in position. Postural hypotension with orthostatic symptoms may follow, especially after prolonged bed rest, dehydration, or cardiovascular drug use, and can cause dizziness and the potential for falls (Mukai & Lipsitz, 2002).

Cardiac assessment of an older adult includes performing an EKG and monitoring heart rate (40–100 bpm within normal limits), rhythm (noting whether it is regular or irregular), heart sounds (S_1, S_2, and extra heart sounds S_3 and S_4), and murmurs (noting location where loudest). The apical impulse is displaced laterally. In palpation of the carotid arteries, asymmetric volumes and decreased pulsations may indicate aortic stenosis and impaired left cardiac output, respectively. Auscultation of a bruit potentially suggests occlusive arterial disease. Peripheral pulses should be assessed bilaterally at a minimum of one pulse point in each extremity. Assessment may reveal asymmetry in pulse volume suggesting insufficiency in arterial circulation (Docherty, 2002). The nurse should examine lower extremities for varicose veins and note dilation or swelling. In addition, dyspnea with exertion and exercise intolerance are critical to note (Mahler, Fierro-Carrion, & Baird, 2003).

BP should be measured at least twice (Kestel, 2005) on the older adult and performed in a comfortably seated position with back supported and feet flat on the floor. The BP should then be repeated after 5 minutes of rest. Measurements in both supine and standing positions evaluate postural hypotension (Mukai & Lipsitz, 2002).

Nursing care strategies include referrals for older adults who have irregularities of heart rhythm and decreased or asymmetric peripheral pulses. The risk of postural hypotension emphasizes the need for safety precautions (Mukai & Lipsitz, 2002) to prevent falls. These include avoiding prolonged recumbency or motionless standing and encouraging the older adult to rise slowly from lying or sitting positions and wait for 1 to 2 minutes after a position change to stand or transfer. Overt signs of hypotension, such as a change in sensorium or mental status, dizziness, or orthostasis, should be monitored, and fall-prevention strategies should be instituted. For optimal cardiac functioning, sufficient fluid intake is advised to ensure adequate hydration and prevent hypovolemia (Docherty, 2002; Watters, 2002).

Older adults should be encouraged to adopt lifestyle practices for cardiovascular fitness with the aim of a healthy body weight (body mass index [BMI] 18.5–24.9 kg/m^2; American Heart Association Nutrition Committee; Lichtenstein et al., 2006) and normal BP (James et al., 2014). These practices involve eating a healthful diet (Knoops et al., 2004), physical activity appropriate for age and health status (Netz, Wu, Becker, & Tenenbaum, 2005), and elimination of the use of and exposure to tobacco products (U.S. Department of Health and Human Services [USDHHS], 2014).

PULMONARY SYSTEM

Respiratory function slowly and progressively deteriorates with age. This decline in ventilatory capacity seldom affects breathing during rest or customary limited physical activity in healthy older adults (Zeleznik, 2003); however, with greater than usual exertional demands, pulmonary reserve against hypoxia is readily exhausted and dyspnea occurs (Imperato & Sanchez, 2006).

Several age-dependent anatomic and physiologic changes combine to impair the functional reserve of the pulmonary system. Respiratory muscle strength and endurance deteriorate to restrict maximal ventilatory capacity (Buchman et al., 2008). Secondary to calcification of rib-cage cartilage, the chest wall becomes rigid (Imperato & Sanchez, 2006), limiting thoracic compliance. Loss of elastic fibers reduces recoil of small airways, which can collapse and cause air trapping, particularly in dependent portions of the lung. Decreases in alveolar surface area, vascularization, and surfactant production adversely affect gaseous exchange (Zeleznik, 2003).

Additional clinical consequences of aging include an increased anteroposterior chest diameter caused by skeletal changes. An elevated respiratory rate of 12 to 24 breaths per minute accompanies reduced tidal volume for rapid, shallow breathing. Limited diaphragmatic excursion and chest/lung expansion can result in less effective inspiration and expiration (Buchman et al., 2008; Mick & Ackerman, 2004). Because of decreased cough reflex effectiveness and deep-breathing capacity, mucus and foreign matter clearance is restricted, predisposing to aspiration, infection, and bronchospasm (Watters, 2002). Furthermore, elevating the risk of infection is a decline in ciliary and macrophage activities and drying of the mucosal membranes with more difficult mucus excretion (Htwe, Mushtaq, Robinson, Rosher, & Khardori, 2007). With the loss of elastic recoil comes the potential for atelectasis. Because of reduced respiratory center sensitivity, ventilatory responses to hypoxia and hypercapnia are blunted (Imperato & Sanchez, 2006), putting the older adult at risk of developing respiratory distress with illness or administration of narcotics (Zeleznik, 2003).

The modifications in ventilatory capacity with age are reflected in changes in pulmonary function tests measuring lung volumes, flow rates, diffusing capacity, and gas exchange. Whereas the total lung capacity remains constant, the vital capacity is reduced and the residual volume is increased. Reductions in all measures of expiratory flow (forced expiratory volume in 1 second [FEV_1], forced vital capacity [FVC], FEV_1/FVC, peak expiratory flow rate [PEFR]) quantify a decline in useful air movement (Imperato & Sanchez, 2006). Because of impaired alveolar function, diffusing capacity of the lung for carbon monoxide (DLCO) declines as does pulmonary arterial oxygen tension (PaO_2), indicating impaired oxygen exchange; however, arterial pH and partial pressure of arterial carbon dioxide ($PaCO_2$) remain constant (Enright, 2009). Reductions in arterial oxygen saturation and cardiac output restrict the amount of oxygen available for use by tissues, particularly in the supine position, although arterial blood gas seldom limits exercise in healthy subjects (Zeleznik, 2003).

Respiratory assessment includes determination of breathing rate, rhythm, regularity, volume (hyperventilation/hypoventilation), depth (shallow, deep; Docherty, 2002), and effort (dyspnea; Mahler et al., 2003). Auscultation of breath sounds throughout the lung fields may reveal decreased air exchange at the lung bases (Mick & Ackerman, 2004). Thorax and symmetry of chest expansion should be inspected. A history of respiratory disease (tuberculosis, asthma), tobacco use (expressed as pack years), and extended exposure to environmental irritants through work or avocation are contributory (Imperato & Sanchez, 2006).

Subjective assessment of cough includes questions on quality (productive/nonproductive), sputum characteristics (note hemoptysis; purulence indicating possible infection), and frequency (during eating or drinking, suggesting dysphagia and aspiration; Smith & Connolly, 2003).

Secretions and decreased breathing rate during sedation can reduce ventilation and oxygenation (Watters, 2002). Oxygen saturation can be followed through arterial blood gases and pulse oximetry (Zeleznik, 2003), whereas breathing rate (greater than 24 respirations per minute), accessory muscle use, and skin color (cyanosis, pallor) should also be monitored (Docherty, 2002). The inability to expectorate secretions, the appearance of dyspnea, and decreased saturation of oxygen (SaO_2) levels suggest the need for suctioning to clear airways (Smith & Connolly, 2003). Optimal positioning to facilitate respiration should be regularly monitored with use of upright positions (Fowler's or orthopneic position) recommended (Docherty, 2002). Pain assessment may be necessary to allow ambulation and deep breathing (Mick & Ackerman, 2004). See Atypical Presentation of Disease section for assessment of pneumonia, tuberculosis, and influenza.

Nursing care strategies useful in facilitating respiration and maintaining patent airways in the older adult include positioning to allow maximum chest expansion through the use of semi- or high-Fowler's or orthopneic position (Docherty, 2002). Additionally, frequent repositioning in bed or encouraging ambulation, if mobility permits, is advised (Watters, 2002). Analgesics may be necessary for ambulation and deep breathing (Mick & Ackerman, 2004).

Hydration is maintained through fluid intake (6–8 oz/d) and air humidification, which prevent desiccation of mucous membranes and loosen secretions to facilitate expectoration (Suhayda & Walton, 2002). Suctioning may be necessary to clear airways of secretions (Smith & Connolly, 2003) and oxygen should be provided as needed (Docherty, 2002). Incentive spirometry, with the use of sustained maximal inspiration (SMIs) devices, can improve pulmonary ventilation, mainly inhalation, as well as loosen respiratory secretions, particularly in older adults who are unable to ambulate or are declining in function (Dunn, 2004).

Deep-breathing exercises, such as abdominal (diaphragmatic) and pursed-lip breathing, in addition to controlled and huff coughing, can further facilitate respiratory function. Techniques for healthy breathing, including sitting and standing erect, nose breathing (Dunn, 2004), and regular exercise (Netz et al., 2005) should be promoted. Education on eliminating the use of and exposure to tobacco problems should be emphasized (USDHHS, 2014).

RENAL AND GENITOURINARY SYSTEMS

In normal aging, the mass of the kidney declines with a loss of functional glomeruli and tubules in addition to a reduction in blood flow. Concomitantly, changes occur in the activity of the regulatory hormones, vasopressin (antidiuretic hormone), atrial natriuretic hormone, and the renin–angiotensin–aldosterone system (Miller, 2009). These alterations combine to result in diminished glomerular filtration rate (GFR), with a 10% decrement per decade starting at age 30 years, as well as impaired electrolyte and water management (Beck, 1998).

Despite these changes, the older adult maintains the ability to regulate fluid balance under baseline conditions; however, with age, the renal system is more limited in its capacity to respond to externally imposed stresses. This reduced functional reserve increases vulnerability to disturbances in fluid homeostasis as well as to renal complications and failure (Lerma, 2009), particularly from fluid/electrolyte overload and deficit, medications, or illness (Miller, 2009).

The decline in functional nephrons emphasizes the risk from nephrotoxic agents including nonsteroidal anti-inflammatory drugs (NSAIDs), beta-lactam antibiotics, and radiocontrast dyes. Reduced GFR impairs the older adult's ability to excrete renally cleared medications, such as aminoglycoside antibiotics (e.g., gentamicin) and digoxin, increasing the risk of adverse drug reactions (Beyth & Shorr, 2002). Dosages should be based on GFR estimated by the Cockcroft–Gault equation for creatinine clearance (Péquignot et al., 2009) or the modification of diet in renal disease (MDRD), rather than by serum creatinine concentration (Miller, 2009; National Kidney Disease Education Program, 2012). Values of serum creatinine remain unchanged despite an age-associated decline in GFR because of the parallel decrease in both older adults' skeletal muscle mass, which produces creatinine, and GFR for creatinine elimination. Thus, serum creatinine levels overestimate GFR to result in potential drug overdose (Beck, 1998).

Increased risk of electrolyte imbalances can result from an age-dependent impairment in the excretion of excessive sodium loads, particularly in heart failure and with NSAID use, leading to intravascular volume overload. Clinical indicators include weight gain (greater than 2%); intake greater than output; edema; change in mental status; tachycardia; bounding pulse; pulmonary congestion with dyspnea, rales; increased BP and central venous pressure (CVP); as well as distended neck/peripheral veins (Beck, 1998).

Conversely, sodium wasting or excess sodium excretion when maximal sodium conservation is needed can occur with diarrhea. Hypovolemia and dehydration may ensue (Stern, 2006), manifesting as acute change in mental status (may be the initial symptom), weight loss (greater than 2%), decreased tissue turgor, dry oral mucosa, tachycardia, decreased BP, postural hypotension, flat neck veins, poor capillary refill, oliguria (less than 30 mL/hr), increased hematocrit and specific gravity of urine, and blood urea nitrogen (BUN): plasma creatinine ratio greater than 20:1, and serum osmolality greater than 300 mOsm/kg (Mentes, 2006).

Impaired potassium excretion puts the older adult at risk for hyperkalemia, particularly in heart failure and with use of potassium supplements, potassium-sparing diuretics, NSAIDs, and angiotensin-converting enzyme (ACE) inhibitors (Mick & Ackerman, 2004). Clinical indicators include diarrhea, change in mental status, cardiac dysrhythmias or arrest, muscle weakness and areflexia, paresthesias and numbness in extremities, EKG abnormalities, and serum potassium greater than 5.0 mEq/L (Beck, 1998).

Limited acid excretion capability can cause metabolic acidosis during acute illness in the older adult. This condition presents as Kussmaul's respirations, change in mental status, nausea, vomiting, arterial blood pH less than 7.35, serum bicarbonate less than 22 mEq/L, and $PaCO_2$ less than 38 mmHg with respiratory compensation (Beck, 1998).

Causes of abnormal water metabolism with age include diminution in maximal urine concentrating ability (Sands, 2012), which, in concert with blunted thirst sensation and total body water, can result in hypertonic dehydration and hypernatremia (Mentes, 2006). Often associated with insensible fluid loss from fever (Miller, 2009), hypernatremia presents with thirst; dry oral mucosa; dry, furrowed tongue; postural hypotension; weakness; lethargy; serum sodium less than 150 mEq/L; and serum osmolality less than 290 mOsm/kg. Disorientation, seizures, and coma occur in severe hypernatremia (Suhayda & Walton, 2002).

Impaired excretion of a water load, exacerbated by ACE inhibitors, thiazide diuretics (Miller, 2009), and selective serotonin reuptake inhibitors (SSRIs; Mentes, 2006), predisposes the older adult to water intoxication and hyponatremia (Beck, 1998). Clinical indicators involve lethargy, nausea, muscle weakness and cramps, serum sodium less than 135 mEq/L, and serum osmolality less than 290 mOsm/kg. Confusion, coma, and seizures are seen in severe hyponatremia (Suhayda & Walton, 2002).

Changes in the lower urinary tract with age include reduced bladder elasticity and innervation, which contribute to decreases in urine flow rate, voided volume, and bladder capacity, as well as increases in postvoid residual and involuntary bladder contractions. A delayed or decreased perception of the signal from the bladder to void and decline in pelvic floor functioning (Ellsworth, Marschall-Kehrel, King, & Lukacz, 2013) translate into urinary urgency (Kevorkian, 2004). Increased nocturnal urine flow, which results from altered regulatory hormone production, impaired ability to concentrate urine (Sands, 2012), and bladder-muscle instability, can lead to nocturnal polyuria (Miller, 2009). In older men, benign prostatic hyperplasia (BPH) can result in urinary urgency, hesitancy, and frequency. All these changes combine to increase the risk of urinary incontinence in the older adult. Furthermore, urgency and nocturia increase the risk of falls. Changes with age in the physiology of the urinary tract, such as increased vaginal pH and decreased antibacterial activity of urine, in addition to the functional changes of the bladder, contribute to the development of bacteriuria, with potential for urinary tract infection (UTI; Htwe et al., 2007; Stern, 2006).

Renal assessment includes monitoring for renal function (GFR) based on creatinine clearance, particularly in acute and chronic illnesses (Lerma, 2009; Miller, 2009; Péquignot et al., 2009). The choice, dose, need, and alternatives for nephrotoxic and renally excreted agents should be considered (Beyth & Shorr, 2002).

Dehydration, volume overload, and electrolyte status are assessed first by screening for risk of fluid and electrolyte imbalances based on the older adult's age, medical and nutritional history, medications, cognitive and functional abilities, psychosocial status, and bowel and bladder patterns. Data on fluid intake and output; daily weights; and vital signs, including orthostatic BP measurements, are needed. Heart rate is a less reliable indicator for dehydration in older adults because of the effects of medications and heart disease (Suhayda & Walton, 2002).

Physical assessment for fluid/electrolyte status focuses on skin for edema and turgor. Note that turgor in older adults is a less reliable indicator for dehydration because of poor skin elasticity, and assessment over the sternum or inner thigh is recommended. Additional assessment involves the oral mucosa for dryness as well as cardiovascular, respiratory, and neurologic systems. Acute changes in mental status, reasoning, memory, or attention may be initial symptoms of dehydration (Suhayda & Walton, 2002). Pertinent laboratory tests include serum electrolytes, serum osmolality, complete blood count (CBC), urine pH and specific gravity, BUN, hematocrit (Mentes, 2006), and arterial blood gases (Beck, 1998).

Evaluations of urinary incontinence, UTI, and nocturnal polyuria using a 72-hour voiding diary are recommended. See Atypical Presentation of Disease section that follows UTI discussion. Voiding history and rectal examination are required to diagnose BPH (see Chapter 21, "Urinary Incontinence"). Fall risk should be addressed when nocturnal or urgent voiding is present (see Chapter 19, "Preventing Falls in Acute Care").

Ongoing care involves monitoring for renal function (Lerma, 2009; Miller, 2009; Péquignot et al., 2009) and for levels of nephrotoxic and renally cleared drugs (Beyth & Shorr, 2002). Maintenance of fluid/electrolyte balance is paramount (Beck, 1998), especially if fluids are given intravenously (Doerflinger, 2009). To prevent dehydration, older adults weighing between 50 and 80 kg (110 and 176 lb) are advised to have a minimum fluid intake of

1,500 to 2,500 mL/d (unless contraindicated by the medical condition; Suhayda & Walton, 2002) from both fluids and food sources, including fruits, vegetables, soups, and gelatin, with avoidance of high salt and caffeine content (Mentes, 2006; Ney, Weiss, Kind, & Robbins, 2009).

Incontinence care and exercise can contribute to management of voiding problems, including reduced incontinence, of older adults (Kim, Suzuki, Yoshida, & Yoshida, 2007; Schnelle et al., 2002). Behavioral interventions recommended for nocturnal polyuria include limited fluid intake in the evening, avoidance of caffeine and alcohol, and a prompted-voiding schedule (Miller, 2009). Institution of safety precautions and fall-prevention strategies are needed in nocturnal or urgent voiding (see Chapter 19).

OROPHARYNGEAL AND GASTROINTESTINAL SYSTEMS

Age-specific alterations in the oral cavity can adversely affect the older adult's nutritional status. Deterioration in the strength of muscles of mastication as well as potential for tooth loss and xerostomia because of dehydration or medications may reduce food intake (Hall, 2009). Contributing to poor appetite are an altered taste perception and a diminished sense of smell (see Chapter 8, "Oral Health Care"; Ney et al., 2009; Visvanathan & Chapman, 2009).

Changes in the esophagus with age include delayed emptying in addition to decreases in upper and lower esophageal sphincter pressures, sphincter relaxation, and peristaltic contractions. Swallowing becomes slower and less efficient (Logemann, Curro, Pauloski, & Gensler, 2013). Although these alterations rarely impair esophageal function and swallowing sufficiently to cause dysphagia or aspiration in normal aging, such conditions can develop in conjunction with disease or medication side effects in older adults (Gregersen, Pedersen, & Drewes, 2008; Ney et al., 2009). Diminished gastric motility with delayed emptying contributes to altered oral-drug passage time and absorption in the stomach; elevated risk of gastroesophageal reflux disease (GERD; Hall, 2009); and decreased postprandial hunger, leading to diminished food intake and possible malnutrition (Visvanathan & Chapman, 2009). Reduced mucin secretion impairs the protective function of the gastric mucosal barrier and increases the incidence of NSAID-induced gastric ulcerations (Newton, 2005). Although the motility and most absorptive functions of the small intestine are preserved with age, absorption of vitamin B_{12}, folic acid, and carbohydrates declines (Hall, 2009). In addition, malabsorption of calcium and vitamin D contributes to the risk of osteoporosis. Supplementation with calcium and vitamins D and B_{12} is now recommended for older adults (U.S. Department of Agriculture [USDA] & USDHHS, 2010; Visvanathan & Chapman, 2009).

Age-dependent weakening of the large-intestine wall predisposes older adults to diverticulosis and may lead to diverticulitis (Hall, 2009). Because motility of the colon appears to be preserved with age, increased self-reports of constipation in older adults may be attributed instead to altered dietary intake, medications, inactivity, or illness. Diminished rectal elasticity, internal anal sphincter thickening, and impaired sensation to defecate contribute to the risk of fecal incontinence in older adults (Gallagher et al., 2008), although this condition is primarily found in combination with previous bowel surgery or disease and not in normal aging (Hall, 2009).

Pancreatic exocrine output of digestive enzymes is preserved to allow normal digestive capacity with aging (Hall, 2009). Regarding endocrine function, aging changes in carbohydrate metabolism allow a genetic predisposition for diabetes to become manifest (Meneilly, 2010). An age-related decrease in gallbladder function increases the risk of gallstone formation. Although liver size and blood flow decline with age, reserve capacity maintains adequate hepatic function, and values of liver function tests remain stable; however, the liver is more susceptible to damage by stressors, including alcohol and tobacco. Associated with changes in the hepatic and intestinal cytochrome P450 system (Hall, 2009), clearance of a range of medications, including many benzodiazepines, declines to result in increased potential for dose-dependent adverse reactions to these drugs (Beyth & Shorr, 2002).

Reductions in antimicrobial activity of saliva and immune response of the gastrointestinal tract with age contribute to a high risk for infectious and inflammatory diseases of this system (Htwe et al., 2007). Furthermore, impaired enteric neuronal function may blunt the older adult's reaction to infection and inflammation and result in atypical presentation of disease (see Atypical Presentation of Disease section; Hall, 2002).

In the gastrointestinal evaluation, the abdomen and bowel sounds are assessed. Liver size, as well as reports of pain, anorexia, nausea, vomiting, and altered bowel habits should be noted (Visvanathan & Chapman, 2009). Assessment of the oral cavity includes dentition and chewing capacity (Chapman, 2007; see Chapter 8).

Weight is monitored with calculation of BMI and compared to recommended values (American Heart Association Nutrition Committee; Lichtenstein et al., 2006; Visvanathan & Chapman, 2009). Deficiencies in diet can be identified through comparisons of dietary intake, using a 24- to 72-hour food intake record, with nutritional guidelines

(Chapman, 2007; Roberts & Dallal, 2005; USDA & USDHHS, 2010). In addition, laboratory values of serum albumin, prealbumin, and transferrin are useful nutritional indicators. Low albumin concentration can also affect efficacy and potential for toxicity of selected drugs, including digoxin and warfarin (Beyth & Shorr, 2002). Several instruments for screening the nutritional status, eating habits, and appetite of older adults are available (see Resources section and Chapter 10, "Nutrition"; Ney et al., 2009).

Signs of dysphagia, such as coughing or choking with solid or liquid food intake, should be reported for further evaluation. If aspiration from dysphagia is suspected, the lungs must be assessed for the presence of infection, typically indicated by unilateral or bilateral basilar crackles in the lungs, dyspnea, tachypnea, and cough (Imperato & Sanchez, 2006). A decline in function or change in mental status may signal atypical presentation of respiratory infection from aspiration (Ney et al., 2009). Evaluation of GERD is based on typical and atypical symptoms (see Atypical Presentation of Disease section; Hall, 2009).

To assess constipation or fecal incontinence, a careful history with a 2-week bowel log noting laxative use is needed. Fecal impaction is assessed by digital examination of the rectum as a hardened mass of feces, which can be palpated. The impaction may also be palpated through the abdomen (Gallagher et al., 2008).

For continuing care, referrals should be provided to a registered dietitian for poor food intake, unhealthy BMI (healthy BMI: 18.5–24.9 kg/m^2; overweight: 25–29.9 kg/m^2; obesity: 30 kg/m^2 or greater; American Heart Association Nutrition Committee; Lichtenstein et al., 2006), and unintentional weight loss of 10% or greater in 6 months (Chapman, 2007; Ney et al., 2009). Drug levels and liver function tests are monitored if drugs are metabolized hepatically (Beyth & Shorr, 2002). Explanation of normal bowel frequency, the importance of diet and exercise, and recommended types of laxatives addresses constipation problems (Gallagher et al., 2008). Mobility should be encouraged to prevent constipation, and prophylactic laxatives should be provided if constipating medications, such as opiates, are prescribed (Stern, 2006). Community-based food and nutrition programs (Visvanathan & Chapman, 2009) and education on healthful diets using the food pyramid for older adults may be useful in improving dietary intake (see Chapter 10; USDA & USDHHS, 2010).

MUSCULOSKELETAL SYSTEM

Musculoskeletal tissues undergo age-associated changes that can negatively impact function in the older adult. Sarcopenia is defined as reduced muscle mass, physical performance, and grip strength (Cederholm & Morley, 2015). A decline in the size, number, and quality of skeletal muscle fibers occurs with aging and lean body mass is replaced by fat and fibrous tissue (Loeser & Delbono, 2009) so that by age 75 years, only 15% of the total body mass is muscle compared to 30% in a young, healthy adult (Matsumura & Ambrose, 2006). These alterations result in diminished contractile muscle force with increased weakness and fatigue plus poor exercise tolerance. Age-specific physiological alterations contributing to sarcopenia include reductions in muscle innervation, insulin activity, and sex steroid (estrogen and testosterone) and growth hormone levels. Additionally, individual factors, such as weight loss, protein deficiency, and physical inactivity, can accelerate development of this condition so it progresses to a clinically significant problem (Jones et al., 2009). Sarcopenia has been documented to affect function adversely in older adults by increasing the risk of disability, falls, unstable gait, and need for assistive devices. Physical activity, particularly strength training, and adequate intake of energy and protein can prevent or reverse sarcopenia (Narici, Maffulli, & Maganaris, 2008).

Age-dependent bone loss occurs in both sexes and at all sites in the skeleton. Whereas bone mass peaks between ages 30 and 35 years, density decreases thereafter at a rate of 0.5% per year. This decrement, caused by reduced osteoblast activity in the deposition of new bone, is accompanied by deterioration in bone architecture and strength. Furthermore, from 5 to 7 years following menopause during estrogen decline, bone loss in women accelerates to a 3% to 5% annual rate (USDHHS, 2004). This loss, resulting from osteoclast activation with elevated bone breakdown or resorption, occurs mainly in cancellous or trabecular bone, such as the vertebral body, and may develop into type I osteoporosis in women aged 51 to 75 years, who risk vertebral fractures. Following this postmenopausal period, bone loss slows again in women and involves cortical bone in the long bones of the extremities. With aging, both women and men may develop type II osteoporosis and are susceptible to hip fractures and kyphosis from vertebral compression fractures in later life (Simon, 2005).

An age-associated decline in the strength of ligaments and tendons, which are integral to normal joint function, predisposes to increased ligament and tendon injury, more limited joint range of motion (ROM), and reduced joint stability, leading to osteoarthritis (Narici et al., 2008). Degeneration of intervertebral disks caused by dehydration and poor nutrient influx elevates the risk of spinal osteoarthritis, spondylosis, and stenosis with aging (Loeser & Delbono, 2009).

Age-related changes in articular cartilage, which covers the bone endings in joints to allow smooth movement, involve increased dehydration, stiffening, crystal formation, calcification, and roughening of the cartilage surface. Although these alterations have a minor effect on joint function under baseline conditions, the aging joint is less capable of withstanding mechanical stress, such as the stress caused by obesity or excess physical activity, and is also more susceptible to diseases, including osteoarthritis (Loeser, 2010).

Age-dependent changes in stature include dorsal kyphosis, reduction in height, flexion of the hips and knees, and a backward tilt of the head to compensate for the thoracic curvature. A shorter stride, reduced velocity, and broader base of support with feet more widely spaced characterize modifications in gait with age (Harris et al., 2008).

The musculoskeletal assessment includes inspection of posture, gait, balance, symmetry of body parts, and alignment of extremities. Kyphosis, bony enlargements, or other abnormalities should be noted. The clinician should palpate bones, joints, and surrounding muscles, evaluating muscle strength on a scale of 0/5, and noting symmetry and signs of atrophy of major upper and lower extremity muscle groups. Active and passive ROM for major joints are evaluated, noting pain, limitation of ROM, and joint laxity. Joint stabilization and slow movements in ROM examinations are advised to prevent injury. Functionality, mobility, fine and gross motor skills, balance, and fall risk should be assessed (see Chapter 7, "Assessment of Physical Function," and Chapter 19; Harris et al., 2008).

For continuing care, referrals to physical or occupational therapy may be appropriate. Increased physical activity, including aerobic (American College of Sports Medicine; Chodzko-Zajko et al., 2009) and ROM (Netz et al., 2005) exercise plus training programs to increase muscle strength and power (i.e., ability to produce force) (Narici et al., 2008), is recommended to maintain maximal function. Interventions to promote such behavior in older adults involve health education, goal setting, and self-monitoring (Conn, Minor, Burks, Rantz, & Pomeroy, 2003). Pain medication may be needed to enhance functionality (see Chapter 18, "Pain Management"; McCleane, 2008). Strategies to prevent falls (see Chapter 19) and avoid physical restraints (see Chapter 23, "Physical Restraints and Side Rails in Acute and Critical Care Settings") are appropriate.

To prevent and treat osteoporosis, adequate daily intake of calcium (1,200 mg for women aged 50 years and older) and vitamin D (400 IU for women aged 50 to 70 years and 600 IU for women aged 71 years and older), physical exercise, and smoking cessation are recommended (USDHHS, 2004). In addition, routine bone mineral density screening for osteoporosis is advised for women aged 65 years and older, as well as for women aged 60 to 64 years at increased risk for osteoporotic fractures (Agency for Healthcare Research and Quality [AHRQ], 2014).

NERVOUS SYSTEM AND COGNITION

Age-related alterations in the nervous system can affect function and cognition in older adults. Changes include a reduced number of cerebral and peripheral neurons (Hall, 2002), modifications in dendrites and glial support cells in the brain, and loss and remodeling of synapses. Decreased levels of neurotransmitters, particularly dopamine, as well as deficits in systems that relay signals between neurons and regulate neuronal plasticity also occur with aging (Mattson, 2009).

Combined, these neurological changes contribute to decrements in general muscle strength; deep tendon reflexes; sensation of touch, pain, and vibration; and nerve conduction velocity (Hall, 2002), which result in slowed coordinated movements and increased response time to stimuli (Matsumura & Ambrose, 2006). These clinical consequences, although relatively mild in normal aging, cause an overall slowing of motor skills with potential deficits in balance, gait, coordination, reaction time, and agility (Harris et al., 2008; Narici et al., 2008). Such decline in function can adversely affect an older adult's daily activities, notably ambulation and driving, and predispose to falls and injury (American College of Sports Medicine; Chodzko-Zajko et al., 2009; Craft, Cholerton, & Reger, 2009).

Neurological changes, along with thinning of the skin, compromise thermoregulation in the older adult. These result in decreased sensitivity to ambient temperature as well as impaired heat conservation, production, and dissipation with predisposition to hypothermia and hyperthermia (Kuchel, 2009). Febrile responses to infection may be blunted or absent (see Atypical Presentation of Disease section; High, 2009; Htwe et al., 2007; Watters, 2002).

With age, the speed of cognitive processing slows (Harada et al., 2013) and some degree of cognitive decline is common (Park, O'Connell, & Thomson, 2003) but not universal in the older adult population (Stewart, 2004). Older adults demonstrate significant heterogeneity in cognitive performance, which may be positively impacted by education, good health, and physical activity (Colcombe & Kramer, 2003).

Specific cognitive abilities exhibit differing levels of stability or decline with age. For example, crystallized intelligence, or the information and skills acquired from experience, remains largely intact, whereas fluid intelligence, or creative reasoning and problem solving, declines (Harada et al., 2013). Sustained attention is unaffected by aging, although divided attention, or the ability to concentrate on multiple tasks concurrently, deteriorates. The mild decline in executive function, which includes the capability of directing behavior and completing multistep tasks, usually has minimal impact on an older adult's ability to manage daily activities. Although language abilities and comprehension appear stable, spontaneous word finding may deteriorate and is often a complaint of older adults. Remote memory, or recalling events in the distant past, and procedural memory, or remembering ways to perform tasks, remain intact but declarative memory, or learning new information, is slowed (Craft et al., 2009). However, despite some deficits, memory functions are adequate for normal life in successful aging (Henry, MacLeod, Phillips, & Crawford, 2004).

Changes in the nervous system increase the risk of sleep disorders (Espiritu, 2008) and delirium in the older adult, especially in acute care (see Chapter 17, "Delirium: Prevention, Early Recognition, and Treatment"). Neural changes affect the perception, tolerance, and response to treatment of pain (McCleane, 2008). In addition, age-specific alterations predispose neurons to degeneration, contributing to Alzheimer's disease (Charter & Alekoumbides, 2004), Parkinson's disease, and Huntington's disease (Mattson, 2009).

Assessment, with periodic reassessment, of baseline functional status (see Chapter 7) should include evaluation of fall risk, gait, and balance (see Chapter 19) as well as basic, instrumental, and advanced activities of daily living (ADL). During acute illness, functional status, pain (see Chapter 18), and symptoms of delirium (see Chapter 17) should be monitored. Evaluation of baseline cognition with periodic reassessment (see Chapter 6, "Assessing Cognitive Function") and sleep disorders (Espiritu, 2008) is warranted. The impact of physical and cognitive changes of aging on an older adult's level of safety and attentiveness in daily tasks should be determined (Craft et al., 2009; Harada et al., 2013; Henry et al., 2004; Park et al., 2003). Temperature indicating hypothermia (less than 95°F or less than 35°C) or hyperthermia (greater than 105°F or greater than 40.6°C) must be closely watched (Kuchel, 2009; Lu, Leasure, & Dai, 2010).

For care of the older adult, fall-prevention strategies should be implemented (see Chapter 19). If delirium is identified, nursing interventions for its treatment are needed (see Chapter 17). Particularly during surgery, procedures, such as the use of warmed intravenous fluids, humidified gases, and temperature-regulating blankets (Doerflinger, 2009), should be instituted to maintain normal temperatures and prevent hypothermia in the older patient (Watters, 2002). Lifestyle modifications recommended to improve cognitive function include regular physical exercise (Colcombe & Kramer, 2003), intellectual stimulation (Harada et al., 2013), and a healthful diet (JNC, 2004; USDA & USDHHD, 2010). Behavioral interventions for sleep disorders may be warranted (Irwin, Cole, & Nicassio, 2006).

IMMUNE SYSTEM AND VACCINATION

Immunosenescence, or the age-related dysfunction in immune response, is characterized by reduced cell-mediated immune function and humoral immune responses (Weiskopf, Weinberger, & Grubeck-Loebenstein, 2009), as well as increased inflammatory response (High, 2009; Hunt, Walsh, Voegeli, & Roberts, 2010). In older adults, immunosenescence is responsible, in part, for the increased susceptibility to and severity of infectious diseases (Htwe et al., 2007), the lower efficacy of vaccination (Weiskopf et al., 2009), and the chronic inflammatory state, which may contribute to chronic disease with age (Hunt et al., 2010).

Infectious diseases are a critical threat to older adults, especially because vaccination efficacy declines with age. Mortality rates for infectious diseases are highest for adults older than 85 years (Htwe et al., 2007), whereas reactivation of viruses, particularly varicella zoster leading to herpes zoster, occurs significantly more frequently in older adults (High, 2009). Immunosenescence, by dampening the induction of adaptive immune responses, results in reduced response rates to vaccination. For example, influenza vaccination has a protection rate of only 56% in older persons. Furthermore, antibody titers following booster vaccinations, such as against tetanus, are lower and decline faster with diminished antibody function in older adults compared to younger individuals (Weiskopf et al., 2009).

Current immunization recommendations for older adults are available from the Centers for Disease Control and Prevention (CDC, 2015). Vaccination with pneumococcal polysaccharide for pneumococcal infections is recommended for individuals 65 years of age and older, with one-time revaccination indicated if the patient was vaccinated 5 or more years previously and was aged younger than 65 years at the time of primary vaccination. For seasonal influenza, all individuals 50 years of age and older should be vaccinated with the inactivated vaccine just prior to influenza season each year. A single dose of zoster vaccine is recommended for all adults 60 years of age and older regardless of prior zoster history. A complete tetanus vaccine series is indicated for individuals having an uncertain history of tetanus immunization or having received fewer than three doses. Boosters should be given at 10-year intervals or more frequently with high-risk injuries. Hepatitis vaccines should also be considered for older adults depending on circumstances such as potential exposure and travel (CDC, 2015; High, 2009).

ATYPICAL PRESENTATION OF DISEASE

Diseases, particularly infections, often manifest with atypical features in older adults. Signs and symptoms are frequently subtle in the very old. These may initially involve nonspecific declines in functional or mental status, anorexia with reduced oral intake, incontinence, falls (Htwe et al., 2007), fatigue (Hall, 2002), or exacerbation of chronic illness such as heart failure or diabetes (High, 2009).

As a presenting sign of infection, fever is often blunted or absent, particularly in very old (High, 2009), frail, or malnourished (Watters, 2002) adults. Compared to young adults with a normal mean baseline body temperature of 98.6°F (37°C), frail older adults have a lower mean oral baseline temperature of 97.4°F (36.3°C; Lu et al., 2010). A blunted response to inflammatory stimuli in combination with lower basal temperature can result in a lack of measurable febrile response. Increasing age is a predisposing factor for the absence of fever (Htwe et al., 2007).

Assessment of the older patient should note any changes from baseline (including those that are subtle and nonspecific) in functioning, mental status and behavior (e.g., increased/new onset confusion), appetite, or exacerbation of chronic illness (High, 2009; Watters, 2002). This is especially important in individuals with cognitive impairment who are unable to describe symptoms.

To detect fever, normal temperature should be established for the older adult and monitored for changes of 2°F to 2.4°F (1.1–1.3°C) above baseline (Htwe et al., 2007). Oral temperatures of 99°F (37.2°C) or greater on repeated measurements also can be used to signify fever. The difficulty of diagnosing infection based on signs and symptoms may result in greater reliance on laboratory and radiologic evaluations (High, 2009).

In the assessment of disease, both typical and atypical symptoms must be considered. Evaluation for pneumococcal pneumonia includes monitoring for typical symptoms, such as productive cough, fever, chills, and dyspnea, as well as insidious, atypical symptoms, including tachypnea, lethargy (Bartlett et al., 2000), weakness, falls, decline in functional status, delirium, or increased/new-onset confusion with absent high fever. Decreased appetite and dehydration may be the only initial symptoms in the older adult (Imperato & Sanchez, 2006). Although chest radiograph is basic to diagnosis, the older adult who is dehydrated may not show infiltrate or consolidation, and these findings may appear only after hydration (Htwe et al., 2007).

Clinical features of tuberculosis in the older person are often atypical and nonspecific. Presenting symptoms may include dizziness, nonspecific pain, or impaired cognition rather than the typical manifestations of fever, night sweats, cough, or hemoptysis (High, 2009). Typical influenza symptoms of cough, fever, and chills may be combined with altered mental status in older adults (Htwe et al., 2007).

In an acute myocardial infarction, the classic presentation of severe chest pain and diaphoresis may be replaced by dyspnea, confusion, and anxiety (Gray-Vickrey, 2010).

UTI in older adults may present with classical symptoms of dysuria, flank or suprapubic discomfort, hematuria, and urinary frequency and urgency, or atypical symptoms of new-onset/worsening incontinence, anorexia, confusion, nocturia, or enuresis (Htwe et al., 2007).

For peritonitis, atypical symptoms, such as confusion and fatigue, may be manifest rather than the typical symptoms of rigidity (Hall, 2002). Evaluation of GERD is based on typical presenting symptoms of heartburn (pyrosis) and acid regurgitation, as well as atypical symptoms in the older adult of dysphagia, chest pain, hoarseness, vomiting, chronic cough, or recurrent aspiration pneumonia (Hall, 2009).

CASE STUDY

Ms. M is an 89-year-old woman presenting with productive cough, dyspnea, fatigue, and increased confusion over the past week. Her vital signs are pulse, 96 bpm; temperature, 98.6°F; respiration, 31 bpm; and BP, 110/55 mmHg. A chest radiograph shows multilobe infiltrates with a diagnosis of pneumonia. How severe is her pneumonia?

Ms. M's symptoms of a respiratory rate greater than 30 respirations per minute, multilobe infiltrates on a chest radiograph, and diastolic BP of less than 60 mmHg characterize her pneumonia as severe (Bartlett et al., 2000), and she is likely to require admission to an intensive care unit. However, several age-related changes affect her symptoms of pneumonia. Pneumonia may present in the older adult with typical symptoms of productive cough, fever, and dyspnea or with more insidious, atypical symptoms of tachypnea, lethargy (Bartlett et al., 2000), weakness, falls, decline in functional status, or increased/new-onset confusion. Decreased appetite and dehydration may be the only initial symptoms (Imperato & Sanchez, 2006).

(continued)

CASE STUDY *(continued)*

Because of reduced sympathetic innervation of the heart with age, the heart rate of an older adult does not increase in response to stress comparable to that of a younger individual (Kitzman & Taffet, 2009). Thus, 96 bpm in an 89-year-old person is tachycardic and indicates a severe stress reaction. Furthermore, because of a blunted febrile response to infection, particularly in a very old, frail, or malnourished adult, a fever may not be manifest even with severe infection (High, 2009; Htwe et al., 2007; Lu et al., 2010; Watters, 2002).

SUMMARY

Changes that occur with age strongly impact the health and functional status of older adults. Thus, recognition of and attention to these alterations are critically important in nursing assessment and care. Armed with knowledge of age-related changes and using the clinical protocol described in this chapter, nurses can play a vital role in improving geriatric standards of practice. Designing interventions that take age-related changes into consideration, educating patients and family caregivers on these alterations, and sharing information with professional colleagues will all serve to ensure optimal care of older adults.

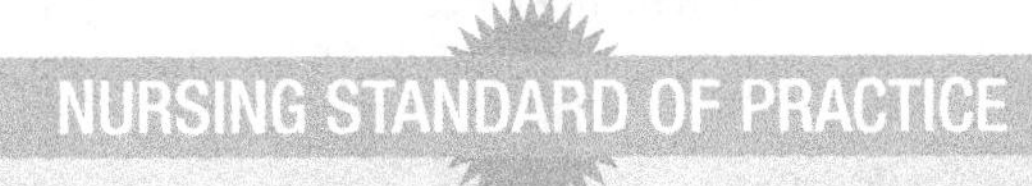

Protocol 3.1: Age-Related Changes in Health

I. GOAL

To identify anatomical and physiological changes, which are attributed to the normal aging process

II. OVERVIEW

Age-associated changes are most pronounced in advanced age of 85 years or older, may alter the older person's response to illness, show great variability among individuals, are often impacted by genetic and long-term lifestyle factors, and commonly involve a decline in functional reserve with reduced response to stressors.

III. STATEMENT OF PROBLEM

Gerontological changes are important in nursing assessment and care because they can adversely affect health and functionality and require therapeutic strategies; must be differentiated from pathological processes to allow development of appropriate interventions; predispose to disease, thus emphasizing the need for risk evaluation of the older adult; and can interact reciprocally with illness, resulting in altered disease presentation, response to treatment, and outcomes.

IV. AGE-ASSOCIATED CARDIOVASCULAR CHANGES

A. Definition
   1. Isolated systolic hypertension: systolic BP 140 mmHg and diastolic BP 90 mmHg
B. Etiology
   1. Arterial wall thickening and stiffening, decreased compliance
   2. Left ventricular and atrial hypertrophy; sclerosis of atrial and mitral valves
   3. Strong arterial pulses, diminished peripheral pulses, cool extremities
C. Implications
   1. Decreased cardiac reserve
      a. At rest: No change in heart rate, cardiac output
      b. Under physiological stress and exercise: Decreased maximal heart rate and cardiac output, resulting in fatigue, shortness of breath, slow recovery from tachycardia
      c. Risk of isolated systolic hypertension; inflamed varicosities
      d. Risk of arrhythmia, postural, and diuretic-induced hypotension; may cause syncope

(continued)

Protocol 3.1: Age-Related Changes in Health *(continued)*

D. Parameters of cardiovascular assessment
   1. Cardiac assessment: EKG; heart rate, rhythm, murmurs, heart sounds; palpate carotid artery and peripheral pulses for symmetry (Docherty, 2002)
   2. Assess BP (lying, sitting, and standing) and pulse pressure (Mukai & Lipsitz, 2002)

V. AGE-ASSOCIATED CHANGES IN THE PULMONARY SYSTEM

A. Etiology
   1. Decreased respiratory muscle strength; stiffer chest wall with reduced compliance
   2. Diminished ciliary and macrophage activity, drier mucous membranes; decreased cough reflex
   3. Decreased response to hypoxia and hypercapnia
B. Implications
   1. Reduced pulmonary functional reserve
      a. At rest: No change
      b. With exertion: Dyspnea, decreased exercise tolerance
   2. Decreased respiratory excursion and chest/lung expansion with less effective exhalation; respiratory rate of 12 to 24 breaths per minute
   3. Decreased cough and mucus/foreign matter clearance
   4. Increased risk of infection and bronchospasm with airway obstruction
C. Parameters of pulmonary assessment
   1. Assess respiration rate, rhythm, regularity, volume, depth (Docherty, 2002), and exercise capacity (Mahler et al., 2003). Ascultate breath sounds throughout lung fields (Mick & Ackerman, 2004).
   2. Inspect thorax appearance, symmetry of chest expansion. Obtain smoking history.
   3. Monitor secretions, breathing rate during sedation, positioning (Docherty, 2002; Watters, 2002), arterial blood gases, pulse oximetry (Zeleznik, 2003).
   4. Assess cough, need for suctioning (Smith & Connolly, 2003).
D. Nursing care strategies
   1. Maintain patent airways through upright positioning/repositioning (Docherty, 2002), suctioning (Smith & Connolly, 2003).
   2. Provide oxygen as needed (Docherty, 2002); maintain hydration and mobility (Watters, 2002).
   3. Incentive spirometry as indicated, particularly if immobile or declining in function (Dunn, 2004)
   4. Educate patient on cough enhancement (Dunn, 2004), smoking cessation (USDHHS, 2014).

VI. AGE-ASSOCIATED CHANGES IN THE RENAL AND GENITOURINARY SYSTEMS

A. Definitions
   1. To determine renal function (GFR):
      a. *Cockcroft–Gault equation*: Calculation of creatinine clearance in older adults (Péquignot et al., 2009)
      For men
      $$\text{Creatinine clearance (mL/min)} = \frac{(140 - \text{Age in years}) \times (\text{Body weight in kg})}{72 \times (\text{Serum creatinine, mg/dL})}$$
      For women, the calculated value is multiplied by 85% (0.85).
      b. *MDRD*: See National Kidney Disease Education Program calculator (National Kidney Disease Education Program, 2012).
B. Etiology
   1. Decreases in kidney mass, blood flow, GFR (10% decrement/decade after age 30 years); decreased drug clearance
   2. Reduced bladder elasticity, muscle tone, capacity
   3. Increased postvoid residual, nocturnal urine production
   4. In males, prostate enlargement with risk of BPH

(continued)

Protocol 3.1: Age-Related Changes in Health *(continued)*

C. Implications
   1. Reduced renal functional reserve; risk of renal complications in illness
   2. Risk of nephrotoxic injury and adverse reactions from drugs
   3. Risk of volume overload (in heart failure), dehydration, hyponatremia (with thiazide diuretics), hypernatremia (associated with fever), and hyperkalemia (with potassium-sparing diuretics); reduced excretion of acid load
   4. Increased risk of urinary urgency, incontinence (not a normal finding), UTI, nocturnal polyuria; potential for falls

D. Parameters of renal and genitourinary assessment
   1. Assess renal function (GFR through creatinine clearance; Lerma, 2009; Miller, 2009; National Kidney Disease Education Program, 2012; Péquignot et al., 2009).
   2. Assess choice/need/dose of nephrotoxic agents and renally cleared drugs (Beyth & Shorr, 2002; see Chapter 20, "Reducing Adverse Drug Events").
   3. Assess for fluid/electrolyte and acid/base imbalances (Suhayda & Walton, 2002).
   4. Evaluate nocturnal polyuria, urinary incontinence, and BPH (Miller, 2009). Assess UTI symptoms (see Atypical Presentation of Disease section; Htwe et al., 2007).
   5. Assess fall risk if nocturnal or urgent voiding (see Chapter 19)

E. Nursing care strategies
   1. Monitor nephrotoxic and renally cleared drug levels (Beyth & Shorr, 2002).
   2. Maintain fluid/electrolyte balance (Doerflinger, 2009). Minimum ingestion of 1,500 to 2,500 mL/d from fluids and foods for 50- to 80-kg adults to prevent dehydration (Suhayda & Walton, 2002).
   3. For nocturnal polyuria: limit fluids in evening, avoid caffeine, use prompted-voiding schedule (Miller, 2009)
   4. Fall prevention for nocturnal or urgent voiding (see Chapter 19)

VII. AGE-ASSOCIATED CHANGES IN THE OROPHARYNGEAL AND GASTROINTESTINAL SYSTEMS

A. Definition(s)
   1. BMI: Healthy, 18.5 to 24.9 kg/m^2; overweight, 25 to 29.9 kg/m^2; obese, 30 kg/m^2 or greater

B. Etiology
   1. Decreases in strength of muscles of mastication, taste, and thirst perception
   2. Decreased gastric motility with delayed emptying
   3. Atrophy of protective mucosa
   4. Malabsorption of carbohydrates, vitamins B_{12} and D, folic acid, calcium
   5. Impaired sensation to defecate
   6. Reduced hepatic reserve; decreased metabolism of drugs

C. Implications
   1. Risk of chewing impairment, fluid/electrolyte imbalances, poor nutrition
   2. Gastric changes: altered drug absorption, increased risk of GERD, maldigestion, NSAID-induced ulcers
   3. Constipation not a normal finding; risk of fecal incontinence with disease (not in healthy aging)
   4. Stable liver function tests; risk of adverse drug reactions

D. Parameters of oropharyngeal and gastrointestinal assessment
   1. Assess abdomen, bowel sounds
   2. Assess oral cavity (see Chapter 8); chewing and swallowing capacity, dysphagia (coughing, choking with food/fluid intake; Ney et al., 2009). If aspiration occurs, assess lungs (rales) for infection and typical/atypical symptoms (Bartlett et al., 2000; High, 2009; see Atypical Presentation of Disease section, www.consultgerirn.org).
   3. Monitor weight, calculate BMI, and compare to standards (American Heart Association Nutrition Committee; Lichtenstein et al., 2006). Determine dietary intake and compare to nutritional guidelines (Chapman, 2007; USDA & USDHHS, 2010; Visvanathan & Chapman, 2009; see Chapter 10).
   4. Assess for GERD, constipation and fecal incontinence, and fecal impaction by digital examination of rectum or palpation of abdomen.

(continued)

Protocol 3.1: Age-Related Changes in Health *(continued)*

E. Nursing care strategies
   1. Monitor drug levels and liver function tests if on medications metabolized by liver. Assess nutritional indicators (Chapman, 2007; USDA & USDHHS, 2010; Visvanathan & Chapman, 2009).
   2. Educate patient on lifestyle modifications and OTC medications for GERD.
   3. Educate patient on normal bowel frequency, diet, exercise, recommended laxatives. Encourage mobility, provide laxatives if on constipating medications (Stern, 2006).
   4. Encourage participation in community-based nutrition programs (Visvanathan & Chapman, 2009); educate on healthful diets (USDA & USDHHS, 2010).

VIII. AGE-ASSOCIATED CHANGES IN THE MUSCULOSKELETAL SYSTEM

A. Definition
   Sarcopenia: Reduced muscle mass, physical performance, and grip strength associated with aging
B. Etiology
   1. Sarcopenia evokes increased weakness and poor exercise tolerance.
   2. Lean body mass replaced by fat with redistribution of fat
   3. Bone loss in women and men after peak mass at age 30 to 35 years
   4. Decreased ligament and tendon strength; intervertebral disc degeneration; articular cartilage erosion; changes in stature with kyphosis, height reduction
C. Implications
   1. Sarcopenia: increased risk of disability, falls, unstable gait
   2. Risk of osteopenia and osteoporosis
   3. Limited ROM, joint instability, risk of osteoarthritis
D. Nursing care strategies
   1. Encourage physical activity through health education and goal setting (Conn et al., 2003) to maintain function (American College of Sports Medicine; Chodzko-Zajko et al., 2009).
   2. Administer pain medication to enhance functionality (see Chapter 18). Implement strategies to prevent falls (see Chapters 19 and 23).
   3. Prevent osteoporosis by adequate daily intake of calcium and vitamin D, physical exercise, and smoking cessation (USDHHS, 2004). Advise routine bone mineral density screening (AHRQ, 2014).

IX. AGE-ASSOCIATED CHANGES IN THE NERVOUS SYSTEM AND COGNITION

A. Etiology
   1. Decrease in neurons and neurotransmitters
   2. Modifications in cerebral dendrites, glial support cells, synapses
   3. Compromised thermoregulation
B. Implications
   1. Impairments in general muscle strength, deep tendon reflexes, nerve conduction velocity; slowed motor skills and potential deficits in balance and coordination
   2. Decreased temperature sensitivity; blunted or absent fever response
   3. Slowed speed of cognitive processing. Some cognitive decline is common but not universal. Most memory functions are adequate for normal life.
   4. Increased risk of sleep disorders, delirium, neurodegenerative diseases
C. Parameters of nervous system and cognition assessments
   1. Assess, with periodic reassessment, baseline functional status (Craft et al., 2009; see Chapters 6 and 19). During acute illness, monitor functional status and delirium (see Chapter 17).
   2. Evaluate, with periodic reassessment, baseline cognition (see Chapter 6) and sleep disorders (Espiritu, 2008).

(continued)

Protocol 3.1: Age-Related Changes in Health *(continued)*

3. Assess impact of age-related changes on level of safely and attentiveness in daily tasks (Henry et al., 2004; Park et al., 2003).
4. Assess temperature during illness or surgery (Kuchel, 2009).

D. Nursing care strategies
1. Institute fall-prevention strategies (see Chapter 19)
2. To maintain cognitive function, encourage lifestyle practices of regular physical exercise (Harada et al., 2013), intellectual stimulation (Mattson, 2009), healthful diet (JNC, 2004)
3. Recommend behavioral interventions for sleep disorders

X. AGE-ASSOCIATED CHANGES IN THE IMMUNE SYSTEM

A. Etiology
1. Immune response dysfunction (Kuchel, 2009) with increased susceptibility to infection, reduced efficacy of vaccination (Htwe et al., 2007), chronic inflammatory state (Hunt et al., 2010)

B. Nursing care strategies
1. Follow CDC immunization recommendations for the older adult for pneumococcal infections, seasonal influenza, zoster, tetanus, and hepatitis (CDC, 2015; High, 2009)

XI. ATYPICAL PRESENTATION OF DISEASE

A. Etiology
1. Diseases, especially infections, may manifest with atypical symptoms in older adults.
2. Symptoms/signs are often subtle and include nonspecific declines in function or mental status, decreased appetite, incontinence, falls (Htwe et al., 2007), fatigue (Hall, 2002), exacerbation of chronic illness (High, 2009).
3. Fever blunted or absent in very old (High, 2009), frail, or malnourished (Watters, 2002) adults. Baseline oral temperature in older adults is 97.4°F (36.3°C) versus 98.6°F (37°C) in younger adults (Lu et al., 2010).

B. Parameters of disease assessment
1. Note any change from baseline in function, mental status, behavior, appetite, chronic illness (High, 2009).
2. Assess fever. Determine baseline and monitor for changes 2°F to 2.4°F (1.1°C–1.3°C) above baseline (Htwe et al., 2007). Oral temperatures above 99°F (37.2°C) or greater also indicate fever (High, 2009).
3. Note typical and atypical symptoms of pneumococcal pneumonia (Bartlett et al., 2000; Htwe et al., 2007; Imperato & Sanchez, 2006), tuberculosis (Kuchel, 2009), influenza (Htwe et al., 2007), acute myocardial infarction (Gray-Vickrey, 2010), UTI (Htwe et al., 2007), peritonitis (Hall, 2002), and GERD (Hall, 2009).

XII. EVALUATION/EXPECTED OUTCOMES (FOR ALL SYSTEMS)

A. The older adult will experience successful aging through appropriate lifestyle practices and health care.

B. Health care provider will
1. Identify normative changes in aging and differentiate these from pathological processes.
2. Develop interventions to correct for adverse effects associated with aging.

C. Institution will
1. Develop programs to promote successful aging.

D. Provide staff education on age-related changes in health.

XIII. FOLLOW-UP MONITORING OF CONDITION

A. Continue to reassess effectiveness of interventions.

B. Incorporate continuous quality-improvement criteria into existing programs.

(continued)

Protocol 3.1: Age-Related Changes in Health *(continued)*

ABBREVIATIONS

AHRQ	Agency for Healthcare Research and Quality
BMI	Body mass index
BP	Blood pressure
BPH	Benign prostatic hyperplasia
CDC	Centers for Disease Control and Prevention
EKG	Electrocardiogram
GERD	Gastroesophageal reflux disease
GFR	Glomerular filtration rate
JNC	Joint National Committee
MDRD	Modification of diet in renal disease
NSAID	Nonsteroidal anti-inflammatory drug
OTC	Over the counter
ROM	Range of motion
USDA	U.S. Department of Agriculture
USDHHS	U.S. Department of Health and Human Services
UTI	Urinary tract infection

RESOURCES

Government Informational Agencies

Administration on Aging
http://www.aoa.gov

Agency for Healthcare Research and Quality
http://www.ahrq.gov

National Institute on Aging
http://www.nia.nih.gov

Non-Profit Organizations

Alliance for Aging Research
http://www.agingresearch.org

American Federation of Aging Research
http://www.afar.org

National Council on Aging
http://www.ncoa.org

Professional Societies

American Geriatrics Society
http://www.americangeriatrics.org

Gerontological Advanced Practice Nurses Association
https://www.gapna.org

National Gerontological Nursing Association
http://www.ngna.org

REFERENCES

Agency for Healthcare Research and Quality (AHRQ). (2014). *Guide to clinical preventive services, 2014: Recommendations of the U.S. preventive services task force.* Rockville, MD. Retrieved from http://www.ahrq.gov/professionals/clinicians-providers/guidelines-recommendations. *Evidence Level I.*

AlGhatrif, M., & Lakatta, E. G. (2015). The conundrum of arterial stiffness, elevated blood pressure, and aging. *Current Hypertension Reports, 17*(2), 12. *Evidence Level II.*

American College of Sports Medicine, Chodzko-Zajko, W. J., Proctor, D. N., Fiatarone Singh, M. A., Minson, C. T., Nigg, C. R.,...Skinner, J. S. (2009). American College of Sports Medicine position stand. Exercise and physical activity for older adults. *Medicine & Science in Sports & Exercise, 41*(7), 1510–1530. *Evidence Level I.*

American Heart Association Nutrition Committee, Lichtenstein, A. H., Appel, L. J., Brands, M., Carnethon, M., Daniels, S., Franch, H. A.,...Wylie-Rosett, J. (2006). Diet and lifestyle recommendations revision 2006: A scientific statement from the American Heart Association Nutrition Committee. *Circulation, 114*(1), 82–96. *Evidence Level I.*

Baltimore Longitudinal Study of Aging. (2015). Retrieved from www.blsa.nih.gov. *Evidence Level I.*

Bartlett, J. G., Dowell, S. F., Mandell, L. A., File, T. M., Jr., Musher, D. M., & Fine, M. J. (2000). Practice guidelines for the management of community-acquired pneumonia in adults. Infectious Diseases Society of America. *Clinical Infectious Diseases, 31*(2), 347–382. *Evidence Level I.*

Beck, L. H. (1998). Changes in renal function with aging. *Clinics in Geriatric Medicine, 14*(2), 199–209. *Evidence Level V.*

Beyth, R. J., & Shorr, R. I. (2002). Principles of drug therapy in older patients: Rational drug prescribing. *Clinics in Geriatric Medicine, 18*(3), 577–592. *Evidence Level V.*

Buchman, A. S., Boyle, P. A., Wilson, R. S., Gu, L., Bienias, J. L., & Bennett, D. A. (2008). Pulmonary function, muscle strength and mortality in old age. *Mechanisms of Ageing and Development, 129*(11), 625–631. *Evidence Level V.*

Cederholm, T., & Morley, J. E. (2015). Sarcopenia: The new definitions. *Current Opinion in Clinical Nutrition and Metabolic Care, 18*(1), 1–4. *Evidence Level II.*

Centers for Disease Control and Prevention (CDC). (2015). *Adult immunization schedules.* Retrieved from www.cdc.gov/vaccines/schedules/hcp/adult.html. *Evidence Level I.*

Chapman, I. M. (2007). The anorexia of aging. *Clinics in Geriatric Medicine, 23*(4), 735–756. *Evidence Level V.*

Charter, R. A., & Alekoumbides, A. (2004). Evidence for aging as the cause of Alzheimer's disease. *Psychological Reports, 95* (3 Pt. 1), 935–945. *Evidence Level I.*

Colcombe, S., & Kramer, A. F. (2003). Fitness effects on the cognitive function of older adults: A meta-analytic study. *Psychological Science, 14*(2), 125–130. *Evidence Level I.*

Conn, V. S., Minor, M. A., Burks, K. J., Rantz, M. J., & Pomeroy, S. H. (2003). Integrative review of physical activity intervention research with aging adults. *Journal of the American Geriatrics Society, 51*(8), 1159–1168. *Evidence Level I.*

Craft, S., Cholerton, B., & Reger, M. (2009). Cognitive changes with normal and pathological aging. In J. B. Halter, J. G. Ouslander, M. E. Tinetti, S. Studenski, K. P. High, & S. Asthana (Eds.), *Hazzard's geriatric medicine and gerontology* (6th ed., pp. 751–765). New York, NY: McGraw-Hill. *Evidence Level V.*

Docherty, B. (2002). Cardiorespiratory physical assessment for the acutely ill: 1. *British Journal of Nursing, 11*(11), 750–758. *Evidence Level I.*

Doerflinger, D. M. C. (2009). Older adult surgical patients: Presentation and challenges. *AORN Journal, 90*(2), 223–244. *Evidence Level V.*

Dunn, D. (2004). Preventing perioperative complications in an older adult. *Nursing, 34*(11), 36–41. *Evidence Level V.*

Ellsworth, P., Marschall-Kehrel, D., King, S., & Lukacz, E. (2013). Bladder health across the life course. *International Journal of Clinical Practice, 67*(5), 397–406. *Evidence Level V.*

Enright, P. L. (2009). Aging of the respiratory system. In J. B. Halter, J. G. Ouslander, M. E. Tinetti, S. Studenski, K. P. High, & S. Asthana (Eds.), *Hazzard's geriatric medicine and gerontology* (6th ed., pp. 983–986). New York, NY: McGraw-Hill. *Evidence Level V.*

Espiritu, J. R. (2008). Aging-related sleep changes. *Clinics in Geriatric Medicine, 24*(1), 1–14. *Evidence Level V.*

Gallagher, P. F., O'Mahony, D., & Quigley, E. M. (2008). Management of chronic constipation in the elderly. *Drugs & Aging, 25*(10), 807–821. *Evidence Level V.*

Gray-Vickrey, P. (2010). Gathering "pearls" of knowledge for assessing older adults. *Nursing, 40*(3), 34–43. *Evidence Level V.*

Gregersen, H., Pedersen, J., & Drewes, A. M. (2008). Deterioration of muscle function in the human esophagus with age. *Digestive Diseases and Sciences, 53*(12), 3065–3070. *Evidence Level II.*

Hall, K. E. (2002). Aging and neural control of the GI tract. II. Neural control of the aging gut: Can an old dog learn new tricks? *American Journal of Physiology: Gastrointestinal and Liver Physiology, 283*(4), G827–G832. *Evidence Level V.*

Hall, K. E. (2009). Effect of aging on gastrointestinal function. In J. B. Halter, J. G. Ouslander, M. E. Tinetti, S. Studenski, K. P. High, & S. Asthana (Eds.), *Hazzard's geriatric medicine and gerontology* (6th ed., pp. 1059–1064). New York, NY: McGraw-Hill. *Evidence Level V.*

Harada, C. N., Natelson Love, M. C., & Triebel, K. (2013). Normal cognitive aging. *Clinics in Geriatric Medicine, 29*(4), 737–752. *Evidence Level V.*

Harris, M. H., Holden, M. K., Cahalin, L. P., Fitzpatrick, D., Lowe, S., & Canavan, P. K. (2008). Gait in older adults: A review of the literature with an emphasis toward achieving favorable clinical outcomes, Part I. *Clinical Geriatrics, 16*(7), 33–42. *Evidence Level I.*

Henry, J. D., MacLeod, M. S., Phillips, L. H., & Crawford, J. R. (2004). A meta-analytic review of prospective memory and aging. *Psychology and Aging, 19*(1), 27–39. *Evidence Level I.*

High, K. P. (2009). Infection in the elderly. In J. B. Halter, J. G. Ouslander, M. E. Tinetti, S. Studenski, K. P. High, & S. Asthana (Eds.), *Hazzard's geriatric medicine and gerontology* (6th ed., pp. 1507–1515). New York, NY: McGraw-Hill. *Evidence Level V.*

Htwe, T. H., Mushtaq, A., Robinson, S. B., Rosher, R. B., & Khardori, N. (2007). Infection in the elderly. *Infectious Disease Clinics of North America, 21*(3), 711–743. *Evidence Level V.*

Hunt, K. J., Walsh, B. M., Voegeli, D., & Roberts, H. C. (2010). Inflammation in aging part I: Physiology and immunological mechanisms. *Biological Research for Nursing, 11*(3), 245–252. *Evidence Level V.*

Imperato, J., & Sanchez, L. D. (2006). Pulmonary emergencies in the elderly. *Emergency Medicine Clinics of North America, 24*(2), 317–338. *Evidence Level V.*

Irwin, M. R., Cole, J. C., & Nicassio, P. M. (2006). Comparative meta-analysis of behavioral interventions for insomnia and their efficacy in middle-aged adults and in older adults 55+ years of age. *Health Psychology, 25*(1), 3–14. *Evidence Level I.*

James, P. A., Oparil, S., Carter, B. L., Cushman, W. C., Dennison-Himmelfarb, C., Handler, J.,... Ortiz, E. (2014). Evidence-based guideline for the management of high blood pressure in adults: Report from the panel members appointed to the Eighth Joint National Committee (JNC). *Journal of the American Medical Association, 311*(5), 507–520. *Evidence Level I.*

Jones, T. E., Stephenson, K. W., King, J. G., Knight, K. R., Marshall, T. L., & Scott, W. B. (2009). Sarcopenia—Mechanisms and treatments. *Journal of Geriatric Physical Therapy, 32*(2), 83–89. *Evidence Level II.*

Kestel, F. (2005). The best BP. *Advance for Nurses, 12*, 33–34. *Evidence Level V.*

Kevorkian, R. (2004). Physiology of incontinence. *Clinics in Geriatric Medicine, 20*(3), 409–425. *Evidence Level V.*

Kim, H., Suzuki, T., Yoshida, Y., & Yoshida, H. (2007). Effectiveness of multidimensional exercises for the treatment of stress urinary incontinence in elderly community-dwelling Japanese women: A randomized, controlled, crossover trial.

Journal of the American Geriatrics Society, 55, 1932–1939. *Evidence Level II.*

Kitzman, D., & Taffet, G. (2009). Effects of aging on cardiovascular structure and function. In J. B. Halter, J. G. Ouslander, M. E. Tinetti, S. Studenski, K. P. High, & S. Asthana (Eds.), *Hazzard's geriatric medicine and gerontology* (6th ed., pp. 883–895). New York, NY: McGraw-Hill. *Evidence Level V.*

Knoops, K. T., de Groot, L. C., Kromhout, D., Perrin, A. E., Moreiras-Varela, O., Menotti, A., & van Staveren, W. A. (2004). Mediterranean diet, lifestyle factors, and 10-year mortality in elderly European men and women: The HALE project. *Journal of the American Medical Association, 292*(12), 1433–1439. *Evidence Level II.*

Kuchel, G. A. (2009). Aging and homeostatic regulation. In J. B. Halter, J. G. Ouslander, M. E. Tinetti, S. Studenski, K. P. High, & S. Asthana (Eds.), *Hazzard's geriatric medicine and gerontology* (6th ed., pp. 621–629). New York, NY: McGraw-Hill. *Evidence Level V.*

Lakatta, E. G. (2000). Cardiovascular aging in health. *Clinics in Geriatric Medicine, 16*(3), 419–444. *Evidence Level V.*

Lerma, E. V. (2009). Anatomic and physiologic changes of the aging kidney. *Clinics in Geriatric Medicine, 25*(3), 325–329. *Evidence Level V.*

Loeser, R. F. (2010). Age-related changes in the musculoskeletal system and the development of osteoarthritis. *Clinics in Geriatric Medicine, 26*(3), 371–386. *Evidence Level V.*

Loeser, R. F., Jr., & Delbono, O. (2009). Aging of the muscles and joints. In J. B. Halter, J. G. Ouslander, M. E. Tinetti, S. Studenski, K. P. High, & S. Asthana (Eds.), *Hazzard's geriatric medicine and gerontology* (6th ed., pp. 1355–1368). New York, NY: McGraw-Hill. *Evidence Level V.*

Logemann, J. A., Curro, F. A., Pauloski, B., & Gensler, G. (2013). Aging effects on oropharyngeal swallow and the role of dental care in oropharyngeal dysphagia. *Oral Diseases, 19*(8), 733–737. *Evidence Level V.*

Lu, S. H., Leasure, A. R., & Dai, Y. T. (2010). A systematic review of body temperature variations in older people. *Journal of Clinical Nursing, 19*(1–2), 4–16. *Evidence Level I.*

Mahler, D. A., Fierro-Carrion, G., & Baird, J. C. (2003). Evaluation of dyspnea in the elderly. *Clinics in Geriatric Medicine, 19*(1), 19–33. *Evidence Level V.*

Matsumura, B. A., & Ambrose, A. F. (2006). Balance in the elderly. *Clinics in Geriatric Medicine, 22*(2), 395–412. *Evidence Level V.*

Mattson, M. (2009). Cellular and neurochemical aspects of the aging human brain. In J. B. Halter, J. G. Ouslander, M. E. Tinetti, S. Studenski, K. P. High, & S. Asthana (Eds.), *Hazzard's geriatric medicine and gerontology* (6th ed., pp. 739–750). New York, NY: McGraw-Hill. *Evidence Level V.*

McCleane, G. (2008). Pain perception in the elderly patient. *Clinics in Geriatric Medicine, 24*(2), 203–211. *Evidence Level V.*

Meneilly, G. S. (2010). Pathophysiology of diabetes in the elderly. *Clinical Geriatrics, 18*, 25–28. *Evidence Level V.*

Mentes, J. (2006). Oral hydration on older adults: Greater awareness is needed in preventing, recognizing, and treating dehydration. *American Journal of Nursing, 106*(6), 40–49. *Evidence Level V.*

Mick, D. J., & Ackerman, M. H. (2004). Critical care nursing for older adults: Pathophysiological and functional considerations. *Nursing Clinics of North America, 39*(3), 473–493. *Evidence Level V.*

Miller, M. (2009). Disorders of fluid balance. In J. B. Halter, J. G. Ouslander, M. E. Tinetti, S. Studenski, K. P. High, & S. Asthana (Eds.), *Hazzard's geriatric medicine and gerontology* (6th ed., pp. 1047–1058). New York, NY: McGraw-Hill. *Evidence Level V.*

Mukai, S., & Lipsitz, L. A. (2002). Orthostatic hypotension. *Clinics in Geriatric Medicine, 18*(2), 253–268.

Narici, M. V., Maffulli, N., & Maganaris, C. N. (2008). Ageing of human muscles and tendons. *Disability and Rehabilitation, 30*(20–22), 1548–1554. *Evidence Level V.*

National Kidney Disease Education Program. (2012). *Resource center: Estimation of kidney function for prescription medication dosage in adults.* Retrieved from http://www.nkdep.nih.gov/resources/CKD-drug-dosing.shtml. *Evidence Level I.*

Netz, Y., Wu, M. J., Becker, B. J., & Tenenbaum, G. (2005). Physical activity and psychological well-being in advanced age: A meta-analysis of intervention studies. *Psychology & Aging, 20*(2), 272–284. *Evidence Level I.*

Newton, J. L. (2005). Effect of age-related changes in gastric physiology on tolerability of medications for older people. *Drugs & Aging, 22*(8), 655–661. *Evidence Level V.*

Ney, D. M., Weiss, J. M., Kind, A. J., & Robbins, J. (2009). Senescent swallowing: Impact, strategies, and interventions. *Nutrition in Clinical Practice, 24*(3), 395–413. *Evidence Level V.*

Park, H. L., O'Connell, J. E., & Thomson, R. G. (2003). A systematic review of cognitive decline in the general elderly population. *International Journal of Geriatric Psychiatry, 18*(12), 1121–1134. *Evidence Level I.*

Péquignot, R., Belmin, J., Chauvelier, S., Gaubert, J. Y., Konrat, C., Duron, E., & Hanon, O. (2009). Renal function in older hospital patients is more accurately estimated using the Cockcroft–Gault formula than the modification diet in renal disease formula. *Journal of the American Geriatrics Society, 57*(9), 1638–1643. *Evidence Level II.*

Roberts, S. B., & Dallal, G. E. (2005). Energy requirements and aging. *Public Health Nutrition, 8*(7A), 1028–1036. *Evidence Level I.*

Sands, J. M. (2012). Urine concentrating and diluting ability during aging. *Journals of Gerontology. Series A, Biological Sciences & Medical Sciences, 67*(12), 1352–1357. *Evidence Level V.*

Schnelle, J. F., Alessi, C. A., Simmons, S. F., Al-Samarrai, N. R., Beck, J. C., & Ouslander, J. G. (2002). Translating clinical research into practice: A randomized controlled trial of exercise and incontinence care with nursing home residents. *Journal of the American Geriatrics Society, 50*(9), 1476–1483. *Evidence Level II.*

Shah, S. J., Nakamura, K., Marcus, G. M., Gerber, I. L., McKeown, B. H., Jordan, M. V., . . . Michaels, A. D. (2008). Association of the fourth heart sound with increased left ventricular end-diastolic stiffness. *Journal of Cardiac Failure, 14*(5), 431–436. *Evidence Level III.*

Simon, L. S. (2005). Osteoporosis. *Clinics in Geriatric Medicine, 21*(3), 603–629. *Evidence Level V.*

Smith, C. M., & Cotter, V. T. (2012). *Want to know more—Geriatric nursing protocol: Age-related changes in health*. Hartford Institute for Geriatric Nursing. Retrieved from http://consultgerirn.org/topics/normal_aging_changes/want_to_know_more. *Evidence Level V.*

Smith, H. A., & Connolly, M. J. (2003). Evaluation and treatment of dysphagia following stroke. *Topics in Geriatric Rehabilitation, 19*(1), 43–59. *Evidence Level V.*

Stern, M. (2006). Neurogenic bowel and bladder in the older adult. *Clinics in Geriatric Medicine, 22*(2), 311–330. *Evidence Level V.*

Stewart, R. (2004). Review: In older people, decline of cognitive function is more likely than improvement, but rate of change is very variable. *Evidence-Based Mental Health, 7*(3), 92. *Evidence Level I.*

Suhayda, R., & Walton, J. C. (2002). Preventing and managing dehydration. *Medsurg Nursing, 11*(6), 267–278. *Evidence Level V.*

Thomas, S., & Rich, M. W. (2007). Epidemiology, pathophysiology, and prognosis of heart failure in the elderly. *Clinics in Geriatric Medicine, 23*(1), 1–10. *Evidence Level V.*

U.S. Department of Agriculture (USDA) & U.S. Department of Health and Human Services (USDHHS). (2010). *Dietary guidelines for Americans, 2010*. Retrieved from www.health.gov/dietaryguidelines/2010.asp. *Evidence Level I.*

U.S. Department of Health and Human Services (USDHHS). (2004). *Bone health and osteoporosis: A report of the surgeon general.* Retrieved from www.surgeongeneral.gov/library/reports. *Evidence Level I.*

U.S. Department of Health and Human Services (USDHHS). (2014). *The health consequences of smoking—50 years of progress: A report of the surgeon general, 2014*. Retrieved from www.surgeongeneral.gov/library/reports/50-years-of-progress. *Evidence Level I.*

Visvanathan, R., & Chapman, I. M. (2009). Undernutrition and anorexia in the older person. *Gastroenterology Clinics of North America, 38*(3), 393–409. *Evidence Level V.*

Watters, J. M. (2002). Surgery in the elderly. *Canadian Journal of Surgery, 45*(2), 104–108. *Evidence Level V.*

Weiskopf, D., Weinberger, B., & Grubeck-Loebenstein, B. (2009). The aging of the immune system. *Transplant International, 22*(11), 1041–1050. *Evidence Level V.*

Zeleznik, J. (2003). Normative aging of the respiratory system. *Clinics in Geriatric Medicine, 19*(1), 1–18. *Evidence Level V.*

4

Health Care Decision Making

Linda Farber Post and Marie Boltz

EDUCATIONAL OBJECTIVES

On completion of this chapter, the reader should be able to:

1. Define *informed consent* and its supporting bioethical and legal principles
2. Understand the role of culture in health care decision making
3. Differentiate between competence and capacity
4. Understand the process of decisional capacity assessment
5. Describe the nurse's role and responsibility as an advocate for the patient's voice in health care decision making

OVERVIEW

Health care is about decisions—how they are made, who makes them, and according to what standards. Until the latter half of the 20th century, patients were told what health care interventions would benefit them and they rarely questioned the doctor's instructions. The rise of the rights movement in most areas of society promoted the idea that patients would benefit from robust participation in decision making affecting their health outcomes. Building on the well-established doctrine of informed consent, as well as statutory and case law, all states came to require that patient goals, values, and preferences be central to health care decision making. The result was a greater degree of clinician–patient collaboration in planning and implementing care decisions.

Although all health care activities deserve principled and thoughtful decision making, the benefit–burden–risk calculus associated with treatment and diagnostic interventions typically requires specific informed consent by or on behalf of the patient. For this reason, the determination of patients' decision-making capacity, authority, and standards becomes a most pressing issue that arises daily in the clinical setting.

BACKGROUND AND STATEMENT OF PROBLEM

Ethical Principles and Professional Obligations

Core ethical principles that underlie the health care decision process and give rise to clinician obligations include:

- Respect for autonomy: supporting and facilitating the capable patient's exercise of self-determination regarding health care
- Beneficence: promoting the patient's best interest and well-being and protecting the patient from harm
- Nonmaleficence: avoiding actions likely to cause the patient harm

For a description of evidence levels cited in this chapter, see Chapter 1, "Developing and Evaluating Clinical Practice Guidelines: A Systematic Approach."

- Justice: allocating fairly the benefits and burdens related to health care delivery and ensuring that decisions are based on clinical need rather than ethically irrelevant characteristics, such as race, religion, or socioeconomic status

The tension between and among these ethical principles can create dilemmas for clinicians when their obligations conflict. For example, care providers have a duty to respect patients' autonomy by honoring their decisions *and* a duty to protect them from the harm of risky choices. Care providers are also expected to provide care to patients who need it *and* be responsible stewards of limited resources. Clinical, legal, and ethically valid decisions by or for patients invoke a careful balancing of information, principles, rights, and responsibilities in light of medical realities, cultural factors, and, increasingly, concerns about resource allocation and access to care.

Autonomy and Capacity

The well-settled right to determine what happens to one's own body has two equally important components: the right to *consent* to treatment and the right to *refuse* treatment. Grounded in the ethical principle of respect for persons, this right to bodily integrity is considered so fundamental that it is protected by the U.S. Constitution, state constitutions, and decisions of the U.S. Supreme Court (*Cruzan v. Director,* 1990). All persons are considered to have the potential for autonomy, expressed in the clinical setting through informed decision making. The threshold question is whether they have the *capacity to exercise* autonomy.

Respect for autonomy is widely considered to be the ethical principle most central to health care decision making because of its emphasis on self-governance and choices that reflect personal values. This heightened emphasis on self-determination is largely a Western phenomenon, however, and is not universally shared. Even capable patients, who are easily confused, exhibit diminished or fluctuating capacity or from cultures that value collective rather than individual decision making come and may not be comfortable with pure autonomous decision making. Instead, they may involve trusted others in planning their care, thus demonstrating *assisted*, *supported*, or *delegated* autonomy as their preferred method of decision making. If this is their customary dynamic and if it appears to be effective for them, there is no reason to encourage them to adopt an unfamiliar decision-making style in the mistaken belief that only self-governance is authentic. For these patients, autonomy may not be reflected in self-determined decision making about treatment, but in expressions of values and goals of care. Drawing on the assistance or support of trusted others does not diminish the integrity of the process. Voluntarily delegating decision-making authority to others is also an autonomous choice but it is one that must be explicitly confirmed, not inferred.

Diminished or fluctuating capacity is not a reason to ignore the patient's voice but is a signal to attend more carefully to what is being communicated. The "what" and "how" of the treatment may be a decision for others to make; the "why" or the rationale in the patient's voice must be heard.

Capacity and Competence

Decisional capacity refers to a set of skills related to health care decision making, including the ability to:

- Understand and process information about diagnosis, prognosis, and treatment options
- Weigh the benefits, burdens, and risks of the proposed options
- Apply a set of personal values to the analysis
- Arrive at a decision that is consistent over time
- Communicate the decision

Capacity runs along a continuum rather than being all on or all off. Some patients are able to make all their own decisions—personal, legal, financial, health care—and some, like infants and adults with profound cognitive impairment, are unable to make any decisions. Because capacity is decision specific rather than global, most people are able to make some decisions and not others.

Although the terms *capacity* and *competence* are often used interchangeably, in the health care setting their distinctions go beyond semantics. Competence is a *legal* presumption that an adult has the mental ability to negotiate various legal tasks, such as entering into a contract, making a will, and standing for trial. Incompetence is a judicial determination that because a person lacks this ability, she or he should be prevented from doing certain things. In contrast, capacity is a *clinical* determination that a person has the ability to understand, make, and take responsibility for the consequences of health care decisions. Because the legal system should rarely be involved in medical decisions, the patient's capacity for decision making is an assessment made by clinicians.

Consent and Refusal

In the clinical setting, the principle of respect for autonomy is most clearly expressed in the doctrine of informed consent and refusal. Because therapeutic and diagnostic interventions typically involve a range of benefits, burdens, and risks, express consent is almost always required before interventions are implemented. Informed consent is a process over time rather than a single event or a signed document. Among adults with a language barrier associated with education and/or ethnicity, comprehension might be limited (Fink et al., 2010). Providing adequate time for the informed consent discussion(s) and the opportunity to ensure understanding and voluntariness are essential to a valid decision about whether to authorize a proposed intervention. As an expression of autonomy, the most effective consent process is a collaborative interaction that includes consultation with clinicians and, possibly, family and trusted others.

Informed consent and refusal engage capable patients or surrogates acting on behalf of patients without capacity in a process that requires:

- Patient decisional capacity
- Disclosure of sufficient material information relevant to the decision in question
- Understanding of the information provided
- Voluntariy choosing among the options
- Consent to or refusal of the proposed intervention (Lo, 2000)

Education can improve decisional capacity to give safe, informed consent even for clinically depressed older adults (Lapid, Rummans, Pankratz, & Appelbaum, 2004). In one study, depressed patients' involvement in health care decision making not only increased the likelihood of their receiving treatment congruent with depression treatment guidelines, but also showed reduced symptoms of depression over an 18-month period (Clever et al., 2006). "Framing" can be persuasive; a clinician's emphasis on the distinctions about the efficacy of a treatment and whether it would be curative or palliative can influence a patient's decision even more than information given about the disease or treatment options (Van Kleffens, van Baarsen, & van Leeuwen, 2004).

Decision-Making Authority

Treatment decisions are typically made by capable patients based on their health goals, values, and preferences in response to information they receive about their diagnosis, prognosis, and therapeutic options. These decisions are, thus, an expression of autonomy, reflecting the view that health care is not something that is *done to* patients; rather, it is a collaborative endeavor in which patients and clinicians contribute to the shared goal of recovery, rehabilitation, or palliation.

Readiness for decision making has a temporal, as well as a contextual, component. Asked in focus groups why they had or had not been involved in any advance care planning (ACP), older adults and their caregivers revealed considerable variability in their readiness for discussion of different components of the ACP process such as advance directive creation, communication with family and physicians, and consideration of their treatment goals (Fried, Bullock, Iannone, & O'Leary, 2009). Participants identified barriers and benefits to ACP and said that it was not the only way to prepare for decline in health or death. Prior experience with health care decision making for others influenced older adults' propensity to engage in ACP. Having an active role in shared decision making is associated with enhanced cancer-specific quality of life, satisfaction, and more likely use of adjuvant therapy for women with breast cancer but not for men with prostate cancer (Hack et al., 2010; Mandelblatt, Kreling, Figeuriedo, & Feng, 2006).

Perceptions of ACP are crucial in determining readiness to engage in the process of proactive consideration of health care options. If "ACP" is perceived as synonymous with "end of life," it is not surprising that individuals, families, and care professionals are reluctant to initiate or participate in "the discussion." The common response is, "No one is dying here, so we don't have to deal with these matters now."

When patients are not capable of making decisions about their treatment, others are asked to choose for them, basing their decisions as much as possible on what is known of the patients' preferences or what is considered to be in their best interest. The determination of decision-making authority is among the most critical tasks in the clinical setting. When patients lack the ability to make treatment decisions, authority to act on their behalf must be vested in others—appointed agents, family, or other surrogates. The threshold determination, then, is of the patient's decisional capacity: an assessment of an individual's ability to make decisions about health care and treatment.

DECISION AIDS

Especially because the elder population is expected to double during the next 20 years, capacity assessments in the geriatric setting are likely to be requested and relied on with increasing frequency. Because decisional capacity is an important marker of an individual's ability to complete specific tasks or make specific decisions, the reliability of capacity assessments is crucial in evaluating what individuals are able to do for themselves. Nevertheless, although decisional capacity is an index of patient ability to make decisions and, therefore, involves cognitive processes, its assessment requires more than a test of mental acuity or a psychiatric examination (Post & Blustein, 2015).

Given the importance of assessing decision-making capacity, the desire for a precise method of measurement is understandable, especially in the geriatric setting. "Decisional capacity assessments are important tools in optimizing safety and autonomy when there are questions about an older adult's ability to make decisions related to healthcare, independent living, financial management, and other areas that are essential to daily functioning" (Braun & Moye, 2010, p. 204).

Decision aids assist, guide, and support a decision-making process that requires consideration of benefits, burdens, risks, and options. Studies indicate that decision aids lead to decisions that are value based, more informed, less conflicted, and characterized by a process that is more participatory than passive compared to standard decision-making approaches (O'Connor et al., 2004). Decision aids made a difference in physician–patient discussion about the use of adjuvant therapy for women with breast cancer (Siminoff, Gordon, Silverman, Budd, & Ravdin, 2006); clarified values and options, and increased knowledge regarding breast and ovarian genetic testing counseling (Wakefield et al., 2008); and improved men's knowledge on the risks and benefits of prostate-specific antigen (PSA) testing (Watson et al., 2006). An "order effect" was discerned regarding the sequence in which information was presented in a decision aid to women with breast cancer (Ubel et al., 2010). The order of presentation of information about the risks and benefits of tamoxifen influenced their perceptions. Bias was eliminated by the simultaneous presentation of information of competing options and risks.

A comprehensive review of several additional capacity assessment instruments (Racine & Billick, 2012) concluded that sensitivity and specificity tend to be in tension with efficiency and ease of use. Some can be administered in less than 10 minutes but may be more general, whereas others, which are more specific and in depth, require considerably more time and complicated scoring systems. Although none of the instruments is considered to be the gold standard, the literature indicates that their use in clinical practice could improve accuracy in capacity determination. Especially in the elder population, where capacity issues may be complex and multifactorial, these tools may be useful adjuncts to clinical interviews, medical record reviews, interviews, neuropsychological testing, and functional assessment.

ASSESSMENT OF THE PROBLEM

Determination of Decision-Making Capacity

The importance of capacity determination resides in the presumption that adults have decisional capacity and, absent contrary evidence, treatment decisions typically defer to patient goals, values, and preferences. This deference usually extends to all decisions made by capable individuals, including those decisions that appear risky or ill advised. Capacity assessment is important because patients who lack the ability to appreciate the implications of, and accept responsibility for, their choices are vulnerable to the risks of deficient decision making. Indeed, the reason capacity determination is considered so important and receives so much attention is that honoring the decisions of a capable patient demonstrates respect for the person, whereas honoring the decisions of a patient without capacity can be seen as an act of abandonment. Thus, clinicians have an obligation to ensure that capable patients have the opportunity to make treatment decisions that will be implemented and that incapacitated patients will be protected by having decisions made for them by others who act in their best interest.

Fulfilling this obligation requires that clinicians appreciate the characteristics of decision-making capacity, the elements of which include the ability to:

- Understand and process information about diagnosis, prognosis, and treatment options
- Weigh the relative benefits, burdens, and risks of the care options
- Apply a set of values to the analysis
- Arrive at a decision that is consistent over time
- Communicate the decision (Roth, Meisel, & Lidz, 1997)

Capacity assessment depends on interaction with the patient over time rather than on specific tests. There is no gold standard instrument or "capacimeter" that assesses decisional capacity (Kapp & Mossman, 1996). The Mini-Mental State Examination (MMSE) estimates orientation, long- and short-term memory, and mathematical and language dexterity. It is not a test of executive function (an assessment more likely to capture reasoning and recall) and is, therefore, less helpful in gauging the patient's ability to understand the implications of a decision (Allen et al., 2003). It has been suggested, however, that an MMSE score less than 19 or more than 23 might be able to distinguish those with and without capacity for decision making (Karlawish, Casarett, James, Xie, & Kim, 2005). The Assessment of Capacity for Everyday Decision-Making (ACED) is a reportedly valid and reliable instrument to assess everyday decisional capacity in those with mild to moderate cognitive impairment (Lai et al., 2008). Its use in facilitating assessment of health care decision-making capacity has not been reported but could be explored in future studies.

Although there is no consistent standardized definition of decisional capacity, there is evidence that safe and sufficient decision making is retained in early-stage dementia (Kim, Karlawish, & Caine, 2002). Persons with mild to moderate dementia can make or at least participate in making treatment decisions, but impaired memory recall might be a barrier to their demonstrating understanding of treatment options (Moye, Karel, Azar, & Gurrera, 2004). Standard assessment of appreciation of diagnostic and treatment information should focus on the patient's ability to state the importance or implications of the choice on his or her future health. Specific neuropsychological tests (e.g., MacArthur Competence Assessment Tool and Hopemont Capacity Assessment Interview) can predict decisional capacity for those with mild to moderate dementia, although reasoning and appreciation might differ among those with mental illness (Gurrera, Moye, Karel, Azar, & Armesto, 2006).

In one study, the standard of decision making most highly valued by a group of geriatricians, psychologists, and ethics committee members was the ability to appreciate the consequences of a decision, followed by the ability to respond "yes" or "no" to a question; the standard least supported was that the decision had to seem reasonable (Volicer & Ganzini, 2003).

Clinical Importance of Decisional Capacity

Accurate and useful capacity assessment depends on the recognition that capacity is decision-specific rather than global and works on a sliding scale based on the notion of risk. The greater the risk attached to a decision, the higher the level of capacity required to make a decision that will be honored. For example, a person with diminished capacity may be able to decide what to have for lunch or when to shower without undue risk of harm. A patient who asks to be removed from life support, however, is someone whose level of capacity would need to be considerably higher, demonstrating comprehension of the risk–benefit ratio and appreciation of the consequences.

Evidence also suggests that adults with mild to moderate mental retardation are able to make and provide a rationale for their treatment decisions and evaluate the risks and benefits of treatment options (Cea & Fisher, 2003). Because most people have the ability to make some decisions and not others, respect for autonomy requires clinicians to identify the widest range of decisions each patient is capable of making. A note in the chart saying, "Patient lacks decision-making capacity" is extremely unhelpful because it implies that the individual is unable to make any decisions about anything. This inhibits the exercise of autonomy by arbitrarily precluding decision making when, in fact, the patient may only lack the ability to make complex treatment decisions. Far more helpful would be an entry that says, "Patient lacks the capacity to make decisions about participation in a drug study" or "Patient lacks the capacity to make decisions about dialysis."

Likewise, decisional capacity may not be constant but may fluctuate, depending on the patient's clinical condition, medication, and/or time of day. Among gerontological nurses, protecting the right of older adults with diminished capacity or physical function to make those health care decisions that they can appropriately make is among their top practice concerns (Alford, 2006). Precisely because decisional capacity is not static, it is imperative for the protection of those with mild to moderate dementia that their understanding and reasoning about treatments and interventions are periodically assessed (Moye et al., 2006). Approaching patients for discussions and decisions when they are at their most capable (e.g., during the patient's "window of lucidity"), enhances their opportunities to participate in planning their health care.

Although disagreement with a proposed care plan or refusal of recommended treatment does not by itself demonstrate incapacity, risky or potentially harmful decisions should be carefully scrutinized to protect vulnerable patients from the consequences of deficient decision making. Because appointing a health care agent requires a lower level of capacity than that needed to make the often complex decisions the agent will make, even patients with diminished capacity may be able to select the persons they want to speak for them (Mezey, Teresi, Ramsey, Mitty, & Bobrowitz, 2002).

Decision Making in the Absence of Capacity

The more difficult clinical scenario is decision making on behalf of patients who have lost or never had the capacity to make decisions for themselves. Two approaches have been developed in response to the needs of incapacitated patients: advance directives and surrogate decision making. Advance directives (see Chapter 39, "Advance Care Planning") include the *instruction directive*, also known as a living will, which is a list of interventions the patient does or does not want in specified circumstances, and the *appointment directive*, also known as a health care proxy or durable power of attorney for health care (DPOAHC), which is the legal designation of a health care agent with the same decision-making authority as the patient. A related type of prospective care planning is the Practitioner/Physician Orders for Life-Sustaining Treatment (POLST) or Medical Orders for Life-Sustaining Treatment (MOLST), which are consolidated sets of medical orders specifically for patients with life-limiting illnesses (Bomba, 2011; Fromme, Zive, Schmidt, Olszewski, & Toll, 2012).

Despite the advantages of ACP, it is estimated that only one third of the adult population in the United States has an advance directive (American Bar Association Commission on Law and Aging, 2014). For that reason, the majority of health care decisions for incapacitated patients are made by surrogates, usually family or others close to the patient, who are asked by the care team to participate in making treatment decisions. Absent explicit instructions from the patient (verbally or in an advance directive), decisions by others are based on either *substituted judgment* (when the patient's wishes are known or can be inferred) or the *best interest standard* (when the patient did not have or articulate treatment preferences). Substituted judgment determines what the *patient* would choose based on prior statements and patterns of decision making. In contrast, the best interest standard invokes the *surrogate's* evaluation of the proposed intervention's benefits and burdens to the patient.

A health care surrogate may be any capable person 18 years of age or older who, although not specifically chosen or legally appointed, assumes the responsibility for making health care decisions on behalf of a person who lacks the capacity to make those decisions. Informal surrogates are individuals, typically family members, who are presumed to know the patient best and to act in his or her best interest. Formal surrogates may be specified by state law in a hierarchy, typically in descending order of relation to the patient. *Family consent laws* are state-specific statutes that set out the state-approved decision-making hierarchy—the order in which persons are authorized to make decisions on behalf of a patient who lacks decisional capacity and has not appointed a health care agent by means of an advance directive or DPOAHC. To gain as much insight as possible into the patient's goals, values, and preferences, and approximate as closely as possible the decisions he or she would make if capable, the ethical imperative is to engage the decision-making efforts of individuals who know the patient best before moving to those with a less vested relationship to him or her. For that reason, a good-faith effort is typically required to contact members in each level of the hierarchy in turn, moving to a lower level only when it has been determined that no one at a higher level is able or willing to assume decision-making responsibilities. Most states accord considerable latitude to surrogates, especially next of kin, in consenting to treatment. Decisions about limiting treatment are more problematic and may be significantly restricted, depending on the state in which the patient is receiving care (see the Resources section, American Bar Association Commission on Law & Aging, for state guidelines).

Context of Health Care Decision Making

Health care goals and the treatment preferences for achieving them typically change as an individual's health and functional status change (Fried et al., 2006). Previously unacceptable conditions may become more or less acceptable as they are experienced. For example, patients already in pain may be less likely to refuse a treatment outcome that includes being in pain than patients who are not currently suffering moderate to severe pain (Fried et al., 2006). Likewise, patients' treatment and comfort goals may differ from those of their family caregivers and professional providers (Steinhauser et al., 2000).

Just as there is the right to learn one's medical information, there is also a right not to be burdened with unwanted information. Older adults or those from cultures that traditionally shield patients from knowledge of their illness may prefer to have information disclosed to a particular family member, the family as a group, or trusted others, who will use it to make decisions on the patient's behalf. With the implementation of the Health Insurance Portability and Accountability Act of 1996 (HIPAA), most hospitals have a form for patients to sign, designating their preferred decision maker(s). Another approach is to ask, "You're here because you're not feeling well. We're going to do some tests and examinations, and then decisions about treatment will need to be made. Some patients like to have all the information; others don't. What would make you comfortable? Who would you like us to talk to? Would you like to be part of those discussions and decisions?"

It is not uncommon for even capable patients to say, "Talk to my daughter. She makes all my decisions about important things. Just do whatever she thinks is right." This is an autonomous decision, delegating a trusted person to be the decision maker and, if this is the dynamic the patient prefers, it would be inappropriate to try to change it. Although it is important to respect patient preferences and cultural traditions, however, a patient's waiver of the right to have information must be explicitly confirmed, not presumed.

Trust is a critical element in the patient–provider relationship, especially in decision-making situations in which information is disclosed and questions are answered. Various factors influence information exchange and shared decision making (Edwards, Davies, & Edwards, 2009). Providers may be influenced by their perceptions of informed patients and their interest in participatory decision making, their limited knowledge of patients' cultures, or a tendency to stereotype patients rather than view them as individuals. Patients may be influenced by their personal motivations to obtain and use information, cultural identity and expression, health literacy, and ability to cope with the possibility of receiving distressing information. Of note, a shared influence reported by providers and patients is the sick-role expectation (Edwards et al., 2009). African American patients have been shown to be significantly more likely than Caucasian patients to report low trust of the U.S. health care system, unrelated to age or socioeconomic status (Halbert, Armstrong, Gandy, & Shaker, 2006), as well as little interest in ACP and advance directives (Cox et al., 2006). This is not, however, an indication that patients of color and minority ethnic populations do not want to participate in health care decision making, including decisions at the end of life.

Quality-of-Life Considerations in Decision Making

Although there is almost universal acknowledgement of the patient's desire to be comfortable (i.e., relieved of pain and suffering) and to achieve a sense of completion, other quality-of-life considerations elicit more varied responses. Attitudes about the importance of clergy, being physically touched, and using all available technology may differ among patients, families, and caregivers. Older adults with varying degrees of functional impairment and past experiences with treatment decision making were found to be more interested in the outcome of a serious medical event than with the curative interventions and whether the intervention could restore or maintain their ability to participate in activities they valued (Rosenfeld, Wenger, & Kagawa-Singer, 2000). Among older adults with end-stage renal disease, the decision to begin dialysis was found to be influenced by their family caregiving responsibilities, feeling that they had no other options, and their current enjoyment of life that inhibited contemplation of their death (Visser et al., 2009). Those who rejected dialysis were more often older, male, widowers compared to those who accepted dialysis. The former group imagined that they would experience a loss of autonomy and a continuing trajectory of functional loss, have difficulty getting to the dialysis center, and have to start thinking about the future—a prospect that was unappealing to them at the time. These findings speak to the contextual and temporal nature of health care decision making that has been explored by others (Fried et al., 2009).

INTERVENTIONS AND CARE STRATEGIES

Assessing the patient's orientation and understanding can provide critical information about decision-making behavior in different circumstances, as well as the ability to articulate care wishes. Reporting that a patient is "disoriented to time and place" is helpful only in establishing the context in which more focused and useful decisional capacity assessment should take place.

Documentation needs to be specific and descriptive. The entry should describe the circumstances or interaction(s) that led to the conclusion about the patient's ability to make decisions. Because capacity is decision specific, accurate and useful statements are "Patient appears to lack the capacity to make decisions about discharge; she is unable to describe how she will cook or get to the bathroom at home" or "Patient lacks the capacity to make decisions about surgery; he was unable to name the type of surgery, what the surgery is supposed to correct, or what is involved or to be expected during recovery."

Communicating information includes determining what the patient and/or surrogate(s) understand, what they need or want to know, and how involved they want to be in decision making. Providing the relevant medical facts in lay language and avoiding medical jargon that creates distance are essential. It is also important to consider the participants in the decision making. Who should be present? What is their relationship to the patient? What is their decisional authority? What information is necessary, at what level of detail, and how will it be used? When is the information to be provided and over what period of time (Popejoy, 2005)?

Whenever language barriers or preferences are identified, certified interpreters are essential. Trained interpreters might be the only health care staff who recognize that patients, families or other surrogates, and the physician or health care professionals have differing interpretations of illness, treatment, and health; inconsistent understandings of the goals and plan of care, and disparate views about death and dying. Moreover, these varied parties may use language and decision-making frameworks differently. An interpreter may realize that truth telling might not only be perceived as disrespectful and dangerous but may potentially shorten the patient's life span, as believed in certain cultures. A trained interpreter is more than a word-for-word translator but, rather, can serve as a mediator, culture broker, patient advocate, witness, educator, and participant who interprets both fact and nuance.

CASE STUDY

Mr. Peters is an 85-year-old man with advanced Alzheimer's disease who has been living in a nursing home for the past 6 months. When he stopped eating several weeks ago, he was hospitalized for placement of a percutaneous endoscopic gastrostomy (PEG) tube to provide artificial nutrition and hydration. He returned to the nursing home briefly but developed uncontrolled diarrhea and apparent abdominal discomfort. Two days ago, his PEG tube fell out and he has been readmitted to the hospital for treatment of the diarrhea and possible replacement of the PEG.

Mr. Peters opens his eyes and responds to painful stimuli but does not interact and appears not to recognize family members. He is clearly incapable of participating in discussions or decisions about his care. His close family includes his son and granddaughter, who are visiting from California, and his grandson, Jason, who has been very involved for several years in providing and deciding about Mr. Peters's care.

A clinical ethics consultation has been convened, including Mr. Peters's family, his two attending physicians, the house and nursing staff who have cared for him most consistently, and the bioethicist. Discussion focuses on clarifying his condition and probable clinical course, the goals of care, and his likely care preferences.

Jason describes his grandfather as very active and fiercely independent until age 78, when his dementia began. With his wife, he had raised Jason and, when she died, he continued to raise the boy alone until Jason left for college. When the dementia worsened several years ago, Jason arranged for his grandfather and a team of 24-hour caregivers to move into an apartment next to his. That arrangement continued until Mr. Peters required care that could best be provided in a skilled nursing facility.

All three family members agree that, given Mr. Peters's personality, values, and lifetime behavior pattern, he would not have wanted to be maintained in his current condition, certainly not dependent on artificial nutrition and hydration. Nevertheless, they express concern about the ethics, legality, and clinical effect of not replacing the PEG tube, and are especially uncomfortable about whether it would be considered "starving" him to death.

According to the care team, Mr. Peters's advanced dementia is not reversible and he will continue to deteriorate mentally and physically until death. The doctors referred to the considerable literature demonstrating that, in patients with advanced dementia, artificial nutrition and hydration can cause gastrointestinal (GI) distress, including nausea, bloating, gas, and diarrhea, which appears to have happened to Mr. Peters. In the opinion of the care team, continued artificial nutrition and hydration would only contribute to the patient's suffering and prolong the dying process. The doctors also explain that, far from suffering, Mr. Peters appears more comfortable because the PEG fell out and the diarrhea has stopped. They assure the family that the patient could be admitted to the nursing home's hospice unit where he will receive comfort care, including pain and other symptom management. The bioethicist addressed the relevant ethical issues discussed here.

Discussion

The ethics analysis of this case focuses on decision making for an incapacitated patient, promoting the patient's best interest and protecting him from harm, and forgoing life-sustaining treatment, specifically artificial nutrition and hydration, at the end of life.

Surrogate decision making on behalf of patients lacking capacity uses the following standards.

- The patient's wishes as expressed directly through discussions with others or in advance directives
- Substituted judgment (when the patient's wishes are known or can be inferred)
- The best interest standard (when the patient's wishes are not known or inferable)

Mr. Peters has not left any explicit instructions but, his family, knowing him very well, is able to predict with confidence what he would and would not have wanted based on his characteristic patterns of behavior and decision making. In this case, the family's substituted judgment is consistent with what was considered by the family and the care team to be in the patient's best interest—protecting him from continued artificial nutrition and hydration that would have increased his suffering without providing benefit, and prolonged his dying. Framing this as *protecting* the patient from the burdens and risks of an intervention rather than *depriving* him of necessary treatment can make this decision more tolerable for distressed families.

One of the most difficult surrogate decisions is forgoing life-sustaining treatment and, because providing nourishment is so intimately associated with love and nurturing, forgoing artificial nutrition and hydration is especially wrenching for families and caregivers. Clinicians, ethicists, and courts have consistently agreed that artificial nutrition and hydration are medical

(continued)

CASE STUDY *(continued)*

treatments, the benefits, burdens, and risks of which should be assessed like those of any other intervention.

Capable patients and the appointed health care agents of incapacitated patients have a well-established right to refuse any unwanted treatment, including those that are life sustaining. Absent capacity or advance directives, the family's authority to make end-of-life decisions, including forgoing artificial nutrition and hydration, depends on the laws of the state in which the patient is treated. Many states permit family and surrogates authorized by case or statutory law to make these decisions based on substituted judgment or their assessment of the patient's best interest in light of the patient's condition and prognosis. Other states require surrogates, even next of kin, to provide explicit evidence that the patient would have refused artificial nutrition and hydration in order to authorize withholding or withdrawing the interventions. Because of the jurisdictional variations, the completion of advance directives, including the legal appointment of health care agents and alternate agents, should be strongly encouraged by health care professionals.

SUMMARY

The notion of "ownership" of one's body applies to health care decision making even in times of crisis. Patients with diminished or fluctuating decisional capacity should not be denied the opportunity to make the specific health care decisions they are capable of making. A vulnerable patient who lacks capacity, despite some social or conversational skills, needs to be protected from the potentially harmful effects of uninformed, poorly reasoned, and potentially risky health care decisions. It is suggested that the best way for nurses to learn older adults' informational needs, avoid undue paternalism, and promote their patients' best interests is to engage them in discussion about their health goals, values, and preferences (Tuckett, 2006). The ethical obligations that must be assumed by health care professionals are skillfully assessing the clinical situation; assessing the benefits, burdens, and risks of the therapeutic options; the patient's capacity to make and take responsibility for the relevant decisions; and the surrogate's need for information, guidance, and support.

NURSING STANDARD OF PRACTICE

Protocol 4.1: Health Care Decision Making

I. GOALS

To ensure nurses in acute care:

A. Understand the supporting bioethical and legal principles of informed consent
B. Are able to differentiate between competence and capacity
C. Understand the issues and processes used to assess decisional capacity
D. Can describe the nurse's role and responsibility as an advocate for the patient's voice in health care decision making

II. OVERVIEW

A. Capable persons (i.e., those with decisional capacity) have a well-established right, grounded in law and Western bioethics, to determine what is done to their bodies.
B. In any health care setting, the exercise of autonomy (self-determination) is seen in the process of informed consent to and refusal of treatment and/or care planning.
C. Determination of decision-making capacity is a compelling clinical issue because treatment and diagnostic interventions have the potential for significant benefit, burden, and/or risk.

(continued)

Protocol 4.1: Health Care Decision Making *(continued)*

D. Honoring the decisions of a capable patient demonstrates respect for the person; honoring the decisions of a patient without capacity is an act of abandonment.

III. BACKGROUND AND STATEMENT OF THE PROBLEM

A. Introduction
   1. Core ethical principles that are the foundation of clinician obligation are the following:
      a. Respect for autonomy, beneficence, nonmaleficence, and distributive justice
      b. Clinically, legally, and ethically valid decisions by or for patients require a careful balancing of information, principles, rights, and responsibilities in light of medical realities, cultural factors and, increasingly, concerns about resource allocation.
      c. Even capable patients, including those who are older adults, easily confused, or from cultures that do not consider autonomy a central value, as well as patients with diminished or fluctuating capacity, may not be capable of or comfortable with exercising purely autonomous decision making.
      d. Care professionals have an obligation to be alert to questionable or fluctuating capacity both in patients who refuse and those who consent to recommended treatment. Capable individuals may choose to make their own care decisions or they may voluntarily delegate decision-making authority to trusted others. Delegation of decisional authority must be explicitly confirmed, not inferred.
      e. The context of decision making can include cultural imperatives and taboos; perceptions of pain, suffering and quality of life, and death; education and socioeconomic status; language barriers; and advance health care planning.

B. Definitions
   1. *Consent*: The informed consent process requires evidence of decisional capacity, disclosure of sufficient information, understanding of the information provided, voluntariness in choosing among the options, and, on those bases, consent to or refusal of the intervention.
   2. *Competence*: A *legal* presumption that an adult has the mental ability to negotiate various legal tasks (e.g., entering into a contract, making a will).
   3. *Incompetence*: A *judicial* determination that a person lacks the ability to negotiate legal tasks and should be prevented from doing so.
   4. *Decisional capacity*: A *clinical* determination that an individual has the ability to understand and to make and take responsibility for the consequences of health decisions. Because capacity is not global but decision specific, patients may have the ability to make some decisions but not others. Capacity may fluctuate according to factors, including clinical condition, time of day, medications, and psychological and comfort status.

C. Essential elements
   1. Decisional capacity reflects the ability to understand the facts, appreciate the implications, and assume responsibility for the consequences of a decision.
   2. The elements of decisional capacity: The ability to understand and process information; weigh the relative benefits, burdens, and risks of each option; apply personal values to the analysis; arrive at a consistent decision; and communicate the decision.
   3. Standards of decision making
      a. Prior explicit articulation: A decision based on the previous expression of a capable person's wishes through oral or written comments or instructions.
      b. Substituted judgment: A decision by others based on the formerly capable person's wishes that are known or can be inferred from prior behaviors or decisions.
      c. Best interests standard: A decision based on what others judge to be in the best interest of an individual who never had or made known health care wishes and whose preferences cannot be inferred.

IV. ASSESSMENT OF DECISIONAL CAPACITY

A. There is no gold standard instrument to assess capacity.

B. Assessment should occur over time, at different times of day, and with attention to the patient's comfort level.

(continued)

Protocol 4.1: Health Care Decision Making *(continued)*

C. The MMSE or Mini-Cog Test are not tests of capacity. Tests of executive function might better approximate the reasoning and recall needed to understand the implications of a decision.
D. Clinicians agree that the ability to understand the consequences of a decision is an important indicator of decisional capacity.
E. Safe and sufficient decision making is retained in early stage of dementia (Kim et al., 2002) and by adults with mild to moderate mental retardation (Cea & Fisher, 2003).

V. NURSING CARE STRATEGIES

A. Communicate with the patient and family or other surrogate decision makers to enhance their understanding of treatment options.
B. Be sensitive to racial, ethnic, religious, and cultural mores and traditions regarding end-of-life care planning, disclosure of information, and care decisions.
C. Be aware of conflict-resolution support and systems available in the care-providing organization.
D. Observe, document, and report the patient's ability to:
   1. Articulate his or her needs and preferences
   2. Follow directions
   3. Make simple choices and decisions (e.g., "Do you prefer the TV on or off?" "Do you prefer orange juice or water?")
   4. Communicate consistent care wishes
E. Observe period(s) of confusion and lucidity; document the specific time(s) when the patient seems more or less "clear." Observation and documentation of the patient's mental state should occur during the day, evening, and at night.
F. Assess the patient's understanding relative to the particular decision at issue. The following probes and statements are useful in assessing the degree to which the patient has the skills necessary to make a health care decision.
   1. "Tell me in your own words what the physician explained to you."
   2. "Tell me which parts, if any, were confusing."
   3. "What do you feel you have to *gain* by agreeing to (the proposed intervention)?
   4. "Tell me what you feel you have to *lose* by agreeing to (the proposed intervention).
   5. "Tell me what you feel you have to gain or lose by refusing (the proposed intervention).
   6. "Tell me why this decision is important (difficult, frightening, etc.) to you."
G. Select (or construct) appropriate decision aids.
H. Help the patient express what he or she understands about the clinical situation, the goals of care, and his or her expectation of the outcomes of the diagnostic or treatment interventions.
I. Help the patient identify who should participate in diagnostic and treatment discussions and decisions.

VI. EVALUATION AND EXPECTED OUTCOME(S)

A. The number of referrals to the ethics committee or ethics consultant in situations of decision-making conflict between any of the involved parties
B. The use of interpreters in communication of, or decision making about, diagnostic and/or treatment interventions
C. Plan of care: instructions regarding frequency of observation to ascertain the patient's lucid periods, if any
D. Documentation
   1. Is the process of the capacity assessment described?
   2. Is the assessment specific to the decision at issue?
   3. Is the informed consent and refusal interaction described?
   4. Are the specifics of the patient's degree or spheres of orientation described?
   5. Is the patient's language used to describe the diagnostic or treatment intervention under consideration recorded?
   6. Is the patient's demeanor during this discussion recorded?

(continued)

Protocol 4.1: Health Care Decision Making *(continued)*

7. Are the patient's questions and the clinician(s) answers recorded?
8. Are appropriate mental status descriptors used consistently?

ABBREVIATION

MMSE Mini-Mental State Examination

ACKNOWLEDGMENT

The author acknowledges the work of Ethel Mitty, PhD, whose knowledge, wisdom, and collaboration enriched the previous iterations of this chapter. Her influence continues to touch and improve the lives of patients, students, and colleagues.

RESOURCES

American Bar Association (ABA)
http://www.americanbar.org

American Bar Association Commission on Law & Aging, Legislative Updates
See link for chart that summarizes the wide variation on how states allocate decisional authority in the absence of patient capacity to make health care decisions, *as well as legislative updates and other relevant information.*
http://www.americanbar.org/groups/law_aging.html

American Society of Bioethics and Humanities
http://www.asbh.org

The Hastings Center
http://www.thehastingscenter.org

Health Insurance Portability and Accountability Act of 1996 (HIPAA)
http://www.hhs.gov/ocr/privacy

The Office for Civil Rights (OCR) enforces the HIPAA Privacy Rule
http://www.hhs.gov/ocr/privacy/hipaa/understanding/summary/index.html

REFERENCES

Alford, D. M. (2006). Legal issues in gerontological nursing—Part 2: Responsible parties and guardianships. *Journal of Gerontological Nursing, 32*(2), 15–18. *Evidence Level VI.*

Allen, R. S., DeLaine, S. R., Chaplin, W. F., Marson, D. C., Bourgeois, M. S., Dijkstra, K., & Burgio, L. D. (2003). Advance care planning in nursing homes: Correlates of capacity and possession of advance directives. *The Gerontologist, 43*(3), 309–317. *Evidence Level IV.*

American Bar Association Commission on Law and Aging. (2014). *Myths and facts about health care advance directives.* Retrieved from www.americanbar.org/content/dam/aba/administrative/law_aging/2011/2011_aging_bk_myths_factshcad.authcheckdam.pdf. *Evidence Level VI.*

Bomba, P. (2011). Landmark legislation in New York affirms benefits of a two-step approach to advance care planning including MOLST: A model of shared, informed medical decision-making and honoring patient preferences for care at the end of life. *Widener Law Review, 17*(475), 475–500. *Evidence Level V.*

Braun, M., & Moye, J. (2010). Decisional capacity assessment: Optimizing safety and autonomy for older adults. *Generations, 34*(2), 102–105. *Evidence Level VI.*

Cea, C. D., & Fisher, C. B. (2003). Healthcare decision-making by adults with mental retardation. *Mental Retardation, 41*(2), 78–87. *Evidence Level IV.*

Clever, S. L., Ford, D. E., Rubenstein, L. V., Rost, K. M., Meredith, L. S., Sherbourne, C. D.,... Cooper, L. A. (2006). Primary care patients' involvement in decision-making is associated with improvement in depression. *Medical Care, 44*(5), 398–405. *Evidence Level IV.*

Cox, C. L., Cole, E., Reynolds, T., Wandrag, M., Breckenridge, S., & Dingle, M. (2006). Implications of cultural diversity in do not attempt resuscitation (DNAR) decision-making. *Journal of Multicultural Nursing and Health, 12*(1), 20–28. *Evidence Level I.*

Cruzan v. Director. (1990). Missouri Department of Health, 497 U.S. 261.

Edwards, M., Davies, M., & Edwards, A. (2009). What are the external influences on information exchange and shared decision-making in healthcare consultations: A meta-synthesis of the literature. *Patient Education and Counseling, 75*(1), 37–52. *Evidence Level I.*

Fink, A. S., Prochazka, A. V., Henderson, W. G., Bartenfeld, D., Nyirenda, C., Webb, A.,... Parmelee, P. (2010). Predictors of comprehension during surgical informed consent. *Journal of the American College of Surgeons, 210*(6), 919–926. *Evidence Level II.*

Fried, T. R., Bullock, K., Iannone, L., & O'Leary, J. R. (2009). Understanding advance care planning as a process of health behavior change. *Journal of the American Geriatrics Society, 57*(9), 1547–1555. *Evidence Level IV.*

Fried, T. R., Byers, A. L., Gallo, W. T., Van Ness, P. H., Towle, V. R., O'Leary, J. R., & Dubin, J. A. (2006). Prospective study of health status preferences and changes in preferences over time in adults. *Archives of Internal Medicine, 166*(8), 890–895. *Evidence Level IV.*

Fromme, E. K., Zive, D., Schmidt, T. A., Olszewski, E., & Toll, S. W. (2012). POLST registry, do-not-resuscitate orders and other patient treatment preferences. *Journal of the American Medical Association, 307*(1), 34–35. *Evidence Level IV.*

Gurrera, R. J., Moye, J., Karel, M. J., Azar, A. R., & Armesto, J. C. (2006). Cognitive performance predicts treatment decisional abilities in mild to moderate dementia. *Neurology, 66*(9), 1367–1372. *Evidence Level IV.*

Hack, T. F., Pickles, T., Ruether, J. D., Weir, L., Bultz, B. D., Mackey, J., & Degner, L. F. (2010). Predictors of distress and quality of life in patients undergoing cancer therapy: Impact of treatment type and decisional role. *Psycho-Oncology, 19*(6), 606–616. *Evidence Level II.*

Halbert, C. H., Armstrong, K., Gandy, O. H., Jr., & Shaker, L. (2006). Racial differences in trust in health care providers. *Archives of Internal Medicine, 166*(8), 896–901. *Evidence Level IV.*

Kapp, M. B., & Mossman, D. (1996). Measuring decisional capacity: Cautions on the construction of a "capacimeter." *Psychology, Public Policy, and Law, 2*(1), 73–95. *Evidence Level VI.*

Karlawish, J. H., Casarett, D. J., James, B. D., Xie, S. X., & Kim, S. Y. (2005). The ability of persons with Alzheimer disease (AD) to make a decision about taking an AD treatment. *Neurology, 64*(9), 1514–1519. *Evidence Level IV.*

Kim, S. Y., Karlawish, J. H., & Caine, E. D. (2002). Current state of research on decision-making competence of cognitively impaired elderly persons. *American Journal of Geriatric Psychiatry: Official Journal of the American Association for Geriatric Psychiatry, 10*(2), 151–165. *Evidence Level V.*

Lai, J. M., Gill, T. M., Cooney, L. M., Bradley, E. H., Hawkins, K. A., & Karlawish, J. H. (2008). Everyday decision-making ability in older persons with cognitive impairment. *American Journal of Geriatric Psychiatry: Official Journal of the American Association for Geriatric Psychiatry, 16*(8), 693–696. *Evidence Level IV.*

Lapid, M. I., Rummans, T. A., Pankratz, V. S., & Appelbaum, P. S. (2004). Decisional capacity of depressed elderly to consent to electroconvulsive therapy. *Journal of Geriatric Psychiatry and Neurology, 17*(1), 42–46. *Evidence Level II.*

Lo, B. (2000). *Resolving ethical dilemmas: A guide for clinicians* (2nd ed.). Philadelphia, PA: Lippincott, Williams, & Wilkins. *Evidence Level VI.*

Mandelblatt, J., Kreling, B., Figeuriedo, M., & Feng, S. (2006). What is the impact of shared decision making on treatment and outcomes for older women with breast cancer? *Journal of Clinical Oncology: Official Journal of the American Society of Clinical Oncology, 24*(30), 4908–4913. *Evidence Level IV.*

Mezey, M., Teresi, J., Ramsey, G., Mitty, E., & Bobrowitz, T. (2002). *Determining a resident's capacity to execute a health care proxy. Voices of decision in nursing homes: Respecting residents' preferences for end-of-life care.* New York, NY: United Hospital Fund. *Evidence Level IV.*

Moye, J., Karel, M. J., Azar, A. R., & Gurrera, R. J. (2004). Capacity to consent to treatment: Empirical comparison of three instruments in older adults with and without dementia. *The Gerontologist, 44*(2), 166–175. *Evidence Level IV.*

Moye, J., Karel, M. J., Gurrera, R. J., & Azar, A. R. (2006). Neuropsychological predictors of decision-making capacity over 9 months in mild-to-moderate dementia. *Journal of General Internal Medicine, 21*(1), 78–83. *Evidence Level IV.*

O'Connor, A. M., Stacey, D., Entwistle, V., Llewellyn-Thomas, D., Rovner, D., Holmes-Rovner, M., . . . Jones, J. (2004). *Decision aids for people facing health treatment or screening decisions.* Chichester, UK: John Wiley & Sons. *Evidence Level I.*

Popejoy, L. (2005). Health-related decision-making by older adults and their families: How clinicians can help. *Journal of Gerontological Nursing, 31*(9), 12–18. *Evidence Level V.*

Post, L. F., & Blustein, J. (2015). *Handbook for health care ethics committees* (2nd ed.). Baltimore, MD: Johns Hopkins University Press. *Evidence Level VI.*

Racine, C. E., & Billick, S. B. (2012). Assessment instruments of decision-making capacity. *Journal of Psychiatry & Law, 40*(2), 243–263. *Evidence Level V.*

Rosenfeld, K. E., Wenger, N. S., & Kagawa-Singer, M. (2000). End-of-life decision making: A qualitative study of elderly individuals. *Journal General Internal Medicine, 15*(9), 620–625. *Evidence Level IV.*

Roth, L. H., Meisel, A., & Lidz, C. W. (1997). Tests of competency to consent to treatment. *American Journal of Psychiatry, 134*(3), 279–284. *Evidence Level VI.*

Siminoff, L. A., Gordon, N. H., Silverman, P., Budd, T., & Ravdin, P. M. (2006). A decision aid to assist in adjuvant therapy choices for breast cancer. *Psycho-Oncology, 15*(11), 1001–1013. *Evidence Level II.*

Steinhauser, K. E., Christakis, N. A., Clipp, E. C., McNeilly, M., McIntyre, L., & Tulsky, J. A. (2000). Factors considered important at the end of life by patients, family, physicians, and other care providers. *Journal of the American Medical Association, 284*(19), 2476–2482. *Evidence Level IV.*

Tuckett, A. G. (2006). On paternalism, autonomy and best interests: Telling the (competent) aged-care resident what they want to know. *International Journal of Nursing Practice, 12*(3), 166–173. *Evidence Level V.*

Ubel, P. A., Smith, D. M., Zikmund-Fisher, B. J., Derry, H. A., McClure, J., Stark, A., . . . Fagerlin, A. (2010). Testing whether decision aids introduce cognitive biases: Results of a randomized trial. *Patient Education and Counseling, 80*(2), 158–163. *Evidence Level II.*

Van Kleffens, T., van Baarsen, B., & van Leeuwen, E. (2004). The medical practice of patient autonomy and cancer treatment refusals: A patients' and physicians' perspective. *Social Science and Medicine, 8*(11), 2325–2336. *Evidence Level IV.*

Visser, A., Dijkstra, G. J., Kuiper, D., de Jong, P. E., Franssen, C. F., Gansevoort, R. T., . . . Reijneveld, S. A. (2009). Accepting or declining dialysis: Considerations taken into account by elderly patients with end-stage renal disease. *Journal of Nephrology, 22*(6), 794–799. *Evidence Level IV.*

Volicer, L., & Ganzini, L. (2003). Health professionals' views on standards for decision-making capacity regarding refusal of medical treatment in mild Alzheimer's disease. *Journal of the American Geriatrics Society, 51*(5), 1270–1274. *Evidence Level IV.*

Wakefield, C. E., Meiser, B., Homewood, J., Taylor, A., Gleeson, M., Williams, R.,... Australian GENetic testing Decision Aid Collaborative Group. (2008). A randomized trial of a breast/ovarian cancer genetic testing decision aid used as a communication aid during genetic counseling. *Psycho-Oncology, 17*(8), 844–854. *Evidence Level II.*

Watson, E., Hewitson, P., Brett, J., Bukach, C., Evans, R., Edwards, A.,... Austoker, J. (2006). Informed decision making and prostate specific antigen (PSA) testing for prostate cancer: A randomised controlled trial exploring the impact of a brief patient decision aid on men's knowledge, attitudes and intention to be tested. *Patient Education and Counseling, 63*(3), 367–379. *Evidence Level II.*

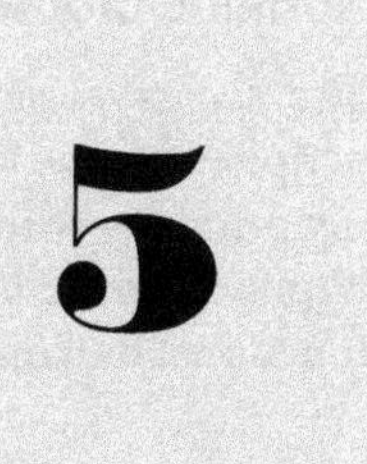

Sensory Changes

Pamela Z. Cacchione

EDUCATIONAL OBJECTIVES

On completion of this chapter, the reader should be able to:

1. Describe the normal changes of aging that affect the senses in the older adult
2. Identify common disorders that impact the senses in the older adult
3. Determine how best to assess the sensory status in the older adult
4. Identify nursing strategies to manage sensory impairment in the older adult
5. Collaborate with interprofessional team members who can assist the older adults with sensory impairment

OVERVIEW

Understanding how to assess for and manage sensory deficits is essential to holistic nursing. A goal of *Healthy People 2020* is to decrease the prevalence and severity of disorders of vision, hearing, balance, smell, and taste, as well as voice, speech, and language (USDHHS, 2010). This chapter on sensory changes addresses common age-related changes associated with the senses as well as disease states and injuries to the senses that occur more commonly with aging. Nursing care related to the *Healthy People 2020* goals regarding sensory changes are also addressed.

BACKGROUND AND STATEMENT OF PROBLEM

Individuals experience and interact with their environments through their senses. Vision, hearing, smell, taste, and peripheral sensation allow us to safely experience and enjoy the world around us. Changes in sensory function (vision, hearing, smell, taste, and peripheral sensation) are common as people age. These sensory changes can negatively impact the older adult's ability to interact with his or her environment, decreasing quality of life. For example, changes in hearing can impact an older person's communication skills; changes in vision can impact his or her health literacy by limiting the ability to take medications safely. Researchers have determined that sensory impairment is more dangerous than previously thought (Cacchione, 2014). More recent, sensory impairment, particularly vision and hearing impairment, has been linked to increased mortality (Cugati et al., 2007; Gopinath et al., 2013; Karpa et al., 2010). *Healthy People 2020* emphasizes the importance of healthy senses, including vision, hearing, balance, smell, and taste. Vision and hearing abilities are essential to language, whether spoken, signed, or read (U.S. Department of Health and Human Services [USDHHS], 2010). Decreases in sense of smell can interfere with an older adult's ability to smell smoke in a fire or recognize spoiled food. Many adults report a decrease in taste that impacts their desire to eat. Decreased peripheral sensation sets up an individual for falls.

For a description of evidence levels cited in this chapter, see Chapter 1, "Developing and Evaluating Clinical Practice Guidelines: A Systematic Approach."

NORMAL CHANGES OF AGING SENSES

The senses—vision, hearing, taste, smell, balance, and peripheral sensation—change with aging, usually presenting primarily with a slowing of function. A summary table is presented describing the changes that occur and the functional outcomes for each sense (Table 5.1).

Vision

There are several changes that occur with vision as people age. The eyelids start lagging, potentially obscuring vision; the pupil takes longer to dilate and contract, slowing accommodation; and presbyopia is widespread.

Presbyopia

A loss of elasticity in the lens and stiffening of the muscle fibers of the lens of the eye leads to a decrease in the eyes' ability to change the shape of the lens to focus on near objects, such as fine print, and decreases ability to adapt to light (National Eye Institute [NEI], 2010; Whiteside, Wallhagen, & Pettengill, 2006).

Hearing

Normal changes of aging impacting hearing acuity include the decrease in function of the hair fibers in the ear canal that normally aid in the natural removal of cerumen and the protection of the ear canal from external elements. Conduction of sound is limited by the ossification of the stapes, decreasing the vibration of the stapes and thickening of the tympanic membrane making it less flexible (Wallhagen, Pettengill, & Whiteside, 2006).

Presbycusis

Presbycusis is the most common form of hearing loss in the United States (Bagai, Thavendiranathan, & Detsky,

TABLE 5.1
Normal Changes of Aging

Sense	Change With Aging	Functional Outcome
Vision	■ Decreased dark adaptation ■ Decreased upward gaze ■ Eyes become drier and produce fewer tears ■ Cornea becomes less sensitive ■ Pupils decrease in size ■ Visual fields become smaller	■ Increased safety risk in changing environmental light ■ Decreased field of vision ■ Dry, irritated eyes ■ Slow to recognize injury to the cornea ■ Inability to adjust to glare and change in lighting conditions ■ Safety risk for driving and maneuvering in the environment
Hearing	■ Ear drum thickens ■ Loss of high-frequency hearing acuity ■ Decreased ability to process sounds after age 50 ■ Increased cerumen impactions ■ Ossification of the stapes	■ Thickened ear drum decreases sound moving across the ear canal ■ Decreased ability to hear sounds, such as /p/, /w/, /f/, /sh/, and women's and children's voices ■ Requires more time to process and respond to auditory stimuli ■ Decreased hearing because of blockage of sound
Smell	■ Decreased ability to identify odors ■ Impacts ability to taste	■ Inability to identify spoiled food or smoke ■ Limits enjoyment in eating
Taste	■ Decreased number of taste buds ■ Limited decrease in taste supported by studies ■ Less saliva production	■ Decreased sensitivity to flavors ■ Dry mouth affects ability to swallow
Sensation	■ Decreased vibratory sense ■ Decreased two-point discrimination ■ Decreased temperature sensitivity ■ Decreased balance ■ Decreased proprioception ■ Changed pain sensation	■ Increases risk for injury ■ Decreased ability to sense pressure ■ Decreased protective response to withdraw from hot objects ■ Risk of falls ■ Decreased protective mechanism

Adapted from Bromley (2000); Linton (2007); Murphy et al. (2002); Schiffman (1997); Seiberling and Conley (2004); Wallhagen et al. (2006); Whiteside et al. (2006).

2006). This high-frequency sensorineural hearing loss is a multifactorial process that varies in severity and is associated with aging (Gates & Mills, 2005). Presbycusis usually has a bilateral progressive onset and is caused by gradual loss of hair cells and fibrous changes in the small blood vessels that supply the cochlea. Risk factors include heredity, environmental exposure, free radicals, and mitochondrial deoxyribonucleic acid (DNA) damage (Huang & Tang, 2010). Clinical presenting symptoms of this irreversible condition include high-frequency hearing loss and difficulty hearing high-pitched sounds such as /t/, /p/, /k/, /s/, /z/, /sh/, and /ch/ (Huang & Tang, 2010; Wallhagen, Strawbridge, Shema, & Kaplan, 2004). Background noise further aggravates this hearing deficit.

Smell

Changes in smell are common as we age, but are not considered a normal part of aging. Frequently, older adults complain of distortions of smell. Factors associated with loss of sense of smell include age and gender, with older males being more prone to smell loss (Hoffman, Cruickshanks, & Davis, 2009). The environment, trauma, diseases, or illness can diminish the sense of smell (Hoffman et al., 2009). Changes in the sense of smell have also been found to correlate with neurological conditions, such as Parkinson's disease, and genetically with Alzheimer's disease (Albers, Tabert, & Devanand, 2006; Oleson & Murphy, 2015; Wilson, Arnold, Schneider, Tang, & Bennett, 2007).

Taste

Common changes in taste include a decreased ability to detect the intensity of taste but not somatic sensations, such as touch and burning pain in the tongue, when compared with younger adults (Fukunaga, Uematsu, & Sugimoto, 2005). However, complete loss of taste is rare and changes in taste are more often related to dental concerns; diseases or illness, such as rhinitis, allergies, or infections; and medications or cancer treatments to the head and neck (Fukunaga et al., 2005; Hoffman et al., 2009).

Peripheral Sensation

Peripheral nerve function that controls the sense of touch declines slightly with age. Two-point discrimination and vibratory sense both decrease with age. The ability to perceive painful stimuli is preserved in aging. However, there may be a slowed reaction time for pulling away from painful stimuli with aging (Linton, 2007).

ASSESSMENT OF THE PROBLEM

Vision

The prevalence of visual impairment increases with age and the settings in which older adults live, with vision impairment affecting approximately 2.6 million adults older than 65 years in the United States (Prevent Blindness America, 2012). According to data from the National Health and Nutrition Examination Survey (NHANES; Dillon, Gu, Hoffman, & Ko, 2010; Schiller, Lucas, & Peregoy, 2012; Swenor, Ramulu, Willis, Friedman, & Lin, 2013), in older adults aged 70 to 79 years, 3.4%, and in older adults 80 years and older, 15.9% were found to be visually impaired (Swenor et al., 2013), but this varied by race and ethnicity with non-Hispanic Whites (13.8%), non-Hispanic Blacks (21.1%), and Mexican Americans (24%). Additionally, a study investigating socioeconomic factors in vision found that increasing age and lower socioeconomic status were associated with vision impairment (Zheng et al., 2012). Adults aged 80 years and older accounted for 7.7% of one study's participants but were 69% of the cases of blindness (Congdon et al., 2004). This is worrisome because this is the fastest growing segment of our population.

Studies evaluating older adults in long-term care settings demonstrate prevalence rates of visual impairment from 27% to 57% of older adults (Bron & Caird, 1997; Cacchione, Culp, Dyck, & Laing, 2003; Swanson, McGwin, Elliott, & Owsley, 2009). Uncorrected refractive error was also found to be common in visually impaired older adults. In one study, of the 8.8% of the older adults found to be visually impaired, 59% were impaired because of an uncorrected refractive error (Vitale, Cotch, & Sperduto, 2006). Leading causes of blindness by race and ethnicity were found to be macular degeneration in Whites, cataracts and open-angle glaucoma in Blacks, and open-angle glaucoma in Hispanic persons (Congdon et al., 2004). Cataracts, one of the leading causes of blindness, are unilateral or bilateral clouding of the crystalline lens that presents as painless, progressive loss of vision (NEI, 2009).

The definition of visual impairment varies by different groups and by country (Agency for Healthcare Research and Quality [AHRQ], 2004). The United States defines low vision as *best corrected visual acuity*:

- Normal vision: visual acuity of 20/20 or better
- Mild vision impairment: 20/25 to 20/50
- Moderate visual impairment: 20/60 to 20/160
- Severe visual impairment (legally blind): 20/200 to 20/400
- Profound vision impairment: 20/400 to 20/1,000

- Near-total vision loss: less than or equal to 20/1,250
- Total blindness: no light perception

Low vision can also be defined based on visual field limitations. *Severe visual impairment* is defined as best corrected field less than or equal to 20° (legal blindness). *Profound visual impairment* is defined as visual field less than or equal to 10 degrees (AHRQ, 2004).

Nursing Assessment of Vision

The health history is an essential part of vision assessment. Several health conditions predispose older adults to visual impairment. In the United States, diabetes is a common cause of disease-related blindness associated with diabetic retinopathy, with 40% to 45% of diabetics having some stage of diabetic retinopathy (NEI, 2015b). Hypertension carries with it the risk of hypertensive retinopathy. Ascertaining a thorough baseline health history with yearly reviews and updates is essential in maintaining visual health. Health questions related to visual health include the questions shown in Table 5.2 (Cacchione, 2007; Wallhagen et al., 2006).

Examination of the Eye

The external structures can cause decreased vision if the lids lag because of laxity of the skin of the upper eyelid. Lid lag can interfere with visual acuity and fields, which may require surgery. A decreased level of tear function can negatively impact visual acuity. In severe cases, cataracts can be visible with the naked eye and appear as a whitish gray pupil instead of black. Cloudiness of the whole cornea of the eye is indicative of a corneal problem, not a cataract. If the person has had cataract surgery, the lens implant may be visible on close inspection.

TABLE 5.2

Vision History Questions

- When was your last eye exam?
- How would you describe your eyesight?
- Any change in your eyesight?
- When did you notice this change?
- Are you experiencing any blurred vision?
- Are you having any double vision?
- Are you bothered by glare?
- Are you experiencing any eye pain?
- Are you using any eye drops for any reason?
- Any history of trauma or injury to your eyes?
- Have you had any eye surgeries?
- Do you have cataracts?
- Any family history of eye problems?

Adapted from Cacchione (2007); Whiteside et al. (2006).

Fundus Exam. Using an ophthalmoscope, a nurse can visualize the red reflex and, with experience and practice, the fundus of the eye. This is often difficult with small pupils. Darkening the room may help with dilating the pupils. Optometrists and ophthalmologists dilate the pupils to allow for a better view of the fundus. Cataracts will appear as a dark shadow in the anterior portion of the lens in front of the retina.

Vision Testing. Vision testing should be completed before the eyes are dilated and assessed in each eye, then both eyes together for both uncorrected and corrected (with glasses) vision.

Distance Vision. The "gold standard" in eye charts, the Snellen chart, is one of the most commonly used to assess distance vision. Visual acuity is tested at 20 feet. The individual is asked to read the letters on the chart until he or she misses more than two on a line of acuity. Acuity equals the line above the line with more than two errors. Acuity measures range from 20/10 to 20/800 on the Snellen chart.

Early Treatment Diabetic Retinopathy Study. The Early Treatment Diabetic Retinopathy Study (ETDRS; Ferris, Kassoff, Bresnick, & Bailey, 1982) eye chart is also used frequently and can be used at a distance of 4 meters. At this distance, the greatest visual acuity measured is 20/200—the equivalent of legal blindness.

Pin-Hole Test. With best vision, with or without glasses, a card with a small pin hole or a multiple pin-hole occluder can be placed in front of the eye, and the vision is tested again at the last line the individual was able to read. This test identifies refractive error of the peripheral cornea of the lens of the eye by allowing only perpendicular light into the lens (Kalinowski, 2008). If the individual can read farther down the chart with the pin hole, his or her vision may be improved with better refraction of his or her eyeglasses or, if he or she does not have glasses, vision could be improved with eyeglasses.

Near Vision. Near vision is important for health literacy, especially regarding reading food or medication labels. There are several ways to assess near vision. Two commonly used tools are the Rosenbaum Pocket Eye Screener and the Lighthouse for the Blind Near Vision Screener. The Rosenbaum Pocket Eye Screener is a noncopyrighted tool based on the Snellen chart that can be useful in assessing near vision in the acute care and primary care settings.

The Rosenbaum is true to scale when compared with the Snellen chart at the 20/200, 20/400, and 20/800 acuity levels. However, the other levels are slightly too large, causing an overestimation of visual acuity (Horton & Jones, 1997).

Lighthouse for the Blind Near Vision Screener (Lighthouse for the Blind). This handheld vision screener has a cord that can be used at 40 and 20 centimeters to measure the proper distance for testing near vision. This near vision screener mimics the ETDRS eye chart in a smaller version but is not pocket size. It does not, however, have the concern over the scale matching of the ETDRS distance acuity level. For research purposes, it has the added feature of the cord for measuring a consistent distance.

Contrast Sensitivity. Contrast sensitivity is often compromised by aging and diseases or conditions of the eye. Decreases in contrast sensitivity occur with cataracts, glaucoma, and retinopathies (Mäntyjärvi & Laitinen, 2001; Owsley, 2011). Contrast sensitivity provides information on how well an individual may perform in real-life conditions. Decline in contrast sensitivity impacts one's ability to distinguish when one step ends and another begins, identify light switches on the wall, read materials not made in high-contrast font, or identify the buttons on the remote. Intact contrast sensitivity is important for day-to-day safety and function within the environment. Impaired contrast sensitivity has been associated with falls, decreased physical function, and nursing home placement in older adults (Swanson et al., 2009).

The Pelli–Robson Contrast Sensitivity Chart (Pelli, Robson, & Wilkins, 1988) is read at the 1- or 3-meter distance. All letters are presented at the 20/200 acuity level but in decreasing shades of black to gray. The Pelli–Robson Contrast Sensitivity Chart is widely used in practice and works well for older adults who are experienced in recognizing letters (Hirvelä & Laatikainen, 1995; Morse & Rosenthal, 1997). The Vistech Contrast Sensitivity Test, another contrast sensitivity measure, has four patches of gray circles with lines in different directions (Kennedy & Dunlap, 1990). The person being examined points to the direction in which the lines within the circle are pointed (Morse & Rosenthal, 1997).

Visual Fields. *Fields of vision* refers to the area of peripheral vision visible when the individual is focusing straight ahead (Cassin & Rubin, 2001). The vision in visual fields can be affected by many eye conditions, specifically glaucoma, macular degeneration, and retinopathies (Jessa, Evans, Thomson, & Rowlands, 2007), as well as neurological disorders that inhibit eye movement or affect the blood supply to the optic nerve. Intact visual fields are necessary to function safely in one's environment. In assessing visual fields by confrontation, a gross clinical measure of visual fields, the examiner faces the patient and determines whether the patient can identify the examiner's moving fingers as they are moving into their field of view (Seidel, Dains, Ball, & Benedict, 2003). Although subjective and dependent on the examiner having normal fields of vision, the confrontation test is useful in quickly identifying large losses in visual fields.

The Humphrey Visual Field Test is completed by an ophthalmologist and assesses visual fields using a static type of perimetry (Gianutsos & Suchoff, 1997). This instrument provides a more reliable measure of functional visual fields. The Goldman VI4e kinetic perimetry visual field testing, on the other hand, assesses kinetic type of functional visual fields (Gillmore, 2002). Kinetic perimetry entails the introduction of a moving stimulus, moving from a nonvisible area toward the fixed point of view. The Goldman VI4e kinetic perimetry visual field testing is hard to standardize because it is operator dependent (Gillmore, 2002). Because these automated methods are more widely used, the location of the visual field deficit may clue the examiner about the type of eye condition. For example, unilateral visual field deficits may be related to a cerebral vascular accident, glaucoma will affect the peripheral fields, and macular degeneration has associated loss of central field of vision.

Stereopsis. Stereopsis is the process in which humans have the ability to use the different viewpoints provided by their eyes to produce a vivid perception of depth and three-dimensional shapes (Norman et al., 2008; Read, Phillipson, Serrano-Pedraza, Milner, & Parker, 2010). There are multiple methods of measuring stereopsis and it is not thought to be affected by aging but may be negatively impacted by distance acuity and eye diseases (Norman et al., 2008).

Visual Function Questionnaire

The NEI Visual Function Questionnaire (VFQ-25) is a 25-item survey that assesses the functional impact of visual impairment. It provides a subjective report on 12 functional subscales: general vision, near vision, distance vision, driving, peripheral vision, color vision, ocular pain, general health, vision-specific role difficulties, dependency, social function, and mental health (Revicki, Rentz, Harnam, Thomas, & Lanzetta, 2010). The NEI VFQ-25 has sound psychometric properties in cognitively intact older adults (Mangione et al., 2001).

Conditions of the Eye

Diseases That Alter Vision Seen More Frequently as People Age

Cataracts. Cataracts are clouding of the crystalline lens that presents either unilaterally or bilaterally as painless, progressive loss of vision (NEI, 2009). Cataracts are usually age related but they can be secondary to glaucoma, diabetes, Alzheimer's disease; congenital; injury related; or related to medications or sunlight exposure (NEI, 2009). The management of cataracts includes early identification and monitoring followed by surgical extraction and lens implantation once vision is affected.

Macular Degeneration. This involves the development of drusen deposits in the retinal pigmented epithelium and is the leading cause of central vision loss and legal blindness in older adults (Revicki et al., 2010). Macular degeneration is more common in fair-haired, blue-eyed individuals. Other risk factors include smoking and excessive sunlight exposure. There are wet and dry forms of macular degeneration. The wet form of macular degeneration is more easily treated than the dry form. Newer treatments of expensive injectable medications are available to slow the progression of dry macular degeneration (NEI, 2015a).

Glaucoma. Glaucoma is a progressive, serious form of eye disease that can damage the optic nerve and result in vision loss and blindness (NEI, 2014). Primary open-angle glaucoma is the most common form of glaucoma in older adults (Linton, 2007). Increased intraocular pressure causes atrophy and cupping of the optic nerve head, which leads to visual field deficits that can progress to blindness. Vision changes include loss of peripheral vision, intolerance to glare, decreased perception of contrast, and decreased ability to adapt to the dark. Treatments are available to delay vision loss, but no cure is available. Glaucoma is the leading cause of blindness all over the world (NEI, 2014). African Americans and Mexican Americans are five times more likely to develop glaucoma (NEI, 2014).

Diabetic Retinopathy. This results from end-organ damage from diabetes causing retinopathy and spotty vision. The risk can be reduced by tight blood sugar control. Almost 9% of diabetics older than 65 years develop diabetic retinopathy (Prevent Blindness America, 2012). Diabetic retinopathy starts as mild nonproliferative retinopathy with microaneurysms on the retina and progresses as moderate to severe nonproliferative retinopathy in which blood vessels in the retina are blocked, depriving the retina of adequate blood supply, then progresses to proliferative retinopathy in which the growth of new abnormal fragile blood vessels that leak can cause blindness (NEI, 2012).

TABLE 5.3
Implications of Vision Changes in Older Adults

Impact on safety
Inability to read medication labels
Difficulty navigating stairs or curbs
Difficulty driving
Difficulty crossing streets
Impact on quality of life
Reduces ability to remain independent
Difficulty or unable to read
Falls

Hypertensive Retinopathy. Similar to diabetic retinopathy, hypertensive retinopathy is caused by end-organ damage from poorly controlled hypertension causing background and, eventually, proliferative retinopathy. Hypertensive retinopathy is usually treated with laser photocoagulation and tight blood pressure control.

Temporal Arteritis. This is an autoimmune disorder that causes inflammation of the temporal artery, also known as *giant cell arteritis*. It presents as malaise, scalp tenderness, unilateral temporal headache, jaw claudication, and sudden vision loss (usually unilateral). This vision loss is a medical emergency but is potentially reversible if identified immediately. The client should see an ophthalmologist or go to the emergency room immediately if symptoms develop.

Detached Retina. This is a condition that can occur in patients with cataracts or recent cataract surgery, trauma, or it can occur spontaneously. A detached retina presents as a curtain coming down across a patient's line of vision. An individual experiencing this should see an ophthalmologist or proceed to the closest emergency room immediately. See Table 5.3 for implications of vision changes on an older adult's function.

INTERVENTIONS AND CARE STRATEGIES

Vision

The nurse should obtain a past medical history to avoid disruption in the management of chronic eye conditions, ensuring continuation of ongoing regimens, such as eye drops for glaucoma. Without the continuation of the individual's eye drops, eye pressures could precipitously increase causing an acute exacerbation of the glaucoma, potentially dramatically limiting vision. If an acute change in an individual's vision occurs, the primary care provider should be notified immediately. Depending on the signs and symptoms present, the individual may need to see an ophthalmologist or go to the emergency room to receive treatment to restore the vision or limit the deterioration. Many cities have ophthalmological emergency rooms.

Lighting is important in an individual's environment. Too little light can limit an individual's vision. Too much light, depending on the individual's eye condition, such as cataracts or macular degeneration, may cause eye pain and glare. It is important to ascertain whether an individual is sensitive to light. If he or she is sensitive to light, indirect light and night lights may be helpful to provide a safe environment. The majority of older adults benefit from improved lighting. To avoid glare, directing incandescent lamps directly on a task, such as sewing or reading, often improves visual acuity and is well tolerated. Glare occurs when a light shines directly into the eye or reflects off a shiny surface. Low-vision specialists recommend trying different positions and wattage of lighting to find what works best for each individual (Community Services for the Blind and Partially Sighted, 2004).

Encourage the use and proper fitting of the person's eyeglasses. Older adults' eyeglasses should be labeled with the person's name so they can be returned to the owner if they are set down and left behind. Even with eyeglasses, magnification may be helpful. Have family provide lighted magnification if needed (large lighted magnifiers are available from low-vision centers). A low-vision optometrist or specialist can assist in recommending the appropriate level of magnifier.

Contrast sensitivity is a problem with several eye conditions, including cataracts, glaucoma, and macular degeneration. Adding contrast to the edge of each step, fixtures in the home, light switches that blend into the wall, or faucets that blend into the sink can create a safer and more functional environment.

Annual screening is not recommended in the older adult (Chou, Dana, & Bougatsos, 2009). However, nurses should encourage an annual dilated eye exam either with an optometrist or ophthalmologist (Robinson, Mairs, Glenny, & Stokes, 2012). More frequent eye exams may be needed for older adults with diabetes or hypertension, glaucoma, and macular degeneration (American Academy of Ophthalmology Preferred Practice Patterns Committee, 2010). Nurses are members of the interprofessional team responsible for preventing unnecessary disability. Therefore, nurses should make sure that there is a mechanism in place to trigger these visits on an annual basis.

Hearing Impairment

Surveys to identify older adults with hearing impairment often suffer from underreporting on self-report instruments. The latest version of the NHANES included audiometric testing in older adults and found a prevalence rate of 25% in those between 65 and 74 years, and 50% of adults older than 75 years have disabling hearing loss (Dillon et al., 2010; National Institute on Deafness and Other Communication Disorders [NIDCD], 2015a). Hearing loss has been found to be greater in men and progresses more quickly than in women (Chao & Chen, 2009; NIDCD, 2015a). Yet, less than a third of those who could benefit from a hearing aid have ever used them (NIDCD, 2015a). This dramatic increase in prevalence rates is magnified in the nursing home population. Prevalence rates of hearing impairment in the nursing home are similar to rates of visual impairment, at approximately 24% (Warnat & Tabloski, 2006). When hearing is tested through audiometry, the prevalence rates increase to 42% to 90% (Bagai et al., 2006; Cacchione et al., 2003; Tolson, Swan, & Knussen, 2002). The American Academy of Audiology defines hearing loss based on decibels or loudness and the Hertz or the pitch of sound. Normal speech is in the 0- to 25-dB level, mild hearing loss is defined as hearing in the 25- to 40-dB level. Hearing between 40 and 70 dB is considered moderate hearing loss. Severe hearing loss is between 70 and 90 dB; greater than 90 dB is considered profound hearing loss (Mehr, 2007). Aging impairs the processing of sound through the ear canal as well as the central nervous system processing of sounds, making it more difficult to hear the higher frequencies, including women's and children's voices (Huang & Tang, 2010).

Assessment of Hearing

Despite the U.S. Preventive Services Task Force not having sufficient evidence to recommend routine hearing screening in older adults, it is essential that older adults are assessed for hearing impairment (Bainbridge & Wallhagen, 2014). Often, it is easy to determine when an older adult is hard of hearing just by having a conversation with him or her. The older adult may lean in closer an attempt to hear better, turn the head to the "good ear," or cup a hand behind the ear. Older adults may have to ask for things to be repeated; they may report having trouble hearing their grandchildren's or other's high-pitched voices. Older adults often complain that people are mumbling. Any or all of these signs may be present. Regardless of whether any of these signs are present, all older adults should have their hearing screened annually at their primary care visit (Bagai et al., 2006). Primary care providers play an important role in screening for hearing loss and making appropriate referrals for older adults (Bainbridge & Wallhagen, 2014). Methods of screening are described herein.

Hearing Handicap Inventory for the Elderly—Screen

The Hearing Handicap Inventory for the Elderly—Screen (HHIE-S; Ventry & Weinstein, 1983) is a 10-item scale used to determine how hearing is impacting an older adult's daily life and to assist in identifying who might benefit from a hearing aid and an audiology referral. The scale takes approximately 5 minutes to complete and is targeted for community-dwelling older adults. This scale is available online through the Hartford Foundation Institute for Geriatric Nursing "Try This Best Practices in Care for Older Adults" (Demers, 2001). The HHIE-S has reported excellent sensitivity and specificity for severe hearing loss, but the sensitivity and specificity decrease as the level of hearing impairment lessens (Adams-Wendling, Pimple, Adams, & Titler, 2008).

Whisper Test

The whisper test involves covering or rubbing one ear canal, and, from a distance of 2 feet, whispering a three-syllable word on an exhale that the patient either correctly or incorrectly repeats back. An incorrect response triggers a repeat attempt to see whether the older adult can identify a different three-syllable word. The consistency of the level of the whispered word makes this test difficult to compare from examiner to examiner. However, despite this difficulty, it has been found to be a valid and reliable test to screen for hearing loss (Bagai et al., 2006).

Handheld Audioscope

The handheld audioscope is a device developed to specifically screen for hearing impairment. It has a test tone that is presented at the 60-dB level. The decibel levels that may be tested include the 20-, 25-, and 40-dB levels at the 500-, 1,000-, 2,000-, and 4,000-Hz levels (Yueh et al., 2007). The audioscope has an otoscope that allows for the direct inspection of the tympanic membrane or cerumen impactions, which can result in conductive hearing loss present in up to 30% of older adults (Lewis-Cullinan & Janken, 1990; Yueh, Shapiro, MacLean, & Shekelle, 2003). Testing using the audioscope should be performed in a quiet setting and may not be as useful in the long-term care environment with high noise levels. Bagai et al. (2006) recommends a basic algorithm for primary care providers to ask whether the individual has any difficulty with his or her hearing; if yes, then refer for audiometry. If he or she denied difficulty with hearing, then screen with an audioscope, if one is available; if not, the whisper test, which is not as reliable as the audioscope. If the question response, whisper test, or audioscope are positive for a hearing impairment, referral is made for full audiometry.

Pure Tone Audiometry

Pure tone audiometry is the gold standard of hearing tests, particularly if completed in a soundproof booth with 92% sensitivity and 94% specificity in detecting sensorineural hearing loss (Frank & Petersen, 1987). Pure tone audiometry allows for testing of a wide range of decibels and Hertz levels, or loudness and pitch or frequencies, allowing for testing at the 5- to 120-dB level and 250 to 4,000 Hz. Portable pure tone audiometers with noise-reduction earphones are available and can be used in the community, outpatient, and long-term care settings when access to an audiologist is limited. This wide range of tones allows for a better understanding of the individual's functional hearing. Pure tone audiometry by an audiologist is the next step after screening has identified a hearing deficit (Yueh et al., 2003).

Tuning Fork Tests

Two tuning fork tests have been used in hearing screenings, although one systematic review discouraged their use because they were found to be unreliable with limited accuracy (Bagai et al., 2006). The tuning fork should be either 256 or 512 Hz (M. I. Wallhagen, personal communication, November 18, 2006). The Rinne test is meant to differentiate whether an older adult hears better by bone or air conduction and can help determine whether an individual had sensorineural or conductive hearing loss. The Weber test is used to help identify unilateral hearing loss.

Hearing Changes Common in Older Adults

Conductive hearing loss usually involves abnormalities of the middle or external ear, including the ear canal, tympanic membrane, and ossicular chain of bones in the middle ear (Marcincuk & Roland, 2002; Yueh et al., 2003). Causes of conductive hearing impairment include cerumen impactions or foreign bodies, ruptured eardrum, otitis media, and otosclerosis (Wallhagen et al., 2006; Yueh et al., 2003).

Sensorineural hearing loss is the most common form of hearing loss in older adults (Linton, 2007); it involves damage to the inner ear, the cochlea, or the fibers of the eighth cranial nerve. Sensorineural hearing loss is usually a bilateral progressive onset and is caused by gradual loss of hair cells, and fibrous changes in the small blood vessels that supply the cochlea. Risk factors include heredity, environmental exposure, free radical, and mitochondrial DNA damage (Huang & Tang, 2010). Additional causes of sensorineural hearing loss include viral or bacterial infections, trauma, tumors, noise exposure, cardiovascular conditions, ototoxic drugs, and Ménière's disease (Wallhagen et al., 2006).

Central auditory processing disorder is an uncommon disorder with prevalence ranging from 0.75% to 14.3% (Gates, Cooper, Kannel, & Miller, 1990; Quaranta et al., 2014) that includes an inability to process incoming signals and is often found in patients with stroke and older adults with neurological conditions such as Alzheimer's disease and Parkinson's disease (Pekkonen et al., 1999). The person's hearing is intact but his or her ability to process the sound is impaired, resulting in impaired speech understanding (Quaranta et al., 2014).

Tinnitus, otherwise known as *ringing in the ear,* is of two types: subjective and objective. Subjective tinnitus is a condition in which there is perceived sound in the absence of acoustic stimulus (Ahmad & Seidman, 2004; Lockwood, Salvi, & Burkard, 2002). Objective tinnitus is considered rare and presents as ringing in the ear that is audible by the individual and others. It is thought to have a vascular or neurological condition or Eustachian tube dysfunction (Crummer & Hassan, 2004). Subjective ringing in the ears may fluctuate and can be caused by noise-induced damage to the hair receptors of the cochlear nerve and age-related changes in the organs of hearing and balance. Tinnitus can also be caused by hormonal changes, thyroid disorders, and tumors (NIDCD, 2014c). Patients with tinnitus should be referred to an ear, nose, and throat (ENT) specialist.

Ménière's disease is characterized by fluctuating hearing loss, dizziness, vertigo, tinnitus, and a sensation of pressure in the affected ear (NIDCD, 2010). Ménière's disease typically begins between ages 40 and 60 years, and sometimes it resolves on its own (NIDCD, 2010). Unfortunately, the fluctuating hearing loss can become permanent hearing loss over time. Possible causes of Ménière's disease include vascular constriction similar to that found in migraines; viral infections, allergies, and autoimmune disorders and may have a genetic component as Ménière's disease tends to run in families (NIDCD, 2010).

Implications of Hearing Changes

Older adults who have hearing impairment experience a decreased quality of communication, social isolation, low self-esteem, and generally lower quality of life. More recent, older adults with hearing impairment have been identified as at higher risk of dementia and higher mortality rates (Karpa et al., 2010; Lin et al., 2013). Decreased hearing impacts an individual's word recognition, decreasing the ability to communicate. This, in turn, can lead to significant safety issues. For example, if patient education about medication administration is provided only verbally, key information can be misheard and misinterpreted. Difficulty understanding the spoken word can lead to fatigue and speech paucity of friends and loved ones.

Speech paucity is described as decreased attempts to have meaningful conversations because of the difficulty in getting the message through to a hearing-impaired loved one. Speech paucity (Wallhagen et al., 2006) leads to social isolation of the hearing impaired because only the necessary information is transferred and no everyday social information is shared (Wallhagen et al., 2004). This can lead to depression and low self-esteem in the hearing-impaired individual and the partner. Other factors that lead to social isolation in hearing-impaired older adults include the inability to hear the phone or the doorbell ringing or knocking at the door.

Ideally, older adults who develop hearing loss will see an audiologist and obtain unilateral or bilateral hearing aids to improve their ability to communicate with the people around them. Unfortunately, the stigma, cost, and delay in pursuing hearing aids are barriers to their success. Hearing aids should be pursued early in the course of hearing impairment. For example, hearing aids can be very helpful when hearing is impaired to the point that background noise interferes with understanding the spoken word. Success in using hearing aids at this level of hearing improves the chance that older adults will continue with hearing aids. Once an individual is offered a hearing aid, hearing rehabilitation should accompany the hearing-aid dispensing; this will increase the use of the hearing aid and positively impact his or her independent living and quality of life (Bainbridge & Wallhagen, 2014; Yueh & Shekelle, 2007). Once older adults become used to the silence, it is hard to adapt to the increased ambient noise heard with hearing aids. Often, older adults require extensive coaching from an audiologist to get through the transition phase of wearing hearing aids. Technology has improved to the point of analog hearing aids that can be finely tuned to the individual's needs (Bainbridge & Wallhagen, 2014). In one intervention group of older adults fitted with hearing aids, 98% experienced benefit and their caregivers perceived significant benefit as well (Tolson et al., 2002). University settings are often the most cost-effective locations to pursue hearing aids. The cost of hearing aids is an important factor because most insurance plans, including Medicare, do not cover hearing aids, but will cover cochlear implants.

Cochlear implants are another technological advancement that has demonstrated positive outcomes in profoundly deaf or severely hard-of-hearing older adults in the areas of speech recognition (NIDCD, 2014a). A cochlear implant works by bypassing the damaged parts of the ear and stimulating the auditory nerve. These impulses are sent to the brain through the auditory nerve and the brain recognizes them as sound (NIDCD, 2014a). Severe hearing impairment must be present unilaterally or bilaterally before this surgical intervention is considered. In one study, cochlear implants were found to improve word recognition and health-related quality of life (Francis, Chee, Yeagle, Cheng, & Niparko, 2002). At this time, there is only evidence for unilateral cochlear implants in profoundly deaf adults rather than bilateral cochlear implants because of cost and limited functional gain (Bond et al., 2009). Despite these improvements, relatively few adults have received this new technology. As of 2012, according to the U.S. Food and Drug Administration, nearly 58,000 adults have received cochlear implants (NIDCD, 2014a). Technological advances will continue to improve our options for hearing-impaired older adults.

Smell and Taste

Smell and taste are two senses that are difficult to separate because they overlap, particularly, when food is involved. Both these senses are dependent on chemosensation, the ability of the nose, mouth, and throat to identify tastes and smells based on chemical reactions that occur when odors or tastes are present in the environment (American Academy of Otolaryngology–Head and Neck Surgery, 2001). Often when people go to their primary care provider as a result of having lost their sense of taste they are surprised to learn that they have a smell disorder instead (NIDCD, 2014b). The sense of smell and ability to identify odors decrease because of normal changes in aging. Up to 50% of octogenarians have smell disorders (Murphy et al., 2002). This can be problematic for safety reasons. An inability to smell smoke, for instance, could put an older adult at risk. Studies have also linked the loss of smell to Alzheimer's disease and Parkinson's disease (Mesholam, Moberg, Mahr, & Doty, 1998; Müller, Reichmann, Livermore, & Hummel, 2002; Oleson & Murphy, 2015; Vasavada et al., 2015). Taste problems are rare, ranging from 0.72% in those aged 65 years and older to 1.7% in those aged 85 years and older (Hoffman et al., 2009).

Changes in Smell and Taste Common to Older Adults

There are four types of olfactory disorders: (a) *hyposmia* is the reduction of the sense of smell, (b) *parosmia* is the distortion in the sense of smelling the presence of an odor, (c) *anosmia* is no sense of smell, and (d) *phantosmia* is the perception of an odor when no odor source is present (Albers et al., 2006; NIDCD, 2015b). Olfactory disorders impact quality of life, and increase mortality in older adults (Pinto, Wroblewski, Kern, Schumm, & McClintock, 2014). Common complaints from people with olfactory disorders include difficulty with cooking, decreased appetite, eating spoiled food, too little perception of body odor, and inability to detect gas leaks or smoke (Albers et al., 2006; Murphy et al., 2002).

Because of the impact on quality of life and mortality, it is important to take a complete history and physical examination with older adults. A thorough cranial nerve exam and head and neck examination should be included. If an older adult has a subjective complaint of decreased sense of smell or if an olfactory disorder is identified, the individual should be referred to an otorhinolaryngologist by the primary care provider (Miwa et al., 2001; NIDCD, 2015b).

Most changes in taste are thought to occur because of an oral condition, xerostomia (dry mouth), decreased sense of smell, medications, diseases, and tobacco use (Seiberling & Conley, 2004). Dysgeusias or taste disorders may resolve spontaneously. The taste sensory system has the capacity to recover function after being damaged (Hoffman et al., 2009; NIDCD, 2014b). Dysgeusia is defined as a condition in which a foul, salty, rancid, or metallic taste sensation persists in the mouth and can be associated with burning mouth syndrome (NIDCD, 2014b). Additional taste disorders include hypogeusia, which is the decreased ability to taste sweet, sour, bitter, salty, or savory tastes; and ageusia, which is the inability to detect any tastes (NIDCD, 2014b). However, because of the poor outcomes for older adults with taste disorders, referral for treatment is indicated either to an otolaryngologist, neurologist, or a subspecialist at a smell and taste center (Bromley, 2000; Hoffman et al., 2009).

As with olfactory disorders, disorders of taste are often identified on history, not by physical examination. There are very few tests to assess for taste disorders. Therefore, the history is essential. Substance abuse, including tobacco, alcohol, and cocaine, should be reviewed. The individual's dietary habits should be reviewed. Questions regarding recent dental work or procedures should also be asked. Ascertaining whether the individual has a history of gastric reflux could reveal manageable conditions impacting taste. Other potential causes of taste disorders include upper respiratory and middle ear infections, radiation therapy for head and neck cancers, exposure to chemical and certain medications, head injury, and poor oral hygiene (NIDCD, 2014b). A thorough review of medications is fundamental in the evaluation of a taste disorder (Bromley, 2000).

Diseases That Alter Taste Seen More Frequently as People Age

Burning Mouth Syndrome

Burning mouth syndrome produces a sensation that one's tongue is tingling or burning. This syndrome is most common in middle-aged and older women (NIDCD, 2014b). There may be several contributing factors: vitamin B deficiencies, local trauma, gastrointestinal disorders causing reflux, allergies, salivary dysfunction, and diabetes.

Xerostomia

Dry mouth is common with many medications used to treat disorders common to older adults, including anticholinergic medications, antidepressants, antihistamines, angiotensin-converting enzyme (ACE) inhibitors, lipid-lowering agents, antiparkinsonian medications, and anticonvulsants, to name a few (Bromley, 2000; Seiberling & Conley, 2004).

Implications of Taste and Smell Changes

Inability to smell limits some of the pleasures of everyday life, decreasing quality of life. The smell of a spring rain, of a Christmas tree, of flowers, or of coffee brewing may not be detectable. Taste is diminished because of the inability to smell. Of significant concern in older adults who have smell and taste disorders is malnutrition. Appetite is detrimentally affected because of the inability to smell and taste the food. Inability to smell is a safety hazard because of the inability to smell smoke in a fire or a gas leak. Decreased sense of taste may also result in inability to recognize spoiled food, resulting in nausea, vomiting, or infectious diarrhea. Because decreased sense of smell is associated with neurodegenerative diseases and increased mortality (Pinto et al., 2014; Vasavada et al., 2015), it is important to investigate potential reversible causes for a person's decreased sense of smell.

Peripheral Sensation

Two percent to 7% of all patients presenting with symptoms of neuropathy in a general medical practice will have peripheral neuropathy (Smith & Singleton, 2004). In older adults in an NHANES study, older than 70 to 79 years, 28% reported the loss of feeling in their feet; this increased to 35% in adults older than 80 years (Dillon et al., 2010). This is important because poor nerve function can impact late-life disability (Ward et al., 2014). A prospective study evaluating older adults for peripheral sensory neuropathy found prevalence rates of 26% for those 65 to 74 years old and 54% for those 85 years and older (Mold, Vesely, Keyl, Schenk, & Roberts, 2004). Common disorders that increase the risk of peripheral neuropathy include diabetes; alcoholism; osteoporosis with compression fractures; peripheral vascular disease; infections; nutritional deficiencies, particularly of vitamins (e.g., thiamine and B_{12}); and malignancies (Mold et al., 2004). Because of the multitude of risk factors for peripheral neuropathy, a neurology consultation is recommended for complicated presentations of peripheral neuropathy to help determine the appropriate evaluation and management of the condition.

Changes in Peripheral Sensation Common to Older Adults

Conditions that alter peripheral sensation are seen more frequently as people age and include peripheral neuropathy, diabetic neuropathy, phantom limb pain, and acute sensory loss.

Peripheral Neuropathy. This is a heterogenous group of disorders (Merkies, Faber, & Lauria, 2015) that present with nerve pain in the distal extremities related to nerve-fiber damage in the motor, large sensory, small sensory, and autonomic nerve fibers from underlying systemic illnesses, neurotoxic drugs, primary disorders of the immune system, and hereditary disorders (Merkies et al., 2015). The most commonly suspected causes are circulatory problems (peripheral vascular disease and diabetes) or vitamin deficiencies. Common vitamin deficiencies that impact peripheral nerves include thiamine and B_{12}.

Diabetic Neuropathy. This is end-organ damage to the peripheral nerves from microvascular changes that occur with diabetes. It often leads to loss of sensation in the feet of diabetics, contributing to undetected trauma to the extremities and subsequent refractory infections because of poor vascular supply to the extremity. It is extremely important to teach diabetics and patients with peripheral neuropathy to provide special attention and care to their feet.

Phantom Limb Pain. This is the experience of pain that can range from dull ache to crushing pain where an amputated limb once was. The sensory cortex of the brain has influence in this mechanism. This pain is often chronic and requires special interventions for control and management, including electronic prosthetics, analgesics, and psychosocial support.

Acute Sensory Loss. Acute sensory loss may be caused by a stroke, acute nerve entrapment in the spine, traumatic nerve damage, or compartment syndrome resulting from trauma to a limb. This sensory loss presents with acute onset of numbness, tingling, severe nerve pain, or lack of sensation and function in the affected extremity.

Implications of Peripheral Sensation Changes

Inability to recognize position sense, pressure, or to ascertain where feet are positioned on the floor can lead to falls, burns, lacerations, calluses, and pressure ulcers. Intact peripheral sensation is essential for remaining safe in the environment.

Nursing Assessment and Care Strategies of Peripheral Sensation

Nurses should take appropriate health histories to ascertain the presence of decreased sensation or pain in limbs. Physical examination should always include a thorough inspection and physical examination of the individual's legs and feet (Hellman, 2002) or the affected extremity. Diabetics and people known to have peripheral neuropathy should have thorough neurological exams, including vibratory sense with a tuning fork over bony prominences and Semmes–Weinstein monofilament testing of the feet along with testing proprioception (Boike & Hall, 2002). A referral to neurology may be necessary for nerve conduction testing, which is the most important tool in the diagnostic workup of older adults with suspected peripheral neuropathy (Merkies et al., 2015).

Semmes–Weinstein Monofilament Test

This inexpensive simple procedure is used to screen for decreased sensation in several plantar sites on the foot. The Semmes–Weinstein monofilament is placed against the sole of the foot in eight different areas on the foot. The individual is asked to report when he or she perceives any sensations (Boike & Hall, 2002). The Semmes–Weinstein nylon monofilament 5.04 gauge buckles at a pressure of 10 g. Loss of sensation at this level of pressure indicates a risk for ulcer development. Identification of this risk is important for improving the vigilance of foot care (Armstrong & Lavery, 1998).

Vibratory Sense

This is assessed by using a 128-Hz vibrating tuning fork on a lower extremity bony prominence. The examiner places the vibrating tuning fork on the bony prominence and asks the individual whether he or she feels any vibration (Boike & Hall, 2002). Older adults should be able to feel the vibration.

Proprioception

This is the ability of individuals to determine where they are in space. To assess for deficits in proprioception in the feet that may set the older adult up for falls and local trauma, the examiner has the individual close his or her eyes, then the examiner holds the large toe on the sides and moves the toe up or down and asks the individual to identify which direction the toe was moved. Inability to correctly identify the direction is an indication of decreased proprioception.

CASE STUDY

Mr. Sweets is a 75-year-old African American male living by himself in the community. He lives in a senior apartment building where he receives housekeeping services and can participate in a meal plan if he likes. He arrives on the acute care of the elderly (ACE) unit in your hospital with a diagnosis of hyperglycemia and a urinary tract infection. He also has a history of hypertension, hyperlipidemia, and osteoarthritis of the left hip. He is widowed and has three children: two live in the area, the other lives out of state. He is a retired aeronautical engineer. His medications include Metformin 1,500 mg daily increased from 1,000 mg; Zocor, 40 mg orally daily; lisinopril, 20 mg daily; hydrochlorothiazide (HCTZ), 25 mg daily; and Tylenol Extra Strength, 1,000 mg three times a day for his hip discomfort.

On your admission assessment, you discover that he remembers receiving verbal instructions to cut his diabetic pills in half. Thus, since that appointment, he has only been taking 500 mg of Metformin instead of 1,500 mg. His primary care provider had instructed him to take one and one half tablets of his Metformin not just half a tablet. You were not sure whether this was just a misunderstanding or whether Mr. Sweets was having difficulty hearing. You are also concerned that his vision may be a problem as well because of his 5-year history of known diabetes.

After you complete taking your history, you gather your supplies to complete your physical exam. Your supplies include an audioscope; Lighthouse for the Blind Near Vision Screener; three plastic bags—one

(continued)

CASE STUDY *(continued)*

full of coffee, baby powder, and peppermint candies—128-Hz tuning fork; and a Semmes–Weinstein monofilament test. The audioscope reveals that Mr. Sweets's ear canals are completely occluded with cerumen and he can only hear the test tone that is delivered at the 60-dB level. On the near vision screener, he scored 20/125 in both eyes with his dirty glasses. Unfortunately, because his blood sugar currently is and has been elevated, it is unclear how much of the decreased vision is caused by his elevated blood sugar and how much is related to possible refractive error or diabetic retinopathy. Mr. Sweets was able to correctly identify each scent in the plastic bags. When you examine his feet, you identify that he has significant sensation loss on the bottom of his feet. He has intact vibratory sense in the ankle, but his vibratory sense is decreased in both great toes. His feet are currently free of any calluses, deformities, or open wounds. He does have some thickened toe nails.

Discussion

These assessments impact the care plan for Mr. Sweets. His sensory deficits most likely precipitated his hospital admission. Written instructions may have helped prevent this, but his near vision may have interfered with the understanding of the written directions as well. He should have written instructions in large font, because of his vision, ideally in 14- to 16-point type. Because of bilateral cerumen impactions, he will need to begin using cerumen softening drops and have the cerumen removed with a cerumen spoon or irrigation after a few days. If this is not successful, he may need to be seen by an otolaryngologist (ear–nose– throat [ENT] physician) to have the cerumen removed. If his hearing is still impaired after the cerumen is removed, Mr. Sweets should see an audiologist.

Based on your history, he was last seen by an ophthalmologist 3 years ago. He should be seen by an ophthalmologist to determine whether any treatments for his diabetic retinopathy are necessary. He should receive anticipatory guidance to see an ophthalmologist every 6 months to yearly because of his diabetes. He would qualify for low-vision services if his acuity remained at 20/125. He would also benefit from increased contrast. Older adults with diabetic retinopathy often need enhanced contrast. This can be achieved by adding red to light-colored fixtures and white to dark-colored fixtures, remote controls, and other electrical devices that are usually solid colors with limited contrast. A low-vision specialist could be very helpful here to make his home environment safe and user friendly.

Mr. Sweets should be evaluated by a diabetic foot nurse and a podiatrist to have his nails trimmed and to learn more about foot care. He will need to learn how to complete daily foot inspections as well as assistance learning what type of footwear is appropriate for his feet. His hip may cause him some difficulty reaching his feet. It will be important for him to use mirrors and palpation to assist him in his self-care. A diabetic nurse educator can assist him with further information on the management of the disease and empower him to ask more questions and clarify when information does not appear compatible with what his symptoms are.

Mr. Sweets was discharged from the hospital after 4 days. His Metformin was increased to 1,500 mg; he is afebrile and discharged on oral antibiotics for his urinary tract infection. He had his glasses cleaned and ears cleaned out over those 4 days so his hearing has improved to where he can hear at the 40-dB level. He has an appointment to see the audiologist. An appointment was also made for ophthalmology. Follow-up appointments have also been made with the endocrine staff, with the diabetic nurse educator, and diabetic foot nurse on the same visit. These appointments were written out on a 4- by 6-inch index card with a black marker that he could read with his glasses. Sensory impairment is an interprofessional health care problem. Good communication among disciplines is essential in maintaining Mr. Sweets's functional status and ability to stay in the community. Nurses are best prepared to help Mr. Sweets navigate and coordinate visits to the other disciplines. Screening completed by nurses either in the community, acute care, or long-term care settings can identify problems that have often been passed off by the older adult as the result of normal aging.

NURSING STANDARD OF PRACTICE

Protocol 5.1: Sensory Changes

I. OVERVIEW

The Individualized Sensory Enhancement of the Elderly (I-SEE) program was developed to tailor nursing interventions to the type and level of sensory impairment experienced by the older adult (Cacchione, 2007). Originally developed to address hearing- and visually impaired older adults, the I-SEE can logically be extended to address sensory impairment in smell, taste, and peripheral sensation. There are three levels to the I-SEE program: nursing assessments, nursing actions, and nursing referrals.

II. NURSING SENSORY ASSESSMENTS

A. History
   1. Ask questions about changes in hearing, vision, sense of smell, and taste, as well as any numbness and tingling in extremities.
   2. Review medications that may be exacerbating the sensory problem, such as anticholinergic medications, antibiotics, aminoglycosides, and high-dose aspirin.
   3. Determine whether symptoms occurred suddenly or gradually.
   4. Clarify whether symptoms are unilateral or bilateral.
   5. Inquire whether the individual has had any prior treatment for sensory conditions.
   6. Ascertain whether sensory conditions interfere with daily function.
   7. Ask about ability to drive; both daytime and nighttime driving can be impacted by visual impairment as well as hearing and the peripheral nervous system.
   8. Determine interest in receiving treatment for these conditions.

B. For each positive symptom reported, gather more information by asking about the following: character, associated symptoms, radiation, location, intensity, and duration, as well as what makes it better, what medications the individual has tried for these symptoms, and what makes it worse. These questions can be easily remembered by using the acronym CAR LID BMW. Answers to these questions provide a better understanding of the individual's concerns.

III. PHYSICAL EXAM FOR ALL SYSTEMS

A. Inspect the external structures of the eyes and ears; examine the ear canal for cerumen using an otoscope.
B. Check visual acuity with a near vision screener and distance acuity measure and contrast sensitivity.
C. Perform whisper test to assess rough hearing. If available in your setting, use a handheld audioscope to assess up to 40-dB hearing. If a greater range of hearing testing is needed, use a portable audiometer with noise-reduction earphones—a referral to audiology may be indicated.
D. Assess the nares; determine whether they are patent using the otoscope.
E. Inspect the mouth and tongue for any obvious lesions, odors, or deviations from normal.
F. Perform a neurosensory exam of the extremities, including a monofilament test.
G. Complete a monofilament test on all diabetics. This test quantifies the level of sensory impairment in the feet of patients with diabetes.
H. Assess vibratory sense of the extremities with a 128-Hz tuning fork and proprioception.

IV. NURSING ACTIONS AND REFERRALS

A. Vision
   1. Avoid disruption in the management of chronic eye conditions by obtaining past history and ensuring continuation of ongoing regimens such as eye drops for glaucoma.
   2. Notify the primary care provider of any acute change in vision.
   3. Encourage the use of good lighting in patient rooms. Avoid glare whenever possible.

(continued)

Protocol 5.1: Sensory Changes *(continued)*

4. Encourage the use of the patient's eyeglasses. Have family provide lighted magnification if needed. (These are the large magnifiers with a light attached; available for purchase on a sliding scale at low-vision centers.)
5. Add contrast to the fixtures and electronics in the room if light switches blend into the wall or faucets blend into the sink. Other low-contrast items in the environment include remote controls, television sets, and radios.
6. Encourage annual eye exams either with an optometrist or ophthalmologist.
7. Schedule an annual dilated exam for patients with diabetes and hypertension by ophthalmologist.
8. Written materials should be provided in at least 14- to 16-point high-contrast fonts with generous white space to improve visual tracking.
9. Encourage use of adaptive equipment.
10. Reinforce referrals for low-vision intervention.

B. Hearing
1. Assess for cerumen impactions. Request cerumen softening drops followed by cerumen removal or ear, nose, and throat consultation.
2. Get the person's attention and face him or her before speaking to assist the individual with lip reading; if female, consider wearing red lipstick to increase the contrast of your lips, a common compensatory mechanism for older adults.
3. Have at least one pocket amplifier on the nursing unit to use with hard-of-hearing individuals.
4. Do not shout at people with hearing impairments, but rather use lower tones of your voice.
5. Provide written instructions (use thick, black marker if person is also visually impaired).
6. Encourage use and ensure appropriate care for hearing aids: remove batteries at night; use brush provided to gently clean the tubes to reduce wax accumulation. Before sending bed linens or clothing to the laundry, determine whether the patient's hearing aid is in his or her ear or in its designated location (bedside table or medication cart).
7. Notify the primary care provider of any sudden change in hearing, including tinnitus or sensations of fullness.
8. Referral to audiologist and/or ENT as indicated (e.g., complicated cerumen impactions, new-onset tinnitus, or vertigo).
9. Encourage use of adaptive equipment, particularly in social settings.

C. Taste and smell
1. Take all complaints of inability or decreased ability to smell or taste seriously. Do not pass them off to medications or poor dentition.
2. Notify the primary care provider of an abrupt change in taste or smell.
3. ENT referral for evaluation for change in smell or taste.
4. Patient teaching should focus on safety issues with odors of gas and spoiled food.
5. Educate seniors to have smoke and carbon monoxide detectors in their homes, date all food in the refrigerator, and evaluate food with methods other than sense of smell and taste.

D. Peripheral sensation
1. Educate every older adult to examine his or her feet daily, as well as to look inside his or her shoes before putting them on each day.
2. Educate older adults to always wear shoes or protective slippers when he or she is ambulating to avoid unintentional injury to his or her feet.
3. The individual should be instructed to inform his or her primary provider of any lesions, calluses, or red areas.
4. Extremities should be kept clean and thoroughly dry before applying lotion.
5. Encourage the individual to bring in footwear for evaluation by the advanced practice nurse if he or she has concerns about safety. Most medical supply companies carry diabetic healing shoes that have wide toe boxes and Velcro straps that can be purchased for less than $50.
6. Refer diabetics to facilities with certified diabetes educator and foot care specialist.
7. Implement fall precautions and initiate referral to physical therapy for all diabetics with peripheral neuropathy.
8. Refer all older adults with decreased sensation or circulation to a podiatrist or foot care specialist for ongoing foot care.
9. Encourage a diet rich in thiamine and B_{12}.

(continued)

Protocol 5.1: Sensory Changes *(continued)*

V. EXPECTED OUTCOMES

A. Baseline visual acuity and hearing acuity for all older patients will be performed before discharge from the hospital, and on admission to home care or nursing home.
B. Fall precautions should be in place for all older patients with sensory impairments. Older adults should avoid falls and injuries to extremities if they have decreased sensation of lower extremities.
C. Accidental exposure to toxins, either in the air or in food because of decreased sense of smell or taste, should be avoided.

VI. FOLLOW-UP MONITORING

A. Annual vision assessment: Medicaid in most states will pay for a new pair of eyeglasses every 2 years.
B. When vision is worse than 20/125, individuals should be referred to a low-vision specialist to provide training in the use of visual assistive devices.
C. Given that hearing can change significantly over time, an audiological evaluation for hearing-impaired older adults every 2 years is important. Primary care annual visits should ask about hearing impairment and complete an audioscope evaluation. And refer to audiology for positive screens for hearing loss. Some states will pay through Medicaid for one hearing aid under limited conditions. Hearing aids have been shown to be better accepted if older adults receive them when they start having difficulty with word finding with background noise. Encouragement and hearing rehabilitation are needed to improve the consistent use of hearing aids. Audiologists can help train older adults and their families in the use of hearing aids.
D. When abrupt changes in smell or taste are reported, a referral to a dentist or ENT is indicated.
E. Long-term adjustments must be made in the home when smell and taste are affected. First, food should be dated and discarded after 48 hours to avoid accidentally eating spoiled food. Smoke and carbon monoxide detectors must be present.
F. When xerostomia (severe dry mouth) is found, a referral to a dentist is indicated.
G. Older adults with decreased peripheral sensation should be referred to neurology for an accurate diagnosis and followed regularly by a podiatrist or foot care specialist.

VII. INTERPROFESSIONAL CARE OF SENSORY CHANGES

A. Care of the aging senses is an interprofessional endeavor. Nurses who frequently have the most contact with clients can take the lead in assessing and screening older adults for decreased sensory function.
B. Once these deficits are identified, it is important to take the appropriate steps and identify the resources available to the older adult.
C. Occupational therapists, low-vision specialists, audiologists, nutritionists, otolaryngologists, and neurologists are just some of the interprofessionals who may be part of the team caring for the sensory-impaired older adult.
D. Good communication among disciplines is essential to assist the older adult in benefitting from each specialist.

ABBREVIATIONS

ENT ear, nose, and throat
I-SEE Individualized Sensory Enhancement of the Elderly

RESOURCES

Related Professional Organizations and Informational Sites

Administration on Aging
http://www.aoa.gov

American Speech–Language-Hearing Association
http://www.asha.org

Assisted Listening Devices: Summary of available assisted listening devices
http://www.asha.org/public/hearing/treatment/assist_tech.htm

Cochlear Implants
General information including video on cochlear implants
http://www.fda.gov/cdrh/cochlear

Hear Now
Will accept donated hearing aids to refit for the underserved
http://www.starkeyhearingfoundation.org/hear-now.php

The Lighthouse for the Blind
Consumer and health professional information on visual impairment and dual impairment; will accept donated hearing aids to refit for the underserved
http://www.lighthouse.org

Lighting Research Center
Consumer, builders, and health professional information on lighting
http://www.lrc.rpi.edu/programs/lightHealth/AARP/index.asp

The National Eye Institute
Contains health information for consumers and health professionals; also has images of eye diseases and eye charts
http://www.nei.nih.gov

National Institute on Aging Information Center
http://www.nia.nih.gov

National Institute on Deafness and Other Communication Disorders
Contains information for health care providers and consumers
http://www.nidcd.nih.gov

Talking Tapes
Access to talking books for visually impaired older adult
http://www.talkingtapes.org

For Patients and Families

Aging in the Know
Your gateway to health and aging resources on the web. Created by the American Geriatrics Society Foundation for Health in Aging (FHA).
http://www.healthinaging.org/agingintheknow

League for Hard of Hearing
http://www.lhh.org

Prentiss Care Networks Project
Care networks for formal and informal caregivers of older adults
http://caregiving.case.edu

REFERENCES

Adams-Wendling, L., Pimple, C., Adams, S., & Titler, M. G. (2008). Nursing management of hearing impairment in nursing facility residents. *Journal of Gerontological Nursing, 34*(11), 9–17. *Evidence Level V.*

Agency for Healthcare Research and Quality (AHRQ). (2004). *Technology assessment: Vision rehabilitation for elderly individuals with low vision and blindness.* Rockville, MD: Author. *Evidence Level VI.*

Ahmad, N., & Seidman, M. (2004). Tinnitus in the older adult: Epidemiology, pathophysiology and treatment options. *Drugs & Aging, 21*(5), 297–305. *Evidence Level VI.*

Albers, M. W., Tabert, M. H., & Devanand, D. P. (2006). Olfactory dysfunction as a predictor of neurodegenerative disease. *Current Neurology and Neuroscience Reports, 6*(5), 379–386. *Evidence Level I.*

American Academy of Ophthalmology Preferred Practice Patterns Committee. (2010). *Comprehensive adult medical eye evaluation.* San Francisco, CA. American Academy of Ophtalmology. Retrieved from www.guideline.gov/content.aspx?id=25644#. *Evidence Level I.*

American Academy of Otolaryngology–Head and Neck Surgery. (2001). *Smell and taste.* Retrieved from http://www.entnet.org/HealthInformation/smellTaste.cfm. *Evidence Level VI.*

Armstrong, D. G., & Lavery, L. A. (1998). Diabetic foot ulcers: Prevention, diagnosis and classification. *American Family Physician, 57*(6), 1325–1332, 1337–1338. *Evidence Level VI.*

Bagai, A., Thavendiranathan, P., & Detsky, A. S. (2006). Does this patient have hearing impairment? *Journal of the American Medical Association, 295*(4), 416–428. *Evidence Level I.*

Bainbridge, K. E., & Wallhagen, M. I. (2014). Hearing loss in an aging American population: Extent, impact and management. *Annual Review of Public Health, 35,* 139–52. *Evidence Level VI.*

Boike, A. M., & Hall, J. O. (2002). A practical guide for examining and treating the diabetic foot. *Cleveland Clinic Journal of Medicine, 69*(4), 342–348. *Evidence Level VI.*

Bond, M., Mealing, S., Anderson, R., Elston, J., Weiner, G., Taylor, R. S.,... Stein, K. (2009). The effectiveness and cost-effectiveness of cochlear implants for severe to profound deafness in children and adults: A systematic review and economic model. *Health Technology Assessment, 13*(44), 1–330. *Evidence Level I.*

Bromley, S. M. (2000). Smell and taste disorders: A primary care approach. *American Family Physician, 61*(2), 427–436, 438. *Evidence Level VI.*

Bron, A. J., & Caird, F. I. (1997). Loss of vision in the ageing eye. Research into Ageing Workshop, London, 10 May 1995. *Age and Ageing, 26*(2), 159–162. *Evidence Level VI.*

Cacchione, P. Z. (2007). Nursing care of older adults with age-related vision loss. In S. Crocker-Houde (Ed.), *Vision loss in older adults: Nursing assessment and care management* (pp. 131–148). New York, NY: Springer Publishing Company. *Evidence Level VI.*

Cacchione, P. Z. (2014). Sensory impairment: A new research imperative. *Journal of Gerontological Nursing, 40*(4), 3–5. *Evidence Level VI.*

Cacchione, P. Z., Culp, K., Dyck, M. J., & Laing, J. (2003). Risk for acute confusion in sensory-impaired, rural, long-term-care elders. *Clinical Nursing Research, 12*(4), 340–355. *Evidence Level III.*

Cassin, B., & Rubin, M. L. (2001). *Dictionary of eye terminology* (4th ed.). Gainesville, FL: Triad Publishing. Retrieved from http://www.eyeglossary.net. *Evidence Level IV.*

Chao, T. K., & Chen, T. H. (2009). Predictive model for progression of hearing loss: Meta-analysis of multi-state outcome. *Journal of Evaluation in Clinical Practice, 15*(1), 32–40. *Evidence Level I.*

Chou, R., Dana, T., & Bougatsos, C. (2009). Screening older adults for impaired visual acuity: A review of the evidence for the U.S. Preventive Services Task Force. *Annals of Internal Medicine, 151*(1), 44–58. *Evidence Level I.*

Community Services for the Blind and Partially Sighted. (2004). *Enhancing low vision: Lighting*. Retrieved from http://www.independentliving.org/donet/217_community_services_for_the_blind_and_partially_sighted.html. *Evidence Level VI.*

Congdon, N., O'Colmain, B., Klaver, C. C., Klein, R., Muñoz, B., Friedman, D. S., . . . Eye Diseases Prevalence Research Group. (2004). Causes and prevalence of visual impairment among adults in the United States. *Archives of Ophthalmology, 122*(4), 477–485. *Evidence Level I.*

Crummer, R. W., & Hassan, G. A. (2004). Diagnostic approach to tinnitus. *American Family Physician, 69*(1), 120–126. *Evidence Level V.*

Cugati, S., Cuming, R. G., Smith, W., Burlutsky, G., Mitchell, P., & Want, J. J. (2007). Visual impairment, age-related macular degeneration, cataract and long-term mortality: The Blue Mountains Eye Study. *Archives of Ophthalmology, 125*, 917–924. *Evidence Level II.*

Demers, K. (2001). *Hearing screening. Try this: Best practices in nursing care for older adults.* Hartford Institute for Geriatric Nursing. Retrieved from consultgeri.org/try-this/general-assessment/issue-12. *Evidence Level V.*

Dillon, C. F., Gu, Q., Hoffman, H. J., & Ko, C. W. (2010, April). *Vision, hearing, balance and sensory impairments in Americans aged 70 years and older: United States, 1999–2006* (NCHS Data Brief No. 31). Hyattsville, MD: National Center for Health Statistics. *Evidence Level II.*

Ferris, F. L., III, Kassoff, A., Bresnick, G. H., & Bailey, I. (1982). New visual acuity charts for clinical research. *American Journal of Ophthalmology, 94*(1), 91–96. *Evidence Level III.*

Francis, H. W., Chee, N., Yeagle, J., Cheng, A., & Niparko, J. K. (2002). Impact of cochlear implants on the functional health status of older adults. *Laryngoscope, 112*(8 Pt. 1), 1482–1488. *Evidence Level III.*

Frank, T., & Petersen, D. R. (1987). Accuracy of a 40 dB HL audioscope and audiometer screening for adults. *Ear and Hearing, 8*(3), 180–183. *Evidence Level II.*

Fukunaga, A., Uematsu, H., & Sugimoto, K. (2005). Influences of aging on taste perception and oral somatic sensation. *Journals of Gerontology. Series A, Biological Sciences and Medical Sciences, 60*(1), 109–113. *Evidence Level II.*

Gates, G. A., Cooper, J. C., Jr., Kannel, W. B., & Miller, N. J. (1990). Hearing in the elderly: The Framingham cohort, 1983–1985. *Ear and Hearing, 11*, 247–256. *Evidence Level II.*

Gates, G. A., & Mills, J. H. (2005). Presbycusis. *Lancet, 366*(9491), 1111–1120. *Evidence Level V.*

Gianutsos, R., & Suchoff, I. B. (1997). Visual fields after brain injury: Management issues for the occupational therapist. In M. Scheiman (Ed.), *Understanding and managing vision deficits: A guide for occupational therapists* (pp. 333–358). Thorogare, NJ: Slack. *Evidence Level VI.*

Gillmore, G. (2002). *Modules 12: Visual field testing. Glaucoma I, continuing education module.* Retrieved from http://www.eyetec.net/group3/M12Start.htm. *Evidence Level VI.*

Gopinath, B., Schneider, J., McMahon, C. M., Burlutsky, G., Leeder, S. R., & Michell, P. (2013). Dual sensory impairment in older adults increases the risk of mortality: A population-based study. *PLoS One, 8*(3), e55054. doi:10.1371/journal.phone.0055054. *Evidence Level II.*

Hellman, C. (2002). Nurse practitioner management of the patient with diabetic foot ulcers. *Clinical Excellence for Nurse Practitioners, 5*(5), 11–15. *Evidence Level VI.*

Hirvelä, H., & Laatikainen, L. (1995). Visual acuity in a population aged 70 years or older; prevalence and causes of visual impairment. *Acta Ophtalmologica Scandinavica, 73*(2), 99–104. *Evidence Level III.*

Hoffman, H. J., Cruickshanks, K. J., & Davis, B. (2009). Perspectives on population-based epidemiological studies of olfactory and taste impairment. *Annals of the New York Academy of Sciences, 1170*, 514–530. *Evidence Level I.*

Horton, J. C., & Jones, M. R. (1997). Warning on inaccurate Rosenbaum cards for testing near vision. *Survey of Ophthalmology, 42*(2), 169–174. *Evidence Level VI.*

Huang, Q., & Tang, J. (2010). Age-related hearing loss or presbycusis. *European Archives of Otorhinolaryngology, 267*(8), 1179–1191. *Evidence Level I.*

Jessa, Z., Evans, B., Thomson, D., & Rowlands, G. (2007). Vision screening of older people. *Ophthalmology, Physiology and Optometry, 27*, 527–546. doi:10.1111/j.1475-1313.2007.00525.x. *Evidence Level I.*

Kalinowski, M. A. (2008). "Eye" dentifying vision impairment in the geriatric patient. *Geriatric Nursing, 29*(2), 125–132. *Evidence Level V.*

Karpa, M. J., Gopinath, B., Beath, K., Rochtchina, E., Cumming, R. G., Wang, J. J., & Mitchell, P. (2010). Associations between hearing impairment and mortality risk in older persons. The Blue Mountains Hearing Study. *Annals of Epidemiology, 20*, 452–459. doi:10.1016/j.an-nepidem. 2010.03.011. *Evidence Level II.*

Kennedy, R. S., & Dunlap, W. P. (1990). Assessment of the Vistech contrast sensitivity test for repeated-measures applications. *Optometry and Vision Science, 67*(4), 248–251. *Evidence Level II.*

Lewis-Cullinan, C., & Janken, J. K. (1990). Effect of cerumen removal on the hearing ability of geriatric patients. *Journal of Advanced Nursing, 15*(5), 594–600. *Evidence Level II.*

Lin, F. R., Yaffe, K., Xia, J., Xue, Q. L., Harris, Purchase-Helzner, E., . . . Simonsick, E. M. (2013). Hearing loss and cognitive decline in older adults *Journal of the American Medical Association, 173*, 293–299. doi:10.1001/jamainternmed.2014.1868 *Evidence Level II.*

Linton, A. D. (2007). Age-related changes in the special senses. In A. D. Linton & H. H. W. Lach (Eds.), *Matteson and McConnell's gerontological nursing, concepts and practice* (3rd ed., pp. 600–630). St. Louis, MO: Saunders Elsevier. *Evidence Level V.*

Lockwood, A. H., Salvi, R. J., & Burkard, R. F. (2002). Tinnitus. *New England Journal of Medicine, 347*(12), 904–910. *Evidence Level V.*

Mangione, C. M., Lee, P. P., Gutierrez, P. R., Spritzer, K., Berry, S., Hays, R. D., & National Eye Institute Visual Function Questionnaire Field Test Investigators. (2001). Development of the 25-item National Eye Institute Visual Function Questionnaire.

Archives of Ophthalmology, 119(7), 1050–1058. *Evidence Level II.*

Mäntyjärvi, M., & Laitinen, T. (2001). Normal values for the Pelli-Robson contrast sensitivity test. *Journal of Cataract and Refractive Surgery, 27*(2), 261–266. *Evidence Level III.*

Marcincuk, M. C., & Roland, P. S. (2002). Geriatric hearing loss. Understanding the causes and providing appropriate treatment. *Geriatrics, 57*(4), 44, 48–50. *Evidence Level VI.*

Mehr, A. S. (2007). *Understanding your audiogram.* Retrieved from http://www.aurorahealthcare.org/yourhealth/healthgate/getcontent.asp?URLhealthgate=%22100920.html%22. *Evidence Level IV.*

Merkies, I. S. J., Faber, C. G., & Lauria, G. (2015). Advances in diagnostics and outcome measures in peripheral neuropathies. *Neuroscience Letters, 596,* 3–13. doi.org/10.1016/jneulet.2015.02.0380304–3940. *Evidence Level I.*

Mesholam, R. I., Moberg, P. J., Mahr, R. N., & Doty, R. L. (1998). Olfaction in neurodegenerative disease: A meta-analysis of olfactory functioning in Alzheimer's and Parkinson's diseases. *Archives in Neurology, 55*(1), 84–90. *Evidence Level I.*

Miwa, T., Furukawa, M., Tsukatani, T., Costanzo, R. M., DiNardo, L. J., & Reiter, E. R. (2001). Impact of olfactory impairment on quality of life and disability. *Archives of Otolaryngology—Head & Neck Surgery, 127*(5), 497–503. *Evidence Level II.*

Mold, J. W., Vesely, S. K., Keyl, B. A., Schenk, J. B., & Roberts, M. (2004). The prevalence, predictors, and consequences of peripheral sensory neuropathy in older patients. *Journal of the American Board of Family Practice, 17*(5), 309–318. *Evidence Level II.*

Morse, A. R., & Rosenthal, B. P. (1997). Vision and vision assessment. In J. A. Teresi, M. P. Lawton, D. Holmes, & M. Ory (Eds.), *Measurement in elderly chronic care populations* (pp. 45–60). New York, NY: Springer Publishing Company. *Evidence Level VI.*

Müller, A., Reichmann, H., Livermore, A., & Hummel, T. (2002). Olfactory function in idiopathic Parkinson's disease (IPD): Results from cross-sectional studies in IPD patients and long-term follow-up of de-novo IPD patients. *Journal of Neural Transmission, 109*(5–6), 805–811. *Evidence Level II.*

Murphy, C., Schubert, C. R., Cruickshanks, K. J., Klein, B. E., Klein, R., & Nondahl, D. M. (2002). Prevalence of olfactory impairment in older adults. *Journal of the American Medical Association, 288*(18), 2307–2312. *Evidence Level III.*

National Eye Institute (NEI). (2004). *Statistics and data: Prevalence of blindness data.* Retrieved from http://www.nei.nih.gov/eyedata/pbd_tables.asp. *Evidence Level VI.*

National Eye Institute (NEI). (2012). *Facts about diabetic eye disease.* Retrieved from http://www.nei.nih.gov/health/diabetic/retinopathy. *Evidence Level VI.*

National Eye Institute (NEI). (2009). Cataracts. Retrieved from https://nei.nih.gov/health/cataract/cataract_facts. *Evidence Level VI.*

National Eye Institute (NEI). (2010). Presbyopia. Retrieved from https://nei.nih.gov/health/errors/presbyopia. *Evidence Level VI.*

National Eye Institute (NEI). (2015a). *Facts about age-related macular degeneration.* Retrieved from http://www.nei.nih.gov/health/maculardegen/armd_facts. *Evidence Level VI.*

National Eye Institute (NEI). (2015b). Facts about diabetic eye disease. Retrieved from https://nei.nih.gov/health/diabetic/retinopathy. *Evidence Level VI.*

National Institute on Deafness and Other Communication Disorders (NIDCD). (2010). *Ménière's disease.* Retrieved from http://www.nidcd.nih.gov/health/balance/meniere.aspx. *Evidence Level VI.*

National Institute on Deafness and Other Communication Disorders (NIDCD). (2014a). *Cochlear implants.* Retrieved from http://www.nidcd.nih.gov/health/hearaing/pages/coch.aspx. *Evidence Level VI.*

National Institute on Deafness and Other Communication Disorders (NIDCD). (2014b). *Taste disorders.* Retrieved from http://www.nidcd.nih.gov/health/smelltaste/pages/taste.aspx. *Evidence Level VI.*

National Institute on Deafness and Other Communication Disorders (NIDCD). (2014c). *Tinnitus.* Retrieved from http://www.nidcd.nih.gov/health/hearaing/Pages/Tinnitus.aspx. *Evidence Level VI.*

National Institute on Deafness and Other Communication Disorders (NIDCD). (2015a). *Quick statistics.* Retrieved from http://www.nidcd.nih.gov/health/statistics/Pages/quick.aspx. *Evidence Level VI.*

National Institute on Deafness and Other Communication Disorders (NIDCD). (2015b). *Smell disorders.* Retrieved from http://www.nidcd.nih.gov/health/smelltaste/pages/smell.aspx. *Evidence Level VI.*

Norman, J. F., Norman, H. F., Craft, A. E., Walton, C. L., Bartholomew, A. N., Burton, C. L.,... Crabtree, C. E. (2008). Stereopsis and aging. *Vision Research, 48*(23–24), 2456–2465. *Evidence Level II.*

Oleson, S., & Murphy, C. (2015). Olfactory dysfunction in ApoE 4/4 homozygotes with Alzhemer's disease. *Journal of Alzheimer's Disease, 46*(3), 791–803. Advance online publication doi:10.3233/JAD-150089. *Evidence Level II.*

Owsley, C. (2011), Aging and vision. *Vision Research, 51,* 1610–1622. doi:10.1016/j.visres.2010.10.020. *Evidence Level I.*

Pekkonen, E., Jääskeläinen, I. P., Hietanen, M., Huotilainen, M., Näätänen, R., Ilmoniemi, R. J., & Erkinjuntti, T. (1999). Impaired preconscious auditory processing and cognitive functions in Alzheimer's disease. *Clinical Neurophysiology, 110*(11), 1942–1947. *Evidence Level II.*

Pelli, D. G., Robson, J. G., & Wilkins, A. J. (1988). The design of a new letter chart for measuring contrast sensitivity. *Clinical Vision Science, 2*(3), 187–199. *Evidence Level III.*

Pinto, J. M., Wroblewski, K. E., Kern, D. W., Schumm, L. P., & McClintock M. K. (2014). Olfactory dysfunction predicts 5-year mortality in older adults. *PLOS one, 9*(10), e107541. doi:10.1371/journal.pone.0107541. *Evidence Level II.*

Prevent Blindness America. (2012). *Vision problems in the US.* Retrieved from www.visionproblemsus.org. *Evidence Level II.*

Quaranta, N., Coppola, F., Casulli, M., Barulli, O., Lanza, F., Tortelli, R.,... Logrosicino, G. (2014). The prevalence of peripheral and central hearing impairment and its relation to cognition in older adults. *Audiology & Neurotology, 19*(Suppl. 1), 10–14. doi:10.1159/000371597. *Evidence Level II.*

Read, J. C., Phillipson, G. P., Serrano-Pedraza, I., Milner, A. D., & Parker, A. J. (2010). Stereoscopic vision in the absence of lateral occipital cortex. *PLoS One, 5*(9), 1–14. *Evidence Level I.*

Revicki, D. A., Rentz, A. M., Harnam, N., Thomas, V. S., & Lanzetta, P. (2010). Reliability and validity of the National Eye Institute Visual Function Questionnaire-25 in patients with age-related macular degeneration. *Investigative Ophthalmology & Visual Science, 51*(2), 712–717. *Evidence Level II.*

Robinson, B. E., Mairs, K., Glenny, C., & Stokes, P. (2012). An evidence-based guideline for frequency of optometric eye examinations. *Primary Health Care Open Access, 2*(4), 1–6. doi:10.4172/2167–1079.1000121. *Evidence Level I.*

Schiffman, S. S. (1997). Taste and smell losses in normal aging and disease. *Journal of the American Medical Association, 278*(16), 1357–1362. *Evidence Level V.*

Schiller, J. S., Lucas, J. W., & Peregoy, J. A. (2012). Summary health statistics for U.S. adults: National health interview survey 2011. *Vital Health Statistics, 10*(256), 1–218. *Evidence Level III.*

Seiberling, K. A., & Conley, D. B. (2004). Aging and olfactory and taste function. *Otolaryngologic Clinics of North America, 37*(6), 1209–1228. *Evidence Level V.*

Seidel, H. M., Dains, J. E., Ball, J. W., & Benedict, G. W. (2003). *Mosby's guide to physical examination* (5th ed., pp. 278–312). St. Louis, MO: Mosby. *Evidence Level VI.*

Smith, A. G., & Singleton, J. R. (2004). The diagnostic yield of a standardized approach to idiopathic sensory-predominant neuropath. *Archives of Internal Medicine, 164*(9), 1021–1025. *Evidence Level III.*

Swanson, M. W., McGwin, G., Jr., Elliott, A. F., & Owsley, C. (2009). The nursing home Minimum Data Set for vision and its association with visual acuity and contrast sensitivity. *Journal of the American Geriatrics Society, 57*(3), 486–491. doi:10.1111/j.1532–5415.2008.02144.x. *Evidence Level III.*

Swenor, B. K., Ramulu, P. Y., Willis, J. R., Friedman, D., & Lin, F. R. (2013). The prevalence of concurrent hearing and vision impairment in the United States. *Journal of the American Medical Association Internal Medicine, 173*(4), 312–313. *Evidence Level III.*

Tolson, D., Swan, I., & Knussen, C. (2002). Hearing disability: A source of distress for older people and carers. *British Journal of Nursing, 11*(15), 1021–1025. *Evidence Level II.*

U.S. Department of Health and Human Services (USDHHS). (2010). *Healthy people 2020.* Retrieved from http://www.healthypeople.gov/2020/topicsobjectives2020/default.aspx. *Evidence Level VI.*

Vasavada, M. M., Wang, J., Eslinger, P. J., Gill, D. J., Sun, X., Karunanayaka, P., & Yang, Q. X. (2015). Olfactory cortex degeneration in Alzheimer's disease and mild cognitive impairment. *Journal of Alzheimer's Disease, 45*(3), 947–958. *Evidence Level II.*

Ventry, I. M., & Weinstein, B. E. (1983). Identification of elderly people with hearing problems. *American Speech and Hearing Association, 25*(7), 37–42. *Evidence Level III.*

Vitale, S., Cotch, M. F., & Sperduto, R. D. (2006). Prevalence of visual impairment in the United States. *Journal of the American Medical Association, 295*(18), 2158–2163. *Evidence Level III.*

Wallhagen, M. I., Pettengill, E., & Whiteside, M. (2006). Sensory impairment in older adults: Part 1. Hearing loss. *American Journal of Nursing, 106*(10), 40–48. *Evidence Level VI.*

Wallhagen, M. I., Strawbridge, W. J., Shema, S. J., & Kaplan, G. A. (2004). Impact of self-assessed hearing loss on a spouse: A longitudinal analysis of couples. *Journals of Gerontology. Series B, Psychological Sciences and Social Sciences, 59*(3), S190–S196. *Evidence Level III.*

Ward, R. E., Boudreau, R. M., Caserotti, P., Harris, T. B., Zivkovic, S., Goodpaster, B. H . . . Strotmeyer, E. S., Health Aging and Body Composition Study. (2014). Sensory and motor peripheral nerve function and incident mobility disability. *Journal of the American Geriatric Society, 62*(12), 2273–2279. *Evidence Level III.*

Warnat, B. M., & Tabloski, P. (2006). Sensation: Hearing, vision, taste, touch, and smell. In P. A. Tabloski (Ed.), *Gerontological nursing* (Vol. 1, pp. 384–420). Upper Saddle River, NJ: Pearson Education. *Evidence Level VI.*

Whiteside, M. M., Wallhagen, M. I., & Pettengill E. (2006). Sensory impairment in older adults: Part 2. Vision loss. *American Journal of Nursing, 106*(11), 52–61. *Evidence Level V.*

Wilson, R. S., Arnold, S. E., Schneider, J. A., Tang, Y., & Bennett, D. A. (2007). The relationship between cerebral Alzheimer's disease pathology and odour identification in old age. *Journal of Neurology, Neurosurgery, and Psychiatry, 78*(1), 30–35. *Evidence Level II.*

Yueh, B., Collins, M. P., Souza, P. E., Heagerty, P. J., Liu, C. F., Boyko, E. J., . . . Hedrick, S. C. (2007). Screening for auditory impairment—Which hearing assessment test (SAI-WHAT): RCT design and baseline characteristics. *Contemporary Clinical Trials, 28*(3), 303–315. *Evidence Level II.*

Yueh, B., Shapiro, N., MacLean, C. H., & Shekelle, P. G. (2003). Screening and management of adult hearing loss in primary care: Scientific review. *Journal of the American Medical Association, 289*(15), 1976–1985. *Evidence Level I.*

Yueh, B., & Shekelle, P. (2007). Quality indicators for the care of hearing loss in vulnerable elders. *Journal of the American Geriatrics Society, 55*(Suppl. 2), S335–S339. *Evidence Level II.*

Zheng, Y., Lamoureux, E. Finkelstein, E., Wu, R., Lavanya, R., Chua, D., . . . Wong, T. Y. (2012). Independent impact of area-level socioeconomic measures on visual impairment. *Investigative Ophthalmology & Visual Science, 52*(12), 8799–8805. doi:10.1167/iovs.11–7700. *Evidence Level III.*

6

Assessing Cognitive Function

Pieter Heeren, Johan Flamaing, Jos Tournoy,
Marquis D. Foreman, and Koen Milisen

EDUCATIONAL OBJECTIVES

On completion of this chapter, the reader should be able to:

1. Discuss the importance of assessing cognitive function
2. Describe the methods of assessing cognitive function
3. Compare and contrast the clinical features of delirium, mild cognitive impairment, dementia, and depression
4. Incorporate the assessment of cognitive function into daily practice

OVERVIEW

Cognitive function comprises perception, memory, and thinking—the processes by which a person perceives, recognizes, registers, stores, and uses information (Foreman & Vermeersch, 2004). Although alterations in cognitive functioning are inherent to aging, there are criteria that define pathological conditions, such as delirium, mild cognitive impairment, dementia, and depression (American Psychiatric Association, 2013). These disorders have diverse clinical features and causes, but are all characterized by decline from a previously attained level (Sachdev et al., 2014). Clinicians often fail to detect these disorders in older adults, when only using routine history and standard examination (Burton et al., 2012; Douzenis et al., 2010; Torisson, Minthon, Stavenow, & Londos, 2012). This might have serious consequences that include missed opportunities to treat correctable conditions and minimize or prevent unfavorable outcomes such as functional decline and death (Bradshaw et al., 2013; Torisson et al., 2012). Assessing cognitive functioning is paramount for the early detection of pathological conditions and for monitoring the effectiveness of interventions (McCarten et al., 2012).

BACKGROUND AND STATEMENT OF PROBLEM

Declines in cognitive function are a hallmark of aging (McEvoy, 2001); however, most declines in cognition with aging have no or minor clinical impact and are not pathological. Examples of nonpathological changes include a diminished ability to learn complex information, a delayed response time, and minor loss of recent memory; declines are especially evident with complex tasks or with those requiring multiple steps for completion (McEvoy, 2001).

Pathological conditions of cognitive impairment that are prevalent with aging include delirium, mild cognitive impairment, dementia, and depression (depression can also be present without cognitive impairment; please see Table 6.1 for a comparison of the clinical features. Chapters 15, 16, and 17 describe these conditions more extensively. Several strategies exist to prevent, treat, or slow these conditions (Inouye, Westendorp, & Saczynski, 2014; Langa &

For a description of evidence levels cited in this chapter, see Chapter 1, "Developing and Evaluating Clinical Practice Guidelines: A Systematic Approach."

TABLE 6.1

A Comparison of the Clinical Features of Delirium, Mild Cognitive Impairment, Dementia, and Depression

Clinical Feature	Delirium	Mild Cognitive Impairment	Dementia	Depression
Onset	Sudden/abrupt; depends on cause; often at twilight	Insidious/slow; often unrecognized, as impairment does not interfere with daily activities	Insidious/slow but recognizable, as impairment interferes with daily activities; depends on cause	Often coincides with major life changes; often abrupt, but can be gradual
Course	Short; diurnal fluctuations in symptoms; worse at night, in darkness, and on awakening	Long; no diurnal effects, symptoms can improve, stabilize, or progress yet relatively stable over time, may see deficits with increased stress	Long; no diurnal effects, symptoms progressive yet relatively stable over time, may see deficits with increased stress	Diurnal effects, typically worse in the morning; situational fluctuations in symptoms, but less than that with delirium
Progression	Abrupt	Variable: possibly absent or slow but uneven	Slow but uneven	Variable, rapid or slow, but generally even
Duration	Several hours to less than 1 month; longer if unrecognized and untreated (sometimes untreatable)	Months to years	Months to years	At least 2 weeks, can be several months to years
Consciousness	Disturbed	Clear	Clear—possibly disturbed in advanced dementia	Clear
Alertness	Fluctuates from stuporous to hypervigilant	Normal	Normal—possibly disturbed in advanced dementia	Often disturbed
Attention	Inattentive, easily distractible; the person cannot focus on an idea or task	Generally normal; if attention is affected, the person might have difficulties with complex-attention tasks (e.g., complex-problem solving)	Generally normal, depending on the cause; shifting from one (rather simple) attention task to another can be problematic	Often disturbed
Orientation	Generally impaired; disoriented to time and place, should not be disoriented to person	Generally normal	Generally disturbed—impaired in advanced dementia	Selective disorientation
Memory	Recent and immediate impairment, unable to recall events of hospitalization and current illness, forgetful, unable to recall instructions	If memory is afflicted, mild declines in memory (misplacing things, repeating questions, having troubles keeping track of dates/appointments)	Major declines in memory (unable to recall recent events)	Selective or "patchy" impairment, "islands" of intact memory, recall better if cued, evaluation often difficult because of low motivation
Thinking	Disorganized; rambling, irrelevant and incoherent conversation; unclear or illogical flow of ideas	If thinking is disturbed, changes in language (e.g., word-finding difficulties) and visuospatial function (e.g., slow to identify roadway hazards) might occur.	Difficulty with abstraction, thoughts impoverished; judgment impaired	Intact but with themes of hopelessness, helplessness, or self-deprecation

(continued)

TABLE 6.1

A Comparison of the Clinical Features of Delirium, Mild Cognitive Impairment, Dementia, and Depression *(continued)*

Clinical Feature	Delirium	Mild Cognitive Impairment	Dementia	Depression
Perception	Perceptual disturbances, such as illusions and visual and auditory hallucinations; misperceptions of common people and objects common	Intact	Misperceptions usually absent	Intact; delusions and hallucinations absent except in severe cases
Psychomotor behavior	Variable; hypoactive, hyperactive, and mixed	Normal	Normal, may have apraxia	Variable; psychomotor retardation or agitation
Associated features	Variable affective changes; symptoms of autonomic hypo-hyperarousal	The person might attempt to conceal or laugh off cognitive deficits	Affect tends to be superficial, inappropriate; attempts to conceal deficits in intellect; personality changes, aphasia, agnosia may be present; often lacks insight	Affect depressed; dysphoric mood, exaggerated and detailed complaints; preoccupied with personal thoughts; insight present; verbal elaboration; somatic complaints, poor hygiene, and neglect of self
Assessment	Distracted from task; fails to remember instructions, frequent errors without notice	Although a person or relative might report failings, these are often difficult to differentiate from declines inherent to aging. Neuropsychological tests have fairly good norms to detect this difference.	Failings highlighted by family, frequent "near miss" answers, struggles with test, great effort to find an appropriate reply, frequent requests for feedback on performance	Failings highlighted by individual; frequent "don't know" answers, little effort; frequently gives up; indifferent toward test: does not care or attempt to find answer

Levine, 2014). However, these opportunities exist mainly when and if these conditions are detected early.

Clinicians often fail to evaluate cognitive function when using routine history and standard examination (Burton et al., 2012; Torisson et al., 2012). Hence, early detection of cognitive impairment exists only when cognitive function is assessed (McCarten et al., 2012). Without assessment, these pathological conditions are often un(der)diagnosed (Torisson et al., 2012), and the individuals with these conditions face much greater, accelerated, and long-term cognitive and functional decline and death (Barry, Murphy, & Gill, 2011; Bradshaw et al., 2013). Yet, it is clear that the assessment of cognitive function is a crucial step in a cascade of strategies to prevent, reverse, halt, or minimize cognitive decline.

ASSESSMENT OF THE PROBLEM

Methods for Assessing Cognitive Function

A two-step approach is recommended for determining the nature of impairment (Cordell et al., 2013; Jackson, Naqvi, & Sheehan, 2013; Simmons, Hartmann, & Dejoseph, 2011). The first step is screening for impairment, the second includes a full evaluation, if necessary. Screening is conducted to briefly determine the presence or absence of impairment. If screening results indicate possible impairment, a full evaluation is necessary to make a diagnosis of dementia, delirium, depression, mild cognitive impairment, or some other health problem. The content of a full evaluation varies depending on the patient's presentation and includes tests to find out the etiologies of impairment and assess its severity (Cordell et al., 2013).

When a diagnosis is made, appropriate reassessment or *monitoring* is necessary to track cognitive and global functioning over time as a means for following the progression or regression of impairment, especially in response to treatment (Cordell et al., 2013; Shenkin, Russ, Ryan, & MacLullich, 2014).

Instruments to Screen for Cognitive Impairment

Numerous instruments are available to assess cognitive functioning, of which Folstein's Mini-Mental State Examination

(MMSE) is the most frequently recommended and best studied (Folstein, Folstein, & McHugh, 1975; Lin, O'Connor, Rossom, Perdue, & Eckstrom, 2013; Tombaugh & McIntyre, 1992). The MMSE consists of 11 items assessing orientation, attention, memory, concentration, language, and constructional ability. Each question is scored as either correct or incorrect; the total score ranges from 0 to 30 and reflects the number of correct responses. A score less than 24 is often considered demonstrative of impaired cognition.

The performance on the MMSE can be influenced by education (individuals with less than an eighth-grade education commit more errors), language (non-native English speakers commit more errors, which is related to sociocultural differences), verbal ability (the MMSE can only be used with individuals who can respond verbally to questioning), and age (older people do less well; Tombaugh & McIntyre, 1992). Furthermore, it is important to stress that the MMSE is not available for public use without cost (Lin et al., 2013).

The Montreal Cognitive Assessment (MoCA) is a new instrument for detecting and monitoring cognitive impairment (Nasreddine et al., 2005). It assesses the following cognitive domains: attention and concentration, executive functions, memory, language, visuoconstructional skills, conceptual thinking, calculations, and orientation. The total score is 30 points and a score of 26 or above is generally considered normal. Validation studies of the MoCA indicate its performance to be equivalent or superior to that of the MMSE, especially in patients with mild cognitive impairment (Dong et al., 2012; Liew, Feng, Gao, Ng, & Yap, 2015). Permission to use or reproduce the MoCA is required in research and commercial settings.

As the administration times of both the MMSE and the MoCA are quite long (approximately 10–15 minutes for trained users), it is recommended to use a briefer test for screening purposes, such as the Mini-Cog (Borson, Scanlan, Brush, Vitaliano, & Dokmak, 2000), to decide whether it is appropriate to conduct the MMSE or the MoCA. The Mini-Cog is a four-item screening test consisting of a three-item recall and a clock-drawing item; for example, draw the face of a clock, number the clock face, and place the hands on the clock face to indicate a specific time such as 11:10. Although the Mini-Cog is widely used and well known, clinicians might select other brief tools to use in their clinical practice, because there is no optimal tool to detect cognitive impairment in all settings and patient populations (Cordell et al., 2013; Lin et al., 2013).

Most cognitive screenings tests, among the ones mentioned earlier, are initially developed as a measure for global cognitive abilities. Because it is often difficult to make a differential diagnosis (Is the impairment delirium, mild cognitive impairment, dementia or depression, or possibly one superimposed on another?), parallel use of other short instruments, such as the Confusion Assessment Method (CAM; Inouye et al., 1990), the Delirium Observation Screening Scale (DOSS; Detroyer et al., 2014; Schuurmans, Shortridge-Baggett, & Duursma, 2003), or the Geriatric Depression Scale (GDS; Yesavage et al., 1982), can be useful to determine the nature of impairment. See Chapters 15, 16, and 17 for a more detailed discussion about which screening tool to choose per condition.

The 4AT is a recently designed screening instrument for detecting both delirium and (moderate to severe) cognitive impairment (Bellelli et al., 2014). Its key features are: brevity (administered in less than 2 minutes), no special training required, allows for assessment of "untestable" patients, does not require supplemental materials, and incorporates brief cognitive test items. The attention item, in which a patient is asked to tell the months of the year in backward order starting from December, was reported to be very predictive for the presence of delirium (inattention was present in persons who were unable to reach July; O'Regan et al., 2014). The 4AT is free to download and use (www.the4AT.com). Although the first results concerning the 4AT are promising, more research is needed to confirm its validity and reliability (Bellelli et al., 2014; Lees et al., 2013).

It is also recommended that formal cognitive testing be supplemented with information from close relatives (Cordell et al., 2013; Langa & Levine, 2014). This information assists in determining the duration of impairment—which is crucial for making a diagnosis—and can be obtained through history taking or the Informant Questionnaire on Cognitive Decline in the Elderly (IQCODE; Jorm & Jacomb, 1989) and/or the Family Confusion Assessment Method (FAM-CAM; Steis et al., 2012). The Neuropsychiatric Inventory (NPI; Kaufer et al., 2000) and caregiver burden assessments (Adelman, Tmanova, Delgado, Dion, & Lachs, 2014) can also be used to obtain information from relatives.

Formal screening is not always possible. When a patient is too sick for formal testing (e.g., inattentive or responding unusually or inappropriately to conversation or questioning), naturally occurring observations during daily and routine contacts with the patient (e.g., during bathing, feeding, transferring the patient) can be used to evaluate an individual's cognitive functioning easily and in a nonthreatening way. The Nurses' Observation Scale for Cognitive Abilities (NOSCA) was developed and validated to standardize the reporting of these observations (Persoon, Banningh, van de Vrie, Rikkert, & van Achterberg, 2011; Persoon et al., 2012).

When time is scarce, at minimum, it is necessary to establish whether a patient fulfills the criteria for delirium

(Inouye et al., 1990), because patients with delirium have the highest risk for severe short-term adverse outcomes (Witlox et al., 2010). Therefore, in expectation of formal screening results, the use of the instruments mentioned earlier should temporarily be substituted by assessment of orientation (to time and place) and attention (e.g., naming of days of the week (no errors should be allowed), or months of the year backward (one error should be allowed), serial sevens (i.e., in subsequently substracting 7 from 100; one error should be allowed for five subtractions), or digit spans backward (i.e., the length of the longest list of digits that a person can recite backward; normally three or more; Inouye et al., 2014). Any suspected or uncertain cases should be handled as delirious until proven otherwise (Inouye et al., 2014).

When screening results indicate impairment, referral to a specialist setting (e.g., memory clinic, neuropsychologist, psychiatrist, advanced practice nurse, etc.) is necessary for more diagnostic workup (i.e., extensive history taking, clinical and neurological examination, extended neuropsychological assessment, brain imaging, blood sampling, etc.). Chapters 15, 16, and 17 describe more extensively how a differential diagnosis can be made.

When to Assess Cognitive Function

As there is insufficient evidence supporting universal screening for cognitive impairment in older patients (Moyer, 2014), screening interventions are usually applied to a smaller group of persons with specific risk factors (i.e., case finding). Recommendations for assessing cognition with standardized and validated tools include: presence of signs, symptoms, or complaints of cognitive impairment (Lin et al., 2013; Moyer, 2014) with behavior that is inappropriate to a situation or unusual for the individual (including functional decline; Foreman & Vermeersch, 2004); when there is no informant to confirm absence of signs or symptoms (Cordell et al., 2013); and before making important treatment decisions as an adjunct to determining an individual's capacity to consent and capacity to adhere to treatment guidelines (Fletcher, 2007).

When and how frequently cognitive functioning needs to be (re-) assessed is in part a function of the purpose for the assessment, the condition of the patient (e.g., unusual/inappropriate behavior), and the results of prior or current testing. Of course, patients with (suspected) delirium need to be monitored frequently (e.g., every 4–8 hours) because of the possible course and risks of this condition. In case of reassessment after onset of treatment, it is important to know that delirium interventions might only need a few hours before effects can be measured, whereas effects of interventions to improve complaints and signs related to depression or dementia might only be measured after 2 or more weeks, if possible.

Cautions for Assessing Cognitive Function

Various characteristics of the physical environment should be considered to ensure that the results of the cognitive assessment accurately reflect the individual's abilities and not extraneous factors. Overall, the ideal assessment environment should maximize the comfort and privacy of both the assessor and the individual. The environment should enhance performance by maximizing the individual's ability to participate in the assessment process (Dellasega, 1998). To accomplish this, the room should be well lit and of comfortable ambient temperature. Lighting must be balanced to be sufficient for the individual to see the examination materials adequately, while not being so bright as to create glare. Also, the environment should be free from distractions that can result from extraneous noise, scattered assessment materials, or brightly colored and/or patterned clothing and flashy jewelry on the assessor (Lezak, Howieson, & Loring, 2004).

It will be vital to prepare the individual for the assessment—explaining what will take place and how long it will take—hence reducing anxiety and creating an emotionally nonthreatening environment and a safe individual–assessor relationship (Engberg & McDowell, 2000). Therefore, it is essential to avoid counterproductive statements that describe the assessment as consisting of "simple," "silly," or "stupid" questions. These tend to diminish motivation to perform and heighten anxiety when errors are committed.

Performing the assessment in the presence of others should be avoided when possible, as the other individual may be distracting. If the other is a relative, additional problems may arise. For example, when the individual fails to respond or responds in error, significant others tend to provide the answer, or to say such things as "Now, you know the answer to that," or "Now, you know that's wrong." Because older adults are especially sensitive to any insinuation that they may have some "memory problem," it is important for the assessor in these cases to stress the importance of the assessment without increasing the individual's anxiety. An informant questionnaire, like the Informant Questionnaire on Cognitive Decline in the Elderly (like the IQCODE; Jorm & Jacomb, 1989), can be a creative solution to deal with disturbing others.

The assessment can be perceived by the individual as intrusive, intimidating, fatiguing, and offensive; characteristics that can seriously and negatively affect performance. Consequently, an initial period to establish rapport with the individual is recommended (Lezak et al., 2004). This period also allows a determination of the individual's capacity for assessment, for example, do conditions exist that could alter the performance of the individual or interpretation of results such as sensory decrements? As a consequence, the assessor can alter the testing environment through simple methods, for example, by taking a position across from the individual or a little to the side. In this position, the individual can readily use the assessor's nonverbal communication as well as read the assessor's lips. Positioning also is important relative to lighting and glare.

Finally, avoid assessment periods immediately on awakening from sleep (wait at least 30 minutes) and immediately before and after meals or medical procedures (Foreman, Fletcher, Mion, & Trygslad, 2003). In addition, it should be said that even in perfect circumstances and in the absence of pathological conditions, patients may perform poorly on cognitive screening tests for other reasons, including acute illness, sleep deprivation, cultural issues, and so on (Shenkin et al., 2014) Therefore, it is paramount that screening results are reported with the appropriate context in which these were obtained. Otherwise, at a future date, patient charts might falsely reflect chronic impairment (Cordell et al., 2013; Shenkin et al., 2014).

CASE STUDY

Before

Mrs. O, a 72-year-old retired farmer's wife, was referred to the emergency department (ED), because her primary care provider (PCP) judged her to be slow in responding. For more than 10 weeks, she has been complaining about intolerable pain in her right hip, which could not be managed effectively by the PCP with acetaminophen and tramadol hydrochloride. An x-ray had revealed that the 15-year-old hip prosthesis needed replacement and surgery had been scheduled in the upcoming week. As a result of to this problem, Mrs. O became dependent on her husband for several activities of daily living (bathing, dressing, toileting, and transferring).

In the ED

The triage nurse in the ED reports to his colleague on the observational ward that Mrs. O is a gentle, cooperative lady who needs upgrading of pain therapy in attendance of surgery. As intolerable pain is her main complaint, he administered an intravenous bolus of 5 mg piritramide.

The admitting nurse of the observational unit decides to assess Mrs. O's cognitive functioning, because her husband reports to be overwhelmed by his wife's condition. He described that his wife's cognitive status was known to be problematic—she was diagnosed with mild cognitive impairment a year ago (MMSE: 22/30), but it worsened dramatically since the funeral of her sister 2 weeks ago. He also added that she had been talking nonsense from time to time since then. In brief, there are arguments for the presence of delirium, depression, and dementia, or possibly one superimposed on another.

Some instances later, Mrs. O starts shouting for help. She is agitated, disoriented to time and place, and fails to recite the months of the year backward. Blood test results show that she was experiencing multiple problems: low sodium levels, high creatinine level, and presence of inflammation. It is likely that the intravenous bolus of piritramide triggered or worsened delirium, as it is known that opiates should be administered with caution in people at risk of delirium (Clegg & Young, 2011)—which was probably not considered by the triage nurse, as he did not assess Mrs. O's cognitive functioning before administering the drug. A transfer to the intensive care unit is necessary owing to tachycardia and surgery needs to be postponed until the aforementioned problems are corrected.

2 Weeks Later

When there were no more arguments for the presence of delirium (e.g., no fluctuating behavior, inattention or disorganized thinking, etc.), Mrs. O's cognitive functioning (MMSE 21/30) and depressive symptoms (GDS: 2/30) were assessed to evaluate her capacity to adhere to rehabilitation following surgery.

Mrs. O had an uncomplicated postoperative course and regained functional independence after participating in a patient-centered rehabilitation program targeting patients with cognitive impairment.

SUMMARY

The determination of an individual's cognitive status is critical in the process and outcomes of illness and its treatment. Being competent in the assessment of cognitive functioning requires (a) knowledge and skill as they relate to the performance of the assessment of cognitive functioning, (b) sensitivity to the issues that can negatively bias the results and interpretation of this assessment, (c) accurate and comprehensive documentation of the assessment, and (d) the incorporation of the results of the assessment in the development of the individual's plan of care.

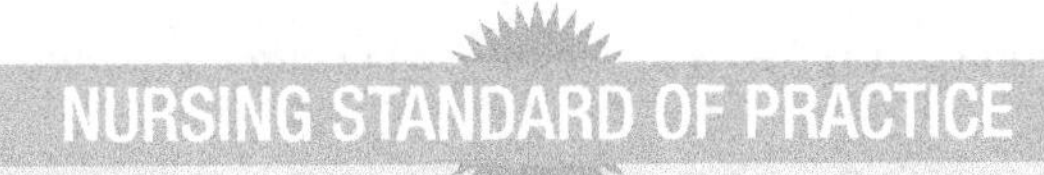

Protocol 6.1: Assessing Cognitive Function

I. GOALS

The goals of cognitive assessment include the following:

A. To determine an individual's cognitive abilities
B. To recognize early and diagnose the presence of cognitive impairment
C. To monitor an individual's cognitive response to various treatments

II. OVERVIEW

A. Detecting cognitive impairment in older patients is important because of the impairment's association with adverse events (Bradshaw et al., 2013).
B. Assessing cognitive function is necessary for early detection and prompt treatment of impairment (McCarten et al., 2012).

III. BACKGROUND AND STATEMENT OF PROBLEM

A. Definition of cognitive functioning includes the processes by which an individual perceives, registers, stores, retrieves, and uses information.
B. The fifth edition of the *Diagnostic and Statistical Manual of Mental Disorders* (*DSM-5*) provides criteria for diagnosing declines from a previously attained level (see *DSM-5* for specific criteria; American Psychiatric Association [APA], 2013; Sachdev et al., 2014).
   1. *Delirium* is a disturbance in attention and awareness that develops over a short period of time and tends to fluctuate in severity during the course of a day, combined with a disturbance in cognition (e.g., disorientation, memory deficit, etc.), neither of which are better explained by another neurocognitive disorder, but by one or multiple physiological effects (APA, 2013).
   2. *Mild neurocognitive disorder* (or *mild cognitive impairment*) is characterized by a modest cognitive decline from a previous level of performance in at least one cognitive domain (e.g., executive function, complex attention, etc.), that does not interfere with capacity for independence in everyday activities if the decline is not exclusively present in the context of a delirium or attributable to another mental disorder (APA, 2013).
   3. *Major neurocognitive disorder* (or *dementia*) is characterized by a significant cognitive decline from a previous level of performance in at least one cognitive domain (e.g., learning and memory, language, etc.) that interferes with independence in everyday activities if the decline is not exclusively present in the context of a delirium or attributable to another mental disorder (APA, 2013).
   4. *Depression* is a disorder represented by several symptoms. At the very least, one symptom needs to be the presence of a depressed mood or loss of interest or pleasure during a 2-week period, which causes clinically significant distress and leads to a decline from previous functioning; these symptoms cannot be attributed to direct physiological effects of a substance or a general medical condition (APA, 2013).

IV. ASSESSMENT OF COGNITIVE FUNCTION

A. Methods for assessing cognitive function
   1. *Screening*: to determine the absence or presence of impairment
   2. *Full evaluation*: to make a diagnosis if screening results indicate impairment
   3. *Monitoring*: to track cognitive status over time, especially in response to treatment
B. Instruments to screen for cognitive impairment
   1. *MMSE* (Folstein et al., 1975) is the most recommended and best studied instrument. It can be used to screen for or monitor cognitive impairment. However, performance on the MMSE is adversely influenced by education, age, language, and verbal ability. The MMSE is not available for public use without cost.

(continued)

Protocol 6.1: Assessing Cognitive Function *(continued)*

2. *MoCA* can both detect and monitor cognitive impairment. Its performance is reported to be equivalent or superior to that of the MMSE, especially in patients with mild cognitive impairment.
3. *Mini-Cog* is a widely used and recommended instrument that is often preferred over MMSE and MoCA for detecting impairment because the administration time of MMSE and MoCA is quite long. Depending on the setting, many other tools are available to briefly screen for the presence or absence of cognitive impairment.
4. *Differential diagnosis*: Parallel use of other short instruments, such as the CAM (Inouye et al., 1990), the DOSS (Schuurmans et al., 2003), or the GDS (Yesavage et al., 1982), can be useful to determine the nature of impairment.
5. *Heteroanamnesis*: Information from relatives assists in determining the duration and nature of impairment. IQCODE, NPI, and FAM-CAM can be used to obtain this information.
6. *Naturally occurring observations*: NOSCA standardizes the reporting of observations and conversations during naturally occurring care interactions (Persoon et al., 2011). The use of NOSCA is especially relevant when a patient's condition does not allow the use of other aforementioned instruments.
7. *When screening results indicate impairment*: Referral to a specialist setting (e.g., memory clinic, neuropsychologist, psychiatrist, advanced practice nurse, etc.) is necessary for more diagnostic workup (i.e., extensive history taking, clinical and neurological examination, extended neuropsychological assessment, brain imaging, blood sampling, etc.).

C. When to assess cognitive function
  1. Presence of signs, symptoms, and/or complaints of cognitive impairment
  2. With behavior that is inappropriate to a situation and/or unusual for the individual (including functional decline)
  3. Lack of an informant to confirm absence of signs or symptoms
  4. Before making important treatment decisions as an adjunct to determining an individual's capacity to consent and capacity to adhere to treatment guidelines

D. Cautions for assessing cognitive function
  1. Physical environment (Dellasega, 1998)
     a. Comfortable ambient temperature
     b. Adequate lighting (not glaring)
     c. Free of distractions (e.g., should preferably be conducted in the absence of others and other activities)
     d. Position self to maximize individual's sensory abilities
  2. Interpersonal environment (Engberg & McDowell, 2000)
     a. Prepare individual for assessment
     b. Initiate assessment within nonthreatening conversation
     c. Let individual set pace of assessment
     d. Be emotionally nonthreatening
  3. Timing of assessment (Foreman et al., 2003)
     a. Select time of assessment to reflect actual cognitive abilities of the individual
     b. Avoid the following times:
        i. Immediately on awakening from sleep (wait at least 30 minutes)
        ii. Immediately before and after meals
        iii. Immediately before and after medical diagnostic or therapeutic procedures
        iv. In the presence of unstable and/or interfering medical conditions (e.g., fever, nausea)
  4. Reporting of assessment results (Shenkin et al., 2014)
     a. Report screening results with the context in which they were obtained.

V. EVALUATION/EXPECTED OUTCOMES

A. Patient
  1. Is assessed at recommended moments
  2. Any impairment detected early

(continued)

Protocol 6.1: Assessing Cognitive Function *(continued)*

3. Care tailored to appropriately address cognitive status/impairment
4. Satisfaction with care improved

B. Health care provider
1. Competent to assess cognitive function
2. Able to differentiate among delirium, mild cognitive impairment, dementia, and depression
3. Uses standardized cognitive assessment protocol
4. Satisfaction with care improved

C. Institution
1. Improved documentation of cognitive assessments
2. Impairments in cognitive function identified promptly and accurately
3. Improved referral to appropriate advanced providers (e.g., geriatricians, geriatric nurse practitioners, neurologists, psychiatrists, memory clinics) for additional assessment and treatment recommendations
4. Decreased overall costs of care

VI. FOLLOW-UP MONITORING

A. Provider competence in the assessment of cognitive function
B. Consistent and appropriate documentation of cognitive assessment
C. Consistent and appropriate care and follow-up in instances of impairment
D. Timely and appropriate referral for diagnostic and treatment recommendations

VII. RELEVANT PRACTICE GUIDELINES

A. United States Preventive Services Task Force. *Cognitive impairment in older adults: Screening*. Retrieved from http://www.uspreventiveservicestaskforce.org/Page/Document/UpdateSummaryFinal/cognitive-impairment-in-older-adults-screening?ds=1&s=cognitive

B. Guidelines and Protocols Advisory Committee (GPAC) guideline. *Cognitive impairment in the elderly—recognition, diagnosis, management*. Retrieved from http://www2.gov.bc.ca/gov/content/health/practitioner-professional-resources/bc-guidelines/cognitive-impairment

C. National Institute for Health and Clinical Excellence (NICE) guideline. *Delirium: Diagnosis, prevention, and management*. Retrieved from http://guidance.nice.org.uk/CG103

D. The Registered Nurse Association of Ontario. *Best practice guideline for screening for delirium, dementia, and depression in older adults*. Retrieved from http://rnao.ca/bpg/guidelines/caregiving-strategies-older-adults-delirium-dementia-and-depression

E. The National Guideline Clearinghouse. *Delirium, dementia, cognitive disorders*. Retrieved from http://www.guideline.gov/search/search.aspx?term=delirium%2c+dementia%2c+cognitive+disorders

ABBREVIATIONS

CAM	Confusion Assessment Method
DOSS	Delirium Observation Screening Scale
DSM-5	*Diagnostic and Statistical Manual of Mental Disorders, Fifth Edition*
FAM-CAM	Family Confusion Assessment Method
GDS	Geriatric Depression Scale
GPAC	Guidelines and Protocols Advisory Committee
IQCODE	Informant Questionnaire on Cognitive Decline in the Elderly
MMSE	Mini-Mental State Examination
MoCA	Montreal Cognitive Assessment
NICE	National Institute for Health and Clinical Excellence
NOSCA	Nurses' Observation Scale for Cognitive Abilities
NPI	Neuropsychiatric Inventory

RESOURCES

Recommended Instruments for Assessing Cognitive Functioning

4AT
www.the4AT.com

Mini-Mental State
www.minimental.com

Montreal Cognitive Assessment
www.mocatest.org

Mini-Cog
http://www.alz.org/documents_custom/minicog.pdf

Additional Online Information About Assessing Cognitive Functioning

ConsultGeriRN
A series of tips on various aspects of assessing and caring for older adults sponsored by the Hartford Institute for Geriatric Nursing at New York University College of Nursing.
www.consultgerirn.org

Geriatric Toolkits
www.gericareonline.net/tools/index.html

ICU Delirium and Cognitive Impairment Study Group
www.icudelirium.org

Iowa Index of Geriatric Assessment Tools (IIGAT)
www.healthcare.uiowa.edu/igec/tools

REFERENCES

Adelman, R. D., Tmanova, L. L., Delgado, D., Dion, S., & Lachs, M. S. (2014). Caregiver burden: A clinical review. *Journal of the American Medical Association, 311*(10), 1052–1060. *Evidence Level V.*

American Psychiatric Association. (2013). *Diagnostic and statistical manual of mental disorders* (5th ed.). Arlington, VA: American Psychiatric Press.

Barry, L. C., Murphy, T. E., & Gill, T. M. (2011). Depression and functional recovery after a disabling hospitalization in older persons. *Journal of the American Geriatrics Society, 59*(7), 1320–1325. *Evidence Level IV.*

Bellelli, G., Morandi, A., Davis, D. H., Mazzola, P., Turco, R., Gentile, S., . . . MacLullich, A. M. J. (2014). Validation of the 4AT, a new instrument for rapid delirium screening: A study in 234 hospitalised older people. *Age and Ageing, 43*(4), 496–502. *Evidence Level IV.*

Borson, S., Scanlan, J., Brush, M., Vitaliano, P., & Dokmak, A. (2000). The Mini-Cog: A cognitive "vital signs" measure for dementia screening in multi-lingual elderly. *International Journal of Geriatric Psychiatry, 15*(11), 1021–1027. *Evidence Level IV.*

Bradshaw, L. E., Goldberg, S. E., Lewis, S. A., Whittamore, K., Gladman, J. R., Jones, R. G., & Harwood, R. H. (2013). Six-month outcomes following an emergency hospital admission for older adults with co-morbid mental health problems indicate complexity of care needs. *Age and Ageing, 42*(5), 582–588. *Evidence Level IV.*

Burton, C. Z., Twamley, E. W., Lee, L. C., Palmer, B. W., Jeste, D. V., Dunn, L. B., & Irwin, S. A. (2012). Undetected cognitive impairment and decision-making capacity in patients receiving hospice care. *American Journal of Geriatric Psychiatry: Official Journal of the American Association for Geriatric Psychiatry, 20*(4), 306–316. *Evidence Level IV.*

Clegg, A., & Young, J. B. (2011). Which medications to avoid in people at risk of delirium: A systematic review. *Age and Ageing, 40*(1), 23–29. *Evidence Level I.*

Cordell, C. B., Borson, S., Boustani, M., Chodosh, J., Reuben, D., Verghese, J., . . . Medicare Detection of Cognitive Impairment Workgroup. (2013). Alzheimer's Association recommendations for operationalizing the detection of cognitive impairment during the Medicare Annual Wellness Visit in a primary care setting. *Alzheimer's & Dementia: Journal of the Alzheimer's Association, 9*(2), 141–150. *Evidence Level VI.*

Dellasega, C. (1998). Assessment of cognition in the elderly: Pieces of a complex puzzle. *Nursing Clinics of North America, 33*(3), 395–405. *Evidence Level VI.*

Detroyer, E., Clement, P. M., Baeten, N., Pennemans, M., Decruyenaere, M., Vandenberghe, J., . . . Milisen, K. (2014). Detection of delirium in palliative care unit patients: A prospective descriptive study of the Delirium Observation Screening Scale administered by bedside nurses. *Palliative Medicine, 28*(1), 79–86. *Evidence Level IV.*

Dong, Y., Lee, W. Y., Basri, N. A., Collinson, S. L., Merchant, R. A., Venketasubramanian, N., & Chen, C. L. (2012). The Montreal Cognitive Assessment is superior to the Mini-Mental State Examination in detecting patients at higher risk of dementia. *International Psychogeriatrics/IPA, 24*(11), 1749–1755. *Evidence Level IV.*

Douzenis, A., Michopoulos, I., Gournellis, R., Christodoulou, C., Kalkavoura, C., Michalopoulou, P. G., . . . Lykouras, L. (2010). Cognitive decline and dementia in elderly medical inpatients remain underestimated and underdiagnosed in a recently established university general hospital in Greece. *Archives of Gerontology and Geriatrics, 50*(2), 147–150. *Evidence Level IV.*

Engberg, S. J., & McDowell, J. (2000). Comprehensive geriatric assessment. In J. T. Stone, J. F. Wyman, & S. A. Salisbury (Eds.), *Clinical gerontological nursing: A guide to advanced practice* (2nd ed., pp. 63–85). Philadelphia, PA: Saunders. *Evidence Level VI.*

Fletcher, K. (2007). Dementia. In E. Capezuti, D. Zwicker, M. Mezey, & T. Fulmer (Eds.), *Evidence-based geriatric nursing protocols* (3rd ed., pp. 83–109). New York, NY: Springer Publishing Company. *Evidence Level VI.*

Folstein, M. F., Folstein, S. E., & McHugh, P. R. (1975). "Mini-mental state." A practical method for grading the cognitive state of patients for the clinician. *Journal of Psychiatric Research, 12*(3), 189–198. *Evidence Level IV.*

Foreman, M. D., Fletcher, K., Mion, L. C., & Trygslad, L. (2003). Assessing cognitive function. In M. Mezey, T. Fulmer, & I. Abraham (Eds.), D. Zwicker (Managing ed.), *Geriatric nursing protocols for best practice* (2nd ed., pp. 99–115). New York, NY: Springer Publishing Company. *Evidence Level VI.*

Foreman, M. D., & Vermeersch, P. E. H. (2004). Measuring cognitive status. In M. Frank-Stromborg & S. J. Olsen (Eds.), *Instruments for clinical health care research* (3rd ed., pp. 100–127). Sudbury, MA: Jones & Bartlett. *Evidence Level I.*

Inouye, S. K., van Dyck, C. H., Alessi, C. A., Balkin, S., Siegal, A. P., & Horwitz, R. I. (1990). Clarifying confusion: The confusion assessment method. A new method for detection of delirium. *Annals of Internal Medicine, 113*(12), 941–948. *Evidence Level IV.*

Inouye, S. K., Westendorp, R. G., & Saczynski, J. S. (2014). Delirium in elderly people. *Lancet, 383*(9920), 911–922. *Evidence Level VI.*

Jackson, T. A., Naqvi, S. H., & Sheehan, B. (2013). Screening for dementia in general hospital inpatients: A systematic review and meta-analysis of available instruments. *Age and Ageing, 42*(6), 689–695. *Evidence Level I.*

Jorm, A. F., & Jacomb, P. A. (1989). The Informant Questionnaire on Cognitive Decline in the Elderly (IQCODE): Socio-demographic correlates, reliability, validity and some norms. *Psychological Medicine, 19*(4), 1015–1022. *Evidence Level IV.*

Kaufer, D. I., Cummings, J. L., Ketchel, P., Smith, V., MacMillan, A., Shelley, T., . . . DeKosky, S. T. (2000). Validation of the NPI-Q, a brief clinical form of the Neuropsychiatric Inventory. *Journal of Neuropsychiatry and Clinical Neurosciences, 12*(2), 233–239. *Evidence Level IV.*

Langa, K. M., & Levine, D. A. (2014). The diagnosis and management of mild cognitive impairment: A clinical review. *Journal of the American Medical Association, 312*(23), 2551–2561. *Evidence Level VI.*

Lees, R., Corbet, S., Johnston, C., Moffitt, E., Shaw, G., & Quinn, T. J. (2013). Test accuracy of short screening tests for diagnosis of delirium or cognitive impairment in an acute stroke unit setting. *Stroke: A Journal of Cerebral Circulation, 44*(11), 3078–3083. *Evidence Level IV.*

Lezak, M. D., Howieson, D. B., & Loring D. W. (2004). *Neuropsychological assessment* (4th ed.). New York, NY: Oxford University Press. *Evidence Level VI.*

Liew, T. M., Feng, L., Gao, Q., Ng, T. P., & Yap, P. (2015). Diagnostic utility of Montreal cognitive assessment in the fifth edition of *diagnostic and statistical manual of mental disorders*: Major and mild neurocognitive disorders. *Journal of the American Medical Directors Association, 16*(2), 144–148. *Evidence Level IV.*

Lin, J. S., O'Connor, E., Rossom, R. C., Perdue, L. A., & Eckstrom, E. (2013). Screening for cognitive impairment in older adults: A systematic review for the U.S. Preventive Services Task Force. *Annals of Internal Medicine, 159*(9), 601–612. *Evidence Level I.*

McCarten, J. R., Anderson, P., Kuskowski, M. A., McPherson, S. E., Borson, S., & Dysken, M. W. (2012). Finding dementia in primary care: The results of a clinical demonstration project. *Journal of the American Geriatrics Society, 60*(2), 210–217. *Evidence Level V.*

McEvoy, C. L. (2001). Cognitive changes in aging. In M. D. Mezey (Ed.), *The encyclopedia of elder care* (pp. 139–141). New York, NY: Springer Publishing Company. *Evidence Level VI.*

Moyer, V. A. (2014). Screening for cognitive impairment in older adults: U.S. Preventive Services Task Force recommendation statement. *Annals of Internal Medicine, 160*(11), 791–797. *Evidence Level VI.*

Nasreddine, Z. S., Phillips, N. A., Bedirian, V., Charbonneau, S., Whitehead, V., Collin, I., . . . Chertkow, H. (2005). The Montreal Cognitive Assessment, MoCA: A brief screening tool for mild cognitive impairment. *Journal of the American Geriatrics Society, 53*(4), 695–699. *Evidence Level IV.*

O'Regan, N. A., Ryan, D. J., Boland, E., Connolly, W., McGlade, C., Leonard, M., . . . Timmons, S. (2014). Attention! A good bedside test for delirium? *Journal of Neurology, Neurosurgery, and Psychiatry, 85*(10), 1122–1131. *Evidence Level IV.*

Persoon, A., Banningh, L. J., van de Vrie, W., Rikkert, M. G., & van Achterberg, T. (2011). Development of the Nurses' Observation Scale for Cognitive Abilities (NOSCA). *ISRN Nursing, 2011*, 895082. *Evidence Level IV.*

Persoon, A., Schoonhoven, L., Melis, R. J., van Achterberg, T., Kessels, R. P., & Rikkert, M. G. (2012). Validation of the NOSCA—Nurses' observation scale of cognitive abilities. *Journal of Clinical Nursing, 21*(21–22), 3025–3036. *Evidence Level IV.*

Sachdev, P. S., Blacker, D., Blazer, D. G., Ganguli, M., Jeste, D. V., Paulsen, J. S., & Petersen, R. C. (2014). Classifying neurocognitive disorders: The *DSM-5* approach. *Nature Reviews Neurology, 10*(11), 634–642. *Evidence Level VI.*

Schuurmans, M. J., Shortridge-Baggett, L. M., & Duursma, S. A. (2003). The Delirium Observation Screening Scale: A screening instrument for delirium. *Research and Theory for Nursing Practice, 17*(1), 31–50. *Evidence Level IV.*

Shenkin, S. D., Russ, T. C., Ryan, T. M., & MacLullich, A. M. (2014). Screening for dementia and other causes of cognitive impairment in general hospital in-patients. *Age and Ageing, 43*(2), 166–168. *Evidence Level VI.*

Simmons, B. B., Hartmann, B., & Dejoseph, D. (2011). Evaluation of suspected dementia. *American Family Physician, 84*(8), 895–902. *Evidence Level V.*

Steis, M. R., Evans, L., Hirschman, K. B., Hanlon, A., Fick, D. M., Flanagan, N., & Inouye, S. K. (2012). Screening for delirium using family caregivers: Convergent validity of the Family Confusion Assessment Method and interviewer-rated Confusion Assessment Method. *Journal of the American Geriatrics Society, 60*(11), 2121–2126. *Evidence Level IV.*

Tombaugh, T. N., & McIntyre, N. J. (1992). The Mini-Mental State Examination: A comprehensive review. *Journal of the American Geriatrics Society, 40*(9), 922–935. *Evidence Level I.*

Torisson, G., Minthon, L., Stavenow, L., & Londos, E. (2012). Cognitive impairment is undetected in medical inpatients: A study of mortality and recognition amongst healthcare professionals. *BMC Geriatrics, 12*, 47. *Evidence Level IV.*

Witlox, J., Eurelings, L. S., de Jonghe, J. F., Kalisvaart, K. J., Eikelenboom, P., & van Gool, W. A. (2010). Delirium in elderly patients and the risk of postdischarge mortality, institutionalization, and dementia: A meta-analysis. *Journal of the American Medical Association, 304*(4), 443–451. *Evidence Level I.*

Yesavage, J. A., Brink, T. L., Rose, T. L., Lum, O., Huang, V., Adey, M., & Leirer, V. O. (1982). Development and validation of a geriatric depression screening scale: A preliminary report. *Journal of Psychiatric Research, 17*(1), 37–49. *Evidence Level IV.*

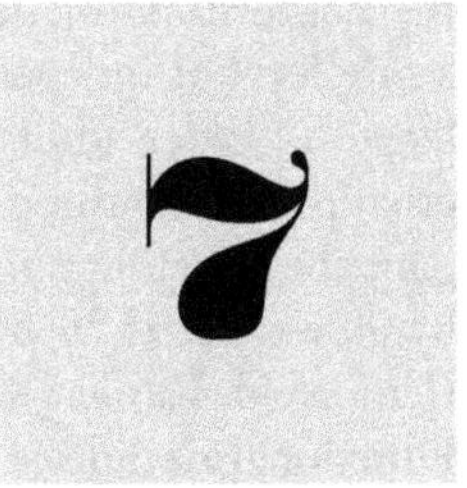

Assessment of Physical Function

Denise M. Kresevic

EDUCATIONAL OBJECTIVES

On completion of this chapter, the reader should be able to:

1. Describe common components of standardized functional assessment instruments for acute care
2. Identify unique challenges to gathering information from older adults regarding functional assessments
3. Describe common nursing care interventions to promote, maintain, and restore functional health in older adults in acute care settings
4. Acknowledge the importance of ongoing functional assessment in planning for transitions of care

OVERVIEW

Physical functioning is a dynamic process of interaction between individuals and their environments. The process is influenced by motivation, physical capacity, illness, cognitive ability, pain, and the external environment, including social supports. Management of these day-to-day activities (e.g., eating, bathing, ambulating, managing money) serves as the foundation for safe, independent functioning of all adults. Functional assessment instruments provide a common language of health for patients, family members, and health care providers across settings, especially for care of older adults. These assessements also serve as important parameters for goal setting and interprofessional collaboration.

The consequences of not assessing for change in status are significant. Acute changes in functional ability often signal an acute illness and an increased need for assistance to maintain safety. Likewise, improvements in function signal recovery and a return to health. These changes have important implications for nursing care across settings, but especially during hospitalization. The ability to assess functional status is critical in accurately identifying normal aging changes, illness, and disability, and in developing an individualized plan for continuity of care across settings. The failure to assess function can lead to increased risk of complications (e.g., malnutrition, falls); hospital readmissions, likelihood of being discharged to a nursing home setting (Fortinsky, Covinsky, Palmer, & Landefeld, 1999); and mortality (Boyd, Xue, Guralnik, & Fried, 2005; Rozzini, Sabatini, & Trabucchi, 2005), as well as decreased functional recovery (Boyd et al., 2005; Boyd, Ritchie, Tipton, Studenski, & Wieland, 2008; Gill, Allore, & Guo, 2004; Volpato et al., 2007) and quality of life.

BACKGROUND AND STATEMENT OF PROBLEM

Physical functioning, the ability to manage day-to-day functioning (e.g., bathing, dressing, ambulating, managing medications), rather than the absence of disease, is

For a description of evidence levels cited in this chapter, see Chapter 1, "Developing and Evaluating Clinical Practice Guidelines: A Systematic Approach."

the cornerstone of health for older adults. Maintaining a safe level of independent functioning may pose a challenge for older adults dealing with acute illness or exacerbations of chronic illnesses. Hospitalization can also contribute to functional decline, with decline experienced by an estimated 20% to 40% of hospitalized older adults (Landefeld, Palmer, Kresevic, Fortinsky, & Kowal, 1995). Functional decline is a common complication in hospitalized older adults, even in those with good baseline function (Gill, Allore, Gahbauer, & Murphy, 2010). The cause of this decline appears multifactorial and includes individual as well as environmental factors. Evidence that targeted interventions are effective in preventing and reversing functional decline continues to mount (Barnes et al., 2012). Hospitalization provides a unique opportunity to assess function, provide evidenced-based interventions, plan for services, and promote "successful aging."

Educational intervention has demonstrated improvements in caregiver knowledge and patient outcome (Resnick, Galik, Boltz, & Pretzer-Aboff, 2011).

Patient risk factors for functional decline include prehospitalization functional loss; the presence of two or more comorbidities; taking five or more prescription medications; having had a hospitalization or emergency room visit in the previous 12 months (McCusker, Kakuma, & Abrahamowicz, 2002); depression (Covinsky et al., 1998); impaired cognition, including delirium (Inouye, Schlesinger, & Lydon, 1999; Narain et al., 1988); pain (Reid, Williams, & Gill, 2005); nutritional problems; adverse medication effects (Graf, 2006); fear of falling (Boltz, Capezuti, & Shabbat, 2011); low self-efficacy and outcome expectations (McAuley et al., 2006; Resnick, 2002); and attitudes toward functional independence and views on hospitalization (Boltz, Capezuti, & Shabbat, 2011; Boltz, Capezuti, Shabbat, & Hall, 2010; Boyd et al., 2008; Brown, Williams, Woodby, Davis, & Allman, 2007).

These risk factors for functional decline are also associated with common risk factors for functional decline, including falls, injuries, acute illness, medication side effects, depression, malnutrition, baseline functional impairment, and decreased mobility associated with iatrogenic complications such as incontinence, falls, and pressure sores (Creditor, 1993). In one randomized clinical trial of hospitalized older adults, the daily nursing assessment of ability to perform bathing, dressing, grooming, toileting, transferring, and ambulation during routine nursing care yielded information necessary for maintenance of function in self-care activities (Landefeld et al., 1995).

Studies over the past 20 years have found that the use of multidisciplinary assesseements and nursing protocols can reduce hospital length of stay and costs while maintaining patient outcomes and not increasing hospital readmission rates (Barnes et al., 2012).

This chapter addresses the need for and goals of functional assessment of older adults in acute care, and it provides a clinical practice protocol to guide nurses in this assessment (Protocol 7.1).

ASSESSMENT OF THE PROBLEM

Assessment of function includes an ongoing systematic process of identifying the older person's physical abilities and need for help or assistance. Functional assessment also provides the opportunity to identify individual strengths and measures of "successful aging" and also promotes maintenance of health. This information is especially important for nurses in planning for transitions of care, including discharge to other facilities or home and evaluating continuity of care. Nurses are in a pivotal position in all care settings, but particularly during hospitalization, to assess the functional status of older adults by direct observation during routine care and through information gathered from the individual patient, the patient's family, and any other long-term caregivers.

Including critical components of functional assessments into routine assessments in the acute care setting can provide (a) baseline functional capacity and recent changes in level of independence indicative of possible illness, especially infections; (b) baseline information to benchmark patients' response to treatment as they move along the continuum from acute care to rehabilitation or from acute to subacute care (e.g., following a new stroke or hip replacement surgery); (c) information regarding care needs and eligibility for services, including safety, physical therapy, and post hospitalization needs; and (d) information on quality of care. The ongoing use of a standardized functional assessment instrument promotes systematic communication of the patient's health status between care settings. It also allows units to compare their level of care with other units in the facility, measure outcomes, and plan for continuity of care (Table 7.1; Campbell, Seymour, Primrose, & ACMEPLUS Project, 2004).

Although gathering information about functional status is a critical indicator of quality care in geriatrics, it requires significant time, skill, and knowledge. Older persons often present to the care setting with multiple medical conditions resulting in fatigue and pain. Acute illnesses may be superimposed on multiple interrelated medical comorbidities. In addition, sensory aging changes, particularly vision and hearing, can threaten the accuracy of responses. Ideally, information regarding functional status should be elicited as part of the routine history of older

TABLE 7.1
Functional Assessment of Older Adults

Dimension	Assessment Parameter	Standardized Instrument	Nursing Strategy
ADL Bathing Dressing Eating Toileting Hygiene Transferring	Self-report of patient Surrogate report Observation during hospitalization	Katz ADL index (Katz et al., 1963)	Orient to environment Encourage active participation in ADL Range-of-motion exercises Encourage to be out of bed Promote continence Consult PT/OT for strengthening exercises
Mobility Balance sitting and standing Gait steadiness Turns	Self-report Surrogate report Observation	"Get Up and Go" test (Mathias et al., 1986)	Ambulate PT/OT consult Mobility aids Community referrals
IADL Housework Finances Driving Shopping Meal preparation Reading Medication adherence Current events awareness Hobbies Employment Volunteer work	Self-report (include normal daily routine) Surrogate report (able to balance check book, traffic violations)	Lawton IADL scale (Gurland et al., 1994; Lawton & Brody, 1969) DAFA—for patients with dementia (Karagiozis et al., 1998)	Assess ability to: ■ Find hospital room ■ Read newspaper ■ Read pill bottles ■ Order hospital meals from menu Facilitate as needed: ■ Community referrals for transportation and/or Meals on Wheels ■ OT consult to assess home management skills (cooking, laundry, etc.) ■ Home care referral, including medication management, follow-up medical care, rehabilitation, home safety management, and ADL support
Frailty	Self-report	Fried Fraility Scale (Fried et al., 2009)	Weight loss, fatigue, handgrip, physical activity and walking speed

ADL, activities of daily living; DAFA, Direct Assessment of Functional Abilities; IADL, instrumental activities of daily living; PT/OT, physical therapist/occupational therapist.

adults and incorporated into daily care routines of all caregivers. In addition, comprehensive assessment of function provides an opportunity to teach patients and families about normal aging as well as indicators of pathology.

Assessment Instruments

Collecting systematic information regarding tasks of daily living (e.g., bathing, dressing, ambulating, using a phone, taking medications, managing finances) can be accomplished by the use of standardized instruments. The use of standardized instruments serves to ensure inclusive assessments, the ability to communicate in a common language, and the ability to benchmark information over time. Several instruments have been developed over the years to measure function. Although all measure components of function, the decision of which instrument to use depends on the primary purpose of the assessment and the institutional preferences and resources (Kane & Kane, 2000). No single instrument will meet the needs of all care settings.

Many performance-based measures and observational instruments can be incorporated into routine care practices without significantly burdening caregivers. Incorporating electronic medical record templates into routine documentation can function as a prompt for providers, decreasing the time and increasing the communication of the results of these assessments.

The Katz Index of Independence in Activities of Daily Living (commonly referred to as the Katz ADL index) assesses activities of daily living (ADL), including bathing, dressing, transferring, toileting, continence, and eating (Katz, Ford, Moskowitz, Jackson, & Jaffe, 1963). This scale is used widely to assess function of older adults in all settings, including during hospitalization (Mezey, Rauckhorst, &

Stokes, 1993). Originally, the Katz ADL index was proposed as an observation tool with scores ranging from 1 to 3, indicating *independent ability*, *limited assistance*, and *extensive assistance* for each activity. Over time, the instrument has evolved into a dichotomized tool with independent versus dependent ability of each task (Kane & Kane, 2000). With established reliability (0.94–0.97), it is easy to use either as an observational or a self-reported measure of level of independence (Kane & Kane, 2000). The Katz ADL index is easily incorporated into history and physical assessment flowsheets and takes little time to complete. Many other tools exist to assess ADL, including the Barthel index for physical functioning and the Older Americans Resources and Services ADL scale (OARS-ADL; Burton, Damon, Dillinger, Erickson, & Peterson, 1978; Mahoney & Barthel, 1965; Mezey et al., 1993).

In addition to ADL tools, instruments to measure more complex physical function called *instrumental activities of daily living* (IADL) have been proposed to be included in a comprehensive assessment of function in older adults. The majority of these instruments assess the individual's function in relation to the environment. Common IADL skills identified include using a phone, shopping, meal preparation, housekeeping, laundry, medication administration, transportation, and money management (Kane & Kane, 2000). Although assessment of ADL provides useful information for nursing care needs both during and after hospitalization, IADL information helps target critical post hospital care needs. Although direct observation of the patient's IADL may not occur during an acute hospitalization, it is important for the nurse to assess this information to plan for the patient's discharge. Common instruments used to measure IADL include the Lawton IADL scale, the Older Americans Resources and Services Instrumental Activities of Daily Living (OARS-IADL) scale, and the Direct Assessment of Functional Abilities (DAFA) scale.

Perhaps the most widely used IADL instrument for hospitalized older adults is the Lawton IADL scale. This scale assesses eight items with each scored from 0 (dependence) to 8 (independent self-care). Reliability coefficients have been reported to be 0.96 for men and 0.93 for women (Kane & Kane, 2000).

More recent, scales that address frailty have been developed to assist in the assessment of at-risk individuals. Frailty is characterized by five components: weight loss, fatigue, handgrip, physical activity, and walking speed (Fried et al., 2009). The most widely used is the Fried Frailty scale (see Chapter 27). This scale uses objective and self-report data.

Assessment of function in individuals with dementia presents a unique challenge. The Direct Assessment of Functional Abilities (DAFA), a 10-item observational measure of IADL, has been found to be useful in assessing function in the presence of dementia (Karagiozis, Gray, Sacco, Shapiro, & Kawas, 1998; see www.consultgerirn.org/resources and the Resources section of this chapter for assessment instruments).

Regardless of the instrument used, basic ADL and IADL function should be assessed for each patient, including capacity for dressing, eating, transferring, toileting, hygiene, ambulation, and medication adherence (see Chapter 20, "Reducing Adverse Drug Events"). Appropriate assessment instruments should be readily available on the acute care unit for reference and/or incorporated into routine documentation instruments for history, daily assessment, and discharge planning. To adequately assess function, sensory and cognitive capacity should be established and environmental adaptations, such as magnifying glasses or hearing amplifiers, may be necessary and should be accessible to nursing staff.

Direct Assessment of Patients

Although nurses often rely on reports of physical functioning and capacity for ADL and IADL from patients and family members, direct observation provides strong evidence for current capacity versus past ability.

Functional assessments are constantly conducted by nurses every time they notice that a patient can no longer pick up a fork or has difficulty walking. A comprehensive functional assessment leads to more than simply noticing a change in activity or ability, however. In a systematic manner, nurses need to assess the ability of a patient to perform ADL in the context of the patient's baseline functional and hospitalization status.

While assessing functional status, the patient should be made as comfortable as possible, with frequent rest periods allowed. Adaptive aids, such as glasses and hearing aids, should be applied. Often, family members accompany the older person and can assist in answering questions regarding function. It is important for patients and family members to understand that baseline functional levels as well as any recent changes in function need to be reported. Many older adults may be reluctant to report decline in function, fearing that such reports will threaten their autonomy and independent living.

Occasionally, the history and physical examination may reveal clues to further identify functional status. Muscle weakness and atrophy of legs may indicate lack of ability to safely ambulate independently. Temporal muscle wasting may indicate moderate to severe malnutrition resulting from inability to shop, prepare meals, or adequately consume sufficient calories. Hand contractures present with arthritis or cerebral vascular accidents alert the nurse to pay particular attention to performance versus self-report of ability to open pill bottles, dial a phone, or write checks. General appearance (e.g., hair, teeth, fingernails) and condition of clothing (e.g., clean and dry versus urine-soaked undergarments) may give rise to information on bathing, dressing, continence, and ability to do laundry.

Specific Functional Assessments

Ambulation

Inherent in both ADL and IADL is ambulation, a critical parameter for functional assessment. Early nursing assessment of the hospitalized patient's ability to walk is very important in order to ensure safety and prevent falls and injuries (see Chapter 19, "Preventing Falls in Acute Care"). The ability to safely ambulate is contingent on the ability to transfer, propel forward, and pivot with sufficient strength and balance. Ambulation is necessary for self-care both in the hospital and after hospital discharge. It is also a very sensitive indicator of acute health changes. Therefore, the ability to ambulate should be assessed by both self- or proxy report and by direct observation.

Some instruments used to assess ambulation, balance, and gait are sensitive measures of mobility (Applegate, Blass, & Franklin, 1990); however, they are also complex and time consuming to use. Therefore, direct observation of an individual's ability to get out of bed, sit in a chair, assume a standing position, and steadily walk a short distance—with or without assistive devices—is much simpler to do yet important to ensure safety (Applegate et al., 1990; Cress et al., 1995).

An efficient performance-based measure of ambulation, balance, and gait that can be observed during routine care of the hospitalized patient is the "Get Up and Go" test (Cress et al., 1995). To do a Get Up and Go test, patients are observed sitting in a chair, standing, walking, and pivoting. Direct observation of the patient should include an assessment of speed of performance, hesitancy, stumbling, swaying, grabbing for support, or unsafe maneuvers such as sitting too close to the edge of a chair or dizziness while pivoting (Tinetti & Ginter, 1998). Performance is scored from 1 (normal balance and steady gait) to 5 (severely abnormal balance and gait), which is clear evidence of fall risk (Kane & Kane, 2000). Assessment of unsafe transfers or ambulation indicates the need to begin immediate restorative therapies to prevent falls and injuries. These can include attention to environmental designs, such as walking paths free of clutter, handrails, and rest areas to encourage daily ambulation, as opposed to bed rest and immobility (Creditor, 1993). Although the Get Up and Go test is easy to perform, it is relatively subjective. Objectivity may be enhanced by timing the tasks (Kane & Kane, 2000).

Sensory Capacity

Evaluation of the potential impact of sensory changes on the performance of ADL is often underestimated. Impaired vision is especially important in medication adherence and safety. A simple test for functional vision is to have older adults read from a newspaper. A moderate impairment can be noted if only the headline can be read (Tinetti & Ginter, 1998). Another way to assess vision is to have older persons read prescription bottles. Functional assessment of safe medication administration includes the ability to read pill bottles and repeat directions for use, potential side effects, and instructions of when to contact a health care provider. Glasses should be available with clean lenses. Inability to read raises questions of literacy, undiagnosed vision difficulties, and safety for medication administration. Often overlooked is the number of older people who may not be able to read but are too embarrassed to reveal that information. As part of routine care, older adults should be encouraged to actively participate each day in learning about medications. In addition, at the time of discharge, nurses need to verify patient and family knowledge and skills regarding medications. This may include discussing medications as well as directly observing older adults opening pill bottles and identifying the correct pills.

Hearing ability is also essential for functioning and cognition. Individuals with decreased hearing may be inaccurately labeled as *cognitively impaired*. Hearing aids may not have been sent to the hospital with the older patient and should be obtained by the family. Hearing acuity may be validated by asking patients to identify the sound of a ticking watch. The "whisper test" may also be used. This is performed by whispering 10 words while standing 6 inches away from the individual. Inability to repeat five of the 10 words indicates a need for further assessment of hearing acuity. Occlusion of the external ear canal by cerumen, an easily treatable cause of decreased hearing acuity, may be evident with visualization (Mathias, Nayak, & Isaacs, 1986). Individuals with hearing deficits detected as part of bedside assessment should be referred for additional assessment and treatment. Amplifier devices may be useful and are an inexpensive item to stock on hospital nursing units.

Cognitive Capacity

Cognitive function is a major factor in a person's functional capacity, and baseline data regarding cognitive function should be gathered. However, such assessments most often initially rely on information provided by family members because acute illness may manifest as acute confusional states and not reflect baseline cognitive function (Kruianski & Gurland, 1976; see Chapter 6, "Assessing Cognitive Function"). Fluctuating attention may indicate an acute, reversible impairment (delirium) or temporary reactions to hospitalization. An acute change in cognition should be evaluated immediately for the presence of a potentially life-threatening, reversible medical condition (see Chapter 17, "Delirium: Prevention, Early Recognition, and Treatment").

Cause of Functional Decline

All instances of functional decline should be assessed for an underlying reversible cause such as acute illness. With the resolution of acute illness (e.g., urinary tract infection [UTI], pneumonia, postoperative recovery), impaired ADL are expected to return to baseline with appropriate care and rehabilitation. Comprehensive musculoskeletal or neurological examination, laboratory tests, or referral for a therapeutic trial of physical or occupational therapy may be needed to boost recovery. In some cases, functional decline may accompany a predictable downward spiral associated with end-stage chronic diseases such as Alzheimer's disease or terminal illnesses. However, even in individuals with these conditions, all potentially reversible causes should be fully explored.

INTERVENTIONS AND CARE STRATEGIES

Functional ability is a sensitive indicator of health in older adults. The need for assistance with ADL is an important nursing assessment to provide safe individualized care during hospitalization and also aids in care planning during and after a hospital stay. Sudden loss of function, including the ability to ambulate, is the hallmark of acute illness in older adults. Although recovery from illness may be associated with improvements in function, early nursing interventions to address care needs, refer to therapy, and modify environments of care help to ensure safety and decrease further loss of function. Therefore, all nurses must be skilled at incorporating a comprehensive functional assessment into all patient care assessments and communicating these assessments to the care team across transitions. Nurses need to be knowledgeable and skilled in assessment of function, implementing supportive environments, and providing geriatric-sensitive care to prevent functional decline. Geriatric-sensitive care incorporates strategies to prevent bed rest, encourage exercise and ambulation, ensure adequate nutrition, and encourage ongoing communication among all team members. Such care is essential in maximizing safe, independent functioning of hospitalized older adults (see Chapter 14, "Preventing Functional Decline in the Acute Care Setting").

Use of Assessment Information

Knowledge of ADL and IADL abilities, including shopping, housework, finances, food preparation, medication administration, and transportation, is an important part of providing individual nursing care for comprehensive discharge planning (Woolf, 1990). In summary, for older people, the evaluation of function represents the cornerstone of good nursing care and affords a sound baseline by which to provide information essential to plan for continued care across settings.

CASE STUDY 1

Mrs. Hope, a 74-year-old retired night nurse and recent widow, is admitted to the hospital from her physician's office. Her admitting diagnosis is pneumonia, dehydration, and weakness. She is accompanied by her daughter. Her past medical history is significant for hypertension, congestive heart failure (CHF), and chronic obstructive pulmonary disease (COPD). She is extremely hard of hearing, but has refused to wear her hearing aid. She smokes approximately 10 cigarettes a day, which she has done for more than 50 years. Her daughter admits that, lately, Mrs. Hope has not been taking most of her pills, although she has been taking aspirin for pain. She has also been losing weight and has poor appetite with little fluid intake. Laboratory values indicate anemia with a very low hematocrit and a urinary tract infection (UTI). A chest x-ray indicates a lung nodule.

Although on the unit, Mrs. Hope prefers to sleep in the recliner, saying she is most comfortable there and prefers to nap during the day. Despite intravenous (IV) fluids, blood transfusions, diuresis for fluid overload, oxygen therapy, occupational therapy for energy conservation, and round-the-clock acetaminophen for "aches and pains," Mrs. Hope continues to be weak and needs assistance with daily bathing and ambulation. She is able to communicate well using a hearing amplifier after her ears are cleaned of wax. She is assessed by the multidisciplinary care team over the next several days. After the team meeting, consultations are obtained for physical therapy, nutrition services,

(continued)

CASE STUDY 1 *(continued)*

pharmacy, geriatric clinical nurse specialist, and social work, the team begins to discuss Mrs. Hope's desires for her advance directives. Over the next few days, with nutritional supplements and therapy, her fatigue improves. Referrals for home care are made for nursing and therapy as well as for telehealth to monitor her CHF. Mrs. Hope's medication regimen is adjusted, substituting acetaminophen, rather than aspirin, for her pain. She and her daughter are instructed on a high-calorie diet and are provided with information on senior care and smoking-cessation programs. She is given vaccines for influenza and pneumonia. A future outpatient appointment for a comprehensive geriatric evaluation is made to for a comprehensive geriatric assessment once her acute conditions resolve, including further testing of her lung nodule, cognitive status, and follow-up on advance directives.

Mrs. Hope is discharged home with her daughter after medications, diet, and exercises are reviewed using a teach-back method of education. The numbers for the home care agency and directions to the outpatient appointment are printed out for her at the time of discharge.

Discussion

This case study indicates the need to assess baseline function, changes in function, and trajectory of function following acute care. Assessment in this case used components from several standardized functional assessment instruments and incorporated them into existing care routines. Care was enhanced by collaboration among multiple disciplines and across settings. Opportunities for assessment and resolution of impairment rely on institutional preferences and resources, as well as the functional level of the patient. Despite Mrs. Hope's impaired function, the hospital staff worked to enhance her physical functioning as much as possible within the current care setting and a context of safety. Although the focus of acute care is on resolving exacerbations of chronic diseases, such as CHF, other issues, such as advance directives, should also be addressed. In this case, follow-up of several issues will need to be done after hospitalization. Given the complexity of many large health care systems, ideally, these appointments can be arranged before the patient leaves the hospital.

CASE STUDY 2

Mr. Goode is an 86-year-old retired college history professor who is well known for his accomplishments as a collegiate football player. His wife of 60 years died last year. He lives alone in a one-floor condominium. His daughter and son live in the same city. He has a cleaning lady who comes once a week. He has been receiving Meals on Wheels; he admits to being a terrible cook. Mr. Goode has been driving only short distances during the daytime since his cataract surgery 15 years ago. He rides his stationary exercise bike daily to keep up his "boyish" figure.

Mr. Goode has a long history of cardiac disease, including two myocardial infarctions and a coronary bypass graft 20 years ago. He has degenerative joint disease that affects his hips and knees, and 10 years ago he underwent bilateral knee replacements. Twenty years ago, he had prostate surgery for enlargement. His current medications include lisinopril 5 mg, furosemide 20 mg, potassium chloride 8 mEq every other day, acetaminophen 650 mg twice a day, and analgesic balm as needed.

Mr. Goode is admitted to the emergency room extremely short of breath; the cleaning lady had called 911. He has crackles in his lungs and 4+ pitting edema of his legs. He is placed on oxygen and given IV Lasix. A Foley catheter is placed, and an IV of $D_5\frac{1}{2}$NS at 50 mL per hour is started. On admission to the nursing unit, he requires assistance to move from the cart to the bed. He complains of nausea, weakness, and knee pain. His physician orders bed rest and Benadryl 25 mg at bedtime as needed for sleep.

On hospital day 2, Mr. Goode refuses to get out of bed because of knee pain. He requests assistance with his bathing and eating. His weight has decreased 2 pounds, and he has decreased crackles in his lungs. His daughter arrives with his glasses, hearing aids with batteries, and pillboxes. His medication boxes are still filled from the previous 5 days. His laboratory results return. His urine is positive for bacteria, red and white cells, and leukoesterase, confirming a UTI. An electrocardiogram is negative for an acute myocardial infarction. A chest x-ray confirms acute CHF and pneumonia. He is placed on antibiotics and his diuretics are increased for 1 day. He cannot recall the last time he had a bowel movement.

During team rounds, his orders are changed to the following: out of bed and ambulate in hallway twice a day, discontinue Foley catheter and Benadryl, and wean oxygen. His nurses review his baseline ADL

(continued)

CASE STUDY 2 *(continued)*

function and current function and request a physical therapy consultation to evaluate safe ambulation and a social work consultation to evaluate self-care ability and home care services. The patient requests analgesic balm for his knees. Fall precautions are initiated, including frequent prompted voiding. He is ordered a bowel stimulant and encouraged to drink warm prune juice for constipation.

On hospital day 4, Mr. Goode ambulates out to the nurse's station and announces that he feels much better and is ready to go home. His progress is reviewed on team rounds. The physical therapy evaluation reveals that he is capable of ambulating and transferring independently and safely, and the therapist recommends a continued home exercise program. He is given information on community arthritis programs, including water aquatics and tai chi. The social worker has shared information with Mr. Goode and his son regarding the "life line" and recommended check-in phone calls every evening. Nutrition services recommended a low-salt diet and used sample menus to practice food choices, and a nurse has reviewed medications with Mr. Goode and his daughter, using a "teach-back method." A pillbox is filled in the pharmacy. The daughter agrees to purchase a scale with large numbers. Mr. Goode's daughter will check the pillbox weekly. Mr. Goode is ready for discharge from the hospital and will return to his condominium because he has returned to his baseline ADL. Before discharge he agrees to updating his vaccines for pneumonia and zooster. He is encouraged to schedule a visit with his primary care provider before he leaves the hospital.

Discussion

Similar to case 1 this case stresses the importance of establishing baseline function and using standardized instruments to assess and communicate levels of function. Again the critical collaboration with a multidisplinary team is evident in planning and evaluating care needs.

This case illustrates the appropriate in-hospital interventions needed to reverse decline, such as early ambulation, attention to sensory needs, treatment of constipation, and judicious use of medications.

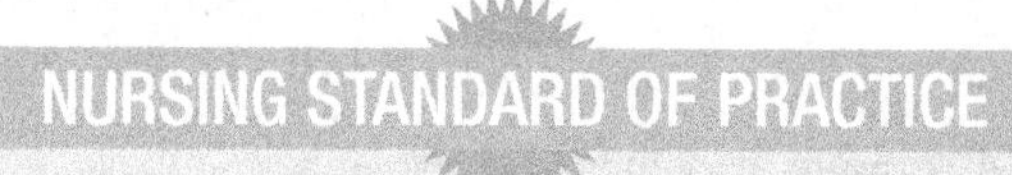

Protocol 7.1: Assessment of Physical Function

I. GOAL

To maximize physical functioning, ensure safety, and prevent or minimize decline in ADL function, and plan for transitions of care.

II. OBJECTIVE

The following nursing care protocol has been designed to help bedside nurses to monitor function in older adults, prevent decline, and maintain the function of older adults during acute hospitalization.

III. BACKGROUND

A. Functional status of individuals describes the capacity and performance of safe ADL and IADL (Applegate et al., 1990; Kane & Kane, 2000; Katz et al., 1963; Lawton & Brody, 1969) and is a sensitive indicator of health or illness in older adults. It is, therefore, a critical nursing assessment (Byles, 2000; Campbell et al., 2004; Kresevic et al., 1998; Mezey et al., 1993).

B. Some functional decline may be prevented or ameliorated with prompt and aggressive nursing intervention (e.g., ambulation, toileting schedules, enhanced communication, adaptive equipment, attention to medications and dosages, and management of pain [Barnes et al., 2012; Bates-Jensen et al., 2004; Counsell et al., 2000; Landefeld et al., 1995; Palmer, Counsell, & Landefeld, 1998]).

(continued)

Protocol 7.1: Assessment of Physical Function *(continued)*

C. Some functional decline may occur progressively and is not reversible. This decline often accompanies chronic and terminal disease states such as degenerative joint disease, Parkinson's disease, dementia, heart failure, and cancer (Hirsch, Sommers, Olsen, Mullen, & Winograd, 1990). Interprofessional team care meetings may be helpful in clarifying the trajectory of illness and referring for appropriate follow-up.
D. Functional status is influenced by physiological aging changes, acute and chronic illness, and adaptation to the physical environment. Functional decline is often the initial symptom of acute illness such as infections (e.g., pneumonia and UTI). These declines are usually reversible and require medical evaluation (Applegate et al., 1990; Sager & Rudberg, 1998). Functional status is contingent on motivation, cognition, and sensory capacity, including vision and hearing (Pearson, 2000).
E. Risk factors for functional decline include injuries, acute illness, medication side effects, pain, depression, malnutrition, decreased mobility, prolonged bed rest (including the use of physical restraints), prolonged use of Foley catheters, and changes in environment or routines (Counsell et al., 2000; Landefeld et al., 1995; McCusker et al., 2002).
F. Additional complications of functional decline include loss of independence, falls, incontinence, malnutrition, decreased socialization, and increased risk for long-term institutionalization and depression (Covinsky et al., 1998; Creditor, 1993; Landefeld et al., 1995). (See related chapters.)
G. Recovery of function can also be a measure of return to health, such as for those individuals recovering from exacerbations of cardiovascular or respiratory diseases and acute infections, recovering from joint replacement surgery, or new strokes (Katz et al., 1963).
H. Functional status evaluation assists in planning future care needs post-hospitalization, such as short-term skilled care, assisted living, home care, and need for community services (Graf, 2006; Landefeld et al., 1995), or long-term residential care.
I. Physical environments of care with attention to the special needs of older adults serve to maintain and enhance function (i.e., chairs with arms, elevated toilet seat, levers versus door knobs, enhanced lighting; Kresevic et al., 1998; Landefeld et al., 1995).

IV. ASSESSMENT PARAMETERS

A. Comprehensive functional assessment of older adults includes independent performance of basic ADL, social activities, or IADL, the assistance needed to accomplish these tasks, and sensory ability, pain level, cognition, and capacity to ambulate (Campbell et al., 2004; Doran et al., 2006; Freedman, Martin, & Schoeni, 2002; Kane & Kane, 2000; Katz et al., 1963; Lawton & Brody, 1969; Lightbody & Baldwin, 2002; McCusker et al., 2002; Tinetti & Ginter, 1998).
   1. Basic ADL (bathing, dressing, grooming, eating, continence, transferring)
   2. IADL (meal preparation, shopping, medication administration, housework, transportation, accounting)
   3. Mobility (ambulation, pivoting)
B. Older adults may view their health in terms of how well they can function rather than in terms of disease alone. Strengths should be emphasized as well as needs for assistance (Depp & Jeste, 2006; Pearson, 2000).
C. The clinician should validate, document, and communicate baseline functional status and recent or progressive decline in function (Graf, 2006).
D. Function should be assessed over time to validate capacity, decline, or progress (Applegate et al., 1990; Callahan, Thomas, Goldhirsh, & Leipzig, 2002; Kane & Kane, 2000).
E. Standard instruments selected to assess function should be efficient to administer and easy to interpret. They should provide useful practical information for clinicians and be incorporated into routine history taking and daily assessments (Kane & Kane, 2000; Kresevic et al., 1998). (See "Function" topic at www.consultgerirn.org for tools.)
F. Interprofessional communication regarding functional status, changes, and expected trajectory should be part of all care settings and should include the patient and family whenever possible (Counsell et al., 2000; Covinsky et al., 1998; Kresevic et al., 1998; Landefeld et al., 1995).
G. Interprofessional rounds support promotion of function by addressing functional assessment (baseline and current), evaluating potential interventions, and helping develop a plan of care with measureable goals.

(continued)

Protocol 7.1: Assessment of Physical Function *(continued)*

V. CARE STRATEGIES

A. Strategies to maximize functional status and to prevent decline
   1. Maintain individual's daily routine. Help to maintain physical, cognitive, and social function through physical activity and socialization. Encourage ambulation, encourage the individual to get out of bed for meals, allow flexible visitation, including pets, and encourage reading the newspaper (Kresevic & Holder, 1998; Landefeld et al., 1995).
   2. Educate older adults, family, and formal caregivers on the value of independent functioning and the consequences of functional decline (Graf, 2006; Kresevic & Holder, 1998; Vass, Avlund, Lauridsen, & Hendriksen, 2005): increased risk for complications such as malnutrition, falls, hospital readmissions, increased likelihood of being discharged to a nursing home setting (Fortinsky et al., 1999); increased mortality (Boyd et al., 2005; Rozzini et al., 2005); and decreased functional recovery (Boyd et al., 2005, 2008; Gill et al., 2004; Volpato et al., 2007), ultimately decreasing quality of life.
      a. Physiological and psychological value of independent functioning
      b. Reversible functional decline associated with acute illness (Hirsch et al., 1990; Sager & Rudberg, 1998)
      c. Strategies to prevent functional decline: exercise, nutrition, pain management, and socialization (Kresevic & Holder, 1998; Landefeld et al., 1995; Siegler, Glick, & Lee, 2002; Tucker, Molsberger, & Clark, 2004)
      d. Sources of assistance to manage decline
   3. Encourage activity, including routine exercise, range of motion, and ambulation to maintain activity, flexibility, and function (Counsell et al., 2000; Landefeld et al., 1995; Pedersen & Saltin, 2006).
   4. Minimize bed rest (Bates-Jensen et al., 2004; Covinsky et al., 1998; Kresevic & Holder, 1998; Landefeld et al., 1995).
   5. Explore alternatives to physical restraint use (e.g., cover tubings; use distraction; Covinsky et al., 1998; Kresevic & Holder, 1998; see Chapter 23, "Physical Restraints and Side Rails in Acute and Critical Care Settings").
   6. Judiciously use medications, especially psychoactive medications, in geriatric dosages (Inouye, Rushing, Foreman, Palmer, & Pompei, 1998; see Chapter 17).
   7. Assess and treat for pain (Covinsky et al., 1998).
   8. Design environments with handrails; wide doorways; raised toilet seats; shower seats; enhanced lighting; low beds; and chairs of various types and height, including recliners and rocking chairs (Cunningham & Michael, 2004; Kresevic et al., 1998).
   9. Help individuals regain baseline function after acute illnesses by using exercise, physical or occupational therapy consultation, nutrition, and coaching (Conn, Minor, Burks, Rantz, & Pomeroy, 2003; Covinsky et al., 1998; Engberg, Sereika, McDowell, Weber, & Brodak, 2002; Forbes, 2005; Hodgkinson, Evans, & Wood, 2003; Kresevic et al., 1998).

B. Strategies to help older individuals cope with functional decline
   1. Help older adults and family members determine realistic functional capacity based on health trajectory with interprofessional consultation (Kresevic & Holder, 1998).
   2. Provide caregiver education and support for families of individuals when decline cannot be ameliorated in spite of nursing and rehabilitative efforts (Graf, 2006). Palliative care consultation may offer the family and team important management strategies, particularly postacute care.
   3. Carefully document all intervention strategies and patient response (Graf, 2006).
   4. Provide information to caregivers on causes of functional decline related to acute and chronic conditions (Covinsky et al., 1998).
   5. Provide education to address safety care needs for falls, injuries, and common complications. Short-term skilled care for physical therapy may be needed; long-term care settings may be required to ensure safety (Covinsky et al., 1998).
   6. Provide sufficient protein and caloric intake to ensure adequate intake and prevent further decline. Liberalize diet to include personal preferences (Edington et al., 2004; Landefeld et al., 1995).

(continued)

Protocol 7.1: Assessment of Physical Function *(continued)*

7. Provide caregiver support and community services, such as senior centers, Meals on Wheels, home care, nursing, and physical and occupational therapy services to manage functional decline (Covinsky et al., 1998; Graf, 2006).

VI. EXPECTED OUTCOMES

A. Patients can
   1. Maintain safe level of ADL and ambulation.
   2. Make necessary adaptations to maintain safety and independence, including assistive devices and environmental adaptations.
   3. Strive to attain highest quality of life despite low functional level.
B. Providers can demonstrate
   1. Increased assessment, identification, and management of patients susceptible to or experiencing functional decline. Provide routine assessment of functional capacity despite level of care.
   2. Ongoing documentation and communication of capacity, interventions, goals, and outcomes
   3. Competence in preventive and restorative strategies for function
   4. Competence in assessing safe environments of care that foster safe independent function
C. Institution will experience
   1. System-wide incorporation of functional assessment into routine assessments
   2. A reduction in incidence and prevalence of functional decline
   3. A decrease in morbidity and mortality rates associated with functional decline
   4. Reduction in the use of physical restraints, prolonged bed rest, and Foley catheters
   5. Decreased incidence of delirium
   6. An increase in prevalence of patients who leave hospital with baseline or improved functional status
   7. Decreased readmission rate
   8. Increased early utilization of nutritional and rehabilitative services (occupational and physical therapy)
   9. Evidence of geriatric-sensitive physical care environments that facilitate safe, independent function such as low beds, comfortable chairs, and caregiver education on safe environmental design and exercise programs
   10. Evidence of continued interprofessional assessments, care planning, and evaluation of care related to function, including post hospital follow-up planning

VII. RELEVANT PRACTICE GUIDELINES

Several resources are now available to guide adoption of evidence-based nursing interventions to enhance function in older adults.

A. Agency for Healthcare Research and Quality and National Guideline Clearinghouse: www.guideline.gov
B. McGill University Health Centre Research and Clinical Resources for Evidence Based Nursing: www.muhc-ebn.mcgill.ca
C. National Quality Forum: www.qualityforum.org/Home.aspx
D. Registered Nurses Association of Ontario. (2005). *Clinical practice guidelines*. Retrieved from www.rnao.org/Page.asp?PageID=861&SiteNodeID=270&BL_ExpandID
E. University of Iowa Hartford Center of Geriatric Nursing Excellence. *Evidence-based practice guidelines*. Retrieved from www.nursing.uiowa.edu

ABBREVIATIONS

ADL	Activities of daily living
IADL	Instrumental activities of daily living
UTI	Urinary tract infection

RESOURCES

Agency for Healthcare Research and Quality and National Guideline Clearinghouse
http://www.guideline.gov

McGill University Health Centre Research and Research and Clinical Resources for Evidence Based Nursing

National Quality Forum
http://www.qualityforum.org/Home.aspx

NICHE: Nurses Improving Care for Health System Elders
http://www.nicheprogram.org

Registered Nurses Association of Ontario. *Clinical Practice Guidelines.*
http://www.rnao.org/Page.asp?PageID=861&SiteNodeID=270&BL_ExpandID

Hartford Center of Geriatric Nursing Excellence. *Evidence-Based Practice Guidelines.*

REFERENCES

Applegate, W. B., Blass, J., & Franklin, T. F. (1990). Instruments for the functional assessment of older patients. *New England Journal of Medicine, 322*(17), 1207–1214. *Evidence Level IV.*

Barnes, D. E., Palmer, R. M., Kresevic, D. M., Fortinsky, R. H., Kowal, J., Chren, M.-M., & Landefeld, C. S. (2012). Acute care for elders units produced shorter hospital stays at lower cost while maintaining patients' functional status. *Health Affairs, 31*(6), 1227–1236. *Evidence Level I.*

Bates-Jensen, B. M., Alessi, C. A., Cadogan, M., Levy-Storms, L., Jorge, J., Yoshii, J., . . . Schnelle, J. F. (2004). The minimum data set bedfast quality indicators: Differences in nursing homes. *Nursing Research, 53*(4), 260–272. *Evidence Level V.*

Boltz, M., Capezuti, E., & Shabbat, N. (2011). Nursing staff perceptions of physical function in hospitalized older adults. *Applied Nursing Research, 24*(4), 215–222. *Evidence Level IV.*

Boltz, M., Capezuti, E., Shabbat, N., & Hall, K. (2010). Going home better not worse: Older adults' views on physical function during hospitalization. *International Journal of Nursing Practice, 16*(**4**), 381–388. *Evidence Level IV.*

Boyd, C. M., Ritchie, C. S., Tipton, E. F., Studenski, S. A., & Wieland, D. (2008). From bedside to bench: Summary from the American Geriatrics Society/National Institute on Aging Research Conference on comorbidity and multiple morbidity in older adults. *Aging Clinical and Experimental Research, 20*(3), 181–188. *Evidence Level V.*

Boyd, C. M., Xue, Q. L., Guralnik, J. M., & Fried, L. P. (2005). Hospitilization and development of dependence in activities of daily living in a cohort of disabled older women: The Women's Health and Aging Study I. *Journals of Gerontology. Series A, Biological Sciences and Medical Sciences, 60*(7), 888–893. *Evidence Level IV.*

Brown, C. J., Williams, B. R., Woodby, L. L., Davis, L. L., & Allman, R. M. (2007). Barriers to mobility during hospitalization from the perspective of older patients, their nurses and physicians. *Journal of Hospitalist Medicine, 2*(5), 305–313. *Evidence Level IV.*

Burton, R. M., Damon, W. W., Dillinger, D. C., Erickson, D. J., & Peterson, D. W. (1978). Nursing home rest and care: An investigation of alternatives. In E. Pfeiffer (Ed.), *Multidimensional functional assessment: The DARS methodology.* Durham, NC: Duke Center for Study of Aging Human Development. *Evidence Level III.*

Byles, J. E. (2000). A thorough going over: Evidence for health assessments for older persons. *Austrialian and New Zealand Journal of Public Health, 24*(2), 117–123. *Evidence Level I.*

Callahan, E. H., Thomas, D. C., Goldhirsh, S. L., & Leipzig, R. M. (2002). Geriatric hospital medicine. *Medical Clinics of North America, 86*(4), 707–729. *Evidence Level VI.*

Campbell, S. E., Seymour, D. G., Primrose, W. R., & ACMEPLUS Project. (2004). A systematic literature review of factors affecting outcome in older medical patients admitted to hospital. *Age and Ageing, 33*(2), 110–115. *Evidence Level I.*

Conn, V. S., Minor, M. A., Burks, K. J., Rantz, M. J., & Pomeroy, S. H. (2003). Integrative review of physical activity intervention research with aging adults. *Journal of the American Geriatrics Society, 51*(8), 1159–1168. *Evidence Level I.*

Counsell, S. R., Holder, C. M., Liebenauer, L. L., Palmer, R. M., Fortinsky, R. H., Kresevic, D. M., . . . Landefeld, C. S. (2000). Effects of a multicomponent intervention on functional outcomes and process of care of hospitalized older patients: A randomized controlled trial of acute care for elders (ACE) in a community hospital. *Journal of the American Geriatrics Society, 48*(12), 1572–1581. *Evidence Level II.*

Covinsky, K. E., Palmer, R. M., Kresevic, D. M., Kahana, E., Counsell, S. R., Fortinsky, R. H., & Landefeld, C. S. (1998). Improving functional outcomes in older patients: Lessons from an acute care for elders unit. *Joint Commission Journal on Quality Improvement, 24*(2), 63–76. *Evidence Level II.*

Creditor, M. C. (1993). Hazards of hospitalization of the elderly. *Annals of Internal Medicine, 118*(3), 219–223. *Evidence Level VI.*

Cress, M. E., Schechtman, K. B., Mulrow, C. D., Fiatarone, M. A., Gerety, M. B., & Buchner, D. M. (1995). Relationship between physical performance and self-perceived physical function. *Journal of the American Geriatrics Society, 43*(2), 93–101. *Evidence Level IV.*

Cunningham, G. O., & Michael, Y. L. (2004). Concepts guiding the study of the impact of the built environment on physical activity for older adults: A review of the literature. *American Journal of Health Promotion, 18*(6), 435–443. *Evidence Level I.*

Depp, C. A., & Jeste, D. V. (2006). Definitions and predictors of successful aging: A comprehensive review of larger quantitative studies. *American Journal of Geriatric Psychiatry, 14*(1), 6–20. *Evidence Level I.*

Doran, D. M., Harrison, M. B., Laschinger, H. S., Hirdes, J. P., Rukholm, E., Sidani, S., . . . Tourangeau, A. E. (2006).

Nursing-sensitive outcomes data collection in acute care and long-term-care settings. *Nursing Research, 55*(Suppl. 2), S75–S81. *Evidence Level VI.*

Edington, J., Barnes, R., Bryan, F., Dupree, E., Frost, G., Hickson, M., . . . Coles, S. J. (2004). A prospective randomised controlled trial of nutritional supplementation in malnourished elderly in the community: Clinical and health economic outcomes. *Clinical Nutrition, 23*(2), 195–204. *Evidence Level II.*

Engberg, S., Sereika, S. M., McDowell, B. J., Weber, E., & Brodak, I. (2002). Effectiveness of prompted voiding in treating urinary incontinence in cognitively impaired homebound older adults. *Journal of Wound, Ostomy, and Continence Nursing, 29*(5), 252–265. *Evidence Level II.*

Forbes, D. A. (2005). An educational programme for primary healthcare providers improved functional ability in older people living in the community. *Evidence-Based Nursing, 8*(4), 122. *Evidence Level VI.*

Fortinsky, R. H., Covinsky, K. E., Palmer, R. M., & Landefeld, C. S. (1999). Effects of functional status changes before and during hospitalization on nursing home admission of older patients. *Journals of Gerontology. Series A, Biological Sciences & Medical Sciences, 54A*, M521–M526. *Evidence Level IV.*

Freedman, V. A., Martin, L. G., & Schoeni R. F. (2002). Recent trends in disability and functioning among older adults in the United States: A systematic review. *Journal of the American Medical Association, 288*(24), 3137–3146. *Evidence Level I.*

Fried, L. P., Xue, Q. L., Cappola, A. R., Ferrucci, L., Chaves, P., Varadhan, R., . . . Bandeen-Roche, K. (2009). Nonlinear multisystem physiological dysregulation associated with frailty in older women: Implications for etiology and treatment. *Journals of Gerontology. Series A, Biological Sciences and Medical Sciences 64*(10), 1049–1057. *Evidence Level IV.*

Gill, T. M., Allore, H. G., Gahbauer, E. A., & Murphy, T. E. (2010). Change in disability after hospitalization or restricted activity in older persons. *Journal of the American Medical Association, 304*(17), 1919–1928. *Evidence Level IV.*

Gill, T. M., Allore, H., & Guo, Z. (2004). The deleterious effects of bed rest among community-living older persons. *Journals of Gerontology. Series A, Biological Sciences and Medical Sciences, 59*(7), 755–761. *Evidence Level IV.*

Graf, C. (2006). Functional decline in hospitalized older adults. *American Journal of Nursing, 106*(1), 58–67. *Evidence Level V.*

Gurland, B. J., Cross, P., Chen, J., Wilder, D. E., Pine, Z. M., Lantigua, R. A., & Fulmer, T. (1994). A new performance test of adaptive cognitive functioning: The Medication Management (MM) test. *International Journal of Geriatric Psychiatry, 9*(11), 875–885. *Evidence Level VI.*

Hirsch, C. H., Sommers, L., Olsen, A., Mullen, L., & Winograd, C. H. (1990). The natural history of functional morbidity in hospitalized older patients. *Journal of the American Geriatrics Society, 38*(12), 1296–1303. *Evidence Level IV.*

Hodgkinson, B., Evans, D., & Wood, J. (2003). Maintaining oral hydration in older adults: A systematic review. *International Journal of Nursing Practice, 9*(3), S19–S28. *Evidence Level I.*

Inouye, S. K., Rushing, J. T., Foreman, M. D., Palmer, R. M., & Pompei. P. (1998). Does delirium contribute to poor hospital outcomes? A three-site epidemiologic study. *Journal of General Internal Medicine, 13*(4), 234–242. *Evidence Level III.*

Inouye, S. K., Schlesinger, M. J., & Lydon, T. J. (1999). Delirium: A symptom of how hospital care is failing older patients and a window to improve quality of hospital care. *American Journal of Medicine, 106*(5), 565–573. *Evidence Level V.*

Kane, R. A., & Kane, R. L. (Eds.). (2000). *Assessing older persons: Measures, meaning, and practical applications.* New York, NY: Oxford University Press. *Evidence Level VI.*

Karagiozis, H., Gray, S., Sacco, J., Shapiro, M., & Kawas C. (1998). The Direct Assessment of Functional Abilities (DAFA): A comparison to an indirect measure of instrumental activities of daily living. *The Gerontologist, 38*(1), 113–121. *Evidence Level III.*

Katz, S., Ford, A. B., Moskowitz, R. W., Jackson, B. A., & Jaffe, M. W. (1963). Studies of illness and the aged. The index of ADL: A standardized measure of biological and psychosocial function. *Journal of the American Medical Association, 185*, 914–919. *Evidence Level I.*

Kresevic, D., & Holder, C. (1998). Interdisciplinary care. *Clinics in Geriatric Medicine, 14*(4), 787–798. *Evidence Level VI.*

Kresevic, D. M., Counsell, S. R., Covinsky, K., Palmer, R., Landefeld, C. S., Holder, C., & Beeler, J. (1998). A patient-centered model of acute care for elders. *Nursing Clinics of North America, 33*(3), 515–527. *Evidence Level VI.*

Kruianski, J., & Gurland, B. (1976). The performance test of activities of daily living. *International Journal of Aging & Human Development, 7*(4), 343–352. *Evidence Level VI.*

Landefeld, C. S., Palmer, R. M., Kresevic, D. M., Fortinsky, R. H., & Kowal, J. (1995). A randomized trial of care in a hospital medical unit especially designed to improve the functional outcomes of acutely ill older patients. *New England Journal of Medicine, 332*(20), 1338–1344. *Evidence Level II.*

Lawton, M. P., & Brody, E. M. (1969). Assessment of older people: Self-maintaining and instrumental activities of daily living. *The Gerontologist, 9*(3), 179–186. *Evidence Level IV.*

Lightbody, E., & Baldwin, R. (2002). Inpatient geriatric evaluation and management did not reduce mortality but reduced functional decline. *Evidence-Based Mental Health, 5*(4), 109. *Evidence Level VI.*

Mahoney, F. I., & Barthel, D. W. (1965). Functional evaluation: The Barthel index. *Maryland State Medical Journal, 14*, 61–65. *Evidence Level III.*

Mathias, S., Nayak, U. S., & Isaacs, B. (1986). Balance in elderly patients: The "Get-Up and Go" test. *Archives of Physical Medicine and Rehabilitation, 67*(6), 387–389. *Evidence Level VI.*

McAuley, E., Konopack, J. F., Morris, K. S., Motl, R. W., Hu, L., Doerksen, S. E., & Rosengren, K. (2006). Physical activity and functional limitations in older women: Influence of self-efficacy. *Journals of Gerontology. Series B, Psychological Sciences and Social Sciences, 61*(5), P270–P277. *Evidence Level IV.*

McCusker, J., Kakuma, R., & Abrahamowicz, M. (2002). Predictors of functional hospitalized elderly patients: A systematic review. *Journals of Geronotology. Series A, Biological Sciences and Medical Sciences, 57*(9), M569–M577. *Evidence Level I.*

Mezey, M. D., Rauckhorst, L. H., & Stokes, S. A. (1993). *Health assessment of the older individual.* New York, NY: Springer Publishing Company. *Evidence Level VI.*

Narain, J. P., Rubenstein, L. Z., Wieland, G. D., Rosbrook, B., Strome, L. S., Pietruszka, F., & Morley, J. E. (1988). Predictors of immediate and 6-month outcomes in hospitalized elderly patients. The importance of functional status. *Journal of the American Geriatrics Society, 36*(9), 775–783. *Evidence Level IV.*

Palmer, R. M., Counsell, S., & Landefeld, C. S. (1998). Clinical interventions trials: The ACE unit. *Clinics in Geriatric Medicine, 14*(4), 831–849. *Evidence Level I.*

Pearson, V. I. (2000). Assessment of function in older adults. In R. I. Kane & R. A. Kane (Eds.), *Assessing older persons: Measures, meanings and practical applications* (pp. 17–34). New York, NY: Oxford University Press. *Evidence Level VI.*

Pedersen, B. K., & Saltin, B. (2006). Evidence for prescribing exercise as therapy in chronic disease. *Scandinavian Journal of Medicine & Science in Sports, 16*(Suppl. 1), 3–63. *Evidence Level I.*

Reid, M. C., Williams, C. S., & Gill, T. M. (2005). Back pain and decline in lower extremity physical function among community-dwelling older persons. *Journals of Gerontology. Series A, Biological Sciences and Medical Sciences, 60*(6), 793–797. *Evidence Level IV.*

Resnick, B. (2002). Geriatric rehabilitation: The influence of efficacy beliefs and motivation. *Rehabilitation Nursing, 27*(4), 152–159. *Evidence Level IV.*

Resnick, B., Galik, E., Boltz, M., & Pretzer-Aboff, I. (2011). *Restorative care nursing for older adults: A guide for all care settings.* New York, NY: Springer Publishing Company. *Evidence Level VI.*

Rozzini, R., Sabatini, T., & Trabucchi, M. (2005). Hospital organization: General internal medical and geriatrics wards. *Journals of Gerontology. Series A, Biological Sciences and Medical Sciences, 60*(4), 535. *Evidence Level IV.*

Sager, M. A., & Rudberg, M. A. (1998). Functional decline associated with hospitalization for acute illness. *Clinics in Geriatric Medicine, 14*(4), 669–679. *Evidence Level II.*

Siegler, E. L., Glick, D., & Lee, J. (2002). Optimal staffing for acute care of the elderly (ACE) units. *Geriatric Nursing, 23*(3), 152–155. *Evidence Level VI.*

Tinetti, M. E., & Ginter, S. F. (1998). Identifying mobility dysfunctions in elderly patients. Standard neuromuscular examination or direct assessment? *Journal of the American Medical Association, 259*(8), 1190–1193. *Evidence Level I.*

Tucker, D., Molsberger, S. C., & Clark, A. (2004). Walking for wellness: A collaborative program to maintain mobility in hospitalized older adults. *Geriatric Nursing, 25*(4), 242–245. *Evidence Level VI.*

Vass, M., Avlund, K., Lauridsen, J., & Hendriksen, C. (2005). Feasible model for prevention of functional decline in older people: Municipality-randomized, controlled trial. *Journal of the American Geriatrics Society, 53*(4), 563–568. *Evidence Level II.*

Volpato, S., Onder, G., Cavalieri, M., Guerra, G., Sioulis, F., Maraldi, C., . . . Fellin, R.; Italian Group of Pharmacoepidemiology in the Elderly Study (GIFI). (2007). Characteristics of nondisabled older patients developing new disability associated with medical illnesses and hospitalization. *Journal of General Internal Medicine, 22*(5), 668–674. *Evidence Level IV.*

Woolf, S. H. (1990). Screening for hearing impairment. In R. B. Goldbloom & R. S. Lawrence (Eds.), *Preventing disease: Beyond the rhetoric* (pp. 331–346). New York, NY: Springer-Verlag. *Evidence Level VI.*

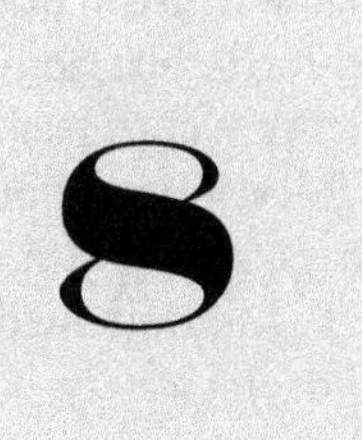

Oral Health Care

Linda J. O'Connor

EDUCATIONAL OBJECTIVES

On completion of this chapter, the reader should be able to:

1. Discuss the consequences of poor oral health
2. Describe a thorough oral assessment in the older adult
3. Describe the oral hygiene plan of care for nonintubated older adults
4. Discuss nursing interventions for oral care

OVERVIEW

Poor oral health is associated with malnutrition, dehydration, cardiovascular disease, pneumonia, aspiration pneumonia, poor glycemic control in type 1 and 2 diabetes, and chronic obstructive pulmonary disease (COPD) exacerbations (Bascones-Martinez, Gonzalez-Febles, & Sanz-Esporin, 2014; Belstrom, Damgaard, Nielsen, & Holmstrup, 2012; Bingham, Ashley, De Jong, & Swift, 2010; Cotti, Dessi, Piras, & Mercuro, 2011; Desvarieux et al., 2010; El-Solh, 2011; Holmlund & Lind, 2012; Jung et al., 2014; Ledic et al., 2013; Liu et al., 2012; Lockhart et al., 2009; Negrato, Tarzia, Jovanovic, & Chinellato, 2013; Nicolosi, Lewin, González, Jara, & Rubio Mdel, 2011; Oliveira et al., 2010; Ozcaka, Becerik, Bicakci, & Kiyak, 2014; Pace & McCullough, 2010; Si et al., 2012; Tada & Miura, 2010; Uyar et al., 2013). Oral health also affects nutritional status, ability to speak, self-esteem, mental wellness, and overall well-being (Haumschild & Haumschild, 2009; Montero, López, Galindo, Vicente, & Bravo, 2009; Naito et al., 2010; Quandt et al., 2010). Many oral diseases are not part of the natural aging process but side effects of medical treatment and medications.

BACKGROUND AND STATEMENT OF PROBLEM

Plaque retention is a problem in older adults who have difficulty in mechanically removing plaque caused by diminished manual dexterity, impaired vision, or chronic illness (Brown, Goryakin, & Finlayson, 2009; Hakuta, Mori, Ueno, Shinada, & Kawaguchi, 2009). An older adult's functional ability and cognitive status affect his or her ability to perform oral care and denture care. Dental plaque harbors microorganisms, including *Streptococcus, Staphylococcus*, gram-positive rods, gram-negative rods, and yeasts (Coulthwaite & Verran, 2007). Dentures also have the potential to harbor *Streptococcus pneumoniae, Haemophilus influenza, Escherichia coli, Klebsiella*, and *Pseudomonas* secondary to spending time in nonhygienic environments (Coulthwaite & Verran, 2007). Dentures have been seen thrown in with patients' clothing, thrown

For a description of evidence levels cited in this chapter, see Chapter 1, "Developing and Evaluating Clinical Practice Guidelines: A Systematic Approach."

in a washbasin or other containers with bathing items, and so forth, instead of being properly cleaned and stored in a denture cup. Lack of good oral hygiene increases the risk of development of secondary infections, extended hospital stays, and significant negative health outcomes.

Multiple medications produce side effects that affect the oral cavity. Cardiac medications can cause salivary dysfunction, gingival enlargement, and lichenoid mucosal reactions. Steroid treatment can predispose a patient to oral candidiasis, and cancer treatments can cause a plethora of oral conditions such as stomatitis, salivary hypofunction, microbial infections, and xerostomia.

The mouth reflects the culmination of multiple stressors over the years and, as the mouth ages, it is less able to tolerate these stressors. With an increase in chronic disease and medication usage as a person ages, the prevalence of root caries, tooth loss, oral cancers, soft-tissue lesions, and periodontal problems increases significantly (Christensen, 2007; Saunders & Friedman, 2007). Many of the oral health problems seen in older adults could be avoided with routine preventive care. Many older adults believe in the myth that a decline in oral health is a normal part of aging.

ASSESSMENT OF THE PROBLEM

Physical Assessment

The promotion of oral health through assessment and good oral hygiene is an essential part of nursing care. Oral assessment is part of the nurse's head-to-toe assessment of the older adult and is done on admission and at the beginning of each shift. The nurse assesses the condition of the oral cavity, which should be pink, moist, and intact; the presence of or absence of natural teeth and/or dentures; ability to function with or without natural teeth and/or dentures; and the patient's ability to speak, chew, or swallow. Natural teeth should be intact, and dentures (partial or full) should fit comfortably and not be moving when the older adult is speaking. Any abnormal findings such as dryness, swelling, sores, ulcers, bleeding, white patches, broken or decayed teeth, halitosis, ill-fitting dentures, difficulty swallowing, signs of aspiration, and pain, are documented by the nurse, and the health care team informed.

Poorly fitting dentures can cause ulcerations and candidiasis (oral fungal infection, masses, and denture stomatitis). Denture stomatitis presents as red, inflamed tissue beneath dentures, caused by fungal infections and insufficient oral hygiene. Some oral mucosal diseases that nursing may see are angular cheilitis (red and white cracked lesions in the corners of the mouth, caused by inflammation and a fungal infection), cicatricial pemphigoid (produces red, inflamed lesions on the gingival, palate, tongue, and cheek tissues), lichen planus (most common form presents as a lacy white appearance on the tongue and/or cheeks), and pemphigus vulgaris (red bleeding tissues resulting from trauma but heal without scarring). Untreated lesions can develop into large, infected regions, which require immediate medical attention. Dental professionals diagnose oral mucosal diseases, but the nurse needs to be aware of any abnormal findings and report them immediately.

The nurse also needs to assess the patient for functional ability and manual dexterity to provide oral hygiene. The nurse needs to observe the older adult providing oral hygiene to make sure that it is effective. The primary focus for nurses is to maintain the older adult's function so that older adults may participate in their daily care. Once the older adult performs his or her oral hygiene, the nurse must follow up as appropriate to complete the oral hygiene.

Assessment Tools

The Oral Health Assessment Tool (OHAT) is an eight-category screening tool that can be used with cognitively intact or impaired older adults. The OHAT provides an organized, efficient method for nurses to document their oral assessment. The eight categories (lips, tongue, gums and tissues, saliva, natural teeth, dentures, oral cleanliness, and dental pain) are scored from 0 (healthy) to 2 (unhealthy). Total scores range from 0 to 16; the higher the score, the poorer the older adult's oral health (Chalmers, King, Spencer, Wright, & Carter, 2005). The OHAT may be implemented in any health care setting. See the Resources section for access to this tool.

INTERVENTION AND CARE STRATEGIES

The gold standard for providing oral hygiene is the toothbrush. It is the mechanical action of the toothbrush that is important for plaque removal. If the older adult has any decrease in function or manual dexterity, the nursing staff needs to assess the older adult's ability to provide effective oral hygiene and provide assistance as needed. Foam swabs are available in numerous facilities to provide oral hygiene. Research has shown that foam swabs cannot remove plaque as well as toothbrushes can (Pace & McCullough, 2010). Foam swabs may be used for cleaning the oral mucus of an edentulous older adult.

Lemon–glycerin swabs or swab sticks cause drying of the oral mucosa and erosion of the tooth enamel. Lemon–glycerin swabs or swab sticks are detrimental to the older adult and are never to be used.

Alcohol-free commercial mouth rinses may be used. Toothpaste with fluoride is currently recommended by the American Dental Association to reduce cavities and to help reduce periodontal disease.

The use of chlorhexidine in the geriatric patient is determined by the dentist. There are some side effects of chlorhexidine (bitter taste; change in the taste of food; mouth irritation; and staining of teeth, mouth, fillings, and dentures) that may have negative outcomes for the older adult (Quagliarello et al., 2009). A good oral assessment by the nurse during each shift is essential for the geriatric patient on chlorhexidine and so is monitoring of the patient's nutritional intake.

Education of the nursing staff is imperative. Two of the major barriers cited by nursing staff are inadequate knowledge of how to assess and provide care and lack of appropriate supplies. Implementation of evidence-based protocols combined with ongoing educational training sessions have been demonstrated to have a positive impact on oral care being provided and on the oral health status of older adults (Gluhak, Arnetzl, Kirmeier, Jakse, & Arnetzl, 2010; Ribeiro et al., 2009; Young, Murray, & Thompson, 2008). Staff needs to be instructed on oral hygiene and the proper care of different appliances. Dentures should be brushed before placing them into a denture cup. Dentures should be removed at night, but some older adults prefer to keep their dentures in continuously. It therefore becomes even more important for the nurse to do an assessment of the oral mucosa. In the acute care and long-term care setting, the older adult may not have dental adhesive and, therefore, there is a high risk for food particles to get caught underneath of their dentures. It is important that staff remember to take the dentures out after each meal, rinse them and the patient's mouth, and place the dentures back in. Complete denture care should be given morning, night, and as needed.

Education of nursing staff, older adults, and families is imperative. Nurses need to be educated in oral assessment and nursing assistants need to be educated in observation of the oral cavity and what to report to the nurse. Both nurses and nursing assistants need to be educated about the proper techniques for providing oral hygiene and caring for oral appliances. Patients and families need to be educated on the importance of good oral health and hygiene and to dispel the oral-health myths that exist about oral health and aging in general.

Education focused on the importance of good oral health and hygiene in the older adult, the myths about oral health and aging, evidence-based practice protocols, implementing these protocols, and the appropriate products for providing oral hygiene to their patients and residents must be provided to administrators. Without the proper supplies, it is impossible for the nursing staff to provide the oral-hygiene care the older adult needs and to properly implement evidence-based protocols for oral health and hygiene in the older adult.

CASE STUDY

Mrs. Smith, an 84-year-old female with a history of Alzheimer's-type dementia, was admitted for recent decreased oral intake and percutaneous endoscopic gastrostomy (PEG) placement. Mrs. Smith was alert, oriented to herself, pleasant, cooperative with care, and able to follow simple directions. She lived at home with her family and received care from a home health aide. The initial oral assessment was done on day 2 of admission and it was found that upper dentures and lower natural teeth were both covered with food particles. Her oral mucosa was noted to be dry. The upper dentures were difficult to remove and caused her pain. The upper denture was being "kept in place" by a collection of old food, which was found on removal. The oral mucosa under the upper denture was covered with sores and ulcers and was bleeding, infected, and very painful. The health team was notified, a dental consultant was called, and an oral hygiene plan of care was implemented. Mrs. Smith's diet was changed to puree while her oral mucosa was healing and the PEG placement was put on hold. On inquiry, it was learned from the family that their long-time aide had just moved, and the new aide had been with them for only a few months. It was during this time that they noticed the decline in Mrs. Smith's nutritional intake. The family chose to hire a new aide, and both the family and the new aide were educated on proper oral hygiene for Mrs. Smith. Once Mrs. Smith's oral mucosa had healed, the upper denture was replaced, and she was returned to her regular diet. Her oral intake returned to baseline, and a PEG was no longer required.

Discussion

This case study illustrates how poor oral care often goes undetected, the importance of good oral care, the need for physical assessment by the nurse, and the need for staff and family education. This patient was being admitted for an invasive procedure secondary to poor oral health caused by poor oral care. Although the family was involved in Mrs. Smith's care (she had no contractures or skin breakdown), her lack of oral care had gone unnoticed by them. The admitting nurse

(continued)

CASE STUDY *(continued)*

documented that the patient had dentures on the admission form but did not do a physical oral assessment. The nurse caring for the patient on day 2 had attended an oral health seminar and included the physical oral assessment in her morning rounds. She also followed up with the nursing assistants to ensure that oral care had been provided to the patient after each meal. The implementation of an oral hygiene plan of care and education of nursing staff, family, and home care staff ensured that Mrs. Smith received the oral care required for her oral mucosa to heal, her nutritional status to return to baseline, and prevented the unnecessary placement of a PEG.

SUMMARY

As previously stated, many of the oral health problems in older adults could be avoided with routine preventive care, but many older adults believe in the myth that a decline in their oral health is a normal part of aging (Allen, O'Sullivan, & Locker, 2009; Borreani, Jones, Scambler, & Gallagher, 2010; McKenzie-Green, Giddings, Buttle, & Tahana, 2009). To dispel this myth and improve the oral health of older adults, it is imperative that health care professionals provide continuing education to patients and families, advocate for oral health prevention, and provide oral care to older adults in all settings. Well-developed evidence-based oral care protocols and educational training sessions have been demonstrated to have a positive impact on the oral health status of older patients.

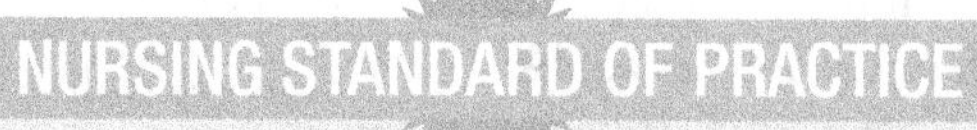

NURSING STANDARD OF PRACTICE

Protocol 8.1: Providing Oral Health Care to Older Adults

I. GOAL

The promotion of oral health through good oral hygiene is an essential part of nursing care. The RN or designee provides regular oral care for functionally dependent and cognitively impaired older adults.

II. BACKGROUND

A. Oral hygiene is directly linked with systemic infections, cardiac disease, cerebrovascular accident, acute myocardial infarction, glucose control in diabetes, nutritional intake, comfort, ability to speak, and the patient's self-esteem and overall well-being.

B. Definitions
   1. *Oral* refers to the mouth (natural teeth, gingival and supporting tissues, hard and soft palate, mucosal lining of the mouth and throat, tongue, salivary glands, chewing muscles, upper and lower jaw, and lips).
   2. *Oral cavity* includes cheeks, hard and soft palate.
   3. *Oral hygiene* is the prevention of plaque-related disease, the destruction of plaque through the mechanical action of tooth brushing and flossing, or use of other oral hygiene aids
   4. *Edentulous* means that natural teeth have been removed.

III. PARAMETERS OF ASSESSMENT

A. The RN conducts an oral assessment or evaluation on admission and on every shift. The nurse assesses the condition of:
   1. The oral cavity; should be pink, moist, and intact
   2. The presence of or absence of natural teeth and/or dentures
   3. Ability to function with or without natural teeth and/or dentures
   4. The patient's ability to speak, chew, or swallow
   5. Any abnormal findings, such as dryness, swelling, sores, ulcers, bleeding, white patches, broken or decayed teeth, halitosis, ill-fitting dentures, difficulty swallowing, signs of aspiration, and pain

B. Assessment tool: The OHAT. See the Resources section for access to this tool.

(continued)

Protocol 8.1: Providing Oral Health Care to Older Adults *(continued)*

IV. NURSING CARE STRATEGIES

A. Oral hygiene plan of care: dependent mouth care of the edentulous patient
   1. Oral care is provided during morning care, evening care, and as needed
   2. Wash hands and don gloves
   3. Remove dentures
   4. Brush dentures with toothbrush/toothpaste and rinse
   5. Brush patient's tongue
   6. Reinsert dentures
   7. Apply lip moisturizer

B. Dependent mouth care: patients with teeth or partial dentures
   1. Oral care is provided during morning care, evening care, and as needed
   2. Wash hands and don gloves
   3. Gently brush teeth in an up-and-down motion with short strokes using the toothbrush
   4. Brush patient's tongue
   5. Apply lip moisturizer

C. For partial dentures, follow procedure for full denture cleaning and insertion.

D. Assisted or supervised care
   1. Oral care is provided during morning care, evening care, and as needed
   2. Assess what patient can do and provide assistance as needed
   3. Set up necessary items

V. EVALUATION OF EXPECTED OUTCOMES

A. Patient will
   1. Receive oral hygiene a minimum of once every 8 hours while in the acute care, long-term care, or home care setting.
   2. Patients and families will be referred to dental services for follow-up treatment.
   3. Patients and families will be educated on the importance of good oral hygiene and follow-up dental services.

B. RN will
   1. Conduct an assessment or evaluation of the oral cavity on admission and every shift
   2. Notify the physician of any abnormalities present in the oral cavity
   3. Assess what each patient can do independently
   4. Observe aspiration precautions while providing care
   5. Provide oral care education to patients and families

C. Institution will
   1. Provide access to dental services as appropriate
   2. Provide ongoing education to health care providers
   3. Provide a yearly oral health and dental care in-service to health care providers

ABBREVIATION

OHAT Oral Health Assessment Tool

RESOURCES

American Academy of Periodontology
www.peno.org

Centers for Disease Control and Prevention
http://www.cdc.gov/OralHealth
http://www.consultgerirn.org

Chalmers, J. M., King, P. L., Spencer, A. J., Wright, F. A., & Carter, K. D. (2005). The oral health assessment tool—Validity and reliability. *Australian Dental Journal, 50*(3), 191–199. *Evidence Level III.*

National Institute of Dental and Craniofacial Research
http://www.nidcr.nih.gov

REFERENCES

Allen, P. F., O'Sullivan, M., & Locker, D. (2009). Determining the minimally important difference for the Oral Health Impact Profile-20. *European Journal of Oral Sciences, 117*(2), 129–134. *Evidence Level IV.*

Bascones-Martinez, A., Gonzalez-Febles, J., & Sanz-Esporin, J. (2014). Diabetes and periodontal disease. Review of the literature. *American Journal of Dentistry, 27*(2), 65–67. *Evidence Level I.*

Belstrom, D., Damgaard, C., Nielsen, C. H., & Holmstrup, P. (2012). Does a causal relation between cardiovascular disease and periodontitis exist? *Microbes and Infection, 14*, 411–418. *Evidence Level I.*

Bingham, M., Ashley, J., De Jong, M., & Swift, C. (2010). Implementing a unit-level intervention to reduce the probability of ventilator-associated pneumonia. *Nursing Research, 59*(Suppl. 1), S40–S47. *Evidence Level IV.*

Borreani, E., Jones, K., Scambler, S., & Gallagher, J. E. (2010). Informing the debate on oral health care for older people: A qualitative study of older people's views on oral health and oral health care. *Gerodontology, 27*(1), 11–18. *Evidence Level IV.*

Brown, T. T., Goryakin, Y., & Finlayson, T. L. (2009). The effect of functional limitations on the demand for dental care among adults 65 and older. *Journal of the California Dental Association, 37*(8), 549–558. *Evidence Level V.*

Chalmers, J. M., King, P. L., Spencer, A. J., Wright, F. A., & Carter, K. D. (2005). The oral health assessment tool—Validity and reliability. *Australian Dental Journal, 50*(3), 191–199. *Evidence Level III.*

Christensen, G. J. (2007). Providing oral care for the aging patient. *Journal of the American Dental Association (1939), 138*(2), 239–242. *Evidence Level V.*

Cotti, E., Dessi, C., Piras, P., & Mercuro, G. (2011). Can a chronic dental infection be considered a cause of cardiovascular disease? *International Journal of Cardiology, 148*, 4–10. *Evidence Level I.*

Coulthwaite, L., & Verran, J. (2007). Potential pathogenic aspects of denture plaque. *British Journal of Biomedical Science, 64*(4), 180–189. *Evidence Level V.*

Desvarieux, M., Demmer, R. T., Jacobs, D. R., Rundak, T., Boden-Albala, B., Sacco, R. L., & Papapanou, P. N. (2010). Periodonal bacteria and hypertension: The oral infections and vascular disease epidemiology study (INVEST). *Journal of Hypertension, 28*(7), 1413–1421. *Evidence Level III.*

El-Solh, A. A. (2011). Association between pneumonia and oral care in nursing home residents. *Lung, 189*, 173–180. *Evidence Level I.*

Gluhak, C., Arnetzl, G. V., Kirmeier, R., Jakse, N., & Arnetzl, G. (2010). Oral status among seniors in nine nursing homes in Styria, Austria. *Gerodontology, 27*(1), 47–52. *Evidence Level IV.*

Hakuta, C., Mori, C., Ueno, M., Shinada, K., & Kawaguchi, Y. (2009). Evaluation of an oral function promotion programme for the independent elderly in Japan. *Gerodontology, 26*(4), 250–258. *Evidence Level IV.*

Haumschild, M. S., & Haumschild, R. J. (2009). The importance of oral health in long-term care. *Journal of the American Medical Directors Association, 10*, 667–671. *Evidence Level V.*

Holmlund, A., & Lind, L. (2012). Number of teeth is related to atherosclerotic plaque in the carotid arteries in an elderly population. *Journal of Periodontology, 83*, 287–291. *Evidence Level IV.*

Jung, Y. S., Shin, M. H., Kim, I. S., Kweon, S. S., Lee, Y. H., Kim, O. J., . . . Kim, O. S. (2014). Relationship between periodontal disease and subclinical atherosclerosis: The Don-gu study. *Journal of Clinical Periodontology, 41*, 262–268. *Evidence Level III.*

Ledic, K., Marinkovic, S., Puhar, I., Spalj, S., Popovic-Grle, S., Ivic-Kardum, M., . . . Plancak, D. (2013). Periodontal disease increases risk for chronic obstructive pulmonary disease. *Collegium Antropologicum, 37*(3), 937–942. *Evidence Level III.*

Liu, Z., Zhang, W., Zhang, J., Zhou, X., Zhang, L., Song, Y., & Wang, Z. (2012). Oral hygiene, periodontal health and chronic obstructive pulmonary disease exacerbations. *Journal of Clinical Periodontology, 39*, 45–52. *Evidence Level III.*

Lockhart, P. B., Brennan, M. T., Thornhill, M., Michalowicz, B. S., Noll, J., Bahrani-Mougeot, F. K., & Sasser, H. C. (2009). Poor oral hygiene as a risk factor for infective endocarditis-related bacteremia. *Journal of the American Dental Association (1939), 140*(10), 1238–1244. *Evidence Level II.*

McKenzie-Green, B., Giddings, L. S., Buttle, L., & Tahana, K. (2009). Older peoples' perceptions of oral health: "It's just not that simple." *International Journal of Dental Hygiene, 7*(1), 31–38. *Evidence Level V.*

Montero, J., López, J. F., Galindo, M. P., Vicente, P., & Bravo, M. (2009). Impact of prosthodontic status on oral wellbeing: A cross-sectional cohort study. *Journal of Oral Rehabilitation, 36*(8), 592–600. *Evidence Level IV.*

Naito, M., Kato, T., Fujii, W., Ozeki, M., Yokoyama, M., Hamajima, N., & Saitoh, E. (2010). Effects of dental treatment on the quality of life and activities of daily living in institutionalized elderly in Japan. *Archives of Gerontology and Geriatrics, 50*(1), 65–68. *Evidence Level V.*

Negrato, C. A., Tarzia, O., Jovanovic, L., & Chinellato, L. E. (2013). Periodontal disease and diabetes mellitus. *Journal of Applied Oral Science, 21*(1), 1–12. *Evidence Level I.*

Nicolosi, L. N., Lewin, P. G., González, N., Jara, L., & Rubio Mdel, C. (2011). Association between oral health and acute coronary syndrome in elderly people. *Acta Odontol Latinoam, 24*(3), 229–234. *Evidence Level III.*

Oliveira, F. J., Vieira, R. W., Coelho, O. R., Petrucci, O., Oliveira, P. P., Antunes, N., . . . Antunes, E. (2010). Systemic inflammation caused by chronic periodontitis in acute ischemic heart attack patients. *Revista Brasileira de Cirurgia Cardiovascular, 25*(1), 51–58. *Evidence Level III.*

Ozcaka, O., Becerik, S., Bicakci, N., & Kiyak, A. H. (2014). Periodontal disease and systemic diseases in an older population. *Archives of Gerontology and Geriatrics, 59*, 474–479. *Evidence Level IV.*

Pace, C. C., & McCullough, G. H. (2010). The association between oral microorganisims and aspiration pneumonia in the institutionalized elderly: Review. *Dysphagia, 25*(4), 307–322. *Evidence Level I.*

Quagliarello, V., Juthani-Mehta, M., Ginter, S., Towle, V., Allore, H., & Tinetti, M. (2009). Pilot testing of intervention protocols to prevent pneumonia in nursing home residents. *Journal of the American Geriatrics Society, 57*(7), 1226–1231. *Evidence Level II.*

Quandt, S. A., Chen, H., Bell, R. A., Savoca, M. R., Anderson, A. M., Leng, X., . . . Arcury, T. A. (2010). Food avoidance and food modification practices of older rural adults: Association with oral health status and implications for service provision. *The Gerontologist, 50*(1), 100–111. *Evidence Level V.*

Ribeiro, D. G., Pavarina, A. C., Giampaolo, E. T., Machado, A. L., Jorge, J. H., & Garcia, P. P. (2009). Effect of oral hygiene education and motivation on removable partial denture wearers: Longitudinal study. *Gerodontology, 26*(2), 150–156. *Evidence Level II.*

Saunders, R., & Friedman, B. (2007). Oral health conditions of community-dwelling cognitively intact elderly persons with disabilities. *Gerodontology, 24*, 67–76. *Evidence Level IV.*

Si, Y., Fan, H., Song, Y., Zhou, X., Zhang, J., & Wang, Z. (2012). Association between periodontitis and chronic obstructive pulmonary disease in a Chinese population. *Journal of Periodontology, 83*, 1288–1296. *Evidence Level III.*

Tada, A., & Miura, H. (2012). Prevention of aspiration pneumonia (AP) with oral care. *Archives of Gerontology and Geriatrics, 55*, 16–21. *Evidence Level I.*

Uyar, I. S., Sahin, V., Akpinar, B. M., Abacilar, F., Okur, F. F., Ozdemir, U., . . . Yasa, E. F. (2013). Does oral hygiene trigger carotid artery intima-media thickness? *Heart Surgery Forum, 16*(4), E232–E236. *Evidence Level III.*

Young, B. C., Murray, C. A., & Thomson, J. (2008). Care home staff knowledge of oral care compared to best practice: A west of Scotland pilot study. *British Dental Journal, 205*(8), E15. *Evidence Level V.*

9

Managing Oral Hydration

Janet C. Mentes

EDUCATIONAL OBJECTIVES

On completion of this chapter, the reader should be able to:

1. Describe older adults at risk of dehydration
2. Identify key aspects of a hydration assessment
3. List specific interventions to promote hydration in older adults across care settings
4. Identify outcomes of a hydration management program

OVERVIEW

Studies using biomarkers (serum sodium, osmolality, and blood urea nitrogen [BUN]/creatinine ratio) for dehydration and volume depletion from the Established Populations for Epidemiologic Studies of the Elderly (EPESE; Stookey, Pieper, & Cohen, 2005) and National Health and Nutrition Examination Survey III (NHANES III; Stookey, 2005) found that the prevalence rate for these conditions in community-dwelling older adults could range from 0.5% to 60% depending on the markers used. Another study found that 48% of older adults presenting with dehydration at an emergency room (ER) unit were from the community (Bennett, Thomas, & Riegel, 2004) and, more recent, El-Sharkawy, Shahota, Maughan, and Lobo (2014) found that 40% of older adults were dehydrated on admission to a hospital and 44% were found to be dehydrated at 48 hours. Maintaining adequate fluid balance is an essential component of health across the life span; older adults are more vulnerable to shifts in water balance—both overhydration and dehydration—because of age-related changes and increased likelihood that an older individual has several medical conditions (Hooper, Bunn, Jimoh, & Fairweather-Tait, 2013). Dehydration is the more frequent occurrence in older adults (Warren et al., 1994; Xiao, Barber, & Campbell, 2004). In fact, avoidable hospitalizations for dehydration in older adults have increased by 40% from 1990 to 2000, at a cost of $1.14 billion (Xiao et al., 2004), and is one of the Agency for Healthcare Research and Quality's 13 ambulatory care-sensitive conditions. When dehydration is considered as a comorbid condition the cost of hospitalizations and rehospitalizations is even higher (Frangeskou, Lopez-Valcarcel, & Serra-Majem, 2014).

For a description of evidence Levels cited in this chapter, see Chapter 1, "Developing and Evaluating Clinical Practice Guidelines: A Systematic Approach."

Careful attention to hydration requirements of older adults will not only help prevent hospitalizations for dehydration but also decrease associated conditions such as acute confusion and delirium (Foreman, 1989; Mentes & Culp, 2003; Mentes, Culp, Maas, & Rantz, 1999; O'Keeffe & Lavan, 1996; Seymour, Henschke, Cape, & Campbell, 1980), adverse drug reactions (Doucet et al., 2002), infections (Beaujean et al., 1997; Masotti et al., 2000), increased morbidity associated with bladder cancer (Michaud et al., 1999), coronary heart disease (Chan, Knutsen, Blix, Lee, & Fraser, 2002; Rasouli, Kiasari, & Arab, 2008), stroke (Lin, Lee, Hung, Chang, & Yang, 2014; Rodriguez et al., 2009), and other thromboembolytic events (Kelly et al., 2004). Furthermore, dehydration has been associated with longer hospital stays for rehabilitation (Frangeskou et al., 2014; Mukand, Cai, Zielinski, Danish, & Berman, 2003) and for readmission to the hospital (Frangeskou et al., 2014; Gordon, An, Hayward, & Williams, 1998). Even in healthy community-dwelling older adults, physical performance and cognitive processing is affected by mild dehydration (Ainslie et al., 2002).

Oral hydration of older adults is particularly complex for a variety of reasons. In the following review, issues of age-related changes, risk factors, assessment measures, and nursing strategies for effective interventions for dehydration are addressed.

BACKGROUND AND STATEMENT OF PROBLEM

Water is an essential component of body composition. Intricate cellular functions, such as gene expression, protein synthesis, and uptake and metabolism of nutrients, are affected by hydration status. Organ systems, specifically the cardiovascular and renal systems, are particularly vulnerable to fluctuating levels of hydration (Metheny, 2000).

Older individuals are at increased risk for hydration problems stemming from several converging age-related factors, including lack of thirst (Ainslie et al., 2002; Phillips, Bretherton, Johnston, & Gray, 1991; Phillips et al., 1984); changes in body composition, specifically loss of fluid-rich muscle tissue (Bossingham, Carnell, & Campbell, 2005); increasing inability to respond efficiently to physiological stressful events through which dehydration results (Farrell et al., 2008; Rolls, 1998); and renal changes, including a reduced renal capacity to handle water and sodium efficiently (Macias-Nuñez, 2008). Additionally, personal, often lifetime hydration habits, may contribute to risk but have not been explored in relation to underhydration. As a result, older adults are often at risk for a chronic state of underhydration. Several studies (Bossingham et al., 2005; Morgan, Masterson, Fahlman, Topp, & Boardley, 2003; Raman et al., 2004) of community-dwelling older adults suggest that under normal conditions, older adults maintain adequate hydration; however, when challenged by environmental stressors—physical or emotional illness, surgery, or trauma—they are at increased risk for dehydration and rapidly become dehydrated if they are already chronically underhydrated.

DEFINITIONS

Dehydration

Dehydration is the depletion in total body water (TBW) content caused by pathological fluid losses, diminished water intake, or a combination of both. It results in hypernatremia (more than 145 mEq/L) in the extracellular fluid compartment, which draws water from the intracellular fluids. The water loss is shared by all body-fluid compartments and relatively little reduction in extracellular fluids occurs. Thus, circulation is not compromised unless the loss is very large.

Underhydration

Underhydration is a precursor condition to dehydration associated with insidious onset and poor outcomes (Mentes, 2006; Mentes & Culp, 2003). Others have referred to this condition as *mild dehydration* (Stookey et al., 2005), *chronic dehydration* (Bennett et al., 2004), or *impending water loss dehydration* (Hooper et al., 2011).

ASSESSMENT OF THE PROBLEM

Assessment of the hydration status consists of determining adequate intake, risk identification with attention to specific populations at increased risk, assessment of hydration habits, and evaluation of specific biochemical and clinical indicators.

Determining Adequate Intake

All older adults should have an individualized fluid goal determined by a documented standard for daily fluid intake. There are many standards that have been developed (Table 9.1). However, Gaspar (2011) has compared four standards and has produced a nomogram based on an individual's weight and height, which is the most individualized standard. Table 9.1 provides examples of daily fluid goal calculations.

Risk Identification

Risk for dehydration in ill or frail older adults across care settings has been studied more frequently. Although there is no outstanding risk factor for dehydration, age, gender,

TABLE 9.1

Daily Fluid Goal Formulas

- 1,600 mL/m^2 of body surface per day (Butler & Talbot, 1944; Gaspar, 1988, 1999); more recent Gaspar (2011) recommended 75% of this standard and has developed a nomogram.
- 30 mL/kg body weight with 1,500 mL/d minimum (Chernoff, 1994)
- 1 mL/kcal fluid for adults (National Research Council, 1989)
- 100 mL fluid/kg for the first 10 kg BW, 50 mL fluid/kg for next 10 kg of BW, and 15 mL fluid/kg for remaining kilograms of weight (Chidester & Spangler, 1997)
- 1,600 mL/d (Hodgkinson, Evans, & Wood, 2003)

BW, body weight.

TABLE 9.2

Dehydration Risk-Appraisal Checklist

The greater the number of characteristics present, the greater the risk for hydration problems. Please check all that apply.

❒ > 85 years	❒ Female
Significant Health Conditions	
❒ MMSE score < 24 (indicating cognitive impairment)	❒ Semi-dependent in ADL
❒ Dementia diagnosis	❒ Repeated infections
❒ GDS score ≥ 6 (indicating depression)	❒ History of dehydration
	❒ Urinary incontinence
Medications	
❒ Laxatives	❒ Psychotropics: antipsychotics, antidepressants, anxiolytics
❒ Diuretics	
Intake Behaviors	
❒ BMI < 21 or > 27	❒ Can drink independently but forgets
❒ Requires assistance to drink	❒ Poor eater
❒ Has difficulty swallowing/chokes	

ADL, activities of daily living; BMI, body mass index; GDS, Geriatric Depression Scale; MMSE, Mini-Mental State Examination.

From Mentes and Wang (2010). Reprinted with permission from Mentes and Kang (2011).

ethnicity, class, and number of medications taken, level of activities of daily living (ADL) dependency, presence of cognitive impairment, presence of medical conditions such as infectious processes, and a prior history of dehydration have all been associated with dehydration in older adults (Mentes & Iowa–Veterans Affairs Nursing Research Consortium [IVANRC], 2000). Therefore, although single risk factors are discussed, it is likely that clusters of risk factors may be more helpful in clinical settings (Leibovitz et al., 2007).

Increasing age is associated with increased likelihood of dehydration (Ciccone, Allegra, Cochrane, Cody, & Roche, 1998; Lavizzo-Mourey, Johnson, & Stolley, 1988; Warren et al., 1994). Ciccone et al. (1998) found that adults aged 85 years and older were three times more likely to have a diagnosis of dehydration on admission to an emergency department than adults aged 65 to 74 years. Older African American and Black adults have higher prevalence rates of dehydration on hospitalization than Caucasian adults (Lancaster, Smiciklas-Wright, Heller, Ahern, & Jensen, 2003; Warren et al., 1994). Female gender has been associated with risk for dehydration in nursing home residents (Lavizzo-Mourey et al., 1988); however, male hospitalized patients had an increased risk for dehydration (Warren et al., 1994) and, more recent, no gender differences were detected in a large database study (Xiao et al., 2004).

In general, individuals in long-term care (LTC) settings are considered to be at increased risk, with one third of residents experiencing a dehydration episode in a 6-month period (Mentes, 2006). However, many of the factors are also characteristic of older adult hospitalized patients as well. See Protocol 9.1 for patient, staff, and family issues that serve as risk factors for dehydration. An example of a tool to determine risk is the Dehydration Risk Appraisal Checklist (Mentes & Wang, 2010) developed to be used by nursing home staff members and based on information that could be retrieved from the Minimum Data Set (MDS; Table 9.2).

At-Risk Populations

Several groups of patients, based on medical diagnosis, are at increased risk of dehydration. These groups include the chronic mentally ill, surgical, stroke, and end-of-life patients.

Chronic Mentally Ill Patients

Special consideration should be given to chronic mentally ill older adults (e.g., individuals with schizophrenia, bipolar disorder, obsessive–compulsive disorder) because they may be at risk of hydration problems. Their antipsychotic medications may blunt their thirst response and put them at increased risk in hot weather for dehydration and heat stroke (Batscha, 1997). In addition, even small increases in their antipsychotic medications may predispose them to neuroleptic malignant syndrome (NMS), of which hyperthermia and dehydration are prominent features (Bristow & Kohen, 1996; Jacobs, 1996; Sachdev, Mason, & Hadzi-Pavlovic, 1997). In these individuals, risks for overhydration stem from a combination of the drying side effects of prescribed psychotropic medications and the individual's compulsive behaviors that result in excessive fluid intake (Cosgray, Davidhizar, Giger, & Kreisl, 1993).

Patients With Stroke

There is increasing evidence that dehydration may play an important part in contributing to early cerebral ischemia (Rodriguez et al., 2009), and in the early recovery from stroke (Kelly et al., 2004; Lin et al., 2014). In fact, Kelly et al. (2004) found that dehydration in patients with stroke was hospital acquired and led to poorer outcomes for recovering patients with stroke. Dehydration, signified by increased serum osmolality, led to a 2.8- to 4.7-fold increase in the risk of hospitalized patients with stroke acquiring a venous thromboembolism (VTE). Lin et al. (2014) found that by managing stroke patients' fluid intake based on their admission BUN/creatinine ratio significantly decreased neurological deficits called "stroke in evolution" in older adults with ischemic stroke (2014). Hospitalized patients recovering from stroke should be carefully and continuously monitored for dehydration. Another sequela of stroke is dysphagia, which can cause dehydration (Whelan, 2001). This appears to be related not only to the dysphagia resulting from the stroke but also the poor palatability of the thickened fluids offered to patients to prevent aspiration.

Surgical Patients

Prolonged nothing by mouth (NPO) status before elective surgery has been linked to increased risk of dehydration and adverse effects, such as thirst, hunger, irritability, headache, hypovolemia, and hypoglycemia, in surgical patients (Smith, Vallance, & Slater,1997; Yogendran, Asokumar, Cheng, & Chung, 1995). Crenshaw and Winslow (2002) have found that despite the formulation of national guidelines developed by the American Society of Anesthesiologist Task Force on Preoperative Fasting, patients were still being instructed to fast too long before surgery (Crenshaw & Winslow, 2002). In fact, patients may safely consume clear liquids up to 2 hours before elective surgery using general anesthesia, regional anesthesia, or sedation anesthesia (American Society of Anesthesiologists, 2011).

End-of-Life Patients

Maintaining or withholding fluids at the end of life remains a controversial issue. Proponents suggest that dehydration in the terminally ill patient is not painful and lessens other noxious symptoms of terminal illness, such as excessive pulmonary secretions, nausea, edema, and pain (dehydration acts as a natural anesthetic; Fainsinger & Bruera, 1997). Some suggest additional benefit from the decreased need to stand up to use the restroom and receive bedpans or diaper changes, which could be difficult or painful for someone at the end of life.

Opponents to this position suggest that associated symptoms of dehydration, such as acute confusion and delirium, are stressful and reduce the quality of life for the terminally ill older adult (Bruera, Belzile, Watanabe, & Fainsinger, 1996). Most research that has been done with terminally ill patients with cancer has examined discomforts of dehydration, including thirst, dry mouth, and agitated delirium. However, research has not demonstrated a link between biochemical markers of dehydration and these various symptoms in terminally ill patients (Burge, 1993; Ellershaw, Sutcliffe, & Saunders, 1995; Morita, Tei, Tsunoda, Inoue, & Chihara, 2001). It is suggested that several confounding factors influence the uncomfortable dehydration-like symptoms that accompany the end of life. These include use and dosage of opiates, type and location of cancer, hyperosmolality, stomatitis, and oral breathing (Morita et al., 2001). On the other hand, Bruera et al. (1996) have determined that small amounts of fluids delivered subcutaneously via hypodermoclysis plus opioid rotation was effective in decreasing delirium and antipsychotic use and did not cause edema in terminally ill patients. A 2-day pilot study of parenteral hydration in terminally ill patients with cancer led to statistically significant decreases in hallucination, myoclonus, fatigue, and sedation (Bruera et al., 2005). However, research suggests that artificial hydration does not prolong life (Bruera et al., 2005, 2012; Meier, Ahronheim, Morris, Baskin-Lyons, & Morrison, 2001; Mitchell, Kiely, & Lipsitz, 1997).

Therefore, it is recommended that maintaining or withholding fluids at the end of life be an individual decision that should be based on the etiology of illness, use of medications, presence of delirium, and family and patient preferences (Fainsinger & Bruera, 1997; Morita et al., 2001; Schmidlin, 2008). Schmidlin (2008) recommended early discussions with patients and family on their wishes as well as educating patients on the current knowledge about artificial hydration so that proper patient-centered care will be provided.

Hydration Habits

Hydration habits may indicate the level of risk for dehydration in older adults. Some hydration habits may have developed over a lifetime, and others are adaptations to current health status. Four major categories of hydration habits have been identified (Mentes, 2006). The categories include those older adults who "can drink," "cannot drink," "will not drink," and older adults who are at the "end of life." For example, older adults who can drink are those who are functionally capable of accessing and consuming fluids but who may not know what is an adequate intake or may forget to drink secondary to cognitive impairment; older adults who cannot drink are those who are physically incapable of accessing or safely consuming fluids related to physical frailty or difficulty in swallowing; older adults who will not drink are those who are capable of consuming fluids safely but who do not because of concerns about being able to reach the toilet with or without assistance or who relate that they have never consumed many fluids; and older adults who are terminally ill comprise the end-of-life category. Understanding hydration habits of older adults can help nurses to plan appropriate interventions to improve or ensure adequate intake (Mentes, 2006).

Indicators of Hydration Status

A priority for nursing, regardless of clinical setting, is the prevention of dehydration. Unfortunately, many of the standard tests for detection of dehydration only confirm a diagnosis of dehydration after it is too late to prevent the episode. In our fast-paced nursing environments, it is difficult to monitor the fluid intake of all our older patients. In using any measure for detection of impending or current dehydration, serial measures offer the greatest likelihood of accuracy (Mentes, 2006). Many studies have used a single test— either biochemical or clinical signs/symptoms— which have insufficient evidence to support diagnostic accuracy (Hooper et al., 2015). Although controversial, urine color and specific gravity have been shown to be reliable indicators of hydration status (not dehydration) in older individuals with adequate renal function in nursing homes and a Veterans Administration Medical Center (Culp, Mentes, & Wakefield, 2003; Mentes, Wakefield, & Culp, 2006). Specifically, the use of urine color, as measured by a urine color chart, can be helpful in monitoring hydration status (Armstrong et al., 1994; Mentes & IVANRC, 2000). The urine color chart has eight standardized colors ranging from *pale straw* (number 1) to *greenish brown* (number 8), approximating urine-specific gravities of 1.003 to 1.029 (Armstrong et al., 1994). The urine color chart is most effective when an individual's average urine color is calculated over several days for an individual referent value. If the older person's urine becomes darker from his or her average color, further assessment into recent intake and health status can be conducted and fluids can be adjusted to improve hydration status before dehydration occurs. Limitations in using urine indices to estimate specific gravity include (a) certain medications and foods can discolor the urine (Mentes, Wakefield, & Culp, 2006; Wakefield, Mentes, Diggelmann, & Culp, 2002), (b) persons must be able to give a urine specimen for color evaluation, and (c) best results in the use of urine color as an indicator have been documented in older adults with adequate renal function (Mentes et al., 2006). In addition, the timing of collection of urine is also important. In a recent study of younger adults, Perrier et al. (2013) found that a late afternoon (between 4:00 and 8:00 p.m.) specimen best reflected overall hydration status as measured by urine osmolality when compared to a 24-hour urine collection. This would need to be tested with a sample of older adults.

Bioelectrical impedance analysis (BIA) is a measurement that has been used mostly in the fitness industry to estimate body composition, including body mass index (BMI), TBW, and intracellular and extracellular water. Several nursing studies have used impedance measurements to estimate TBW and intracellular and extracellular water (Culp et al., 2003, 2004). Although mostly used in research, BIA is a noninvasive, reliable method used to estimate body water (Ritz & Source Study, 2001). Because TBW is dependent on weight and body composition, this measure is best used after a baseline value of TBW, intracellular, and extracellular fluid in liters has been documented. Then, deviations from the individual baseline can be noted. In a recent Cochrane Review for diagnostic accuracy, a single measure of bioelectrical impedance with resistance at 50 Hz was found to be diagnostic of impending dehydration in two studies and equivocal in two studies (Hooper et al., 2015).

Salivary osmolality is an emerging clinical indicator of hydration status that is sensitive in younger healthy adults (Oliver, Laing, Wilson, Bilzon, & Walsh, 2008) and has been tested in a small sample of nursing home residents (Woods & Mentes, 2011) and older hospitalized adults with a mean age of 78 years (Fortes et al., 2015). Salivary osmolality demonstrated 70% sensitivity and 68% specificity for water-loss dehydration as well as 78% sensitivity and 72% specificity for water and solute dehydration in this study (Fortes et al., 2015).

Indicators of Dehydration

Dehydration is the loss of body water from intracellular and interstitial fluid compartments that is associated with hypertonicity (Mange et al., 1997). Therefore, the most reliable indicators of dehydration are elevated serum sodium, serum osmolality, and BUN/creatinine ratio

TABLE 9.3

Approximate Ranges of Laboratory Tests for Hydration Status

Test	Value Ranges for	
	Impending Dehydration	Dehydration
BUN/creatinine ratio	20–24	> 25
Serum osmolality	normal 280–300 mmol/kg	> 300 mmol/kg
Serum sodium		> 150 mEq/L
Urine osmolality		> 1,050 mmol/kg
Urine-specific gravity	1.020–1.029	> 1.029
Urine color	dark yellow	greenish brown
Amount of urine	800–1,200 mL/d	> 800 mL/d

BUN, blood urea nitrogen.

Sources: Armstrong et al. (1994, 1998); Mentes, Wakefield, and Culp (2006); Metheny (2000); Wakefield, Mentes, Diggelmann, and Culp (2002); Wallach (2000). Adapted with permission from Mentes and Kang (2011).

(Table 9.3). The most common clinical assessments of dehydration include the presence of dry oral mucous membranes, tongue furrows, decreased saliva, sunken eyes, decreased urine output, upper body weakness, a rapid pulse (Gross et al., 1992), and tongue dryness (Vivanti, Harvey, & Ash, 2010; Vivanti, Harvey, Ash, & Battististutta, 2008). Decreased axillary sweat production as a clinical sign of dehydration has produced contradictory results, making it an unreliable indicator of dehydration (Eaton, Bannister, Mulley, & Connolly, 1994; Gross et al., 1992). Assessment of sternal skin turgor as a sign of dehydration has been a mainstay in nursing practice; however, it is also an ambiguous indicator for dehydration in older individuals, with some researchers finding it unreliable because of age-related changes in skin elasticity (Gross et al., 1992) and others finding it reliable (Chassagne, Druesne, Capet, Ménard, & Bercoff, 2006; Vivanti et al., 2008). From a systematic review, Hooper et al. (2015) found that the clinical symptoms/signs of "expressing fatigue" and "missing drinks between meals" were the only measures with the ability to diagnose impending and current dehydration.

In conclusion, Hooper at al. (2015) found that three single tests versus serial testing showed ability to diagnose impending and current dehydration, including expressing fatigue, missing drinks between meals, and BIA with a resistance of 50 Hz. It was further concluded that a combination of two tests—fatigue and missing drinks—further increased diagnostic accuracy.

CASE STUDY

Mrs. Chung is an 87-year-old Chinese American woman who was admitted to the hospital for observation secondary to an episode of dehydration. She has resided at Sunny Days Assisted Living Facility for the past month. Staff describe her as fiercely independent despite experiencing some declines in her health recently. Her medical diagnoses include hypertension, for which she receives atenolol 25 mg daily and enalapril 20 mg daily; status post–mild cerebrovascular accident (CVA) with residual left-sided weakness, for which she is taking 80 mg of aspirin daily; osteoarthritis, for which she takes Tylenol Extra Strength twice daily; and cataracts, for which she is reluctant to have surgery. She is cognitively intact and requires only minor assistance with bathing.

Before hospitalization, Mrs. Chung had become more withdrawn and concerned about her health. Her family noticed that she has altered some of her daily routines. For example, she eliminated her daily tea because she finds it difficult to use the new microwave at the assisted care facility (ACF) to heat her water because of unfamiliarity. She stays in her bed much of the day, complaining that she does not have any energy. When questioned, she reluctantly admits that she has been having more problems with her long-standing urinary incontinence and she is afraid to leave her room because she is fearful that she will not be able to make it to a bathroom on time. Consequently, she has further restricted the amount of fluid that she consumes on a daily basis.

Mrs. Chung is at high risk of dehydration given that she has recently begun to restrict her fluids because of unfamiliarity with the microwave to heat her water for tea. Older adults from different cultures may wish to have their beverages served at different temperatures. Especially when ill, ethnic older adults may prefer to have warmed beverages. In addition, Mrs. Chung is "treating" her urinary incontinence by restricting her fluids, which places her at risk for dehydration and urinary tract infections. This scenario is not uncommon in older adults struggling to maintain independence. One of the major reasons for admission to a nursing home is the presence of urinary incontinence. Finally, there is some evidence that Mrs. Chung is depressed, which would also place her at risk for dehydration often secondary to decreased food and fluid intake. Additional risk

(continued)

CASE STUDY *(continued)*

factors include her age (87 years old), gender, and use of an angiotensin-converting enzyme (ACE) inhibitor, which acts on the renin–angiotensin–aldosterone (RAA) system.

Discussion

Interventions to prevent dehydration in Mrs. Chung would include evaluating her for a urinary tract infection and offering her an evaluation for her urinary incontinence that could include use of medications, if indicated; use of behavioral strategies, including urge inhibition (strategies to prolong urge to urinate) and/or Kegel exercises. Education around the importance of maintaining adequate fluid intake to minimize urinary incontinence is indicated, which should include a discussion about the amount of daily fluids required and the provision of a graduated cup to help her ascertain appropriate amounts. Helping her simplify the use of the microwave and/or attendance at social events at the ACF where fluids are provided could be implemented. Lastly, an evaluation for depression may be indicated if the previous interventions do not improve her mood.

SUMMARY

Dehydration in older adults is a costly yet preventable health problem. Best practices for hydration management have been identified primarily in the nursing home population. They include providing access to fluids at all times, regularly offering fluids throughout the day, assessing fluid preferences and providing the fluid of choice, and appropriate supervision of personnel who will be providing the fluids. Nursing personnel should assess the older adult's ability to self-manage hydration habits as well as preventing extended periods of time when the older adult does not have access to fluids (as in fasting for a diagnostic test). Regularly offering fluids through fluid rounds, a beverage cart, or other novel means, such as tea time, is another principle of good hydration practices. Accommodating older peoples' preferences for type of beverage and appropriate temperature of beverage has been shown to increase fluid intake. Lastly, appropriate supervision of how much fluid per day is required and how assistance is given to older adults who are not capable of drinking themselves to ensure that required amounts are consumed is also the key in maintaining adequate hydration. Attention to concerns about toileting is another important issue in helping older adults to maintain adequate hydration. The hydration practices of healthier, community-dwelling older adults are less well known and require further study.

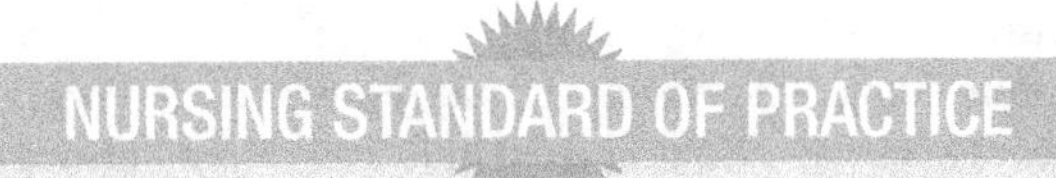

Protocol 9.1: Managing Oral Hydration

I. GOAL

Minimize episodes of dehydration in older adults

II. OVERVIEW

Maintaining adequate fluid balance is an essential component of health across the life span; older adults are more vulnerable to shifts in water balance, both overhydration and dehydration, because of age-related changes and increased likelihood that an older individual has several medical conditions. Dehydration is the more frequently occurring problem.

III. BACKGROUND AND STATEMENT OF THE PROBLEM

A. Definitions
   1. *Dehydration* is depletion in TBW content caused by pathological fluid losses, diminished water intake, or a combination of both. It results in hypernatremia (more than 145 mEq/L) in the extracellular fluid compartment, which draws water from the intracellular fluids (Metheny, 2000). The water loss is shared by all body-fluid compartments and relatively little reduction in extracellular fluids occurs. Thus, circulation is not compromised unless the loss is very large.

(continued)

Protocol 9.1: Managing Oral Hydration *(continued)*

2. *Underhydration* is a precursor condition to dehydration associated with insidious onset and poor outcomes (Mentes & Culp, 2003). Others have referred to this condition as *mild dehydration* (Stookey, 2005; Stookey et al., 2005) or *chronic dehydration* (Bennett et al., 2004).

B. Etiologic factors associated with dehydration
   1. Age-related changes in body composition with resulting decrease in TBW (Bossingham et al., 2005; Lavizzo-Mourey et al., 1988; Metheny, 2000)
   2. Decreasing renal function (Lindeman, Tobin, & Shock, 1985)
   3. Lack of thirst (Farrell et al., 2008; Kenney & Chiu, 2001; Mack et al., 1994; Miescher & Fortney, 1989; Phillips et al., 1991, 1984)
   4. Poor tolerance for hot weather (Josseran et al., 2009)

C. Risk factors
   1. Patient characteristics
      a. Older than 85 years of age (Ciccone et al., 1998; Gaspar, 1999; Lavizzo-Mourey et al., 1988)
      b. Female (Gaspar, 1988; Lavizzo-Mourey et al., 1988)
      c. Semi-dependent in eating (Gaspar, 1999)
      d. Functionally more independent (Gaspar, 1999; Mentes & Culp, 2003)
      e. Few fluid ingestion opportunities (Gaspar, 1988, 1999)
      f. Inadequate nutrient intake (Gaspar, 1999)
      g. Alzheimer's disease or other dementias (Albert, Nakra, Grossberg, & Caminal, 1989, 1994)
      h. Four or more chronic conditions (Lavizzo-Mourey et al., 1988)
      i. Four medications (Lavizzo-Mourey et al., 1988)
      j. Fever (Pals et al., 1995; Weinberg et al., 1994)
      k. Vomiting and diarrhea (Wakefield, Mentes, Holman, & Culp, 2008)
      l. Individuals with infections (Warren et al., 1994)
      m. Individuals who have had prior episodes of dehydration (Mentes, 2006)
      n. Diuretics: thiazide (Wakefield et al., 2008), loop and thiazide (Lancaster et al., 2003)
   2. Staff and family characteristics
      a. Inadequate staff and professional supervision (Kayser-Jones, Schell, Porter, Barbaccia, & Shaw, 1999)
      b. Depression or loneliness associated with decreased fluid intake as identified by nursing staff (Mentes, Chang, & Morris, 2006)
      c. Family or caregivers not spending time with patient (Mentes et al., 2006)

IV. PARAMETERS OF ASSESSMENT

A. Health history (Mentes & IVANRC, 2000)
   1. Specific disease states: dementia, congestive heart failure, chronic renal disease, malnutrition, and psychiatric disorders such as depression (Albert et al., 1989; Gaspar, 1988; Warren et al., 1994)
   2. Presence of comorbidities: more than four chronic health conditions (Lavizzo-Mourey et al., 1988)
   3. Prescription drugs: number and types (Lavizzo-Mourey et al., 1988)
   4. Past history of dehydration, repeated infections (Mentes, 2006)

B. Physical assessments (Mentes & IVANRC, 2000)
   1. Vital signs
   2. Height and weight
   3. BMI (Vivanti et al., 2008)
   4. Review of systems
   5. Indicators of hydration
   6. Chief complaint of fatigue (Hooper et al., 2015)

C. Laboratory tests
   1. Urine-specific gravity (Mentes, 2006; Wakefield et al., 2002)

(continued)

Protocol 9.1: Managing Oral Hydration *(continued)*

2. Urine color (Mentes, 2006; Wakefield et al., 2002)
3. BUN/creatinine ratio
4. Serum sodium
5. Serum osmolality and a serum osmolality estimation equation based on serum measures of urea, glucose, sodium, and potassium (Siervo, Bunn, Prado, & Hooper, 2014)
6. Salivary osmolality (Fortes et al., 2015)

D. Individual fluid-intake behaviors (Mentes, 2006)
  1. Won't drink subcategory of hydration patterns (Mentes, 2006)
  2. Missing drinks between meals (Hooper et al., 2015)

V. NURSING CARE STRATEGIES

A. Risk identification (Mentes & IVANRC, 2000)
  1. Identify acute situations: vomiting, diarrhea, or febrile episodes
  2. Use a tool to evaluate risk: Dehydration Risk Appraisal Checklist (Mentes & Wang, 2010)

B. Acute hydration management
  1. Monitor input and output (Weinberg et al., 1994).
  2. Provide additional fluids as tolerated (Weinberg et al., 1994).
  3. Minimize fasting times for diagnostic and surgical procedures ("Practice Guidelines for Preoperative Fasting," 1999).

C. Ongoing hydration management
  1. Calculate a daily fluid goal (see Table 9.3; Mentes & IVANRC, 2000).
  2. Compare current intake to fluid goal (Mentes & IVANRC, 2000).
  3. Provide fluids consistently throughout the day (Ferry, 2005; Simmons, Alessi, & Schnelle, 2001).
  4. Plan for at-risk individuals:
     a. Fluid rounds (Robinson & Rosher, 2002)
     b. Provide two 8-oz glasses of fluid, one in the morning the other in the evening (Robinson & Rosher, 2002).
     c. "Happy hours" to promote increased intake (Musson et al., 1990)
     d. "Tea time" to increase fluid intake (Mueller & Boisen, 1989)
     e. Offer a variety of fluids throughout the day (Simmons et al., 2001) with attention to resident's preferred beverage (Bunn, Jimoh, Wilsher, & Hooper, 2015).
  5. Increase staff awareness of the importance of adequate hydration (Bunn et al., 2015).
  6. Encourage staff to provide increased assistance with drinking and reminders as well as assistance with toileting (Bunn et al., 2015).
  7. Fluid regulation and documentation
     a. Teach able individuals to use a urine color chart to monitor hydration status (Armstrong et al., 1994, 1998; Mentes, 2006).
     b. Document a complete intake recording, including hydration habits (Mentes & IVANRC, 2000).
     c. If resident is cognitively intact (MMSE > 27 consider using the Drinks Diary (Jimoh, Bunn, & Hooper, 2015).
     d. Know volumes of fluid containers to accurately calculate fluid consumption (Burns, 1992; Hart & Adamek, 1984).

VI. EVALUATION AND EXPECTED OUTCOMES

A. Maintenance of body hydration (Mentes & Culp, 2003; Robinson & Rosher, 2002; Simmons et al., 2001)
B. Decreased infections, especially urinary tract infections (McConnell, 1984; Mentes & Culp, 2003; Robinson & Rosher, 2002)
C. Improvement in urinary incontinence (Spangler, Risley, & Bilyew, 1984)
D. Lowered urinary pH (Hart & Adamek, 1984)

(continued)

Protocol 9.1: Managing Oral Hydration *(continued)*

E. Decreased constipation (Robinson & Rosher, 2002)
F. Decreased acute confusion (Mentes et al., 1999)

VII. FOLLOW-UP MONITORING OF CONDITION

A. Urine color chart monitoring in patients with better renal function (Armstrong et al., 1994, 1998; Wakefield et al., 2002)
B. Urine-specific gravity checks (Armstrong et al., 1994, 1998; Wakefield et al., 2002)
C. Twenty-four-hour intake recording (Metheny, 2000)
D. Drinks Diary to document fluid intake in individuals who are cognitively intact (Jimoh et al., 2015)

VIII. RELEVANT PRACTICE GUIDELINES

A. Hydration management evidence-based protocol available from the University of Iowa College of Nursing Gerontological Nursing Interventions Research Center, Research Dissemination Core. Author: Janet Mentes, revised 2010.

ABBREVIATIONS

BMI	Body mass index
BUN	Blood urea nitrogen
IVANRC	Iowa–Veterans Affairs Nursing Research Consortium
MMSE	Mini-Mental State Examination
TBW	Total body water

NOTE

1. Portions of this chapter were adapted with permission from Mentes, J. C., & Kang, S. (2011). Evidence-based protocol: Hydration management. In M. G. Titler (Series Ed.), *Series on evidence-based practice for older adults*. Iowa City, IA: University of Iowa College of Nursing Gerontological Nursing Interventions Research Center, Research Translation and Dissemination Core.

RESOURCES

Evidence-based website for geriatric nursing sponsored by the Hartford Institute for Geriatric Nursing
www.consultgerirn.org

Hydration for Health sponsored by Danone Waters
www.healthyhydrationcoach.com

Dr. Lee Hooper's study website
driestudy.appspot.com

University of Iowa Evidence-Based Protocols
www.nursing.uiowa.edu/excellence/evidence-based-practice-guidelines

REFERENCES

Ainslie, P. N., Campbell, I. T., Frayn, K. N., Humphreys, S. M., MacLaren, D. P., Reilly, T., & Westerterp, K. R. (2002). Energy balance, metabolism, hydration, and performance during strenuous hill walking: The effect of age. *Journal of Applied Physiology, 93*(2), 714–723. *Evidence Level III.*

Albert, S. G., Nakra, B. R., Grossberg, G. T., & Caminal, E. R. (1989). Vasopressin response to dehydration in Alzheimer's disease. *Journal of the American Geriatrics Society, 37*(9), 843–847. *Evidence Level III.*

Albert, S. G., Nakra, B. R., Grossberg, G. T., & Caminal, E. R. (1994). Drinking behavior and vasopressin responses to hyperosmolality in Alzheimer's disease. *International Psychogeriatrics, 6*(1), 79–86. *Evidence Level III.*

American Society of Anesthesiologists. (1999). Practice guidelines for preoperative fasting and the use of pharmacologic agents to reduce the risk of pulmonary aspiration: Application to health patients undergoing elective procedures: A report by the American Society of Anesthesiologist Task Force on Preoperative Fasting. *Anesthesiology, 90*(3), 896–905. *Evidence Level I.*

American Society of Anesthesiologists. (2011). Practice guidelines for preoperative fasting and the use of pharmacologic agents to reduce the risk of pulmonary aspiration: Application to healthy patients undergoing elective procedures: An updated report by the American Society of Anesthesiologists Committee on Standards and Practice Parameters. *Anesthesiology, 114,* 495–511. doi:10.1097/ALN.0b013e3181fcbfd9. *Evidence Level I.*

Armstrong, L. E., Maresh, C. M., Castellani, J. W., Bergeron, M. F., Kenefick, R. W., LaGasse, K. E., & Riebe, D. (1994). Urinary indices of hydration status. *International Journal of Sport Nutrition, 4*(3), 265–279. *Evidence Level IV.*

Armstrong, L. E., Soto, J. A., Hacker, F. T., Jr., Casa, D. J., Kavouras, S. A., & Maresh, C. M. (1998). Urinary indices during dehydration, exercise, and rehydration. *International Journal of Sport Nutrition, 8*(4), 345–355. *Evidence Level IV.*

Batscha, C. L. (1997). Heat stroke. Keeping your clients cool in the summer. *Journal of Psychosocial Nursing and Mental Health Services, 35*(7), 12–17. *Evidence Level V.*

Beaujean, D. J., Blok, H. E., Vandenbroucke-Grauls, C. M., Weersink. A. J., Raymakers, J. A., & Verhoef, J. (1997). Surveillance of nosocomial infections in geriatric patients. *Journal of Hospital Infection, 36*(4), 275–284. *Evidence Level IV.*

Bennett, J. A., Thomas, V., & Riegel, B. (2004). Unrecognized chronic dehydration in older adults: Examining prevalence rate and risk factors. *Journal of Gerontological Nursing, 30*(11), 22–28; quiz 52–23. *Evidence Level IV.*

Bossingham, M. J., Carnell, N. S., & Campbell, W. W. (2005). Water balance, hydration status, and fat-free mass hydration in younger and older adults. *American Journal of Clinical Nutrition, 81*(6), 1342–1350. *Evidence Level II.*

Bristow, M. F., & Kohen, D. (1996). Neuroleptic malignant syndrome. *British Journal of Hospital Medicine, 55*(8), 517–520. *Evidence Level V.*

Bruera, E., Belzile, M., Watanabe, S., & Fainsinger, R. L. (1996). Volume of hydration in terminal cancer patients. *Supportive Care in Cancer, 4*(2), 147–150. *Evidence Level IV.*

Bruera, E., Hui, D., Dalal, S., Torres-Vigil, I., Trumble, J. Roosth, J., . . . Tarleton, K. (2012). Parenteral hydration in patients with advanced cancer: A multi-center, double-blind, placebo-controlled randomized trial. *Journal of Clinical Oncology, 31,* 111–118. doi:10.1200/JCO.2012.44.6518. *Evidence Level II.*

Bruera, E., Sala, R., Rico, M. A., Moyano, J., Centeno, C., Willey, J., & Palmer, J. L. (2005). Effects of parenteral hydration in terminally ill cancer patients: A preliminary study. *Journal of Clinical Oncology, 23*(10), 2366–2371. *Evidence Level III.*

Bunn, D., Jimoh, F., Wilsher, S. H., & Hooper, L. (2015). Increasing fluid intake and reducing dehydration risk in older people living in long-term care: A systematic review. *Journal of the American Medical Directors Association, 16,* 101–113. doi:10.1016/j.jamda.2014.10.016. *Evidence Level I.*

Burge, F. I. (1993). Dehydration symptoms of palliative care cancer patients. *Journal of Pain Symptom Management, 8*(7), 454–464. *Evidence Level IV.*

Burns, D. (1992). Working up a thirst. *Nursing Times, 88*(26), 44–45. *Evidence Level IV.*

Butler, A. M., & Talbot, N. B. (1944). Parenteral fluid therapy. *New England Journal of Medicine, 231,* 585–590. *Evidence Level VI.*

Chan, J., Knutsen, S. F., Blix, G. G., Lee, G. W., & Fraser, G. E. (2002). Water, other fluids, and fatal coronary heart disease: The Adventist Health Study. *American Journal of Epidemiology, 155*(9), 827–833. *Evidence Level IV.*

Chassagne, P., Druesne, L., Capet, C., Ménard, J. F., & Bercoff, E. (2006). Clinical presentation of hypernatremia in elderly patients: A case control study. *Journal of the American Geriatrics Society, 54*(8), 1225–1230. *Evidence Level IV.*

Chernoff, R. (1994). Meeting the nutritional needs of the elderly in the institutional setting. *Nutrition Reviews, 52*(4), 132–136. *Evidence Level VI.*

Chidester, J. C., & Spangler, A. A. (1997). Fluid intake in the institutionalized elderly. *Journal of the American Dietetic Association, 97*(1), 23–28; quiz 29–30. *Evidence Level IV.*

Ciccone, A., Allegra, J. R., Cochrane, D. G., Cody, R. P., & Roche, L. M. (1998). Age-related differences in diagnoses within the elderly population. *American Journal of Emergency Medicine, 16*(1), 43–48. *Evidence Level IV.*

Cosgray, R., Davidhizar, R., Giger, J. N., & Kreisl, R. (1993). A program for water-intoxicated patients at a state hospital. *Clinical Nurse Specialist, 7*(2), 55–61. *Evidence Level V.*

Crenshaw, J. T., & Winslow, E. H. (2002). Preoperative fasting: Old habits die hard. *American Journal of Nursing, 102*(5), 36–44. *Evidence Level IV.*

Culp, K., Mentes, J., & Wakefield, B. (2003). Hydration and acute confusion in long-term care residents. *Western Journal of Nursing Research, 25*(3), 251–266; discussion 267–273. *Evidence Level IV.*

Culp, K. R., Wakefield, B., Dyck, M. J., Cacchione, P. Z., DeCrane, S., & Decker, S. (2004). Bioelectrical impedance analysis and other hydration parameters as risk factors for delirium in rural nursing home residents. *Journals of Gerontology. Series A, Biological Sciences and Medical Sciences, 59*(8), 813–817. *Evidence Level II.*

Doucet, J., Jego, A., Noel, D., Geffroy, C. E., Capet, C., Couffin, E., . . . Bercoff, E. (2002). Preventable and non-preventable risk factors for adverse drug events related to hospital admission in the elderly: A prospective study. *Clinical Drug Investigations, 22*(6), 385–392. *Evidence Level IV.*

Eaton, D., Bannister, P., Mulley, G. P., & Connolly, M. J. (1994). Axillary sweating in clinical assessment of dehydration in ill elderly patients. *British Medical Journal, 308*(6939), 1271. *Evidence Level IV.*

Ellershaw, J. E., Sutcliffe, J. M., & Saunders, C. M. (1995). Dehydration and the dying patient. *Journal of Pain Symptom Management, 10*(3), 192–197. *Evidence Level IV.*

El-Sharkawy, A. M., Shahota, O., Maughan, R. J., & Lobo, D. W. (2014). Hydration in the older hospital patient—Is it a problem? *Age & Ageing, 43,* i33–i35. doi:10.1093/ageing/afu046. *Evidence Level IV.*

Fainsinger, R. L., & Bruera, E. (1997). When to treat dehydration in a terminally ill patient? *Supportive Care in Cancer, 5*(3), 205–211. *Evidence Level VI.*

Farrell, M. J., Zamarripa, F., Shade, R., Phillips, P. A., McKinley, M., Fox, P. T., . . . Egan, G. F. (2008). Effect of aging on regional cerebral blood flow responses associated with osmotic thirst and its satiation by water drinking: A PET study. *Proceedings of the National Academy of Sciences of the United States of America, 105*(1), 382–387. *Evidence Level III.*

Ferry, M. (2005). Strategies for ensuring good hydration in the elderly. *Nutrition Reviews, 63*(6 Pt. 2), S22–S29. *Evidence Level VI.*

Foreman, M. D. (1989). Confusion in the hospitalized elderly: Incidence, onset, and associated factors. *Research in Nursing & Health, 12*(1), 21–29. *Evidence Level III.*

Fortes, M. B., Owen, J. A., Raymond-Barker, P., Bishop, C., Elghenzai, S., Oliver, S. J., & Walsh, N. P. (2015). Is this elderly patient dehydrated? Diagnostic accuracy of hydration assessment using physical signs, urine and saliva markers. *Journal of American Medical Directors Association, 16,* 221–228. doi:10.1016/j.jamda.2014.09.012. *Evidence Level IV.*

Frangeskou, M., Lopez-Valcarcel, B., & Serra-Majem, L. (2015). Dehydration in the elderly: A review focused on economic burden. *Journal of Nutrition Health and Aging, 19*(6), 619–627. *Evidence Level V.*

Gaspar, P. M. (1988). What determines how much patients drink? *Geriatric Nursing, 9*(4), 221–224. *Evidence Level IV.*

Gaspar, P. M. (1999). Water intake of nursing home residents. *Journal of Gerontological Nursing, 25*(4), 23–29. *Evidence Level IV.*

Gaspar, P. M. (2011). Comparison of four standards for determining adequate water intake of nursing home residents. *Research and Theory for Nursing Practice: An International Journal, 25*(1), 11–22. doi:10.1891/0889-7182.25.1.11. *Evidence Level IV.*

Gordon, J. A., An, L. C., Hayward, R. A., & Williams, B. C. (1998). Initial emergency department diagnosis and return visits: Risk versus perception. *Annals of Emergency Medicine, 32*(5), 569–573. *Evidence Level IV.*

Gross, C. R., Lindquist, R. D., Woolley, A. C., Granieri, R., Allard, K., & Webster, B. (1992). Clinical indicators of dehydration severity in elderly patients. *Journal of Emergency Medicine, 10*(3), 267–274. *Evidence Level IV.*

Hart, M., & Adamek, C. (1984). Do increased fluids decrease urinary stone formation? *Geriatric Nursing, 5*(6), 245–248. *Evidence Level III.*

Hodgkinson, B., Evans, D., & Wood, J. (2003). Maintaining oral hydration in older adults: A systematic review. *International Journal of Nursing Practices, 9*(3), S19–S28. *Evidence Level I.*

Hooper, L., Attreed, N. J., Campbell, W. W., Channell, A. M., Chassagne, P., Culp, K., . . . Hunter, P. (2011). Clinical and physical signs for identification of impending and current water-loss dehydration in older people [Protocol]. *Cochrane Database of Systematic Reviews, 2011*(2), CD009647. doi:10.1002/14651858.CD009647. *Evidence Level I.*

Hooper, L., Attreed, N. J., Campbell, W. W., Channell, A. M., Chassagne, P., Culp, K. R., . . . Hunter, P. (2015). Clinical symptoms, signs and tests for identification of impending and current water loss dehydration in older adults (1007). *Cochrane Database of Systematic Reviews, (4),* CD009647. doi:10.1002/14651858CD009647.Pub2. *Evidence Level I.*

Hooper, L., Bunn, D., Jimoh, F. O., & Fairweather-Tait, S. J. (2013). Water-loss dehydration and aging. *Mechanisms of Aging and Development, 136–137,* 50–58. doi:10.1016/jmad.2013.11.009. *Evidence Level V.*

Jacobs, L. G. (1996). The neuroleptic malignant syndrome: Often an unrecognized geriatric problem. *Journal of the American Geriatrics Society, 44*(4), 474–475. *Evidence Level V.*

Jimoh, F. O., Bunn, D., & Hooper, L. (2015). Assessment of a self-reported drinks diary for the estimation of drinks intake by care home residents: Fluid intake study in the elderly (FISE). *Journal of Nutrition, Health and Aging, 19*(5), 491–496. Advance online publication. Retrieved from http://download.springer.com/static/pdf/256/art%253A10.1007%252Fs12603-015-0458-3.pdf?auth66=1426368021_a358fe3ba2bbbe43e4f822e2e04eebb7&ext=.pdf. *Evidence Level IV.*

Josseran, L., Caillère, N., Brun-Ney, D., Rottner, J., Filleul, L., Brucker, G., & Astagneau, P. (2009). Syndromic surveillance and heat wave morbidity: A pilot study based on emergency departments in France. *BMC Medical Informatics and Decision Making, 9,* 14. *Evidence Level IV.*

Kayser-Jones, J., Schell, E. S., Porter, C., Barbaccia, J. C., & Shaw, H. (1999). Factors contributing to dehydration in nursing homes: Inadequate staffing and lack of professional supervision. *Journal of the American Geriatrics Society, 47*(10), 1187–1194. *Evidence Level IV.*

Kelly, J., Hunt, B. J., Lewis, R. R., Swaminathan, R., Moody, A., Seed, P. T., & Rudd, A. (2004). Dehydration and venous thromboembolism after acute stroke. *QJM: Monthly Journal of the Association of Physicians, 97*(5), 293–296. *Evidence Level IV.*

Kenney, W. L., & Chiu, P. (2001). Influence of age on thirst and fluid intake. *Medicine and Science in Sports and Exercise, 33*(9), 1524–1532. *Evidence Level V.*

Lancaster, K. J., Smiciklas-Wright, H., Heller, D. A., Ahern, F. M., & Jensen, G. (2003). Dehydration in black and white older adults using diuretics. *Annals of Epidemiology, 13*(7), 525–529. *Evidence Level IV.*

Lavizzo-Mourey, R., Johnson, J., & Stolley, P. (1988). Risk factors for dehydration among elderly nursing home residents. *Journal of the American Geriatrics Society, 36*(3), 213–218. *Evidence Level IV.*

Leibovitz, A., Baumoehl, Y., Lubart, E., Yaina, A., Platinovitz, N., & Segal, R. (2007). Dehydration among long-term care elderly patients with oropharyngeal dysphagia. *Gerontology, 53*(4), 179–183. *Evidence Level IV.*

Lin, L., Lee, J., Hung, Y., Chang, C., & Yang, J. (2014). BUN/creatinine ratio-based hydration for preventing stroke-in-evolution after acute ischemic stroke. *American Journal of Emergency Medicine, 32,* 709–712. doi:10.1016/j.ajem.2014.03.045. *Evidence Level III.*

Lindeman, R. D., Tobin, J., & Shock, N. W. (1985). Longitudinal studies on the rate of decline in renal function with age. *Journal of the American Geriatrics Society, 33*(4), 278–285. *Evidence Level IV.*

Macias-Nuñez, J. F. (2008). The normal ageing kidney–morphology and physiology. *Reviews in Clinical Gerontology, 18,* 175–197. *Evidence Level V.*

Mack, G. W., Weseman, C. A., Langhans, G. W., Scherzer, H., Gillen, C. M., & Nadel, E. R. (1994). Body fluid balance in dehydrated healthy older men: Thirst and renal osmoregulation. *Journal of Applied Physiology, 76*(4), 1615–1623. *Evidence Level III.*

Mange, K., Matsuura, D., Cizman, B., Solo, H., Ziyadeh, F. N., Goldfarb, S., & Neilson, E. G. (1997). Language guiding therapy: The case of dehydration versus volume depletion. *Annals of Internal Medicine, 127*(9), 848–853. *Evidence Level V.*

Masotti, L., Ceccarelli, E., Cappelli, R., Barabesi, L., Guerrini, M., & Forconi, S. (2000). Length of hospitalization in elderly patients with community-acquired pneumonia. *Aging, 12*(1), 35–41. *Evidence Level IV.*

McConnell, J. (1984). Preventing urinary tract infections. *Geriatric Nursing, 5*(8), 361–362. *Evidence Level III.*

Meier, D. E., Ahronheim, J. C., Morris, J., Baskin-Lyons, S., & Morrison, R. S. (2001). High short-term mortality in hospitalized patients with advanced dementia: Lack of benefit of tube feeding. *Archives of Internal Medicine, 161*(4), 594–599. *Evidence Level III.*

Mentes, J. C. (2006). A typology of oral hydration problems exhibited by frail nursing home residents. *Journal of Gerontological Nursing, 32*(1), 13–19, quiz 20–21. *Evidence Level IV.*

Mentes, J. C., Chang, B. L., & Morris, J. (2006). Keeping nursing home residents hydrated. *Western Journal of Nursing Research, 28*(4), 392–406; discussion 407–418. *Evidence Level IV.*

Mentes, J. C., & Culp, K. (2003). Reducing hydration-linked events in nursing home residents. *Clinical Nursing Research, 12*(3), 210–225; discussion 226–228. *Evidence Level III.*

Mentes, J. C., Culp, K., Maas, M., & Rantz, M. (1999). Acute confusion indicators: Risk factors and prevalence using MDS data. *Research in Nursing & Health, 22*(2), 95–105. *Evidence Level IV.*

Mentes, J. C., & Iowa–Veterans Affairs Research Consortium (2000). Hydration management protocol. *Journal of Gerontological Nursing, 26*(10), 6–15. *Evidence Level I.*

Mentes, J. C., & Kang, S. (2011). Evidence-based protocol: Hydration management. In M. G. Titler (Series Ed.), *Series on evidence-based practice for older adults.* Iowa City, IA: University of Iowa College of Nursing Gerontological Nursing Interventions Research Center, Research Translation and Dissemination Core.

Mentes, J. C., Wakefield, B., & Culp, K. (2006). Use of a urine color chart to monitor hydration status in nursing home residents. *Biological Research for Nursing, 7*(3), 197–203. *Evidence Level IV.*

Mentes, J. C., & Wang, J. (2010). Measuring risk for dehydration in nursing home residents. *Research in Gerontological Nursing, 31*, 1–9. *Evidence Level IV.*

Metheny, N. (2000). *Fluid and electrolyte balance: Nursing considerations* (4th ed.). St. Louis, MO: Lippincott, Williams, & Wilkins. *Evidence Level VI.*

Michaud, D. S., Spiegelman, D., Clinton, S. K., Rimm, E. B., Curhan, G. C., Willett, W. C., & Giovannucci, E. L. (1999). Fluid intake and the risk of bladder cancer in men. *New England Journal of Medicine, 340*(18), 1390–1397. *Evidence Level IV.*

Miescher, E., & Fortney, S. M. (1989). Responses to dehydration and rehydration during heat exposure in young and older men. *American Journal of Physiology, 257*(5 Pt. 2), R1050–1056. *Evidence Level III.*

Mitchell, S. L., Kiely, D. K., & Lipsitz, L. A. (1997). The risk factors and impact on survival of feeding tube placement in nursing home residents with severe cognitive impairment. *Archives of Internal Medicine, 157*(3), 327–332. *Evidence Level III.*

Morgan, A. L., Masterson, M. M., Fahlman, M. M., Topp, R. V., & Boardley, D. (2003). Hydration status of community-dwelling seniors. *Aging Clinical and Experimental Research, 15*(4), 301–304. *Evidence Level IV.*

Morita, T., Tei, Y., Tsunoda, J., Inoue, S., & Chihara, S. (2001). Determinants of the sensation of thirst in terminally ill cancer patients. *Supportive Care in Cancer, 9*(3), 177–186. *Evidence Level IV.*

Mueller, K. D., & Boisen, A. M. (1989). Keeping your patient's water level up. *RN, 52*(7), 65–68. *Evidence Level V.*

Mukand, J. A., Cai, C., Zielinski, A., Danish, M., & Berman, J. (2003). The effects of dehydration on rehabilitation outcomes of elderly orthopedic patients. *Archives of Physical Medicine and Rehabilitation, 84*(1), 58–61. *Evidence Level IV.*

Musson, N. D., Kincaid, J., Ryan, P., Glussman, B., Varone, L., Gamarra, N., . . . Silverman, M. (1990). Nature, nurture, nutrition: Interdisciplinary programs to address the prevention of malnutrition and dehydration. *Dysphagia, 5*(2), 96–101. *Evidence Level V.*

National Research Council. (1989). *Recommended dietary allowances* (10th ed.). Washington, DC: The National Academies Press. *Evidence Level IV.*

O'Keeffe, S. T., & Lavan, J. N. (1996). Predicting delirium in elderly patients: Development and validation of a risk-stratification model. *Age and Ageing, 25*(4), 317–321. *Evidence Level IV.*

Oliver, S. J., Laing, S. J., Wilson, S., Bilzon, J. L., & Walsh, N. P. (2008). Saliva indices track hypohydration during 48h of fluid restriction or combined fluid and energy restriction. *Archives of Oral Biology, 53*(10), 975–980. *Evidence Level II.*

Pals, J. K., Weinberg, A. D., Beal, L. F., Levesque, P. G., Cunnungham, T. J., & Minaker, K. L. (1995). Clinical triggers for detection of fever and dehydration. Implications for long-term care nursing. *Journal of Gerontological Nursing, 21*(4), 13–19. *Evidence Level IV.*

Perrier, E., Demazieres, A., Girard, N., Pross, N., Osbild, D., Metzger, D., . . . Klein, A (2013). Circadian variation and responsiveness of hydration biomarkers to changes in daily water intake. *European Journal of Applied Physiology, 113*, 2143–2151. doi:10.1007/s00421-013-2649-0. *Evidence Level III.*

Phillips, P. A., Bretherton, M., Johnston, C. I., & Gray, L. (1991). Reduced osmotic thirst in healthy elderly men. *American Journal of Physiology, 261*(1 Pt. 2), R166–R171. *Evidence Level III.*

Phillips, P. A., Rolls, B. J., Ledingham, J. G., Forsling, M. L., Morton, J. J., Crowe, M. J., & Wollner, L. (1984). Reduced thirst after water deprivation in healthy elderly men. *New England Journal of Medicine, 311*(12), 753–759. *Evidence Level III.*

Raman, A., Schoeller, D., Subar, A. F., Troiano, R. P., Schatzkin, A., Harris, T., . . . Tylavsky, F. A. (2004). Water turnover in 458 American adults 40–79 yr of age. *American Journal of Physiology. Renal Physiology, 286*(2), F394–F401. *Evidence Level IV.*

Rasouli, M., Kiasari, A. M., & Arab, S. (2008). Indicators of dehydration and haemoconcentration are associated with the prevalence and severity of coronary artery disease. *Clinical and Experimental Pharmacology & Physiology, 35*(8), 889–894. *Evidence Level IV.*

Ritz, P., & Source Study. (2001). Bioelectrical impedance analysis estimation of water compartments in elderly diseased patients: The source study. *Journals of Gerontology, Series A, Biological Sciences and Medical Sciences, 56*(6), M344–M348. *Evidence Level IV.*

Robinson, S. B., & Rosher, R. B. (2002). Can a beverage cart help improve hydration? *Geriatric Nursing, 23*(4), 208–211. *Evidence Level IV.*

Rodriguez, G. J., Cordina, S. M., Vazquez, G., Suri, M. F., Kirmani, J. F., Ezzeddine, M. A., & Qureshi, A. I. (2009). The hydration influence on the risk of stroke (THIRST) study. *Neurocritical Care, 10*(2), 187–194. *Evidence Level IV.*

Rolls, B. J. (1998). Homeostatic and non-homeostatic controls of drinking in humans. In M. J. Arnaud (Ed.), *Hydration throughout life* (pp. 19–28). Montrouge, France: John Libbey Eurotext. *Evidence Level II.*

Sachdev, P., Mason, C., & Hadzi-Pavlovic, D. (1997). Case-control study of neuroleptic malignant syndrome. *American Journal of Psychiatry, 154*(8), 1156–1158. *Evidence Level IV.*

Schmidlin, E. (2008). Artificial hydration: The role of the nurse in addressing patient and family needs. *International Journal of Palliative Nursing, 14*(10), 485–489. *Evidence Level IV.*

Seymour, D. G., Henschke, P. J., Cape, R. D., & Campbell, A. J. (1980). Acute confusional states and dementia in the elderly: The role of dehydration/volume depletion, physical illness and age. *Age and Ageing, 9*(3), 137–146. *Evidence Level IV.*

Siervo, M., Bunn, D., Prado, C. M., & Hooper, L. (2014). Accuracy of prediction equations for serum osmolarity in frial older people with and without diabetes. *American Journal of Clinical Nutrition, 100*, 867–876. doi:10.3945/ajcn.114.086769. *Evidence Level IV.*

Simmons, S. F., Alessi, C., & Schnelle, J. F. (2001). An intervention to increase fluid intake in nursing home residents: Prompting and preference compliance. *Journal of the American Geriatrics Society, 49*(7), 926–933. *Evidence Level II.*

Smith, A. F., Vallance, H., & Slater, R. M. (1997). Shorter preoperative fluid fasts reduce postoperative emesis. *British Medical Journal, 314*(7092), 1486. *Evidence Level II.*

Spangler, P. F., Risley, T. R., & Bilyew, D. D. (1984). The management of dehydration and incontinence in nonambulatory geriatric patients. *Journal of Applied Behavior Analysis, 17*(3), 397–401. *Evidence Level III.*

Stookey, J. D. (2005). High prevalence of plasma hypertonicity among community-dwelling older adults: Results from NHANES III. *Journal of the American Dietetic Association, 105*(8), 1231–1239. *Evidence Level IV.*

Stookey, J. D., Pieper, C. F., & Cohen, H. J. (2005). Is the prevalence of dehydration among community-dwelling older adults really low? Informing current debate over the fluid recommendation for adults aged 70+ years. *Public Health Nutrition, 8*(8), 1275–1285. *Evidence Level IV.*

Vivanti, A., Harvey, K., & Ash, S. (2010). Developing a quick and practical screen to improve the identification of poor hydration in geriatric and rehabilitative care. *Archives of Gerontology and Geriatrics, 50*(2), 156–164. *Evidence Level IV.*

Vivanti, A., Harvey, K., Ash, S., & Battistutta, D. (2008). Clinical assessment of dehydration in older people admitted to hospital: What are the strongest indicators? *Archives of Gerontology and Geriatrics, 47*(3), 340–355. *Evidence Level IV.*

Wakefield, B., Mentes, J., Diggelmann, L., & Culp, K. (2002). Monitoring hydration status in elderly veterans. *Western Journal of Nursing Research, 24*(2), 132–142. *Evidence Level IV.*

Wakefield, B. J., Mentes, J., Holman, J. E., & Culp, K. (2008). Risk factors and outcomes associated with hospital admission for dehydration. *Rehabilitation Nursing, 33*(6), 233–241. *Evidence Level IV.*

Wallach, J. (2000). *Interpretation of diagnostic tests* (7th ed., pp. 135–141). Philadelphia, PA: Lippincott, Williams, & Wilkins. *Evidence Level VI.*

Warren, J. L., Bacon, W. E., Harris, T., McBean, A. M., Foley, D. J., & Phillips, C. (1994). The burden and outcomes associated with dehydration among US elderly, 1991. *American Journal of Public Health, 84*(8), 1265–1269. *Evidence Level IV.*

Weinberg, A. D., Pals, J. K., Levesque, P. G., Beal, L. F., Cunningham, T. J., & Minaker, K. L. (1994). Dehydration and death during febrile episodes in the nursing home. *Journal of the American Geriatrics Society, 42*(9), 968–971. *Evidence Level IV.*

Whelan, K. (2001). Inadequate fluid intakes in dysphagic acute stroke. *Clinical Nutrition, 20*(5), 423–428. *Evidence Level II.*

Woods, D. L., & Mentes, J. C. (2011). Spit: Saliva in nursing research, uses and methodological consideration. *Biological Research for Nursing, 13*, 320–327. *Evidence Level VI.*

Xiao, H., Barber, J., & Campbell, E. S. (2004). Economic burden of dehydration among hospitalized elderly patients. *American Journal of Health System Pharmacy, 61*(23), 2534–2540. *Evidence Level IV.*

Yogendran, S., Asokumar, B., Cheng, D. C., & Chung, F. (1995). A prospective randomized double-blinded study of the effect of intravenous fluid therapy on adverse outcomes on outpatient surgery. *Anesthesia and Analgesia, 80*(4), 682–686. *Evidence Level II.*

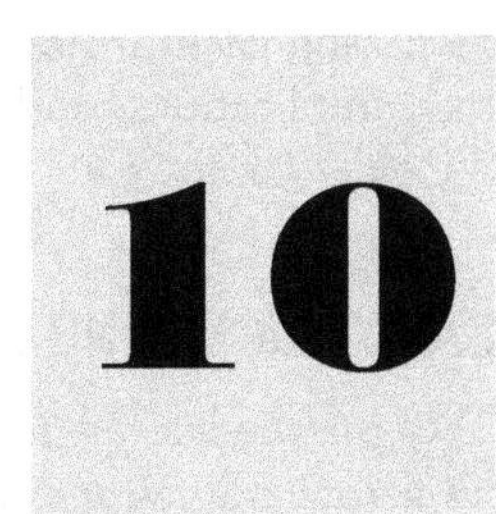

Nutrition

Rose Ann DiMaria-Ghalili

EDUCATIONAL OBJECTIVES

On completion of this chapter, the reader should be able to:

1. Recognize factors that place the older adult at risk for malnutrition
2. Discuss methods to screen and assess nutritional status in the older adult
3. Use appropriate nursing interventions in the hospitalized older adult who is either at risk for malnutrition or has malnutrition
4. Identify the importance of screening for nutrition risk during transitions in care

OVERVIEW

Nutritional status is the balance of nutrient intake, physiological demands, and metabolic rate (DiMaria-Ghalili, 2002). However, older adults are at risk of poor nutrition (DiMaria-Ghalili & Amella, 2005). Furthermore, malnutrition, a recognized geriatric syndrome (Institute of Medicine [IOM], 2008), is of concern because it can often be unrecognizable and impacts morbidity, mortality, and quality of life (Chen, Schilling, & Lyder, 2001), and is a precursor for frailty in the older adult. Malnutrition in older adults is defined as "faulty or inadequate nutritional status; undernourishment characterized by insufficient dietary intake, poor appetite, muscle wasting, and weight loss" (Chen et al., 2001, p. 139). In the older adult, malnutrition exists along the continuum of care (Furman, 2006). Older adults admitted to acute care settings from either the community or long-term care settings may already be malnourished or may be at risk for the development of malnutrition during hospitalization. A diagnosis of malnutrition during an acute care stay increases the length of stay (12.6 ± 5 vs. 4.4 ±1 days), cost of hospitalization ($26,944 vs. $9,485), and services needed on discharge (e.g., home care, long-term care; Corkins et al., 2014). Bed rest is common during hospital stay, and the associated loss of lean mass that accompanies bed rest can impact the already vulnerable nutritional status of older adults (English & Paddon-Jones, 2010). The IOM notes that although malnutrition is a problem in older adults, most health care professionals, including nurses, have little training concerning the nutritional needs of older adults (IOM, 2008). Therefore, it is imperative that acute care nurses carefully assess and monitor the nutritional status of older adults to identify the risk factors of malnutrition so that appropriate interventions are instituted in a timely fashion. The focus of this nursing protocol is the

For a description of evidence levels cited in this chapter, see Chapter 1, "Developing and Evaluating Clinical Practice Guidelines: A Systematic Approach."

discussion of nutrition in aging as it relates to risk factors, implications, and interventions for malnutrition in the older adults.

BACKGROUND AND STATEMENT OF PROBLEM

The prevalence of malnutrition in older adults varies across studies and settings. Using a large probability sample of community-dwelling older adults (60 years and older), 5.9% were malnourished and 56.3% were at risk of malnutrition (DiMaria-Ghalili, Michael, & Rosso, 2013). Researchers report the prevalence of malnutrition in older adults in nursing homes between 1.5% and 67% (Bell, Lee, & Tamura, 2015) and between 12% and 70% in hospitals (Heersink, Brown, DiMaria-Ghalili, & Locher, 2010). Limited information is currently available on the prevalence of malnutrition as older adults transition from the hospital to the home. However, older adults do experience declines in nutrition and health status after hospital discharge, which impact the ability to shop and prepare meals, placing them at further nutritional risk after discharge from the hospital (Anyanwu, Sharkey, Jackson, & Sahyoun, 2011).

Marasmus, kwashiorkor, and *mixed marasmus–kwashiorkor* originally described the subtypes of malnutrition associated with famine, and these terms eventually characterized disease-related malnutrition. In 2012, the Academy of Nutrition and Dietetics and the American Society for Parenteral and Enteral Nutrition published criteria for the identification of adult malnutrition (undernutrition; White et al., 2012). Inflammation is the cornerstone of the new adult disease-related malnutrition subtypes and include "starvation-related malnutrition" in the context of social and environmental circumstances (without inflammation), "chronic disease-related malnutrition" (with chronic inflammation of a mild to moderate degree; e.g., rheumatoid arthritis), and "acute disease or injury-related malnutrition" (with acute inflammation of a severe degree; e.g., major infections or trauma). Defining characteristics focus on energy intake, weight loss, physical findings (loss of body fat, muscle mass, and presence of fluid accumulation), and reduced grip strength. Visceral proteins (e.g., albumin, prealbumin) are negative acute phase proteins, typically suppressed during an inflammatory state, and are not indicative of nutritional status during inflammation. Consequently, albumin is no longer recommended to identify malnutrition (White et al., 2012). The new adult malnutrition categories underscore the impact of a loss of lean body mass and skeletal muscle associated with the catabolic nature of the inflammatory process (Jensen et al., 2010). Although *sarcopenia* is an age-related loss of muscle mass and muscle strength (Rolland, Van Kan, Gillette-Guyonnet, & Vellas, 2011), bed rest during hospitalization is also associated with a loss of lean body mass, which adversely impacts functional capacity (Rowell & Jackson, 2010).

The risk factors for malnutrition in the older adult are multifactorial and include dietary, economic, psychosocial, and physiological factors (DiMaria-Ghalili & Amella, 2005). Dietary factors include little or no appetite (Carlsson, Tidermark, Ponzer, Söderqvist, & Cederholm, 2005), problems with eating or swallowing (Serra-Prat et al., 2012), eating inadequate servings of nutrients, and eating fewer than two meals a day (Ramic et al., 2011). Limited income may cause restriction in the number of meals eaten per day or dietary quality of meals eaten (Lee & Berthelot, 2010; Samuel et al., 2012). Isolation is also a risk factor as older adults who live alone may lose their desire to cook because of loneliness, and appetite often decreases after the loss of a spouse (Ramic et al., 2011; Stroebe, Schut, & Stroebe, 2007). Impairment in functional status can place the older adult at risk of malnutrition (Oliveira, Fogaca, & Leandro-Merhi, 2009) because adequate functioning is needed to secure and prepare food (DiMaria-Ghalili, 2014). Difficulty in cooking is related to disabilities, and disabilities can hinder the ability to prepare or ingest food (Anyanwu et al., 2011; DiMaria-Ghalili, 2014). Chronic conditions can negatively influence nutritional intake as well as cognitive impairment (Inelmen, Sergi, Coin, Girardi, & Manzato, 2010). Psychological factors are known risk factors of malnutrition. For example, depression is related to unintentional weight loss (Chen, Baik, Huang, & Tang, 2007; Engel et al., 2011). Furthermore, poor oral health (Palacios & Joshipuro, 2015) and xerostomia (dry mouth caused by decreased saliva) can impair the ability to lubricate, masticate, and swallow food (Palacios & Joshipuro, 2015). Antidepressants, antihypertensives, and bronchodilators can contribute to xerostomia (DiMaria-Ghalili & Amella, 2005). Change in taste (from medications, nutrient deficiencies, or taste bud atrophy) can also alter nutritional intake (DiMaria-Ghalili & Amella, 2005).

Body composition changes in normal aging include increase in body fat, visceral fat stores, and a decrease in lean body mass (Janssen, Heymsfield, Allison, Kotler, & Ross, 2002). Furthermore, the low skeletal muscle mass associated with aging is related to functional impairment and physical disability (Janssen, Heymsfield, & Ross, 2002).

The impact of malnutrition on the health of the hospitalized older adult is well documented. In this population, malnutrition is related to prolonged hospital stay, poor health status, institutionalization, and death (Corkins et al., 2014). Malnutrition is also related to frailty and impaired functional status (Litchford, 2014).

ASSESSMENT OF THE PROBLEM

Areas of nutrition status assessment in the hospitalized older adult should focus on identification of malnutrition and risk factors for malnutrition not only during hospitalization, but also on hospital discharge. The Joint Commission mandates a nutrition screening be performed within 24 hours of hospital admission for all patients (The Joint Commission, 2009). In a recent survey of nurses' nutrition screening and assessment practices (*n* = 545), nurses reported they are primarily responsible for the initial nutrition screening (Guenter & DiMaria-Ghalili, 2013). Thirty-one percent reported using a validated nutrition assessment tool, the most frequently reported were the Mini-Nutritional Assessment (MNA; 49.1%) and the Subjective Global Assessment (32.4%).

The MNA (Guigoz, Vellas, & Garry, 1994) is a comprehensive two-level tool that can be used to screen and assess the older hospitalized patient for malnutrition by evaluating the presence of risk factors for malnutrition in this age group (DiMaria-Ghalili & Guenter, 2008). The MNA-SF (short form) is based on the full MNA, the original 18-item questionnaire. The MNA-SF consists of six questions on food intake, weight loss, mobility, psychological stress or acute disease, presence of dementia or depression, and body mass index (BMI; Kaiser et al., 2010), and can be used as a screening tool. The full MNA provides a more detailed assessment. The validity and reliability of the MNA for use in hospitalized older adults is well documented (Salva, Corman, Andrieu, Salas, Porras, & Vellas, 2004). If a patient scores less than 12 on the screen (MNA-SF), then the assessment section should be completed in order to compute the malnutrition indicator score. The MNA-SF is easy to administer and is comprised of six questions. The assessment section requires measurement of midarm muscle and calf circumference. Although these anthropometric measurements are relatively easy to obtain with a tape measure, nurses may first require training in these procedures before incorporating the MNA as part of a routine nursing assessment. Protocols should be established to identify interventions to be implemented once the screening and assessment data are obtained and should include consultation with a dietitian. See "Nutrition in the Elderly" in the Resources section for the topic of MNA in nutrition and consultgerirn .org/resources for *Assessing Nutrition in Older Adults* (DiMaria-Ghalili & Amella, 2012).

Additional assessment strategies include proper measurement of height and weight and a detailed weight history. Height should always be directly measured and never recorded via patient self-report. An alternative way of measuring standing height is knee height (Salva et al., 2004) with special calipers. An alternative to knee height measures is a demi-span measurement, meaning half the total arm span. (For directions on estimating height based on demi-span measurement, see Appendix 2 in *A Guide to Completing the Mini Nutritional Assessment* from the Nestle Nutrition Institute at www.mna-elderly.com/mna_forms.html.)

A calorie count or dietary intake analysis is a good way to quantify the type and amount of nutrients ingested during hospitalization (DiMaria-Ghalili & Amella, 2005). Traditionally, laboratory indicators of nutritional status included measures of visceral proteins such as serum albumin, transferrin, and prealbumin (DiMaria-Ghalili & Amella, 2005). However, these visceral proteins are also negative acute phase reactants and are decreased during a stressed inflammatory state, limiting the ability to predict malnutrition in the acutely ill hospitalized patient. Monitoring inflammatory markers, such as C-reactive protein (Jensen, Hsiao, & Wheeler, 2012) or interleukin 6 (Jensen & Wheeler, 2012), can help to determine if depleted albumin reflects malnutrition or an inflammatory response. In spite of this, albumin is a strong prognostic marker for morbidity and mortality in the older hospitalized patient (Sullivan, Roberson, & Bopp, 2005).

INTERVENTIONS AND CARE STRATEGIES

The nursing interventions outlined in the protocol focus on enhancing or promoting nutritional intake and range in complexity from basic fundamental nursing care strategies to the administration of artificial nutrition via parenteral or enteral routes. Before initiating targeted nutritional interventions in the hospitalized older adult, it must first be determined whether the older adult cannot eat, should not eat, or will not eat (Sobotka et al., 2009; Ukleja et al., 2010; Volkert et al., 2006). Factors to consider include the gastrointestinal tract (starting with the mouth) working properly without any functional, mechanical, or physiological alterations that would limit the ability to adequately ingest, digest, and/or absorb food. Also, does the older adult have any chronic or acute health condition in which the normal intake of food is contraindicated? Or, is the older adult simply not eating, or is the appetite decreased? If the gastrointestinal tract is functional and can be used to provide nutrients, then nutritional interventions should be targeted at promoting adequate oral intake.

Nursing care strategies focus on ways to increase food intake as well as ways to enhance and manage the environment to promote increased food intake. When functional or mechanical factors limit the ability to take in nutrients, nurses should obtain interdisciplinary consultations from speech therapists, occupational therapists, physical therapists, psychiatrists, and/or dietitians to collaborate on strategies that would enhance the ability of the older adult to feed himself or herself or to eat. Oral nutritional supplementation has been shown to improve nutritional status in malnourished hospitalized older adults (Joanna Briggs Institute, 2007; Volkert et al., 2006) and should be considered in the hospitalized older adult who is malnourished or is at risk of malnutrition. When used, oral liquid nutritional supplements should be given at least 60 minutes before meals (Wilson, Purushothaman, & Morley, 2002). Specialized nutritional support should be reserved for select situations. If the provision of nutrients via the gastrointestinal tract is contraindicated, then parenteral nutrition via the central or peripheral route should be initiated (Ukleja et al., 2010). If the gastrointestinal tract can be used, then nutrients should be delivered via enteral tube feeding (Ukleja et al., 2010). The exact location of the tube and type of feeding tube inserted depend on the disease state, length of time tube feeding is required, and risk of aspiration. Patients started on specialized nutritional support should be routinely reassessed for the continued need for specialized nutrition support and transitioned to oral feeding when feasible. Also, advance directives, if not completed, should be addressed before initiating specialized nutrition support (see Chapter 4, "Health Care Decision Making" and Chapter 39, "Advance Care Planning").

CASE STUDY

Mrs. V. H. is a 75-year-old female admitted to the hospital with a myocardial infarction and is on a telemetry unit for further workup before coronary artery bypass grafting surgery. On admission, her standing height is 5 feet 8 inches and she weighs 140 pounds. Her BMI is 21.33. Her past medical history is significant for rheumatoid arthritis. She describes herself as generally in good health until she was admitted to the hospital. Medications include 400 mg of ibuprofen every 6 hours, as needed. Mrs. V. H. is the primary caregiver for her 80-year-old husband, who has altered cognitive functioning and is bedridden after a stroke 3 years ago. She complained of being tired and lacking energy before admission. Her weight history is significant for a 10-pound weight loss in the past 3 months. Mrs. V. H. said she started taking oral energy drinks because she was often too tired to cook a complete dinner for herself and lacked energy and was concerned about weight loss. She reported regaining 2 pounds after taking three cans of an oral nutritional supplement per day for about 4 weeks. She reported having more strength after regaining some of her weight back. Although she is married, she is isolated because she does not have any social support systems to rely on. Her only living relative is a cousin who is 70 years old and lives 60 miles away and visits twice a month. During the assessment, Mrs. V. H. continually complained of being physically exhausted from caring for her husband at home and being too tired to eat or cook a nutritious meal for herself. She is worried about how she will care for her husband on discharge from surgery and hopes that she can recover in the same nursing home that her husband was admitted to.

Mrs. V. H. does have chronic inflammatory conditions (rheumatoid arthritis and cardiovascular diseases) that along with the recent weight loss could place her at risk for chronic inflammatory malnutrition. Furthermore, her social history is significant and could contribute to starvation-related malnutrition. As the sole caregiver for her disabled husband, she is isolated, tired, and has a decreased appetite. Her MNA-SF score is 7 based on moderate loss of appetite, weight loss greater than 6.6 pounds during the last 3 months, goes out, has suffered an acute event, has no psychological problems, and has a BMI of 21.33. Because her score is below 11, she is at risk for malnutrition, and a complete assessment level of the MNA is performed. Her total MNA assessment score is 17.5 based on an assessment score of 10.5 and a screening score of 7.0, indicating she is at risk for malnutrition. Although she is on a regular diet, she only takes in about 50% of her meals. Oral nutritional supplements are ordered twice daily between meals. Consultations obtained from the social worker, dietitian, and physical therapist are warranted.

SUMMARY

Hospitalized older adults are at risk of malnutrition. Nurses should carefully assess and monitor the nutritional status of the older hospitalized patient so that appropriate nutrition-related interventions can be implemented in a timely fashion.

NURSING STANDARD OF PRACTICE

Protocol 10.1: Nutrition in Aging

I. GOAL

Improve in indicators of nutritional status in order to optimize functional status and general well-being and promote positive nutritional status

II. OVERVIEW

Older adults are at risk of malnutrition, with 39% to 47% of hospitalized older adults being malnourished or at risk of malnutrition (Kaiser et al., 2010).

III. BACKGROUND/STATEMENT OF PROBLEM

A. Definition(s)
   1. Malnutrition: Any disorder of nutritional status, including disorders resulting from a deficiency of nutrient intake, impaired nutrient metabolism, or overnutrition
B. Etiology and/or epidemiology: Older adults are at risk for undernutrition because of dietary, economic, psychosocial, and physiological factors (DiMaria-Ghalili & Amella, 2005).
   1. Dietary intake
      a. Little or no appetite (Carlsson et al., 2005; Ramic et al., 2011)
      b. Problems with eating or swallowing (Serra-Prat et al., 2012)
      c. Eating inadequate servings of nutrients (Ramic et al., 2011)
      d. Eating fewer than two meals a day (Ramic et al., 2011)
   2. Limited income may cause restriction in the number of meals eaten per day or dietary quality of meals eaten (Samuel et al., 2012).
   3. Isolation
      a. Older adults who live alone may lose desire to cook because of loneliness (Ramic et al., 2011; Stroebe et al., 2007)
      b. Appetite of widows decreases (DiGiacomo, Lewis, Lolan, Phillips, & Davidson, 2013)
      c. Difficulty cooking because of disabilities (Anyanwu et al., 2011)
      d. Lack of access to transportation to buy food (DiMaria-Ghalili & Amella, 2005)
   4. Chronic illness
      a. Chronic conditions can affect intake (DiMaria-Ghalili, 2014).
      b. Disability can hinder ability to prepare or ingest food (Anyanwu et al., 2011; Litchford, 2014).
      c. Depression can cause decreased appetite (Engel et al., 2011).
      d. Poor oral health (cavities, gum disease, and missing teeth), and xerostomia, or dry mouth impairs ability to lubricate, masticate, and swallow food (Palacios & Joshipura, 2015).
      e. Antidepressants, antihypertensives, and bronchodilators can contribute to xerostomia (DiMaria-Ghalili & Amella, 2005).
   5. Physiological changes
      a. Decrease in lean body mass and redistribution of fat around internal organs lead to decreased caloric requirements (Janssen, Heymsfield, Allison, et al., 2002)
      b. Change in taste (from medications, nutrient deficiencies, or taste bud atrophy) can also alter nutritional status (DiMaria-Ghalili & Amella, 2005)

IV. PARAMETERS OF ASSESSMENT

A. General: During routine nursing assessment, any alterations in general assessment parameters that influence intake, absorption, or digestion of nutrients should be further assessed to determine whether the older adult is at nutritional risk. These parameters include:
   1. General assessment, including present history, assessment of symptoms, past medical and surgical history, and comorbidities (DiMaria-Ghalili, 2014)

(continued)

Protocol 10.1: Nutrition in Aging *(continued)*

2. Social history (DiMaria-Ghalili, 2014)
3. Drug–nutrient interactions: Drugs can modify the nutrient needs and metabolism of older people. Restrictive diets, malnutrition, changes in eating patterns, alcoholism, and chronic disease with long-term drug treatment are some of the risk factors in older adults that place them at risk for drug–nutrient interactions (DiMaria-Ghalili, 2014).
4. Functional limitations (DiMaria-Ghalili, 2014)
5. Psychological status (DiMaria-Ghalili, 2014)
6. Physical assessment: Physical examination with emphasis on oral examination (see Chapter 8, "Oral Health Care"); loss of subcutaneous fat, muscle wasting, and BMI (DiMaria-Ghalili, 2014); and dysphagia.

B. Dietary intake: In-depth assessment of dietary intake during hospitalization may be documented with a dietary intake analysis (calorie count; DiMaria-Ghalili & Amella, 2005).

C. Risk assessment tool: The MNA should be performed to determine whether an older hospitalized patient is either at risk of malnutrition or has malnutrition. The MNA determines risk based on food intake, mobility, BMI, history of weight loss, psychological stress, or acute disease, and dementia or other psychological conditions. If score on the MNA-SF is 11 points or less, the in-depth MNA assessment should be performed (DiMaria-Ghalili & Guenter, 2008). See the Resources section or go to consultgerirn.org/resources for nutrition information.

D. Anthropometry
1. Obtain an accurate weight and height through direct measurement. Do not rely on patient recall. If the patient cannot stand erect to measure height, then either a demi-span measurement or a knee-height measurement should be taken to estimate height using special knee-height calipers (DiMaria-Ghalili & Amella, 2005). Height should never be estimated or recalled because of shortening of the spine with advanced age; self-reported height may be off by as much as 2.4 cm (DiMaria-Ghalili & Amella, 2005).
2. Weight history: A detailed weight history should be obtained along with current weight. Detailed weight history should include a history of weight loss, whether the weight loss was intentional or unintentional, and during what period. A loss of 10 pounds. over a 6-month period, whether intentional or unintentional, is a critical indicator for further assessment (DiMaria-Ghalili & Amella, 2005).
3. Calculate BMI to determine whether weight for height is within normal range: 23 to 30. A BMI below 23 is a sign of undernutrition (Centers for Medicare & Medicaid Services, 2011).

E. Visceral proteins: Serum albumin, transferrin, and prealbumin are visceral proteins traditionally used to assess and monitor nutritional status (DiMaria-Ghalili & Amella, 2005). However, keep in mind that these proteins are negative acute-phase reactants, so during a stress state, the production is usually decreased. In the older hospitalized patient, albumin levels may be a better indicator of prognosis than nutritional status (White et al., 2012). Consider using inflammatory markers (C-reactive protein or interleukin-6) to ascertain whether the changes in albumin are caused by nutritional alterations or an inflammatory state (Jensen et al., 2012; Jensen & Wheeler, 2012).

F. Functional status: Measure handgrip strength using a hand dynamometer (White et al., 2012); review ability to perform ADL and IADL (DiMaria-Ghalili, 2014).

G. Transitional care needs determine the ability of the patient to shop, cook, and feed self after discharge (DiMaria-Ghalili, 2014).

V. NURSING CARE STRATEGIES

A. Collaboration (DiMaria-Ghalili & Amella, 2005)
1. Refer to a dietitian if the patient is at risk of undernutrition or has undernutrition.
2. Consult with a pharmacist to review the patient's medications for possible drug–nutrient interactions.
3. Consult with a multidisciplinary team specializing in nutrition.
4. Consult with a social worker, an occupational therapist, and a speech therapist as appropriate.

(continued)

Protocol 10.1: Nutrition in Aging *(continued)*

B. Alleviate dry mouth
   1. Avoid caffeine; alcohol and tobacco; and dry, bulk, spicy, salty, or highly acidic foods.
   2. If the patient does not have dementia or swallowing difficulties, offer sugarless hard candy or chewing gum to stimulate saliva.
   3. Keep lips moist with petroleum jelly.
   4. Take frequent sips of water.

C. Maintain adequate nutritional intake
   Daily requirements for healthy older adults include 30 kcal/kg of body weight, and 1 to 1.2 g/kg of protein per day (Bauer et al., 2013), with no more than 30% of calories from fat. Caloric, carbohydrate, protein, and fat requirements may differ depending on degree of malnutrition and physiological stress.

D. Improve oral intake
   1. Assess each patient's ability to eat within 24 hours of admission (Jefferies, Johnson, & Ravens, 2011).
   2. Engage in mealtime rounds to determine how much food is consumed and whether assistance is needed (Jefferies et al., 2011)
   3. Limit staff breaks to before or after patient mealtimes to ensure that adequate staff are available to help with meals (Jefferies et al., 2011).
   4. Encourage family members to visit at mealtimes.
   5. Ask family to bring favorite foods from home when appropriate.
   6. Ask about patient food preferences and honor them.
   7. Suggest small, frequent meals with adequate nutrients to help patients regain or maintain weight (Joanne Briggs Institute, 2007).
   8. Provide nutritious snacks (Joanne Briggs Institute, 2007).
   9. Help patient with mouth care and placement of dentures before food is served (Jefferies et al., 2011).

E. Provide conducive environment for meals
   1. Remove bedpans, urinals, and emesis basins from rooms before mealtime.
   2. Administer analgesics and antiemetics on a schedule that will diminish the likelihood of pain or nausea during mealtimes.
   3. Serve meals to patients in a chair if they can get out of bed and remain seated.
   4. Create a more relaxed atmosphere by sitting at the patient's eye level and making eye contact during feeding.
   5. Order a late food tray or keep food warm if the patients are not in their rooms during mealtimes.
   6. Do not interrupt patients for round and nonurgent procedures during mealtimes.

F. Specialized nutritional support (Sobotka et al., 2009; Ukleja et al., 2010; Volkert et al., 2006)
   1. Start specialized nutritional support when a patient cannot, should not, or will not eat adequately and if the benefits of nutrition outweigh the associated risks.
   2. Before initiation of specialized nutritional support, review the patient's advance directives regarding the use of artificial nutrition and hydration.

G. Provide oral supplements
   1. Supplements should not replace meals but should be provided between meals and not within the hour preceding a meal and at bedtime (Joanne Briggs Institute, 2007; Wilson et al., 2002).
   2. Ensure that oral supplement is at the appropriate temperature (Joanne Briggs Institute, 2007).
   3. Ensure that the patient can open oral supplement packaging (Joanne Briggs Institute, 2007).
   4. Monitor the intake of the prescribed supplement (Joanne Briggs Institute, 2007).
   5. Promote a sip style of supplement consumption (Joanne Briggs Institute, 2007).
   6. Include supplements as part of the medication protocol (Joanne Briggs Institute, 2007).

H. NPO orders
   1. Schedule older adults for tests or procedures early in the day to decrease the length of time they are not allowed to eat and drink.
   2. If testing late in the day is inevitable, ask the physician whether the patient can have an early breakfast.

(continued)

Protocol 10.1: Nutrition in Aging *(continued)*

3. See ASA practice guideline regarding recommended length of time patients should be kept NPO for elective surgical procedures.

VI. EVALUATION/EXPECTED OUTCOMES

A. Patient will
   1. Experience improvement in indicators of nutritional status.
   2. Improve functional status and general well-being.
B. Provider should
   1. Ensure that care includes food and fluid of adequate quantity and quality in an environment conducive to eating, with appropriate support (e.g., modified eating aids) for people who can potentially chew and swallow but are unable to feed themselves.
   2. Continue to reassess patients who are malnourished or at risk for malnutrition.
   3. Monitor for refeeding syndrome.
C. Institution will
   1. Ensure that all health care professionals who are directly involved in patient care should receive education and training on the importance of providing adequate nutrition.
D. QA/QI
   1. Establish QA/QI measures surrounding nutritional management in aging patients.
E. Educational
   1. Provided education and training includes
      a. Nutritional needs and indications for nutrition support
      b. Options for nutrition support (oral, enteral, and parenteral)
      c. Ethical and legal concepts
      d. Potential risks and benefits
      e. When and where to seek expert advice
   2. Patient and/or caregiver education includes how to maintain or improve nutritional status as well as how to administer, when appropriate, oral liquid supplements, enteral tube feeding, or parenteral nutrition.

VII. FOLLOW-UP MONITORING

A. Monitor for gradual increase in weight over time.
   1. Weigh patient weekly to monitor trends in weight.
   2. Daily weights are useful for monitoring fluid status.
B. Monitor and assess for refeeding syndrome (Skipper, 2012).
   1. Carefully monitor and assess patients the first week of aggressive nutritional repletion.
   2. Assess and correct the following electrolyte abnormalities: hypophosphatemia, hypokalemia, hypomagnesemia, hyperglycemia, and hypoglycemia.
   3. Assess fluid status with daily weights and strict intake and output.
   4. Assess for congestive heart failure in patients with respiratory or cardiac difficulties.
   5. Ensure caloric goals will be reached slowly, over more than 3 to 4 days to avoid refeeding syndrome when repletion of nutritional status is warranted.
   6. Be aware that refeeding syndrome is not only exclusive to patients started on aggressive artificial nutrition, but may also be found in older adults with chronic comorbid medical conditions and poor nutrient intake started with aggressive nutritional repletion via oral intake.

VIII: RELEVANT GUIDELINES

A. Preoperative nutrition assessment
   1. ACS NSQIP®/AGS (2012)

(continued)

Protocol 10.1: Nutrition in Aging *(continued)*

B. Preoperative fasting
   1. ASA (1999)
   2. Lambert and Carey (2015)
C. Nutrition interventions
   1. Bauer et al. (2013)
   2. Sobotka et al. (2009)
   3. Ukleja et al. (2010)
   4. Volkert et al. (2006)

ABBREVIATIONS

ACS	American College of Surgeons
ADL	Activities of daily living
AGS	American Geriatrics Society
ASA	American Society of Anesthesiologists
BMI	Body mass index
IADL	Instrumental activities of daily living
MNA	Mini-Nutritional Assessment
NPO	Nothing by mouth
NSQIP	National Surgical Quality Improvement Program
QA/QI	Quality assurance/quality improvement

NOTE

1. This chapter is based on the geriatric nursing protocol series. See http://consultgerirn.org/topics/nutrition_in_the_elderly/want_to_know_more

RESOURCES

Academy of Nutrition and Dietetics
Resources for Older Adults
www.eatright.org/resources/for-seniors

Resources for Professionals
www.eatrightpro.org/resources/advocacy/lifecycle-nutrition/nutrition-for-older-adults

Regulatory/Authoritative Sites

Academy of Nutrition and Dietitics
www.eatright.org

American Geriatrics Society
www.americangeriatrics.org

American Medical Directors Association: Clinical Tools and Products
www.amda.com/tools/index.cfm

American Society for Parenteral and Enteral Nutrition
www.nutritioncare.org

The Gerontological Society of America
www.geron.org

National Conference of Gerontological Nurse Practitioners
www.acnpweb.org/i4a/pages/Index.cfm?pageID=3697

National Gerontological Nursing Association
www.ngna.org

National Institutes of Health
www.nlm.nih.gov/medlineplus/nutritionforseniors.html

U.S. Department of Health and Human Services
www.hhs.gov

Mini-Nutritional Assessment

Nestle Nutrition Institute
www.mna-elderly.com

Nutrition in the Elderly

ConsultGeriRN website of the Hartford Institute for Geriatric Nursing
consultgerirn.org/resources

Knee-Height Measurement

Florida International University's Long-term Care Institute Resource Materials
nutritionandaging.fiu.edu/about_long_materials.asp

REFERENCES

Anyanwu, U. O., Sharkey, J. R., Jackson, R. T., & Sahyoun, N. R. (2011). Home food environment of older adults transitioning from hospital to home. *Journal of Nutrition in Gerontology and Geriatrics, 30,* 105–121. *Evidence Level IV.*

ACS NSQIP®/AGS. (2012). Best Practice Guidelines: Optimal Preoperative Assessment of the Geriatric Surgical Patient. Retrieved from www.americangeriatrics.org. *Evidence Level VI.*

ASA. (1999). Practice guidelines for preoperative fasting and the use of pharmacologic agents to reduce the risk of pulmonary aspiration: Application to healthy patients undergoing elective procedures: A report by the American Society of Anesthesiologist Task Force on Preoperative Fasting. *Anesthesiology, 90,* 896–905. *Evidence Level VI.*

Bauer, J., Biolo, G., Cederholm, T., Cesari, M., Cruz-Jentoft, A. J., Morley, J. E.,...Boirie, Y. (2013). Evidence-based recommendations for optimal dietary protein intake in older people: A position paper from the PROT-AGE Study Group. *Journal of the American Medical Directors Association, 14*(8), 542–559. *Evidence Level I.*

Bell, C. L., Lee, A. S. W., & Tamura, B. K. (2015). Malnutrition in the nursing home. *Current Opinion in Clinical Nutrition and Metabolic Care, 18,* 17–23. *Evidence Level VI.*

Carlsson, P., Tidermark, J., Ponzer, S., Söderqvist, A., & Cederholm, T. (2005). Food habits and appetite of elderly women at the time of a femoral neck fracture and after nutritional and anabolic support. *Journal of Human Nutrition and Dietetics, 18,* 117–120. *Evidence Level II.*

Centers for Medicare & Medicaid Services. (2011). *Physician quality reporting system measures specification manual for claims and registry: Reporting of individual measures.* Chicago, IL: American Medical Association. *Evidence Level VI.*

Chen, C. C., Bai, Y. Y., Huang, G. H., & Tang, S. T. (2007). Revisiting the concept of malnutrition in older people. *Journal of Clinical Nursing, 16*(11), 2015–2026. *Evidence Level IV.*

Chen, C. C., Schilling, L. S., & Lyder, C. H. (2001). A concept analysis of malnutrition in the elderly. *Journal of Advance Nursing, 36,* 131–142. *Evidence Level V.*

Corkins, M. R., Guenter, P., DiMaria-Ghalili, R. A., Jensen, G. L., Malone, A., Miller, S.,...Enteral, N. (2014). Malnutrition diagnoses in hospitalized patients: United States, 2010. *Journal of Parenteral and Enteral Nutrition, 38*(2), 186–195. *Evidence Level IV.*

DiGiacomo, M., Lewis, J., Nolan, M. T., Phillips, J., & Davidson, P. M. (2013). Health transitions in recently widowed older women: A mixed methods study. *BMC Health Service Research, 13,* 143. *Evidence Level IV.*

DiMaria-Ghalili, R. A. (2002). Changes in nutritional status and postoperative outcomes in elderly CABG patients. *Biological Research for Nursing, 4,* 73–84. *Evidence Level IV.*

DiMaria-Ghalili, R. A. (2014). Integrating nutrition in the comprehensive geriatric assessment. *Nutrition in Clinical Practice, 29*(4), 420–427. *Evidence Level V.*

DiMaria-Ghalili, R. A., & Amella, E. J. (2005). Nutrition in older adults. *American Journal of Nursing, 105*(3), 40–50. *Evidence Level V.*

DiMaria-Ghalili, R. A., & Amella, E. J. (2012). Assessing nutrition in older adults. In S. Greenberg (Ed.), *Try this: Best practices in nursing care for hospitalized older adults.* Issue #9. Retrieved from http://consultgerirn.org/uploads/File/trythis/try_this_9.pdf. *Evidence Level V.*

DiMaria-Ghalili, R. A., & Guenter, P. A. (2008). The mini nutritional assessment. *American Journal of Nursing, 108*(2), 50–59. *Evidence Level V.*

DiMaria-Ghalili, R. A., Michael, Y. L., & Rosso, A. L. (2013). Malnutrition in a sample of community-dwelling older Pennsylvanians. *Journal of Aging Research and Clinical Practice, 2*(1), 39–45. *Evidence Level IV.*

Engel, J. H., Siewerdt, F., Jackson, R., Akobundu, U., Wait, C., & Sahyoun, N. (2011). Hardiness, depression, and emotional well-being and their association with appetite in older adults. *Journal of the American Geriatrics Society, 59*(3), 482–487. *Evidence Level IV.*

English, K. L., & Paddon-Jones, D. (2010). Protecting muscle mass and function in older adults during bed rest. *Current Opinion in Clinical Nutrition and Metabolic Care, 13,* 34–39. *Evidence Level VI.*

Furman, E. F. (2006). Undernutrition in older adults across the continuum of care: Nutritional assessment, barriers, and interventions. *Journal of Gerontological Nursing, 32,* 22–27. *Evidence Level VI.*

Guenter, P., & DiMaria-Ghalili, R. A. (2013). Survey of nurses' nutrition screening and assessment practices in hospitalized patients. *Medical Surgery Nursing, 22*(5), 10–13. *Evidence Level IV.*

Guigoz, Y., Vellas, B., & Garry, P. J. (1994). Mini nutritional assessment: A practical assessment tool for grading the nutritional state of elderly patients. *Facts and Research in Gerontology, 4*(Suppl. 2), 15–59. *Evidence Level IV.*

Heersink, J. T., Brown, C. J., Dimaria-Ghalili, R. A., & Locher, J. L. (2010). Undernutrition in hospitalized older adults: Patterns and correlates, outcomes, and opportunities for intervention with a focus on processes of care. *Journal of Nutrition in the Elderly, 29*(1), 4–41. *Evidence Level V.*

Inelmen, E. M., Sergi, G., Coin, A., Girardi, A., & Manzato, E. (2010). An open-ended question: Alzheimer's disease and involuntary weight loss: Which comes first? *Aging Clinical and Experimental Research, 22,* 192–197. *Evidence Level V.*

Institute of Medicine. (2008). *Retooling for an aging America: Building the health care workforce.* Washington, DC: National Academies Press. *Evidence Level VI.*

Janssen, I., Heymsfield, S. B., Allison, D. B., Kotler, D. P., & Ross, R. (2002). Body mass index and waist circumference independently contribute to the prediction of nonabdominal, abdominal subcutaneous, and visceral fat. *American Journal of Clinical Nutrition, 75,* 683–688. *Evidence Level IV.*

Janssen, I., Heymsfield, S. B., & Ross, R. (2002). Low relative skeletal muscle mass (sarcopenia) in older persons is associated with functional impairment and physical disability. *Journal of the American Geriatrics Society, 50,* 889–896. *Evidence Level IV.*

Jefferies, D., Johnson, M., & Ravens, J. (2011). Nurturing and nourishing: The nurses' role in nutritional care. *Journal of Clinical Nursing, 20*, 317–330. *Evidence Level I.*

Jensen, G. L., Hsiao, P. Y., & Wheeler, D. (2012). Adult nutrition assessment tutorial. *Journal of Parenteral and Enteral Nutrition, 36*, 267–274. *Evidence Level VI.*

Jensen, G. L., Mirtallo, J., Compher, C., Dhaliwal, R., Forbes, A., Grijalba, R. F., . . . Waitzberg, D. (2010). Adult starvation and disease-related malnutrition: A proposal for etiology-based diagnosis in the clinical practice setting from the International Consensus Guideline Committee. *Journal of Parenteral and Enteral Nutrition, 34*, 156–159. *Evidence Level VI.*

Jensen, G. L., & Wheeler, D. (2012). A new approach to defining and diagnosing malnutrition in adult critical illness. *Current Opinion in Critical Care, 18*, 206–211. *Evidence Level VI.*

Joanna Briggs Institute. (2007). Effectiveness of interventions for undernourished older inpatients in the hospital setting. *The JBI Database of Best Practice Information Sheets and Technical Reports, 11*(2), 1–4. *Evidence Level I.*

Kaiser, M. J., Bauer, J. M., Rämsch, C., Uter, W., Guigoz, Y., Cederholm, T., . . . Sieber, C. C. (2010). Frequency of malnutrition in older adults: A multinational perspective using the Mini Nutritional Assessment. *Journal of the American Geriatrics Society, 58*, 1734–1738. doi:10.1111/j.1532-5415.2010.03016.x. *Evidence Level I.*

Lambert, E., & Carey, S. (2015). Practice guideline recommendations on perioperative fasting: A systematic review. *Journal of Parenteral and Enteral Nutrition*. Advance online publication. *Evidence Level I.*

Lee, M. R., & Berthelot, E. R. (2010). Community covariates of malnutrition based mortality among older adults. *Annals of Epidemiology, 20*(5), 371–379. *Evidence Level IV.*

Litchford, M. D. (2014). Counteracting the trajectory of frailty and sarcopenia in older adults. *Nutrition in Clinical Practice, 29*(4), 428–434. *Evidence Level VI.*

Oliveira, M. R., Fogaca, K. C., & Leandro-Merhi, V. A. (2009). Nutritional status and functional capacity of hospitalized elderly. *Nutrition Journal, 8*, 54. *Evidence Level IV.*

Palacios, C., & Joshipura, K. J. (2015). Nutrition and oral health: A two-way relationship. In C. W. Bales, J. L. Locher, & E. Saltzman (Eds.), *Handbook of clinical nutrition and aging* (3rd ed., pp. 81–98). New York, NY: Humana Press. *Evidence Level VI.*

Ramic, E., Pranjic, N., Batic-Mujanovic, O., Karic, E., Alibasic, E., & Alic, A. (2011). The effect of loneliness on malnutrition in elderly population. *Medical Archives, 65*(2), 92–95. *Evidence Level IV.*

Rolland, Y., Van Kan, G. A., Gillette-Guyonnet, S., & Vellas, B. (2011). Cachexia versus sarcopenia. *Current Opinion in Clinical Nutrition and Metabolic Care, 14*, 15–21. *Evidence Level VI.*

Rowell, D. S., & Jackson, T. J. (2010). Additional costs of inpatient malnutrition, Victoria, Australia, 2003–2004. *European Journal of Health Economics, 12*, 353–361. *Evidence Level IV.*

Salva, A., Corman, B., Andrieu S, Salas, J., Porras, C., & Vellas, B. (2004). Minimum data set for nutritional intervention studies in the elderly IAG/ IANA task force consensus. *Journal of Nutrition Health and Aging, 8*, 202–206. *Evidence Level V.*

Samuel, L. J., Szanton, S. L., Weiss, C. O., Thorpe, R. J., Jr., Semba, R. D., & Fried, L. P. (2012). Financial strain is associated with malnutrition risk in community-dwelling older women. *Epidemiological Research International, 2012*, 696518. *Evidence Level IV.*

Serra-Prat, M., Palomera, M., Gomez, C., Sar-Shalom, D., Saiz, A., Montoya, J. G., . . . Clave, P. (2012). Oropharyngeal dysphagia as a risk factor for malnutrition and lower respiratory tract infection in independently living older persons: A population-based prospective study. *Age and Ageing, 41*(3), 376–381. *Evidence Level IV.*

Skipper, A. (2012). Refeeding syndrome or refeeding hypophosphatemia: A systematic review of cases. *Nutrition in Clinical Practice, 27*, 34–40. *Evidence Level I.*

Sobotka, L., Schneider, S. M., Berner, Y. N., Cederholm, T., Krznaric, Z., Shenkin, A., . . . ESPEN. (2009). ESPEN guidelines on parenteral nutrition: Geriatrics. *Clinical Nutrition, 28*(4), 461–466. *Evidence Level I.*

Stroebe, M., Schut, H., & Stroebe, W. (2007). Health outcomes of bereavement. *Lancet, 370*(9603), 1960–1973. *Evidence Level IV.*

Sullivan, D. H., Roberson, P. K., & Bopp, M. M. (2005). Hypoalbuminemia 3 months after hospital discharge: Significance for long-term survival. *Journal of the American Geriatrics Society, 53*, 1222–1226. *Evidence Level IV.*

The Joint Commission. (2009). *The comprehensive accreditation manual for hospitals: The official handbook.* Oakbrook Terrace, IL: Joint Commission Resources. *Evidence Level VI.*

Ukleja, A., Freeman, K. L., Gilbert, K., Kochevar, M., Kraft, M. D., Russell, M. K., . . . American Society for Parenteral and Enteral Nutrition Board of Directors. (2010). Standards for nutrition support: Adult hospitalized patients. *Nutrition in Clinical Practice, 25*(4), 403–414. *Evidence Level I.*

Volkert, D., Berner, Y. N., Berry, E., Cederholm, T., Coti Bertrand, P., Milne, A., . . . ESPEN. (2006). ESPEN guidelines on enteral nutrition: Geriatrics. *Clinical Nutrition, 25*(2), 330–360. *Evidence Level I.*

White, J. V., Guenter, P., Jensen, G., Malone, A., Schofield, M., Academy of Nutrition and Dietitics Directors, & A. S. P. E. N. Board of Directors. (2012). Consensus statement of the Academy of Nutrition and Dietetics/American Society for Parenteral and Enteral Nutrition: Characteristics recommended for the identification and documentation of adult malnutrition (undernutrition). *Journal of the Academy of Nutrition and Dietitics, 112*(5), 730–738. *Evidence Level VI.*

Wilson, M. M., Purushothaman, R., & Morley, J. E. (2002). Effect of liquid dietary supplements on energy intake in the elderly. *American Journal of Clinical Nutrition, 75*, 944–947. *Evidence Level IV.*

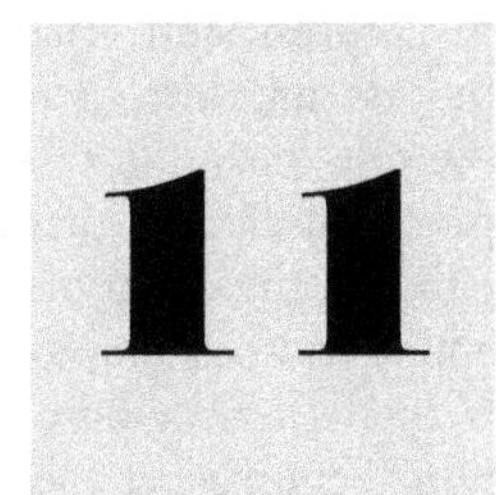

Family Caregiving

Deborah C. Messecar

EDUCATIONAL OBJECTIVES

On completion of this chapter, the reader should be able to:

1. Describe characteristics and factors that put family caregivers at risk of unhealthy transitions into the caregiving role
2. Identify key aspects of a family caregiving preparedness assessment
3. List specific interventions to support family caregivers of older adults to take on their caregiving duties
4. Identify family caregiver outcomes expected from the implementation of this protocol

OVERVIEW

Family caregivers are a key link in providing safe and effective transitional care to frail older adults as they move across levels of care (e.g., acute to subacute) or across settings (e.g., hospital to home; Bauer, Fitzgerald, Haesler, & Manfrin, 2009; Coleman & Boult, 2003; Naylor, 2003; Naylor & Keating, 2008; Naylor, Kurtzman, & Pauly, 2009). Frail older adults coping with complex chronic conditions are vulnerable to problems with care as they typically have multiple providers and move frequently between and among health care settings. Incomplete communication among providers and across health care agencies is linked to high-risk care transitions with adverse outcomes and an increased risk of hospital readmission and or length of hospital stay (Bauer et al., 2009; Geary & Schumacher, 2012; Jencks, Williams, & Coleman, 2009). Nurses in collaboration with family caregivers can bridge the gap between the care provided in hospital and other settings and the care needed in the community. Transitional care for frail older people can be improved if interventions address family inclusion and education, communication exists between health care workers and family, and interprofessional communication and ongoing support after the transition.

Helping Caregivers Take on the Caregiving Role

Helping the caregiver with the role-acquisition process is a critical nursing function that facilitates good transitional care. Indicators of a healthy assumption of the caregiving role are those factors that either indicate a robust and positive role-acquisition process or signal potential difficulty with assuming the caregiver role. When trying to ascertain what those indicators might be, the following questions about the caregiver role-acquisition process can be posed: What constitutes health during the role-acquisition process? What indicates a positive state of health during

For a description of evidence levels cited in this chapter, see Chapter 1, "Developing and Evaluating Clinical Practice Guidelines: A Systematic Approach."

this process? and What threats to health may occur as the process unfolds? (Schumacher, 1995, p. 219). Because the role-transition process unfolds over time, identifying process indicators that move patient and family members either in the direction of health or on the way to vulnerability and risk allows early assessment and intervention to facilitate healthy outcomes of the caregiving role acquisition (Schumacher, Beck, & Marren, 2006). If unhealthy role-taking transitions can be identified, then they can either be prevented or ameliorated.

Who Is Likely to Be or Become a Caregiver?

Being a family caregiver is a widespread experience in the United States. Depending on how family caregiving is defined, national surveys estimate that up to 65 million people or 29% of the U.S. population provide care for a chronically ill, disabled family member or friend during any given year (National Alliance for Caregiving [NAC] & AARP, 2009). Reflecting an increasing trend, 38% of all family caregivers of adults older than 18 years are men, 62% are women, and the majority is older than 48 years (NAC & AARP, 2009). Among the primary family caregivers of disabled or ill adults older than 65 years, the proportion of male caregivers is lower (about 32%), but this number has increased from prior years (Wolff & Kasper, 2006). Primary family caregivers usually take care of relatives (86%), and of these, most care for a parent (36%), an in-law (8%), or grandparent or grandparent-in-law (7%; NAC & AARP, 2009). Older caregivers who are 65 years or older are more likely to be caring for a spouse than younger caregivers (19% vs. 3%), whereas younger caregivers are more likely to be caring for a parent or parent-in-law (48% vs. 23%). For frail older adults, it is estimated that 41.3% of caregivers are adult children and 38.4% are spouses (Wolff & Kasper, 2006). The most common caregiver arrangement remains that of an adult female child providing care to an elderly female parent (NAC & AARP, 2009). Many caregivers are older and are at risk of chronic illness themselves. In addition, national surveys indicate a trend in the United States of care recipients being older and more disabled, and more caregivers acting as the primary source of care (NAC & AARP, 2009; Wolff & Kasper, 2006). Family and friends continue to provide more than 80% of all long-term care services in the country.

Impact of Unhealthy Caregiving Transitions on Caregiver

Caregiving has documented negative consequences for the caregiver's physical and emotional health. Caregiving-related stress in a chronically ill spouse results in a 63% higher mortality rate than their noncaregiving peers (Schulz & Beach, 1999). The impact of caregiving on health increases over time. Among caregivers providing care for 5 years or more, 23% report that their health is fair or poor (NAC & AARP, 2009). Stress from caring for an older adult with dementia has been shown to impact the caregiver's immune system for up to 3 years after their caregiving ends (Kiecolt-Glaser et al., 2003). Caregivers who live with their care recipients report poorer health (28%) versus 13% for those who live apart. Caregivers who report high burden and/or provide more hours of care per week say their health has suffered (NAC & AARP, 2009). Spouse caregivers who provide heavy care (36 or more hours per week) are six times more likely than noncaregivers to experience symptoms of depression or anxiety; for child caregivers, the rate is twice as high (Cannuscio et al., 2002). In addition to mental health morbidity, family caregivers also experience physical health deterioration. Family caregivers have chronic conditions at more than twice the rate of noncaregivers (NAC & AARP, 2009). Family caregivers experiencing extreme stress have also been shown to age prematurely. It is estimated that this stress can take as much as 10 years off a family caregiver's life (Arno, 2006).

BACKGROUND AND STATEMENT OF PROBLEM

Definitions

Family Caregiving

Family caregiving is broadly defined and refers to a broad range of unpaid care provided in response to illness or functional impairment to a chronically ill or functionally impaired older family member, partner, friend, or neighbor that exceeds the support usually provided in family relationships (Arno, 2006; Schumacher, Beck, et al., 2006).

Caregiving Roles

Caregiving roles can be classified into a hierarchy according to who takes on the bulk of responsibilities versus only intermittent supportive assistance. Historically, primary caregivers have been defined as those caregivers who tend to provide most of the everyday aspects of care, whereas secondary caregivers were defined as those who help out as needed to fill the gaps (Cantor & Little, 1985; Penning, 1990; Tennstedt, McKinlay, & Sullivan, 1989). Among caregivers who live with their care recipients, spouses account for the bulk of primary caregivers, whereas adult children are more likely to be secondary caregivers. The range of the family caregiving role includes protective caregiving, like "keeping an eye on" an older adult who is currently independent but at risk, to full-time, round-the-clock care for a severely impaired family member. Health care providers may fail to assess the full scope of the family caregiving role if they associate family caregiving only with the performance of tasks.

Caregiver Role Transition

Caregiver role acquisition is a family role transition that occurs through situated interaction as part of a role-making process (Schumacher, 1995). This is the process of taking on the caregiving role at the beginning of caregiving or when a significant change in the caregiving context occurs. Role transitions occur when a role is added to or deleted from the role set of a person—or when the behavioral expectations for an established role change significantly. Role transitions involve changes in the behavior expectations along with the acquisition of new knowledge and skills (Schumacher, Beidler, Beeber, & Gambino, 2006; Schumacher, Stewart, Archbold, Dodd, & Dibble, 2000). Examples of major role transitions are becoming a new parent, getting a divorce, and changing careers. The acquisition of the family caregiving role is a specific type of role transition that occurs within families in response to the changes in health of a family member who has suffered a decline in his or her self-care ability or health.

Indicators of Healthy Caregiver Role Transitions

The broad categories of indicators of healthy transitions include subjective well-being, role mastery, and well-being of relationships. These are the subjective, behavioral, and interpersonal parameters of health most likely to be associated with healthy role transitions (Schumacher, 1995). *Subjective well-being* is defined as "subjective responses to caregiving role transition" (Schumacher, 1995, p. 219). Subjective well-being includes any pattern of subjective reactions that arise from assuming the caregiver role within the boundary of the caregiving situation. Examples of some of the more important possible threats to subjective well-being could include role strain and depression. Role mastery is associated with accomplishment of skilled role performance and comfort with the behavior required in a new health-related care situation. Examples of threats to role mastery, which indicate a vulnerability and risk of unhealthy transitions, are role insufficiency and lack of preparedness. *Well-being of relationships* refers to the quality of the relationship between the caregiver and older adult. Examples of threats to well-being of relationships are family conflict or a poor quality of relationship with the care receiver.

Family Caregiving Activities

Family caregiving activities include assistance with day-to-day activities, illness-related care, care management, and invisible aspects of care. Day-to-day activities include personal care activities (bathing, eating, dressing, mobility, transferring from bed to chair, and using the toilet) and instrumental activities of daily living (IADL; meal preparation, grocery shopping, making telephone calls, and money management; NAC & AARP, 2009; Walker, Pratt, & Eddy, 1995). Illness-related activities include managing symptoms, coping with illness behaviors, carrying out treatments, and performing medical or nursing procedures that include an array of medical technologies (Schumacher, Beidler, et al., 2006; Schumacher et al., 2000). Care management activities include accessing resources, communicating with and navigating the health care and social services systems, and acting as an advocate (Schumacher, Beidler, et al., 2006; Schumacher et al., 2000). Invisible aspects of care have been defined as protective actions the caregiver takes to ensure the older adult's safety and well-being without his or her knowledge (Bowers, 1987).

Caregiver Assessment

Caregiver assessment refers to an ongoing iterative process of gathering information that describes a family caregiving situation and identifies the particular issues, needs, resources, and strengths of the family caregiver.

Risk Factors for Unhealthy Caregiving Transitions

Gender

Female caregivers are more likely to provide a higher level of care than men, which is defined as helping with at least two activities of daily living (ADL) and providing more than 40 care hours per week. Male caregivers are more likely to provide care at the lowest level, which is defined as no ADL and devoting very few hours of care per week (NAC & AARP, 2009; Pinquart & Sörensen, 2006a). A number of studies have found that female caregivers are more likely than males to suffer from anxiety, depression, and other symptoms associated with emotional stress caused by caregiving (Davies, Sridhar, Newkirk, Beaudreau, & O'Hara, 2012; Mahoney, Regan, Katona, & Livingston, 2005; Yee & Schulz, 2000); lower levels of physical health and subjective well-being than caregiving men (Pinquart & Sörensen, 2006a); and are at a higher risk of adverse outcomes (Schulz, Martire, & Klinger, 2005). In the pooled analysis from the Resources for Enhancing Alzheimer's Caregiver Health (REACH) trials, females had higher initial levels of burden and depression (Gitlin et al.,

2003). However, Freedman, Cornman, and Carr (2014) found that there are positive aspects of spousal caregiving for older wives that offset other unpleasant aspects of the role. Female spouse caregivers responded to nursing home placement of their care recipient with decreased burden and depression compared with their male counterparts in the New York University caregiver intervention (Gaugler, Roth, Haley, & Mittelman, 2011).

Ethnicity

Rates of caregiving vary somewhat by ethnicity. Among the U.S. adult population older than 18 years, 17% of White and 15% of African American families provide informal care, whereas a slightly lower percentage of Asian Americans (14%) and Hispanic Americans (13%) are engaged in caregiving for persons older than 50 years (NAC & AARP, 2009). These prevalence rates are not significantly different from those seen in 2004. However, in another national survey, which looked only at people older than 70 years, 44% of Latinos were found to receive informal home care compared with 34% of African Americans and 25% of non-Hispanic Whites (Weiss, González, Kabeto, & Langa, 2005). Ethnic differences are also found regarding the care recipient. Among people aged older than 70 years who require care, Whites are the most likely to receive help from their spouses, Hispanics are the most likely to receive help from their adult children, and African Americans are the most likely to receive help from a nonfamily member (National Academy on an Aging Society, 2000).

Studies show that ethnic minority caregivers provide more care (Pinquart & Sörenson, 2005) and report worse physical health than White caregivers (Dilworth-Anderson, Williams, & Gibson, 2002; Pinquart & Sörenson, 2005). African American caregivers experience less stress and depression and get more rewards related to caregiving when compared with White caregivers (Cuellar, 2002; Dilworth-Anderson et al., 2002; Gitlin et al., 2003; Haley et al., 2004; Pinquart & Sörenson, 2005). However, the interaction between minority status and relationship to the care receiver on caregiving responses in a recent study on impact of attachment and model of self indicates the possibility that interaction moderates the relation between relationship factors and caregiving responses in African American caregivers (Morse, Shaffer, Williamson, Dooley, & Schulz, 2012). Other trials have reported similar differential effects for African American, Hispanic or Latino, and White caregivers (Belle et al., 2006; Lee, Czaja, & Schulz, 2010). Hispanic and Asian American caregivers exhibit more depression than White caregivers (Gitlin et al., 2003; Pinquart & Sörensen, 2005). In addition, formal services are rarely used by ethnic minorities, which puts them at further risk of negative outcomes (Dilworth-Anderson et al., 2002; Pinquart & Sörensen, 2005). A meta-analysis of three qualitative studies examined African American, Chinese, and Latino caregiver impressions of their clinical encounters around their care receiver's diagnosis of Alzheimer's disease (Mahoney, Cloutterbuck, Neary, & Zhan, 2005). The primary issues identified in the analysis by Mahoney, Cloutterbuck, et al. (2005) were disrespect for concerns as noted by African American caregivers, stigmatization of persons with dementia as noted by Chinese caregivers, and fear that home care would not be supported as noted by Latino caregivers. Goins et al. (2011) found among American Indian adults that greater cultural identity and engagement in traditional healing practices are associated with greater likelihood of taking on the caregiving role. These findings indicate a need for greater culturally sensitive communications from health care providers.

Age

Several recent studies have found that younger age caregivers compared with their older counterparts are more prone to depressive symptoms and burden from caregiving (Morse et al., 2012; Shankar, Hirschmanm, Hanlon, & Naylorm, 2014). In a subsequent analysis from the REACH I trials, being younger was associated with higher levels of depression for Black and White caregivers but not for Hispanic caregivers (Sörensen & Pinquart, 2005). In the 2009 California Health Interview Survey, self-identified baby boomer caregivers reported engaging in poor health behaviors due to the demands of providing care (Hoffman, Lee, & Mendez-Luck, 2012). These findings are in contrast to past research that has indicated that spouse caregivers, who tend to be older, have more burden. In REACH II subgroup follow-up analyses of minority caregivers, older Black caregivers experienced a decrease in burden with the intervention compared with younger Black caregivers (Lee et al., 2010), a finding that could be a result of the fact that older caregivers were more likely to be spouses.

Income and Educational Level

Low income is also related to being an ethnic minority and being "non-White," and the latter are risk factors for poorer health outcomes. Persons who become caregivers may be more likely to have incomes below the poverty level and be in poorer health, independent of caregiving (Vitaliano, Zhang, & Scanlan, 2003). Usually, educational level has been combined with income in most caregiving studies, so there is a lack of data on this variable. One study

(Buckwalter et al., 1999) reported that caregivers who were less educated tended to report as slightly more depressed than those who were better educated. This is consistent with the findings from the REACH trial meta-analysis (Gitlin et al., 2003). In the meta-analysis completed by Schulz et al. (2005), caregivers with low incomes and low levels of education were more at risk of adverse outcomes. In one recent study, limited finances were associated with greater burden among caregivers of cognitively impaired elderly adults at the time of hospitalization (Shankar et al., 2014).

Relationship (Spouse, Nonspouse)

Past research conducted primarily among non-Hispanic White samples has shown that caregiving outcomes differ between nonspouse (who are mostly adult children) and spouse caregivers (Morse et al., 2012; Pinquart & Sörensen, 2004; Shankar et al., 2014). In a meta-analytic comparison study of differences in spouse, adult children, and children-in-law as caregivers of older adults, spouses had more depression, greater burden, and lower well-being. Greater psychological distress among spouses was explained primarily by higher levels of providing care (Pinquart & Sörensen, 2011). Children-in-law viewed the caregiving relationship less positively and had fewer rewards from caregiving (Pinquart & Sörensen, 2011). In other reviews of the literature, authors noted that spousal caregivers have reported higher levels of depression than nonspouses (Gitlin, Corcoran, Winter, Boyce, & Hauck, 2001; Pruchno & Resch, 1989) and that spouses reported less "upset" with the care receiver's behavior than nonspouses, who showed no decrease in "upset." A prior meta-analysis of caregiving studies found that spousal caregivers benefited less from existing interventions than adult children (Sörensen, Pinquart, & Duberstein, 2002).

Quality of Caregiver–Care Receiver Relationship

Disruption in the caregiver and care receiver relationship (Croog, Burleson, Sudilovsky, & Baume, 2006; Flannery, 2002) and/or a poor quality of relationship (Archbold, Stewart, Greenlick, & Harvath, 1990, 1992; Shim, Landerman, & Davis, 2011) can make caregiving seem more difficult even if the objective caregiving situation (e.g., hours devoted to caregiving and number of tasks performed) does not seem to be too demanding. Archbold et al. (1992) reported that the deleterious effects of the lack of preparedness on caregiver strain faded after 9 months; however, a poor relationship with the care receiver remained strongly related to caregiver strain. Reporting a poorer quality of relationship with the care receiver was associated with a 23.5% prevalence of anxiety and 10% prevalence of depression in the Mahoney, Regan, et al. (2005) descriptive study.

Lack of Preparedness

Most caregivers are not prepared for the many responsibilities they face and receive no formal instruction in caregiving activities (NAC & AARP, 2009). New duties can include complex tasks such as administering medications, managing side effects, monitoring complex chronic conditions, and/or assuming responsibility for new tasks like handling insurance claims and doing personal care. Moorman and Macdonald (2013) found that medical complexity of the care recipients' care is an important contributor to caregiving strain. Yet, although caregivers are called on to take on these many new responsibilities, they often lack the skills needed to do so (Schumacher, Beck, et al., 2006). Stewart, Archbold, Harvath, and Nkongho (1993) reported that although health care professionals were a caregiver's main source of information on providing physical care, the caregiver received no preparation on how to care for the patient emotionally or deal with the stresses of caregiving. Lack of preparedness can significantly increase the caregiver's perceptions of strain, especially during times of transition from hospital to home (Archbold et al., 1990, 1992).

Baseline Levels of Burden and Depressive Scores

In a meta-analysis of 84 caregiving studies, Pinquart and Sörensen (2003) found that caregivers have higher levels of stress and depression as well as lower levels of subjective well-being, physical health, and self-efficacy than noncaregivers. The strongest negative effects of caregiving were observed for clinician-rated depression. Differences in perceived stress and depression between caregivers and noncaregivers were larger in spouses than in adult children (Pinquart & Sörensen, 2003). Caregivers of care receivers who have dementia (Pinquart & Sörensen, 2006a) have more problems with symptom management (Butler et al., 2005; Grande, Farquhar, Barclay, & Todd, 2004) and problematic communication (Tolson, Swan, & Knussen, 2002) and have also reported increased burden, strain, and depression across studies.

Physical Health Problems

Vitaliano et al.'s (2003) quantitative review of 23 studies from North America, Europe, and Australia examined relationships of caregiving with several health outcomes. They found that caregivers are at greater risk of health problems than are noncaregivers. These studies included 1,594 caregivers of persons with dementia and 1,478 noncaregivers who were similar in age (mean: 65.6 years old) and sex ratio (65% women, 35% men). In this review, six physiological and five self-reported categories were examined that are indicators of illness risk and illness. The physiological categories included level of stress hormones, antibodies, immune counts/functioning, and cardiovascular and metabolic variables. Caregivers had a 23% higher level of stress hormones (adrenocorticotropic hormone, catecholamines, cortisol, etc.) and a 15% lower level of antibodies (Epstein–Barr virus, herpes simplex, immunoglobulin G test) than did noncaregivers. Comorbid medical illnesses are important because many caregivers are middle-aged to older adults, and they may be ill before they become caregivers. It is interesting to note that the relationship between caregiver status and physiological risk was stronger for men than women (Vitaliano et al., 2003). High perceived strain was associated with increased mortality, which did not differ by race, gender, or type of caregiving relationship (i.e., child, spouse; Perkins et al., 2013). Zarit et al. found that how caregivers who managed their own health poorly were at greater risk of increased stress-related caregiving outcomes (Zarit, Femia, Kim, & Whitlatch, 2010).

ASSESSMENT OF THE PROBLEM

Although systematic assessment of the patient is a routine element of clinical practice, assessment of the family caregiver is rarely carried out to determine what help the caregiver may need. Effective intervention strategies for caregivers should be based on an accurate assessment of caregiver risk and strengths. According to a broad consensus of researchers and family caregiving organizations (Schumacher, Beck, et al., 2006; Stewart et al., 1993), assessing the caregiver should involve addressing the following topics. These are applicable across settings (e.g., home, hospital) but may not need to be measured in every assessment.

- Initial assessments compared to reassessments (the latter focus on what has changed over time)
- New versus continuing care situations
- An acute episode prompting a change in caregiving versus an ongoing need requiring a focus on services (Family Caregiver Alliance [FCA], 2006)

Caregiving Context

The caregiving context includes the background on the caregiver and the caregiving situation. The caregiver's relationship to the care recipient (spouse or nonspouse) is important because spouse and nonspouse caregivers have different risks and needs (Gitlin et al., 2003; Pinquart & Sörensen, 2011; Sörensen et al., 2002). The caregiver's various roles and responsibilities can either take away from or enhance his or her ability to provide care. For example, working caregivers may have to develop strategies to juggle family and work responsibilities, so we need to know what their employment status is (work/home/volunteer; Pinquart & Sörensen, 2006a). The duration of caregiving (Sörensen et al., 2002) can give the clinician clues about how new caregiving is for the caregiver, or alert the clinician to possibility of caregiver exhaustion with the role. Questions about household status, such as how many people are in the home and the existence and involvement of extended family and social support (Pinquart & Sörensen, 2006a), can give the clinician clues about how much support the caregiver has readily available. Depending on the type of impairment of the care receiver, the physical environment of the home or facility where care takes place can be very important (Vitaliano et al., 2003). Determine what the caregiver's financial status is; for example, is he or she getting by, or is the caregiver short of funds to provide for everyday necessities (Vitaliano et al., 2003)? Ask about potential resources that the caregiver could choose to use and list these (Pinquart & Sörensen, 2006a). Explore the family's cultural background (Dilworth-Anderson et al., 2002; Goins et al., 2011) and look for clues on how to use this as a resource.

Caregiver's Perception of Recipient's Health and Functional Status

List activities the care receiver needs help with; include both ADL and IADL (Pinquart & Sörensen, 2003, 2006a). Determine whether the care recipient has any cognitive impairment. If the answer to this question is "yes," ask whether there are any behavioral problems (Gitlin et al., 2003; Sörensen et al., 2002). The presence of mobility problems can also make caregiving more difficult. Assess this by simply asking whether the care recipient has problems with getting around (Archbold et al., 1990; see Chapter 7, "Assessment of Physical Function").

Lack of Caregiver Preparedness

Does the caregiver have the skills, abilities, or knowledge to provide the care recipient with needed care? To assess preparedness, use questions from the Preparedness for Caregiving Scale (PCGS) (see consultgerirn.org/resources). The PCGS was developed by Archbold et al. (1990, 1993). The concept of preparedness derives from role theory, in which socialization to a role is assumed to be important for role enactment and performance. The questions prompt caregivers to rate how well prepared they think they are for caregiving in four perspectives of domain-specific preparedness: physical needs, emotional needs, resources, and stress. The clinician can interview the caregiver or ask the caregiver to complete the scale like a survey. The responses to the scale items can also be tallied and averaged for an overall score. If pressed for time, the clinician can simply ask, overall, how well prepared the caregiver thinks he or she is to care for a family member, and then follow this with more specific questions if the response indicates preparedness is low. The PCGS was evaluated in a longitudinal correlational study of family caregivers ($N = 103$) of older patients with chronic diseases (Archbold et al., 1990, 1992). The scale has five Likert-type items with possible responses ranging from 1 (not at all prepared) to 4 (very well prepared). Overall scores are computed by averaging responses to the five items. Scores range from 1.00 to 4.00; the lowest score correlating with least preparedness. Archbold et al. (1992) reported internal reliability (Cronbach's alpha) of 0.72 at 6 weeks and 0.71 at the 9-month interview.

Quality of Family Relationships

The caregiver's perception of the quality of the relationship with the care receiver is a key predictor of the presence or absence of strain from caregiving (Archbold et al., 1990). The quality of the relationship can be assessed using the Mutuality scale (Messecar, Parker-Walsch, & Lindauer, 2011) developed by Archbold et al. (1990, 1992). *Mutuality* is defined as the caregiver's perceived quality of the relationship with the care receiver. Questions include: How close do you feel to him or her? and How much does he or she express feelings of appreciation for you and the things you do? An overall score can be obtained by calculating the mean across all items—or the questions can be used in an open-ended interview format in which the clinician then probes for more information and history about the relationship. This scale can also be completed via self-administration and then reviewed by the clinician with the caregiver (interview the caregiver apart from the care receiver). For this scale, there is no item that asks about the relationship overall; instead, the items explore several key features of the relationship such as conflict, shared positive past memories, felt positive regard, and positive reciprocity between the caregiver and the care receiver. The questions open the door for the clinician to probe in a gentle way the quality of the relationship. Caregivers rate how they feel about the care recipient with possible responses ranging from 0 (not at all) to 4 (a great deal). The caregiver's mutuality score is computed by taking the average of the scores on the 15 items. Internal reliability and consistency (Cronbach's alpha) of the scale was 0.91 at both 6 weeks and 9 months from discharge from the hospital (Archbold et al., 1990).

Indicators of Problems With Quality of Care

In Cooper, Selwood, and Livingston's (2008) systematic review of the prevalence of elder abuse and neglect, they concluded that one in four vulnerable elders are at risk of abuse and only a small percentage of these cases are detected. Indicators of problems with the quality of care can include the following: evidence of an unhealthy environment, inappropriate management of finances, and demonstration of a lack of respect for older adult. The nurse's observations can be guided by the Elder Mistreatment Assessment (Fulmer, 2002), which helps the nurse identify elder abuse and neglect issues (see Elder Mistreatment Assessment instrument at consultgerirn.org/resources). This assessment instrument comprised seven sections that reviews signs, symptoms, and subjective complaints of elder abuse, neglect, exploitation, and abandonment (Fulmer, Paveza, Abraham, & Fairchild, 2000; Fulmer, Street, & Carr, 1984; Fulmer & Wetle, 1986). There is no "score," but the older adult should be referred to social services if there is evidence of mistreatment, a complaint by the older adult, or if there is high risk or probable abuse, neglect, exploitation, or abandonment of the older adult. Please also refer to Chapter 13, "Mistreatment Detection."

Caregiver's Physical and Mental Health Status

The caregiver's perception of his or her own health (Pinquart & Sörensen, 2006a, 2007) is one of the most reliable indicators of a physical health problem. Depression or other emotional distress (e.g., anxiety) can be assessed using the Center for Epidemiological Studies—Depression Scale Revised (CESD-R; see cesd-r.com/about-cesdr/; Eaton, Muntaner, Smith, Tien, & Ybarra, 2004; Pinquart & Sörensen, 2006a, 2007; Sörensen et al., 2002). The CESD-R was initially designed as a screen for the community dwelling at risk for developing major depressive symptomatology. It has been used widely in intervention studies with family caregivers, where it has been self-administered. In 2004, the tool was revised; however, the revised scale has been scored so that the same range of values still applies. The CESD-R website contains all the information needed to use the tool, which is in the public domain. For each of the 20 items, participants rate frequency of occurrence during the past week on a 4-point scale from 0 (not at all or less than 1 day) to 3 (nearly every day for 2 weeks). In order to have the same range as the original, the values for the top two responses (5–7 days and nearly every day) give the same value of 3. Scores range from 0 to 60, with a higher score indicating the presence of a greater number and frequency of depressive symptoms. A score of 16 or higher has been identified as discriminatory between groups with clinically relevant and nonrelevant depressive symptoms (Fulmer et al., 2000; Radloff, 1977).

Burden or strain can be assessed using the modified Caregiver Strain Index (CSI; see consultgerirn.org/resources, Family Caregiving; Sullivan, 2002). Preexisting burden or strain places caregivers at greater risk for poor outcomes, such as depression and poor health, and may prevent them from benefiting from interventions (Perkins et al., 2013; Schulz & Beach, 1999; Sullivan, 2002; Vitaliano et al., 2003). The modified CSI is a tool that can be used to quickly identify families with potential caregiving concerns. It is a 13-question tool that measures strain related to care provision. There is at least one item for each of the following major domains: financial, physical, psychological, and social and personal. Positive responses to seven or more items on the index indicate a greater level of strain. Internal consistency reliability is high (Cronbach's alpha = 0.86) and construct validity is supported by correlations with the physical and emotional health of the caregiver and with subjective views of the caregiving situation. A positive screen (seven or more items positive) on the CSI indicates a need for more in-depth assessment to facilitate appropriate intervention.

Rewards of Caregiving

Although early family caregiving research focused almost exclusively on negative outcomes of caregiving, clearly, there are many positive aspects of providing care. Spouses can be drawn closer together by caregiving, which can be an expression of love. Caregivers caring for a parent with Parkinson's or Alzheimer's who had positive experiences in caregiving reported fewer feelings of being overwhelmed or distressed by their situations (Habermann, Hines, & Davis, 2013) Child caregivers can feel a sense of accomplishment from helping their adult parents. Caregivers should be encouraged to explore and list their perceived benefits of caregiving (Archbold et al., 1995). These can include the satisfaction of helping a family member, developing new skills and competencies, and/or improved family relationships.

Self-Care Activities for the Caregiver

Self-care activities can include things like setting aside time to exercise, having time for oneself, and obtaining respite. Even if the caregiver does not use this strategy, ask him or her think about strategies that would work for him or her. Caregivers need to be reminded that self-care is not a luxury; it is a necessity. At a minimum, caregivers need to learn how to put themselves first, manage stress, socialize, and get help.

INTERVENTIONS AND CARE STATEGIES

Definitions

Psychoeducational Interventions

Psychoeducational interventions involve a structured program geared toward providing information about the care receiver's disease process and about resources and services, and training caregivers to respond effectively to disease-related problems, such as memory and behavior problems in patients with dementia or depression and anger in patients with cancer. Use of lectures, group discussions, and written materials is always led by a trained leader. Support may be part of a psychoeducational group, but it is secondary to the educational content. Use of technology such as phones, Internet, video contact, and interactive voice recognition to support caregivers as they take on new caregiving responsibilities is included in this category.

Supportive Interventions

This category subsumes both professionally led and peer-led unstructured support groups focused on building rapport among participants and creating a space in which to discuss problems, successes, and feelings regarding caregiving.

Respite or Adult Day Care

Respite care is given either in-home or as site-specific supervision, assistance with ADL, or skilled nursing care designed to give the caregiver time off.

Psychotherapy

This type of intervention involves a therapeutic relationship between the caregiver and a trained professional. Most psychotherapeutic interventions with caregivers follow a cognitive behavioral approach.

Interventions to Improve Care Receiver Competence

These interventions include memory clinics for patients with dementia and activity therapy programs designed to improve affect and everyday competence.

Multicomponent Interventions

Interventions in this group included various combinations of educational interventions, support, psychotherapy, and respite in Sörensen et al.'s (2002) and Pinquart and Sörensen's (2006a) meta-analyses. Individual studies carried out after the 2002 meta-analysis include nursing management and interprofessional care interventions and REACH II.

Overview

Past reviews of caregiver interventions, such as support groups, individual counseling, and education confirm that there is no single, easily implemented, and consistently effective method for eliminating the stresses and/or strain of being a caregiver (Knight, Lutzky, & Macofsky-Urban, 1993; Toseland & Rossiter, 1989). In 2002, Sörensen and colleagues performed a meta-analysis on the effects of a second generation of 78 caregiver intervention studies. The most consistent significant improvements in all outcome domains (burden, depression, well-being, ability and knowledge, and care receiver symptoms) assessed in the meta-analysis resulted from psychotherapy and caregiver psychoeducational interventions aimed at improving caregiver knowledge and abilities or skill building. They followed this up with a meta-analysis of 127 studies with 5,930 participants to examine what works in caregiving interventions (Pinquart & Sörensen, 2006b) and found significant effects for psychoeducational, supportive and counseling, and multicomponent interventions. Another systematic review of respite interventions demonstrated only small effects on caregivers with clear benefits for only certain subgroups (Mason et al., 2007). Multicomponent interventions, which combined features of psychotherapy and knowledge or skill building, had the largest effect on burden and, in addition, were effective in improving well-being, ability, and knowledge. The effects of different types of interventions on selected indicators of unhealthy caregiver transitions from the meta-analyses and studies completed since 2002 are presented in Table 11.1.

Other studies of psychotherapy and psychoeducational interventions fit the same pattern of results (Akkerman & Ostwald, 2004; Berry, Grant, Elliott, Edwards, & Fine, 2012; Bishop et al., 2014; Burns et al., 2005; Coon, Thompson, Steffen, Sorocco, & Gallagher-Thompson, 2003; Gitlin, Winter, Dennis, Hodgson, & Hauck, 2010; Harris, Durkin, Allen, DeCoster, & Burgio, 2011; Hébert et al., 2003; Hepburn et al., 2005; Judge, Yarry, Looman, & Bass, 2013; Lavretsky et al., 2013; Martire et al., 2010; Mittelman, Roth, Clay, & Haley, 2007; Mittelman, Roth, Coon, & Haley, 2004; Mittelman, Roth, Haley, & Zarit, 2004; Rodriguez-Sanchez et al., 2013; Zarit et al., 2011). All of these interventions address key negative aspects of caregiving: being overwhelmed with the physical demands of care, feeling isolated, not having time for oneself, having difficulties with the care recipient's behavior, and dealing with one's own negative responses.

There are several characteristics across interventions that seem to have a moderating effect on caregiving outcomes. Focusing the caregiver training exclusively on the care receiver to alter his or her symptoms has almost no effect on the caregiver (Agren, Evangelista, Hjelm, & Stromberg, 2012; Flynn Longmire et al., 2014; Pinquart & Sörensen, 2006b; Sörensen et al., 2002; Sherwood et al., 2012). Agren et al.'s (2012) psychoeducation intervention had no impact on caregiver's perceived control, health, depression, or burden. In the Sörensen (2002) meta-analysis, group interventions were less effective in improving caregiver burden than individual and mixed interventions, which is consistent with Knight et al. (1993) but inconsistent with the meta-analysis performed by Yin, Zhou, and Bashford (2002). Length of an intervention appears to be important in alleviating caregiver depression and care receiver symptoms. Caregivers do less well with shorter interventions regarding depression because they lose the supportive aspects of prolonged contact with a group or a professional before they can benefit.

Characteristics of the caregiver are also associated with intervention effectiveness. Some caregivers benefit less from interventions than others do. For example, Sörensen et al. (2002) found that spouse caregivers benefited less from interventions than did adult children. Table 11.2 presents caregiver characteristics associated with various indicators of unhealthy caregiver transitions.

Interventions With Little Effect

Some intervention approaches have been consistently disappointing, showing either no significant effects or limited responses. In Lee and Cameron's (2004) update of the Cochrane Database Review, reanalysis of three trials of respite care found no significant effects of respite on any outcome variable. Interventions focused on medication management of the care receiver's dementing condition (Lingler, Martire, & Schulz, 2005) and/or targeted to managing problematic behavior (Livingston, Johnston, Katona, Paton, & Lyketsos, 2005) were similarly disappointing. A meta-analysis of habit training for the management of urinary incontinence interventions showed that not only were there no significant differences in incontinence between the intervention and control groups, but

TABLE 11.1
Effects of Different Types of Interventions on Indicators of Unhealthy Caregiver Transitions

Type of Intervention	Burden or Strain	Depression, Distress, or Lack of Well-Being	Lack of Preparedness
Psychoeducation	Significant effect (Pinquart & Sörensen, 2006b; Sörensen, Pinquart, & Duberstein, 2002).	Significant effect (Pinquart & Sörensen, 2006b; Sörensen et al., 2002)	Significant effect (Pinquart & Sörensen, 2006b; Sörensen et al., 2002)
Skill building	Decreased burden—six studies (Acton & Winter, 2002)	Decreased depression—six studies (Acton & Winter, 2002)	Increased knowledge—nine studies (Acton & Winter, 2002)
		Significant reduction in depressive symptoms (Gallagher-Thompson et al., 2003)	14% improved reaction to CR symptoms (Hébert et al., 2003)
		Decreased bother, anxiety, depression (Mahoney, Tarlow, & Jones, 2003)	
		Decreased depression (Coon et al., 2003)	
		Decreased distress (Hepburn et al., 2005)	
		Improved quality of life (Bishop et al., 2014)	
		Improved depression when the caregiver reports engaging in exemplary care activities (Harris, Durkin, Allen, DeCoster, & Burgio, 2011)	
	Improved strain (Judge, Yarry, Looman, & Bass, 2013)	Improved psychosocial outcomes (Judge et al., 2013)	
		Decreased depressive symptoms (Berry, Grant, Elliott, Edwards, & Fine, 2012)	
Supportive interventions	Significant effect (Sörensen et al., 2002; Pinquart & Sörensen, 2006b)		Significant effect (Pinquart & Sörensen, 2006b; Sörensen et al., 2002)
		Preserved self-rated health (Mittelman, Roth, Clay, & Haley, 2007)	
Psychotherapy	Significant effect (Pinquart & Sörensen, 2006b; Sörensen et al., 2002)	Significant effect (Pinquart & Sörensen, 2006b; Sörensen et al., 2002)	Significant effect (Pinquart & Sörensen, 2006b; Sörensen et al., 2002)
	Decreased objective burden	Decreased anxiety (Akkerman & Ostwald, 2004)	Some improved reaction to CR symptoms (A. Burns et al., 2005)
		Decreased depression with yogic meditation (Lavretsky et al., 2013)	
		Improved mental health (Rodriguez-Sanchez et al., 2013)	
Respite	Significant effect (Pinquart & Sörensen, 2006b; Sörensen et al., 2002)	Significant effect (Pinquart & Sörensen, 2006b; Sörensen et al., 2002)	
		Decreased depression—three studies (Acton & Winter, 2002)	

(continued)

TABLE 11.1
Effects of Different Types of Interventions on Indicators of Unhealthy Caregiver Transitions *(continued)*

Type of Intervention	Burden or Strain	Depression, Distress, or Lack of Well-Being	Lack of Preparedness
	Small effect (Mason et al., 2007)	Small effect (Mason et al., 2007)	
		Stress lowered on days respite used (Zarit et al., 2011)	
Focus on CR		Significant effect (Sörensen et al., 2002)	
		COPE: functioning improved for CR but no significant CG improvement (Gitlin, Winter, Dennis, Hodgson, & Hauck, 2010)	COPE: no significant CG improvement in confidence (Gitlin et al., 2010)
		Treating CR depression decreased burden (Martire et al., 2010)	
	No effect (Agren et al., 2012)	No effect (Agren et al., 2012)	
	No effect (Flynn Longmire et al., 2014)	Distress decreased (Flynn Longmire et al., 2014)	
		No improvement in emotional health (Sherwood et al., 2012)	
Multicomponent—added to this category	Large significant effect (Pinquart & Sörensen, 2006b; Sörensen et al., 2002)	Improved distress and depression (Bass, Clark, Looman, McCarthy, & Eckert, 2003; Callahan et al., 2006)	Significant effect (Pinquart & Sörensen, 2006b; Sörensen et al., 2002)
	REACH II interventions decreased burden (Elliott, Burgio, & Decoster, 2010)	REACH II interventions decreased depression levels, improved self-rated health (Elliott et al., 2010)	
	Significant decrease in burden in TCARE (Montgomery, Kwak, Kosloski, & O'Connell Valuch, 2011)	Significant decrease in depression in TCARE (Montgomery et al., 2011)	
Nursing and interprofessional care management—includes hospital or rehabilitation at-home and primary care	Improved carer strain (Burton & Gibbon, 2005)	Less burden (Crotty, Whitehead, Miller, & Gray, 2003)	
	Decreased burden/strain—two studies (Acton & Winter, 2002)	Less strain (R. Harris, Ashton, Broad, Connolly, & Richmond, 2005)	
	REACH interventions overall decreased burden (Gitlin et al., 2003)	More strain after intervention (Wade et al., 2003)	
	Decreased burden (Kalra et al., 2004)	Significant decrease in depressive symptoms (Eisdorfer et al., 2003)	
	Burden and strain were responsive to intervention (Schulz, Martire, & Klinger, 2005)	Decreased depression, distress, anxiety—four studies (Acton & Winter, 2002)	
		Decreased anxiety and depression (Kalra et al., 2004)	
		Decreased depression (Mittelman, Roth, Coon, et al., 2004)	
		Decreased reaction ratings (Mittelman, Roth, Haley, et al., 2004)	

(continued)

TABLE 11.1
Effects of Different Types of Interventions on Indicators of Unhealthy Caregiver Transitions ***(continued)***

Type of Intervention	Burden or Strain	Depression, Distress, or Lack of Well-Being	Lack of Preparedness
		Clinically significant decreases in depression and anxiety (Schulz et al., 2005)	
		Significant effect (Pinquart & Sörensen, 2006b; Sörensen et al., 2002)	
		Higher role rewards (Li et al., 2003)	
		Caregiver affect improved (Gitlin, Hauck, Dennis, & Winter, 2005)	
		Well-being worse in control group (Burns, Nichols, Martindale-Adams, Graney, & Lummus, 2003)	
Focus on physical or emotional health of CG		Decreased psychological distress (King, Baumann, O'Sullivan, Wilcox, & Castro, 2002)	
		Decreased depression and anxiety (Waelde, Thompson, & Gallagher-Thompson, 2004)	

CG, caregiver; COPE, Care of Persons With Dementia in Their Environments; CR, care receiver; REACH, Resources for Enhancing Alzheimer's Caregiver Health; TCARE, Tailored Caregiver Assessment and Referral.

TABLE 11.2
Effects of Different Types of Caregiver Characteristics on Indicators of Unhealthy Caregiver Transitions

Characteristics of Caregiving Situation	Burden	Depression or Lack of Well-Being	Lack of Preparedness
CR has dementia	Less effective (Sörensen, Pinquart, & Duberstein, 2002)	Less effective (Sörensen et al., 2002)	Less effective (Sörensen et al., 2002)
Adult child CGs	Greater improvement (Sörensen et al., 2002)	Greater improvement (Sörensen et al., 2002)	Greater improvement (Sörensen et al., 2002)
		Nonspouses did better (Gitlin et al., 2003)	
Spouse CGs	Smaller improvement (Sörensen et al., 2002)	Smaller improvement (Sörensen et al., 2002)	Smaller improvement (Sörensen et al., 2002)
		Wives with low mastery and high anxiety benefited the most (D. F. Mahoney, Tarlow, & Jones, 2003)	
		Cuban husbands improved more on depressive symptoms (Eisdorfer et al., 2003)	
	REACH II spouse CGs improved quality of life (burden) for African Americans only (Belle et al., 2006)	REACH II spouse CGs improved quality of life (depression) for African Americans only (Belle et al., 2006)	

(continued)

TABLE 11.2

Effects of Different Types of Caregiver Characteristics on Indicators of Unhealthy Caregiver Transitions (*continued*)

Characteristics of Caregiving Situation	Burden	Depression or Lack of Well-Being	Lack of Preparedness
		Wives improved more on burden and depression after CR nursing home placement (Gaugler et al., 2011)	
Older CGs	Greater improvement (Pinquart & Sörensen, 2006b; Sörensen et al., 2002)	No effects (Sörensen et al., 2002)	Greater improvement (Pinquart & Sörensen, 2006b; Sörensen et al., 2002)
	Higher risk for burden (Schulz et al., 2005)	Higher risk for depression (Schulz et al., 2005)	
	Older African American CGs improved more (Sörensen et al., 2005; C. C.Lee, Czaja, & Schulz, 2010)	Older African American CGs improved more (Sörensen et al., 2005; Lee et al., 2010)	
		Greater improvement in well-being (Sörensen et al., 2002)	
Female CGs	Greater improvement (Pinquart & Sörensen, 2006b; Sörensen et al., 2002)	Females benefit more (Gallagher-Thompson et al., 2003; Pinquart & Sörensen, 2006b)	Greater improvement (Sörensen et al., 2002)
	Better improvement (Gitlin et al., 2003)	Cuban daughters improved more on depressive symptoms (Eisdorfer et al., 2003)	
	Higher risk for burden (Schulz et al., 2005)	Higher risk for depression (Schulz et al., 2005)	
Ethnicity	African American CGs had lower levels of caregiver burden (Pinquart & Sörensen, 2005)	Latinos benefit as much (Eisdorfer et al., 2003)	Hispanic and Asian American CGs were more depressed; African American CGs had lower levels of depression (Pinquart & Sörensen, 2005)
		Cuban husbands and daughters improved more on depressive symptoms (Eisdorfer et al., 2003)	
		Hispanics did better (Gitlin et al., 2003)	
	REACH II Hispanics and Whites decreased burden compared to African Americans though all groups improved (Elliott, Burgio, & Decoster, 2010)	REACH II Hispanics and Whites decreased depression compared to African Americans though all groups improved (Elliott et al., 2010)	
Lower education	Better improvement (Gitlin et al., 2003)	Better improvement (Gitlin et al., 2003)	
	Higher risk for burden (Schulz et al., 2005)	Higher risk for depression (Schulz et al., 2005)	

CG, caregiver; CR, care receiver; REACH, Resources for Enhancing Alzheimer's Caregiver Health.

that caregivers found the intervention labor intensive (Ostaszkiewicz, Johnston, & Roe, 2004).

In Acton and Winter's (2002) meta-analysis of dementia, caregiving studies; small, diverse samples; lack of intervention specificity; diversity in the length, duration, and intensity of the intervention strategies; and problematic outcome measures led to nonsignificant results for many tested interventions (Cooke, McNally, Mulligan, Harrison, & Newman, 2001). They also reported that two thirds of the interventions they examined did not show any improvement in any outcome measures. Their analysis was hampered by lack of detailed description of the interventions in the studies they examined. Study limitations have also been a factor leading to disappointing results for some innovative caregiving interventions for caregivers of care receivers with other long-term, debilitating illnesses.

For example, interventions designed to teach arthritis management as a couple (Martire et al., 2003) to decrease the gap between caregiver's expectations and care receiver's actual functional abilities with skill-building and nurse-coached pain management all had disappointing results because of either small sample sizes or the complexity of the problems they were designed to address (Martin-Cook, Davis, Hynan, & Weiner, 2005; Schumacher et al., 2002). According to Price, Hermans, and Grimley Evans (2000), modification interventions for wandering have never been adequately tested because of the many flaws identified in the existing published research; outcome measurement has also been problematic. More distal outcomes, such as depression, perceived stress, caregiver strain, and self-efficacy less directly related to the actual intervention, are less likely to change significantly (Bourgeois, Schulz, Burgio, & Beach, 2002; Burgio, Stevens, Guy, Roth, & Haley, 2003) than outcomes that are more specific to the intervention (Hébert et al., 2003).

Caregivers caring for care receivers who have conditions that worsen substantially over time (dementia, heart failure, Parkinson's disease, and stroke) have reported either less improvement, no improvement, or increased strain after intervention (Agren et al., 2012; Forster et al., 2001; Pinquart & Sörensen, 2006b; Sörensen et al., 2002; Wright, Litaker, Laraia, & DeAndrade, 2001). Across many studies, Sörensen et al. (2002) reported that interventions with caregivers of dementia patients are less successful than for other caregivers. They also noted that if levels of caregiving are relatively high and cannot be reduced, as is the case for dementia caregivers, then burden and depression are less amenable to change as well. A multidisciplinary rehabilitation program for patients with Parkinson's disease resulted in no improvement in depression for caregivers after treatment (Trend, Kaye, Gage, Owen, & Wade, 2002). A meta-analysis of hospital-at-home care for patients with stroke reported no evidence from clinical trials to support a radical shift in the care of patients with acute stroke from hospital-based care (Langhorne et al., 2000). Individual studies that examined other psychoeducational and/or support and counseling interventions for stroke caregivers (albeit with relatively small samples) found no significant changes between the intervention and control groups (Clark, Rubenach, & Winsor, 2003; Gräsel, Biehler, Schmidt, & Schupp, 2005; Larson et al., 2005). Only an intensive, multicomponent skills-training intervention significantly decreased burden anxiety and depression for this category of caregivers (Kalra et al., 2004). A number of family-based and symptom-management interventions for patients with cancer have also found no significant intervention effects (Hudson, Aranda, & Hayman-White, 2005; Kozachik et al., 2001; Kurtz, Kurtz, Given, & Given, 2005; Northouse, Kershaw, Mood, & Schafenacker, 2005; Wells, Hepworth, Murphy, Wujcik, & Johnson, 2003), or the effects were not sustainable (Northouse et al., 2013). In several of these studies, there was a large dropout rate among the intervention participants because of the rapidly deteriorating condition of the care receivers.

Resources for Enhancing Alzheimer's Caregiver Health

The REACH project was designed to test promising interventions for enhancing family caregiving for persons with dementia and overcome several of the limitations of prior research (Schulz et al., 2003). More than 1,200 caregivers participated at six sites nationwide. The sample was more diverse than most caregiving studies because of the multisite design: participants were 56% White, 24% African American, and 19% Latino (Wisniewski et al., 2003). Five sites participated in this trial nationwide. The following five interventions were tested:

1. A 12-month, computer-mediated automated interactive voice response intervention designed to assist family caregivers managing care receivers with dementia (Mahoney, Tarlow, & Jones, 2003)
2. A psychoeducational (skill-building) approach modeled after community-based support groups tailored to be sensitive to ethnic groups tested (Gallagher-Thompson et al., 2003)
3. A manual-guided care-recipient–focused behavior management skill training and caregiver-focused, problem-solving training intervention tailored on cultural preferences of White and African American caregivers (Burgio et al., 2003)
4. A family therapy intervention designed to enhance communication between caregivers and other family members by identifying existing problems in communication and facilitating changes in interaction patterns (Eisdorfer et al., 2003)
5. Two primary care interventions delivered over a period of more than 24 months, which included patient behavior management only and patient behavior management plus caregiver stress and coping (Burns, Nichols, Martindale-Adams, Graney, & Lummus, 2003)
6. In-home occupational therapy visits designed to help families modify the environment to reduce caregiver burden (Gitlin, Hauck, Dennis, & Winter, 2005)

When the results from the REACH interventions were pooled, overall interventions decreased burden significantly compared to the control conditions (Gitlin et al., 2003). Only the family therapy with computer technology intervention was effective in reducing depressive symptoms. Interventions were superior to control conditions on burden for women and caregivers with lower education. Interventions had greater impact on depression among Hispanics, nonspouses, and caregivers with lower education.

REACH II followed up on REACH I, but, unlike the first set of studies, which implemented a variety of interventions at six sites, REACH II implemented the same two interventions at each of five participating sites. REACH II specifically implemented a multicomponent intervention and tested new tools for assessing caregivers at risk of adverse outcomes. Intervention participants received individual risk profiles and the REACH intervention through nine in-home and three telephone sessions for more than 6 months. Caregivers receiving REACH II reported better self-rated health, sleep quality, physical health, and emotional health than for those caregivers not receiving the intervention. Findings supported using a structured, multicomponent skills-training intervention that targeted caregiver self-care behaviors as one of five target areas. Overall, REACH II improved self-reported health status and decreased burden and bother in racially and ethnically diverse caregivers of people with dementia (Elliott, Burgio, & Decoster, 2010). An analysis of the findings by sociodemographic groups indicated that caregiver's age and religious coping moderated the effects of the intervention for Hispanics and Blacks. The older Hispanic and Black caregivers who received the intervention reported a decrease in caregiver burden from baseline to follow-up (Lee et al., 2010). Findings from the REACH studies support use of multicomponent interventions tailored for specific caregiving characteristics.

Aspects of Interventions That Improve Effectiveness

A key conclusion of the REACH I and II trials and several of the meta-analyses (Elliott et al., 2010; Gitlin et al., 2003; Pinquart & Sörensen, 2006b; Schulz et al., 2005; Sörensen et al., 2002) reviewed in this chapter was that family caregiver interventions need to be multicomponent and tailored. Multicomponent interventions have the potential to include a repertoire of various strategies that target different aspects of the caregiving experience. In focus groups conducted during a caregiving clinical trial, Farran et al. (2004) identified and cataloged the information and skills caregivers reported they needed to respond to their own needs or the caregiving process. This included care receiver issues such as managing difficult behaviors, worrisome symptoms, personal care problems, and caregiver concerns such as managing competing responsibilities and stressors, finding and using resources, and handling their emotional and physical responses to care (Farran et al., 2004). *Tailored interventions* are interventions that are crafted to match a specific target population; for example, spouse caregivers of patients with Alzheimer's disease and their specific caregiving issues and concerns identified through assessment (Archbold et al., 1995; Beeber & Zimmerman, 2012; Horton-Deutsch, Farran, Choi, & Fogg, 2002). The Tailored Caregiver Assessment and Referral (TCARE) protocol is a manualized care management protocol specifically designed for care managers working with caregivers (Montgomery, Kwak, Kosloski, & O'Connell Valuch, 2011). Shifting from a traditional focus on the patient to a more family-centered approach and assessment is more helpful (Beeber & Zimmerman, 2012; Bowen, Maclehose, & Beaumont, 2011). Interventions that are individualized or tailored in combination with skill building demonstrated the best evidence of effectiveness (Gitlin et al., 2008, 2010; Pusey & Richards, 2001). Among the psychoeducation interventions, some of the most effective were predicated on a skill-building approach (Gallagher-Thompson et al., 2003; Hepburn, Tornatore, Center, & Ostwald, 2001). Collaboration or a partnership model with the caregiver is also a key component of making the tailoring process more effective (Harvath et al., 1994). Programs that work collaboratively with care receivers and their families and are more intensive and modified to the caregiver's needs are also more successful (Brodaty, Green, & Koschera, 2003). Clinicians interested in the translation of evidence-based programs into sustainable community-based programs should review reports of the ongoing challenges to be expected with such projects (Teri et al., 2012).

Nursing Care Strategies

1. *Identify content and skills needed to increase preparedness for caregiving.*
   Psychoeducational skill-building interventions include information about the care needed by the care receiver and how to provide it, as well as coaching on how to manage the caregiving role. Tasks associated with taking on the caregiving role include dealing with change, juggling competing responsibilities and stressors, providing and managing care, finding and using resources, and managing the physical and emotional responses to care (Acton & Winter, 2002; Farran, Loukissa, Perraud, & Paun, 2003; Farran et al., 2004; Gitlin et al., 2003; Pinquart & Sörensen, 2006b; Sörensen et al., 2002).

2. *Form a partnership with the caregiver before generating strategies to address issues and concerns.*
   The goal of this partnership is blending the nurse's knowledge and expertise in health care with the caregiver's knowledge of the family member and the caregiving situation. Each party brings essential knowledge to the process of mutual negotiation between the family and the nurse. Together, they develop ideas to address the issues and concerns that are most salient for the caregiver and care receiver. One strategy that can be used in the hospital setting is to interview the caregiver using the Family Preferences Index developed by Li et al. (2003) to assess family member's preferences to participate in care while the older adult is hospitalized (Brodaty et al., 2003; Gitlin et al., 2005; Harvath et al., 1994; Nolan, 2001). A checklist to elicit and engage the perspectives of older adults and their caregivers at medical visits can be used to enhance communication (Wolff et al., 2014).
3. *Identify the caregiving issues and concerns on which the caregiver wants to work and generate strategies.*
   Multiple strategies should be generated for each caregiving issue and concern. One of the most important findings from the review of literature on caregiving is that multicomponent interventions are superior to narrow, single-approach problem solving (Acton & Winter, 2002; Gitlin et al., 2005; Sörensen et al., 2002). Several Level II individual studies are presented in Table 11.1.
4. *Assist the caregiver in identifying strengths in the caregiving situation.*
   Not all outcomes from caregiving are negative, and caregiving can be rewarding for some caregivers who derive pride and satisfaction from the important role they are filling. Incorporating pleasurable activities into the daily routine or incorporating something that is either fun or meaningful into some caregiving task is a way of enhancing caregiving. Even in really difficult situations there may be some positive benefit derived such as satisfaction in meeting an important commitment and/or recognition of personal growth (Archbold et al., 1995).
5. *Assist the caregiver in finding and using resources.*
   Navigating the health care system is one of the most difficult skills caregivers have to master (Archbold et al., 1995; Farran et al., 2004; Schumacher et al., 2002). Caregivers rarely know how to translate a need that they have into a request for help from the health care system. Learning how to speak to health care providers, how to negotiate billing, and how to request help with transportation—all of these tasks can be overwhelming. For some caregivers, Internet and other online sources of support and information can be helpful.
6. *Help caregivers identify and manage their physical and emotional responses to caregiving.*
   We know that caregiving is sometimes associated with deterioration of the caregiver's health or significant depression (Schulz et al., 2005). Generating strategies to take care of the caregiver is just as important as the strategies for caring for the care recipient.
7. *Use an interprofessional approach when working with family caregivers.*
   Multicomponent interventions have the strongest record in terms of alleviating some of the global negative consequences of caregiving. Involving a team of other health professionals helps the nurse and family generate new ideas for strategies and brings a fresh perspective to the idea-generating process (Acton & Winter, 2002; Belle et al., 2006; Elliott et al., 2010; Farran et al., 2003, 2004; Gitlin et al., 2003; Sörensen et al., 2002). Several Level II studies are presented in Table 11.1.

CASE STUDY

Alison Walsh is the oldest of two children and the only one who still lives in the same city as her widowed mother. She describes her relationship with her mother as very strained and without much love—only discipline. Her mother, who recently suffered a stroke and is considered marginal for staying home by her neurologist, is expecting that Alison will move in and take care of her. In fact, Alison's mother has virtually no resources for any other option. Alison's mother is being discharged today from the hospital. Alison says she would feel hard-pressed to take on all of the new care that her mother will require, including having to do baths and many, if not all, of her ADL. In addition,

(continued)

CASE STUDY *(continued)*

she feels her relationship with her mother is so poor she does not understand why she should have to be the caregiver at this time when she has her own problems. Adding to her difficulties, Alison has only one other sibling to call on for help, and he lives more than 2,000 miles away in another city. Her husband has health problems as well and his care takes considerable time.

As a child caregiver, Alison is at higher risk of depression or anxiety. The goal of intervention with Alison will be to identify and address aspects of her caregiving situation amenable to modification. The possible targets for intervention will vary from one caregiver to another, and it is important that the approach be tailored. Addressing aspects of caregiving that are strong predictors of unhealthy caregiver transitions, such as a lack of preparedness, stress and strain in the relationship, and overall burden, can help the nurse tailor the caregiver interventions. In this case study, only three parameters of assessment (lack of preparedness, poor relationship quality, and need to find rewards of caregiving) will be addressed along with some suggested strategies for addressing the concerns indicated.

First, in Alison's case, caregivers may be reluctant to raise concerns about their lack of preparedness to the nurse. They may connect lack of preparedness with being embarrassed about their own lack of understanding, or they may simply not know what it is they do not know. For example, in Alison's case, she may not realize that formal resources could be tapped to provide some of the personal care that she feels unable or unwilling to perform. Exploration of her readiness to provide care will help Alison raise her concerns so that they can be fully addressed.

Second, a lack of mutuality (the positive quality of the relationship between caregiver and care recipient) is very predictive of future and sustained reported difficulty with caregiving. Alison has a difficult relationship with her mother now and a history of a poor quality relationship from childhood. This puts her at risk of experiencing more strain from caregiving. Alison is aware that her relationship with her mother is difficult, but she may not realize how much this is adding to her strain. Alison will need to think about strategies to get support and help to deal with her feelings.

Third, although in Alison's situation there might not seem to be any rewards of caregiving, it is important to ask about these anyway. There are two very important reasons for nurses exploring positive aspects of caregiving with the caregiver; caregivers want to talk about them, and these factors will be an important indicator of the quality of care provided to the care recipient. Nurses need to encourage an increase in positive affect (i.e., feelings such as gratitude, forgiveness, and the like) while at the same time working on decreasing negative feelings such as depression, anxiety, and guilt.

SUMMARY

Outcomes Specific to Caregiving

The goal of the guideline is to reduce the likelihood of unhealthy transitions to the caregiving role by lowering caregiver strain, depression, and poor physical health for caregivers. Indicators of problems with this include reports of depression and/or fatigue, increased use of over-the-counter and prescription medications, increased use of health services, neglect of own health, and substance abuse. Increased focus on the caregiver system as the unit of service should increase the nurse's confidence in working with family caregivers.

Outcomes Specific to Patient

These include improvement (where possible) in patient functional status, nutrition, and hygiene. Improved symptom management for care recipients with significant chronic disease is also a desired outcome. This could include better pain management for care recipients with cancer, improved glycemic control for care recipients with diabetes, and/or diminished problematic behaviors for care recipients with dementia. The emotional well-being of the care recipient should also be an outcome of interventions to aid the caregiver. Decreased use of emergency services and increased use of formal care supports are system outcomes that might be expected.

NURSING STANDARD OF PRACTICE

Protocol 11.1: Family Caregiving

I. GOAL

To identify viable strategies to monitor and support family caregivers

II. OVERVIEW

Family caregivers provide more than 80% of the long-term care for older adults in this country. Caregiving can be difficult, time-consuming work added on top of job and other family responsibilities. If the caregiver suffers negative consequences from the caregiving role and these are not mitigated, increased morbidity and mortality may result for the caregiver. Not all outcomes from caregiving are negative; there are many caregivers who report rewards from caregiving.

III. BACKGROUND AND STATEMENT OF PROBLEM

A. Definitions
   1. *Family caregiving* is broadly defined and refers to a broad range of unpaid care provided in response to illness or functional impairment to a chronically ill or functionally impaired older family member, partner, friend, or neighbor that exceeds the support usually provided in family relationships (Schumacher, Beck, et al., 2006).
   2. Caregiver role transitions: *Caregiver role acquisition* is a family role transition that occurs through situated interaction as part of a role-making process (Schumacher, 1995). This is the process of taking on the caregiving role at the beginning of caregiving or when a significant change in the caregiving context occurs. Role transitions occur when a role is added to or deleted from the role set of a person, or when the behavioral expectations for an established role change significantly (NAC & AARP, 2009).
   3. Indicators of healthy caregiver role transitions: The broad categories of indicators of healthy transitions include subjective well-being, role mastery, and well-being of relationships. These are the subjective, behavioral, and interpersonal parameters of health most likely to be associated with healthy role transitions (NAC & AARP, 2009).
   4. Family caregiving activities include assistance with day-to-day activities, illness-related care, care management, and invisible aspects of care. Day-to-day activities include personal care activities (bathing, eating, dressing, mobility, transferring from bed to chair, and using the toilet) and IADL (meal preparation, grocery shopping, making telephone calls, and money management; Walker et al., 1995). Illness-related activities include managing symptoms, coping with illness behaviors, carrying out treatments, and performing medical or nursing procedures that include an array of medical technologies (Schumacher, Beidler et al., 2006; Schumacher et al., 2000). Care management activities include accessing resources, communicating with and navigating the health care and social services systems, and acting as an advocate (Schumacher et al., 2000). Invisible aspects of care are protective actions the caregiver takes to ensure the older adult's safety and well-being without the elders knowledge (Bowers, 1987).
   5. Caregiving roles can be classified into a hierarchy according to who takes on the bulk of responsibilities versus only intermittent supportive assistance. Primary caregivers tend to provide most of the everyday aspects of care, whereas secondary caregivers help out as needed to fill the gaps (Cantor & Little, 1985; Penning, 1990; Tennstedt et al., 1989). Among caregivers who live with their care recipients, spouses account for the bulk of primary caregivers, whereas adult children are more likely to be secondary caregivers. The range of the family caregiving role includes protective caregiving, like "keeping an eye on" an older adult who is currently independent but at risk, to full-time, around-the-clock care for a severely impaired family member. Health care providers may fail to assess the full scope of the family caregiving role if they associate family caregiving only with the performance of tasks.
   6. *Caregiver assessment* refers to an ongoing iterative process of gathering information that describes a family caregiving situation and identifies the particular issues, needs, resources, and strengths of the family caregiver.

B. Etiology and/or epidemiology of risk factors associated with unhealthy caregiving transitions
   1. Just being a caregiver puts an individual at increased risk of higher levels of stress and depression and lower levels of subjective well-being and physical health (Pinquart & Sörensen, 2006a, 2007; Vitaliano et al., 2003).

(continued)

Protocol 11.1: Family Caregiving *(continued)*

2. Female caregivers on average provide more direct care and report higher levels of burden and depression (Gitlin et al., 2003).
3. Ethnic minority caregivers provide more care, use less formal services, and report worse physical health than White caregivers (Dilworth-Anderson et al., 2002; Pinquart & Sörensen, 2006a, 2007).
4. African American caregivers experience less stress and depression and get more rewards from caregiving than White caregivers (Cuellar, 2002; Dilworth-Anderson et al., 2002; Gitlin et al., 2003; Haley et al., 2004; Pinquart & Sörensen, 2004), but younger or nonspouse caregivers do not respond as well to interventions (Belle et al., 2006; Lee et al., 2010).
5. Hispanic and Asian American caregivers exhibit more depression (Gitlin et al., 2003; Pinquart & Sörensen, 2004) particularly among young Hispanic caregivers (Lee et al., 2010).
6. Less-educated caregivers report more depression (Buckwalter et al., 1999; Gitlin et al., 2003).
7. Spouse caregivers report higher levels of depression than nonspouse caregivers (Pinquart & Sörensen, 2004; Pruchno & Resch, 1989), but appear to benefit more from interventions (Elliott et al., 2010).
8. Caregivers who have a poor-quality relationship with the care recipient report more strain (Archbold et al., 1990; Croog et al., 2006; Flannery, 2002).
9. Caregivers who lack preparedness for the caregiving role also have increased strain (Archbold et al., 1990, 1992).
10. Caregivers of care recipients who have dementia have more strain and burden (Pinquart & Sörensen, 2003).

IV. PARAMETERS OF ASSESSMENT

A. Caregiving context
  1. Caregiver relationship with care recipient (spouse, nonspouse; Elliott et al., 2010; Gitlin et al., 2003; Sörensen et al., 2002)
  2. Caregiver roles and responsibilities
    a. Duration of caregiving (Sörensen et al., 2002)
    b. Employment status (work/home/volunteer; Pinquart & Sörensen, 2004)
    c. Household status (number in home, etc.; Pinquart & Sörensen, 2004)
    d. Existence and involvement of extended family and social support (Pinquart & Sörensen, 2004)
  3. Physical environment (home, facility; Gitlin et al., 2010; Vitaliano et al., 2003)
  4. Financial status (Vitaliano et al., 2003)
  5. Potential resources that caregiver could choose to use—list (Pinquart & Sörensen, 2004)
  6. Family's cultural background (Dilworth-Anderson et al., 2002; Goins et al., 2011)

B. Caregiver's perception of health and functional status of care recipient
  1. List activities care receiver needs help with; include both ADL and IADL (Pinquart & Sörensen, 2004)
  2. Presence of cognitive impairment—if yes, any behavioral problems (Gitlin et al., 2003; Sörensen et al., 2002)
  3. Presence of mobility problems—assess with single question (Archbold et al., 1990)

C. Caregiver preparedness for caregiving
  1. Does caregiver have the skills, abilities, or knowledge to provide care recipient with needed care (see PCGS at consultgerirn.org/resources)?

D. Quality of family relationships
  1. The caregiver's perception of the quality of the relationship with the care receiver (see Mutuality Scale; Archbold et al., 1990; Messecar et al., 2011)

E. Indicators of problems with quality of care
  1. Unhealthy environment
  2. Inappropriate management of finances
  3. Lack of respect for older adult (see EAI at www.consultgerirn.org/resources)

F. Caregiver's physical and mental health status
  1. Self-rated health: single item—asks what the caregiver's perception of his or her health is (Pinquart & Sölensen, 2006a, 2007).

(continued)

Protocol 11.1: Family Caregiving *(continued)*

2. Health conditions and symptoms
    a. Depression or other emotional distress (e.g., anxiety; Pinquart & Sörensen, 2003, 2006a, 2007; Sörensen et al., 2002; see cesd-r.com/cesdr)
    b. Reports of burden or strain (Schulz & Beach, 1999; Vitaliano et al., 2003; see Caregiver Stain Index at www.consultgerirn.org/resources—Family Caregiving topic)
3. Rewards of caregiving
    a. List perceived benefits of caregiving (Archbold et al., 1995)
    b. Satisfaction of helping family member
    c. Developing new skills and competencies
    d. Improved family relationships
4. Self-care activities for caregiver
    a. Attending to own health care needs
    b. Getting exercise
    c. Taking time off
    d. Seeking support
    e. Getting proper rest and nutrition

V. NURSING CARE STRATEGIES

A. Identify content and skills needed to increase preparedness for caregiving (Acton & Winter, 2002; Farran et al., 2003; Gitlin et al., 2003; Pusey & Richards, 2001; Schumacher, Beidler et al., 2006; Schumacher et al., 2000; Sörensen et al., 2002).
B. Form a partnership with the caregiver before generating strategies to address issues and concerns (Brodaty et al., 2003; Gitlin et al., 2003; Harvath et al., 1994).
C. Invite participation in care while in the hospital using the Family Preferences Index, a 14-item approach to exploring caregivers' personal choices for participating in the care of hospitalized older adult family members to determine preferences to provide care (Messecar, Powers, & Nagel, 2008).
D. Identify the caregiving issues and concerns on which the caregiver wants to work and generate strategies (Acton & Winter, 2002; Gitlin et al., 2003; Schumacher, Beidler et al., 2006; Sörensen et al., 2002).
E. Assist the caregiver in identifying strengths in the caregiving situation (Archbold et al., 1995).
F. Assist the caregiver in finding and using resources (Archbold et al., 1995; Farran et al., 2004; Schumacher et al., 2002).
G. Help caregivers identify and manage their physical and emotional responses to caregiving (Schulz & Beach, 1999).
H. Use an interprofessional approach when working with family caregivers (Acton & Winter, 2002; Farran et al., 2003, 2004; Gitlin et al., 2003; Sörensen et al., 2002).

VI. EVALUATION OR EXPECTED OUTCOMES

A. Outcomes specific to caregiving transitions
    1. Lower caregiver strain
    2. Decreased depression
    3. Improved physical health
B. Outcomes specific to patient
    1. Quality of family caregiving
    2. Care recipient's functional status, nutrition, hygiene, and symptom management
    3. Care recipient's emotional well-being
    4. Decreased occurrence of adverse events such as increased frequency of emergent care

ABBREVIATIONS

ADL Activities of daily living
EAI Elder Assessment Instrument
IADL Instrumental activities of daily living
PCGS Preparedness for Caregiving Scale

ACKNOWLEDGMENTS

The author wishes to gratefully acknowledge the assistance of Patricia Archbold and Barbara Stewart, the developers of the Caregiver Preparedness and Mutuality scales, for their assistance in providing information and access to these valuable caregiving assessment tools. This protocol also benefited from the perspective provided by Hong Li, the developer of the Family Preference Index, on the critical importance of involving family caregivers early in the hospital care process to facilitate a healthy transition into the caregiving role.

RESOURCES

Caregiver Strain Index
http://consultgerirn.org/uploads/File/trythis/try_this_14.pdf

CESD-R
http://cesd-r.com/cesdr

Elder Assessment Instrument (EAI)
http://consultgerirn.org/uploads/File/trythis/try_this_15.pdf

Preparedness Scale
http://consultgerirn.org/uploads/File/trythis/try_this_28.pdf

REFERENCES

Acton, G. J., & Winter, M. A. (2002). Interventions for family members caring for an elder with dementia. *Annual Review of Nursing Research, 20*, 149–179. *Evidence Level I.*

Agren, S., Evangelista, L. S., Hjelm, C., & Stromberg, A. (2012). Dyads affected by chronic heart failure: A randomized study evaluating effects of education and psychosocial support to patients with heart failure and their partners. *Journal of Cardiac Failure, 18*, 359–366. doi:10.1016/j.cardfail.2012.01.014. *Evidence Level II.*

Akkerman, R. L., & Ostwald, S. K. (2004). Reducing anxiety in Alzheimer's disease family caregivers: The effectiveness of a nine-week cognitive-behavioral intervention. *American Journal of Alzheimer's Disease and Other Dementias, 19*(2), 117–123. *Evidence Level II.*

Archbold, P. G., Stewart, B. J., Greenlick, M. R., & Harvath, T. A. (1990). Mutuality and preparedness as predictors of caregiver role strain. *Research in Nursing & Health, 13*(6), 375–384. *Evidence Level II.*

Archbold, P. G., Stewart, B. J., Greenlick, M. R., & Harvath, T. A. (1992). Clinical assessment of mutuality and preparedness in family caregivers to frail older people. In S. G. Funk, E. M. Tornquist, M. T. Champagne, & L. A. Copp (Eds.), *Key aspects of elder care* (pp. 332–337). New York, NY: Springer Publishing Company. *Evidence Level II.*

Archbold, P. G., Stewart, B. J., Miller, L. L., Harvath, T. A., Greenlick, M. R., Van Buren, L., . . . Schook J. E. (1995). The PREP system of nursing interventions: A pilot test with families caring for older members. Preparedness (PR), enrichment (E) and predictability (P). *Research in Nursing & Health, 18*(1), 3–16. *Evidence Level II.*

Arno, P. S. (2006, January). *Economic value of informal caregiving.* Presented at the Care Coordination and the Caregiving Forum, Department of Veterans Affairs, NIH, Bethesda, MD. *Evidence Level IV.*

Bass, D. M., Clark, P. A., Looman, W. J., McCarthy, C. A., & Eckert, S. (2003). The Cleveland Alzheimer's managed care demonstration: Outcomes after 12 months of implementation. *The Gerontologist, 43*(1), 73–85. *Evidence Level II.*

Bauer, M., Fitzgerald, L., Haesler, E., & Manfrin, M. (2009). Hospital discharge planning for frail older people and their family. Are we delivering best practice? A review of the evidence. *Journal of Clinical Nursing, 18*(18), 2539–2546. *Evidence Level V.*

Beeber, A. S., & Zimmerman, S. (2012). Adapting the family management style framework for families caring for older adults with dementia. *Journal of Family Nursing, 18*, 123–145. doi:10.1177/1074840711427144. *Evidence Level IV.*

Belle, S. H., Burgio, L., Burns, R., Coon, D., Czaja, S. J., Gallagher-Thompson, D., . . . Zhang, S; Resources for Enhancing Alzheimer's Caregiver Health (REACH) II Investigators. (2006). Enhancing the quality of life of dementia caregivers from different ethnic or racial groups: A randomized, controlled trial. *Annals of Internal Medicine, 145*(10), 727–738. *Evidence Level II.*

Berry, J., Grant, J., Elliott, T., Edwards, G., & Fine, P., (2012). Does problem-solving training for family caregivers benefit their care recipients with severe disabilities? A latent growth model of the project CLUES randomized clinical trial. *Rehabilitation Psychology, 57*(2), 98–112. *Evidence Level II.*

Bishop, D., Miller, I., Weiner, D., Guilmette, T., Mukand, J., Feldmann, E., . . . Springate, B. (2014). Family intervention: telephone tracking (FITT): A pilot stroke outcome study. *Topics in Stroke Rehabilitation, 21*(Suppl. 1), S63–S74. doi:10.1310/tsr21S1-S63. *Evidence Level II.*

Bourgeois, M. S., Schulz, R., Burgio, L. D., & Beach, S. (2002). Skills training for spouses of patients with Alzheimer's disease: Outcomes of an intervention study. *Journal of Clinical Geropsychology, 8*(1), 53–73. *Evidence Level II.*

Bowen, C., MacLehose, A., & Beaumont, J. G. (2011). Advanced multiple sclerosis and the psychosocial impact on families. *Psychology & Health, 26*, 113–127. doi:10.1080/08870440903287934. *Evidence Level IV.*

Bowers, B. J. (1987). Intergenerational caregiving: Adult caregivers and their aging parents. *Advances in Nursing Science, 9*(2), 20–31. *Evidence Level IV.*

Brodaty, H., Green, A., & Koschera, A. (2003). Meta-analysis of psychosocial interventions for caregivers of people with dementia. *Journal of the American Geriatrics Society, 51*(5), 657–664. *Evidence Level I.*

Buckwalter, K. C., Gerdner, L., Kohout, F., Hall, G. R., Kelly, A., Richards, B., & Sime, M. (1999). A nursing intervention to decrease depression in family caregivers of persons with dementia. *Archives of Psychiatric Nursing, 13*(2), 80–88. *Evidence Level II.*

Burgio, L., Stevens, A., Guy, D., Roth, D. L., & Haley, W. E. (2003). Impact of two psychosocial interventions on white and African American family caregivers of individuals with dementia. *The Gerontologist, 43*(4), 568–579. *Evidence Level II.*

Burns, A., Guthrie, E., Marino-Francis, F., Busby, C., Morris, J., Russell, E.,... Byrne, J. (2005). Brief psychotherapy in Alzheimer's disease: Randomised controlled trial. *British Journal of Psychiatry, 187*(2), 143–147. *Evidence Level II.*

Burns, R., Nichols, L. O., Martindale-Adams, J., Graney, M. J., & Lummus, A. (2003). Primary care interventions for dementia caregivers: 2-year outcomes from the REACH study. *The Gerontologist, 43*(4), 547–555. *Evidence Level II.*

Burton, C., & Gibbon, B. (2005). Expanding the role of the stroke nurse: A pragmatic clinical trial. *Journal of Advanced Nursing, 52*(6), 640–650. *Evidence Level II.*

Butler, L. D., Field, N. P., Busch, A. L., Seplaki, J. E., Hastings, T. A., & Spiegel, D. (2005). Anticipating loss and other temporal stressors predict traumatic stress symptoms among partners of metastatic/recurrent breast cancer patients. *Psycho-Oncology, 14*(6), 492–502. *Evidence Level II.*

Callahan, C. M., Boustani, M. A., Unverzagt, F. W., Austrom, M. G., Damush, T. M., Perkins, A. J.,... Hendrie, H. C. (2006). Effectiveness of collaborative care for older adults with Alzheimer disease in primary care: A randomized controlled trial. *Journal of the American Medical Association, 295*(18), 2148–2157. *Evidence Level II.*

Cannuscio, C. C., Jones, C., Kawachi, I., Colditz, G. A., Berkman, L., & Rimm, E. (2002). Reverberation of family illness: A longitudinal assessment of informal caregiving and mental health status in the nurses' health study. *American Journal of Public Health, 92*(8), 1305–1311. *Evidence Level IV.*

Cantor, M. H., & Little, V. (1985). Aging and social care. In R. H. Binstock & E. Shanas (Eds.), *Handbook of aging and the social sciences* (2nd ed., pp. 745–781). New York, NY: Van Nostrand Reinhold. *Evidence Level V.*

Clark, M. S., Rubenach, S., & Winsor, A. (2003). A randomized controlled trial of an education and counseling intervention for families after stroke. *Clinical Rehabilitation, 17*(7), 703–712. *Evidence Level II.*

Coleman, E. A., & Boult, C. (2003). Improving the quality of transitional care for persons with complex care needs. *Journal of the American Geriatrics Society, 51*(4), 556–557. *Evidence Level VI.*

Cooke, D. D., McNally, L., Mulligan, K. T., Harrison, M. J., & Newman, S. P. (2001). Psychosocial interventions for caregivers of people with dementia: A systematic review. *Aging & Mental Health, 5*(2), 120–135. *Evidence Level I.*

Coon, D. W., Thompson, L., Steffen, A., Sorocco, K., & Gallagher-Thompson, D. (2003). Anger and depression management: Psychoeducational skill training interventions for women caregivers of a relative with dementia. *The Gerontologist, 43*(5), 678–689. *Evidence Level II.*

Croog, S. H., Burleson, J. A., Sudilovsky, A., & Baume, R. M. (2006). Spouse caregivers of Alzheimer patients: Problem responses to caregiver burden. *Aging & Mental Health, 10*(2), 87–100. *Evidence Level IV.*

Cooper, C., Selwood, A., & Livingston, G. (2008). The prevalence of elder abuse and neglect: A systematic review. *Age and Ageing, 37*(2), 151. *Evidence Level I.*

Crotty, M., Whitehead, C., Miller, M., & Gray, S. (2003). Patient and caregiver outcomes 12 months after home-based therapy for hip fracture: A randomized controlled trial. *Archives of Physical Medicine and Rehabilitation, 84*(8), 1237–1239. *Evidence Level II.*

Cuellar, N. G. (2002). A comparison of African American & Caucasian American female caregivers of rural, post-stroke, bedbound older adults. *Journal of Gerontological Nursing, 28*(1), 36–45. *Evidence Level IV.*

Davies, H. D., Sridhar, S. B., Newkirk, L. A., Beaudreau, S. A., & O'Hara, R. (2012). Gender differences in sexual behaviors of AD patients and their relationship to spousal caregiver well-being. *Aging & Mental Health, 16*, 89–101. doi:10.1080/13607863.2011.609532. *Evidence Level II.*

Dilworth-Anderson, P., Williams, I. C., & Gibson, B. E. (2002). Issues of race, ethnicity, and culture in caregiving research: A 20-year review (1980–2000). *The Gerontologist, 42*(2), 237–272. *Evidence Level I.*

Eaton, W. W., Muntaner, C., Smith, C., Tien, A., & Ybarra, M. (2004). Center for epidemiologic studies depression scale: Review and revision (CESD and CESD-R). In M. E. Maruish (Ed), *The use of psychological testing for treatment planning and outcomes assessment* (3rd ed., pp. 363–377). Mahwah, NJ: Lawrence Erlbaum. *Evidence Level II.*

Eisdorfer, C., Czaja, S. J., Loewenstein, D. A., Rubert, M. P., Argüelles, S., Mitrani, V. B., & Szapocznik, J. (2003). The effect of a family therapy and technology-based intervention on caregiver depression. *The Gerontologist, 43*(4), 521–531. *Evidence Level II.*

Elliott, A. F., Burgio, L. D., & Decoster, J. (2010). Enhancing caregiver health: Findings from the resources for enhancing Alzheimer's caregiver health II intervention. *Journal of the American Geriatrics Society, 58*(1), 30–37. *Evidence Level II.*

Family Caregiver Alliance (FCA). (2006). *Caregiver assessment: Principles, guidelines and strategies for change. Report from a national consensus development conference* (Vol. I). San Francisco, CA: Author. *Evidence Level VI.*

Farran, C. J., Gilley, D. W., McCann, J. J., Bienias, J. L., Lindeman, D. A., & Evans, D. A. (2004). Psychosocial interventions to reduce depressive symptoms of dementia caregivers: A randomized clinical trial comparing two approaches. *Journal of Mental Health and Aging, 10*(4), 337–350. *Evidence Level II.*

Farran, C. J., Loukissa, D., Perraud, S., & Paun, O. (2003). Alzheimer's disease caregiving information and skills. Part I: Care recipient issues and concerns. *Research in Nursing & Health, 26*(5), 366–375. *Evidence Level IV.*

Flannery, R. B., Jr. (2002). Disrupted caring attachments: Implications for long-term care. *American Journal of Alzheimer's Disease and Other Dementias, 17*(4), 227–231. *Evidence Level VI.*

Flynn Longmire, C. V., Drye, L. T., Frangakis, C. E., Martin, B. K., Meinert, C. L., Mintzer, J. E.,... Lyketsos, C. G.; DIADS-2 Research Group. (2014). Is sertraline treatment or depression remission in depressed Alzheimer patients associated with improved caregiver well being? Depression in Alzheimer's Disease Study 2. *American Journal of Geriatric Psychiatry, 22*, 14–24. doi:10.1016/j.jagp.2013.02.014. *Evidence Level II.*

Forster, A., Smith, J., Young, J., Knapp, P., House, A., & Wright, J. (2001). Information provision for stroke patients and their caregivers. *Cochrane Database of Systematic Reviews, 2001*(3), CD001919. *Evidence Level I.*

Freedman, V. A., Cornman, J. C., & Carr, D. (2014). Is spousal caregiving associated with enhanced well-being? New evidence from the panel study of income dynamics. *Journals of Gerontology. Series B, Psychological Sciences & Social Sciences, 69*, 861–869. doi:10.1093/geronb/gbu004. *Evidence Level IV.*

Fulmer, T. (2002). *Elder abuse and neglect assessment. Try this: Best practices in nursing care to older adults.* Retrieved from http://consultgerirn.org/resources. *Evidence Level VI.*

Fulmer, T., & Wetle, T. (1986). Elder abuse screening and intervention. *Nurse Practitioner, 11*(5), 33–38. *Evidence Level II.*

Fulmer, T., Paveza, G., Abraham, I., & Fairchild, S. (2000). Elder neglect assessment in the emergency department. *Journal of Emergency Nursing, 26*(5), 436–443. *Evidence Level II.*

Fulmer, T., Street, S., & Carr, K. (1984). Abuse of the elderly: Screening and detection. *Journal of Emergency Nursing, 10*(3), 131–140. *Evidence Level II.*

Gallagher-Thompson, D., Coon, D. W., Solano, N., Ambler, C., Rabinowitz, Y., & Thompson, L. W. (2003). Changes in indices of distress among Latino and Anglo female caregivers of elderly relatives with dementia: Site-specific results from the REACH national collaborative study. *The Gerontologist, 43*(4), 580–591. *Evidence Level II.*

Gaugler, J. E., Roth, D. L., Haley W. E., & Mittelman, M. S. (2011). Modeling trajectories and transitions: Results from the New York University caregiver intervention. *Nursing Research, 60*, S28–S37. doi:10.1097/NNR.0b013e318216007d. *Evidence Level IV.*

Geary, C. R., & Schumacher, K. L. (2012). Care transitions: Integrating transition theory and complexity science concepts. *Advances in Nursing Science, 35*, 236–248. doi:10.1097/ANS.0b013e31826260a5. *Evidence Level VI.*

Gitlin, L. N., Belle, S. H., Burgio, L. D., Czaja, S. J., Mahoney, D., Gallagher-Thompson, D.,... Ory, M. G. (2003). Effect of multicomponent interventions on caregiver burden and depression: The REACH multisite initiative at 6-month follow-up. *Psychology & Aging, 18*(3), 361–374. *Evidence Level I.*

Gitlin, L. N., Corcoran, M., Winter, L., Boyce, A., & Hauck, W. W. (2001). A randomized, controlled trial of a home environmental intervention: Effect on efficacy and upset in caregivers and on daily function of persons with dementia. *The Gerontologist, 41*(1), 4–14. *Evidence Level II.*

Gitlin, L. N., Hauck, W. W., Dennis, M. P., & Winter, L. (2005). Maintenance of effects of the home environmental skill-building program for family caregivers and individuals with Alzheimer's disease and related disorders. *Journals of Gerontology. Series A, Biological Sciences and Medical Sciences, 60*(3), 368–374. *Evidence Level II.*

Gitlin, L. N., Winter, L., Burke, J., Chernett, N., Dennis, M. P., & Hauck, W. W. (2008). Tailored activities to manage neuropsychiatric behaviors in persons with dementia and reduce caregiver burden: A randomized pilot study. *American Journal of Geriatric Psychiatry, 16*(3), 229–239. *Evidence Level II.*

Gitlin, L. N., Winter, L., Dennis, M. P., Hodgson, N., & Hauck, W. W. (2010). A biobehavioral home-based intervention and the well-being of patients with dementia and their caregivers: The COPE randomized trial. *Journal of the American Medical Association, 22*, 983–991. doi:10.1001/jama.2010.1253. *Evidence Level II.*

Goins, R. T., Spencer, S. M., McGuire, L. C., Goldberg, J., Wen, Y., & Henderson J. A. (2011). Adult caregiving among American Indians: The role of cultural factors. *The Gerontologist, 51*, 310–320. doi:10.1093/geront/gnq101. *Evidence Level IV.*

Grande, G. E., Farquhar, M. C., Barclay, S. I., & Todd, C. J. (2004). Caregiver bereavement outcome: Relationship with hospice at home, satisfaction with care, and home death. *Journal of Palliative Care, 20*(2), 69–77. *Evidence Level II.*

Gräsel, E., Biehler, J., Schmidt, R., & Schupp, W. (2005). Intensification of the transition between inpatient neurological rehabilitation and home care of stroke patients. Controlled clinical trial with follow-up assessment six months after discharge. *Clinical Rehabilitation, 19*(7), 725–736. *Evidence Level III.*

Habermann, B., Hines, D., & Davis, L. (2013). Caring for parents with neurodegenerative disease: a qualitative description. *Clinical Nurse Specialist, 27*, 182–187. doi:10.1097/NUR.0b013e318295576b. *Evidence Level IV.*

Haley, W. E., Gitlin, L. N., Wisniewski, S. R., Mahoney, D. F., Coon, D. W., Winter, L.,... Ory, M. (2004). Well-being, appraisal, and coping in African-American and Caucasian dementia caregivers: Findings from the REACH study. *Aging & Mental Health, 8*(4), 316–329. *Evidence Level II.*

Harris, R., Ashton, T., Broad, J., Connolly, G., & Richmond, D. (2005). The effectiveness, acceptability and costs of a hospital-at-home service compared with acute hospital care: A randomized controlled trial. *Journal of Health Services Research & Policy, 10*(3), 158–166. *Evidence Level II.*

Harris, G. M., Durkin, D. W., Allen, R. S., DeCoster, J., & Burgio, L. D. (2011). Exemplary care as a mediator of the effects of caregiver subjective appraisal and emotional outcomes. *The Gerontologist, 51*, 332–342. doi:10.1093/geront/gnr003. *Evidence Level II.*

Harvath, T. A., Archbold, P. G., Stewart, B. J., Gadow, S., Kirschling, J. M., Miller, L.,... Schook, J. (1994). Establishing partnerships with family caregivers: Local and cosmopolitan knowledge. *Journal of Gerontological Nursing, 20*(2), 29–35. *Evidence Level V.*

Hébert, R., Lévesque, L., Vézina, J., Lavoie, J. P., Ducharme, F., Gendron, C.,... Dubois, M. F. (2003). Efficacy of a psychoeducative group program for caregivers of demented persons living at home: A randomized controlled trial. *Journals of Gerontology. Series B, Psychological Sciences and Social Sciences, 58*(1), S58–S67. *Evidence Level II.*

Hepburn, K. W., Lewis, M., Narayan, S., Center, B., Tornatore, J., Bremer, K., & Kirk, L. (2005). Partners in caregiving: A psychoeducation program affecting dementia family caregivers' distress and caregiving outlook. *Clinical Gerontologist, 29*(1), 53–69. *Evidence Level II.*

Hepburn, K. W., Tornatore, J., Center, B., & Ostwald, S. W. (2001). Dementia family caregiver training: Affecting beliefs about caregiving and caregiver outcomes. *Journal of the American Geriatrics Society, 49*(4), 450–457. *Evidence Level II.*

Hoffman, G. J., Lee, J., & Mendez-Luck, C. A. (2012). Health behaviors among baby boomer informal caregivers. *The Gerontologist, 52*, 219–30. doi:10.1093/geront/gns003. *Evidence Level IV.*

Horton-Deutsch, S. L., Farran, C. J., Choi, E. E., & Fogg, L. (2002). The PLUS intervention: A pilot test with caregivers of depressed older adults. *Archives of Psychiatric Nursing, 16*(2), 61–71. *Evidence Level III.*

Hudson, P. L., Aranda, S., & Hayman-White, K. (2005). A psycho-educational intervention for family caregivers of patients receiving palliative care: A randomized controlled trial. *Journal of Pain and Symptom Management, 30*(4), 329–341. *Evidence Level II.*

Jencks, S. F., Williams, M. V., & Coleman, E. A. (2009). Rehospitalizations among patients in the Medicare fee-for-service program. *New England Journal of Medicine, 360*, 1418–1428. *Evidence Level II.*

Judge, K. S., Yarry, S. J., Looman, W. J., & Bass, D. M. (2013). Improved strain and psychosocial outcomes for caregivers of individuals with dementia: Findings from project ANSWERS. *The Gerontologist, 53*, 280–292. doi:10.1093/geront/gns076. *Evidence Level II.*

Kalra, L., Evans, A., Perez, I., Melbourn, A., Patel, A., Knapp, M., & Donaldson, N. (2004). Training carers of stroke patients: Randomised controlled trial. *British Medical Journal, 328*(7448), 1099. *Evidence Level II.*

Kiecolt-Glaser, J. K., Preacher, K. J., MacCallum, R. C., Atkinson, C., Malarkey, W. B., & Glaser, R. (2003). Chronic stress and age-related increases in the proinflammatory cytokine IL-6. *Proceedings of the National Academy of Sciences of the United States of America, 100*(15), 9090–9095. *Evidence Level III.*

King, A. C., Baumann, K., O'Sullivan, P., Wilcox, S., & Castro, C. (2002). Effects of moderate-intensity exercise on physiological, behavioral, and emotional responses to family caregiving: A randomized controlled trial. *Journals of Gerontology. Series A, Biological Sciences and Medical Sciences, 57*(1), M26–M36. *Evidence Level II.*

Knight, B. G., Lutzky, S. M., & Macofsky-Urban, F. (1993). A meta-analytic review of interventions for caregiver distress: Recommendations for future research. *The Gerontologist, 33*(2), 240–248. *Evidence Level I.*

Kozachik, S. L., Given, C. W., Given, B. A., Pierce, S. J., Azzouz, F., Rawl, S. M., & Champion, V. L. (2001). Improving depressive symptoms among caregivers of patients with cancer: Results of a randomized clinical trial. *Oncology Nursing Forum, 28*(7), 1149–1157. *Evidence Level II.*

Kurtz, M. E., Kurtz, J. C., Given, C. W., & Given, B. (2005). A randomized, controlled trial of a patient/caregiver symptom control intervention: Effects on depressive symptomatology of caregivers of cancer patients. *Journal of Pain and Symptom Management, 30*(2), 112–122. *Evidence Level II.*

Langhorne, P., Dennis, M. S., Kalra, L., Shepperd, S., Wade, D. T., & Wolfe, C. D. (2000). Services for helping acute stroke patients avoid hospital admission. *Cochrane Database of Systematic Reviews, 2000*(2), CD000444. *Evidence Level I.*

Larson, J., Franzén-Dahlin, A., Billing, E., Arbin, M., Murray, V., & Wredling, R. (2005). The impact of a nurse-led support and education programme for spouses of stroke patients: A randomized controlled trial. *Journal of Clinical Nursing, 14*(8), 995–1003. *Evidence Level II.*

Lee, C. C., Czaja, S. J., & Schulz, R. (2010). The moderating influence of demographic characteristics, social support, and religious coping on the effectiveness of a multicomponent psychosocial caregiver intervention in three racial ethnic groups. *Journals of Gerontology. Series B, Psychological Sciences & Social Sciences, 65B*(2), 185–194. *Evidence Level II.*

Lee, H., & Cameron, M. (2004). Respite care for people with dementia and their carers. *Cochrane Database of Systematic Reviews, 2004*(2), CD004396. *Evidence Level I.*

Lavretsky, H., Epel, E. S., Siddarth, P., Nazarian, N., Cyr, N. S., Khalsa, D. S, ... Irwin, M. R. (2013). A pilot study of yogic meditation for family dementia caregivers with depressive symptoms: Effects on mental health, cognition, and telomerase activity. *International Journal of Geriatric Psychiatry, 28*, 57–65. doi:10.1002/gps.3790. *Evidence Level IV.*

Li, H., Melnyk, B. M., McCann, R., Chatcheydang, J., Koulouglioti, C., Nichols, L. W., ... Ghassemi, A. (2003). Creating avenues for relative empowerment (CARE): A pilot test of an intervention to improve outcomes of hospitalized elders and family caregivers. *Research in Nursing & Health, 26*(4), 284–299. *Evidence Level I.*

Lingler, J. H., Martire, L. M., & Schulz, R. (2005). Caregiver-specific outcomes in antidementia clinical drug trials: A systematic review and meta-analysis. *Journal of the American Geriatrics Society, 53*(6), 983–990. *Evidence Level I.*

Livingston, G., Johnston, K., Katona, C., Paton, J., & Lyketsos, C. G. (2005). Systematic review of psychological approaches to the management of neuropsychiatric symptoms of dementia. *American Journal of Psychiatry, 162*(11), 1996–2021. *Evidence Level I.*

Mahoney, D. F., Cloutterbuck, J., Neary, S., & Zhan L. (2005). African American, Chinese, and Latino family caregivers' impressions of the onset and diagnosis of dementia: Cross-cultural similarities and differences. *Gerontologist, 45*(6), 783–792. *Evidence Level I.*

Mahoney, D. F., Tarlow, B. J., & Jones, R. N. (2003). Effects of an automated telephone support system on caregiver burden and anxiety: Findings from the REACH for TLC intervention study. *The Gerontologist, 43*(4), 556–567. *Evidence Level II.*

Mahoney, R., Regan, C., Katona, C., & Livingston, G. (2005). Anxiety and depression in family caregivers of people with Alzheimer disease: The LASER-AD study. *American Journal of Geriatric Psychiatry, 13*(9), 795–801. *Evidence Level IV.*

Martin-Cook, K., Davis, B. A., Hynan, L. S., & Weiner, M. F. (2005). A randomized, controlled study of an Alzheimer's caregiver skills training program. *American Journal of Alzheimer's Disease and Other Dementias, 20*(4), 204–210. *Evidence Level II.*

Martire, L. M., Schulz, R., Keefe, F. J., Starz, T. W., Osial, T. A., Jr., Dew, M. A., & Reynolds, C. F., III. (2003). Feasibility of a dyadic intervention for management of osteoarthritis: A pilot study with older patients and their spousal caregivers. *Aging & Mental Health, 7*(1), 53–60. *Evidence Level II.*

Martire, L. M., Schulz, R., Reynolds, C. F., III, Karp, J. F., Gildengers, A. G., & Whyte, E. M. (2010). Treatment of late-life depression alleviates caregiver burden. *Journal of the American Geriatrics Society, 58*(1), 23–29. *Evidence Level II.*

Mason, A., Weatherly, H., Spilsbury, K., Golder, S., Arksey, H., Adamson, J., . . . Drummond, M. (2007). The effectiveness and cost-effectiveness of respite for caregivers of frail older people. *Journal of the American Geriatrics Society, 55*(2), 290–299. *Evidence Level I.*

Messecar, D., Powers, B. A., & Nagel, C. L. (2008). The Family Preferences Index: Helping family members who want to participate in the care of a hospitalized older adult. *American Journal of Nursing, 108*(9), 52–59. *Evidence Level VI.*

Messecar, D. C., Parker-Walsch, C., & Lindauer, A. (2011). Family caregiving. In V. Hirth (Ed.), *Case-based geriatrics: A global approach.* Burr Ridge, IL: McGraw-Hill. *Evidence Level VI.*

Mittelman, M. S., Roth, D. L., Clay, O. J., & Haley, W. E. (2007). Preserving health of Alzheimer caregivers: Impact of a spouse caregiver intervention. *American Journal of Geriatric Psychiatry, 15*(9), 780–789. *Evidence Level II.*

Mittelman, M. S., Roth, D. L., Coon, D. W., & Haley, W. E. (2004). Sustained benefit of supportive intervention for depressive symptoms in caregivers of patients with Alzheimer's disease. *American Journal of Psychiatry, 161*(5), 850–856. *Evidence Level II.*

Mittelman, M. S., Roth, D. L., Haley, W. E., & Zarit, S. H. (2004). Effects of a caregiver intervention on negative caregiver appraisals of behavior problems in patients with Alzheimer's disease: Results of a randomized trial. *Journals of Gerontology. Series B, Psychological Sciences and Social Sciences, 59*(1), P27–P34. *Evidence Level II.*

Moorman, S. M., & Macdonald, C. (2013). Medically complex home care and caregiver strain. *The Gerontologist, 53*, 407–417. doi:10.1093/geront/gns067. *Evidence Level IV.*

Montgomery, R. J., Kwak, J., Kosloski, K., & O'Connell Valuch, K. (2011). Effects of the TCARE intervention on caregiver burden and depressive symptoms: Preliminary findings from a randomized controlled study. *Journals of Gerontology. Series B, Psychological Sciences & Social Sciences, 66*, 640–647. doi:10.1093/geronb/gbr088. *Evidence Level II.*

Morse, J. Q., Shaffer, D. R., Williamson, G. M., Dooley, W. K., & Schulz, R. (2012). Models of self and others and their relation to positive and negative caregiving responses. *Psychology & Aging, 27*, 211–218. doi:10.1037/a0023960. *Evidence Level II.*

National Academy on an Aging Society. (2000). *Caregiving: Helping the elderly with activity limitations. Challenges for the 21st century: Chronic and disabling conditions*, No. 7. Washington, DC: Author. *Evidence Level V.*

National Alliance for Caregiving (NAC) & AARP. (2009). *Caregiving in the U.S.* Bethesda, MD: National Alliance for Caregiving. *Evidence Level IV.*

Naylor, M. D. (2003). Nursing intervention research and quality of care: Influencing the future of healthcare. *Nursing Research, 52*(6), 380–385. *Evidence Level VI.*

Naylor, M., & Keating, S. A. (2008). Transitional care. *American Journal of Nursing, 108*(Suppl. 9), 58–63. *Evidence Level VI.*

Naylor, M. D., Kurtzman, E. T., & Pauly, M. V. (2009). Transitions of elders between long-term care and hospitals. *Policy, Politics, & Nursing Practice, 10*, 187–194. doi:10.1177/1527154409355710. *Evidence Level VI.*

Nolan, M. (2001). Working with family carers: Towards a partnership approach. *Reviews in Clinical Gerontology, 11*(1), 91–97. *Evidence Level V.*

Northouse, L., Kershaw, T., Mood, D., & Schafenacker, A. (2005). Effects of a family intervention on the quality of life of women with recurrent breast cancer and their family caregivers. *Psycho-Oncology, 14*(6), 478–491. *Evidence Level II.*

Northouse, L. L., Mood, D. W., Schafenacker, A., Kalemkerian, G., Zalupski, M., LoRusso, P., . . . Kershaw, T. (2013). Randomized clinical trial of a brief and extensive dyadic intervention for advanced cancer patients and their family caregivers. *Psycho-Oncology, 22*, 555–563. doi:10.1002/pon.3036. *Evidence Level II.*

Ostaszkiewicz, J., Johnston, L., & Roe, B. (2004). Habit retraining for the management of urinary incontinence in adults. *Cochrane Database of Systematic Reviews, 2004*(2), CD002801. doi:10.1002/14651858.CD002801.pub2. *Evidence Level I.*

Penning, M. J. (1990). Receipt of assistance by elderly people: Hierarchical selection and task specificity. *The Gerontologist, 30*, 220–227. *Evidence Level IV.*

Perkins, M., Howard, V. J., Wadley, V. G., Crowe, M., Safford, M. M., Haley, W. E., . . . Roth, D. L. (2013). Caregiving strain and all-cause mortality: Evidence from the REGARDS study. *Journals of Gerontology. Series B, Psychological Sciences & Social Sciences, 68*, 504–512. doi:10.1093/geronb/gbs084. *Evidence Level II.*

Pinquart, M., & Sörensen, S. (2003). Differences between caregivers and noncaregivers in psychological health and physical health: A meta-analysis. *Psychology and Aging, 18*(2), 250–267. *Evidence Level I.*

Pinquart, M., & Sörensen, S. (2004). Associations of caregiver stressors and uplifts with subjective well-being and depressive mood: A meta-analytic comparison. *Aging & Mental Health, 8*(5), 438–449. *Evidence Level I.*

Pinquart, M., & Sörensen, S. (2005). Ethnic differences in stressors, resources, and psychological outcomes of family caregiving: A meta-analysis. *The Gerontologist, 45*(1), 90–106. *Evidence Level I.*

Pinquart, M., & Sörensen, S. (2006a). Gender differences in caregiver stressors, social resources, and health: An updated meta-analysis. *Journals of Gerontology. Series B, Psychological Sciences and Social Sciences, 61*(1), P33–P45. *Evidence Level I.*

Pinquart, M., & Sörensen, S. (2006b). Helping caregivers of persons with dementia: Which interventions work and how large are their effects? *International Psychogeriatrics, 18*(4), 577–595. *Evidence Level I.*

Pinquart, M., & Sörensen, S. (2007). Correlates of physical health of informal caregivers: A meta-analysis. *Journals of Gerontology. Series B, 62*(2), P126–P137. *Evidence Level I.*

Pinquart, M., & Sörensen, S. (2011). Spouses, adult children, and children-in-law as caregivers of older adults: A meta-analytic comparison. *Psychology & Aging, 26*, 1–14. doi:10.1037/a0021863. *Evidence Level I.*

Price, J. D., Hermans, D. G., & Grimley Evans, J. (2000). Subjective barriers to prevent wandering of cognitively impaired people. *Cochrane Database of Systematic Reviews, 2000*(4), CD001932. doi:10.1002/14651858.CD001932. *Evidence Level I.*

Pruchno, R. A., & Resch, N. L. (1989). Mental health of caregiving spouses: Coping as mediator, moderator, or main effect? *Psychology and Aging, 4*(4), 454–463. *Evidence Level I.*

Pusey, H., & Richards, D. (2001). A systematic review of the effectiveness of psychosocial interventions for carers of people with dementia. *Aging & Mental Health, 5*(2), 107–119. *Evidence Level I.*

Radloff, L. (1977). The CES-D scale: A self-report depression scale for research in the general population. *Applied Psychological Measurement, 1*(3), 385–401. *Evidence Level II.*

Rodriguez-Sanchez, E., Patino-Alonso, M. C., Mora-Simon, S., Gomez-Marcos, M. A., Perez-Penaranda, A., Losada-Baltar, A., & García-Ortiz, L. (2013). Effects of a psychological intervention in a primary health care center for caregivers of dependent relatives: A randomized trial. *The Gerontologist, 53,* 397–406. doi:10.1093/geront/gns086. *Evidence Level II.*

Schulz, R., & Beach, S. R. (1999). Caregiving as a risk factor for mortality: The caregiver health effects study. *Journal of the American Medical Association, 282*(23), 2215–2219. *Evidence Level II.*

Schulz, R., Burgio, L., Burns, R., Eisdorfer, C., Gallagher-Thompson, D., Gitlin, L. N., & Mahoney, D. F. (2003). Resources for Enhancing Alzheimer's Caregiver Health (REACH): Overview, site-specific outcomes, and future directions. *The Gerontologist, 43*(4), 514–520. *Evidence Level V.*

Schulz, R., Martire, L. M., & Klinger, J. N. (2005). Evidence-based caregiver interventions in geriatric psychiatry. *Psychiatric Clinics of North America, 28*(4), 1007–1038. *Evidence Level I.*

Schumacher, K., Beck, C. A., & Marren, J. M. (2006). Family caregivers: Caring for older adults, working with their families. *American Journal of Nursing, 106*(8), 40–49. *Evidence Level VI.*

Schumacher, K. L., Beidler, S. M., Beeber, A. S., & Gambino, P. (2006). A transactional model of cancer family caregiving skill. *Advances in Nursing Science, 29*(3), 271–86. *Evidence Level II.*

Schumacher, K. L. (1995). Family caregiver role acquisition: Role-making through situated interaction. *Scholarly Inquiry for Nursing Practice, 9*(3), 211–226. *Evidence Level IV.*

Schumacher, K. L., Koresawa, S., West, C., Hawkins, C., Johnson, C., Wais, E.,... Miaskowski, C. (2002). Putting cancer pain management regimens into practice at home. *Journal of Pain and Symptom Management, 23*(5), 369–382. *Evidence Level IV.*

Schumacher, K. L., Stewart, B. J., Archbold, P. G., Dodd, M. J., & Dibble, S. L. (2000). Family caregiving skill: Development of the concept. *Research in Nursing & Health, 23*(3), 191–203. *Evidence Level IV.*

Shankar, K. N., Hirschmanm, K. B., Hanlon, A. L., & Naylorm, M. D. (2014). Burden in caregivers of cognitively impaired elderly adults at time of hospitalization: A cross-sectional analysis. *Journal of the American Geriatrics Society, 62,* 276–284. doi:10.1111/jgs.12657. *Evidence Level II.*

Sherwood, P. R., Givenm B. A., Given, C. W., Sikorskii, A., You, M., & Prince, J. (2012). The impact of a problem-solving intervention on increasing caregiver assistance and improving caregiver health. *Supportive Care in Cancer, 20,* 1937–1947. doi:10.1007/s00520–011-1295–5. *Evidence Level II.*

Shim, B., Landerman, L. R., & Davis, L. L. (2011). Correlates of care relationship mutuality among carers of people with Alzheimer's and Parkinson's disease. *Journal of Advanced Nursing, 67,* 1729–1738. doi:10.1111/j.1365–2648.2011.05618.x. *Evidence Level IV.*

Sörensen, S., Pinquart, M., & Duberstein, P. (2002). How effective are interventions with caregivers? An updated meta-analysis. *The Gerontologist, 42*(3), 356–372. *Evidence Level I.*

Sörensen, S., & Pinquart M. (2005). Racial and ethnic differences in the relationship of caregiving stressors, resources, and sociodemographic variables to caregiver depression and perceived physical health. *Aging & Mental Health, 9,* P482–P495. *Evidence Level I.*

Stewart, B. J., Archbold, P., Harvath, T., & Nkongho, N. (1993). Role acquisition in family caregivers of older people who have been discharged from the hospital. In S. G. Funk, E. M. Tornquist, M. T. Champagne, & R. A. Wiese (Eds.), *Key aspects of caring for the chronically ill: Hospital and home* (pp. 219–230). New York, NY: Springer Publishing Company. *Evidence Level IV.*

Sullivan, M. T. (2002). *Caregiver strain index (CSI). Try this: Best practices in nursing care to older adults.* Retrieved from http://consultgerirn.org/resources. *Evidence Level VI.*

Tennstedt, S. L., McKinlay, J. B., & Sullivan, L. M. (1989). Informal care for frail elders: The role of secondary caregivers. *The Gerontologist, 29*(5), 677–683. *Evidence Level IV.*

Teri, L., McKenzie, G., Logsdon, R. G., McCurry, S. M., Bollin, S., & Mead, J. (2012). Translation of two evidence-based programs for training families to improve care of persons with dementia. *The Gerontologist, 52,* 452–459. doi:10.1093/geront/gnr132. *Evidence Level V.*

Tolson, D., Swan, I., & Knussen, C. (2002). Hearing disability: A source of distress for older people and carers. *British Journal of Nursing, 11*(15), 1021–1025. *Evidence Level II.*

Toseland, R. W., & Rossiter, C. M. (1989). Group interventions to support family caregivers: A review and analysis. *The Gerontologist, 29*(4), 438–448. *Evidence Level I.*

Trend, P., Kaye, J., Gage, H., Owen, C., & Wade, D. (2002). Short-term effectiveness of intensive multidisciplinary rehabilitation for people with Parkinson's disease and their carers. *Clinical Rehabilitation, 16*(7), 717–725. *Evidence Level III.*

Vitaliano, P. P., Zhang, J., & Scanlan, J. M. (2003). Is caregiving hazardous to one's physical health? A meta-analysis. *Psychological Bulletin, 129*(6), 946–972. *Evidence Level I.*

Wade, D. T., Gage, H., Owen, C., Trend, P., Grossmith, C., & Kaye, J. (2003). Multidisciplinary rehabilitation for people with Parkinson's disease: A randomised controlled study. *Journal of Neurology, Neurosurgery, and Psychiatry, 74*(2), 158–162. *Evidence Level II.*

Waelde, L. C., Thompson, L., & Gallagher-Thompson, D. (2004). A pilot study of a yoga and meditation intervention for dementia caregiver stress. *Journal of Clinical Psychology, 60*(6), 677–687. *Evidence Level III.*

Walker, A., Pratt, C. C., & Eddy, L. (1995). Informal caregiving to aging family members: A critical review. *Family Relations, 44,* 404–411. *Evidence Level I.*

Weiss, C. O., González, H. M., Kabeto, M. U., & Langa, K. M. (2005). Differences in amount of informal care received by non-Hispanic Whites and Latinos in a nationally representative sample of older Americans. *Journal of the American Geriatric Society, 53*(1), 146–151. *Evidence Level IV.*

Wells, N., Hepworth, J. T., Murphy, B. A., Wujcik, D., & Johnson, R. (2003). Improving cancer pain management through patient and family education. *Journal of Pain and Symptom Management, 25*(4), 344–356. *Evidence Level II.*

Wisniewski, S. R., Belle, S. H., Coon, D. W., Marcus, S. M., Ory, M. G., Burgio, L. D., . . . Schulz, R. (2003). The Resources for Enhancing Alzheimer's Caregiver Health (REACH): Project design and baseline characteristics. *Psychology and Aging, 18*(3), 375–384. *Evidence Level II.*

Wolff, J. L., & Kasper, J. D. (2006). Caregivers of frail elders: Updating a national profile. *The Gerontologist, 46*(3), 344–356. *Evidence Level I.*

Wolff, J. L., Roter, D. L., Barron, J., Boyd, C. M., Leff, B., & Finucane, T. E. (2014). A tool to strengthen the older patient–companion partnership in primary care: Results from a pilot study. *Journal of the American Geriatrics Society, 62*, 312–319. doi:10.1111/jgs.12639. *Evidence Level II.*

Wright, L. K., Litaker, M., Laraia, M. T., & DeAndrade, S. (2001). Continuum of care for Alzheimer's disease: A nurse education and counseling program. *Issues in Mental Health Nursing, 22*(3), 231–252. *Evidence Level II.*

Yee, J. L., & Schulz, R. (2000). Gender differences in psychiatric morbidity among family caregivers: A review and analysis. *The Gerontologist, 40*(2), 147–164. *Evidence Level I.*

Yin, T., Zhou, Q., & Bashford, C. (2002). Burden on family members: Caring for frail elderly: A meta-analysis of interventions. *Nursing Research, 51*(3), 199–208. *Evidence Level I.*

Zarit, S. H., Femia, E. E., Kim, K., & Whitlatch, C. J. (2010). The structure of risk factors and outcomes for family caregivers: Implications for assessment and treatment. *Aging & Mental Health, 14*(2), 220–231. *Evidence Level II.*

Zarit, S. H., Kim, K., Femia, E. E., Almeida, D. M., Savla, J., & Molenaar. P. C. (2011). Effects of adult day care on daily stress of caregivers: A within-person approach. *Journals of Gerontology. Series B, Psychological Sciences & Social Sciences, 66*, 538–546. doi:10.1093/geronb/gbr030. *Evidence Level IV.*

12

Issues Regarding Sexuality

Elaine E. Steinke

EDUCATIONAL OBJECTIVES

On completion of this chapter, the reader should be able to:

1. Describe an older adult's interest in sexuality
2. Identify barriers and challenges to sexual health among older adults
3. Discuss normal and pathological changes of aging and their influence on sexual health
4. Identify interventions that may help older adults achieve sexual health

OVERVIEW

Sexuality is an innate quality present in all human beings and is extremely important to an individual's self-identity and general well-being (Wallace, 2008). Sexuality is the expression of basic human needs that includes "intimacy, emotional expression, and love" (World Health Organization [WHO], 2010, p. 1). Moreover, it encompasses both gender roles and sexual orientation, and influencing factors include the "interaction of biological, psychological, cognitive, social, political, cultural, ethical, legal, historical, religious, and spiritual factors" (WHO, 2010, p. 4). *Sexual health* "requires a positive, responsible approach to sexuality and sexual relationships as well as pleasurable, safe sexual experiences that are free from coercion, discrimination or violence" (WHO, 2010, p. 1). Sexual health contributes to the satisfaction of physical needs; however, sexual contact fulfills many social, emotional, and psychological components of life as well. This is evidenced by the fact that human touch and a healthy sex life may evoke feelings of joy, romance, affection, passion, and intimacy, whereas despondency and depression often result from an inability to express one's sexuality (Buttaro, Koeniger-Donohue, & Hawkins, 2014). When this occurs, *sexual dysfunction*, defined as impairment in normal sexual functioning during desire, excitation, and/or orgasmic phases of the sexual response cycle, may result (Steinke, 2014). There are several subtypes of sexual dysfunction, including delayed ejaculation, erectile disorder, female orgasmic disorder, female sexual interest/arousal disorder, genito-pelvic pain/penetration disorder, male hypoactive sexual desire disorder, premature ejaculation, and substance/medication-induced sexual dysfunction (American Psychiatric Association, 2013).

It is frequently assumed that sexual desires and the frequency of sexual encounters begin to diminish later in life. In today's youth-focused society, sexuality in the context of aging is often believed to be impossible and is not openly discussed. The 77 million baby boomers who

For a description of evidence levels cited in this chapter, see Chapter 1, "Developing and Evaluating Clinical Practice Guidelines: A Systematic Approach."

were part of the sexual revolution now face an interesting paradox, in that "the ignorance, prejudice, and silence about sex and sexuality that they fought so hard to upend are still alive and well in old age" (Connolly et al., 2012, p. 43). Despite the negative stereotypes, sexual identity and the need for intimacy do not disappear with increasing age, and older adults do not morph into celibate, asexual beings. Physical intimacy is an important individual right, including in older age. Likewise, safety and protection from sexual abuse are key issues that are often underrecognized (Buttaro et al., 2014; Connolly et al., 2012). This presents both ethical and legal issues, and it is important for nurses to recognize the potential for sexual abuse in all older adults, and particularly in those who are less able to resist such abuses because of physical incapacity, psychological vulnerability, or cognitive impairment.

Recognizing that older adults have a need for physical intimacy and that many wish to remain sexually active as they age is essential in promoting sexual quality of life. In a study of 3,005 U.S. older adults, current sexual activity was reported in 73% of adults aged 57 to 64 years, 53% of adults aged 65 to 74 years, and 26% of adults aged 75 to 84 years (Lindau et al., 2007). Being sexually active has been associated with better health, higher sexual desire scores, and erectile function (Killinger, Boura, & Diokno, 2014).

BACKGROUND AND STATEMENT OF PROBLEM

Despite the persistence of sexual patterns throughout the life span, there is limited research and information to assist nurses assess or intervene to promote sexual health among older adults. Contributing to this disconnect is the lack of societal recognition of sexuality as a continuing human need and a factor that perpetuates lack of sexual assessment and intervention among the older population. Other factors impacting sexual health include the presence of normal and pathological aging changes; environmental barriers to sexual health; special problems of the older adult that interfere with sexual fulfillment, such as cognitive impairment; and comorbid conditions that may impair the ability to be sexually active. Although sexuality in aging has often been overlooked in general, some literature addresses sexual activity and sexual concerns across the adult life span for diagnoses such as heart disease and cancer. For example, two scientific statements from the American Heart Association are available to help nurses and other providers in sexual counseling of cardiac patients and their partners (Levine et al., 2012; Steinke et al., 2013). Although resources are available for selected medical conditions, the widespread adoption of sexual counseling in practice remains problematic.

Nurses' Views Toward Sexuality and Aging

Nurses' hesitancy to discuss sexuality with older adults has a significant impact on the sexual health of this population. Maes and Louis (2011) reported that only 2% of nurse practitioners (N = 500) always conducted a sexual history, and 23.4% never or seldom did so in patients aged 50 years and older, although most reported comfort and confidence in sexual history taking. Nurse practitioners expressed greater hesitancy to discuss sex with patients of the opposite sex, similar to a prior report of general practitioners (Gott, Hinchliff, & Galena, 2004). Besides the barriers of lack of time (59%), interruptions (30%), and limited communication skills, some nurse practitioners (21%) cited the inability to respond to issues that arose from sexual history taking, indicating that increasing providers' knowledge may be an important strategy (Maes & Louis, 2011). Similarly, only 22% of general practitioners reported routine sexual history taking and 15.5% proactively asked patients about sexual dysfunction (Ribeiro et al., 2014). In contrast, a qualitative study evaluating transcribed audio recordings of 483 periodic health exam visits in adults aged 50 to 80 years by physicians revealed that about one half of visits included some discussion of sexual health, and the majority of these discussions was initiated by the physician (Ports, Barnack-Tavlaris, Syme, Perera, & Lafata, 2014).

General discomfort with discussing sexuality by nurses, lack of experience in assessment and management of sexual dysfunction among older adults, and lack of confidence (East & Hutchinson, 2013) often prevent nurses from addressing the sexual needs of this population. A disparity exists between nurses' readiness and willingness to discuss sexual needs and concerns with clients (East & Hutchinson, 2013). Various factors influence sexual discussions such as lack of privacy, personal attitudes, and embarrassment. Although inadequate knowledge by nurses has been reported, a study of nurses' attitudes and beliefs revealed that 92% of nurses understood the impact of diseases and treatment on sexual function, and nearly two thirds stated that they felt both comfortable and responsible for such discussions, but the majority did not discuss sexual concerns in practice (80%) and most lacked confidence (60%) to do so (Saunamäki, Andersson, & Engstrm, 2010). Moreover, the sexuality of older adults is generally excluded from sparse gerontological curricula, and sexual assessment is viewed as less important than other assessments (Dattilo & Brewer, 2005). A study of senior nursing students revealed that most had positive attitudes and acceptance regarding sexual expressions, but most were hesitant in regard to sexual counseling interventions

(Huang, Tsai, Tseng, Li, & Lee, 2013). Without education and experience in managing sensitive issues around sexuality, health professionals are often not comfortable discussing sexual issues with older adults. Health care providers may lessen discomfort when addressing sexual issues by increasing their knowledge on the subject, practicing effective communication strategies to increase comfort in sexual discussions, and routinely introducing this dimension of health into routine assessment and management protocols.

Nurses' understanding of sexuality should be broadened beyond that of a relationship between just men and women. Many clients within various health care systems are lesbian, gay, bisexual, and transgender (LGBT) adults, and these alternative sexual preferences require respect and consideration. Negative media portrayals and gender stereotying are pervasive not only in regard to older adult sexuality, but particularly for those who are gay (Garrett, 2014). In addition, those who are gay and living in rural areas may be further marginalized (Fenge & Jones, 2012). Nurses are in key positions as first-line care providers to focus on health promotion in those who are LGBT, and to proactively work to reduce and eliminate health care disparities and barriers. Health-promotion strategies should address the areas of HIV/AIDS; safe sex; hepatitis immunization and screening; alcohol use and substance abuse; sexually transmitted infections (STIs); physical abuse, anxiety, and depression; as well as wellness exams such as prostate, testicular, breast, cervical, and colon cancer (Lim, Brown, & Justin Kim, 2014). Prevention focused on heart health, physical fitness, tobacco cessation, and diet are important for all older adults.

Older adults in the United States who live with HIV/AIDS face considerable challenges, including stereotyping, prejudice, and discrimination related to real or perceived sexual orientation, and this contributes to anxiety, depression, and higher risk sexual behaviors (Cahill & Valadéz, 2013). Conversely, older gay men with a same-sex domestic or married partner have a more positive affect and less depression (Cahill & Valadéz, 2013). Proactive screening and assessment are critical in the older HIV population, as is effective management that includes treatment of any mental health conditions and comorbidities.

Normal and Pathological Aging Changes

The "sexual response cycle," or the organized pattern of physical response to sexual stimulation, changes with age in both women and men. After menopause, a loss of estrogen in women results in significant sexual changes. This deficiency frequently results in the thinning of the vaginal walls and decreased or delayed vaginal lubrication, which may lead to pain during intercourse (Lobo, 2007; Syme, 2014). Additionally, the labia atrophies, the vagina shortens, and the cervix may descend downward into the vagina and cause further pain and discomfort. Moreover, vaginal contractions are fewer and weaker during orgasm, and after sexual intercourse is completed, women return to the prearoused stage faster than they would at an earlier age. The result of these physiological age-related changes in women is the potential for significant alterations in sexual health that have traditionally received little attention from research or individual health care providers. The pain resulting from anatomical changes and vaginal dryness may result in the avoidance of sexual relationships in order to prevent painful intercourse. In addition, the intensity of postmenopausal symptoms has been associated with greater disruption of sexual function, particularly for those with postsurgically induced menopause compared to natural menopause (Topatan & Yildiz, 2012).

Men also experience decreased hormone levels, mainly a gradual decline in testosterone, which has been associated with decreased frequency and weaker orgasms, a longer refractory period between erections, less forceful and reduced amount of ejaculate, and erectile dysfunction (Syme, 2014; Yeap, Araujo, & Wittert, 2012). Men may experience fatigue, loss of muscle mass, depression, and a decline in libido. As a result of normal aging changes, older men require more direct stimulation of the penis to experience erection, which is somewhat weaker as compared to that experienced in earlier ages. Declining levels of testosterone in the aging man has more far-reaching implications, having been associated with reduced sexual activity, frailty, atherosclerosis, vascular disease, insulin resistance, metabolic syndrome, cardiovascular events, and overall mortality, although further study is needed to establish causal relationships (Yeap et al., 2012). Frailty in an older population has been associated with impaired sexual functioning and distress, and erectile dysfunction (Lee et al., 2013), illustrating the importance of evaluating sexual health and sexual activity, as well as managing comorbid conditions with the goal of improving both overall and sexual health.

Bodily changes, such as wrinkles and sagging skin, may cause both older women and men to feel insecure about initiating a sexual encounter and maintaining emotionally secure relationships. Perceptions of body image and sexual self-esteem often influence sexual interest and sexual activity, perhaps even more so for women than men (Syme, 2014). In addition, attitudes, beliefs, and lack of knowledge contribute to misperceptions about sexuality, changes in sexual function, sexual risk taking, and prevention. Cultural influences on attitudes and beliefs are often grounded in Western beliefs that youth and beauty are of higher value, and that sexuality in older adulthood is nonexistent, shameful, or disgusting (Syme, 2014). Taken together, bodily changes and negative attitudes and beliefs serve to hinder sexual expression among older adults. As noted, the aging baby boomer generation has been at the forefront of promoting sexual expression from their youth; thus, a greater openness to the importance of sexual expression throughout one's life may result, along with greater societal recognition of the role of sexual health promotion in overall health.

In addition to normal aging changes, both chronic illness and a number of medical conditions have been associated with poor sexual health and functioning in the older population. A study of 100 women with chronic illness presenting at internal medicine clinics, revealed that 65% had sexual dysfunction, including painful intercourse, reluctance to engage in sex, orgasmic problems, and sexual dissatisfaction. Predictors of sexual dysfunction included older age; menopausal; unemployed; and experiencing fatigue, sleep problems, and pain and weakness in extremities (Mollaoğlu, Tuncay, & Fertelli, 2013). Diabetic women treated with insulin were more likely to report problems with vaginal lubrication and orgasm than nondiabetic women (Copeland et al., 2012). In 200 men with type 2 diabetes mellitus, 60% had erectile dysfunction, which was significantly associated with older age, fasting plasma glucose, hemoglobin A1c (HbA1c), creatinine level, and systolic blood pressure (Sharifi, Asghari, Jaberi, Salehi, & Mirzamohammadi, 2012). In addition, significant predictors of erectile dysfunction were older age and taking calcium channel blocker medications.

Sexual dysfunction is prevalent in cancer survivors, with 41% reporting a decline in sexual function and 52% with altered body image (Averyt & Nishimoto, 2014). In colorectal cancer, rates may be higher because of the impact of surgery, radiation, and chemotherapy on sexual function. Changes in sensation, vascular scarring, decreased vaginal lubrication, urinary or fecal incontinence, erectile dysfunction, and symptoms, such as fatigue or nausea, may interfere with sexual function. In men with postradical prostatectomy, sexual dysfunction often includes erectile dysfunction, reduced sexual frequency, diminished sexual desire, and orgasmic difficulties; both psychoeducational and psychotherapeutic interventions have positively impacted coping and sexual function in several studies cited in this systematic review (Lassen, Gattinger, & Saxer, 2013).

The presence of depression among older adults impacts sexual health, in that depression often causes a decline in desire and ability to perform exacerbated by its treatment. Lee et al. (2013) found that men who were prefrail or frail had higher depression scores and more erectile dysfunction, and depression mediated almost half of the total effect related to frailty and sexual distress. In a systematic review, those with urgency urinary incontinence faced considerable challenges in maintaining sexuality and overall quality of life, impacting psychological well-being (anxiety and depression), daily activities, sexual function, and work productivity (Coyne et al., 2013). The presence of anxiety and depression should be assessed among older adults and considered for the impact of these emotional and psychological factors on sexual health (see Chapter 15, "Late-Life Depression" and Chapter 21, "Urinary Incontinence").

Medications used to treat commonly occurring medical illnesses among older adults also impact sexual function. Two of the major groups of medications include antidepressants and antihypertensives. Selective serotonin reuptake inhibitors (SSRI) are commonly used to treat depression, and have been linked with sexual dysfunction, although this is likely underreported (Trenque et al., 2013). A meta-analysis of data extracted from 63 studies and more than 26,000 patients treated for major depressive disorder with second-generation antidepressants revealed that citalopram and paroxetine contributed to statistically significant higher risk of sexual dysfunction, whereas buproprion conferred lower risk of sexual dysfunction (Reichenpfader et al., 2014). Cardiac medications that contribute to sexual dysfunction include beta blockers (exception: nebivolol), cardiac glycosides, and diuretics, with mixed results in studies related to alpha blockers, angiotensin-converting enzyme inhibitors (ACEI), and calcium channel blockers; certain drugs exert a negative effect and others have a positive impact on sexual function in some studies (Nicolai et al., 2013). Overall, angiotensin receptor blockers (ARBs) and statins do not appear to contribute to sexual problems in most studies. Combinations of drugs may negatively influence sexual function, for example, those cardiac patients taking a beta blocker alone or in combination with an ACEI had greater than three times the odds of sexual dysfunction (Cook et al., 2008). In a small study of those with heart failure, the number of medications taken significantly negatively impacted sexual activity, particularly for those of older age, who used tobacco or alcohol, and had diabetes (Steinke, Mosack, Wright, Chung, & Moser, 2009).

Special Issues Related to Older Adults and Sexuality

Cognitively impaired older adults continue to have sexual needs and desires that may present a challenge to nurses.

A review of older adults' cognitive functioning and sexual behavior indicated that those older adults engaging in sexual activity tended to have better overall cognitive function; the ability to think abstractly may be important in continuing a sexual relationship (Hartmans, Comijs, & Jonker, 2014). Conversely, forgetfulness, poor decision making, and problems with cognitive sequencing may negatively affect sexual function. Hypersexuality appears to be rare among cognitively impaired elderly, and apathy or indifference toward sexual acitivty may be more prominent (Hartmans et al., 2014).

Continuing sexual needs often manifest in inappropriate sexual behavior. Sexual behaviors common to cognitively impaired older adults may include cuddling, touching of the genitals, sexual remarks, propositioning, grabbing and groping, using obscene language, masturbating without shame, aggression, and irritability. In a small study of 10 patients admitted to an inpatient geriatric psychiatric ward, right frontal lobe stroke was significantly associated with inappropriate sexual behaviors, illustrating that organic causes can contribute to these symptoms (Bardell, Lau, & Fedoroff, 2011). Inappropriate sexual behavior can also lead to elder abuse, and those most likely to be victims are those who are cognitively impaired, although research is limited and such behavior likely underreported (Rosen, Lachs, & Pillemer, 2010). Nurses have an ethical responsibility to be cognizant of the potential for abuse, and to report and intervene promptly to maintain the safety of the older adult victim.

Masturbation is a method by which cognitively impaired men and women may become sexually fulfilled. Nurses in long-term care facilities may assist older adults to improve sexual health by providing an environment in which the older adult may masturbate in private. Accurate assessment and documentation of the ability of cognitively impaired older adults to make competent decisions regarding sexual relationships with others while in long-term care are essential. If the resident has been determined to be incapable of decision making, then the health care staff must prevent the cognitively impaired resident from unsolicited sexual advances by a spouse, partner, or other residents.

Environmental settings may also influence sexuality among older adults. Normally, engaging in sexual intercourse occurs within the privacy of one's bedroom; however, for some older adults, extended care facilities are the substitute for what one called *home*. Residents of extended care facilities state that many of the obstacles they face regarding their sexuality include lack of opportunity, lack of available partner, poor health, feeling sexually undesirable, and guilt for having these sexual feelings (Benbow & Beeston, 2012). In a study of Polish nursing home residents ($N = 85$), mutual respect and being able to depend on one's partner were important relationship factors (Mroczek, Kurpas, Gronowska, Kotwas, & Karakiewicz, 2013). Those reporting sexual tension that occurred occasionally or once per week or less, relieved sexual tension through sexual contact with long-term partners, masturbation, watching erotic videos, walking, and engaging in diversionary activities. Sexual intercourse was reported by 34% of respondents (Mroczek et al., 2013) Negative staff attitudes and beliefs regarding residents' sexual activity often interfere with the expression of sexuality in long-term care settings. Often, only married couples receive the privacy needed for sexual activity (Mroczek et al., 2013)

Health care providers are in a unique position to assess and manage HIV among the older population. The shift in focus of HIV/AIDS care is in managing this chronic condition and its related comorbidities. Negative attitudes and stereotypes often result in greater social isolation and lack of social support by family and friends, with the older adult often more reliant on formal care providers (Cahill & Valadéz, 2013). In addition, greater attention to sexual health education regarding HIV risk in the older population is needed among elders and health care providers.

ASSESSMENT OF THE PROBLEM

A model to guide sexual assessment and intervention is available and has been well used among younger populations since the 1970s. The Permission, Limited Information, Specific Suggestion, Intensive Therapy (PLISSIT) model (Annon, 1976) begins by first seeking permission (P) to discuss sexuality with the older adult. Because many sexual disorders originate in feelings of anxiety or guilt, asking permission may put the client in control of the discussion and facilitate communication between the health care provider and client. This permission may be gained by asking general questions such as "I would like to begin to discuss your sexual health; what concerns would you like to share with me about this area of function?" Questions to guide the sexual assessment of older adults are available on many health care assessment forms. The next step of the model affords an opportunity for the nurse to share limited information (LI) with the older adult. In the case of older adults, this part of the model affords health care providers the opportunity to dispel myths of aging and sexuality and to discuss the impact of normal and pathological aging changes, as well as medications on sexual health. The next part of the model guides the nurse to provide specific suggestions (SS) to improve sexual health. In so doing, nurses may implement several of the interventions recommended for improved sexual health, such as safe sex practices, more effective management of acute and chronic diseases, removal or substitution of causative medications, environmental adaptations, or need for discussions with partners and families. The final part of the model calls for intensive therapy (IT) when needed for clients whose sexual dysfunction goes beyond the scope of nursing management. In these cases, referral to a sexual therapist is appropriate.

Sexual assessments will be most effective using open-ended questions such as "Can you tell me how you express your sexuality?" "What concerns you about your sexuality?" "How has your sexuality changed as you have aged?" "What changes have you noticed in your sexuality since you have been diagnosed or treated for disease?" "What thoughts have you had about ways in which you would like to enhance your sexual health?" The loss of relationships with significant, intimate partners is unfortunately common among older adults and often ends communication about the importance of self to the person experiencing the loss. This greatly impacts the older adult's sexual health. Asking the older adult about past and present relationships in his or her life will help to aid this assessment.

Barriers to sexual health should be assessed, including normal and pathological changes of aging, medications, and psychological problems such as depression. Moreover, lack of knowledge and understanding about sexuality, loss of partners, and family influence on sexual practice often present substantial barriers to sexual health among older adults. Nurses should assess for the presence of physiological changes through a health history, review of systems, and physical examination for the presence of normal and aging changes that impact sexual health. Older adults may view the normal changes of aging and their subsequent impact on appearance as embarrassing or indicative of illness. This may result in a negative body image and a reluctance to pursue sexual health. It is important for nurses to consider the impact of normal and pathological changes of aging on body image and assess their impact frequently.

As discussed earlier, there are a number of medical conditions that have been associated with poor sexual health and functioning including depression, cardiac disease, diabetes, stroke, osteoporosis, cancer, and chronic obstructive pulmonary disease (Hyde et al., 2010; Steinke, 2013). Effective assessment of these illnesses using open-ended health history questions, review of systems, physical examination, and appropriate lab testing will provide necessary information for appropriate disease management and improved sexual function.

Assessing the impact of medications among older adults, especially those commonly used to treat medical illnesses, such as antidepressants and antihypertensives, are essential. Potential medications should be identified by reviewing the client's medication bottles and the client should be questioned about the potential impact of these medications on sexual health. If the medication is found to have an impact on sexual health, alternative medications should be considered. The older adult should also be questioned regarding the use of alcohol because this substance also has a potential impact on sexual response.

INTERVENTIONS AND CARE STRATEGIES

Following a thorough assessment of normal and pathological aging changes, as well as environmental factors, a number of interventions may be implemented to promote the sexual health of older adults. These interventions fall into several broad categories, including (a) education regarding age-associated change in sexual function, (b) compensation for normal aging changes, (c) effective management of acute and chronic illness effecting sexual function, (d) removal of barriers associated with difficulty in fulfilling sexual needs, and (e) special interventions to promote sexual health in cognitively impaired older adults.

Client Education

The most important intervention to improving sexuality among the older population is education. It is important to remember that sexuality was likely not addressed in formal educational systems as the older adults developed and was rarely discussed informally. Older adults may possess dated values that impact sexual action, freedom, and desires and lead to both sexual frustration and conflict. Masters (1986) reported in his seminal work on the sexuality of older adults that older women were raised to believe that when menstruation ceased, they would cease to be feminine. Knowledge is essential to the successful fulfillment of sexuality for all people.

The incidence of HIV and AIDS infection is rising among older adults, and 19% of those aged 55 years and older were living with HIV infection in the United States in 2010, with older adults often diagnosed later in the disease process (Centers for Disease Control and Prevention [CDC], n.d.). There were 2,500 new infections in this age group, with higher rates among men than women and variations among ethnicities. This underscores the significant risk of HIV transmission in the older age group and the need for effective teaching regarding safe-sex practices. Teaching about the use of condoms to prevent the transmission of sexually transmitted diseases is essential. In response to this rise in HIV cases and the presence of other sexually transmitted diseases, it is essential to provide older adults with safe-sex information provided by the CDC.

Compensating for Normal Aging Changes

Assisting older adults to compensate for normal aging changes related to sexual dysfunction will greatly lessen the impact of these changes on sexual health. Among women, the discussion of anatomical changes in sexual anatomy will help them anticipate these changes in sexuality. For example, atrophic vaginitis is often treated with topical or systemic estrogen therapy or dehydroepiandrosterone (DHEA; Buster, 2012), and increased vaginal dryness among women may require the use of artificial water-based lubricants or topical estrogen agents. In men, delayed response and the increased length of time needed for erections and ejaculations are among normal changes of aging, which older adults may not be aware of. When older adults understand the impact of normal aging changes, they then understand the need to plan for more time and direct stimulation in order to become aroused.

One of the most important preventive measures that older adults may undertake to reduce the impact of normal aging changes on sexual health is to continue to engage in sexual activity. In a study of midlife in older men and women across five countries, frequent kissing, cuddling, caressing, and partner touching significantly predicted sexual satisfaction, and sexual frequency was related to sexual satisfaction (Heiman et al., 2011). Planning for more time during sexual activities; being sensitive to changes in one another's bodies; the use of aids to increase stimulation and lubrication; the exploration of foreplay, masturbation, sensual touch, and different sexual positions along with education about these common changes associated with sex and aging may help immensely. By doing so, changes in sexual response patterns are less likely to occur. Eating healthy foods, getting adequate amounts of sleep, exercising, using stress-management techniques, and not smoking are also very important to sexual health.

Effective Management of Acute and Chronic Illness

Effective management of both acute and chronic illnesses that impair sexual health is also important. Interventions that improve sexual health are frameworked within the current interventions to treat disease. In other words, effective disease management using primary, secondary, and tertiary interventions will not only effectively treat the disease but also result in improved sexual health. Consequently, better glucose control among diabetics enhances circulation and may increase arousal and sexual response. Appropriate treatment of depression with medication and psychotherapy will enhance desire and sexual response. Although treatment of depression may help to improve libido and sexual dysfunctions, such as orgasmic disorders, medications to treat depression often impact sexual function by lowering libido and causing orgasmic disorders. Choosing antidepressants with less impact on sexual function, when possible, is an important consideration. For example, mirtazapine supported normal sexual function at 6 months in patients with major depression and sexual dysfunction at baseline (Saiz-Ruiz et al., 2005), and has been successfully used in SSRI-related sexual dysfunction (Ozmenler et al., 2008). Antidepressants more likely to contribute to sexual problems are those in the drug classes of SSRIs or serotonin norepinephrine reuptake inhibitors (SNRIs; Clayton, Croft, & Handiwala, 2014). When considering medication within any class of drug for those older adults who continue to be sexually active, choosing a drug with less sexual side effects, or using the lowest dose of a medication with known sexual side effects may help support sexual function.

Phosphodiesterase-5 inhibitors (PDE5-I), such as sildenafil citrate (Viagra), vardenafil HCl (Levitra), tadalafil (Cialis), and avanafil (Stendra), play a significant role in the treatment of erectile dysfunction that occurs with aging and are effective and well-tolerated treatments (Huang & Lie, 2013). Low-dose PDE5-I on a continuing basis has benefited those with postradical prostatectomy, diabetes mellitus, or after radiotherapy (Huang & Lie, 2013). This may be useful when intermittent dosing of PDE5-I is not effective. As noted previously, a number of medications may adversely affect sexual function in the older adult. Thorough evaluation of prescribed and over-the-counter medications is important in providing optimal medication management with the least sexual side effects and in patient education.

Both older adults and nurses may be hesitant to discuss sexual problems so it is important for nurses to be proactive and bring up the topic of sex. A few targeted questions are often all that is needed to determine interest in sexual activity, sexual concerns, and sexual problems experienced, either related to medications or to a particular chronic disease. For example, a nurse might ask: "What concerns do you have about resuming sexual activity?" "How important is it for you to engage in sexual activity with your partner?" "What sexual activities are most important to you?" "Are there sexual activities that you have been unable to engage in?" and/or "Have you noticed any change in sexual desire that has affected your ability to be sexually active?" Asking these and similar questions is an important step in guiding management of sexual problems (also see Assessment of the Problem section for other suggested questions). Recognition of the continuing sexual needs of older adults among nurses is essential to ongoing dialogue about sexual problems.

Removal of Barriers to Sexual Health

One of the greatest barriers to sexual health among older adults lies with nurses' persistent beliefs that older adults are not sexual beings. Nurses should be encouraged to open lines of communication in order to effectively assess and manage the sexual health needs of aging individuals with the same consistency as other bodily systems and treat alterations in sexual health with available evidence-based strategies.

An essential intervention to promoting sexual health in this population is to educate nurses regarding the continuing sexual needs and desires persisting throughout the life span. Education regarding older adult sexuality as a continuing human need should be included in multidisciplinary education and staff development programs. Educational sessions may begin by discussing prevalent societal myths around older adult sexuality. Nurses should be encouraged to discuss their own feelings about sexuality and its role in the life of older adults. Moreover, the development of policies and procedures to manage sexual issues of older adult clients is important throughout environments of care.

Environmental adaptations to ensure privacy and safety among long-term care and community-dwelling residents are essential. Arrangements for privacy must be made so the dignity of older adults is protected during sexual activity. For example, nurses may assist in finding other activities for the resident's roommate so that privacy may be obtained or in securing a common room that may be used by the older adults for private visits. Call lights or telephones should be kept within reach during sexual activity and adaptive equipment, such as positioning devices or trapezes, may need to be obtained. Interventions, such as providing rooms for privacy and offering consultations for residents regarding evaluation and treatment of their sexual problems, are a few of the many ways this may be accomplished (Wallace, 2008).

Families are an integral part of the interdisciplinary team. However, for older couples, especially those in relationships with new partners, it is often difficult for families to understand that their older relative may have a sexual relationship with anyone other than the person they are accustomed to them being with. A family meeting, with a counselor if needed, is appropriate in order to help the family understand and accept the older adult's decisions about the relationship.

Special Interventions to Promote the Sexual Health of Cognitively Impaired Older Adults

Cognitively impaired older adults continue to have sexual needs and desires but may lack the capacity to make appropriate decisions regarding sexual relationships. Accurate assessment and documentation of the ability to make informed decisions regarding sexual relationships must be conducted by the interdisciplinary team (Benbow & Beeston, 2012). If the older adult is not capable of making competent decisions, participation in sexual relationships may be considered abusive and must be prevented. On the other end of the spectrum, nurses should not attempt to prevent sexual relationships and may play an important role in promoting sexual health among older adults who are cognitively competent to make decisions regarding sexual relationships. In these cases, nurses should implement all necessary interventions to promote the sexual health of older adult clients.

Inappropriate sexual behavior, such as public masturbation, disrobing, or making sexually explicit remarks to other patients or health care professionals, may be a warning sign of unmet sexual needs among older adults. In these situations, a full sexual assessment should be conducted using clear communication and limit setting. Following this, a plan should be developed to manage this behavior while providing the utmost respect and preserving the dignity of the client. Providing an environment in which the older adult may pursue his or her sexuality in private may be a simple solution to a difficult problem. Nonpharmacologic management includes redirecting behavior, reorientation, adapting the environment, seating the resident making sexual advances in a different area during social gatherings, pants without zippers for male residents who tend to expose or fondle themselves in public, education and explanation that behavior is inappropriate, counseling, and using same-sex caregivers (Benbow & Beeston, 2012; Rosen et al., 2010). Supportive strategies include encouraging family members to hug, kiss, and hold hands with their loved one, and the use of pets for sensory stimulation (Rosen et al., 2010). Medication management might be considered, and it includes antidepressants, antipsychotics, anticholinesterases, and anticonvulsants after first evaluating the benefit versus risk (see Chapter 20, "Reducing Adverse Drug Events"). In addition, supportive management in an institutional setting is crucial. Having established policies regarding sexual behavior for those who are cognitiviely intact as well as those who are cognitively impaired, an environment that facilitates open discussion, and education and support of staff are clearly important strategies (Benbow & Beeston, 2012).

CASE STUDY

Mrs. Jones is a highly functioning 79-year-old widow, recently admitted to a nursing home with mild cognitive impairment (MCI). Mrs. Jones began a friendship with Mr. Carl, who is cognitively intact and wheelchair bound. Mr. Carl is married to a woman who resides outside the facility. The nursing staff has noticed more and more intimate touches among the two residents and is concerned about Mrs. Jones's competency to make the decision to participate in this increasingly intimate relationship. Moreover, general concern about the sexual relationship within a long-term care setting prevails among the nursing staff.

The first step in this situation is to conduct a full assessment to determine Mrs. Jones's capacity to participate in this intimate relationship. The right to Mrs. Jones's autonomy is complicated by the presence of MCI and must be explored further. The question remains: Does Mrs. Jones have the decisional capacity to participate in an intimate relationship?

The actual and projected outcomes of the intimate relationship would require assessment to determine what nursing actions are required regarding this relationship. If an assessment of Mrs. Jones finds that she is incapable of understanding the consequences of her relationship with Mr. Carl, then she must be protected from unsolicited sexual advances by a spouse, partner, or other residents. However, if the assessment leads nurses to believe that Mrs. Jones and Mr. Carl understand the risks and consequences of their relationship, then the right to autonomy prevails.

Discussion

If clinicians determine that the older adults have the decisional capacity to consent to a sexual relationship, then a comprehensive health history, review of systems, and physical examination to determine normal and pathological changes of aging that may play a role in this sexual relationship must be conducted. Appropriate lab work for the potential presence of sexually transmitted diseases should be included. A care plan focusing the need to promote sexual health for this couple should be developed. Teaching regarding normal and pathological aging changes and the impact of these changes, as well as medications on sexual function, should be conducted. Normal changes of aging must be compensated for and diseases effecting sexual response should be treated with medications that will not impact sexual health. Safety from the transmission of sexually transmitted diseases and privacy should be provided for the residents, ensuring that their dignity is respected at all times.

SUMMARY

One of the most prevalent myths of aging is that older adults are no longer interested in sex. It is commonly believed that older adults no longer have any interest or desire to participate in sexual relationships. Because sexuality is mainly considered a young person's activity, often associated with reproduction, society does not usually associate older adults with sex. In the youth-oriented society of today, many consider sexuality among older adults to be distasteful and prefer to assume that sexuality among the older population does not exist. However, despite popular belief, sexuality continues to be important, even in the lives of older adults.

Although the sexual health of older adults has been largely ignored in the past decades, evolving images of older adults as healthy and vibrant members of society may result in a decrease in prevalence of myths of this population as nonsexual beings. Changes in the societal image of older adults as asexual celibate beings will greatly enhance removal of barriers to sexual health in the older population. Improved assessment and management of normal and pathological changes of aging and appropriate environmental adaptations and management of special issues of sexuality and aging will also result in improved sexual health in the older population. Oral erectile agents also play a substantial role in enhanced sexual health among older adults.

The fulfillment of sexual needs may be just as satisfying for older adults as it is for younger people. However, several normal and pathological changes of aging complicate sexuality among older adults. Environmental changes may create further barriers to sexual expression among older adults. Despite the many barriers to achieving sexual health among an aging population, nurses are in a critical position to understand sexual needs and capabilities in later life and assist older adults in developing compensatory strategies for improving sexual health in order to have the best possible sexual life. If these strategies and interventions are undertaken, increased awareness and acceptance of older adults' sexuality will ultimately take place, and the concept of sex in old age will no longer be such a shocking topic.

NURSING STANDARD OF PRACTICE

Protocol 12.1: Sexuality in the Older Adult

I. GOAL

To enhance the sexual health of older adults

II. OVERVIEW

Although it is generally believed that sexual desires decrease with age, researchers have identified that sexual desires, thoughts, and actions continue throughout all decades of life. Human touch and healthy sex lives evoke feelings of joy, romance, affection, passion, and intimacy, whereas despondency and depression often result from an inability to express one's sexuality. Health care providers play an important role in assessing and managing normal and pathological aging changes in order to improve the sexual health of older adults.

III. BACKGROUND AND STATEMENT OF THE PROBLEM

A. Definitions
   1. *Sexuality* is a central aspect of being human throughout life that encompasses intimacy, emotional expression, gender identities and roles, and sexual orientation, and is influenced by biological, psychological, cognitive, and other factors (WHO, 2010).
   2. *Sexual health* is a state of physical, emotional, mental, and social well-being related to sexuality, with a positive, responsible approach to sexuality and sexual relationships (WHO, 2010).
   3. *Sexual dysfunction* is an impairment in normal sexual functioning.
B. Etiology and/or epidemiology
   1. Despite the continuing sexual needs of older adults, many barriers prevent sexual health among older adults.
   2. Health care providers often lack knowledge and comfort in discussing sexual issues with older adults (Maes & Louis, 2011; Ribeiro et al., 2014).
   3. The older population is more susceptible to many disabling medical conditions. A number of chronic conditions are associated with poor sexual health and functioning, including depression, cardiac disease, stroke and aphasia, cancer, and diabetes that make sexuality difficult.
   4. Medications used among older adults, especially those commonly used to treat medical illnesses, also impact sexuality such as cardiac medications and antidepressants (Nicolai et al., 2013; Reichenpfader et al., 2014; Trenque et al., 2013).
   5. Normal aging changes make sexual health difficult to achieve such as a higher frequency of vaginal dryness in women and erectile dysfunction in men (Syme, 2014; Topatan & Yildiz, 2012; Yeap et al., 2012).
   6. Environmental barriers also present barriers to sexual health among older adults (Benbow & Beeston, 2012).

IV. ASSESSMENT

A. The PLISSIT model (Annon, 1976) begins by first seeking permission (P) to discuss sexuality with the older adult. The next step of the model affords an opportunity for the nurse to share limited informaion (LI) with the older adult. Specific suggestions (SS) and interventions to improve health are then provided. Referral to intensive therapy (IT) may be needed for those with more complex sexual problems.
B. Ask open-ended questions such as "Can you tell me how you express your sexuality?" or "What concerns you about your sexuality?" and "How has your sexuality changed as you have aged?"
C. Assess for presence of physiological changes through a health history, review of systems, and physical examination for the presence of normal and aging changes that impact sexual health.
D. Review medications among older adults, especially those commonly used to treat medical illnesses that also impact sexuality such as antidepressants and antihypertensives.
E. Assess medical conditions that have been associated with poor sexual health and functioning, including depression, cardiac disease, stroke, cancer, and diabetes.

(continued)

Protocol 12.1: Sexuality in the Older Adult *(continued)*

V. NURSING CARE STRATEGIES

A. Communication and education
   1. Discuss normal age-related physiological changes.
   2. Address how the effects of medications and medical conditions may affect one's sexual function.
   3. Facilitate communication with older adults and their families regarding sexual health as desired, including the following:
      a. Encourage family meetings with open discussion of issues if desired.
      b. Teach about safe-sex practices.
      c. Discuss use of condoms to prevent transmission of STIs and HIV.

B. Health management
   1. Perform a thorough patient assessment.
   2. Conduct a health history, review of systems, and physical examination.
   3. Effectively manage chronic illness.
   4. Improve glucose monitoring and control among diabetics.
   5. Ensure appropriate treatment of depression and screening for depression (see Chapter 15, "Late-Life Depression").
   6. Discontinue and substitute medications that may result in sexual dysfunction, or try lower doses or a different drug class (e.g., ARB instead of ACEI).
   7. Accurately assess and document older adults' ability to make informed decisions (see Chapter 4, "Health Care Decision Making").
   8. Participation in sexual relationships may be considered abusive if the older adult is not capable of making decisions or sexual activity is not consensual.

C. Sexual enhancement
   1. Compensate for normal changes of aging, including engaging in regular sexual activity (Heiman et al., 2011).
      a. Females
         i. Use of artificial water-based lubricants
         ii. Use of topical estrogen (Buster, 2012)
      b. Males
         i. Recognizing the possibility for more time and direct stimulation for arousal caused by aging changes; use of oral erectile agents for erectile dysfunction (Huang & Lie, 2013)
   2. Environmental adaptations
      a. Ensure privacy and safety among long-term care and community-dwelling residents (Wallace, 2008).

VI. EXPECTED OUTCOMES

A. Patients will:
   1. Report high quality of life as measured by a standardized quality-of-life assessment.
   2. Be provided with privacy, dignity, and respect surrounding their sexuality.
   3. Receive communication and education regarding sexual health as desired.
   4. Be able to pursue sexual health free of pathological and problematic sexual behaviors.

B. Nurses will:
   1. Include sexual health questions in their routine history and physical.
   2. Frequently reassess patients for changes in sexual health.

C. Institutions will:
   1. Include sexual health questions on intake and reassessment measures.
   2. Provide education on the ongoing sexual needs of older adults and appropriate interventions to manage these needs with dignity and respect.
   3. Provide a supportive environment that facilitates sexual discussions among staff and clients.
   4. Provide needed privacy for individuals to maintain intimacy and sexual health (e.g., in long-term care).

(continued)

Protocol 12.1: Sexuality in the Older Adult *(continued)*

VII. FOLLOW-UP MONITORING OF CONDITION

Sexual outcomes are difficult to directly assess and measure. However, with the demonstrated link between sexual health and quality of life, quality-of-life measures, such as the Medical Outcomes Study SF-36 Health Survey (RAND Health, 2009), may be used to determine the effectiveness of interventions to promote sexual health. Retrieved from http://www.rand.org/health/surveys_tools/mos/mos_core_36item.html

ABBREVIATIONS

ACEI	Angiotensin-converting enzyme inhibitor
ARB	Angiotensin receptor blocker
PLISSIT	Permission, limited information, specific suggestion, intensive therapy
STIs	Sexually transmitted infections

RESOURCES

American Association of Sexuality Educators Counselors and Therapists
http://www.aasect.org

MedlinePlus
http://www.nlm.nih.gov/medlineplus/sexualhealthissues.html

National Institutes on Aging
http://www.nia.nih.gov/HealthInformation/Publications/sexuality.htm

Prentiss Care Networks Project
Care networks for formal and informal caregivers of older adults
http://caregiving.case.edu

Urology Care Foundation
http://www.urologyhealth.org

World Health Organization
http://www.who.int/reproductivehealth/en

REFERENCES

American Psychiatric Association. (2013). *Diagnostic and statistical manual of mental disorder (*5th ed.*).* Arlington, VA: American Psychiatric Press. *Evidence Level VI.*

Annon, J. (1976). The PLISSIT model: A proposed conceptual scheme for behavioral treatment of sexual problems. *Journal of Sex Education Therapy, 2*(2), 1–15. *Evidence Level VI.*

Averyt, J. C., & Nishimoto, P. W. (2014). Addressing sexual dysfunction in colorectal cancer survivorship and care. *Journal of Gastrointestinal Oncology, 5*(5), 388–394. doi:10.3978/j.issn.2078–6891.2014.059. *Evidence Level V.*

Bardell, A., Lau, T., & Fedoroff, J. P. (2011). Inappropriate sexual behavior in a geriatric population. *International Psychogeriatrics, 23*(7), 1182–1188. doi:10.1017/S1041610211000676. *Evidence Level IV.*

Benbow, S. M., & Beeston, D. (2012). Sexuality, aging, and dementia. *International Psychogeriatrics, 24*(7), 1026–1033. *Evidence Level V.*

Buster, J. E. (2012). Sex and the 50-something woman: Strategies for restoring satisfaction. *Contemporary OB/GYN, 57*(8), 32–39. *Evidence Level V.*

Buttaro, T. M., Koeniger-Donohue, R., & Hawkins, J. (2014). Sexuality and quality of life in aging: Implications for practice. *Journal for Nurse Practitioners, 10*(7), 480–485. *Evidence Level V.*

Cahill, S., & Valadéz, R. (2013). Growing older with HIV/AIDS: New public health challenges. *American Journal of Public Health, 103*(3), e7–e15. *Evidence Level V.*

Centers for Disease Control and Prevention (CDC). (n.d.). *HIV among older Americans.* Retrieved from http://www.cdc.gov/hiv/risk/age/olderamericans/index.html. *Evidence Level V.*

Clayton, A. H., Croft, H. A., & Handiwala, L. (2014). Antidepressants and sexual dysfunction: Mechanisms and clinical implications. *Postgraduate Medicine, 126*(2), 91–99. doi:10.3810/pgm.2014.03.2744. *Evidence Level V.*

Connolly, M., Breckman, R., Callahan, J., Lachs, M., Ramsey-Klawsnik, H., & Solomon, J. (2012). The sexual revolution's last frontier: How silence about sex undermines health, well-being, and safety in old age. *Generations, 36*(3), 43–52. *Evidence Level V.*

Cook, S. C., Arnott, L. M., Nicholson, L. M., Cook, L. R., Sparks, E. A., & Daniels, C. J. (2008). Erectile dysfunction in men with congenital heart disease. *American Journal of Cardiology, 102*(12), 1728–1730. *Evidence Level IV.*

Copeland, K. L., Brown, J. S., Creasman, J. M., Van Den Eeden, S. K., Subak, L. L., Thom, D. H.,...Huang, A. J. (2012). Diabetes mellitus and sexual function in middle-aged and older women. *Obstetrics & Gynecology, 120*(2), 331–340. doi:10.1097/AOG.0b013e31825ec5fa. *Evidence Level IV.*

Coyne, K. S., Wein, A., Nicholson, S., Kvasz, M., Chen, C.-I., & Milsom, I. (2013). Comorbidities and personal burden of urgency urinary incontinence: A systematic review. *International Journal of Clinical Practice, 67*(10), 1015–1033. *Evidence Level IV.*

Dattilo, J., & Brewer, M. K. (2005). Assessing clients' sexual health as a component of nursing practice. *Journal of Holistic Nursing, 23*(2), 208–219. *Evidence Level IV.*

East, L., & Hutchinson, M. (2013). Moving beyond the therapeutic relationship: A selective review of intimacy in the sexual health encounter in nursing practice. *Journal of Clinical Nursing, 22*(23–24), 3568–3576. doi:10.1111/jocn.12247. *Evidence Level V.*

Fenge, L.-A., & Jones, K. (2012). Gay and pleasant land? Exploring sexuality, ageing and rurality in a multi-method, performative project. *British Journal of Social Work, 42*, 300–317. doi:10.1093/bjsw/bcr058. *Evidence Level IV.*

Garrett, D. (2014). Psychosocial barriers to sexual intimacy for older people. *British Journal of Nursing, 23*(6), 327–331. *Evidence Level V.*

Gott, M., Hinchliff, S., & Galena, E. (2004). General practitioner attitudes to discussing sexual health issues with older people. *Social Science & Medicine, 58*(11), 2093–2103. *Evidence Level IV.*

Hartmans, C., Comijs, H., & Jonker, C. (2014). Cognitive functioning and its influence on sexual behavior in normal aging and dementia. *International Journal of Geriatric Psychiatry, 29*, 441–446. doi:10.1002/gps.4025. *Evidence Level V.*

Heiman, J. R., Long, J. S., Smith, S. N., Fisher, W. A., Sand, M. S., & Rosen, R. C. (2011). Sexual satisfaction and relationship happiness in midlife and older couples in five countries. *Archives of Sexual Behavior, 40*, 741–753. doi:10.1007/s10508-010-9703-3. *Evidence Level IV.*

Huang, C.-Y., Tsai, L.-Y., Tseng, T.-H., Li, C.-R., & Lee, S. (2013). Nursing students' attitudes towards the provision of sexual health care in clinical nursing practice. *Journal of Clinical Nursing, 22*(23–24), 3577–3586. *Evidence Level IV.*

Huang, S. A., & Lie, J. D. (2013). Phosphodiesterase-5 (PDE5) inhibitors in the management of erectile dysfunction. *Pharmacy & Therapeutics, 38*(7), 407, 414–419. *Evidence Level V.*

Hyde, Z., Flicker, L., Hankey, G. J., Almeida, O. P., McCaul, K. A., Chub, S. A., & Yeap, B. B. (2010). Prevalence of sexual activity and associated factors in men aged 75 to 95 years. *Annals of Internal Medicine, 153*, 693–702. *Evidence Level IV.*

Killinger, K. A., Boura, J. A., & Diokno, A. C. (2014). Exploring factors associated with sexual activity in community-dwelling older adults. *Research in Gerontological Nursing, 7*(6), 256–263. *Evidence Level IV.*

Lassen, B., Gattinger, H., & Saxer, S. (2013). A systematic review of physical impairments following radical prostatectomy: Effect of psychoeducational interventions. *Journal of Advanced Nursing, 69*(12), 2602–2612. doi:10.1111/jan.12186. *Evidence Level I.*

Lee, D. M., Tajar, A., Ravindrarajah, R., Pye, S. R., O'Connor, D. B., Corona, G., . . . O'Neill, T. W. (2013). Frailty and sexual health in older European men. *Journals of Gerontology: Medical Sciences, 68*(7), 837–844. *Evidence Level IV.*

Levine, G. N., Steinke, E. E., Bakaeen, F. G., Bozkurt, B., Cheitlin, M. D., Conti, J. B., . . . Stewart, W. J. (2012). Sexual activity and cardiovascular disease: A scientific statement from the American Heart Association. *Circulation, 125*, 1058–1072. doi:10.1161/CIR.0b013e3182447787. *Evidence Level I.*

Lim, F. A., Brown, D. V., Jr., & Justin Kim, S. M. (2014). Addressing health care disparities in the lesbian, gay, bisexual, and transgender population: A review of best practices. *American Journal of Nursing, 114*(6), 24–34. doi:10.1097/01.NAJ.0000450423.89759.36. *Evidence Level V.*

Lindau, S. T., Schumm, L. P., Laumann, E. O., Levinson, W., O'Muircheartaigh, C. A., & Waite, L. J. (2007). A study of sexuality and health among older adults in the United States. *New England Journal of Medicine, 357*(8), 762–744. doi:10.1056/NEJMoa067423. *Evidence Level IV.*

Lobo, R. A. (2007). Menopause: Endocrinology, consequences of estrogen deficiency, effects of hormone replacement therapy, treatment regimens. In V. L. Katz, G. M. Lentz, R. A. Lobo, & D. M. Gershenson (Eds.), *Comprehensive gynecology* (5th ed.). Philadelphia, PA: Mosby Elsevier. *Evidence Level VI.*

Maes, C. A., & Louis, M. (2011). Nurse practitioners' sexual history-taking practices with adults 50 and older. *Journal for Nurse Practitioners, 7*(3), 216–222. *Evidence Level IV.*

Masters, W. H. (1986). Sex and aging—Expectations and reality. *Hospital Practice, 21*(8), 175–198. *Evidence Level VI.*

Mollaoğlu, M., Tuncay, F. O., & Fertelli, T. K. (2013). Investigating the sexual function and its associated factors in women with chronic illness. *Journal of Clinical Nursing, 22*(23–24), 3484–3491. doi:10.1111/jocn.12170. *Evidence Level IV.*

Mroczek, B., Kurpas, D., Gronowska, M., Kotwas, A., & Karakiewicz, B. (2013). Psychosexual needs and sexual behaviors of nursing home residents. *Archives of Gerontology and Geriatrics, 57*, 32–38. *Evidence Level IV.*

Nicolai, M. P. J., Liem, S. S., Both, S., Pelger, R. C. M., Putter, H., Schalij, M. J., & Elzevier, H. W. (2013). A review of the positive and negative effects of cardiovascular drugs on sexual function: A proposed table for use in clinical practice. *Netherlands Heart Journal, 22*, 11–19. *Evidence Level V.*

Ozmenler, N. K., Karlidere, T., Bozkurt, A., Yetkin, S., Doruk, A., Sutcigil, L., . . . Ozsahin, A. (2008). Mirtazapine augmentation in depressed patients with sexual dysfunction due to selective seratonin reuptake inhibitors. *Human Psychopharmacology, 23*, 321–326. doi:10.1002/hup.929. *Evidence Level III.*

Ports, K. A., Barnack-Tavlaris, J. L., Syme, M. L., Perera, R. A., & Lafata, J. E. (2014). Sexual health discussions with older adult patients during periodic health exams. *Journal of Sexual Medicine, 11*(4), 901–908. doi:10.1111/jsm.12448. *Evidence Level IV.*

Rand Health. (2009). *36-item short form survey from the RAND Medical Outcomes Study.* Retrieved from http://www.rand.org/health/surveys_tools/mos/mos_core_36item.html

Reichenpfader, U., Gartlehner, G., Morgan, L. C., Greenblatt, A., Nussbaumer, B., Hansen, R. A., . . . Gaynes, B. N. (2014). Sexual dysfunction associated with second-generation antidepressants in patients with major depressive disorder: Results from a systematic review with network meta-analysis. *Drug Safety, 37*, 19–31. doi:10.1007/s40264-013-0129-4. *Evidence Level I.*

Ribeiro, S., Alarcão, V., Simões, R., Miranda, F. L., Carreira, M., & Galvão-Teles, A. (2014). General practitioners' procedures for sexual history taking and treating sexual dysfunction in primary care. *Journal of Sexual Medicine, 11*(2), 386–393. doi:10.1111/jsm.12395. *Evidence Level IV.*

Rosen, T., Lachs, M. S., & Pillemer, K. (2010). Sexual aggression between residents in nursing homes: Literature synthesis of an underrecognized problem. *Journal of the American Geriatrics Society, 58*(10), 1070–1079. *Evidence Level V.*

Saiz-Ruiz, J., Montes, J. M., Ibáñez, Á., Díaz, M., Vicente, F., Pelegrín, C., . . . Ferrando, L. (2005). Assessment of sexual functioning in depressed patients treated with mirtazapine: A naturalistic 6-month study. *Human Psychopharmacology, 20,* 435–440. *Evidence Level IV.*

Saunamäki, N., Andersson, M., & Engstrm, M. (2010). Discussing sexuality with patients: Nurses' attitudes and beliefs. *Journal of Advanced Nursing, 66*(6), 1308–1316. doi:10.1111/j.1365-2648.2010.05260.x. *Evidence Level IV.*

Sharifi, F., Asghari, M., Jaberi, Y., Salehi, O., & Mirzamohammadi, F. (2012). Independent predictors of erectile dysfunction in type 2 diabetes mellitus: Is it true what they say about risk factors? *International Scholarly Research Network, ISRN Endocrinology*, Article ID 502353. doi:10.402/2012/502353. *Evidence Level IV.*

Steinke, E. E. (2013). Sexuality and chronic illness. *Journal of Gerontological Nursing, 39*(11), 18–27. doi:10.3928/00989134-20130916-01. *Evidence Level V.*

Steinke, E. E. (2014). Sexual dysfunction. In B. J. Ackley & G. B. Ladwig (Eds.), *Nursing diagnosis handbook: An evidence-based guide to planning care* (10th ed., pp. 717–724). Maryland Heights, MO: Mosby Elsevier. *Evidence Level V.*

Steinke, E. E., Jaarsma, T., Barnason, S. A., Byrne, M., Doherty, S., Dougherty, C. M., . . . Moser, D. K. (2013). Sexual counseling for individuals with cardiovascular disease and their partners: A consensus document from the American Heart Association and ESC Council on Cardiovascular Nursing and Allied Professions (CCNAP). *Circulation, 128*(18), 2075–2096. doi:10.1161/CIR.0b013e31829c2e53. *Evidence Level I.*

Steinke, E. E., Mosack, V., Wright, D. W., Chung, M. L., & Moser, D. K. (2009). Risk factors as predictors of sexual activity in heart failure, *Dimensions of Critical Care Nursing, 28*(3), 123–129. doi:10.1097/DCC.0b013e31819af08d. *Evidence Level IV.*

Syme, M. L. (2014). The evolving concept of older adult sexual behavior and its benefits. *Generations—Journal of the American Society on Aging, 38*(1), 35–41. *Evidence Level V.*

Topatan, S., & Yildiz, H. (2012). Symptoms experienced by women who enter into natural and surgical menopause and their relation to sexual functions. *Health Care for Women International, 33,* 525–539. doi:10.1080/07399332.2011.646374. *Evidence Level V.*

Trenque, T., Maura, G., Herlem, E., Vailet, C., Sole, E., Auriche, P., & Drame, M. (2013). Reports of sexual disorders related to serotonin reuptake inhibitors in the French pharacovigilance database: An example of underreporting. *Drugs & Safety, 36,* 515–519. doi:10.1007/s40264-013-0069-z. *Evidence Level IV.*

Wallace, M. (2008). How to try this; Sexuality assessment. *American Journal of Nursing, 108*(7), 40–48. *Evidence Level V.*

World Health Organization (WHO). (2010). *Measuring sexual health: Conceptual and practical considerations and related indicators.* Geneva, Switzerland: Author. *Evidence Level VI.*

Yeap, B. B., Araujo, A. B., & Wittert, G. A. (2012). Do low testosterone levels contribute to ill-health during male ageing? *Critical Reviews in Clinical Laboratory Sciences, 49*(5–6), 168–182. doi:10.3109/10408363.2012.725461. *Evidence Level V.*

13

Mistreatment Detection

Billy A. Caceres and Terry Fulmer

EDUCATIONAL OBJECTIVES

On completion of this chapter, the reader should be able to:

1. Educate nurses and other health care professionals about elder mistreatment (EM)
2. Identify risk factors that make older adults vulnerable for mistreatment
3. Discuss the deleterious effects EM may have on older adults' overall health status
4. Provide a framework for identifying, reporting, and managing cases of EM

OVERVIEW

In 2014, the U.S. Department of Justice consulted 750 stakeholders to enhance public and private response to elder mistreatment. Experts increasingly recognize the human, social, and economic impact of EM (U.S. Department of Justice, 2014). Most nurses in the acute care setting (and other settings) have likely provided care for an older adult suffering from EM without knowing it. By 2030, the population of Americans aged 65 years or older is expected to double and comprise 20% of the U.S. population (Centers for Disease Control and Prevention [CDC], 2013). Cases of EM are expected to become more prevalent given this expected surge of older adults. This drastic increase in the older adult population may exacerbate rates of EM. Technological advances of the past century have increased the life span of individuals with chronic diseases. However, older adults with chronic diseases require greater assistance in activities of daily living (ADL) and management of care (CDC, 2013). Also, the population of adults older than 90 years is expected to quadruple by 2050 (He & Muenchrath, 2011). The oldest old are at the greatest risk for EM because of increased disability and dependence on others to meet basic care needs (He & Muenchrath, 2011).

Furthermore, the impact of abuse, neglect, and exploitation has a serious fiscal cost. The direct medical costs associated with violent injuries to older adults are estimated by the National Center on Elder Abuse (NCEA) to add more than $5.3 billion to the nation's annual health expenditures, and the annual financial loss by victims of elder financial exploitation was estimated to be $2.9 billion in 2009, a 12% increase from 2008 (Mouton et al., 2004; National Committee for the Prevention of Elder Abuse, Virginia Tech, MetLife Mature Market Institute, 2011). EM researchers agree that as the population continues to age, cases of EM will reach epidemic levels (National Research Council [NRC], 2003). Now, more than ever before, it is imperative for nurses to become better educated about EM and its complexities.

For a description of evidence levels cited in this chapter, see Chapter 1, "Developing and Evaluating Clinical Practice Guidelines: A Systematic Approach."

Nurses in the inpatient setting serve an important role in recognizing EM as they are often the first health care professional to perform a detailed medical history or physical assessment. Nursing's presence at the bedside affords the opportunity to have direct contact with caregivers, observe caregiver–patient interactions, and identify red flags (Cohen, Halevi-Levin, Gagin, & Friedman, 2006). By virtue of the size of the workforce, which is the largest of any of the health professions, nurses are in a unique and optimal position to assess, identify, and intervene in cases of EM more often than other members of the interdisciplinary health care team.

The identification of EM should be a regular part of any geriatric assessment, and nursing curricula need to include the requisite content to ensure that all graduates have adequate knowledge and skills to assess and detect mistreatment. Many have suggested that mandatory EM training be a prerequisite for relicensure. EM is often multifactorial, so it is important to recognize it as the interplay among characteristics of the abused, the perpetrator, and environmental factors (Killick & Taylor, 2009). Physical markers of EM are often incorrectly attributed to physiological changes in the elderly or symptoms of chronic disease (Wiglesworth et al., 2009). Cases of EM may be challenging for nurses as they are often complicated by denial on the part of the perpetrator and older adult, refusal of services by victims, and fears that an accusation of EM may actually worsen EM. Significant ethical dilemmas may arise because nurses may struggle between their obligation to ensure patient well-being and uncertainty over the presence of EM (Beaulieu & Leclerc, 2006; Daly, Schmeidel Klein, & Jogerst, 2012). The development of EM protocols that are grounded in evidence-based research is crucial to ensure that EM cases are properly handled by nurses and other health care professionals.

BACKGROUND AND STATEMENT OF PROBLEM

Data from the NRC (2003) suggest that more than 2 million older adults suffer from at least one form of EM annually. The National Elder Abuse Incidence Study estimated that more than 500,000 new cases of EM occurred in 1996 (NCEA, 1998). A study by Acierno et al. (2010) estimated the prevalence of EM within a 1-year period to be approximately 11%. Although 44 states and the District of Columbia have legally required mandated reporting, EM is severely underreported. It should be noted that nurses, as mandatory reporters, have an obligation to report *suspected* cases of EM and all reports made in good faith are confidential. There is a lack of consistency across the United States regarding how cases of EM are reported and managed. Cases of EM are dealt with differently, with varying methods of investigation and intervention, state by state (Jogerst et al., 2003). NCEA (1998) estimates that only 16% of cases of EM are actually reported. In a systematic review, one third of health care professionals believe they detected a case of EM; however, only about 50% of that group actually reported the case (Cooper, Selwood, & Livingston, 2009). Similarly, another study found that despite 68% of emergency medical services staff stated they felt they had encountered a case of EM in the past year, only 27% of that group actually made a report (Jones, Walker, & Krohmer, 1995). Despite mandatory reporting on the part of health care professionals, it is believed that many are not reporting all cases of EM detected (Killick & Taylor, 2009). This, coupled with a lack of awareness of EM among older adults (Naughton, Drennan, & Lafferty, 2014), creates barriers for obtaining an accurate sense of the scope of EM and may have serious detrimental effects for victims of EM. In some instances, it may be that EM is addressed internally without reporting; for example, when a hospital administrator calls the police directly but there are no good data on internal processes that agencies use to independently handle EM cases.

Conflicting theories of causation and lack of uniform screening approaches may further impede EM detection. Understandably, it has been difficult for nurses to adequately respond to cases of EM when they are unclear about its manifestations, causes, appropriate screening techniques, and reporting laws. A lack of universally accepted definitions for different types of EM has hampered efforts to ascertain what constitutes EM. In an effort to establish a clear consensus, the NRC (2003) defined EM as either "intentional actions that cause harm or create serious risk of harm (whether harm is intended) to a vulnerable elder by a caregiver or other person who is in a trust relationship to the elder," or "failure by a caregiver to satisfy the elder's basic needs or to protect himself or herself from harm."

Types of EM

Six types of mistreatments are generally included under the umbrella term of EM. Table 13.1 describes each form of EM as well as offers examples of each.

EM is the outcome of the actions of abuse, neglect, exploitation, or abandonment, and can be further classified as intentional or unintentional. For example, intentional neglect is a conscious disregard for caretaking duties that are inherent for the well-being of an older adult. Unintentional neglect might occur when caregivers lack the knowledge and resources to provide quality

TABLE 13.1
Forms of Elder Mistreatment

Type of EM	Definition	Examples
Physical abuse	The use of physical force that may result in bodily injury, physical pain, or impairment	Hitting, beating, pushing, shoving, shaking, slapping, kicking, burning, inappropriate use of drugs, and physical restraints
Sexual abuse	Any form of sexual activity or contact without consent, including with those unable to provide consent	Unwanted touching, rape, sodomy, coerced nudity, and sexually explicit photographing
Emotional/ psychological abuse	The infliction of anguish, pain, or distress through verbal or nonverbal acts	Verbal assaults, insults, threats, intimidation, humiliation, harassment, and enforced social isolation
Financial abuse/ exploitation	The illegal or improper use of an elder's funds, property, or assets	Cashing a person's checks without authorization or permission; forging a signature; misusing or stealing money or possessions; coercing or deceiving a person into signing any document; and the improper use of conservatorship, guardianship, or power of attorney
Caregiver neglect	The refusal or failure to fulfill any part of a person's obligations or duties to an older adult, including social stimulation	Refusal or failure to provide life necessities such as food, water, clothing, shelter, personal hygiene, medicine, comfort, and personal safety
Self-neglect	The behavior of an elderly person that threatens his or her own health or safety; disregard of one's personal well-being and home environment	Refusal or failure to provide oneself with adequate food, water, clothing, shelter, personal hygiene, medication (when indicated), and safety precautions

EM, elder mistreatment.
Adapted from Fulmer and Greenberg (n.d.).

care (Cooper, Dow, Hay, Livingston, & Livingston, 2013; Jayawardena & Liao, 2006).

Neglect, whether intentional or unintentional, is recognized as the most common form of EM. NCEA (1998) revealed that neglect accounts for approximately half of all cases of EM reported to Adult Protective Services (APS). About 39.3% of these cases were classified as self-neglect and 21.6% attributed to caregiver neglect, including both intentional and unintentional. More than 70% of cases received by APS are attributed to cases of self-neglect with those older than 80 years thought to represent more than half of these cases (Lachs & Pillemer, 1995).

There is debate as to whether self-neglect should be included as a type of EM. Although other types of EM occur because of the action or inaction of a perpetrator, in self-neglect, the perpetrator and victim are one and the same (Anthony, Lehning, Austin, & Peck, 2009). Caregiver neglect is frequently identified as the most common and accepted form of EM internationally (Daskalopoulos & Borrelli, 2006; Mercurio & Nyborn, 2006; Oh, Kim, Martins, & Kim, 2006; Stathopoulou, 2004; Tareque, Ahmed, Tiedt, & Hoque, 2014; Yan & Tang, 2003). Most participants identified family members as the most likely perpetrators. Shockingly, neglect was seen as a "quasi-acceptable" form of abuse, whereas physical and emotional/psychological EM was viewed as extreme and harsh.

Theories of EM

The concept of vulnerability has been central to the discussion of EM. Fulmer et al. (2005) conducted a study of older adult patients recruited through emergency departments in two major cities. The purpose of this study was to identify factors within the older adult–caregiver relationship that may predispose some older adults to be victims of neglect over others. The theoretical framework used in this study was the risk-and-vulnerability model, which posits that neglect is caused by the interaction of factors within the older adult or in his or her environment. The risk and vulnerability model was adapted to EM by Frost and Willette (1994) and provides an appropriate lens through which to examine EM (Frost & Willette, 1994; Fulmer et al., 2005). *Vulnerability* is determined by characteristics within the older adult that may make him or her more likely to be a victim of EM such as poor health status, impaired cognition, and history of EM (Frost & Willette, 1994). *Risks* refer to factors in the environment that may predispose an older adult to EM and may include characteristics of caregivers such as health and functional status, as well as a lack of resources and social isolation (Fulmer et al., 2005). It is the interaction between risk and vulnerability that can predispose some older adults to EM (Killick & Taylor, 2009; Paveza, Vandeweerd, & Laumann, 2008).

The risk and vulnerability model and other models have been adapted from the health and social sciences literature in an effort to generate plausible theories of EM. However, there has been no clear consensus on one theory that explains EM (Fulmer, Guadagno, Bitondo Dyer, & Connolly, 2004). The development of interventions and strategies that cross multiple theoretical frameworks is likely to be the most clinically appropriate strategy (NRC, 2003).

Theories of EM, many of which emerged from the fields of family and interpersonal violence, include but are not limited to the following:

1. *Situational theory*: This theory was first used to explain causes of child abuse. The situational theory promotes the idea that stressful family conditions contribute to mistreatment. Thus, EM may be viewed as a consequence of caregiver strain resulting from the overwhelming tasks of caring for a vulnerable or frail older adult (Strauss, 1971).
2. *Psychopathology of the abuser*: This posits that mistreatment stems from a perpetrator's own battle with psychological illness such as substance use, depression, and other mental disorders (Gelles & Strauss, 1979).
3. *Social exchange theory*: This theory speculates that the long-established dependencies present in the victim–perpetrator relationship are responses developed within the family that then continue into adulthood (Gelles, 1983).
4. *Social learning theory*: Developed by Bandura (1978), this theory attributes mistreatment to learned behavior on the part of the perpetrator or victim from either his or her family life or the environment.
5. *Political economy theory*: This theory focuses on how older adults are often disenfranchised in society as their prior responsibilities and even their self-care are shifted onto others (Walker, 1981).

Dementia and EM

Older adults with dementia are particularly vulnerable to EM. As the population of older adults increases, it is expected that so will the number of older adults with dementia (Wiglesworth et al., 2010). The number of older adults with dementia is anticipated to increase threefold by 2050 (Hebert, Weuve, Scherr, & Evans, 2013). Because of the cognitive deficits associated with dementia, it is difficult to screen for EM in this population. The older adult with dementia may not be able to provide a reliable history, and signs of EM may be masked or mimicked by disease (Fulmer et al., 2005). Those providing care for older adults with dementia are at particular risk for caregiver strain and burnout. Disruptive behavior, such as screaming or wailing, physical aggression, or crying, can be exhausting for caregivers in any setting (Lachs, Becker, Siegal, Miller, & Tinetti, 1992).

As many as 47% of older adults with dementia are victims of some form of EM (Wiglesworth et al., 2010). Similarly, in a systematic review, one third of caregivers of older adults with dementia disclosed some form of EM, whereas 5% reported committing physical abuse (Cooper, Selwood, & Livingston, 2008). In a community-based study of caregivers of older adults with dementia, 51% of caregivers reported verbal abuse and 16% reported physical abuse (Cooney, Howard, & Lawlor, 2006). The implications of these data are sobering. However, these figures are likely underestimates of the true prevalence of EM as many cases are not reported.

Objective assessment alone cannot capture all cases of EM and, thus, policies are needed that combine objective measures and interviews with both the older adult and caregiver (Cooper et al., 2008). Some caregivers may be forthcoming with admission of EM and many may ask for help in developing coping strategies and plans of care to provide better care for care recipients (Wiglesworth et al., 2010).

EM in Racial/Ethnic Minorities

Research suggests that racial/ethnic differences might exist in the prevalence of EM; however, these differences are poorly understood (Laumann, Leitsch, & Waite, 2008). The CDC (2013) estimates that, by 2050, racial/ethnic minorities will account for 42% of all older adults. The health of racial/ethnic minority older adults continues to lag behind the health of non-Hispanic Whites as a result of language barriers, poverty, and differing cultural norms (CDC, 2013). DeLiema, Gassoumis, Homeier, and Wilber (2012) and Strasser, Smith, Weaver, Zheng, and Cao (2013) found high rates of EM in Latino older adults. The prevalence of sexual abuse was high at 9% (DeLiema et al., 2012). Risk factors for EM identified in this sample of Latino older adults included younger age, higher education level, and prior history of abuse, whereas years living in the United States were associated with higher risk of caregiver neglect (DeLiema et al., 2012). In addition, several studies indicate that EM may be higher in Blacks (Beach, Schulz, Castle, & Rosen, 2010; Dong, Simon, & Evans, 2013; Laumann et al., 2008). EM seems to be a problem among Asian older adults as well. Dong, Chang, Wong, Wong, and Simon (2011) conducted a qualitative study that revealed that Chinese older adults have limited knowledge of community resources for EM. The most common forms of EM experienced by Chinese and Korean older adults were caregiver neglect and emotional/psychological EM (Dong et al., 2011; Lai, 2011; Lee, Kaplan, & Perez-Stable, 2014). There is a need for more research on the prevalence of EM and culturally appropriate strategies for addressing EM among racial/ethnic minority older adults.

ASSESSMENT OF THE PROBLEM

The American Medical Association (AMA, 1992) released a set of guidelines and recommendations on the management of EM. The AMA urges providers to screen all older adults for EM. Many hospitals already include EM screening as part of the admission process for all patients older than 65 years. Assessment of EM is not easy as subtle signs of EM are hard to identify and may be difficult to substantiate (Anthony et al., 2009; Sandmoe & Kirkevold, 2011). Reporting of EM by health care professionals remains low because of a lack of education and training on the assessment, detection, and reporting of EM (Daly & Coffey, 2010; Thomson, Beavan, Lisk, McCracken, & Myint, 2010; Wagenaar, Rosenbaum, Page, & Herman, 2010). Unsubstantiated fears exist that increasing education on assessment of EM will lead to higher rates of false-positive cases and, therefore, expense and disruption in the system. However, a systematic review of 32 studies revealed that health care professionals educated about EM were not more likely to detect EM cases. However, these health care professionals were more inclined to report detected cases of EM than those who had little or no education (Cooper et al., 2009).

The complexity and variation within most cases of EM make it difficult to describe the profile of a perpetrator or victim. Some researchers suggest that victims of EM may be less likely to meet their own care needs because of cognitive and physical deficits (Cannell, Manini, Spence-Almaguer, Maldonado-Molina, & Andresen, 2014; Dong et al., 2013; Dong, Simon, & Evans, 2012; Dyer, Pavlik, Murphy, & Hyman, 2000). This supports findings on factors that impact mortality of victims of EM (Lachs, Williams, O'Brien, Pillemer, & Charlson, 1998; Schofield, Powers, & Loxton, 2013). Others (Brozowski & Hall, 2010; Draper et al., 2008; Fulmer et al., 2005; McDonald & Thomas, 2013) identified a link between childhood abuse or abuse in young adulthood and physical and sexual EM later in life. Similarly, Brozowski and Hall (2010) found that individuals who were sexually abused before age 60 years were 294% more likely to be victims of physical and sexual abuse in late life. A lack of social support and social isolation increases the risk for EM in older adults (Acierno et al., 2010; Cannell et al., 2014; Dong, Beck, & Simon, 2010; Dong & Simon, 2008; Fulmer et al., 2005). Recent findings suggest that victims of EM report poor overall health (Cannell et al., 2014; Cisler, Amstadter, Begle, Hernandez, & Acierno, 2010). Overall, perpetrators are more likely to be family members, report greater caregiver strain, live with the victim, have a history of mental illness and/or depression, have a history of substance abuse, have lived with the victim for an extended time (approximately 9.5 years), have decreased social support, and report a long history of conflicts with the victim (Giurani & Hasan, 2000; Johannesen & LoGiudice, 2013; Wiglesworth et al., 2010).

While assessing for EM, it is recommended to separate the older adult from the caregiver to obtain a detailed history and physical assessment (Heath & Phair, 2009). Special attention should be paid to both physical and psychological signs of EM. Discrepancies between injury presentation or severity and the report of how the injury occurred as well as discrepancies between explanations from the caregiver and older adult should be paid close attention. Physically abused older adults are more likely to have significantly larger bruises and identify the cause of their injuries. Furthermore, Wiglesworth et al. (2009) assert that abused older adults are more likely to display bruising on the face, lateral aspect of the right arm, and the posterior torso (including back, chest, lumbar, and gluteal regions). Other possible indicators of physical abuse include bruises at various stages of healing, unexplained frequent falls, fractures, dislocations, burns, and human bite marks (Cowen & Cowen, 2002).

It is important to distinguish that signs and symptoms of EM may vary depending on the type of abuse. Table 13.2 provides strategies for assessment of each type of EM. Victims of sexual abuse are more likely to be female and exhibit "genital or urinary irritation or injury; sleep disturbance; extreme upset when changed, bathed, or examined; aggressive behaviors; depression; or intense fear reaction to an individual" (Chihowski & Hughes, 2008, p. 381). Ageist attitudes among health care professionals may limit the cases of sexual abuse that are identified as older adults are rarely thought of as the usual victims of sexual abuse (Vierthaler, 2008). Cannell et al. (2014) estimate that the prevalence of sexual abuse among older adults is low at approximately 0.9%. Victims of financial abuse are harder to identify; however, they share similar traits as victims of emotional/psychological abuse and neglect, including social isolation, physical dependency, and mental disorders (Peisah et al., 2009).

TABLE 13.2
Assessment of Elder Mistreatment

Type of Mistreatment	Questions Used to Assess Type of EM	Physical Assessment and Signs and Symptoms
Physical abuse	Has anyone ever tried to hurt you in any way? Have you had any recent injuries? Are you afraid of anyone? Has anyone ever touched you or tried to touch you without permission? Have you ever been tied down? Suspected evidence of physical abuse (i.e., black eye) ask: – How did that get there? – When did it occur? – Did someone do this to you? – Are there other areas on your body like this? – Has this ever occurred before?	Assess for: Bruises (more commonly bilaterally to suggest grabbing), black eyes, welts, lacerations, rope marks, fractures, untreated injuries, bleeding, broken eyeglasses, use of physical restraints, sudden change in behavior Note whether a caregiver refuses an assessment of the older adult alone. Review any laboratory tests. Note any low- or high-serum prescribed drug levels. Note any reports of being physically mistreated in any way.
Emotional/ psychological abuse	Are you afraid of anyone? Has anyone ever yelled at you or threatened you? Has anyone been insulting you and using degrading language? Do you live in a household where there is stress and/or frustration? Does anyone care for you or provide regular assistance to you? Are you cared for by anyone who abuses drugs or alcohol? Are you cared for by anyone who was abused as a child?	Assess cognition, mood, affect, and behavior. Assess for: Agitation, unusual behavior, level of responsiveness, and willingness to communicate. Delirium Dementia Depression Note any reports of being verbally or emotionally mistreated.
Sexual abuse	Are you afraid of anyone? Has anyone ever touched you or tried to touch you without permission? Have you ever been tied down? Has anyone ever made you do things you did not want to do? Do you live in a household where there is stress and/or frustration? Does anyone care for you or provide regular assistance to you? Are you cared for by anyone who abuses drugs or alcohol? Are you cared for by anyone who was abused as a child?	Assess for: Bruises around breasts or genital area; sexually transmitted diseases; vaginal and/or anal bleeding or discharge; torn, stained, or bloody clothing/ undergarments Note any reports of being sexually assaulted or raped.
Financial abuse/ exploitation	Who pays your bills? Do you ever go to the bank with him or her? Does this person have access to your account(s)? Does this person have power of attorney? Have you ever signed documents you did not understand? Are any of your family members exhibiting a great interest in your assets? Has anyone ever taken anything that was yours without asking? Has anyone ever talked with you before about this?	Assess for: Changes in money handling or banking practice, unexplained withdrawals or transfers from patient's bank accounts, unauthorized withdrawals using the patient's bank card, addition of names on bank accounts/cards, sudden changes to any financial document/will, unpaid bills, forging of the patient's signature, appearance of previously uninvolved family members Note any reports of financial exploitation.

(continued)

TABLE 13.2

Assessment of Elder Mistreatment ***(continued)***

Type of Mistreatment	Questions Used to Assess Type of EM	Physical Assessment and Signs and Symptoms
Caregiver neglect	Are you alone a lot? Has anyone ever failed you when you needed help? Has anyone ever made you do things you did not want to do? Do you live in a household where there is stress and/or frustration? Does anyone care for you or provide regular assistance to you? Are you cared for by anyone who abuses drugs or alcohol? Are you cared for by anyone who was abused as a child?	Assess for: Dehydration, malnutrition, untreated pressure ulcers, poor hygiene, inappropriate or inadequate clothing, unaddressed health problems, nonadherence to medication regimen, unsafe and/or unclean living conditions, animal/insect infestation, presence of lice and/or fecal/urine smell, and soiled bedding Note any reports of feeling mistreated.
Self-neglect	How often do you bathe? Have you ever refused to take prescribed medications? Have you ever failed to provide yourself with adequate food, water, or clothing?	Assess for: Dehydration, malnutrition, poor personal hygiene, unsafe living conditions, animal/insect infestation, fecal/urine smell, inappropriate clothing, nonadherence to medication regimen

EM, elder mistreatment.

Adapted from Fulmer and Greenberg (n.d.).

Since the 1970s, a number of screening instruments have been developed to detect EM. However, few instruments are deemed appropriate for the inpatient setting. Most instruments have had limited testing in the inpatient setting and tend to focus on in-home assessments or extensive questions that are better suited for outpatient and community settings.

The Elder Assessment Instrument (EAI) developed by Fulmer et al. (2004) is a 41-item screening instrument that requires training on administration, but has been shown to be effective in busy inpatient settings (Perel-Levin, 2008). The most recent version of the EAI-R is considered more appropriate for inpatient and outpatient clinics because it relies on objective assessment by the clinician. This assessment includes a survey of general appearance, assessment for dehydration, physical and psychological markers, or pressure ulcers in addition to subjective information reported by the older adult.

The Hwalek–Sengstock Elder Abuse Screening Test (HS-EAST) is a 15-item instrument that relies on self-report from older adults and is documented as appropriate for detecting physical abuse, vulnerability, and high-risk situations. Some instruments focus on the caregiver, but an advantage of HS-EAST is the focus on the older adult's history. It is regarded as appropriate for use in the hospital setting and can be easily administered by nurses (Fulmer et al., 2004; Perel-Levin, 2008). If a positive screen is noted, a detailed physical assessment and medical history should be completed to substantiate possible EM. Referral to experts in trauma or geriatrics should take place for the most comprehensive assessment.

In addition to these screening instruments for EM, there are a number of other reliable and valid instruments that can aide nurses in identifying older adults at risk for EM. Victims of EM tend to have lower physical and cognitive function than their peers (Dong et al., 2012; Fulmer et al., 2005). The Katz Index of Independence in ADL and/or the Lawton Instrumental Activities of Daily Living (IADL) scale may help in identifying older adults with functional deficits (Dong et al., 2012; Graf, 2007). Similarly, with higher rates of depression in victims of EM, the Geriatric Depression Scale (GDS) may be a useful instrument for nurses to use in the inpatient setting (Greenberg, 2012). The GDS is an easy-to-administer 15-item screening instrument that is effective at distinguishing depressed older adults (Greenberg, 2012). Perpetrators of EM often report higher levels of caregiver strain. The Modified Caregiver Strain Index (CSI) is a reliable and self-administered instrument that can assist in assessing caregivers that may benefit from interventions to alleviate stress involved with caregiving demands (Onega, 2013).

The process of identifying cases of self-neglect is oftentimes more daunting than other cases of EM. Assessing self-neglect is further complicated by a lack of standardized screening instruments or markers for detection (Dyer et al., 2006; Kelly, Dyer, Pavlik, Doody, & Jogerst, 2008; Mosqueda et al., 2008). Most instruments require in-depth assessments of home life and rely on objective findings. Nevertheless, data suggest that detection of self-neglect in the inpatient setting is unfortunately made easier because by the time these cases reach the hospital, they are often very severe (Mosqueda et al., 2008). Signs of self-neglect may include lack of adequate nutrition; dehydration; changes in weight; poor hygiene and appearance such as soiled clothing, uncombed hair, debris in teeth; poor adherence to medical treatments such as unfilled prescriptions; refusing to perform dressing changes; poor glucose monitoring; and so forth (Cohen et al., 2006; Naik, Teal, Pavlik, Dyer, & McCullough, 2008; Turner, Hochschild, Burnett, Zulfiqar, & Dyer, 2012). Objective measures as well as questioning of the older adult about health patterns and activities of self-care are also important factors in detecting self-neglect because they can provide important information about the older adult's attitudes and opinions.

INTERVENTIONS AND CARE STRATEGIES

Detailed screening of older adults at risk for EM is the first step in identifying cases of EM (Perel-Levin, 2008). There are various screening instruments that can help in identifying older adults and caregivers at risk for EM. Dedicating time to meet with the older patient and his or her caregiver(s) separately is an important aspect of the screening process. These strategies can highlight any inconsistencies in depictions of how injuries occurred, allowing the nurse to develop a closer relationship with each individual, and express his or her willingness to help each party.

Nurses should not work alone in detecting cases of EM, instead, they should work with professionals from other disciplines as much as possible. The use of interdisciplinary teams with health care professionals from both the inpatient and outpatient settings is the best approach to managing cases of EM (Wiglesworth, Mosqueda, Burnight, Younglove, & Jeske, 2006). Institutions should develop clear guidelines for practitioners to follow when cases of EM are identified (Donder et al., 2012; Perel-Levin, 2008; Sandmoe & Kirkevold, 2011). Referral to appropriate community organizations is vital to ensure safe discharges for suspected victims of EM. Interdisciplinary teams work most effectively when they include team members with expertise in various disciplines, including nursing, social work, medicine, law, and so forth. It is this diversity of skills that allows for innovative approaches to managing cases of EM (Jayawardena & Liao, 2006).

Educating older adults, staff, and caregivers about the nature of EM is key. It is crucial to educate older adults who have the cognitive capacity to accept or refuse interventions about patterns of EM such that EM tends to increase in severity over time (Phillips, 2008). For individuals who lack the cognitive capacity to consent to interventions, it is important to report these cases to APS and develop a plan for safe discharge. Older adults should receive emergency contact information as well as community resources (Lachs & Pillemer, 1995).

Services should be offered not only to victims of EM but also to their suspected perpetrators. Interdisciplinary teams should also recognize the difficulties caregivers may experience in caring for older adults with diminished physical and/or cognitive function and provide these caregivers with support services to assist them in providing the best care they can (Lowenstein, 2009). Helping caregivers gain a better understanding of proper care techniques may help alleviate cases of neglect in particular.

Because of the brief nature of hospital stays, most of the long-term interventions occur in the community setting. A systematic review revealed that community-based interventions tend to concentrate on the situational theory of EM by focusing on education, counseling, and social support for perpetrators of EM to help them cope with stressors of caregiving (Ploeg, Fear, Hutchison, MacMillan, & Bolan, 2009). However, even these community-based interventions have shown mixed results in terms of effectiveness in addressing risk of EM recurrence; depression and self-esteem in older adults; and levels of caregiver strain, stress, and depression in caregivers (Ploeg et al., 2009). In a study of EM referral cases, only 84% of older adults with suspected EM were offered services (Clancy, McDaid, O'Neill, & O'Brien, 2011). The most common services offered were additional monitoring, home support, and counseling. Older adults were generally willing to accept additional services with 75% of those suspected of being victims of EM agreeing to further intervention (Clancy et al., 2011). This suggests that older adults may be open to additional support in cases of suspected EM. However, Jackson and Hafemeister (2013) found that older adults might continue to experience EM even after the close of an APS investigation. This may be because of continued contact with the perpetrator or the perpetrator receiving no legal consequences following investigation. Similarly, a social worker–lawyer intervention for EM victims found that EM was more likely to continue in female victims, married victims, and those who lived with the perpetrator (Rizzo, Burnes, & Chalfy, 2015).

In the inpatient setting, patients are assumed to have the autonomy to refuse medical treatments and participate in the management of their own care as long as they are deemed to be able to provide informed consent. However, what can be done if the older adult is refusing to perform activities considered essential for his or her health and well-being? The answer, at the moment, is very little. There is currently no rigorously tested screening instrument to assess cognitive capacity in this population (Naik et al., 2008). Naik et al. (2008) discuss the ethical dilemma that arises when an older adult is suspected of self-neglect. If the older adult has the cognitive capacity to make decisions about his or her own self-care, there is very little that health care professionals can do to intervene. Interdisciplinary teams are thought to be the most effective way of identifying self-neglect. Although it may seem difficult and costly to use interdisciplinary health care teams to adequately care for this group of older adults, the costs of not connecting these individuals to proper resources can be much greater as their health conditions can go undiagnosed and untreated for a longer time, therefore creating greater health care costs (Lowenstein, 2009).

It is difficult to evaluate the success of interventions implemented in inpatient settings. The nature of discharges reduces the ability of hospital staff to follow-up on cases of EM. Not all suspected victims of EM will return to the same acute care institution for repeat visits, and confidentiality issues can restrict information sharing among health care professionals.

CASE STUDY

Mr. Campo is an 83-year-old male admitted to a medical unit for change in mental status. His 79-year-old wife is at his bedside. On admission assessment, the nurse notices Mr. Campo is confused, weak, and pale. He is also underweight with a body mass index (BMI) of 16.4 kg/m^2. When asked about the change in his cognitive status, Mrs. Campo reports that Mr. Campo was diagnosed with early Alzheimer's dementia and gastric cancer last year. He has become more confused in the past 2 days. Mrs. Campo states she would have brought her husband to the emergency department sooner but their son, José, said she should not worry about it because of his dementia.

His vital signs are as follows: blood pressure of 93/52 mmHg, heart rate of 115 beats per minute, respiratory rate of 23 breaths per minute, and a temperature of 100.8°F. He is unable to verbalize a pain score; however, he does not appear to be in pain at this moment.

On performing an EM assessment, the nurse gathers the following information from Mrs. Campo: Her husband has lost a total of 25 pounds in recent months and has been refusing to eat for the past week. Mrs. Campo's mobility is limited because of multiple sclerosis and their neighbor who used to accompany them to medical visits has moved away. Their son, José, had to move in with them a year ago after he lost his job. Mr. Campo and his son have never had a good relationship and often argue about their living arrangement. This has the entire family very depressed. Mrs. Campo also reveals that José is frequently inebriated but denies having a drinking problem. Moreover, José refuses to take Mr. Campo to see his primary care provider stating that these health changes are "just because he's so old."

Mr. Campo is now on intravenous hydration and is being followed by a dietitian. His vital signs and mental status have improved. Further testing reveals that Mr. Campo has an esophageal tumor, which may be the cause of his anorexia.

Discussion

This may be considered a case of neglect and/or psychological/emotional abuse. José knows that Mr. Campo's health has deteriorated, yet he refuses to seek proper medical attention for his father. He also argues with his father often and may be abusing alcohol. From Mrs. Campo's report, there is no evidence of other forms of EM; however, the case should be investigated further. Although the nurse has yet to meet José, there are a number of signs to indicate that neglect or psychological/emotional abuse may be occurring in this home. As a mandated reporter, the nurse should report this case if he or she suspects any form of EM is present.

A number of risk factors are present in this family to alert the nurse of possible EM. For example, Mr. Campo has cognitive deficits because of dementia and is frail because of his cancer diagnosis. In addition, his wife has functional deficits because of her multiple sclerosis. Also, she reports feeling depressed by her current situation and lacks a strong support system.

The nurse should discuss the case with Mr. Campo's medical team as well as his social worker. The dietitian could provide the family with information about Mr. Campo's nutritional needs. The nurse should collaborate with the family and interdisciplinary team to identify community services for this family.

SUMMARY

With a rapidly aging population, it is likely that cases of EM will become more prevalent. Although most research on EM has focused on EM in the community and long-term care settings, the inpatient setting is ideal for the identification of those at risk for EM. EM prevalence is hard to estimate, yet most experts believe that it is heavily underreported. As the largest health care profession, it is nursing's responsibility to develop an understanding and appreciation for the complexities of detecting and addressing cases of EM. The recognition of markers of EM is an important step in guaranteeing that older adults receive high-quality care. The different manifestations and types of EM often make it challenging for nurses to determine the best strategies for intervention. However, the strategies in this chapter serve as a framework to help nurses navigate these situations. These strategies include best practices from the extant literature on EM that is applicable for acute care nurses.

Nurses serve as advocates for older adults who may not be able to protect themselves from EM. Therefore, nurses should encourage their institutions to develop guidelines for managing suspected cases of EM and establish interdisciplinary teams to determine how to best respond in these circumstances (Daly et al., 2012; Donder et al., 2012). EM detection should be embedded within admission and nursing assessments of older adults. There is no telling how many older adults and caregivers may benefit from a greater focus on EM. It is only through education and the use of interdisciplinary teams to respond to EM cases that nurses can ensure the safety and well-being of older adults in their care.

NURSING STANDARD OF PRACTICE

Protocol 13.1: Detection of Elder Mistreatment

I. GOAL

Determine best practices in identifying and responding to cases of EM

II. OVERVIEW

With the projected increase in the population of older adults worldwide and the rise in medical and technological advances, it is anticipated that older adults will continue to live longer. Therefore, it is expected that cases of EM, although currently underreported, will rise. As patient advocates and providers of care, nurses serve an important function in the screening and treatment of cases of EM. However, current data show that nurses and other health care professionals do not report all cases of EM they encounter either because of lack of knowledge about manifestations of EM or how reporting and investigation by state agencies function.

III. BACKGROUND/STATEMENT OF PROBLEM

A. Definitions
   1. *Elder mistreatment*: "Intentional actions that cause harm or create serious risk of harm (whether harm is intended) to a vulnerable elder by a caregiver or other person who is in a trust relationship to the elder," or "failure by a caregiver to satisfy the elder's basic needs or to protect himself or herself from harm" (NRC, 2003, p. 1). There are conflicting casual theories of EM.
   2. *Physical abuse:* The use of physical force that may result in bodily injury, physical pain, or impairment (NCEA, 2008).
   3. *Sexual abuse:* Any form of sexual activity or contact without consent, including with those unable to provide consent (NCEA, 2008).
   4. *Emotional/psychological abuse*: The infliction of anguish, pain, or distress through verbal or nonverbal acts (NCEA, 2008).
   5. *Financial abuse/exploitation:* The illegal or improper use of an elder's funds, property, or assets (Naik et al., 2008).

(continued)

Protocol 13.1: Detection of Elder Mistreatment *(continued)*

6. *Caregiver neglect:* The refusal or failure to fulfill any part of a person's obligations or duties to an older adult, including social stimulation (NCEA, 2008).
7. *Self-neglect:* The behavior of an older adult that threatens his or her own health or safety. Disregard of one's personal well-being and home environment (NCEA, 2008).
8. *Risk-vulnerability model:* This model posits that neglect is caused by the interaction of factors within the older adult and his or her environment. The risk and vulnerability model adapted to EM by Frost and Willette (1994) provides a good lens through which to examine EM. *Vulnerability* is determined by characteristics within the older adult that increase his or her risk of being abused by caregivers, such as poor health status, impaired cognition, and history of abuse. *Risks* refer to factors in the environment that may predispose an older adult to EM and may include characteristics of caregivers, such as health and functional status, as well as a lack of resources and social isolation (Fulmer et al., 2005).
9. *Situational theory:* This theory was first used to explain causes of child abuse. The situational theory promotes the idea that stressful family conditions contribute to mistreatment. Thus, EM may be viewed as a consequence of caregiver strain because of the overwhelming tasks of caring for a vulnerable or frail older adult (Strauss, 1971).
10. *Psychopathology of the abuser:* This posits that mistreatment stems from a perpetrator's own battle with psychological illness, such as substance use, depression, and other mental disorders (Gelles & Strauss, 1979).
11. *Social exchange theory:* This theory speculates that the long-established dependencies present in the victim–perpetrator relationship are responses developed within the family and then continue into adulthood (Gelles, 1983).
12. *Social learning theory:* This was developed by Bandura (1978), and this theory attributes mistreatment to learned behavior on the part of the perpetrator or victim from either family life or the environment.
13. *Political economy theory:* This theory focuses on how older adults are often disenfranchised in society as their prior responsibilities and even their self-care are shifted onto others (Walker, 1981).

B. Characteristics of victims
   1. Decreased ability to complete ADL and more physically frail (Dyer et al., 2000; Frost & Willette, 1994; Peisah et al., 2009)
   2. Cognitive deficits such as dementia (Dong et al., 2012; Fulmer et al., 2005; Gorbien & Eisenstein, 2005; Naik et al., 2008)
   3. History of trauma earlier in life (Brozowski & Hall, 2010; DeLiema et al., 2012; Draper et al., 2008; Fulmer et al., 2005; Lachs et al., 1998; McDonald & Thomas, 2013)
   4. Depression and other mental disorders, as well as an increased sense of hopelessness (Dong et al., 2012; Dyer et al., 2000; Fulmer et al., 2005; Johannesen & LoGiudice, 2013)
   5. Social isolation and lack of support systems (Acierno et al., 2010; Cannell et al., 2014; Dong et al., 2010; Draper et al., 2008; Dyer et al., 2000; Peisah et al., 2009)
   6. History of substance abuse (Dyer et al., 2000; Peisah et al., 2009)

C. Characteristics of perpetrators
   1. Most commonly family members
   2. Long history of conflict with the victim (Krienert, Walsh, & Turner, 2009)
   3. Lived with victim for an extended time (Rizzo et al., 2015; Wiglesworth et al., 2010)
   4. Higher rates of caregiver strain (Lachs et al., 1992; Strasser et al., 2013; Wiglesworth et al., 2010)
   5. History of mental illness and substance abuse (Jackson & Hafemeister, 2013; Wiglesworth et al., 2010)
   6. Depression and other mental disorders (Giurani & Hasan, 2000; Johannesen & LoGiudice, 2013; Wiglesworth et al., 2010)
   7. Social isolation and lack of support systems (Wiglesworth et al., 2010)

D. Etiology and/or epidemiology
   1. Data from the National Research Council (2003) suggest that more than 2 million older adults suffer from at least one form of EM annually.
   2. The National Elder Abuse Incidence Study estimates that more than half a million new cases of EM occurred in 1996 (NCEA, 1998).

(continued)

Protocol 13.1: Detection of Elder Mistreatment *(continued)*

3. Even though 44 states and the District of Columbia have legally required mandated reporting, EM is severely underreported. There is a lack in uniformity across the United States on how cases of EM are handled (NCEA, 1998).
4. NCEA (1998) estimates that only 16% of cases of abuse are actually reported.
5. The National Council on Elder Abuse revealed that neglect accounts for approximately half of all cases of EM reported to APS. About 39.3% of these cases were classified as self-neglect and 21.6% were attributed to caregiver neglect, including both intentional and unintentional (NRC, 2003).
6. More than 70% of cases received by APS are attributed to cases of self-neglect with those older than 80 years thought to represent more than half of these cases (Lachs & Pillemer, 1995).

IV. PARAMETERS OF ASSESSMENT

A. See Table 13.2.

V. NURSING CARE STRATEGIES

A. Detailed screening to assess for risk factors for EM using a combination of physical assessment, subjective information, and data gathered from screening instruments (Perel-Levin, 2008)
B. Strive to develop a trusting relationship with the older adult as well as the caregiver. Set aside time to meet with each individually (Perel-Levin, 2008).
C. Use of interdisciplinary teams with a diversity of experience, knowledge, and skills can lead to improvements in the detection and management of cases of EM. Early intervention by interdisciplinary teams can help lower risk for worsening abuse and further deficits in health status (Jayawardena & Liao, 2006; Rizzo et al., 2015; Wiglesworth et al., 2010).
D. Institutions should develop guidelines for responding to cases of EM (Donder et al., 2012; Perel-Levin, 2008; Sandmoe & Kirkevold, 2011, Wiglesworth et al., 2010)
E. Institutions should implement culturally appropriate strategies for identifying and addressing EM in racial/ethnic minority older adults (Horsford, Parra-Cardona, Schiamberg, & Post, 2011).
F. Educate victims about patterns of EM such that EM tends to worsen in severity over time (Phillips, 2008).
G. Provide older adults with emergency contact numbers and community resources (Lachs & Pillemer, 1995).
H. Refer to appropriate regulatory agencies.

VI. EVALUATION AND EXPECTED OUTCOMES

A. Reduction of harm through referrals, use of interdisciplinary interventions, and/or relocation to a safer situation and environment (Jackson & Hafemeister, 2013; Rizzo et al., 2015)
B. Victims of EM verbalize an understanding of how to access appropriate services.
C. Caregivers use services, such as respite care or treatment, for mental illness or substance use.
D. If possible, evaluate progress in relationships between caregiver and older adult through screening instruments such as the Modified CSI and GDS among other tools freely available at consultgerirn.org.
E. Institutional establishment of clear and evidence-based guidelines for management of EM cases.

VII. FOLLOW-UP MONITORING OF CONDITION

A. Follow-up monitoring in the acute care setting is limited compared to the follow-up that may be performed in the community or long-term care settings.

VIII. RELEVANT PRACTICE GUIDELINES

A. American Medical Association (AMA). (1992). *Diagnostic and treatment guidelines on elder abuse and neglect*. Chicago, IL: Author.

(continued)

Protocol 13.1: Detection of Elder Mistreatment *(continued)*

ABBREVIATIONS

ADL	Activities of daily living
APS	Adult Protective Services
CSI	Caregiver Strain Index
EM	Elder mistreatment
GDS	Geriatric Depression Scale
NCEA	National Center on Elder Abuse
NRC	National Research Council

RESOURCES

Administration on Aging
http://www.aoa.gov

Elder Justice Roadmap
http://ncea.aoa.gov/Library/Gov_Report/docs/EJRP_Roadmap.pdf

Elder Mistreatment Assessment
http://consultgerirn.org/resources

Journal of Elder Abuse & Neglect
http://www.informaworld.com/smpp/title~content=t792303995~db=all

National Center on Elder Abuse
http://www.ncea.aoa.gov/ncearoot/Main_Site/index.asp

REFERENCES

Acierno, R., Hernandez, M. A., Amstadter, A. B., Resnick, H. S., Steve, K., Muzzy, W., & Kilpatrick, D. G. (2010). Prevalence and correlates of emotional, physical, sexual, and financial abuse and potential neglect in the United States: The National Elder Mistreatment Study. *American Journal of Public Health, 100*(2), 292–297. *Evidence Level IV.*

American Medical Association (AMA). (1992). *Diagnostic and treatment guidelines on elder abuse and neglect.* Chicago, IL: Author. *Evidence Level VI.*

Anthony, E. K., Lehning, A. J., Austin, M. J., & Peck, M. D. (2009). Assessing elder mistreatment: Instrument development and implications for adult protective services. *Journal of Gerontological Social Work, 52*(8), 815–836. *Evidence Level V.*

Aravanis, S. C., Adelman, R. D., Breckman, R., Fulmer, T. T., Holder, E., Lachs, M., . . . Sanders, A. B. (1993). Diagnostic and treatment guidelines on elder abuse and neglect. *Archives of Family Medicine, 2,* 371–388. *Evidence Level VI.*

Bandura, A. (1978). Social learning theory of aggression. *Journal of Communication, 28*(3), 12–29. *Evidence Level V.*

Beach, S. R., Schulz, R., Castle, N. G., & Rosen, J. (2010). Financial exploitation and psychological mistreatment among older adults: Differences between African Americans and non-African Americans in a population-based survey. *The Gerontologist, 50,* 744–757. *Evidence Level IV.*

Beaulieu, M., & Leclerc, N. (2006). Ethical and psychosocial issues raised by the practice in cases of mistreatment of older adults. *Journal of Gerontological Social Work, 46*(3–4), 161–186. *Evidence Level IV.*

Brozowski, K., & Hall, D. R. (2010). Aging and risk: Physical and sexual abuse of elders in Canada. *Journal of Interpersonal Violence, 25*(7), 1183–1199. doi:10.1177/0886260509340546. *Evidence Level V.*

Cannell, M. B., Manini, T., Spence-Almaguer, E., Maldonado-Molina, M., & Andresen, E. M. (2014). U.S. population estimates and correlates of sexual abuse of community-dwelling older adults. *Journal of Elder Abuse & Neglect, 26*(4), 398–413. doi:10.1080/08946566.2013.879845. *Evidence Level IV.*

Centers for Disease Control and Prevention (CDC). (2013). *The state of aging and health in America 2013.* Atlanta, GA: U.S. Department of Health and Human Services. *Evidence Level V.*

Chihowski, K., & Hughes, S. (2008). Clinical issues in responding to alleged elder sexual abuse. *Journal of Elder Abuse & Neglect, 20*(4), 377–400. *Evidence Level V.*

Cisler, J. M., Amstadter, A. B., Begle, A. M., Hernandez, M., & Acierno, R. (2010). Elder mistreatment and physical health among older adults: The South Carolina elder mistreatment study. *Journal of Traumatic Stress, 23*(4), 461–467. doi:10.1002/jts. *Evidence Level IV.*

Clancy, M., McDaid, B., O'Neill, D., & O'Brien, J. G. (2011). National profiling of elder abuse referrals. *Age and Ageing, 40*(3), 346–352. doi:10.1093/ageing/afr023. *Evidence Level IV.*

Cohen, M., Halevi-Levin, S. H., Gagin, R., & Friedman, G. (2006). Development of a screening tool for identifying elderly people at risk of abuse by their caregivers. *Journal of Aging and Health, 18*(5), 660–685. *Evidence Level IV.*

Cooney, C., Howard, R., & Lawlor, B. (2006). Abuse of vulnerable people with dementia by their carers: Can we identify those most at risk? *International Journal of Geriatric Psychiatry, 21*(6), 564–571. *Evidence Level V.*

Cooper, C., Dow, B., Hay, S., Livingston, D., & Livingston, G. (2013). Care workers' abusive behavior to residents in care homes: A qualitative study of types of abuse, barriers, and facilitators to good care and development of an instrument for reporting of abuse anonymously. *International Psychogeriatrics, 25*(5), 733–741. doi:10.1017/S104161021200227X. *Evidence Level IV.*

Cooper, C., Selwood, A., & Livingston, G. (2008). The prevalence of elder abuse and neglect: A systematic review. *Age and Ageing, 37*(2), 151–160. *Evidence Level I.*

Cooper, C., Selwood, A., & Livingston, G. (2009). Knowledge, detection, and reporting of abuse by health and social care professionals: A systematic review. *American Journal of Geriatric Psychiatry, 17*(10), 826–838. *Evidence Level I.*

Cowen, H. J., & Cowen, P. S. (2002). Elder mistreatment: Dental assessment and intervention. *Special Care in Dentistry, 22*(1), 23–32. *Evidence Level V.*

Daly, J., & Coffey, A. (2010). Staff perceptions of elder abuse. *Nursing Older People, 22*(4), 33–37. doi:10.7748/nop2010.05.22.4.33.c7735. *Evidence Level IV.*

Daly, J. M., Schmeidel Klein, A. N., & Jogerst, G. J. (2012). Critical care nurses' perspectives on elder abuse. *Nursing in Critical Care, 17*(4), 172–179. doi:10.1111/j.1478–5153.2012.00511.x. *Evidence Level IV.*

Daskalopoulos, M. D., & Borrelli, S. E. (2006). Definitions of elder abuse in an Italian sample. *Journal of Elder Abuse & Neglect, 18*(2–3), 67–85. *Evidence Level IV.*

DeLiema, M., Gassoumis, Z. D., Homeier, D. C., & Wilber, K. H. (2012). Determining prevalence and correlates of elder abuse using promotores: Low-income immigrant Latinos report high rates of abuse and neglect. *Journal of the American Geriatrics Society, 60*(7), 1333–1339. doi:10.1111/j.1532–5415.2012.04025.x. *Evidence Level IV.*

Donder, L. D., Lang, G., Luoma, M.-L., Penhale, B., Alves, J. F., Tamutiene, I., . . . Verté, D. (2011). Perpetrators of abuse against older women: A multi-national study in Europe. *Journal of Adult Protection, 13*(6), 302–314. doi:10.1108/14668201111194212. *Evidence Level IV.*

Dong, X., Beck, T., & Simon, M. A. (2010). The associations of gender, depression and elder mistreatment in a community-dwelling Chinese population: The modifying effect of social support. *Archives of Gerontology and Geriatrics, 50*, 202–208. doi:10.1016/j.archger.2009.03.011. *Evidence Level IV.*

Dong, X., Chang, E. S., Wong, E., Wong, B., & Simon, M. A. (2011). How do U.S. Chinese older adults view elder mistreatment?: Findings from a community-based participatory research study. *Journal of Aging and Health, 23*(2), 289–312. doi:10.1177/0898264310385931. *Evidence Level IV.*

Dong, X., & Simon, M. A. (2008). Is greater social support a protective factor against elder mistreatment? *Gerontology, 54*(6), 381–388. *Evidence Level IV.*

Dong, X., Simon, M., & Evans, D. (2012). Decline in physical function and risk of elder abuse reported to social services in a community-dwelling population of older adults. *Journal of the American Geriatrics Society, 60*(10), 1922–1928. doi:10.1111/j.1532–5415.2012.04147.x. *Evidence Level IV.*

Dong, X., Simon, M., & Evans, D. (2013). Elder self-neglect is associated with increased risk for elder abuse in a community-dwelling population: findings from the Chicago health and aging project. *Journal of Aging and Health, 25*(1), 80–96. doi:10.1177/0898264312467373. *Evidence Level IV.*

Draper, B., Pfaff, J. J., Pirkis, J., Snowdon, J., Lautenschlager, N. T., Wilson, I., & Almeida, O. P. (2008). Long-term effects of childhood abuse on the quality of life and health of older people: Results from the depression and early prevention of suicide in general practice project. *Journal of the American Geriatrics Society, 56*(2), 262–271. *Evidence Level IV.*

Dyer, C. B., Kelly, P. A., Pavlik, V. N., Lee, J., Doody, R. S., Regev, T., . . . Smith, S. M. (2006). The making of a self-neglect severity scale. *Journal of Elder Abuse & Neglect, 18*(4), 13–23. *Evidence Level IV.*

Dyer, C. B., Pavlik, V. N., Murphy, K. P., & Hyman, D. J. (2000). The high prevalence of depression and dementia in elder abuse or neglect. *Journal of the American Geriatrics Society, 48*(2), 205–208. *Evidence Level IV.*

Frost, M. H., & Willette, K. (1994). Risk for abuse/neglect: Documentation of assessment data and diagnoses. *Journal of Gerontological Nursing, 20*(8), 37–45. *Evidence Level V.*

Fulmer, T., & Greenberg, S. (n.d.). *Elder mistreatment and abuse.* Retrieved from http://consultgerirn.org/resources. *Evidence Level V.*

Fulmer, T., Guadagno, L., Bitondo Dyer, C., & Connolly, M. T. (2004). Progress in elder abuse screening and assessment instruments. *Journal of the American Geriatrics Society, 52*(2), 297–304. *Evidence Level V.*

Fulmer, T., Paveza, G., VandeWeerd, C., Fairchild, S., Guadagno, L., Bolton-Blatt, M., & Norman, R. (2005). Dyadic vulnerability and risk profiling in elder neglect. *The Gerontologist, 45*(4), 525–534. *Evidence Level IV.*

Gelles, R. J. (1983). An exchange/social control theory. In D. Finkelhor, R. Gelles, M. Straus, & G. Hotaling (Eds.), *The dark side of families: Current family violence research.* (pp. 300–308). Newbury Park, CA: Sage. *Evidence Level V.*

Gelles, R. J., & Strauss, M. A. (1 979). Determinants of violence in the family: Toward a theoretical integration. In W. R. Burr, R. Hill, F. I. Nye, & I. L. Reiss (Eds.), *Contemporary theories about the family* (pp. 549–581). New York, NY: Free Press. *Evidence Level V.*

Giurani, F., & Hasan, M. (2000). Abuse in elderly people: The granny battering revisited. *Archives of Gerontology and Geriatrics, 31*(3), 215–220. *Evidence Level V.*

Gorbien, M. J., & Eisenstein, A. R. (2005). Elder abuse and neglect: An overview. *Clinics in Geriatric Medicine, 21*(2), 279–292. *Evidence Level V.*

Graf, C. (2007). *The Lawton instrumental activities of daily living scale.* Retrieved from http://consultgerirn.org/resources. *Evidence Level V.*

Greenberg, S. (2012). *The geriatric depression scale.* Retrieved from http://consultgerirn.org/uploads/File/trythis/try_this_4.pdf. *Evidence Level V.*

He, W., & Muenchrath, M. N. (2011). *American community survey reports, ACS-17, 90+ in the United States: 2006–2008. Evidence Level V.*

Heath, H., & Phair, L. (2009). The concept of frailty and its significance in the consequences of care or neglect for older people: An analysis. *International Journal of Older People Nursing, 4*(2), 120–131. doi:10.1111/j.1748–3743.2009.00165.x. *Evidence Level V.*

Hebert, L. E., Weuve, J., Scherr, P. A., & Evans, D. L. (2013). Alzheimer disease in the United States (2010–2050) estimated using the 2010 census. *Neurology, 80,* 1778–1783. *Evidence Level IV.*

Horsford, S. R., Parra-Cardona, J. R., Schiamberg, L., & Post, L. A. (2011). Elder abuse and neglect in African American families: Informing practice based on ecological and cultural frameworks. *Journal of Elder Abuse & Neglect, 23*(1), 75–88. doi:10.1080/08946566.2011.534709. *Evidence Level V.*

Jackson, S. L., & Hafemeister, T. L. (2013). Enhancing the safety of elderly victims after the close of an APS investigation. *Journal of Interpersonal Violence, 28*(6), 1223–1239. doi:10.1177/0886260512468241. *Evidence Level IV.*

Jayawardena, K. M., & Liao, S. (2006). Elder abuse at end of life. *Journal of Palliative Medicine, 9*(1), 127–136. *Evidence Level V.*

Jogerst, G. J., Daly, J. M., Brinig, M. F., Dawson, J. D. Schmuch, G. A., & Ingram, J. G. (2003). Domestic elder abuse and the law. *American Journal of Public Health, 93*(12), 2131–2136. *Evidence Level IV.*

Johannesen, M., & LoGiudice, D. (2013). Elder abuse: A systematic review of risk factors in community-dwelling elders. *Age and Ageing, 42*(3), 292–298. doi:10.1093/ageing/afs195. *Evidence Level I.*

Jones, J., Dougherty, J., Schelble, D., & Cunningham, W. (1988). Emergency department protocol for the diagnosis and evaluation of geriatric abuse. *Annals of Emergency Medicine, 17*(10), 1006–1015. *Evidence Level VI.*

Jones, J. S., Walker, G., & Krohmer, J. R. (1995). To report or not to report: Emergency services response to elder abuse. *Prehospital and Disaster Medicine, 10*(2), 96–100. *Evidence Level IV.*

Kelly, P. A., Dyer, C. B., Pavlik, V., Doody, R., & Jogerst, G. (2008). Exploring self-neglect in older adults: Preliminary findings of the self-neglect severity scale and next steps. *Journal of the American Geriatrics Society, 56*(Suppl. 2), S253–S260. *Evidence Level IV.*

Killick, C., & Taylor, B. J. (2009). Professional decision making on elder abuse: Systematic narrative review. *Journal of Elder Abuse & Neglect, 21*(3), 211–238. *Evidence Level I.*

Krienert, J. L., Walsh, J. A., & Turner, M. (2009). Elderly in America: A descriptive study of elder abuse examining national incident-based reporting system (NIBRS) data, 2000–2005. *Journal of Elder Abuse & Neglect, 21*(4), 325–345. *Evidence Level IV.*

Lachs, M. S., Becker, M., Siegal, A. P., Miller, R. L., & Tinetti, M. E. (1992). Delusions and behavioral disturbances in cognitively impaired elderly persons. *Journal of the American Geriatrics Society, 40*(8), 768–773. *Evidence Level IV.*

Lachs, M. S., & Pillemer, K. (1995). Abuse and neglect of elderly persons. *New England Journal of Medicine, 332*(7), 437–443. *Evidence Level V.*

Lachs, M. S., Williams, C. S., O'Brien, S., Pillemer, K. A., & Charlson, M. E. (1998). The mortality of elder mistreatment. *Journal of the American Medical Association, 280*(5), 428–432. *Evidence Level IV.*

Lai, D. W. L. (2011). Abuse and neglect experienced by aging Chinese in Canada. *Journal of Elder Abuse & Neglect, 23*(4), 326–347. doi:10.1080/08946566.2011.584047. *Evidence Level IV.*

Laumann, E. O., Leitsch, S. A., & Waite, L. J. (2008). Elder mistreatment in the United States: Prevalence estimates from a nationally representative study. *Journals of Gerontology. Series B, Psychological Sciences and Social Sciences, 63,* S248–S254. *Evidence Level IV.*

Lee, Y.-S., Kaplan, C. P., & Perez-Stable, E. J. (2014). Elder mistreatment among Chinese and Korean immigrants: The role of sociocultural contexts on perceptions and help-seeking behaviors. *Journal of Elder Abuse & Neglect, 26*(3), 244–269. doi:10.1080/08946566.2013.820656. *Evidence Level IV.*

Lowenstein, A. (2009). Elder abuse and neglect—"Old phenomenon": New directions for research, legislation, and service developments. *Journal of Elder Abuse & Neglect, 21*(3), 278–287. *Evidence Level V.*

McDonald, L., & Thomas, C. (2013). Elder abuse through a life course lens. *International Psychogeriatrics, 25*(8), 1235–1243. doi:10.1017/S104161021300015X. *Evidence Level IV.*

Mercurio, A. E., & Nyborn, J. (2006). Cultural definitions of elder maltreatment in Portugal. *Journal of Elder Abuse & Neglect, 18*(2–3), 51–65. *Evidence Level IV.*

Mosqueda, L., Brandl, B., Otto, J., Stiegel, L., Thomas, R., & Heisler, C. (2008). Consortium for research in elder self-neglect of Texas research: Advancing the field for practitioners. *Journal of the American Geriatrics Society, 56*(Suppl. 2), S276–S280. *Evidence Level VI.*

Mouton, C. P., Rodabough, R. J., Rovi, S. L., Hunt, J. L., Talamantes, M. A., Brzyski, R. G., & Burge, S. K. (2004). Prevalence and 3-year incidence of abuse among postmenopausal women. *American Journal of Public Health, 94,* 605–612. *Evidence Level IV.*

Naik, A. D., Teal, C. R., Pavlik, V. N., Dyer, C. B., & McCullough, L. B. (2008). Conceptual challenges and practical approaches to screening capacity for self-care and protection in vulnerable older adults. *Journal of the American Geriatrics Society, 56*(Suppl. 2), S266–S270. *Evidence Level V.*

National Center on Elder Abuse (NCEA). (1998). *The national elder abuse incidence study: Final report.* Retrieved from http://aoa.gov/AoARoot/AoA_Programs/Elder_Rights/Elder_Abuse/docs/ABuseReport_Full.pdf. *Evidence Level IV.*

National Center on Elder Abuse (NCEA). (2008). *Information about laws related to elder abuse.* Retrieved from http://www.ncea.aoa.gov/NCEAroot/Main_Site/Library/Laws/InfoAboutLaws_08_08.aspx. *Evidence Level V.*

National Committee for the Prevention of Elder Abuse, Virginia Tech, MetLife Mature Market Institute (2011). *The MetLife study of elder financial abuse: Crimes of occasion, desperation and predation against America's elders.* Westport, CT: Author. *Evidence Level IV.*

National Research Council (NRC). (2003). Elder mistreatment: Abuse, neglect, and exploitation in an aging America. Panel to Review Risk and Prevalence of Elder Abuse and Neglect. In R. J. Bonnie & R. B. Wallace (Eds.), *Committee on National Statistics and Committee on Law and Justice, Division of Behavioral and Social Sciences and Education.* Washington, DC: National Academies Press. *Evidence Level V.*

Naughton, C., Drennan, J., & Lafferty, A. (2014). Older people's perceptions of the term elder abuse and characteristics associated with a lower level of awareness. *Journal of Elder Abuse & Neglect, 26*(3), 300–318. doi:10.1080/08946566.2013.867242. *Evidence Level IV.*

Neale, A., Hwalek, M., Scott, R., Sengstock, M., & Stahl, C. (1991). Validation of the Hwalek-Sengstock elder abuse screening test. *Journal of Applied Gerontology, 10*, 406–418. *Evidence Level IV.*

Oh, J., Kim, H. S., Martins, D., & Kim, H. (2006). A study of elder abuse in Korea. *International Journal of Nursing Studies, 43*(2), 203–214. *Evidence Level IV.*

Onega, L. L. (2013). *The modified caregiver strain index.* Retrieved from http://consultgerirn.org/uploads/File/trythis/try_this_14.pdf. *Evidence Level V.*

Paveza, G., Vandeweerd, C., & Laumann, E. (2008). Elder self-neglect: A discussion of a social typology. *Journal of the American Geriatrics Society, 56*(Suppl. 2), S271–S275. *Evidence Level V.*

Peisah, C., Finkel, S., Shulman, K., Melding, P., Luxenberg, J., Heinik, J., . . . Bennett, H. (2009). The wills of older people: Risk factors for undue influence. *International Psychogeriatrics, 21*(1), 7–15. *Evidence Level V.*

Perel-Levin, S. (2008). *Discussing screening for elder abuse at the primary health care level.* Retrieved from http://www.who.int/ageing/publications/Discussing_Elder_Abuseweb.pdf. *Evidence Level V.*

Phillips, L. R. (2008). Abuse of aging caregivers: Test of a nursing intervention. *Advances in Nursing Science, 31*(2), 164–181. *Evidence Level III.*

Phillips, L. R., & Rempusheski, V. F. (1985). A decision-making model for diagnosing and intervening in elder abuse and neglect. *Nursing Research, 34*(3), 134–139. *Evidence Level IV.*

Ploeg, J., Fear, J., Hutchison, B., MacMillan, H., & Bolan, G. (2009). A systematic review of interventions for elder abuse. *Journal of Elder Abuse & Neglect, 21*(3), 187–210. *Evidence Level I.*

Rizzo, V. M., Burnes, D., & Chalfy, A. (2015). A systematic evaluation of a multidisciplinary social work–lawyer elder mistreatment intervention model. *Journal of Elder Abuse & Neglect, 27*(1), 1–18. doi:10.1080/08946566.2013.792104. *Evidence Level IV.*

Sandmoe, A., & Kirkevold, M. (2011). Nurses' clinical assessments of older clients who are suspected victims of abuse: An exploratory study in community care in Norway. *Journal of Clinical Nursing, 20*(1–2), 94–102. doi:10.1111/j.1365-2702.2010.03483.x. *Evidence Level IV.*

Schofield, M. J., Powers, J. R., & Loxton, D. (2013). Mortality and disability outcomes of self-reported elder abuse: A 12-year prospective investigation. *Journal of the American Geriatrics Society, 61*(5), 679–685. doi:10.1111/jgs.12212. *Evidence Level IV.*

Shelkey, M., & Wallace, M. (2012). *Katz index of independence in activities of daily living.* Retrieved from http://consultgerirn.org/uploads/File/trythis/try_this_2.pdf. *Evidence Level V.*

Stathopoulou, G. (2004). Greece. In K. Malley-Morrison (Ed.), *International perspectives on family violence and abuse: A cognitive ecological approach* (pp. 131–149). Mahwah, NJ: Lawrence Erlbaum. *Evidence Level V.*

Strasser, S. M., Smith, M., Weaver, S., Zheng, S., & Cao, Y. (2013). Screening for Elder Mistreatment among older adults seeking legal assistance services. *Western Journal of Emergency Medicine, 14*(4), 309–315. doi:10.5811/westjem.2013.2.15640. *Evidence Level IV.*

Strauss, M. A. (1971). Some social antecedents of physical punishment: A linkage theory interpretation. *Journal of Marriage and the Family, 33*, 658–663. *Evidence Level IV.*

Tareque, M. I., Ahmed, M. M., Tiedt, A. D., & Hoque, N. (2014). Can an active aging index (AAI) provide insight into reducing elder abuse? A case study in Rajshahi district, Bangladesh. *Archives of Gerontology and Geriatrics, 58*(3), 399–407. doi:10.1016/j.archger.2013.11.003. *Evidence Level IV.*

Thomson, A. M., Beavan, J. R., Lisk, R., McCracken, L. C., & Myint, P. K. (2010). Training in elder abuse: The experience of higher specialist trainees in geriatric medicine in the UK. *Archives of Gerontology and Geriatrics, 51*(3), 257–259. doi:10.1016/j.archger.2009.11.012. *Evidence Level IV.*

Turner, A., Hochschild, A., Burnett, J., Zulfiqar, A., & Dyer, C. B. (2012). High prevalence of medication non-adherence in a sample of community-dwelling older adults with adult protective services-validated self-neglect. *Drugs & Aging, 29*(9), 741–749. doi:10.1007/s40266-012-0007-2. *Evidence Level IV.*

United Nations. (2007). *World population prospects: The 2006 revision.* Retrieved from http://www.un.org/esa/population/publications/wpp2006/English.pdf. *Evidence Level V.*

U.S. Department of Justice. (2014). *The elder justice roadmap: A stakeholder initiative to respond to an emerging health, justice, financial and social crisis.* Retrieved from http://ncea.aoa.gov/Library/Gov_Report/docs/EJRP_Roadmap.pdf. *Evidence Level V.*

Vierthaler, K. (2008). Best practices for working with rape crisis centers to address elder sexual abuse. *Journal of Elder Abuse & Neglect, 20*(4), 306–322. *Evidence Level VI.*

Wagenaar, D. B., Rosenbaum, R., Page, C., & Herman, S. (2010). Primary care physicians and elder abuse: Current attitudes and practices. *Journal of the American Osteopathic Association, 110*(12), 703–711. Retrieved from http://www.ncbi.nlm.nih.gov/pubmed/21178151. *Evidence Level IV.*

Walker, A. (1981). Towards a political economy of old age. *Ageing and Society, 1*(1), 73. doi:10.1017/S0144686X81000056. *Evidence Level VI.*

Wiglesworth, A., Austin, R., Corona, M., Schneider, D., Liao, S., Gibbs, L., & Mosqueda, L. (2009). Bruising as a marker of physical elder abuse. *Journal of the American Geriatrics Society, 57*(7), 1191–1196. *Evidence Level IV.*

Wiglesworth, A., Mosqueda, L., Mulnard, R., Liao, S., Gibbs, L., & Fitzgerald, W. (2010). Screening for abuse and neglect of people with dementia. *Journal of the American Geriatrics Society, 58*(3), 493–500. *Evidence Level IV.*

Yan, E., & Tang, C. S. (2003). Proclivity to elder abuse: A community study on Hong Kong Chinese. *Journal of Interpersonal Violence, 18*(9), 999–1017. *Evidence Level IV.*

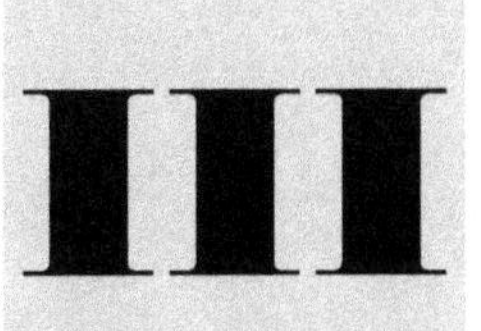

Clinical Interventions

14

Preventing Functional Decline in the Acute Care Setting

Marie Boltz, Barbara Resnick, and Elizabeth Galik

EDUCATIONAL OBJECTIVES

On completion of this chapter, the reader should be able to:

1. Discuss the functional trajectory of the hospitalized older adult
2. Identify risk factors for functional decline
3. Describe the influence of the care environment on physical function
4. Discuss interventions to optimize physical function of hospitalized older adults

OVERVIEW

As described in Chapter 7, "Assessment of Physical Function," functional decline is a common complication in hospitalized older adults, even in those with good baseline function (Gill, Allore, Gahbauer, & Murphy, 2010). Loss of physical function is associated with poor long-term outcomes, including increased likelihood of being discharged from a hospital to a nursing home setting (Fortinsky, Covinsky, Palmer, & Landefeld, 1999), increased morbidity and mortality (Rozzini et al., 2005), increased rehabilitation costs, and decreased long-term functional recovery (Boyd, Xue, Guralik, & Fried, 2005; Boyd et al., 2008; Volpato et al., 2007). The immobility associated with functional decline results in infections, pressure ulcers, falls, and nonelective rehospitalizations (Gill, Allore, & Guo, 2004).

The promotion of function is a basic gerontological tenet, and functional recovery is perceived by older adults as a quality outcome of hospitalization (Boltz, Capezuti, Shabbat, & Hall, 2010). Moreover, older adults expect that an acute care stay will not result in functional decline but instead promote the resumption of normal roles and activities post-hospitalization. Although the acute care setting, with its focus on correcting the admitting medical problem, typically prioritizes nursing tasks, such as medication administration, coordination of care, and documentation over the promotion of function as a clinical outcome, there is growing awareness of the need to attend to the functional status of the hospitalized older adult (Nolan & Thomas, 2008; Resnick, Galik, Wells, Boltz, & Holtzman, 2015). This chapter addresses the trajectory of change in physical function during the acute care stay, the factors associated with functional decline, and function-promoting interventions that can potentially modify these factors. Finally, a clinical practice protocol to guide a unit-level approach to function-focused care (FFC; Protocol 14.1: Function-Focused Care Interventions) is provided.

For a description of evidence levels cited in this chapter, see Chapter 1, "Developing and Evaluating Clinical Practice Guidelines: A Systematic Approach."

PHYSICAL FUNCTION AS A CLINICAL MEASURE

Functional decline may result from the acute illness and can begin from preadmission and continue after discharge. In a seminal study, Covinsky et al. (2003) evaluated the changes in performing of activities of daily living (ADL) prior to and after hospitalizations of older adults with medical illness. More than one third declined in ADL function between baseline (2 weeks before admission) and discharge. This included the 23% of patients who declined between baseline and admission, and failed to recover to baseline function between admission and discharge, and the 12% of patients who did not decline between baseline and admission but declined between hospital admission and discharge. Older adults aged 85 years and older comprised the age cohort demonstrating the most functional loss, with rates exceeding 50%.

In their examination of the functional trajectory of hospitalized older adults, Wakefield and Holman (2007) also assessed function at baseline, as well as on admission and day 4. The largest change in functional status was a decline in ADL from baseline to the time of admission; ADL did not return to baseline during the first 4 days in the hospital. The older adults whose ADL scores declined during hospitalization (regardless of the baseline status) were more likely than others to die within 3 months of discharge.

The results of these studies demonstrate that ADL status is unstable in a large percentage of older adults during an acute illness (Covinsky, Pierluissi, & Johnston, 2011). Consequently, Covinsky et al. suggest that an older adult's functional trajectory is a critical "vital sign," an important prognostic marker, and indicator to guide care delivery and transitional care. Baseline function may serve as a useful benchmark when developing discharge goals. Older adults who have sustained loss of ADL function prior to admission would ideally have rehabilitation as a goal of their hospital care. For those patients who have acquired ADL disability from admission to discharge, aggressive postacute rehabilitation plans could be mobilized with the goal of promoting return to baseline function.

PATIENT RISK FACTORS FOR FUNCTIONAL DECLINE

Intrinsic vulnerabilities to functional decline include prehospitalization functional status (McCusker Kakuma, & Abrahamowicz, 2002; Zisberg et al., 2011), the presence of two or more comorbidities, and having had a hospitalization or emergency room visit in the previous 12 months (Covinsky et al., 2011; McCusker et al., 2002). Symptoms of depression both before and during hospitalization have also been associated with dependence in basic ADL at discharge, and 30 and 90 days after discharge (Covinsky, Fortinsky, Palmer, Kresevic, & Landefeld, 1997). Cognitive impairment, including delirium, increases the risk of functional decline in the older adults during and after hospitalization (Boltz, Resnick, Capezuti, Shuluk, & Secic, 2012; Inouye, Schlesinger, & Lydon, 1999; McCusker et al., 2002).

The aggregate number of geriatric conditions present at hospital admission determines a patient's individual risk of functional deterioration (Buurman, van Munster, Korevaar, de Haan, & de Rooij, 2011). Polypharmacy, fall risk, use of an indwelling urinary catheter, urinary incontinence, vision impairment, and hearing loss (Buurman et al., 2012) are associated with a high risk of functional decline that persists 12 months after hospitalization. The patient's fear of falling (Boltz, Resnick, Capezuti, & Shuluk, 2014), self-efficacy, outcome expectations (McAuley et al., 2006), and views on physical activity during hospitalization (Boltz, Capezuti, & Shabbat, 2011; Brown et al., 2007) influence the level of engagement in physical activity and mobility in older adults in general and thus may influence acute care functional outcomes.

THE CARE ENVIRONMENT AND FUNCTION

A social ecological perspective assumes that the physical, social, and organizational environments contribute to patient outcomes, including functional measures (Galik, 2010). The hospital environment, with its emphasis on biomedical interventions for acute medical and surgical problems, is challenged to "fit" the complex physical, social, and psychological circumstances, which predisposes the hospitalized older adult to functional decline. Parke and Chappell (2010) recommend that the older adult–hospital environment fit be viewed through four dimensions: care processes, social climate, policy and procedure, and physical design.

Hospital Care Processes

Hospitalization is associated with significantly greater loss of total, lean, and fat mass as well as strength in older persons. These effects appear particularly important in persons hospitalized for 8 days or more per year (Alley et al., 2010). Hospitalization itself may also pose risks for functional decline because of the deleterious effects of bed rest and restricted activity (Gill, Allore, Holford, & Guo, 2004). Bed rest results in loss of muscle strength and lean muscle mass (Kortebein et al., 2007), decreased aerobic capacity (Kortebein, Symons, & Ferrando, 2008), diminished pulmonary ventilation, altered sensory awareness, reduced appetite and thirst, and decreased plasma volume (Creditor, 1993; Harper, & Lyles, 1988; Hoenig & Rubenstein, 1999). Brown, Redden, Flood, and Allman (2009) describe bed rest and low mobility as an "underrecognized epidemic." In their study of hospitalized older veterans, they used accelerometers to measure activity level. Despite the fact that the majority was able to walk independently (78%), 83% of the measured hospital stay was spent lying in bed.

Another study (Brown, Friedkin, & Inouye, 2004) that evaluated the outcomes associated with mobility found that bed rest in older adults was ordered at some point during hospitalization in 33% of the patients. Almost 60% of the observations indicated no documented medical reason for the bed rest. Physician's orders for bed rest were present on the date of bed rest for only 92 (52%) of the 176 observations. Low mobility (defined as having an average mobility level of bed rest or bed to chair for the entire hospitalization) was compared to high mobility (ambulation two or more times with partial or no assistance, on average). The low mobility group had a statistically significant higher rate of ADL decline, new institutionalization, and death. Similarly, Zisberg et al. (2011) found that low versus high in-hospital mobility was associated with worse functional status at discharge and at 1-month follow-up, even in older adults who were functionally stable prior to admission.

Doherty-King, Yoon, Pecanac, Brown, and Mahoney (2014) shadowed RNs for two to three 8-hour periods using hand-held computer tablets to collect data on frequency and duration of mobility events (standing, transferring, walking to and from the patient bathroom, walking in the patient room, and walking in the hallway) that occurred in the nurse's presence. They found that nurses infrequently initiated mobility events for hospitalized older patients and most often engaged patients in low-level activity (standing and transferring). Other research indicated that illness severity and reason for admission did not explain low levels of mobility, measured by a step-activity monitor (Fisher et al., 2011).

Care processes associated with immobility include physical restraints and "tethering devices," such as catheters, intravenous lines, and medication, which contribute to delirium and/or cause sedation (Boltz, Resnick, Capezuti, Shabbat, & Secic, 2011; Brown, Roth, Peel, & Allman, 2006). Additionally, there is a tendency for staff to perform ADL for patients who could participate or do it for themselves, placing older adults at risk of loss of self-care ability (Boltz, Resnick, Capezuti, Shabbat, & Secic, 2011). This "doing for" as opposed to promoting functional independence is often associated with a lack of understanding of the patient's underlying capability (Resnick, Galik, Boltz, & Pretzer-Aboff, 2011). Interprofessional rounds support a functional approach, with the goal of preventing functional decline and discharging the older adult to the least restrictive setting. Key elements to be addressed include functional assessment (baseline, admission, current ADL status, and physical capability), alternatives to the use of potentially restrictive devices and agents, and a plan for progressive mobility and engagement in ADL (Boltz, Resnick, Chippendale, & Galvin, 2014). Additionally, protocols that support delirium prevention and abatement, and optimize nutrition, while minimizing adverse effects of selected procedures (e.g., urinary catheterization) and medications (e.g., sedative-hypnotic agents) contribute to positive functional outcomes (Kleinpell, 2007).

Social Climate

Leadership commitment to rehabilitative values is essential to support a social climate conducive to the promotion of function (Boltz, Capezuti, & Shabbat, 2011; King & Bowers, 2013). Older adults have identified that respectful, encouraging communication and engagement in decision making as important to facilitating independence (Boltz et al., 2010; Jacelon, 2004). Staff education that addresses the physiology, manifestations and prevention of hospital-acquired deconditioning, assessment of physical capability, rehabilitative techniques, use of adaptive equipment, interprofessional collaboration, and communication that motivates are required to support a function-promoting philosophy (Boltz, Capezuti, & Shabbat, 2011; Gillis, MacDonald, & MacIsaac, 2008; Resnick, Galik, Boltz, & Pretzer-Aboff, 2011). Nursing staff have also described the need for well-defined roles, including areas of accountability for follow-through for function-promoting activities (Boltz, Capezuti, & Shabbat; King & Bowers, 2011). Clear communication of patient needs among staff, and dissemination of data (e.g., compliance with treatment plans and functional outcomes) also support these activities (Resnick et al., 2015).

Policy and Procedure

To foster function-promoting care, policies are needed that clearly define staff roles in assessing physical function and cognition and that implement identified interventions. Other supporting policies address identification and storage of sensory devices (e.g., glasses, hearing aids/amplifiers) and mobility and other assistive devices (Boltz, Capezuti, & Shabbat, 2011; Boltz, Capezuti, Shabbat, & Secic, 2011). Indicative of the low priority placed on mobility promotion is the common process of restricting the patients' ability to walk to tests and procedures within the hospital.

Environment

Acute care environments directly impact patient function and physical activity. The bed is often the only accessible furniture in the room and the height of toilets, beds, and available chairs do not always fall within the range in which transfers and function are optimized (Capezuti et al., 2008). Accessible functional seating and safe walking areas with relevant destination areas promote functional mobility. Adequate lighting, nonglare flooring, door levers, and handrails (including in the patient room) are basic requirements to promote safe mobility (Betrabet Gulwadi & Calkins, 2008; Ulrich et al., 2008). Environmental enhancements to promote orientation include large-print calendars and clocks (Kleinpell, 2007) and control of ambient noise levels, especially in critical care units (Gabo, 2003).

INTERVENTIONS TO PROMOTE PHYSICAL FUNCTION

Support for Cognition

Cognition and physical function are closely linked in older adults. The ability to engage in ADL and physical activity requires varying types and degrees of cognitive capability, including memory, executive function, and visual-spatial ability. Therefore, an appraisal of the older adult's cognition (baseline, admission, and ongoing) is an essential activity associated with promoting physical function (see Chapter 6, "Assessing Cognitive Function") in order to develop, implement, and evaluate a plan to promote maximum physical functioning (Coelho, Santos-Galduroz, Gobbi, & Stella, 2009; Yu, Kolanowski, Strumpf, & Eslinger, 2006).

Interventions to prevent, detect, and manage delirium are associated with improved cognition and thus are integral components of a plan to prevent functional decline (Foreman, Wakefield, Culp, & Milisen, 2004). Liberal visiting hours and familiar items brought in from home (e.g., photos, blankets) provide meaningful sensory input, and along with control of excessive noise and attention to sleep hygiene enhance function-promoting interventions (Landefeld, Palmer, & Kresevic, Fortinsky, & Kowal, 1995). Diversional activities, such as TV, movies, and word games, are associated with "keeping the mind active" and engagement in self-care and physical activity (Boltz et al., 2010). For patients with cognitive challenges, including dementia, activity kits that include tactile, auditory, and visual items enhance cognitive integration, perceptual processing, and neuromuscular strength as well as provide solace and an opportunity for emotional expression and relief from boredom. Activity kits can include a wide range of items such as audiotapes and nontoxic art supplies. In addition, items, such as pieces of textured fabric, clothes to fold, tools, and key-and-lock boards are included for the person with more advanced dementia (Conedera & Mitchell, n.d; Glantz & Richman, 2007). For more information, see Chapter 17, "Delirium: Prevention, Early Recognition, and Treatment."

Older adults with cognitive impairment can benefit from function-promoting interventions with demonstrated improvements in physical and cognitive function (Boltz, Chippendale, Resnick, & Galvin, 2015b). An understanding of the person's values, past experiences, and relationships supports meaningful communication to motivate them, along with the use of humor and verbal cues (Galik, Resnick, & Pretzer-Aboff, 2009). In addition, teamwork with other nursing staff, rehabilitative staff, medical providers, and families was considered a key component in facilitating self-care and physical activity (Boltz, Resnick, Chippendale, & Galvin, 2014; Boltz, Chippendale, Resnick, & Galvin, 2015a).

In addition, adapted communication techniques are necessary to accommodate receptive difficulties associated with cognitive impairment, including dementia. The ability to participate in ADL is often more preserved than clinicians believe, as activities, such as washing the face, brushing one's teeth, and walking, rely on psychomotor memory, which is preserved even in those with moderate to severe cognitive impairment. Communicating with short simple verbal requests, visual cues, and modeling the activity can be helpful in promoting independence in ADL (e.g., assist the person to the sink, set them up to brush their teeth, hand them a toothbrush, and model the behavior; Resnick, Galik, Boltz, & Pretzer-Aboff, 2011).

Physical Therapy and Exercise

Interventions, such as physical therapy and individualized, targeted exercise programs as soon as possible post-admission, have all been tested as ways in which physical activity could be increased and deconditioning and functional decline in hospitalized older adults could be prevented. A single-blinded randomized controlled trial was conducted in a tertiary metropolitan hospital involving 180 acute general medical patients aged 65 years or older (Jones et al., 2006). In addition to usual physiotherapy care, the intervention group performed an exercise program for 30 minutes, twice daily, with supervision and assistance provided by an allied health assistant (AHA). In older adults with low admission ADL scores (modified Barthel Index score less than or equal to 48), there was improvement in function among individuals exposed to the exercise interventions versus those who were not.

Similarly, an individually tailored exercise program to maintain functional mobility, prescribed and progressed by a physical therapist, and supervised by an AHA, provided in addition to usual physiotherapy care, was associated with reduced likelihood of referral for nursing home admissions (Nolan & Thomas, 2008). Despite the known benefit of staying engaged in function and physical activity when hospitalized, a 2007 Cochrane review (de Morton, Keating, & Jeffs, 2007) concluded that, in general, patient participation in these programs has been poor. Challenges to feasibility and implementation of these interventions include competing care demands (e.g., test schedules), illness severity, short hospital stays, a general unwillingness of patients to consent to or actively participate in exercise interventions, and a persistent belief among patients that bed rest will assure recovery (Brown, Peel, Bamman, & Allman, 2006; de Morton et al., 2007; de Morton, Keating, Berlowitz, Jackson, & Lim, 2007).

Functional Mobility Programs

One of the most common forms of physical activity encouraged in acute care settings are functional mobility programs. Mobility is conceptualized as a continuum progressing from bedbound to independent walking (Callen, Mahoney, Wells, Enloe, & Hughes, 2004). The benefits of interventions aimed at promoting functional mobility have recently received growing attention. A literature review conducted by Kalisch, Soohee, and Dabney (2013) identified benefits of mobility programs in four areas: (a) physical outcomes (less delirium, pain, urinary discomfort, difficulty voiding, urinary tract infection, deep vein thrombosis, fatigue, and pneumonia, as well as increased walking and ADL performance, and ventilator-free days), (b) psychological outcomes (less depression, anxiety, and symptom distress, as well as increased comfort and satisfaction), (c) social outcomes (improved quality of life and independence), and (d) organizational outcomes (decreased length of stay, mortality, and cost).

Tucker, Molsberger, and Clark (2004) demonstrated the feasibility of a "Walking for Wellness" program that consisted of a patient education program, a screening process to identify patients who would benefit from physical therapy, and daily walking assistance from cross-trained transportation staff. Walking opportunities included "walking trails" marked inside the hospital, with markers placed every 10 feet at the baseboard of the hallways providing a measure of walking distance, as well as a visual incentive for patients walking in the halls. Unless otherwise indicated by the medical provider, the goal for participants was to walk in the hallways two to three times a day with trained escorts, nursing staff, family, or friends. Weitzel and Robinson (2004) developed an educational program for nursing assistants on a medical unit that emphasized promoting the functional status of hospitalized elders. Content included therapeutic communication, promotion of functional mobility, skin care, and eating/feeding problems. Discharge destination (home or nursing home) and length of stay were compared for patients pre- and postimplementation. There was a significant reduction in length of stay (2.4 days) and increase in the percentage of patients discharged to the home setting.

The positive association between mobility and shorter lengths of stay was also supported in an acute care for elderly (ACE) unit, where ambulation was measured by a step monitor (Fisher et al., 2011). Patients on the ACE unit who had shorter stays tended to ambulate more on the first complete day of hospitalization and had a markedly greater increase in mobility on the second day than patients with longer lengths of stay.

To address motivational issues, Mudge, Giebel, and Cutler (2008) evaluated a functional mobility program enhanced with cognitive interventions. This research team used an individualized, graduated exercise and mobility program with an activity diary, progressive encouragement of functional independence by nursing staff and other members of the multidisciplinary team, and cognitive stimulation sessions in older adults aged 70 years and older on a medical unit. The intervention group had greater improvement in functional status than the control group, with a median modified Barthel Index improvement of 8.5 versus 3.5 points ($p = .03$). In the intervention group, there was a reduction in delirium (19.4% vs. 35.5%, $p = .04$) and a trend toward reduced falls (4.8% vs. 11.3%, $p = .19$; Mudge et al., 2008).

In patients recovering from hip surgery, functional mobility programs are enhanced with measures to prevent postoperative complications. Siu, Penrod, et al. (2006) and Siu, Boockvar, et al. (2006) found that positive processes related to mobilization (including time from admission to surgery, mobilization to and beyond the chair, use of anticoagulants and prophylactic antibiotics, pain control, physical therapy, catheter and restraint use, and active clinical issues) were associated with improved locomotion and self-care at 2 months post-discharge. Patients who experienced no hospital complications and no readmissions retained benefits in locomotion at 6 months. Olson and Karlsson (2007) demonstrated that interventions focused on skin care, pain control, and progressive ambulation yielded improved functional discharge outcomes. See Chapter 34, "Care of the Older Adult With Fragility Hip Fracture."

Critical Care Initiatives to Prevent Functional Decline

The geriatric imperative to support physical function has also been recognized in critical care, and studies are emerging that examine mobility promotion in the critically ill patient, including older adults. A study conducted in a respiratory intensive care unit (RICU) examined the feasibility of early mobility as well as its safety in six activity-related adverse events: fall to knees, tube removal, systolic blood pressure greater than 200 mmHg, systolic blood pressure less than 90 mmHg, oxygen desaturation less than 80%, and extubation. There were less than 1% activity-related adverse events; the majority of survivors (69%) were able to ambulate farther than 100 feet at RICU discharges (Bailey et al., 2007).

Nurse-led mobility protocols have increased the rate of ambulation of patients in critical care units. A multidisciplinary team developed and implemented a mobility order set with an embedded algorithm to guide nursing assessment of mobility potential. Based on the assessments, the protocol empowers the nurse to consult physical therapists or occupational therapists when appropriate. Daily ambulation status reports were reviewed each morning to determine each patient's activity level (Drolet et al., 2013). Similarly, a mobility team (critical care nurse, nursing assistant, physical therapist) in a medical intensive care unit initiated a mobility protocol for patients with acute respiratory failure. The protocol consisted of progressive mobility interventions ranging from passive range of motion for unconscious patients, to active, assistive, and active range-of-motion exercises, to functional activities such as transfer to edge of bed; safe transfers to and from bed, chair, or commode; seated balance activities; pregait standing activities (forward and lateral weight shifting, marching in place); and ambulation. As compared to usual care (passive range-of-motion only), protocol patients were out of bed earlier (5 vs. 11 days, $p \leq .001$), had therapy initiated more frequently in the intensive care unit (91% vs. 13%, $p \leq .001$), and had similar low complication rates. For protocol patients, the intensive care unit length of stay was 5.5 versus 6.9 days for usual care ($p = .025$) and the length of hospital stay for protocol patients was 11.2 versus 14.5 days for usual care ($p = .006$). (The intensive care unit/length of hospital stay was adjusted for body mass index, acuity, and use of a vasopressor.) There were no adverse events during an intensive care unit mobility session and no cost difference between the protocol and usual care costs (Morris et al., 2008).

FFC: A Multimodal Intervention

FFC is a comprehensive, system-level approach that prioritizes the preservation and restoration of functional capability. It is predicated on the philosophy that physical function is as important a treatment goal as correcting the acute admitting problem, and recognizes the multifactorial nature of functional decline (Resnick, Galik, & Boltz, 2013). FFC utilizes a philosophy of care in which nurses acknowledge older adults' physical and cognitive capabilities with regard to function and integrate functional and physical activities into all care interactions. The components of FFC are:

- Assessment of environment and policy/procedures for function and physical activity
- Education of nursing staff, other members of the interprofessional team (e.g., social work, physical therapy) on rehabilitative approaches
- Education of patients and families regarding FFC
- Establishing FFC goals, including discharge goals based on capability assessments, communication with other members of the team (e.g., medicine, physical therapy) and input from patients
- Interprofessional team addresses risk factors that impact goal achievement (e.g., cognitive status, anemia, nutritional status, pain, fear of falling, fatigue, medications, and drug side effects such as somnolence) to optimize patient participation in functional and physical activity
- Mentoring and motivation provided by a nurse change agent (e.g., geriatric resource nurse) using theoretically based interventions that monitoring and motivate the nursing staff to provide FFC and thereby help the nurses to motivate patients to engage in functional and physical activities

Resnick et al. demonstrated that nurses were willing to be engaged in an FFC educational intervention on both medical–surgical (Resnick, Galik, Enders, Sobol, Ham-mersla, Dustin, . . . Trotman, 2011) and trauma units (Resnick et al., 2015) and showed improvements in knowledge and outcome expectations associated with FFC. FFC interactions between patient and nurses have demonstrated a decrease in the overall loss of ADL function from baseline to discharge (Boltz et al., 2012).

Given that family caregivers play a significant role in influencing the physical activity of hospitalized older adults (Boltz, Resnick, Capezuti, Shabbat, & Secic, 2011), FFC has been expanded to actively engage the family caregiver in the planning, implementation, and evaluation of care aimed at promoting functional recovery. The goal of this educational empowerment model (family-centered FFC [Fam-FFC]) is to improve functional outcomes of the patient and prepare the family caregiver for discharge, without increasing caregiver strain or negatively affecting the relationship with the patient (mutuality) or the family affective response. Fam-FFC demonstrated feasibility in a pilot study of 97 patient and family caregiver (FCG) dyads. Patients exposed to Fam-FFC demonstrated improved ADL performance, walking performance, and delirium severity, and less 30-day hospital readmissions. FCGs who participated in Fam-FFC reported better preparedness for caregiving, less anxiety, and less depression from admission to 2 months post-discharge, with no significant increases in strain or decreased mutuality (Boltz, Resnick, Chippendale, et al., 2014). A second pilot study (N = 86) found that patients with dementia who were exposed to Fam-FFC demonstrated improvements in ADL performance and less delirium symptoms at 2 months post-discharge (Boltz et al., 2015b). FCGs who participated in Fam-FFC showed a significant increase in preparedness for caregiving and less anxiety but no significant differences in depression, strain, and mutuality.

CASE STUDY

TS is an 80-year-old man who was admitted from an assisted living (AL) facility to the emergency department (ED) after he was found on the floor. His workup is negative for fractures and head trauma. His admitting diagnoses include pneumonia, anemia, and dehydration. His past medical history, per his daughter's report, is remarkable for mild hypertension, treated with Hydrochlorothiazide (HCTZ) and Captopril, and dementia. On admission, TS was somnolent but able to respond to his name. He is receiving intravenous (IV) antibiotics and hydration. As an alternative to the use of a restraint, the IV site is "camouflaged" with dressing wrap and covered with his sweater so as to not cue him to remove it.

The admitting nurse learns from his daughter and the staff at the AL facility that TS's normal or baseline function is that he is independent in ambulation, continent, (though, at times, he has trouble in way-finding), and needs verbal cues ("prompting") to get dressed and bathe. After hydration, TS becomes more alert. He is able to respond to one-step commands and is moving all extremities, with good range of motion. The primary nurse keeps the daughter informed of his condition and the need to promote mobility and self-care. The interprofessional team makes rounds that afternoon, and with his daughter's and TS's involvement, develops the following plan:

- Monitor confusion assessment method (CAM) and mental status when he is able to respond.
- Daughter is to bring in familiar robe, shoes, and family photo; she also plans to complete social profile, "all about me," to be shared with hospital staff.
- Glasses were labeled with his name and placed on TS.
- No restraints; adjustable-height low bed, in low position, then adjusted to lower leg length to promote safe transfers
- Switch to oral antibiotics; cap IV when able to take sufficient fluids by mouth.
- Assist out of bed for meals, starting that evening.
- In the morning, attempt to ambulate to bathroom, not to be left unattended. Ambulate as tolerated in room and progress to hallway ambulation three times a day.
- Use pressure-reducing mattress.
- Assist, cue, and redirect as needed during meal; monitor for aspiration.
- Encourage self-care during bathing; cue as needed.
- Anemia workup.
- Plan to discharge back to AL at baseline level of function; estimated discharge in 48 to 72 hours.
- The staff at the AL facility will receive a full report on his condition and progress. A plan for a structured routine that includes planned walking, self-care, and involvement in his preferred activities will be developed.

Discussion

The case study demonstrates decision making that recognizes the potential of TS to return to his baseline physical function. The interprofessional team implements measures to correct his delirium and prevent avoidable complications (falls and pressure ulcers) that could negatively impact his function. The plan to promote physical activity and independence in ADL is adapted to his cognitive impairment. His daughter is engaged in his care and the nurse leverages this support to benefit TS.

SUMMARY

Hospitalization poses many challenges to the functional health of older adults. However, functional decline is not inevitable. Interventions formerly perceived to be relevant only for the rehabilitation setting are slowly being recognized as integral to the care and treatment of the older adult in the acute setting. FFC employs nursing care practices that acknowledge the older person's capabilities and potential, while positively modifying the care environment to prevent avoidable functional decline.

NURSING STANDARD OF PRACTICE

Protocol 14.1: Function-Focused Care Interventions

I. GOAL

To help nurses collaborate with the interdisciplinary team to implement interventions that maximize the older adult's functional abilities and performance. This protocol can be used in combination with Protocol 7.1.

II. OBJECTIVE

As stated in Chapter 3, "Age-Related Changes in Health,": To restore or maximize physical functioning, prevent or minimize decline in ADL function and plan for transitions of care.

III. BACKGROUND

A. Functional decline is a common complication in hospitalized older adults, even in those with good baseline function (Gill et al., 2010).
B. Loss of physical function is associated with poor long-term outcomes, including increased likelihood of being discharged to a nursing home setting (Fortinsky et al., 1999), increased mortality (Boyd et al., 2005; Rozzini et al., 2005), increased rehabilitation costs, and decreased functional recovery (Boyd et al., 2005, 2008; Volpato et al., 2007). The immobility associated with functional decline results in infections, pressure ulcers, falls, a persistent decline in function and physical activity, and nonelective rehospitalizations.
C. Functional decline may result from the acute illness and can begin pre-admission (Fortinsky et al., 1999) and continue after discharge. Baseline function serves as a useful benchmark when developing discharge goals (Wakefield & Holman, 2007).
D. Patient risk factors for functional decline include pre-hospitalization functional loss; the presence of two or more comorbidities; taking five or more prescription medications; having had a hospitalization or emergency room visit in the previous 12 months; depression; impaired cognition, including delirium; pain; nutritional problems; adverse medication effects; fear of falling; low self-efficacy, outcome expectations, and attitudes toward functional independence; and views on hospitalization (Boltz, Resnick, Capezuti, Shabbat, & Secic, 2014; Brown et al., 2007; Buurman et al., 2011, 2012; Inouye et al., 1999; McAuley et al., 2006; McCusker et al., 2002).
E. Bed rest results in loss of muscle strength and lean muscle mass, decreased aerobic capacity, diminished pulmonary ventilation, altered sensory awareness, reduced appetite and thirst, and decreased plasma volume (Creditor, 1999; Harper & Lyles, 1988; Hoenig & Rubenstein, 1999; Kortebein et al., 2007, 2008). Care processes, such as curtailing mobility, imposing restraints, and tethering devices which are associated with low mobility, lead to a higher rate of ADL decline, new institutionalization, and death (Boltz et al., 2010, 2011; Brown et al., 2004, 2009; Zisberg et al., 2011).
F. Interprofessional rounds support promotion of function by addressing functional assessment (baseline and current), evaluate potentially restrictive devices and agents, and yield a plan for progressive mobility (Boltz, Resnick, Chippendale, & Galvin, 2014).
G. Leadership commitment to rehabilitative values is essential to support a social climate conducive to the promotion of function (Boltz, Capezuti, & Shabbat, 2011; King & Bowers, 2013).
H. FFC educational intervention on medical–surgical units has shown improvements in knowledge and outcome expectations associated with function-promoting care (Resnick, Galik, Enders, et al., 2011; Resnick, Galik, Boltz, et al., 2011, 2015).

IV. FUNCTION-FOCUSED CARE INTERVENTIONS

A. Hospital care processes (Boltz, Resnick, Chippendale, & Galvin, 2014; Jacelon, 2004; Resnick, Galik, Boltz, Capezuti, & Shabbat, 2011; Resnick, Galik, Enders, et al., 2011)
   1. Evaluation of leadership commitment to rehabilitative values

(continued)

Protocol 14.1: Function-Focused Care Interventions *(continued)*

2. Interprofessional rounds that address functional assessment (baseline and current), evaluate potentially restrictive devices and agents, and yield a plan for progressive mobility
3. Well-defined roles, including areas of accountability for assessment and follow-through for function-promoting activities
4. Method of evaluating communication of patient needs among staff
5. Process of disseminating data (e.g., compliance with treatment plans and functional outcomes)

B. Policy and procedures to support function promotion (Boltz et al., 2010, 2011, 2015b; Kleinpell, 2007)
1. Protocols that minimize adverse effects of selected procedures (e.g., urinary catheterization) and medications (e.g., sedative-hypnotic agents) contribute to positive functional outcomes.
2. Supporting policies: identification and storage of sensory devices (e.g., glasses, hearing aids/amplifiers), mobility devices, and other assistive devices
3. Discharge policies that address the continuous plan for function promotion

C. Physical design (Betrabet Gulwadi & Calkins, 2008; Boltz et al., 2015b; Boltz, Resnick, et al., 2014a; Capezuti et al., 2008; Kleinpell, 2004; Ulrich et al., 2008)
1. Toilets, beds, and chairs at appropriate height to promote safe transfers and function
2. Functional and accessible functional furniture and safe walking areas with relevant/interesting destination areas with distance markers
3. Adequate lighting, nonglare flooring, door levers, and handrails (including in the patient room)
4. Large-print calendars and clocks to promote orientation
5. Control of ambient noise levels
6. Policy on storage of glasses and hearing aids, access to sensory aids, hearing amplifiers and magnifiers

D. Education of nursing staff, other members of the interdisciplinary team (for example, social work, physical therapy) regarding (Boltz et al., 2010; Boltz, Capezuti, & Shabbat, 2011; Gillis et al., 2008; Resnick, Galik, Enders, et al., 2011):
1. The physiology, manifestations, and prevention of hospital-acquired deconditioning
2. Assessment of physical capability
3. Rehabilitative techniques, use of adaptive equipment
4. Interprofessional collaboration
5. Engagement in decision making
6. Communication that motivates is associated with a function-promoting philosophy.

E. Education of patients and families regarding FFC, including the benefits of FFC, the safe use of equipment, and self-advocacy (Boltz et al., 2010; Boltz, Resnick, Chippendale, & Galvin, 2014; Boltz et al., 2015b; Resnick et al., 2015)

F. Clinical assessment and interventions (Boltz, Capezuti, & Shabbat, 2011, Boltz et al., 2015b; Boltz, Resnick, Chippendale, & Galvin, 2014; Nolan & Thomas, 2008; Resnick, Galik, Enders, et al., 2011; Wakefield & Holman, 2007)
1. Assessment of physical function and capability (baseline, at admission, and daily) and cognition (at a minimum daily)
2. Establishing functional goals based on assessments and communication with other members of the team and input from patients
3. Social assessment: history, roles, values, living situation, methods of coping
4. Addressing risk factors that impact goal achievement (e.g., cognitive status, anemia, nutritional status, pain, fear of falling, fatigue, medications, and drug side effects such as somnolence) by the interprofessional team optimizes patient participation in functional and physical activities
5. Developing discharge plans that include carryover of functional interventions, and addressing the unique preferences and needs of the patient

V. EXPECTED OUTCOMES

A. Patients will:
1. Be discharged functioning at their maximum level

(continued)

Protocol 14.1: Function-Focused Care Interventions *(continued)*

B. Providers can demonstrate:
   1. Competence in assessing physical function and developing an individualized plan to promote function, in collaboration with the patient and the interprofessional team
   2. Physical and social environments that enable optimal physical function for older adults
   3. Individualized discharge plans

C. Institution will experience:
   1. A reduction in incidence and prevalence of functional decline
   2. Reduction in the use of physical restraints, prolonged bed rest, and Foley catheters
   3. Decreased incidence of delirium and other adverse events (pressure ulcers and falls)
   4. An increase in prevalence of patients who leave hospital at baseline or with improved functional status
   5. Physical environments that are safe and enabling
   6. Increased patient satisfaction
   7. Enhanced staff satisfaction and teamwork

VI. RELEVANT PRACTICE GUIDELINES

Several resources are now available to guide adoption of evidence-based nursing interventions to enhance function in older adults.

1. Agency for Healthcare Research and Quality (AHRQ). *National guideline clearinghouse.* Retrieved from http://www.guideline.gov
2. McGill University Health Centre Research & Clinical Resources for Evidence Based Nursing (EBN). Retrieved from http://www.muhc-ebn.mcgill.ca
3. National Quality Forum. Retrieved from http://www.qualityforum.org/Home.aspx
4. Registered Nurses Association of Ontario (RNAO). *Clinical practice guidelines.* Retrieved from http:/www.rnao.org/Page.asp?PageID=861&SiteNodeID=270&BL_ExpandID
5. University of Iowa Hartford Center of Geriatric Nursing Excellence (HCGNE). *Evidence-based practice guidelines.* Retrieved from http://www.nursing.uiowa.edu/hartford/nurse/ebp.htm

ABBREVIATIONS

ADL Activities of daily living
FFC Function-focused care

REFERENCES

Alley, D. E., Koster, A., Mackey, D., Cawthon, P., Ferrucci, L., Simonsick, E. M.,... Harris, T. (2010). Hospitalization and change in body composition and strength in a population-based cohort of older persons. *Journal of the American Geriatrics Society, 58*, 2085–2091. *Evidence Level IV.*

Bailey, P., Thomsen, G. E., Spuhler, V. J., Blair, R., Jewkes, J., Bezdjian, L.,... Hopkins, R. O. (2007). Early activity is feasible and safe in respiratory failure patients. *Critical Care Medicine, 35*(1), 139–145. *Evidence Level IV.*

Betrabet Gulwadi, G., & Calkins, M. (2008). *The impact of healthcare environmental design on falls.* Concord CA: Center for Healthcare Design. *Evidence Level V.*

Boltz, M., Capezuti, E., & Shabbat, N. (2011). Nursing staff perceptions of physical function in hospitalized older adults. *Applied Nursing Research, 24*(4), 215–222. *Evidence Level IV.*

Boltz, M., Capezuti, E., Shabbat, N., & Hall, K. (2010). Going home better not worse: Older adults' views on physical function during hospitalization. *International Journal of Nursing Practice, 16*(4), 381–388. *Evidence Level V.*

Boltz, M., Chippendale, T., Resnick, B., & Galvin, J. (2015a). Anxiety in family caregivers of hospitalized persons with dementia: Contributing factors and responses. *Alzheimer Disease & Associated Disorders, 29*(3), 236–241. *Evidence Level IV.*

Boltz, M., Chippendale, T., Resnick, B., & Galvin, J. (2015b). Testing family centered, function-focused care in hospitalized persons with dementia. *Neurodegenerative Disease Management, 5*(3), 203–215. *Evidence Level III.*

Boltz, M., Resnick, B., Capezuti, E., Shabbat, N., & Secic, M. (2011). Function-focused care and changes in physical function in Chinese American and non-Chinese American hospitalized older adults. *Rehabilitation Nursing, 36*(6), 233–240. *Evidence Level IV.*

Boltz, M., Resnick, B., Capezuti, E., & Shuluk, J. (2014). Activity restriction vs. self-direction: Hospitalized older adults' response to fear of falling. *International Journal of Older People Nursing, 9*(1), 44–53. *Evidence Level IV.*

Boltz, M., Resnick, B., Capezuti, E., Shuluk, J., & Secic, M. (2012). Functional decline in hospitalized older adults: Can nursing make a difference? *Geriatric Nursing, 33*(4), 272–279. *Evidence Level IV.*

Boltz, M., Resnick, B., Chippendale, T., & Galvin, J. (2014). Testing a family-centered intervention to promote functional and cognitive recovery in hospitalized older adults. *Journal of the American Geriatrics Society, 62*(12), 2398–2407. doi:10.1111/jgs.13139. *Evidence Level III.*

Boyd, C. M., Landefeld, C. S., Counsell, S. R., Palmer, R. M., Fortinsky, R. H., Kresevic, D.,... Covinsky, K. (2008). Recovery of activities of daily living in older adults after hospitalization for acute medical illness. *Journal of the American Geriatrics Society, 56*, 2171–2179. *Evidence Level IV.*

Boyd, C. M., Xue, Q., Guralik, J. M., & Fried, L. P. (2005). Hospitalization and development of dependence in activities of daily living in a cohort of disabled older women: The Women's Health and Aging Study. *Journal of Gerontology Biological Sciences & Medical Science, 60A*, 888–893. *Evidence Level IV.*

Brown, C. J., Friedkin, R. J., & Inouye, S. K. (2004). Prevalence and outcomes of low mobility in hospitalized older patients. *Journal of the American Geriatrics Society, 52*, 1263–1270. *Evidence Level IV.*

Brown, C. J., Peel, C., Bamman, M. M., & Allman R. (2006). Exercise program implementation proves not feasible during acute care hospitalization. *Journal of Rehabilitation Research Development, 43*(7), 939–946. *Evidence Level III.*

Brown, C. J., Redden, D. T., Flood, K. L., & Allman, R. M. (2009). The underrecognized epidemic of low mobility during hospitalization of older adults. *Journal of the American Geriatrics Society, 57*(9), 1660–1665. *Evidence Level IV.*

Brown, C. J., Roth, D. L., Peel, C., & Allman, R. M. (2006). Predictors of regaining ambulatory ability during hospitalization. *Journal of Hospital Medicine, 1*, 277–284. *Evidence Level IV.*

Brown, C. J., Williams, B. R., Woodby, L. L., Davis, L. L., & Allman, R. M. (2007). Barriers to mobility during hospitalization from the perspective of older patients, their nurses and physicians. *Journal of Hospitalist Medicine, 2*(5), 305–313. *Evidence Level IV.*

Buurman, B. M., Hoogerduijn, J. G., van Gemert, E. A., de Haan, R. J., Marieke J. Schuurmans, M. J., & de Rooij, S. E., (2012). Clinical characteristics and outcomes of hospitalized older patients with distinct risk profiles for functional decline: A prospective cohort study. *PLoS One, 7*(1), e29621. *Evidence Level IV.*

Buurman, B. M., van Munster, B. C., Korevaar, J. C., de Haan, R. J., & de Rooij, S. E. (2011). Variability in measuring (instrumental) activities of daily living functioning and functional decline in hospitalized older medical patients: A systematic review. *Journal of Clinical Epidemiology, 64*, 619–627. *Evidence Level I.*

Callen, B. L., Mahoney, J. E., Wells, T. J., Enloe, M., & Hughes, S. (2004). Admission and discharge mobility of frail hospitalized older adults. *MEDSURG Nursing, 13*(3), 156–164. *Evidence Level III.*

Capezuti, E., Wagner, L. M., Brush, B. L., Boltz, M., Renz, S., & Secic, M. (2008). Bed and toilet heights as potential environmental risk factors. *Clinical Nursing Research, 17*(1), 50–66. *Evidence Level IV.*

Coelho, F. G., Santos-Galduroz, R. F., Gobbi, S., & Stella, F. (2009). Systematized physical activity and cognitive performance in elderly with Alzheimer's dementia: A systematic review. *Review Brasilian Psiquitr, 31*(2), 163–170. *Evidence Level I.*

Conedera, F., & Mitchell, L. (n.d.). *Try this: Therapeutic activity kits*: Retrieved from http://consultgerirn.org/uploads/File/trythis/theraAct.pdf. *Evidence Level VI.*

Covinsky, K. E., Palmer, R. M., Fortinsky, R. H., Counsell, S. R., Stewart, S., Kresevic, D., & Landefeld, S. (2003). Loss of independence in activities of daily living in older adults hospitalized with medical illness: Increased vulnerability with age. *Journal of the American Geriatrics Society, 51*, 451–458. *Evidence Level IV.*

Covinsky, K. E., Fortinsky, R. H., Palmer, R. M., Kresevic, D., & Landefeld, S. (1997). Relation between symptoms of depression and health status outcomes in acutely ill hospitalized older persons. *Annals of Internal Medicine, 126*, 417–425. *Evidence Level IV.*

Covinsky, K. E., Pierluissi, E., & Johnston, C. B. (2011). Hospitalization-associated disability. *Journal of the American Medical Association, 306*, 1782–1784. *Evidence Level V.*

Creditor, M. V. (1993). Hazards of hospitalization of the elderly. *Annals of Internal Medicine, 118*(3), 219–223. *Evidence Level VI.*

de Morton, N. A., Keating, J. L., Berlowitz, D. J., Jackson, B., & Lim, W. K. (2007). Additional exercise does not change hospital or patient outcomes in older medical patients: A controlled clinical trial. *Australian Journal of Physiotherapy, 53*(2), 105–111. *Evidence Level III.*

de Morton, N., Keating, J. L., & Jeffs, K. (2007). The effect of exercise on outcomes for older acute medical inpatients compared with control or alternative treatments: A systematic review of randomized controlled trials. *Clinical Rehabilitation, 1*, 3–16. *Evidence Level I.*

Doherty-King, B., Yoon, J. Y., Pecanac, K., Brown, R., & Mahoney, J. (2014). Frequency and duration of nursing care related to older patient mobility. *Journal of Nursing Scholarship, 46*(1) 20–27. *Evidence Level IV.*

Drolet, A., DeJuilio, P., Harkless, S., Henricks, S., Kamin, E., Leddy, E. A.,... Williams, S. (2013). Move to improve: The feasibility of using an early mobility protocol to increase ambulation in the intensive and intermediate care settings physical therapy *Physical Therapy, 93*(2), 197–207. *Evidence Level III.*

Fisher, S. R., Goodwin, J. S., Protas, E. J., Kuo, Y. F., Graham, J. E., Ottenbacher, K. J.,... Ostir, G. V. (2011). Ambulatory activity of older adults hospitalized with acute medical illness. *Journal of the American Geriatrics Society, 59*, 91–95. *Evidence Level IV.*

Foreman, M. D., Wakefield, B., Culp, K., & Milisen, K. (2001). Delirium in elderly patients: An overview of the state of the science. *Journal of Gerontological Nursing, 27*, 12–20. *Evidence Level V.*

Fortinsky, R. H., Covinsky, K. E., Palmer, R. M., & Landefeld, C. S. (1999). Effects of functional status changes before and during hospitalization on nursing home admission of older patients.

Journals of Gerontology. Series A, Biological Sciences & Medical Sciences, 54A, M521–M526. *Evidence Level IV.*

Gabo, J. Y. (2003). Contribution of the intensive care unit environment to sleep disruption in mechanically ventilated patients and healthy subjects. *American Journal of Respiratory and Critical Care Medicine, 167*(5), 708. *Evidence Level III.*

Galik, E. (2010). Function focused care for long-term care residents with moderate to severe cognitive impairment: A social ecological approach. *Annals of Long-Term Care, 18*(6), 27–33. *Evidence Level V.*

Galik, E., Resnick, B., & Pretzer-Aboff, I. (2009). Knowing what makes them tick: Motivating cognitively impaired older Adults to participate in restorative care. *International Journal of Nursing Practice, 15*(1), 48–55. *Evidence Level IV.*

Gill, T. M., Allore, H. G., & Guo, Z. (2004). The deleterious effects of bed rest among community living older persons. *Journals of Gerontology. Series A, Biological Sciences & Medical Sciences, 59A,* 755–761. *Evidence Level IV.*

Gill, T. M., Allore, H. G., Gahbauer, E. A., & Murphy, T. E. (2010). Change in disability after hospitalization or restricted activity in older persons. *Journal of the American Medical Association, 304*(17), 1919–1928. *Evidence Level IV.*

Gill, T. M., Allore, H. G., Holford, T. R., & Guo, Z. (2004). Hospitalization, restricted activity, and the development of disability among older persons. *Journal of the American Medical Association, 292,* 2115–2124. *Evidence Level IV.*

Gillis, A., MacDonald, B., & MacIsaac, A. (2008). Nurses' knowledge, attitudes, and confidence regarding preventing and treating deconditioning in older adults. *Journal of Continuing Education in Nursing, 39*(12), 547–554. *Evidence Level IV.*

Glantz, C., & Richman, N. (2007). Occupation-based ability centered care for people with dementia. *OT Practice, 12*(2), 10–16. *Evidence Level VI.*

Harper, C. M., & Lyles, Y. M. (1988). Physiology and complications of bed rest. *Journal of the American Geriatrics Society, 36,* 1047–1054. *Evidence Level VI.*

Hoenig, H. M., & Rubenstein, L. Z. (1999). Hospital-associated deconditioning and dysfunction. *Journal of the American Geriatrics Society, 39,* 220–222. *Evidence Level IV.*

Inouye, S., Schlesinger, M., & Lydon, T. (1999). Delirium: A symptom of how hospital care is failing older persons and a window to improve quality of hospital care. *American Journal of Medicine, 106,* 565–573. *Evidence Level VI.*

Jacelon, C. S. (2004). Managing personal integrity: The process of hospitalization for elders. *Journal of Advanced Nursing, 46*(5), 549–557. *Evidence Level IV.*

Jones, C. T., Lowe, A. J., MacGregor, L., Brand C. A., Tweddle, N., & Russell, D. M. (2006). A randomised controlled trial of an exercise intervention to reduce functional decline and health service utilisation in the hospitalised elderly. *Australasian Journal on Ageing, 25*(3), 126–133. *Evidence Level II.*

Kalisch, B. J., Soohee, L., & Dabney, B. W. (2013). Outcomes of inpatient mobilization: A literature review. *Journal of Nursing Scholarship, 23,* 1486–1501. *Evidence Level V.*

King, B., & Bowers, B. (2011). How nurses decide to ambulate hospitalized older adults: Development of a conceptual model. *The Gerontologist, 51,* 786–797. *Evidence Level IV.*

King, B., & Bowers, B. J. (2013). Attributing the responsibility for ambulating patients. *International Journal of Nursing Studies, 50,* 1240–1246. *Evidence Level IV.*

Kleinpell, R. (2007). Supporting independence in hospitalized elders in acute care. *Critical Care Nursing Clinics of North America, 19*(3), 247–252. *Evidence Level V.*

Kortebein, P., Ferrando, A., Lombeida, J., Wolfe, R., & Evans, W. J. (2007). Effect of 10 days of bed rest on skeletal muscle in healthy older adults. *Journal of the American Medical Association, 297,* 1772–1774. *Evidence Level III.*

Kortebein, P., Symons, T. B., Ferrando, A., Paddon-Jones, D., Ronsen, O., Protas, E., ... Evans, W. J. (2008). Functional impact of 10 days of bed rest in healthy older adults. *Journals of Gerontology. Series A, Biological Sciences & Medical Sciences, 63*(10), 1076–1081. *Evidence Level III.*

Landefeld, C. S., Palmer, R. M., Kresevic, D. M., Fortinsky, R. H., & Kowal, J. (1995). A randomized trial of care in a hospital medical unit especially designed to improve the functional outcomes of acutely ill older patients. *New England Journal of Medicine, 332,* 1338–1344. *Evidence Level II.*

McAuley, E., Konopack, J. F., Motl, R. W., Morris, K. S., Doerksen, S. E., & Rosengren, K. R. (2006). Physical activity and quality of life in older adults: Influence of health status and self-efficacy. *Annals of Behavioral Medicine, 31,* 91–103. *Evidence Level IV.*

McCusker, J., Kakuma, R., & Abrahamowicz, M. (2002). Predictors of functional decline in hospitalized elderly patients: A systematic review. *Journals of Gerontology. Series A, Medical Sciences, 57A,* M569–M577. *Evidence Level I.*

Morris, P. E., Goad, A., Thompson, C., Taylor, K., Harry, B., Passmore, L., ... Haponik E. (2008). Early intensive care unit mobility therapy in the treatment of acute respiratory failure. *Critical Care Medicine, 36*(8), 2238–2243. *Evidence Level III.*

Mudge, A. M., Giebel, A. J., & Cutler, A. J. (2008). Exercising body and mind: An integrated approach to functional independence in hospitalized older people. *Journal of the American Geriatrics Society, 56*(4), 630–651. *Evidence Level III.*

Nolan, J., & Thomas, S. (2008). Targeted individual exercise programmes for older medical patients are feasible, and may change hospital and patient outcomes: A service improvement project. *BMC Health Services Research, 8,* 250. *Evidence Level V.*

Olson, L.-E., & Karlsson, J. (2007). Effects of an integrated care pathway with hip fracture. *Journal of Advanced Nursing, 58*(2), 116–125. *Evidence Level III.*

Parke, B., & Chappell, N. L. (2010). Transactions between older people and the hospital environment: A social ecological analysis. *Journal of Aging Studies, 24,* 115–124. *Evidence Level IV.*

Resnick, B., Galik, E., Boltz, M., & Pretzer-Aboff, I. (2011). *Restorative care nursing for older adults: A guide for all care settings.* New York, NY: Springer Publishing Company. *Evidence Level VI.*

Resnick, B., Galik, E., Enders, H., Sobol, K., Hammersla, M., Dustin, I., ... Trotman, S. (2011). Impact nursing care of older adults: Pilot testing of function focused care-acute care intervention. *Journal of Nursing Care Quality,* (2), 169–177. *Evidence Level III.*

Resnick, B., Galik, E., Wells, C., Boltz, M., & Holtzman, C. (2015). Optimizing function and physical activity post trauma: Overcoming system and patient challenges. *International Journal of Orthopaedic and Trauma Nursing, 19*(4), 194–206. *Evidence Level V.*

Rozzini, R., Sabatini, T., Cassinadri, A., Boffelli, S., Ferri, M., Barbisoni, P., . . . Trabucchi, M. (2005). Relationship between functional loss before hospital admission and mortality in elderly persons with medical illness. *Journals of Gerontology. Series A, Biological Sciences & Medical Sciences, 60A*, 1180–1183. *Evidence Level IV.*

Siu, A. L., Boockvar, K. S., Penrod, J. D., Morrison, R. S., Halm, E. A., Litke, A., . . . Magaziner, J. (2006). Effect of inpatient quality of care on functional outcomes in patients with hip fracture. *Medical Care, 44*(9), 799–889. *Evidence Level IV.*

Siu, A. L., Penrod, J. D., Boockvar, K. S., Koval, K., Strauss, E., & Morrison, R. S. (2006). Early ambulation after hip fracture: Effects on function & mortality. *Archives of Internal Medicine, 166*, 766–771. *Evidence Level IV.*

Tucker, D., Molsberger, S. C., & Clark, A. (2004). Walking for Wellness: A collaborative program to maintain mobility in hospitalized older adults. *Geriatric Nursing, 25*(4), 242–245. *Evidence Level V.*

Ulrich, R., Zimring, C., Zhu, X., DuBose, J., Seo, H. B., Choi, Y. S., . . . Joseph, A. (2008). A review of the research literature on evidence-based health care design. *Health Environments Research and Design Journal, 1*(3), 61–125. *Evidence Level V.*

Volpato, S., Onder, G., Cavalieri, M., Guerra, G., Sioulis, F., Maraldi, C., . . . Fellin, R.; Italian Group of Pharmacoepidemiology in the Elderly Study (GIFA). (2007). Characteristics of nondisabled older patients developing new disability associated with medical illnesses and hospitalization. *Journal of General Internal Medicine, 22*(5), 668–674. *Evidence Level IV.*

Wakefield, B. J., & Holman, J. E. (2007). Functional trajectories associated with hospitalization in older adults. *Western Journal of Nursing Research, 29*(2), 161–177. *Evidence Level IV.*

Weitzel, T., & Robinson, S. B. (2004). A model of nurse assistant care to promote functional status in hospitalized elders. *Journal for Nurses in Staff Development, 20*(4), 181–186. *Evidence Level V.*

Yu, F., Kolanowski, A. M., Strumpf, N. E., & Eslinger, P. (2006). Improving cognition and function through exercise intervention in Alzheimer's disease. *Journal of Nursing Scholarship, 38*(4), 358–365. *Evidence Level I.*

Zisberg, A., Shadmi, E., Sinoff, G., Gur-Yaish, N., Srulovici, E., & Admi, H. (2011). Low mobility during hospitalization and functional decline in older adults. *Journal of the American Geriatrics Society, 59*(2), 266–273. *Evidence Level IV.*

15

Late-Life Depression

Glenise L. McKenzie and Theresa A. Harvath

EDUCATIONAL OBJECTIVES

On completion of this chapter, the reader should be able to:

1. Discuss the major risk factors for late-life depression
2. Discuss the consequences of late-life depression
3. Identify the core competencies of a systematic nursing assessment for depression with older adults
4. Identify nursing strategies for older adults with depression

OVERVIEW

Contrary to popular belief, depression is not a normal part of aging. Although depression is less likely in older adults when compared to younger adults it has serious consequences for the individual, his or her family, and our society. Depression in late life interferes with a person's ability to function, decreases quality of life, increases risk of morbidity and mortality (including suicide), and increases use of health care services (Taylor, 2014). The prevalence of major depression and clinically significant depressive symptoms in adults older than 60 years of age varies depending on the clinical context (community-dwelling older adults: 5%–16%; primary care: 5%–10%; post–critical care hospitalization: up to 37%; first year in a nursing home: up to 54%; Hybels & Blazer, 2003; Jackson et al., 2014; Neufeld, Freeman, Joling, & Hirdes, 2014). The numbers of older adults with a diagnosis of clinical depression is increasing (Akincigil et al., 2011).

Late-life depression is common in individuals with coexisting medical conditions and in individuals with physical and/or cognitive disability, which contribute to the challenge of timely identification and treatment of depression in older adults (Lyness et al., 2007). Nurses in all health care settings are pivotal to the early recognition of depression and the facilitation of older patients' access to mental health care. This chapter presents an overview of unipolar late-life depression, with emphasis on age-related assessment considerations, clinical decision making, and nursing intervention strategies. A standard-of-practice protocol for use by nurses in practice settings is presented.

BACKGROUND AND STATEMENT OF PROBLEM

What Is Late-Life Depression?

Late-life depression is a term that includes older adults with a history of depressive disorders in earlier years as well as those who develop symptoms for the first time

For a description of evidence levels cited in this chapter, see Chapter 1, "Developing and Evaluating Clinical Practice Guidelines: A Systematic Approach."

in later life. Depression may range in severity from mild symptoms (subsyndromal) to severe symptoms (major depressive episode), both of which can persist over time with negative consequences for the older patient. Suicidal ideation, psychotic features (especially delusions), and excessive somatic concerns (hypochondriasis) frequently accompany more severe depression in older adults when compared to younger adults with depression (Grayson & Thomas, 2013). Symptoms of anxiety may also coexist with depression in many older adults (Beattie, Pachana, & Franklin, 2010). In fact, comorbid anxiety and depression have been associated with more severe symptoms, decreases in memory, poorer treatment outcomes (Beattie et al., 2010; DeLuca et al., 2005), and increased rates of suicidal ideation (Sareen et al., 2005).

Major Depression

The *Diagnostic and Statistical Manual of Mental Disorders* (5th ed.; *DSM-5*; American Psychiatric Association [APA], 2013) lists the criteria for the diagnosis of a major depressive disorder, the most severe form of depression. These criteria are frequently used as the standard by which older patients' depressive symptoms are assessed in clinical settings. Five criteria (or more) from a list of nine must be present nearly every day during the same 2-week period and must represent a change from previous functioning: (a) depressed, sad, or irritable mood; (b) anhedonia or diminished pleasure in usually pleasurable people or activities; (c) feelings of worthlessness, self-reproach, or excessive guilt; (d) difficulty with thinking or diminished concentration; (e) suicidal thinking or attempts; (f) fatigue and loss of energy; (g) changes in appetite and weight; (h) disturbed sleep; and (i) psychomotor agitation or retardation. For this diagnosis, at least one of the five symptoms must include either depressed mood, by the patient's subjective account or observation of others, or markedly diminished pleasure in almost all people or activities. Concurrent medical conditions are frequently present in older patients and should not preclude a diagnosis of depression; indeed, there is a high incidence of medical comorbidity. The *DSM-5* also provides criteria for persistent depressive disorder (dysthymia), which increases the risk of developing a major depression and manifests with depressive symptoms that occur on a majority of days for at least 2 years.

Major depression seems to be as common among older as younger cohorts. A recent review found diagnostic thresholds (number and type of symptoms) to be consistent between older adults (age 60 years and older) and middle-aged adults (age 40 years and older; Anderson, Slade, Andrews, & Sachdev, 2009). However, older adults may more readily report somatic or physical symptoms than depressed mood (Grayson & Thomas, 2013; Pfaff & Almeida, 2005). The somatic or physical symptoms of depression, however, are often difficult to distinguish from somatic or physical symptoms associated with acute or chronic physical illness, especially in the hospitalized older patient, or the somatic symptoms that are part of common aging processes (Kurlowicz, 1994). For instance, disturbed sleep may be associated with chronic lung disease or congestive heart failure. Diminished energy or increased lethargy may be caused by an acute metabolic disturbance or drug response. Therefore, a challenge for nurses in acute care hospitals and other clinical settings is to not overlook or disregard somatic or physical complaints while also "looking beyond" such complaints to assess the full spectrum of depressive symptoms in older patients.

Minor depression or subsyndromal depression is diagnosed in patients with clinically significant symptoms (causing impairment or distress) that do not meet *DSM-5* standard criteria for major depression or persistent depressive disorder. The *DSM-5* (APA, 2013, p. 183) classifies minor depression as an "other specified depressive disorder with insufficient symptoms" (depressed mood plus 1–3 other symptoms of major depression with at least 2 weeks of duration). Minor depression is at least two to three times as common as major depression for older adults in the community and is most prevalent for older adults residing in long-term care settings (Meeks, Vahia, Lavretsky, Kulkarni, & Jeste, 2011). Additionally, 8% to 10% of older adults with untreated minor depression develop major depression within 1 year and less than one third with minor depression have a remission of symptoms after 1 year (Meeks et al., 2011). Minor depression is serious and the majority of older adults will not improve without treatment.

Depression in Late Life Is Serious

Depression (major, persistent, and minor) is associated with serious negative consequences for older adults, especially for frail older patients, such as those recovering from a severe medical illness or those in nursing homes (Mezuk et al., 2012). Consequences of late-life depression include heightened pain and disability, delayed recovery from medical illness or surgery, worsening of medical symptoms, risk of physical illness, increased health care use, alcoholism, cognitive impairment, worsening social impairment, protein–calorie subnutrition, loss of bone mineral density, functional decline, and increased rates of suicide- and non-suicide-related death (Hoogerduijn, Schuurmans, Duijnstee, de Rooij, & Grypdonck, 2007; Smalbrugge et al., 2006; Wu,

Magnus, Liu, Bencaz, & Hentz, 2009). The "amplification" hypothesis proposed by Katz, Streim, and Parmelee (1994) stated that depression can "turn up the volume" on several aspects of physical, psychosocial, and behavioral functioning in older patients, ultimately accelerating the course of medical illness. For example, Gaynes, Burns, Tweed, and Erickson (2002) found that major depression and comorbid medical conditions interacted to adversely affect health-related quality of life in older adults, and Courtney, O'Reilly, Edwards, and Hassall (2009) identified depression as one of the factors most often associated with poorer quality of life for older adults in nursing homes. For older nursing home residents, depression is also associated with poor adjustment to the nursing home, resistance to daily care, treatment refusal, inability to participate in activities, and further social isolation (Achterberg et al., 2003).

Mortality by suicide is higher among older persons with depression than among their counterparts without depression (Juurlink, Herrmann, Szalai, Kopp, & Redelmeier, 2004). Rates of suicide among older adults (15–20 per 100,000) are the highest of any age group and even exceed rates among adolescents (American Association of Suicidology, 2012; McKeowen, Cuffe, & Schulz, 2006). This is, in large part, caused by the fact that White men older than the age of 85 years are at the greatest risk for suicide, when rates of suicide are estimated to be 80 to 113 per 100,000 (American Association of Suicidology, 2012; Erlangsen, Vach, & Jeune, 2005). In the oldest old (80 years and older), men and women had higher suicide rates than nonhospitalized older adults in the same age range, this age group had significantly higher rates of hospitalization than younger cohorts; three or more medical diagnoses were associated with increased suicide risk (Erlangsen et al., 2005). Among older psychiatric inpatients, increased risk for suicide was associated with affective disorders and first versus later admission (Erlangsen, Zarit, Tu, & Conwell, 2006).

Predictors of late-life suicide include: depressive symptoms (Rorup, Deeg, Poppelaars, Kerkhof, & Onwuteaka-Philipsen, 2011), previous suicide attempt (Wiktorsson, Runeson, Skoog, Ostling, & Waern, 2010), poor self-reported quality of life (Chen et al., 2011), perception of lower health status, poor sleep quality (Bernert, Turvey, Cornwell, & Joiner, 2014), and absence of a confidant (Turvey et al., 2002). Although physical illness and functional impairment increase risk for suicide in older adults, it appears that this relationship is strengthened by comorbid depression (Conwell, Duberstein, & Caine, 2002; Rorup et al., 2011). Disruption of social support (Conwell et al., 2002; Szanto et al., 2012), perceived burdensomeness (Cukrowicz, Cheavens, Van Orden, Ragain, & Cook, 2011; Jahn & Cruckowiz, 2011; Jahn, Cukrowicz, Linton, & Prabhu, 2011), family conflict, and loneliness (Waern, Rubenowitz, & Wilhelmson, 2003) are also significantly associated with suicide in late life.

Recent research has also identified a growing list of cognitive and psychological variables associated with increased risk for suicide among older adults. Decreased decision-making skills (Clark, Dombrovski, Sahakian, & Szanto, 2011), dysfunctional coping skills and poor cognitive control (Richard-Devantoy, Szanto, Butters, Kalkus, & Dombrowski, 2014) have all been correlated with increased risk for suicide. In addition, several social factors may place some older adults at greater risk: lower income and financial strain (Gilman 2012; Rorup et al., 2011), history of childhood physical and sexual abuse (Sachs-Ericsson, Corsention, Rushing, & Sheffler, 2013), and low receipt of filial piety (Simon, Chen, Chang, & Dong, 2014) are associated with increased suicidal ideation in older adults.

Studies have also shown that contact between suicidal older adults and their primary care provider is common (Luoma, Martin, & Pearson, 2002). Almost half of older suicide victims had seen their primary care provider within 1 month of committing suicide (Luoma et al., 2002), whereas 20% had seen a mental health provider. Most of the suicidal patients experienced their first episode of major depression, which was only moderately severe, yet the depressive symptoms went unrecognized and untreated. Older adults with clinically significant depressive symptomatology presented with physical rather than psychological symptoms, including patients who, when asked, admitted having suicidal ideation (Pfaff & Almeida, 2005).

Although the risk for suicide increases with advancing age (Hybels & Blazer, 2003), a growing body of evidence suggests that depression is also associated with higher rates of nonsuicide mortality in older adults (Kronish, Rieckmann, Schwartz, Schwartz, & Davidson, 2009; Schulz, Drayer, & Rollman, 2002); however, evidence is inclusive regarding depression as predictive of mortality in hospitalized older adults (Cole, 2007). Depression can also influence decision-making capacity and may be the cause of indirect life-threatening behavior such as refusal of food, medications, or other treatments in older patients (McDade-Montez, Christensen, Cvengros, & Lawton, 2006; Stapleton, Nielsen, Engelberg, Patrick, & Curtis, 2005). Furthermore, depressive symptoms in older adults have been associated with cognitive impairment and, in some cases, progression to dementia (Walker & Steffens, 2010). These observations suggest that accurate diagnosis and treatment of depression in older patients may reduce the mortality rate in this population. It is in the clinical setting, therefore, that screening procedures and assessment protocols have the most direct impact.

Depression in Late Life Is Misunderstood

Despite its prevalence and associated negative outcomes, depression in older adults continues to be underrecognized, misdiagnosed, and subsequently undertreated (Licht-Strunk et al., 2009; Unützer, 2007). Barriers to care for older adults with depression exist at many levels. In particular, some older adults refuse to seek help because of perceived stigma of mental illness. Others may simply accept their feelings of profound sadness without realizing that they are clinically depressed. Lack of care-provider training in the identification and diagnosis of depression in older adults is also a barrier to timely recognition and treatment (Ayalon, Fialová, Areán, & Onder, 2010). Depressive disorders may also be missed due to overlapping anxiety disorders and/or various somatic or dementia-like symptoms or because patient or provider believe that depression is a "normal" response to medical illness, hospitalization, relocation to a nursing home, or other stressful life events (Taylor, 2014). However, depression—major, persistent, or minor—is not a necessary or normative consequence of life adversity (Snowdon, 2001). When depression occurs after an adverse life event, it represents pathology that should be treated.

Treatment Works for Late-Life Depression

The goals of treating depression in older patients are to decrease depressive symptoms, reduce relapse and recurrence, improve functioning and quality of life, improve medical health, and reduce mortality and health care costs. Significant and equivalent improvements in depressive symptoms occur with both pharmacotherapy and psychotherapy interventions (individually or in combination) in older adult populations (Pinquart, Duberstein, & Lyness, 2006). In addition, treatment of depression improves pain and functional outcomes in older adults (Lin et al., 2003). Recurrence of depression is a serious problem and has been associated with reduced responsiveness to treatment and higher rates of cognitive and functional decline (Driscoll et al., 2005). When compared to younger patients, older adults demonstrate comparable treatment response rates; however, they tend to have higher rates of relapse following treatment (Mitchell & Subramaniam, 2005). Therefore, continuation of treatment to prevent early relapse and longer term maintenance treatment to prevent later occurrences is important. Even in those patients with depression who have a comorbid medical illness or dementia, treatment response can be good (Iosifescu, 2007). Depressed older patients who have mild cognitive impairment may be at greater risk of developing dementia if their depression goes untreated (Modrego & Ferrandez, 2004).

CAUSE AND RISK FACTORS

Several biological and psychosocial factors have been associated with increased risk for late-life depression. Medical comorbidity is a hallmark of depression in older patients and this factor represents a major difference from depression in younger populations (Alexopoulos, Schultz, & Lebowitz, 2005) (see Table 15.1). Biological contributors to depression in late life include vascular disease (myocardial infarction, coronary heart disease, cerebrovascular accident), general health (obesity, pain, new medical illness, insomnia, prior depression, history of suicide attempt, and poor health status), dementia (Alzheimer and vascular dementia), diabetes mellitus, Parkinson's disease, arthritis, and urological problems (Aziz & Steffens, 2013; Cole & Dendukuuri, 2003; Hasin & Grant, 2002; Huang, Dong, Lu, Yue, & Liu, 2010; Vink, Aartsen, & Schoevers, 2008). Genetic factors seem to play more of a role when older adults have had depression throughout their lives versus older adults with onset in later life (Blazer & Hybels, 2005). Neuroanatomic correlates (volume reduction in hippocampus, orbitofrontal cortex, putamen, and thalamus), and the presence of apolipoprotein E have also been associated with late-life depression (Butters et al., 2003; Sexton, Mackay, & Ebmeier, 2013). The link between late-life depression and cognitive impairment is thought to be bidirectional. For example, a history of depression doubles the risk of developing dementia in late life and cognitive symptoms of severe depression can be misinterpreted as symptoms of an early-stage dementia (Morimoto & Alexopoulous, 2013). In an evidence-based review, Cole (2005) found that disability, older age, new medical diagnosis, and poor health status were among the most robust and consistent of all correlates of depression among older medical patients. Those with functional disabilities, especially those with new functional loss, are also at risk.

Psychosocial risk factors for depression in late life include personality attributes (personality disorder, low self-efficacy), life stressors (trauma, low income, less education, poor functional status, disability), and social stressors (bereavement, loneliness, lack of a confidante, impaired social support, being a caregiver; Aziz & Steffens, 2013; Cole, 2007; Cole & Dendukuuri, 2003; Heisel, Links, Conn, van Reekum, & Flett, 2007; Onrust & Cuijpers, 2006; Pinquart & Sorensen, 2004; Vink et al., 2008). It is interesting to note that in a meta-analysis of the impact of negative life events on depression in older adults, Kraaij, Arensman, and Spinhoven (2002) found that although specific negative life events (e.g., death of significant others, illness in self or spouse, or negative relationship events) were moderately associated with increases in depression, the total number of negative life events and daily hassles had the strongest relationships with depression in older adults. This suggests that clinicians should pay close attention to the accumulation of negative life events and daily hassles when developing programs and targeting interventions to mitigate depression in older adults who are at risk for developing depression.

Depression Among Minority Older Adults

Rates of depression among minority older adults are not well understood. Beals et al. (2005) found that the rates of major depressive episodes among older American Indians were 30% of the national average. In a review, Kales and Mellow (2006) found lower rates of depression and higher rates of psychotic diagnoses among African American older adults. In a systematic review of studies of older Asian immigrants, Kuo, Chong, and Joseph (2008) found that the prevalence of depression among Asian Americans ranged from 18% to 20% with significant variability among different Asian minority groups. For example, studies of Vietnamese older adults estimated depression at 50%, whereas studies of older Japanese Americans estimated depression at 3%. Depression was linked to gender, recent immigration status, English proficiency, acculturation, service barriers, and social support.

Baker and Whitfield (2006) reported that depressive symptoms were significantly associated with increased

TABLE 15.1

Physical Illnesses Associated With Depression in Older Patients

Metabolic disturbances
- Dehydration
- Azotemia, uremia
- Acid–base disturbances
- Hypoxia
- Hyponatremia and hypernatremia
- Hypoglycemia and hyperglycemia
- Hypocalcemia and hypercalcemia

Endocrine disorders
- Hypothyroidism and hyperthyroidism
- Hyperparathyroidism
- Diabetes mellitus
- Cushing's disease
- Addison's disease

Infections
- Viral
  - Pneumonia
  - Encephalitis
- Bacterial
- Pneumonia
- Urinary tract
- Meningitis
- Endocarditis
- Other
  - Tuberculosis
  - Brucellosis
  - Fungal meningitis
  - Neurosyphilis

Cardiovascular disorders
- Congestive heart failure
- Myocardial infarction, angina

Pulmonary disorders
- Chronic obstructive lung disease
- Malignancy

Gastrointestinal disorders
- Malignancy (especially pancreatic)
- Irritable bowel
- Other organic causes of chronic abdominal pain, ulcer, diverticulosis
- Hepatitis

Genitourinary disorders
- Urinary incontinence

Musculoskeletal disorders
- Degenerative arthritis

Osteoporosis with vertebral compression or hip fractures
- Polymyalgia rheumatica
- Paget's disease

Neurological disorders
- Cerebrovascular disease
- Transient ischemic attacks
- Stroke
- Dementia (all types)
- Intracranial mass
- Primary or metastatic tumors
- Parkinson's disease

Other Illness
- Anemia (of any cause)
- Vitamin deficiencies
- Hematologic or other systemic malignancy
- Immune disorders

Sources: Alexopoulos et al. (2005); Cole (2005); Holmes and House (2000).

physical impairment among older Blacks. Williams et al. (2007) found that when African American and Caribbean Blacks experience a major depressive disorder, it is usually untreated, more severe, and more disabling than for non-Hispanic Whites. Furthermore, significant disparities exist in the quality of mental health services received by minority older adults (Virnig et al., 2004). A study of managed care enrollees revealed that minority older adults received substantially less follow-up for mental health problems following hospitalization (Virnig et al., 2004).

Although misdiagnosis and subsequent inappropriate treatment can lead to poor health outcomes for minority older adults (Kales & Mellow, 2006), it is not clear that "simple" bias alone can explain the disparities in depression management that exist. For example, Beals et al. (2005) point out that differences in the social construction of depressive experiences may confound the measurement of depression in ethnic older adults. Older American Indians may be reluctant to endorse symptoms of depression because cultural norms associate these complaints with weakness (Beals et al., 2005). In a thoughtful analysis of health disparities, Cooper, Beach, Johnson, and Inui (2006) explore the complex interactions and relationships between patients and providers that frame the context in which disparities can occur. They point out that many historical, cultural, and class-related factors can influence the development of therapeutic relationships between providers and patients. Until more research clarifies the symptom pattern of late-life depression in minority populations (Sadule-Rios, 2012), it is important that clinicians be culturally sensitive and open to atypical presentations of depression that warrant closer scrutiny.

ASSESSMENT OF THE PROBLEM

Protocol 15.1 presents a standard-of-practice protocol for depression in older adults that emphasizes a systematic assessment guide for early recognition of depression by nurses in hospitals and other clinical settings. Early recognition of depression is enhanced by targeting high-risk groups of older adults for assessment methods that are routine, standardized, and systematic by use of both a depression screening tool and individualized depression assessment or interview (Smith, Haedtke, & Shibley, 2015).

It can be challenging to differentiate depression symptoms from dementia symptoms because cognitive impairment is frequently a symptom of depression and significant cognitive impairment in older depressed adults has been implicated in later development of dementia. Therefore, assessment for presenting symptoms indicative of both depression and dementia requires focused attention on the historical progression of symptoms, getting collateral information from a reliable informant (family or caregiver), and using a screening tool sensitive to change in mood symptoms in cognitively impaired individuals (Steffens, 2008).

Depression Screening Tools

Because older adults may not present with the same symptoms as younger adults (Pfaff & Almeida, 2005), it is important that screening for depression among older adults is incorporated into routine health assessments. In a recent meta-analysis (comparing 11 studies with a combined sample of 2,000 subjects) the authors reported that depressed symptoms in older adults are more likely to include agitation, somatic complaints (especially gastrointestinal symptoms), and hypochondriasis and less likely to include feelings of guilt or low sexual interest compared with younger adults with depression (Hegeman, Kok, Van der Mast, & Giltay, 2012). Nursing assessment of depression in older patients can be facilitated by the use of a screening tool designed to detect symptoms of depression. Several depression screening tools have been developed for use with older adults; this review focuses on two common screening tools used with cognitively intact older adults in hospital, clinic, and long-term care settings and one common tool for older adults with cognitive impairment. The Geriatric Depression Scale—Short Form (GDS-SF; Sheikh & Yesavage, 1986) takes a few minutes to complete and was developed specifically for older adults. The GDS-SF is ritten in a simple yes/no format with 15 items that can be self-administered or administered by a clinician; a score of 5 or more is considered positive screen for depression. The GDS has been shown to be valid in inpatient and outpatient settings, with an 84% sensitivity and 95% specificity (Glover & Srinivasan, 2013). Given the brevity, focus, and validity of GDS-SF, it is a good choice for either inpatient or outpatient populations (Mitchell et al., 2010). The GDS-SF has been a reliable screening tool for depressive symptoms in mild cognitive impairment but not in older adults with moderate to severe dementia (Debruyne et al., 2009).

The Patient Health Questionnaire-9 (PHQ-9) is evidence based and was originally designed for use in primary care settings (Kroenke & Spitzer, 2002). The PHQ-9 is recommended for screening cognitively intact older adults for depressive symptoms in primary care, nursing homes, and community settings and can be either self- or clinician administered (Richardson, He, Podgorski, Tu, & Conwell, 2010; Smith et al., 2015). The nine items of the PHQ-9 correspond with the *DSM-5* (APA, 2013) major depressive disorder criteria and scores are based on frequency as well as number of symptoms (scores less than 5 suggest no depression; 5–9 = mild depression; 10–14 = moderate depression; and 20–27 = severe depression). Sensitivity and specificity of the PHQ-9 have both been reported to be more than 80%. The PHQ-9 has also been abbreviated to include just the first two items (PHQ-2) that ask about depressed mood and loss of pleasure (anhedonia); the PHQ-2 has similar sensitivity and specificity to the PHQ-9 (Kroenke, Spitzer, & Williams, 2003; Richardson et al., 2010). Overall, the PHQ is easy to administer, valid in cognitively intact older adults in different settings, and can also be used to monitor response to treatment (Richardson et al., 2010; Smith et al., 2015). The PHQ is not recommended for screening older adults with cognitive impairment.

The Cornell Scale for Depression in Dementia (CSDD) is an interviewer-rated scale that was developed specifically to detect symptoms of depression in older adults with dementia (Alexopoulos, Abrams, Young, & Shamoianl, 1988). The CSDD contains 19 items and a score of 12 or greater suggests depression in an individual with dementia. Screening tools are helpful in identifying depressive symptoms in older adults but do not replace the need for a comprehensive nursing assessment.

Individualized Assessment and Interview

Central to the individualized depression assessment and interview is a focused assessment of the full spectrum of symptoms (nine) for major depression as delineated by the *DSM-5* (APA, 2013). Furthermore, patients should be asked directly and specifically if they have been having suicidal ideation—that is, thoughts that life is not worth living—or if they have been contemplating or have attempted suicide. The number of symptoms, type, duration, frequency, and patterns of depressive symptoms, as well as a change from the patient's normal mood of functioning, should be noted. Additional components of the individualized depression assessment include evidence of psychotic thinking (especially delusional thoughts), anniversary dates of previous losses or stressful events, previous coping style (specifically alcohol or other substance abuse), relationship changes, physical health changes, a history of depression or other psychiatric illness that required some form of treatment, a general loss and crises inventory, and any concurrent life stressors. Subsequent questioning of the family or caregiver is recommended to obtain further information about the older adult's verbal and nonverbal expressions of depression.

DIFFERENTIATION OF MEDICAL OR IATROGENIC CAUSES OF DEPRESSION

Once depressive symptoms are recognized, medical- and drug-related causes should be explored. As part of the initial assessment of depression in the older patient, it is important to obtain and review the medical history and physical and/or neurological examinations. Key laboratory tests should also be obtained and/or reviewed and include thyroid-stimulating hormone levels, chemistry screen, complete blood count, and medication levels, if needed. An electrocardiogram, serum B_{12}, a urinalysis, and serum folate should also be considered to assess for coexisting medical conditions. These conditions may contribute to depression or might complicate treatment of the depression (Alexopoulos, Katz, Reynolds, Carpenter, & Docherty, 2001; Taylor, 2014; Table 15.2). In medically ill older patients, who frequently have multiple medical diagnoses and are prescribed with multiple medications, these "organic" factors in the cause of depression are a major issue in nursing assessment. In collaboration with the patient's physician, efforts should be directed toward treatment, correction, or stabilization of associated metabolic or systemic conditions. When medically feasible, depressogenic medications should be eliminated, minimized, or

TABLE 15.2

Drugs Used to Treat Physical Illness That Can Cause Symptoms of Depression in Patients

Antihypertensives	**Antiparkinsonian agents**
■ Reserpine	■ L-Dopa
■ Methyldope	**Antimicrobials**
■ Propranolol	■ Sulfonamides
■ Clonidine	■ Isoniazid
■ Hydralazine	**Cardiovascular agents**
■ Guanethidine	■ Digitals
■ Diuretics[a]	■ Lidocaine[b]
Analgesics	**Hypoglycemic agents[c]**
■ Narcotic	■ Steroids
■ Morphine	■ Corticosteroids
■ Codeine	■ Estrogens
■ Meperidine	**Others**
■ Pentazocine	■ Cimetidine
■ Propoxphene	■ Cancer chemotherapeutic agents
Nonnarcotic	
■ Indomethacin	

[a]By causing dehydration or electrolyte imbalance.
[b]By causing toxicity.
[c]By causing hypoglycemia.
Adapted from Dhondt et al. (1999).

substituted with those that are less depressogenic (Dhondt et al., 1999; Taylor, 2014). Even when an underlying medical condition or medication is contributing to the depression, treatment of that condition or discontinuation or substitution of the offending agent alone is often not sufficient to resolve the depression, and antidepressant medication is often needed.

INTERVENTIONS AND CARE STRATEGIES

Clinical Decision Making and Treatment

Regardless of the setting, older patients who exhibit the number of symptoms indicative of a major depression, specifically suicidal thoughts or psychosis, and who score *above* the established cutoff score for depression on a depression screening tool (e.g., 5 on the GDS-SF or 8–10 on the GHQ-9) should be referred for a comprehensive psychiatric evaluation. Older patients with less severe depressive symptoms without suicidal thoughts or psychosis but who also score more than the cutoff score on the depression screening tool (e.g., 5 on the GDS-SF or 8–10 on the GHQ-9) should be referred to available psychosocial services (i.e., psychiatric liaison nurses, geropsychiatric advanced practice nurses, social workers, psychologists, a clergy member) for psychotherapy or other psychosocial therapies, as well as to determine whether medication for depression is warranted. It is also important to note that older adults at risk for depression may benefit from brief psychosocial interventions that focus on preventing the development of major depression (Forsman, Jane-Llopis, Schierenbeck, & Wahlbeck, 2009; Lee et al., 2012) with increased social activity interventions being most effective (Forsman, Nordmyr, & Wahlbeck, 2011). Findings have been mixed for prevention efforts focused specifically on minor depression (Krishna et al., 2013).

The type and severity of depressive symptoms influence the type of treatment approach. In general, more severe depression, especially with suicidal thoughts or psychosis, requires intensive psychiatric treatment, including hospitalization, medication with an antidepressant or antipsychotic drug, electroconvulsive therapy (ECT), and intensive psychosocial support (Taylor, 2014)). Less severe depression without suicidal thoughts or psychosis may require treatment with psychotherapy or medication, often on an outpatient basis. Collectively, these data also suggest that patients who have depression complicated by multiple medical and psychiatric comorbidities may benefit from a referral to an interdisciplinary treatment team with specific expertise in geropsychiatry.

The four major categories of treatment for depression in older adults are lifestyle change (exercise and diet); somatic therapies (e.g., pharmacotherapy ECT, and light therapy), psychosocial interventions (e.g., cognitive-behavioral, psychodynamic, social engagement, and reminiscence therapy), and collaborative care interventions. A compelling body of evidence supports the efficacy of these diverse treatment modalities for older adults with depression.

Lifestyle-Change Interventions

In less severe depression, lifestyle change may be effective and carries less risk of adverse effects compared to those related to pharmacological interventions. Physical exercise has been established as an effective treatment for depression in the general population, and this includes older adults who are physically able to participate. Two recent systematic reviews of physical exercise interventions concluded that exercise programs decrease depressive symptoms and quality of life in older adults with major and minor depression (Seong-Hi, Kuem Sun, & Chang-Bum, 2014; Sjosten & Kivela, 2006). Tai chi and qigong are specific meditative exercise methods that also may decrease depressive symptoms and reduce stress (Rogers, Larkey, & Keller, 2009; Wang et al., 2010). Studies showing potential benefits of improved nutrition and diet supplements on depression in late life are building (Nyer et al., 2013; Sanhueza, Ryan, & Foxcroft, 2013). For example, a systematic review on 10 studies on the relationship between vitamin D_3 supplementation and depressive symptoms in older adults reported positive results but more studies are required to make any solid recommendations (Farrington & Moller, 2013). Fish oil and folic acid supplementation have also shown promising results in studies that include older adults (Nyer et al., 2013). Although lifestyle changes (increase in exercise and a healthy diet) are reasonable recommendations, they may be inadequate in older adults who have disabilities and more significant depressive symptoms. Additional interventions, such as pharmacotherapy and psychotherapy, may also be necessary.

Somatic Therapy in Treatment of Late-Life Depression

Somatic therapy for remission of the symptoms of late-life depression includes pharmacotherapy, ECT, and light therapy. Pharmacotherapy or ECT are both shown to be very effective and are recommended for more severe depression. Pharmacotherapy and light therapy may also be recommended for older adults with less severe symptoms and for individuals who have not responded to nonpharmacological treatments (Kok, 2013).

In a recent meta-analysis of 80 controlled trails, antidepressants were found effective for treating depression in older adults and all classes of antidepressants were reported to be superior to placebo (Kok, Nolen, & Heeren, 2012). This meta-analysis also showed a response rate for antidepressants in older adults of 48% and a remission rate of 33.7%, which are similar to rates found in younger adults (Kok et al., 2012). The selective serotonin-reuptake inhibitors (SSRIs) are considered the first-line pharmacotherapy for late-life depression, based on their relatively low side-effect profile and low cost (Kok, 2013; Taylor, 2014). SSRIs have been effective in treating poststroke depression (Chen, Guo, Zhan, & Patel, 2006; Hackett, Anderson, House, & Xia, 2008) and depression in persons with Alzheimer's disease (Thompson, Herrmann, Rapoport, & Lanctôt, 2007). In a systematic review of the literature, Wilson, Mottram, and Vassilas (2008) found that although SSRIs are generally well tolerated in older adults, a significant minority experience serious side effects, including nausea, vomiting, dizziness, and drowsiness. Judicious use of tricyclic antidepressants (TCAs) may be an effective alternative for older adults who cannot tolerate SSRIs (Kok, 2013; Wilson et al., 2008).

Older patients should be closely monitored for therapeutic response to and potential side effects of antidepressant medication to assess whether dose adjustment of antidepressant medication may be warranted. Kok, Nolen, and Heeren (2012) reported that about two thirds of older adults with depression require a change or augmentation to initial treatment to achieve remission. Although, in general, it is advised to start antidepressant medication at low doses in older patients, it is also necessary to increase doses to ensure that older adults with persistent depressive symptoms receive adequate treatment and appropriate follow-up (Kok, 2013).

Research that has suggested that the use of SSRIs in adolescents can increase suicidality has raised concerns about a similar dynamic with older adults. Several studies, however, have found that the use of SSRI antidepressants to treat late-life depression is not associated with increases in suicidal ideation (Barbui, Esposito, & Cipriani, 2009; Nelson, Delucchi, & Schneider, 2008; Stone et al., 2009). In fact, treatment of late-life depression with SSRIs has been shown to significantly reduce suicidal ideation and behavior in older adults (Barbui et al., 2009; Nelson et al., 2008; Stone et al., 2009).

Electroconvulsive Therapy

When older adults are not able to take antidepressants for treatment of late-life depression, clinicians are increasingly looking to the use of ECT to reduce symptoms of depression and improve function. ECT involves the induction of a mild, therapeutic seizure under general anesthesia. For many individuals, the use of ECT conjures up images of barbaric treatments that leave patients severely cognitively impaired. However, ECT is becoming a more widely accepted treatment option for older adults with depression, especially older adults with severe depression that is resistant to pharmacotherapy or has psychotic features (Greenberg & Kellner, 2005; Navarro et al., 2008; Spaans et al., 2015; Van der Wurff, Stek, Hoogendijk, & Beekman, 2003). In fact, because of the relatively low side-effect profile, some researchers suggest that ECT should be considered a front-line treatment (Plakiotis, Barson, Vengadasalam, Haines, & O'Connor, 2013). In a recent systematic review of literature on maintenance of ECT, Van Shaik et al. (2010) found that long-term ECT use was not associated with increases in cognitive impairment and was well tolerated in older adults, even older adults with cardiac conditions.

Light Therapy

The efficacy of bright light therapy to decrease depressive symptoms in older adults with major depression was tested in a recent clinical trial (Lieverse et al., 2011). This 3-week randomized trial compared bright light treatment with placebo (dim light) in 89 older adults with nonseasonal affective disorder. The intervention was well tolerated and showed a positive treatment response (58% vs. 34%). A small pilot study in long-term care also reported significant improvement in mood when comparing bright light treatment versus placebo effects (Royer et al., 2012). This is a promising area for further research and consideration when working with older adults who are depressed.

PSYCHOSOCIAL APPROACHES

The term *psychosocial* encompasses a wide array of approaches. This section provides an overview of the three major psychosocial approaches used in studies with older adult populations: (a) cognitive behavioral, (b) psychodynamic, and (c) reminiscence or life-review therapy.

Cognitive behavioral therapies (CBTs) seek to change the cognitive and/or behavioral context in which depression occurs through the use of various specific techniques such as providing new information, teaching problem-solving strategies, correcting skills deficits, modifying ineffective communication patterns, or changing the physical environment. Although specific treatment protocols vary, CBT approaches tend to be active and focused on solving specific, current day-to-day problems, rather than seeking global personality change in the client. Based on a large and growing evidence base, CBT has been shown to be effective in decreasing depression in clinically depressed older adults with major, dysthymic, and minor depression (Gould, Coulson, & Howard, 2012). Studies of computerized delivery of CBT with older adults are limited; however, there are promising findings, and older individuals may be less likely to drop out than younger individuals (Crabb et al., 2012). Training caregivers (family or paid caregivers) to use CBT approaches (improved communication, increasing pleasant events, and problem-solving behaviors) has also been shown to decrease depression and related behaviors in older adults with dementia (Teri, McKenzie, & LaFazia, 2005). Gallagher-Thompson and Coon (2007) also identified CBT interventions as effective in decreasing depression in the older adults who are caregivers for family members with dementia. A meta-analysis of nonpharmacological treatments reported that individual and group CBT interventions compared to usual treatment significantly reduced depression for people with chronic physical health conditions (Rizzo, Creed, Goldberg, Meader, & Pilling, 2011).

Psychodynamic approaches focus on establishing a therapeutic relationship as a mechanism of change, as well as the historical causes of current client mood and behavior. The client's psychological insight and ongoing emotional experience are considered critical for psychological progress. The evidence for effectiveness of psychodynamic approaches with older adults has increased over the past 5 years. In a recent meta-analysis, a medium effect size was reported for psychotherapy in reducing symptoms of depression in older adults who reside in residential care settings (Cody & Drysdale, 2013). A systematic review of the impact of psychotherapy on symptoms of community-dwelling older adults with minor (subthreshold) depression also found psychotherapy to be effective, safe, and cost-effective (Lee et al., 2012). Additionally, Bharucha, Dew, Miller, Borson, and Reynolds (2006) reviewed 18 studies of psychodynamic approaches ("talk therapy") with residents of long-term care settings and reported significant positive outcomes on measures of depression, hopelessness, and self-esteem. Marital and family therapy may also be beneficial in treating older adults with depression, especially older spouses engaged in caregiving (Buckwalter et al., 1999).

It is important to note that positive social relationships (Neufeld, Hirdes, Perlman, & Rabinowitz, 2015) and church attendance (Rushing, Corsentino, Hames, Sachs-Ericsson, & Steffens, 2013) may provide protection against suicidal ideation for some older adults. Treatment of depression rapidly decreased suicidal ideation in older adults (Bruce et al., 2004; Szanto, Mulsant, Houck, Dew, & Reynolds, 2003). However, older adults in higher risk groups (male, older) needed a significantly longer response time to demonstrate a decrease in suicidal ideation (Szanto et al., 2003).

In a systematic review by Lapierre et al. (2011) it was found that most efforts at suicide prevention target the reduction of risk factors (e.g., through screening and treatment of depression). The authors found that few studies focused on improving protective factors (e.g., resilience) that may be useful in reducing depression in older adults. A recent study by Van Orden et al. (2014) suggests that the desire for death and a sense that life is not worth living is not a normative finding among older adults. This suggests that assessment for a desire for death may be an important part of mental status assessment for older adults in order to identify those individuals who may be at risk for suicide.

In reminiscence therapy, older adults are encouraged to remember the past and to share their memories, either with a therapist or with peers, as a way of increasing self-esteem and social intimacy. It is often highly directive and structured, with the therapist picking each session's reminiscence topic. According to a recent meta-analysis that included 128 trials with older adults participants, reminiscence interventions showed moderate improvement in depression when compared to control groups and effects were maintained at 6-month follow-up (Pinquart & Forstmeier, 2012). In another meta-analysis, group delivery of reminiscence was analyzed and the results showed significant improvement in depressive symptoms when compared to control interventions; however, the effect disappeared after 6 months (Song, Shen, Xu, & Sun, 2014). Nursing interventions to encourage reminiscence include asking patients directly about their past or by linking events in history with the patient's life experience. The use of photographs, old magazines, scrapbooks, and other objects can also stimulate discussion.

In summary, psychosocial treatment has been found effective and safe in decreasing depression in cognitively intact older adults. There is also empirical evidence for the efficacy of cognitive behavioral-based therapies and reminiscence therapy in decreasing depression in individuals with dementia and for the older adults who are caregivers of individuals with dementia. Current meta-analysis also demonstrated the utility of working closely with caregivers—whether family or staff—to introduce psychosocial interventions with resulting reduction in depression in persons with dementia (Orgeta et al., 2014). There is also a small but growing body of evidence related to the use of psychodynamic approaches aimed at decreasing depression in older adults associated with specific comorbid illnesses such as heart disease (Kang-Yi & Gellis, 2010)

Collaborative Care

Collaborative depression care programs focus on multiprofessional teams that include nurses trained as care or case depression managers and have been effective in improving outcomes for older adults with depression (Dreizler, Koppitz, Probst, & Mahrer-Imhof, 2014). A recent meta-analysis that included 14 studies (4,440 participants) comparing nurse-delivered collaborative depression care approaches to usual care for older adults with chronic illness found a moderate impact on depression severity that remained at follow-up (Ekers et al., 2013)

Ethnic minority older adults experienced improved treatment of depression when treated by an interdisciplinary treatment team (Areán et al., 2005) as did low-income older adults (Areán, Gum, Tang, & Unützer, 2007). Similarly, patients with multiple comorbid medical conditions responded positively to a collaborative approach to depression management (Harpole et al., 2005; Unützer et al., 2002). Although older adults with comorbid anxiety disorders took longer to respond to treatment, they experienced greater reductions in depression when treated by a multiprofessional team than similar patients receiving usual primary care (Hegel et al., 2005).

Individualized Nursing Interventions for Depression

Psychosocial and behavioral nursing interventions can be incorporated into the plan of care, based on the patient's individualized need. Provision of safety precautions for patients with suicidal thinking is a priority. In acute medical settings, patients may require transfer to the psychiatric service when suicidal risk is high and staffing is not adequate to provide continuous observation of the patient. In outpatient settings, continuous surveillance of the patient should be provided while an emergency psychiatric evaluation and disposition is obtained.

Promotion of nutrition, elimination, sleep/rest patterns, physical comfort, and pain control has been recommended specifically for depressed medically ill older adults (Voyer & Martin, 2003). Relaxation strategies should be offered to relieve anxiety as an adjunct to pain management. Nursing interventions should also focus on enhancement of the older adult's physical function through structured and regular activity and exercise; referral to physical, occupational, and recreational therapies; and the development of a daily activity schedule (Barbour & Blumenthal, 2005). Enhancement of social support is also an important function of the nurse. This may be done by identifying, mobilizing, or designating a support person, such as a family member, a confidant, friend, volunteer or other hospital resource, church member, support group, patient or peer visitor, and particularly by accessing appropriate clergy for spiritual support.

Nurses should maximize the older adult's autonomy, personal control, self-efficacy, and decision making about clinical care, daily schedules, and personal routines (Lawton, Moss, Winter, & Hoffman, 2002). The use of a graded task assignment in which a larger goal or task is subdivided into several small steps can be helpful in enhancing function, assuring successful experiences, and building older patients' confidence in their performance of various activities (Areán & Cook, 2002). Participation in regular, predictable, and pleasant activities can result in more positive mood changes for older adults with depression (Koenig, 1991). A pleasant-events inventory, elicited from the patient, can be used to incorporate pleasurable activities into the older patient's daily schedule (Koenig, 1991). Music therapy customized to the patient's preference is also recommended to reduce depressive symptoms (Siedliecki & Good, 2006).

Nurses should provide emotional support for depressed older patients by providing empathetic, supportive listening; encouraging patients to express their feelings in a focused manner on issues such as grief or role transition; supportive adaptive coping strategies; identifying and reinforcing strengths and capabilities; maintaining privacy and respect; and instilling hope. In particular, it is important to increase the patient's and family's awareness of the symptoms as part of a depression that is treatable and not the person's fault as a result of personal inadequacies.

CASE STUDY AND DISCUSSION

Ray Stimson is an 87-year-old man with multiple medical problems. He has a history of coronary artery disease (CAD) and had triple-bypass surgery 4 years ago. He also has hypertension, type 2 diabetes, and is hard of hearing. He was admitted to the hospital for surgical repair of a hip fracture following a fall in his home. Mr. Stimson is widowed (11 months) and has two adult children who do not live locally. Before his fall, he was living independently in the community; however, his children were growing increasingly concerned about his safety. Following surgery, Mr. Stimson was irritable and resisted efforts by the nursing staff to participate in self-care activities (e.g., walking, bathing). They often found him laying stoically in bed, staring into space. The nurses also observed that he was occasionally confused and would ask about his deceased wife.

A subsequent referral to the geropsychiatric consultation liaison nurse revealed that Mr. Stimson was experiencing a great deal of postoperative pain that was not well treated on his current medicine regimen. Nursing staff had charted concerns that his opioid analgesic was contributing to his mental confusion. The geropsychiatric evaluation also revealed that Mr. Stimson had been growing increasingly depressed over the past few months and was still actively grieving the loss of his wife of 62 years. As his health had failed and his independent living was threatened, he admitted he had contemplated suicide, stating, "Life is just not worth living anymore." Further assessment revealed that he did not have a specific plan in mind and admitted that he did not really think that was a solution to his problems, but that he could not see that he had many options.

The liaison nurse worked with the medical team to develop a more aggressive plan for pain management. She also arranged for a family conference to discuss discharge-planning issues. During the family conference, the liaison nurse spoke to Mr. Stimson's children about long-term planning. She explained how important it was for Mr. Stimson to participate in any placement decisions that they may be contemplating and to have a sense of control. Although his children were able to express their reservations and concerns about safety, they agreed to explore the kinds of community support services that could be activated to help support their father in his own home for as long as possible.

Mr. Stimson was able to participate in rehabilitation and gained enough strength to return to his home. Arrangements were made for follow-up with mental health services. He was started on an antidepressant and agreed to participate in the senior lunch program twice a week to increase the opportunity for socialization. Several months after his discharge, Mr. Stimson reported that he still missed his wife terribly and that he still was lonely at times. However, he had developed some friendships at the senior center and was getting out one to two times each week. His children called more often and had, for the time being, stopped sending him brochures for assisted living facilities. He acknowledged that he may need to move to a more supervised setting in the future, but for now, he was content to stay in the home where he had many pleasant memories to keep him company.

SUMMARY

Depression significantly threatens the personal integrity, health, and "experience of life" of many older adults. Depression is often reversible with prompt and appropriate treatment. Early recognition can be enhanced by training health care personnel in the use of a standardized protocol that outlines a systematic method for depression assessment adapted for older adults in various settings and with diverse comorbid conditions. Early identification of depression and successful treatment demonstrates to society that depression is the most treatable mental problem in late life. As Blazer (1989) stated, "When there is depression, hope remains" (p. 166).

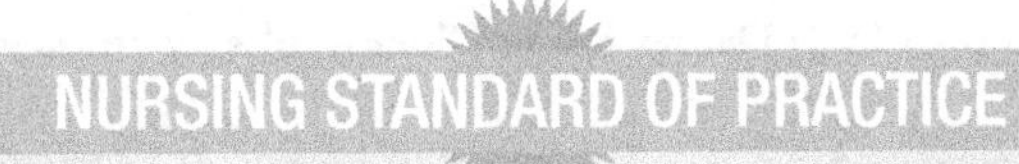

Protocol 15.1: Depression in Older Adults

I. BACKGROUND[a]

A. Depression—both major and minor depressive disorders—is highly prevalent in community-dwelling, medically ill, and institutionalized older adults.
B. Depression is not a natural part of aging or a normal reaction to acute illness hospitalization.
C. Consequences of depression include amplification of pain and disability, delayed recovery from illness and surgery, worsening of drug side effects, excess use of health services, cognitive impairment, subnutrition, and increased suicide- and nonsuicide-related death.
D. Depression (major, persistent, and minor) tends to be long lasting and recurrent. Therefore, a wait-and-see approach is undesirable, and immediate clinical attention is necessary. If recognized, treatment response is good.
E. Somatic symptoms and agitation may be more prominent than depressed mood in late-life depression.
F. Mixed depression and anxiety features may be evident among many older adults.
G. Recognition of depression is hindered by the coexistence of physical illness, cognitive decline, and social and economic problems common in late life. Early recognition, intervention, and referral by nurses can reduce the negative effects of depression.

II. ASSESSMENT PARAMETERS

Identify risk factors/high-risk groups (Aziz & Steffens, 2013; Smith et al., 2015).

A. Biological contributors
   1. Vascular disease (MI, CAD, CVA)
   2. General health (new medical illness, pain, insomnia, prior depression, history of suicide attempt, concomitant substance abuse)
   3. Dementia (vascular and Alzheimer's disease)
   4. Other chronic or disabling medical conditions (diabetes, Parkinson's disease, arthritis, low vision, COPD)
   5. Psychosocial contributors
   6. Personality attributes (personality disorder, low self-efficacy)
   7. Life stressors (trauma, low income, impaired function, disability)
   8. Social stressors (bereavement, loneliness, impaired social support, caregiving)
B. Screen all at-risk groups using a standardized depression screening tool and document score (Smith et al., 2015).
   1. The GDS-SF is recommended for its brevity, validity, and extensive use with medically ill older adults, and inclusion of *few* somatic items that may be confounded with physical illness.
   2. The PHQ-9 and PHQ-2 are recommended for their brevity, validity with older as well as younger adults, and availability in hospital and primary care settings.
C. Perform a *focused* depression assessment on all at-risk groups and document results. Note the number of symptoms; onset; frequency/patterns; duration (especially 2 weeks); and change from normal mood, behavior, and functioning (APA, 2013; Taylor, 2014).
   1. Depressive symptoms
   2. Depressed or irritable mood, frequent crying

[a]Somatic symptoms, also seen in many physical illnesses, are frequently associated with A and B; therefore, the full range of depressive symptoms should be assessed.

(continued)

Protocol 15.1: Depression in Older Adults *(continued)*

3. Loss of interest or pleasure (in family, friends, hobbies, sex)
4. Weight loss or gain (especially loss)
5. Sleep disturbance (especially insomnia)
6. Fatigue/loss of energy
7. Psychomotor slowing/agitation
8. Diminished concentration
9. Feelings of worthlessness/guilt
10. Suicidal thoughts or attempts, hopelessness
11. Psychosis (i.e., delusional/paranoid thoughts, hallucinations)
12. History of depression, current substance abuse (especially alcohol), previous coping style
13. Recent losses or crises (e.g., death of spouse, friend, pet; retirement; anniversary dates; move to another residence, nursing home); change in physical health status, relationships, roles

D. Obtain/review medical history and physical/neurological examination
E. Assess for depressogenic medications (e.g., steroids, narcotics, sedative/hypnotics, benzodiazepines, antihypertensives, H_2 antagonists, beta blockers, antipsychotics, immunosuppressive, cytotoxic agents).
F. Assess for related systematic and metabolic processes (e.g., infection, anemia, hypothyroidism or hyperthyroidism, hyponatremia, hypercalcemia, hypoglycemia, congestive heart failure, kidney failure).
G. Assess for cognitive dysfunction.
H. Assess level of functional disability and quality of life.

III. CARE PARAMETERS

Based on guidelines and reviews (APA, 2010; Pinquart et al., 2006; Taylor, 2014)

A. For severe depression (GDS-SF score of 11 or greater, five to nine depressive symptoms [must include depressed mood or loss of pleasure] plus other positive responses on individualized assessment [especially suicidal thoughts or psychosis and comorbid substance abuse]), refer for psychiatric evaluation. Treatment options may include medication or cognitive behavioral, interpersonal, or brief psychodynamic psychotherapy/counseling (individual, group, family); hospitalization; or electroconvulsive therapy.
B. For less severe depression (GDS-SF score 6 or greater, less than five depressive symptoms, plus other positive responses on individualized assessment), refer to mental health services for psychotherapy/counseling (see previous types), especially for specific issues identified in individualized assessment and to determine whether medication therapy may be warranted. Consider resources such as psychiatric liaison nurses, geropsychiatric advanced practice nurses, social workers, psychologists, and other community and institution-specific mental health services. If suicidal thoughts, psychosis, or comorbid substance abuse are present, a referral for a comprehensive psychiatric evaluation should always be made.
C. For all levels of depression, develop an *individualized* plan integrating the following nursing interventions:
    1. Institute safety precautions for suicide risk as per institutional policy (in outpatient settings, ensure continuous surveillance of the patient while obtaining an emergency psychiatric evaluation and disposition).
    2. Remove or control etiologic agents.
        a. Avoid/remove/change depressogenic medications
        b. Correct/treat metabolic/systemic disturbances
    3. Monitor and promote nutrition, elimination, sleep/rest patterns, physical comfort (especially pain control).
    4. Enhance physical function (i.e., structure regular exercise/activity; refer to physical, occupational, or recreational therapies); develop a daily activity schedule.
    5. Enhance social support (i.e., identify/mobilize a support person(s) [e.g., family, confidant, friends, hospital resources, support groups, patient visitors]); ascertain need for spiritual support and contact appropriate clergy.
    6. Maximize autonomy/personal control/self-efficacy (e.g., include patient in active participation in making daily schedules, short-term goals).

(continued)

Protocol 15.1: Depression in Older Adults *(continued)*

7. Identify and reinforce strengths and capabilities.
8. Structure and encourage daily participation in relaxation therapies, pleasant activities (conduct a pleasant activity inventory), and music therapy.
9. Monitor and document response to medication and other therapies; readminister depression screening tool.
10. Provide practical assistance; assist with problem solving.
11. Provide emotional support (i.e., empathic, supportive listening, encourage expression of feelings, hope instillation), support adaptive coping, and encourage pleasant reminiscences.
12. Provide information about the physical illness and treatment(s) and about depression (i.e., that depression is common, treatable, and not the person's fault). Include attention to addressing potential fear and stigma associated with depression.
13. Educate about the importance of adherence to prescribed treatment regimen for depression (especially medication) to prevent recurrence; educate about *specific* antidepressant side effects.
14. Ensure mental health community link-up; consider collaborative care programs.

IV. EVALUATION OF EXPECTED OUTCOMES

A. Patient
   1. Patient safety will be maintained.
   2. Patients with severe depression will be evaluated by psychiatric services.
   3. Patients will report a reduction of symptoms that are indicative of depression. A reduction in the GDS score will be evident and suicidal thoughts or psychosis will resolve.
   4. Patient's daily functioning will improve.

B. Health care provider
   1. Early recognition of patients at risk, referral, and interventions for depression, and documentation of outcomes will be improved.
   2. Provide support and depression-specific education to patients and their families (and other caregivers) via written and verbal information on depression and its management, including how families or carers can support the person.

C. Institution
   1. The number of patients identified with depression will increase.
   2. The number of in-hospital suicide attempts will not increase.
   3. The number of referrals to mental health services will increase.
   4. The number of referrals to psychiatric nursing home care services will increase.
   5. Staff will receive ongoing education on depression recognition, assessment, and interventions.
   6. Develop collaborative depression care management programs.

V. FOLLOW-UP TO MONITOR CONDITION

A. Continue to track prevalence and documentation of depression in at-risk groups.
B. Show evidence of transfer of information to postdischarge mental health service delivery system.
C. Educate caregivers to continue assessment and management strategies.

ABBREVIATIONS

APA	American Psychiatric Association
CAD	Coronary artery disease
COPD	Chronic obstructive pulmonary disease
CVA	Cerebrovascular accident
GDS-SF	Geriatric Depression Scale–Short Form
MI	Myocardial infarction
PHQ	Patient Health Questionnaire

ACKNOWLEDGMENTS

This chapter is based partly on Chapter 5 of the third edition, coauthored by Dr. Lenore H. Kurlowicz, who died on September 21, 2007. The authors and coeditors acknowledge her tremendous contributions to the field of geropsychiatric nursing.

RESOURCES

Recommended Instruments for Screening for Depression

Cornell Scale for Depression in Dementia (CSDD)

A 19-item clinician-administered tool designed to assess depression in older adults with dementia. Scores are based on caregiver interview and direct observation.

champ-program.org/static/Cornell_Scale.pdf

Geriatric Depression Scale-Short Form (GDS-SF)

A 15-item screening measure for depression in older adults

www.stanford.edu/~yesavage/GDS.html

Patient Health Questionnaire (PHQ-9)

A nine-item scale recommended for screening in older adults. The first two questions of the PHQ- 9 are referred to as the PHQ-2 and may be used to identify the need for a more complete assessment of depressive symptoms using the PHQ-9 or GDS-SF.

www.phqscreeners.com

Additional Online Information About Assessing Depression

Assessing Care of Vulnerable Elders (ACOVE)

www.rand.org/health/projects/acove.html

Portal of Geriatric Online Education

Provides resources for assessment and management of geriatric health issues

https://www.pogoe.org

"Try This"

A series of tips on various aspects of assessing and caring for older adults sponsored by the Hartford Institute for Geriatric Nursing at New York University College of Nursing.

consultgerirn.org/resources

Guidelines

American Psychiatric Association. (2010). *Practice guideline for the treatment of patients with major depressive disorder* (3rd ed.). Arlington, VA: Author. p. 152. Retrieved from www.guideline.gov/content.aspx?id=24158#Section420

NICE Clinical Guidelines, No. 90 (2010). *Depression: The treatment and management of depression in adults* (updated edition). National Collaborating Centre for Mental Health (UK). Leicester, UK: British Psychological Society. Retrieved from www.ncbi.nlm.nih.gov/pubmedhealth/PMH0016629

NICE Clinical Guidelines, No. 91 (2010). *Depression in adults with a chronic physical health problem: Treatment and management. National Collaborating Centre for Mental Health (UK).* Leicester (UK): British Psychological Society. Retrieved from www.ncbi.nlm.nih.gov/pubmedhealth/PMH0033598

REFERENCES

Achterberg, W., Pot, A. M., Kerkstra, A., Ooms, M., Muller, M., & Ribbe, M. (2003). The effect of depression on social engagement in newly admitted Dutch nursing home residents. *The Gerontologist, 43*(2), 213–218. *Evidence Level IV.*

Akincigil, A., Olfson, M., Walkup, J. T., Siegel, M. J., Kalay, E., Amin, S.,... Crystal, S. (2011). Diagnosis and treatment of depression in older community-dwelling adults: 1992–2005. *Journal of the American Geriatrics Society, 59*(6), 1042–1051. *Evidence Level IV.*

Alexopoulos, G. S., Abrams, R. C., Young, R. C., & Shamoian, C. A. (1988). Cornell scale for depression in dementia. *Biological Psychiatry, 23*(3), 271–284. *Evidence Level III.*

Alexopoulos, G. S., Katz, I. R., Reynolds, C. F., III, Carpenter, D., & Docherty, J. P. (2001). The expert consensus guidelines series: Pharmacotherapy of depressive disorders in older patients [Special report]. *Postgraduate Medicine,* 1–86. *Evidence Level VI.*

Alexopoulos, G. S., Schultz, S. K., & Lebowitz, B. D. (2005). Late-life depression: A model for medical classification. *Biological Psychiatry, 58,* 283–289. *Evidence Level IV.*

American Association of Suicidology. (2012). *Elderly suicide fact sheet.* Retrieved from http://www.suicidology.org/Portals/14/docs/Resources/FactSheets/Elderly2012.pdf. *Evidence Level V.*

American Psychiatric Association. (2010). *Practice guideline for the treatment of patients with major depressive disorder* (3rd ed.). Arlington, VA: American Psychatric Press. *Evidence Level IV.*

American Psychiatric Association. (2013). *Diagnostic and statistical manual of mental disorders* (5th ed.). Arlington, VA: American Psychiatric Press. *Evidence Level IV.*

Anderson, T. M., Slade, T., Andrews, G., & Sachdev, P. S. (2009). *DSM-IV* major depressive episode in the elderly: The relationship between the number and the type of depressive symptoms and impairment. *Journal of Affective Disorders, 117*(1–2), 55–62. *Evidence Level IV.*

Areán, P. A., Ayalon, L., Hunkeler, E., Lin, E. H., Tang, L., Harpole, L.,... Unützer J. (2005). Improving depression care for older minority patients in primary care. *Medical Care, 43*(4), 381–390. *Evidence Level VI.*

Areán, P. A., & Cook, B. L. (2002). Psychotherapy and combined psychotherapy/pharmacotherapy for late life depression. *Biological Psychiatry, 52*(3), 293–303. *Evidence Level VI.*

Areán, P. A., Gum, A. M., Tang, L., & Unützer, J. (2007). Service use and outcomes among elderly persons with low incomes being treated for depression. *Psychiatric Services, 58*(8), 1057–1064. *Evidence Level II.*

Ayalon, L., Fialová, D., Areán, P. A., & Onder, G. (2010). Challenges associated with the recognition and treatment of depression in older recipients of home care services. *International Psychogeriatrics, 22*(4), 514–522. *Evidence Level V.*

Aziz, R., & Steffens, D. C. (2013). What are the causes of late-life depression? *Psychiatric Clinics of North America, 36*(4), 497–516. *Evidence Level V.*

Baker, T. A., & Whitfield, K. E. (2006). Physical functioning in older blacks: An exploratory study identifying psychosocial and clinical predictors. *Journal of the National Medical Association, 98*(7), 1114–1120. *Evidence Level III.*

Barbour, K. A., & Blumenthal, J. A. (2005). Exercise training and depression in older adults. *Neurobiology of Aging, 26*(Suppl. 1), S119–S123. *Evidence Level VI.*

Barbui, C., Esposito, E., & Cipriani, A. (2009). Selective serotonin reuptake inhibitors and risk of suicide: A systematic review of observational studies. *Canadian Medical Association Journal, 180*(3), 291–297. *Evidence Level I.*

Beals, J., Manson, S. M., Whitesell, N. R., Mitchell, C. M., Novins, D. K., Simpson, S., & Spicer, P. (2005). Prevalence of major depressive episode in two American Indian reservation populations: Unexpected findings with a structured interview. *American Journal of Psychiatry, 162*, 1713–1722. *Evidence Level VI.*

Beattie, E., Pachana, N. A., & Franklin, S. J. (2010). Double jeopardy: Comorbid anxiety and depression in late life. *Research in Gerontological Nursing, 3*(3), 209–220. *Evidence Level V.*

Bernert, R. A., Turvey, C. L., Cornwell, Y., & Joiner, T. E. (2014). Association of poor subjective sleep quality with risk for death by suicide during a 10-year period: A longitudinal, population-based study of late life. *JAMA Psychiatry, 71*(10), 1129–1137. *Evidence Level IV.*

Bharucha, A. J., Dew, M. A., Miller, M. D., Borson, S., & Reynolds, C., III. (2006). Psychotherapy in long-term care: A review. *Journal of the American Medical Directors Association, 7*(9), 568–580. *Evidence Level I.*

Blazer, D. G. (1989). Depression in the elderly. *New England Journal of Medicine, 320*, 164–166. *Evidence Level V.*

Blazer, D. G., & Hybels, C. F. (2005). Origins of depression in late life. *Psychological Medicine, 35*(9), 1241–1252. *Evidence Level VI.*

Bruce, M. L., Ten Have, T. R., Reynolds, C. F., III, Katz, I. I., Schulberg, H. C., Mulsant, B. H., . . . Alexopoulos, G. S. (2004). Reducing suicidal ideation and depressive symptoms in depressed older primary care patients: A randomized controlled trial. *Journal of the American Medical Association, 291*(9), 1081–1091. *Evidence Level I.*

Buckwalter, K. C., Gerdner, L., Kohout, F., Hall, G. R., Kelly, A., Richards, B., & Sime, M. (1999). A nursing intervention to decrease depression in family caregivers of persons with dementia. *Archives of Psychiatric Nursing, 13*(2), 80–88. *Evidence Level IV.*

Butters, M. A., Sweet, R. A., Mulsant, B. H., Ilyas Kamboh, M., Pollock, B. G., Begley, A.E., . . . DeKosky, S. T. (2003). APOE is associated with age-of-onset, but not cognitive functioning, in late-life depression. *International Journal of Geriatric Psychiatry, 18*, 1075–1081. *Evidence Level IV.*

Chen, W. J., Chen, C. C., Ho, C. K., Chou, F. H. C., Lee, M. B., Lung, F., . . . Sun, F. C. (2011). The relationships between quality of life, psychiatric illness, and suicidal ideation in geriatric veterans living in a veterans' home: A structural equation modeling approach. *American Journal of Geriatric Psychiatry, 19*(6), 597–601. *Evidence Level IV.*

Chen, Y., Guo, J. J., Zhan, S., & Patel, N. C. (2006). Treatment effects of antidepressants in patients with post-stroke depression: A meta-analysis. *Annals of Pharmacotherapy, 40*(12), 2115–2122. *Evidence Level I.*

Clark, L., Dombrovski, A. Y., Sahakian, B. J., & Szanto, K. (2011). Impairment in risk-sensitive decision-making in older suicide attempters with depression. *Psychology and Aging, 26*(2), 321–330. *Evidence Level IV.*

Cody, R. A., & Drysdale, K. (2013). The effects of psychotherapy on reducing depression in residential aged care: A meta-analytic review. *Clinical Gerontologist, 36*(1), 46–69. doi:10.1080/07317115.2012.731474. *Evidence Level I.*

Cole, M. G. (2005). Evidence-based review of risk factors for geriatric depression and brief preventive interventions. *Psychiatric Clinics of North America, 28*(4), 785–803. *Evidence Level I.*

Cole, M. G. (2007). Does depression in older medical inpatients predict mortality? A systematic review. *General Hospital Psychiatry, 29*(5), 425–430. *Evidence Level I.*

Cole, M. G., & Dendukuuri, N. (2003). Risk factors for depression among elderly community subjects: A systematic review and meta-analysis. *American Journal of Psychiatry, 160*(6), 1147–1156. *Evidence Level I.*

Conwell, Y., Duberstein, P. R., & Caine, E. D. (2002). Risk factors for suicide in later life. *Biological Psychiatry, 52*(3), 193–204. *Evidence Level VI.*

Cooper, L. A., Beach, M. C., Johnson, R. L., & Inui, T. S. (2006). Delving below the surface: Understanding how race and ethnicity influence relationships in health care. *Journal of General Internal Medicine, 21*(Suppl. 1), S21–S27. *Evidence Level VI.*

Courtney, M., O'Reilly, M., Edwards, H., & Hassall, S. (2009). The relationship between clinical outcomes and quality of life for residents of aged care facilities. *Australian Journal of Advanced Nursing, 26*(4), 49–57. *Evidence Level IV.*

Crabb, R. M., Cavanagh, K., Proudfoot, J., Learmonth, D., Rafie, S., & Weingardt, K. R. (2012). Is computerized cognitive-behavioural therapy a treatment option for depression in late-life? A systematic review. *British Journal of Clinical Psychology, 51*(4), 459–464. *Evidence Level I.*

Cukrowicz, K. C., Cheavens, J. S., Van Orden, K. A., Ragain, R. M., & Cook, R. L. (2011). Perceived burdensomeness and suicide ideation in older adults. *Psychology and Aging, 26*(2), 331–338. *Evidence Level IV.*

Debruyne, H., Van Buggenhout, M., Le Bastard, N., Aries, M., Audenaert, K., De Deyn, P. P., & Engelborghs, S. (2009). Is the Geriatric Depression Scale a reliable screening tool for depressive symptoms in elderly patients with cognitive impairment? *International Journal of Geriatric Psychiatry, 24*(6), 556–562. *Evidence Level IV.*

DeLuca, A. K., Lenze, E. J., Mulsant, B. H., Butters, M. A., Karp, J. F., Dew, M. A., . . . Reynolds, C. F., III. (2005). Comorbid anxiety disorder in late life depression: Association with memory decline over four years. *International Journal of Geriatric Psychiatry, 20*, 848–854. *Evidence Level III.*

Dhondt, T., Derksen, P., Hooijer, C., Van Heycop Ten Ham, B., Van Gent, P. P., & Heeren, T. (1999). Depressogenic medication as an aetiological factor in major depression: An analysis in a clinical population of depressed elderly people. *International Journal of Geriatric Psychiatry, 14*, 875–881. *Evidence Level IV.*

Dreizler, J., Koppitz, A., Probst, S., & Mahrer-Imhof, R. (2014). Including nurses in care models for older people with mild to moderate depression: An integrative review. *Journal of Clinical Nursing, 23*(7–8), 911–926. *Evidence Level V.*

Driscoll, H. C., Basinski, J., Mulsant, B. H., Butters, M. A., Dew, M. A., Houck, P. R., . . . Reynolds, C. F., III. (2005). Late-onset major depression: Clinical and treatment-response variability. *International Journal of Geriatric Psychiatry, 20*, 661–667. *Evidence Level IV.*

Ekers, D., Murphy, R., Archer, J., Ebenezer, C., Kemp, D., & Gilbody, S. (2013). Nurse-delivered collaborative care for depression and long-term physical conditions: A systematic review and meta-analysis. *Journal of Affective Disorders, 149*(1), 14–22. *Evidence Level I.*

Erlangsen, A., Vach, W., & Jeune, B. (2005). The effect of hospitalization with medical illnesses on the suicide risk in the oldest old: A population-based register study. *Journal of the American Geriatrics Society, 53*(5), 771–776. *Evidence Level III.*

Erlangsen, A., Zarit, S. H., Tu, X., & Conwell, Y. (2006). Suicide among older psychiatric inpatients: An evidence-based study of a high-risk group. *American Journal of Geriatric Psychiatry, 14*(9), 734–741. *Evidence Level III.*

Farrington, E., & Moller, M. (2013). Relationship of vitamin D3 deficiency to depression in older adults: A systematic review of the literature from 2008–2013. *Journal for Nurse Practitioners, 9*(8), 506–515. doi:10.1016/j.nurpra.2013.05.011. *Evidence Level I.*

Forsman, A., Jane-Llopis, E., Schierenbeck, I., & Wahlbeck, K. (2009). Psychosocial interventions for prevention of depression in older people (protocol). *Cochrane Database of Systematic Reviews, 2009*(2), CD007804. doi:10.1002/14651858.CD007804. *Evidence Level I.*

Forsman, A. K., Nordmyr, J., & Wahlbeck, K. (2011). Psychosocial interventions for the promotion of mental health and the prevention of depression among older adults. *Health Promotion International, 26*(Suppl. 1), i85–i107. *Evidence Level I.*

Gallagher-Thompson, D., & Coon, D. W. (2007). Evidence-based psychological treatments for distress in family caregivers of older adults. *Psychology and Aging, 22*(1), 37–51. *Evidence Level I.*

Gaynes, B. N., Burns, B. J., Tweed, D. L., & Erickson, P. (2002). Depression and health-related quality of life. *Journal of Nervous and Mental Disease, 190*(12), 799–806. *Evidence Level III.*

Gilman, S. E., Bruce, M. L., Have, T. T., Alexopoulos, G. S., Mulsant, B. H., Reynolds, C. F., & Cohen, A. (2012). Social inequalitites in depression and suicidal ideation among older primary care patients. *Social Psychiatry and Psychiatric Epidemiology, 48*(1), 59–69. *Evidence Level II.*

Glover, J., & Srinivasan, S. (2013). Assessment of the person with late-life depression. *Psychiatric Clinics of North America, 36*(4), 545–560. *Evidence Level IV.*

Gould, R. L., Coulson, M. C., & Howard, R. J. (2012). Cognitive behavioral therapy for depression in older people: A meta-analysis and meta-regression of randomized controlled trials. *Journal of the American Geriatrics Society, 60*(10), 1817–1830. doi:10.1111/j.1532–5415.2012.04166.x. *Evidence Level I.*

Grayson, L., & Thomas, A. (2013). A systematic review comparing clinical features in early age at onset and late age at onset late-life depression. *Journal of Affective Disorders, 150*(2), 161–170. *Evidence Level I.*

Greenberg, R. M., & Kellner, C. H. (2005). Electroconvulsive therapy: A selected review. *American Journal of Geriatric Psychiatry, 13*, 268–281. *Evidence Level V.*

Hackett, M. L., Anderson, C. S., House, A., & Xia, J. (2008). Interventions for treating depression after stroke. The Cochrane Library. Retrieved from onlinelibrary.wiley.com/doi/10.1002/1 4651858.CD003437.pub3. *Evidence Level I.*

Harpole, L. H., Williams, J. W., Jr., Olsen, M. K., Stechuchak, K. M., Oddone, E., Callahan, C. M., . . . Unützer, J. (2005). Improving depression outcomes in older adults with comorbid medical illness. *General Hospital Psychiatry, 27*(1), 4–12. *Evidence Level II.*

Hasin, D. S., & Grant, B. F. (2002). Major depression in 6050 former drinkers: Association with past alcohol dependence. *Archives of General Psychiatry, 59*, 794–800. *Evidence Level III.*

Hegel, M. T., Unützer, J., Tang, L., Areán, P. A., Katon, W., Noël, P. H., . . . Lin, E. H. (2005). Impact of comorbid panic and posttraumatic stress disorder on outcomes of collaborative care for late-life depression in primary care. *American Journal of Geriatric Psychiatry, 13*(1), 48–58. *Evidence Level II.*

Hegeman, J. M., Kok, R. M., Van Der Mast, R. C., & Giltay, E. J. (2012). Phenomenology of depression in older compared with younger adults: Meta-analysis. *British Journal of Psychiatry, 200*(4), 275–281. *Evidence Level I.*

Heisel, M. J., Links, P. S., Conn, D., van Reekum, R., & Flett, G. L. (2007). Narcissistic personality and vulnerability to late-life suicidality. *American Journal of Geriatric Psychiatry, 15*(9), 734–741. *Evidence Level IV.*

Holmes, J. D., & House, A. O. (2000). Psychiatric illness in hip fracture. *Age and Ageing, 29*(6), 537–546. *Evidence Level I.*

Hoogerduijn, J. G., Schuurmans, M. J., Duijnstee, M. S., de Rooij, S. E., & Grypdonck, M. F. (2007). A systematic review of predictors and screening instruments to identify older hospitalized patients at risk for functional decline. *Journal of Clinical Nursing, 16*(1), 46–57. *Evidence Level I.*

Huang, C. Q., Dong, B. R., Lu, Z. C., Yue, J. R., & Liu, Q. X. (2010). Chronic diseases and risk for depression in old age: A meta-analysis of published literature. *Ageing Research Reviews, 9*(2), 131–141. *Evidence Level I.*

Hybels, C. F., & Blazer, D. G. (2003). Epidemiology of late-life mental disorders. *Clinical Geriatric Medicine, 15*, 663–696. *Evidence Level IV.*

Iosifescu, D. V. (2007). Treating depression in the medically ill. *Psychiatric Clinics of North America, 30*, 77–99. *Evidence Level V.*

Jackson, J. C., Pandharipande, P. P., Girard, T. D., Brummel, N. E., Thompson, J. L., Hughes, C. G.,... Ely, E. W. (2014). Depression, post-traumatic stress disorder, and functional disability in survivors of critical illness in the BRAIN-ICU study: A longitudinal cohort study. *Lancet Respiratory Medicine, 2*(5), 369–379. *Evidence Level III.*

Jahn, D. R., & Cukrowicz, K. C. (2011). The impact of the nature of relationships on perceived burdensomeness and suicide ideation in a community sample of older adults. *Suicide and Life-Threatening Behavior, 41*(6), 635–649. *Evidence Level IV.*

Jahn, D. R., Cukrowicz, K. C., Linton, K., & Prabhu, F. (2011). The mediating effect of perceived burdensomeness on the relationship between depressive symptoms and suicide ideation in a community sample of older adults. *Aging & Mental Health, 15*(2), 214–220. *Evidence Level IV.*

Juurlink, D. N., Herrmann, N., Szalai, J. P., Kopp, A., & Redelmeier, D. A. (2004). Medical illness and the risk of suicide in the elderly. *Archives of Internal Medicine, 164*(11), 1179–1184. *Evidence Level IV.*

Kales, H. C., & Mellow, A. M. (2006). Race and depression: Does race affect the diagnosis and treatment of late-life depression? *Geriatrics, 61*(5), 18–21. *Evidence Level VI.*

Kang-Yi, C., & Gellis, Z. D. (2010). A systematic review of community-based health interventions on depression for older adults with heart disease. *Aging & Mental Health, 14*(1), 1–19. *Evidence Level I.*

Katz, I. R., Streim, J., & Parmelee, P. (1994). Prevention of depression, recurrences, and complications in late life. *Preventive Medicine, 23*, 743–750. *Evidence Level I.*

Koenig, H. G. (1991). Depressive disorders in older medical inpatients. *American Family Practice, 44*, 1243–1250. *Evidence Level VI.*

Kok, R. M. (2013). What is the role of medications in late life depression? *Psychiatric Clinics of North America, 36*(4), 597–605. *Evidence Level IV.*

Kok, R. M., Nolen, W. A., & Heeren, T. J. (2012). Efficacy of treatment in older depressed patients: A systematic review and meta-analysis of double-blind randomized controlled trials with antidepressants. *Journal of Affective Disorders, 141*(2), 103–115. *Evidence Level I.*

Kraaij, V., Arensman, E., & Spinhoven, P. (2002). Negative life events and depression in elderly persons: A meta-analysis. *Journals of Gerontology. Series B, Psychological Sciences and Social Sciences, 57*(1), P87–P94. *Evidence Level I.*

Krishna, M., Honagodu, A., Rajendra, R., Sundarachar, R., Lane, S., & Lepping, P. (2013). A systematic review and meta-analysis of group psychotherapy for sub-clinical depression in older adults. *International Journal of Geriatric Psychiatry, 28*(9), 881–888. *Evidence Level I.*

Kroenke, K., & Spitzer, R. L. (2002). The PHQ-9: A new depression diagnostic and severity measure. *Psychiatric Annals, 32*(9), 1–7. *Evidence Level III.*

Kroenke, K., Spitzer, R. L., & Williams, J. B. (2003). The Patient Health Questionnaire-2: Validity of a two-item depression screener. *Medical Care, 41*(11), 1284–1292. *Evidence Level III.*

Kronish, I. M., Rieckmann, N., Schwartz, J. E., Schwartz, D. R., & Davidson, K. W. (2009). Is depression after an acute coronary syndrome simply a marker of known prognostic factors for mortality? *Psychosomatic Medicine, 71*(7), 697–703. *Evidence Level II.*

Kuo, B., Chong, V., & Joseph, J. (2008). Depression and its psychosocial correlates among older Asian immigrants in North America: A critical review of two decades' research. *Journal of Aging & Health, 20*(6), 615–652. *Evidence Level I.*

Kurlowicz, L. H. (1994). Depression in hospitalized medically ill elders: Evolution of the concept. *Archives in Psychiatric Nursing, 8*, 124–126. *Evidence Level VI.*

Lapierre, S., Erlangsen, A., Waern, M., DeLeo, D., Oyama, H., Scocco, P., ... Quinnett, P. (2011). A systematic review of elderly suicide prevention programs. *Crisis, 32*(2), 88–89. *Evidence Level I.*

Lawton, M. P., Moss, M. S., Winter, L., & Hoffman, C. (2002). Motivation in later life: Personal projects and well-being. *Psychology & Aging, 17*(4), 539–547. *Evidence Level IV.*

Lee, S. Y., Franchetti, M. K., Imanbayev, A., Gallo, J. J., Spira, A. P., & Lee, H. B. (2012). Non-pharmacological prevention of major depression among community-dwelling older adults: A systematic review of the efficacy of psychotherapy interventions. *Archives of Gerontology and Geriatrics, 55*(3), 522–529. *Evidence Level I.*

Licht-Strunk, E., Van Marwijk, H. W. J., Hoekstra, T. B. M. J., Twisk, J. W. R., De Haan, M., & Beekman, A. T. F. (2009). Outcome of depression in later life in primary care: Longitudinal cohort study with three years' follow-up. *British Medical Journal*, 338, 1–7. Retrieved from http://www.bmj.com/content/bmj/338/bmj.a3079.full.pdf. *Evidence Level III.*

Lieverse, R., Van Someren, E. J., Nielen, M. M., Uitdehaag, B. M., Smit, J. H., & Hoogendijk, W. J. (2011). Bright light treatment in elderly patients with nonseasonal major depressive disorder: A randomized placebo-controlled trial. *Archives of General Psychiatry, 68*(1), 61–70. *Evidence Level II.*

Lin, E. H., Katon, W., Von Korff, M., Tang, L., Williams, J. W., Jr., Kroenke, K.,... Unützer, J. (2003). Effect of improving depression care on pain and functional outcomes among older adults with arthritis: A randomized controlled trial. *Journal of the American Medical Association, 290*(18), 2428–2434. *Evidence Level II.*

Luoma, J. B., Martin, C. E., & Pearson, J. L. (2002). Contact with mental health and primary care providers before suicide: A review of the evidence. *American Journal of Psychiatry, 159*, 909–916. *Evidence Level V.*

Lyness, J. M., Kim, J., Tang, W., Tu, X., Conwell, Y., King, D. A., & Caine, E. D. (2007). The clinical significance of subsyndromal depression in older primary care patients. *American Journal of Geriatric Psychiatry, 15*(3), 214–223. *Evidence Level III.*

McDade-Montez, E. A., Christensen, A. J., Cvengros, J. A., & Lawton, W. J. (2006). The role of depression symptoms in dialysis withdrawal. *Health Psychology, 25*(2), 198–204. *Evidence Level IV.*

McKeowen, R. E., Cuffe, S. P., & Schulz, R. M. (2006). U.S. suicide rates by age group, 1970–2002: An examination of recent trends. *American Journal of Public Health, 96*(10), 1744–1751. *Evidence Level V.*

Meeks, T. W., Vahia, I. V., Lavretsky, H., Kulkarni, G., & Jeste, D. V. (2011). A tune in "a minor" can "b major": A review of epidemiology, illness course, and public health implications of subthreshold depression in older adults. *Journal of Affective Disorders, 129*(1), 126–142. *Evidence Level I.*

Mezuk, B., Edwards, L., Lohman, M., Choi, M., & Lapane, K. (2012). Depression and frailty in later life: A synthetic review. *International Journal of Geriatric Psychiatry, 27*(9), 879–892. *Evidence Level V.*

Mitchell, A. J., Bird, V., Rizzo, M., & Meader, N. (2010). Diagnostic validity and added value of the Geriatric Depression Scale for depression in primary care: A meta-analysis of GDS 30 and GDS 15. *Journal of Affective Disorders, 125*(1), 10–17. *Evidence Level I.*

Mitchell, A. J., & Subramaniam, H. (2005). Prognosis of depression in old age compared to middle age: A systematic review of comparative studies. *American Journal of Psychiatry, 162*(9), 1588–1601. *Evidence Level I.*

Modrego, P. J., & Ferrandez, J. (2004). Depression in patients with mild cognitive impairment increases the risk of developing dementia of Alzheimer type: A prospective cohort study. *Archives in Neurology, 61*, 1290–1293. *Evidence Level IV.*

Morimoto, S. S., & Alexopoulos, G. S. (2013). Cognitive deficits in geriatric depression: Clinical correlates and implications for current and future treatment. *Psychiatric Clinics of North America, 36*(4), 517–531. *Evidence Level V.*

Navarro, V., Gastó, C., Torres, X., Masana, G., Penadés, R., Guarch, J.,... Catalán, R. (2008). Continuation/maintenance treatment with nortriptyline versus combined nortriptyline and ECT in late-life psychotic depression: A two-year randomized study. *American Journal of Geriatric Psychiatry, 16*(6), 498–505. *Evidence Level II.*

Nelson, J. C., Delucchi, K., & Schneider, L. S. (2008). Efficacy of second generation antidepressants in late-life depression: A meta-analysis of the evidence. *American Journal of Geriatric Psychiatry, 16*(7), 558–567. *Evidence Level I.*

Neufeld, E., Freeman, S., Joling, K., & Hirdes, J. P. (2014). "When the golden years are blue": Changes in depressive symptoms over time among older adults newly admitted to long-term care facilities. *Clinical Gerontologist, 37*(3), 298–315. *Evidence Level III.*

Neufeld, E., Hirdes, J. P., Perlman, C. M., & Rabinowitz, T. (2015). Risk and protective factors associated with intentional self-harm among older community-residing home care clients in Ontario, Canada. *International Journal of Geriatric Psychiatry, Advance online publication, 30*(10), 1032–1040. *Evidence Level IV.*

Nyer, M., Doorley, J., Durham, K., Yeung, A. S., Freeman, M. P., & Mischoulon, D. (2013). What is the role of alternative treatments in late-life depression? *Psychiatric Clinics of North America, 36*(4), 577–596. *Evidence Level VI.*

Onrust, S. A., & Cuijpers, P. (2006). Mood and anxiety disorders in widowhood: A systematic review. *Aging & Mental Health, 10*(4), 327–334. *Evidence Level I.*

Orgeta, V., Qazi, A., Spector, A. E., & Orrell, M. (2014). Psychological treatments for depression and anxiety in dementia and mild cognitive impairment. *Cochrane Library*, (1), 1–62. *Evidence Level I.*

Pfaff, J. J., & Almeida, O. P. (2005). Detecting suicidal ideation in older patients: Identifying risk factors within the general practice setting. *British Journal of General Practice, 55*(513), 261–262. *Evidence Level IV.*

Pinquart, M., Duberstein, P. R., & Lyness, J. M. (2006). Treatments for later-life depressive conditions: A meta-analytic comparison of pharmacotherapy and psychotherapy. *American Journal of Psychiatry, 163*(9), 1493–1501. *Evidence Level I.*

Pinquart, M., & Forstmeier, S. (2012). Effects of reminiscence interventions on psychosocial outcomes: A meta-analysis. *Aging & Mental Health, 16*(5), 541–558. *Evidence Level I.*

Pinquart, M., & Sorensen, S. (2004). Associations of caregiver stressors and uplifts with subjective well-being and depressive mood: A meta-analytic comparison. *Aging & Mental Health, 8*(5), 438–449. *Evidence Level I.*

Plakiotis, C., Barson, F., Vengadasalam, B., Haines, T. P., & O'Connor, D. W. (2013). Balance and gain in older electroconvulsive therapy recipients: A pilot study. *Neuropsychiatric Disease and Treatment, 3*(9), 805–812. *Evidence Level III.*

Richard-Devantoy, S., Szanto, K., Butters, M. A., Kalkus, J., & Dombrowski, A. Y. (2014). Cognitive inhibition in older high-lethality suicide attempts. *International Journal of Geriatric Psychiatry, 30*, 274–283. *Evidence Level IV.*

Richardson, T. M., He, H., Podgorski, C., Tu, X., & Conwell, Y. (2010). Screening depression aging services clients. *American Journal of Geriatric Psychiatry, 18*(12), 1116–1123. *Evidence Level III.*

Rizzo, M., Creed, F., Goldberg, D., Meader, N., & Pilling, S. (2011). A systematic review of non-pharmacological treatments for depression in people with chronic physical health problems. *Journal of Psychosomatic Research, 71*(1), 18–27. *Evidence Level I.*

Rogers, C. E., Larkey, L. K., & Keller, C. (2009). A review of clinical trials of tai chi and qigong in older adults. *Western Journal of Nursing Research, 31*(2), 245–279. *Evidence Level I.*

Rorup, M. L., Deeg, D. J. H., Poppelaars, J. L., Kerkhof, A. J. F. M., & Onwuteaka-Philipsen, B. D. (2011). Wishes to die in older people: A quantitative study of prevalence and associated factors. *Crisis, 32*(4), 194–203. *Evidence Level IV.*

Royer, M., Ballentine, N. H., Eslinger, P. J., Houser, K., Mistrick, R., Behr, R., & Rakos, K. (2012). Light therapy for seniors in long term care. *Journal of the American Medical Directors Association, 13*(2), 100–102. *Evidence Level III.*

Rushing, N. C., Corsentino, E., Hames, J. L., Sachs-Ericsson, N., & Steffens, D. (2013). The relationship of religious involvement indicators and social support to current and past suicidality among depressed older adults. *Aging & Mental Health, 17*(3), 366–374. *Evidence Level IV.*

Sachs-Ericsson, N., Corsention, E., Rushing, N. C., & Sheffler, J. (2013). Early childhood abuse and later-life suicidal ideation. *Aging & Mental Health, 17*(4), 489–494. *Evidence Level IV.*

Sadule-Rios, N. (2012). A review of the literature about depression in late life among Hispanics in the United States. *Issues in Mental Health Nursing, 33*(7), 458–468. doi:10.3109/01612840.2012.675415. *Evidence Level V.*

Sanhueza, C., Ryan, L., & Foxcroft, D. R. (2013). Diet and the risk of unipolar depression in adults: Systematic review of cohort studies. *Journal of Human Nutrition & Dietetics, 26*(1), 56–70. doi:10.1111/j.1365-277X.2012.01283.x. *Evidence Level I.*

Sareen, J., Cox, B. J., Afifi, T. O., de Graaf, R., Asmundson, G. J., ten Have, M., & Stein, M. B. (2005). Anxiety disorders and risk for suicidal ideation and suicide attempts: A population-based longitudinal study of adults. *Archives of General Psychiatry, 62*(11), 1249–1257. *Evidence Level IV.*

Schulz, R., Drayer, R. A., & Rollman, B. L. (2002). Depression as a risk factor for non-suicide mortality in the elderly. *Biological Psychiatry, 52*(3), 205–225. *Evidence Level IV.*

Seong-Hi, P., Kuem Sun, H., & Chang-Bum, K. (2014). Effects of exercise programs on depressive symptoms, quality of life, and self-esteem in older people: A systematic review of randomized controlled trials. *Applied Nursing Research, 27*(4), 219–226. doi:10.1016/j.apnr.2014.01.004. *Evidence Level I.*

Sexton, C., Mackay, C., & Ebmeier, K. (2013). A systematic review and meta-analysis of magnetic resonance imaging studies in late-life depression. *American Journal of Geriatric Psychiatry, 21*(2), 184–195. doi:10.1016/j.jagp.2012.10.019. *Evidence Level I.*

Sheikh, J. I., & Yesavage, J. A. (1986). Geriatric depression scale (GDS) recent evidence and development of a shorter version. *Clinical Gerontologist, 5*, 165–173. *Evidence Level V.*

Siedliecki, S. L., & Good, M. (2006). Effect of music on power, pain, depression, and disability. *Journal of Advanced Nursing, 54*(5), 553–562. *Evidence Level IV.*

Simon, M. A., Chen, R., Chang, E. S., & Dong, X. (2014). The association between filial piety and suicidal ideation: Findings from a community-dwelling Chinese aging population. *Journals of Gerontology. Series A, Biological Sciences and Medical Sciences, 69*(2), S90–S97. *Evidence Level IV.*

Sjosten, N., & Kivela, S. L. (2006). The effects of physical exercise on depressive symptoms among the aged: A systematic review. *International Journal of Geriatric Psychiatry, 21*(5), 410–418. *Evidence Level I.*

Smalbrugge, M., Pot, A. M., Jongenelis, L., Gundy, C. M., Beekman, A. T., & Eefsting, J. A. (2006). The impact of depression and anxiety on well being, disability and use of health care services in nursing home patients. *International Journal of Geriatric Psychiatry, 21*(4), 325–332. *Evidence Level IV.*

Smith, M., Haedtke, C., & Shibley, B. (2015). Late-life depression detection. *Journal of Gerontological Nursing,* 41(2), 18–25. *Evidence Level V.*

Snowdon, J. (2001). Is depression more prevalent in old age? *Australian and New Zealand Journal of Psychiatry, 35*, 782–787. *Evidence Level VI.*

Song, D., Shen, Q., Xu, T. Z., & Sun, Q. H. (2014). Effects of group reminiscence on elderly depression: A meta-analysis. *International Journal of Nursing Sciences, 1*(4), 416–422. *Evidence Level I.*

Spaans, H. P., Sienaert, P., Bouckaert, F., van den Berg, J. F., Verwijk, E., Kho, K. H., . . . Kok, R. M. (2015). Speed of remission in elderly patients with depression: Electroconvulsive therapy v. medication. *British Journal of Psychiatry, 206*, 67–71. *Evidence Level II.*

Stapleton, R. D., Nielsen, E. L., Engelberg, R. A., Patrick, D. L., & Curtis, J. R. (2005). Association of depression and life-sustaining treatment. *Chest, 127*(1), 328–334. *Evidence Level III.*

Steffens, D. C. (2008). Separating mood disturbance from mild cognitive impairment in geriatric depression. *International Review of Psychiatry, 20*(4), 374–381. *Evidence Level V.*

Stone, M., Laughren, T., Jones, M. L., Levenson, M., Holland, P. C., Hughes, A., . . . Rochester G. (2009). Risk of suicidality in clinical trials of antidepressants in adults: Analysis of proprietary data submitted to US Food and Drug Administration. *British Medical Journal, 339*, b2880. doi:10.1136/bmj.b2880. *Evidence Level I.*

Szanto, K., Dombrovski, A. Y., Sahakian, B. J., Mulsant, B. H., Houck, P. R., Reynolds, C. F., . . . Phil, D. (2012). Social emotion recognition, social functioning, and attempted suicide in late-life depression. *American Journal of Geriatric Psychiatry, 20*(3), 257–265. *Evidence Level IV.*

Szanto, K., Mulsant, B. H., Houck, P., Dew, M. A., & Reynolds, C. F., III. (2003). Occurrence and course of suicidality during short-term treatment of late-life depression. *Archives of General Psychiatry, 60*(6), 610–617. *Evidence Level IV.*

Taylor, W. D. (2014). Depression in the elderly. *New England Journal of Medicine, 371*(13), 1228–1236. *Evidence Level IV.*

Teri, L., Mckenzie, G., & LaFazia, D. (2005). Psychosocial treatment of depression in older adults with dementia. *Clinical Psychology: Science and Practice, 12*(3), 303–316. *Evidence Level I.*

Thompson, S., Herrmann, N., Rapoport, M. J., & Lanctôt, K. L. (2007). Efficacy and safety of antidepressants for treatment of depression in Alzheimer's disease: A meta-analysis. *Canadian Journal of Psychiatry. Revue Canadienne De Psychiatrie, 52*(4), 248–255. *Evidence Level I.*

Turvey, C. L., Conwell, Y., Jones, M. P., Phillips, C., Simonsick, E., Pearson, J. L., & Wallace, R. (2002). Risk factors for late-life suicide: A prospective, community-based study. *American Journal of Geriatric Psychiatry, 10*(4), 398–406. *Evidence Level III.*

Unützer, J. (2007). Late-life depression. *New England Journal of Medicine, 357*(22), 2269–2276. *Evidence Level IV.*

Unützer, J., Katon, W., Callahan, C. M., Williams, J. W., Jr., Hunkeler, E., Harpole, L., . . . Langston, C. (2002). Collaborative care management of late-life depression in the primary care setting: A randomized controlled trial. *Journal of the American Medical Association, 288*(22), 2836–2845. *Evidence Level II.*

Van der Wurff, F. B., Stek, M., Hoogendijk, W. J. G., & Beekman, A. T. (2003). The efficacy and safety of ECT in depressed older adults: A literature review. *International Journal of Geriatric Psychiatry, 34*, 894–904. *Evidence Level V.*

Van Orden, K. A., O'Riley, A. A., Simning, A., Padgorski, C., Richardson, T. M. & Conwell, Y. (2014). Passive suicide ideation: An indicator of risk among older adults seeking aging services? *The Gerontologist, Advance online publication 55*(6), 972–980. Retrieved from http://gerontologist.oxfordjournals.org/content/early/2014/04/04/geront.gnu026.full. *Evidence Level IV.*

Van Shaik, A. M., Comijs, H. C., Sonnenberg, C. M., Beekman, A. T., Sienaert, P., & Stek, M. L. (2010). Efficacy and safety of continuation and maintenance electroconvulsive therapy in depressed elderly patients: A systematic review. *Geriatric Psychiatry, 20*(1), 5–17. *Evidence Level I.*

Vink, D., Aartsen, M. J., & Schoevers, R. A. (2008). Risk factors for anxiety and depression in the elderly: A review. *Journal of Affective Disorders, 106*(1–2), 29–44. *Evidence Level I.*

Virnig, B., Huang, Z., Lurie, N., Musgrave, D., McBean, A. M., & Dowd, B. (2004). Does Medicare managed care provide equal treatment for mental illness across races? *Archives of General Psychiatry, 61*, 201–205. *Evidence Level IV.*

Voyer, P., & Martin, L. S. (2003). Improving geriatric mental health nursing care: Making a case for going beyond psychotropic medications. *International Journal of Mental Health Nursing, 12*(1), 11–21. *Evidence Level VI.*

Waern, M., Rubenowitz, E., & Wilhelmson, K. (2003). Predictors of suicide in the old elderly. *Gerontology, 49*(5), 328–334. *Evidence Level V.*

Walker, E. M., & Steffens, D. C. (2010). Understanding depression and cognitive impairment in the elderly. *Psychiatric Annals, 40*(1), 29–40. *Evidence Level IV.*

Wang, C., Bannuru, R., Ramel, J., Kupelnick, B., Scott, T., & Schmid, C. H. (2010). Tai chi on psychological well-being: systematic review and meta-analysis. *BMC Complementary and Alternative Medicine, 10*(1), 23. *Evidence Level I.*

Wiktorsson, S., Runeson, B., Skoog, I., Ostling, S., & Waern, M. (2010). Attempted suicide in the elderly: Characteristics of suicide attempters 70 years and older and a general population comparison group. *American Journal of Geriatric Psychiatry, 18*(1), 57–67. *Evidence Level IV.*

Williams, D. R., González, H. M., Neighbors, H., Nesse, R., Abelson, J. M., Sweetman, J., & Jackson, J. S. (2007). Prevalence and distribution of major depressive disorder in African Americans, Caribbean blacks, and non-Hispanic Whites: Results from the National Survey of American Life. *Archives in General Psychiatry, 64*(3), 305–315. *Evidence Level IV.*

Wilson, K. C., Mottram, P. G., & Vassilas, C. A. (2008). Psychotherapeutic treatments for older depressed people. *Cochrane Database of Systematic Reviews, 2008*(1), CD004853. *Evidence Level I.*

Wu, Q., Magnus, J. H., Liu, J., Bencaz, A. F., & Hentz, J. G. (2009). Depression and low bone mineral density: A meta-analysis of epidemiologic studies. *Osteoporosis International: A Journal Established as Result of Cooperation Between the European Foundation for Osteoporosis and the National Osteoporosis Foundation of the USA, 20*(8), 1309–1320. *Evidence Level I.*

16

Dementia: A Neurocognitive Disorder

Kathleen Fletcher

EDUCATIONAL OBJECTIVES

On completion of this chapter, the reader should be able to:

1. Describe the spectrum of dementia syndromes
2. Recognize the clinical features of dementia
3. Discuss pharmacological and nonpharmacological approaches in the management of dementia
4. Develop a nursing plan of care for an older adult with dementia

OVERVIEW

Dementia is most commonly defined as a clinical syndrome of cognitive decline. The term *dementia* was eliminated and replaced with "major or minor neurocognitive disorder" in the latest *Diagnostic and Statistical Manual on Mental Health Disorders* (5th ed.; *DSM-5*; American Psychiatric Association, 2013). It was felt that the term dementia was stigmatizing and the focus should be on decline rather than deficit. Because these changes are confusing to many health care professionals and the term dementia remains established in the literature, the terms dementia and *neurocognitive disorder* are used interchangeably in this chapter. In addition to disruptions in cognition, dementia is associated with a gradual decline in function and changes in mood and behavior.

There are many causes of dementia and dementia-like presentations. Differentiating these changes early in the course of illness is important because condition-specific assessment, monitoring, and management strategies can be employed. Differential diagnoses among conditions that cause cognitive impairment are confounded by the fact that these conditions may coexist and disparate neurocognitive disorders may be similarly clinically expressed.

Major goals in the clinical approach to a person presenting with cognitive impairments are identification and resolution of potentially reversible conditions (e.g., delirium, depression), recognition, and control of comorbid conditions, early diagnosis and management of a neurocognitive disorder, and the provision of caregiver support. The focus of this chapter is on assessment and management of the major neurocognitive disorders.

BACKGROUND AND STATEMENT OF PROBLEM

Global estimates reflect that 44.4 million people have dementia today, which will increase to 75.6 million by 2030 and 135.5 million by 2050 (Alzheimer's Disease International, 2013). The rapid growth of the older adult population in the United States is associated with a significant increase in the prevalence of dementia. Dementia affects about 11% of individuals 65 years and older (Alzheimer's Association, 2015). The prevalence increases exponentially with age, rising to

For a description of evidence levels cited in this chapter, see Chapter 1, "Developing and Evaluating Clinical Practice Guidelines: A Systematic Approach."

nearly 32% in individuals 85 years and older (Hebert, Weuve, Scherr, & Evans, 2013). More than 4.7 million individuals in the United States have the most common form of dementia, Alzheimer's disease (AD), a number that is projected to increase to 13.8 million by 2050 (Hebert et al., 2013).

This chapter discusses the most common forms of progressive dementia, AD, vascular dementia (VaD), dementia with Lewy bodies (DLB), and frontotemporal dementia (FTD). Less common, though not less significant, is progressive dementia associated with Parkinson's disease (PDD), dementias associated with HIV, and Creutzfeldt–Jacob disease.

AD, the most common form of dementia, accounts for more than 80% of all cases. A chronic neurodegenerative disease, first described by Alos Alzheimer in 1907, it is characterized by neurofibrillary plaques and "tangles" in the brain. The extracellular accumulation of amyloid beta proteins in the neuritic plaques is one of the hallmarks of AD (Ariga, Miyatake, & Yu, 2010). The variation in the clinical presentation of the disease depends on the area of the brain that is affected. Classic features of AD include progressive loss of memory, deterioration of language and other cognitive functions, decline in the ability to perform activities of daily living (ADL), and changes in personality and behavior and judgment dysfunction (Castellani, Rolston, & Smith, 2010). Mild cognitive impairment (MCI) represents a transitional state between healthy aging and dementia and is characterized by cognitive impairment out of proportion to the age of the individual yet the individual does not meet the criteria for dementia (Yanhong, Chandra, & Venkitesh, 2013). Incidence rates of MCI are 51 to 76.8 per 1,000 person-years with a higher incidence in advanced age, lower education, and hypertension (Luck, Luppa, Briel, & Riedel-Heller, 2010). About 35% of MCI patients progress to AD, with an annual conversion rate of 5% to 10% (Mitchell, 2009). Cerebrospinal fluid (CSF) biomarkers' performance is the most convenient test predicting conversion yet it remains suboptimal (Ferreira et al., 2014).

VaD, sometimes referred to as vascular cognitive impairment (VCI) and previously known as multi-infarct dementia (MID), refers to dementia resulting from cerebrovascular disease. It is the second most common cause of dementia among older adults and represents approximately 20% of all cases of dementia in the United States (Román, 2003). The link between AD and VaD is strong yet not entirely clear (de la Torre, 2012). There are many types of VaD and lumping them under a single rubric causes some diagnostic confusion (Kirshner, 2009). The onset of VaD is usually more acute than AD and the diagnosis of VaD is based on the association between a cerebrovascular event and the onset of clinical features of dementia, including evidence of focal deficits, gait disturbances, personality and mood changes, and impairments in executive function. As compared with AD, memory may not be impaired or is more mildly affected. It is not uncommon that AD and VaD pathology coexist and this, often referred to as a mixed dementia, is likely to increase as the population ages (Langa, Foster, & Larson, 2004).

DLB accounts for about one in 25 diagnosed cases of dementia (Vann Jones & O'Brien, 2014). DLB is a neurodegenerative dementia that results when Lewy bodies form in the brain. Lewy bodies are pathological aggregations of alpha-synuclein found in the cytoplasma of neurons (McKeith et al., 2003). Clinical features include cognitive and behavioral changes in combination with features of parkinsonism. Disorders of executive function occur early. Hallucinations, visual–spatial disturbances and sleep disorders are prominent. Rigidity and unsteady gait are common. Many (but not all) patients with PDD develop a dementia years after the motor symptoms appear. Distinctions have been made clinically between DLB and the dementia associated with PDD based on the sequence of the appearance of symptoms over the time course. In PDD, motor symptoms precede cognitive impairment, while DLB begins with fluctuations in cognition (Mayo & Bordelon, 2014). DLB and PDD may represent the same pathological process along a disease spectrum (Hanson & Lippa, 2009).

FTD, with a prevalence of 15 per 100,000, refers to a group of progressive brain diseases with clinical manifestations dominated by behavioral changes and/or impairments in language (Riedl, MacKenzie, Forsti, Kurz, & Diehl-Schmid, 2014). A growing body of evidence indicates that FTD and amyotrophic lateral sclerosis (ALS) share some clinical, pathological, and molecular features as part of a common neurogenerative spectrum disorder (Gascon & Gao, 2014).

The National Alzheimer's Project Act of 2011 mandates a national plan to address AD and related dementias (specifically VaD, mixed dementia, DLB, and FTD; Montine et al., 2014).

ASSESSMENT OF THE PROBLEM

Goals of Assessment

Early identification of cognitive impairment is the most important goal in assessment. Cognitive impairment resulting from conditions like dementia, delirium, or depression represents critically serious pathology and requires urgent assessment and tailored interventions. Yet, diminished or altered cognitive functioning is often perceived by health care professionals as a normal consequence of aging and opportunities for timely intervention are too often missed

(Milisen, Braes, Fick, & Foreman, 2006). Although distinctions have been made comparing the clinical features of the common cognitive impairments associated with delirium, dementia, and depression, this is difficult to do clinically because these conditions often coexist and older adults can demonstrate atypical features in any of these conditions.

The second most important assessment goal is to identify a potentially reversible primary or contributing cause of a cognitive impairment. The common causes of reversible cognitive impairment (delirium) in the older adult are covered in Chapter 17, "Delirium: Prevention, Early Recognition, and Treatment."

History Taking

Complaints from the patient or observations made by others of memory loss, problems with decision making and/or judgment, or a decline in function in an activity of daily living should alert the health care professional that a progressive form of dementia might exist. Collecting an accurate history is the cornerstone to the assessment process, yet this obviously is a challenge in the individual presenting with cognitive impairment. The assessment domains covered in history taking include functional, cognitive, and behavioral queries and observations. The history-taking process involves first interviewing the patient followed, perhaps, by clarifying, elaborating, and validating information with the family or others familiar with the capabilities and expressions of the patient. An informant questionnaire on cognitive decline can also provide utility with the commonly used tool being the Informant Questionnaire on Cognitive Decline in the Elderly (IQCODE). Although the accuracy is reasonable its use alone may result in misdiagnosis or false reassurance (Quinn et al., 2014), underscoring the need for a comprehensive evaluation.

Even when a diagnosis of dementia has been made, it is often not communicated well across care settings. The easiest way to increase recognition of dementia in older hospital patients is to add the items "severe memory problems," "Alzheimer's disease," and "dementia" to the list of diseases and conditions patients and families are routinely asked about on intake forms and in intake interviews.

Functional Assessment

Dementia is characterized by deterioration in the ability to perform ADL. Because cognitive assessment can be embarrassing and/or threatening it may be more respectful to initiate the conversation around the patient's functional domain. Asking the patient to elaborate on his or her functional abilities in ADL as well as instrumental activities of daily living (IADL) and eliciting any identified decline with specified chronology can provide some insight. The reader is referred to Chapter 6, "Assessing Cognitive Function" for a general approach and tools for functional assessment. Several functional tools have been tested specifically in individuals with dementia.

The Functional Activities Questionnaire (FAQ) is an informant-based measure of functional ability and has been recognized for its ability to discriminate early dementia. An informant, typically the primary caregiver, is asked to rate the performance of the patient in 10 different activities. The Functional Assessment Staging Test (FAST) has been used to effectively discriminate among normal cognition, MCI, and dementia and has proven to be useful in measuring functional performance (Rikkert et al., 2011; Teng et al., 2010). The Alzheimer's Disease Cooperative Study (ADCS)–ADL inventory is a specific functional tool used primarily in clinical drug trials to assess and monitor patients with moderate to severe AD (Galasko et al., 1997). Clinical studies using this scale have indicated that cholinesterase inhibitors offer an effective approach to treating functional decline in certain forms of dementia (Potkin, 2002) and lower scores on ADCS-ADL are predictive of nursing home placement (Miller, Schneider, & Rosenheck, 2011). The patient's daily caregiver is asked to rate the older adult's usual performance on the more basic measures of function over the previous month to identify progression of functional decline. It has been recognized that individuals with a frontotemporal behavioral-variant form of dementia may have greater functional impairment than those with other forms of dementia (Lima-Silva, Bahia, Nitrini, & Yassuda, 2013). In addition to looking for potential treatments this rating helps to provide an explanation to the patient and family for advance care planning while the patient is still capable of decision making. As technology continues to advance, the manually based functional assessments may be replaced by technology-based ones (Lowe et al., 2013).

Cognitive Assessment

The cognitive domain is assessed as part of a broader mental status evaluation, the components of which are listed in Table 16.1. Although some of the parameters of a mental status evaluation (such as memory or cognition) might be measured with a standardized tool, such as the Mini-Mental State Exam (MMSE), others require specific inquiry or direct or indirect observation by the health care professional and/or caregiver. The measure of mood is totally subjective and is based on self-report status. The evaluation always provides the opportunity to identify sensory impairments (vision and hearing loss), which can further impact cognition, function,

TABLE 16.1
Components of Mental Status Evaluation

State of consciousness: quality or state of awareness
General appearance and behavior: appropriately groomed and interactive
Orientation: person, place, time
Attention and concentration: ability to attend and concentrate
Memory: ability to register, recall, retain
Judgment and insight: ability to make appropriate decisions
Executive control functions: ability to abstract, plan, sequence, and use feedback to guide performance
Visual–spatial function: ability to mentally manipulate a figure
Speech and language: ability to communicate ideas and receive and express a message
Thought content: presence of delusions, hallucinations
Mood and affect: how individual feels most days and at a given moment and the appropriateness of behavior demonstrated

and behavior. There are a variety of tools for assessing cognitive impairment, some more sensitive to mild dementia and others to moderate to severe dementia.

The gold standard of tools that measure cognition is the MMSE, which was developed over 30 years ago (Folstein, Folstein, & McHugh, 1975). Used extensively in clinical trials as well as in a variety of clinical settings, it is relatively easy to administer and score and can be used to assess cognitive changes over time. The annual rate of decline on the MMSE in AD is 3.3 points annually (Han, Cole, Bellavance, McCusker, & Primeau, 2000). The MMSE has established validity and reliability although concerns continue to be expressed by clinicians that it is time-consuming and in some circumstances the relevancy of selected questions has been raised. The MMSE score is strongly related to education with high false-positive rates for those with little education; predictive power is also significantly influenced by language (Parker & Philp, 2004). It is insensitive to executive dysfunction and has been criticized for a lack of sensitivity in detecting early or mild dementia (Liefer, 2003). As has been suggested with other measures of cognitive testing, the MMSE may have a cultural bias (Manly & Espino, 2004). Clinicians must remain aware that a high score on the MMSE does not rule out cognitive decline or the possibility of dementia particularly in high-functioning individuals with cognitive complaints (Manning, 2004). The tool is no longer in the public domain and copyright permission must be secured. A tool with comparable sensitivity and specificity for detecting dementia is the St. Louis University Mental Status Exam (SLUMS) and it is available for free (Tariq, Tumosa, Chibnall, Perry, & Morley, 2006).

Instruments, such as the Mini-Cog (Borson, 2003), Memory Impairment Screen (Buschke, 1999), and General Practitioner Assessment of Cognition (Brodaty, 2002), have all been recognized for utility, whereas the Clock Draw test (CDT, Shulman, 2000) and newer instruments, such as the Montreal Cognitive Assessment (MoCA, Nasrredine et al., 2005), have greater sensitivity, address frontotemporal executive function and have less educational and cultural bias (Ismail, Rajji, & Shulman, 2010). Unlike the more language-based tools described earlier, the CDT assesses cognition focused on executive function. A systematic review of the literature identified the CDT's usefulness in predicting future cognitive impairment (Peters & Pinto, 2008). Scoring is based on the ability to free-hand draw the face of a clock, insert the hour numbers in the appropriate location, and then set the hands of the clock to the time designated by the examiner. The CDT is strongly correlated with executive function (i.e., the ability to execute complex behaviors and to solve problems) and is useful in the detection of mild dementia (Peters & Pinto, 2008). It also correlates moderately with driving performance, as the CDT score drops the number of driving errors increases (Freund, Gravenstein, Ferris, Burke, & Shaheen, 2005; Freund, Gravenstein, Ferris, & Shaheen, 2002).

A clinically useful tool that combines the CDT with measures of cognition (three-word recall) is the Mini-Cognitive (Mini-Cog; Borson, Scanlan, Brush, Vitaliano, & Dokmak, 2000). The Mini-Cog detected cognitive impairment in a community sample of predominately ethnic minority better than primary care physician assessment (84% vs. 41%) particularly in milder stages of the disease (Borson, Scanlan, Watanabe, Tu, & Lessig, 2005).

A systematic review of the Mini-Cog for screening for dementia in primary care demonstrated that it was brief; easy to administer; clinically acceptable and effective; and minimally affected by education, gender, and ethnicity (Milne, Culverwell, Guss, Tuppen, & Whelton, 2008) with psychometric properties similar to the MMSE (Brodaty, Low, Gibson, & Burns, 2006).

Behavioral Assessment

Behavioral changes occur both in early-stage and throughout dementia (Kilik et al., 2008), and are also seen in MCI; commonly these include depression, anxiety, and irritability (Monastero, Mangialasche, Camarda, Ercolani, & Camarda, 2009). Regular assessment and monitoring can help identify the triggers of disruptive behavior and early manifestations of the behavior. Timely interventions that result in de-escalation of the behavior can help decrease the level of distress experienced both by the patient and caregiver. Behavioral management can help maintain functionality and safety. Commonly demonstrated behaviors are those associated with agitation and psychosis. Asking the patient about levels of restlessness, anxiety, and irritability is important, as at times these emotional/behavioral states occur even earlier than cognitive changes. Aggression, wandering, delusions and hallucinations, and resistance to care are manageable with nonpharmacological and pharmacological treatment options.

The literature on the link between psychosis and aggression in people with dementia is mixed (Shub, Ball, Abbas, Gottumukkala, & Kunik, 2010). The Neuropsychiatric Inventory (NPI, Cummings, 1994) measures frequency and severity of psychiatric symptoms and behavioral manifestations in individuals with dementia. The NPI takes about 10 minutes to administer during which the caregiver is asked screening and probing questions related to the presence and degree of behaviors such as agitation, anxiety, irritability, apathy, and disinhibition. The NPI also includes a measure of caregiver stress. It has established validity and reliability though it does not discriminate between disorder types (Lai, 2014).

Because as many as 50% of individuals with dementia have coexisting depressive symptoms (Lee & Lyketsos, 2003), it is important to conduct an adjunctive assessment of depression. Recognizing depressive symptoms in older adults is challenging and using an interviewer-rated instrument is recommended in addition to using clinical judgment (Onega, 2006). The Geriatric Depression Scale (GDS) is a screening instrument that takes only a few minutes to administer and is discussed along with appropriate depression-management strategies in detail in a Chapter 15, "Late-Life Depression."

Referral of the patient to a neuropsychologist for more extensive neuro psychological testing is often indicated in order to provide more specific diagnostic information associated with neurodegenerative disease states and areas of brain dysfunction. This kind of assessment can identify subtle cognitive impairments in higher functioning individuals, distinguish MCI from dementia, and can provide direction and support for care providers and the family (Adelman & Daly, 2005).

Physical Examination and Diagnostics

Once the functional, cognitive, and behavioral domains in progressive dementia have been established through history taking of the patient and caregiver, a thorough review of systems is undertaken followed by the physical examination. The history-taking process narrows the differential diagnosis of reversible and irreversible causes for dementia. A thorough neurological and cardiovascular examination will help to specify the etiology of a single type or combined dementia, which will direct the need for laboratory and imaging tests. Cardiovascular findings, such as hypertension, arrhythmias, extra heart sounds or murmurs, along with focal neurological findings, such as weakness and sensory deficit, may favor a diagnosis of VaD, pathological reflexes, gait disorders, and abnormal cerebellar findings that may be indicative of AD, and parkinsonian signs that might indicate dementia associated with either Lewy bodies or PDD (Kane, Ouslander, Abrass, & Resnick, 2013).

There are no specific laboratory tests for the diagnosis of progressive dementia other than those that can primarily indicate a potentially reversible or contributing cause (see Table 16.1 and Chapter 17). The American Academy of Neurology (AAN) recommends two specific laboratory tests (thyroid function and B_{12}) in the initial evaluation of suspected dementia (Knopman et al., 2001). The AAN similarly recommends that all patients with suspected dementia have an MRI study or non-contrast CT as part of the initial workup. Once dementia has become clinically relevant and a cause apparent, there is no further diagnostic yield afforded by imaging.

Caregiver Assessment

It is important to remember that the caregiver is a patient too in that he or she suffers, as does the patient with dementia. Caregiver need and burden refer to the psychological, physical, and financial burden associated with caregiving. Caregivers are at risk of depression, physical illness, and anxiety (Cooper, Balamurali, & Livingston, 2007; Schoenmakers, Buntinx, & Delepeleire, 2010). Behavioral problems are determinants of burden yet feeling confident and positive self-efficacy can diminish caregiver burden (van der Lee, Bakker, Dunenvooden, & Droes, 2014). The Zarit Burden Interview (ZBI) can be used to identify the degree of burden experienced by the caregiver. The ZBI is a four-item screening followed by an additional 12 items; the test has good reliability and validity (Higginson, Gao, Jackson, Murray, & Harding, 2010). Administration of this tool to a community-dwelling caregiver can indicate the extent of impact caregiving has on the caregiver's health, social and emotional well-being, and finances. The Modified Caregiver Strain Index (CSI) is another tool that has been used to identify families with caregiving concerns (Onega, 2008). There is a growing body of literature that describes the relationship between people with dementia and the family members who care for them (Ablitt, Jones, & Muers, 2009).

INTERVENTIONS AND CARE STRATEGIES

There is no cure for progressive dementia. The management of individuals with dementia requires pharmacological and nonpharmacological interventions.

Pharmacological Interventions

The goals of pharmacological therapy in dementia include preserving what the disease destroys in cognitive and functional ability, minimizing what the disease imposes in the way of behavior disturbances, and slowing the progression of the disease effects brought on by the destruction of neurons (Geldmacher, 2003). Nurses, regardless of whether they are the prescribers of drug therapy, need to be informed about the variety of drugs used in managing dementia and the evidence supporting their pharmacological approaches. Although there is substantial evidence that adults with mild to severe AD would benefit from drug therapy, there are no solid data in support for drug therapy for individuals with other forms of dementia (Schwarz, Froelich, & Burns, 2012).

Acetyl cholinesterase inhibitors (AChEIs) are the mainstay of treatment in AD. Three are currently available in the United States: donepezil hydrochloride (Aricept), rivistigmine tartrate (Exelon), and galantamine hydrobromide (Razadyne) with tacrine hydrochloride (Cognex)—the oldest and less favored drug taken off the market in 2013 because of its adverse effect on the liver and multiple daily dosing. A combination drug, memantine/donepezil (Namzaric), is also available. Cognitive improvements in patients with mild to moderate AD have been shown for all three of the AChEIs agents available in the United States (Tan et al., 2014). The acetyl cholinesterase inhibitors are safe and well tolerated; however, they may have gastrointestinal side effects (nausea, anorexia, and diarrhea). There is insufficient evidence at this time that pharmacological therapy for dementia can improve the quality of life for the patient and the caregiver and delay nursing home placement.

Memantine (Namenda), approved for moderate to severe dementia, has a different mechanism of action than the acetyl cholinesterase inhibitors. This *N*-methyl-D-aspartate receptor antagonist has neuroprotective effects that prevent excitatory neurotoxicity. Individuals with AD have improved cognition and behavior on this drug (McShane, Areosa Sastre, & Minakaran, 2006). Side effects of memantine, although uncommon, include diarrhea, insomnia, and agitation. In combined administration of cholinesterase inhibitors with memantine the research is mixed. Some studies (Atri et al., 2013; Riepe et al., 2007) demonstrated increased efficacy in advanced AD as compared to cholinesterase inhibitors alone, whereas another demonstrated that the combined treatment had no benefit (Howard et al., 2012).

Pharmacological Therapy for Problematic Behaviors

Behavior changes are common in the mid- to later stages of progressive dementia and although nonpharmacological interventions are preferred, supplementation with a tailored drug regimen is sometimes necessary. Psychotropic medications, primarily antipsychotics, can be administered to help the individual regain control and be less disruptive—positive outcomes for the caregiver as well as the patient. Drugs must be prescribed in the lowest effective dose for the shortest amount of time. The patient needs to be closely monitored for effectiveness and adverse side effects. Psychotropic medications have a high risk of adverse drug events and this is covered in Chapter 20, "Reducing Adverse Drug Events."

Psychotropic therapy for different behaviors is always short term. Once the target symptoms are relieved or abbreviated, then consideration must be given to terminate therapy. Health care professionals and families are often hesitant to stop antipsychotics fearing a return or worsening of neuropsychiatric symptoms, although the literature reflects that these can generally be withdrawn without detrimental effects (Declercq et al., 2013). Long-term psychotropic drug therapy should be considered only if the symptoms reoccur. Psychotic symptoms (such as delusions and hallucinations) frequently occur in the later stages of progressive dementia and are often associated with agitation and aggression (Ropacki & Jeste, 2005). The conventional antipsychotic, haloperidol (Haldol), has been used for decades and remains the most commonly used drug for rapid tranquilization and control of psychotic symptoms in individuals with dementia. A Cochrane Review (Lonergan, Luxenberg, & Colford, 2002) validated the useful role of haldol in managing aggression but did not find evidence for its role in managing agitation for patients with dementia. The side effects of conventional antipsychotics are considerable and include extrapyramidal symptoms, tardive dyskinesia, sedation, orthostatic hypotension, and falls.

Although not FDA approved, the atypical antipsychotics are often prescribed for use in patients with dementia. Evidence indicates that they may benefit people with dementia but the risks of adverse events (cardiovascular, extrapyramidal symptoms) may outweigh the benefit, especially with long-term treatment (Maher et al., 2011). Agents available on the market include risperidone, olanzapine, quetiapine, ziprasidone, aripiprazole, and paliperidone. There are little to no published data on the efficacy and safety of the last three drugs listed. Additional research is needed to determine when and how to use psychotropic medications to address behaviors in individuals with dementia. Other drug categories are sometimes used to control behavioral symptoms.

Benzodiazepines (lorazepan, oxazepan, alprazolam) are sometimes used to manage agitation and aggression; however, the risk–benefit ratio is often unsatisfactory. Although the benzodiazepines may be useful in rapidly sedating the agitated patient with dementia, the potential for falls and worsening of cognition limit long-term use. Again, nonpharmacological interventions to treat behavioral manifestations of distress are preferred.

Although antidepressants (Seitz et al., 2011) and anticonvulsants are sometimes used to treat agitation in dementia, there is insufficient evidence to support their use. Behavioral disturbances should not necessarily be interpreted as depression.

Supplemental Drugs

Anti-inflammatory drugs and estrogen; herbals, such as gingko; and vitamins, such as B_{12}, folate, and vitamin E—although sometimes touted and commonly used—have no proven efficacy for dementia although some isolated studies have demonstrated a benefit. Dementia associated with VaD requires appropriate control of hypertension, hyperlipidemia, and aspirin therapy. Parkinsonism (rigidity), seen with DLB, may benefit from dopaminergic therapy. Selective antidepressants and amphetamines may be effective in reducing the behavioral symptoms in FTD (Nardell & Tanjo, 2014).

Nonpharmacologic Interventions

Nonpharmacological strategies, including those from the cognitive, behavioral, and environmental domains, in combination with staff support and education are effective. Physical/functional, environmental, psychosocial, behavioral, and end-of-life (EOL) care interventions are discussed as follows.

Physical/Functional Interventions

Maintaining physical and functional well-being of the individual with progressive dementia facilitates independence, maintains health status, and can ease the caregiving burden. Interventions include adequate nutrition and hydration, regular exercise, maintenance of ADL, proper rest and sleep, appropriate bowel and bladder routines, proper dental hygiene and care, and current vaccinations. As comorbidities are common (Lyketsos et al., 2005) regular assessment, vigilant monitoring, and aggressive management of acute and chronic conditions are necessary. Vehicular-driving safety might need to be examined as recent evidence indicates that individuals with dementia pose a risk in driving safety (Man-Son-Hing, Marshall, Molnar, & Wilson, 2007). There is insufficient evidence to support or refute the benefit of neuropsychiatric testing or intervention strategies for drivers with dementia (Iverson et al., 2010).

Environmental Interventions

A specialized ecological model of care, which facilitates interaction between the person and environment in a more homelike atmosphere, has proven to be beneficial for individuals with dementia. This model affords greater privacy, encourages meaningful activities, and permits more choice than the traditional model of care. It also demonstrates that individuals with dementia experience less decline in ADL and are more engaged with the environment with no measurable differences found in cognitive measures, depression, or social withdrawal (Reimer, Slaughter, Donaldson, Currie, & Eliasziw, 2004). A study examining social engagement of residents before and after conversion to a household model (culture change) was highly significant (Morgan-Brown, Newton, & Ormerod, 2013).

A systematic review reported inclusive results and suggested that more research is needed with regard to the use of bright light in fostering better sleep and reducing behavior problems in dementia (Forbes et al., 2009). The use of aromatherapy to reduce disturbed behavior, promote sleep, and stimulate motivation also shows promise but needs more study (Thorgrimsen, Spector, Wiles, & Orrell, 2003). Manipulation of the environment (alarms, circular hallways, visual, or structural barriers) to minimize wandering has not been conclusively demonstrated to be effective (Futrell & Melillo, 2002). There is a lack of robust evidence supporting nonpharmacological interventions for wandering (Robinson et al., 2007).

Psychosocial Interventions

Mental and social engagement is important to the well-being of all older adults. Meaningful activity and involvement are no less important in individuals with dementia. Although the effectiveness of counseling or procedural memory stimulation is not supported in mild-stage dementia, reality orientation does appear to be effective (Bates,

Boote, & Beverley, 2004). The evidence suggests that cognitive therapy is more beneficial than no therapy at all but it may be patient specific (Carrion, Aymerich, Bailles, & Lopez-Bermejo, 2013; Woods, Aguirre, Spector, & Orrell, 2012). Validation therapy, based on caregiver acceptance of the reality of the person with dementia's experience, may be of value but the evidence is lacking (Neal & Barton Wright, 2003).

Recreational therapies, including music, have been shown to reduce psychological symptoms in dementia with limited efficacy and questionable duration of action (O'Connor, Ames, Gardner, & King, 2009) and more research is needed to explore the effects of music therapy on the behavior and well-being of individuals with dementia (Wall & Duffy, 2010). A growing body of evidence shows that individuals with dementia enjoy music but there is little scientific investigation within this area (Baird & Samson, 2015; Samson, Clement, Narme, Schiaratura, & Ehrle, 2015). In addition to music, other cultural arts (poetry, storytelling, dance) have reflected positive social and behavioral changes though there are some study design issues that limit inclusion in a systematic review (de Medeiros & Basting, 2014). Structured nonpharmacological short-term occupational therapy interventions were more useful in improving apathy in patients with dementia than activities of the patient's choice (Ferrero-Arias et al., 2011).

Support groups, counseling, and education for individuals with early AD and their caregivers are essential. Caregivers often experience physical, financial, social, and emotional losses and providing information through a structured education program and engaging them in the care-planning process is essential (Battaglini, 2013). Areas for caregiver education are detailed in Table 16.2.

TABLE 16.2
Education Content for Caregivers

Information about the disease and its progression
Strategies to maintain function and independence
Preservation of cognitive and physical vitality in dementia
Maintaining a safe and comfortable environment
Giving physical and emotional care
Communicating with the individual with dementia
Managing behavioral problems
Advance planning: health care and finances
Caregiver survival tips
Building a caregiver support network

Behavioral Interventions

Behavioral and psychosocial symptoms of dementia are common with every form of progressive dementia, particularly in the moderate stage. The three most troublesome symptoms are agitation, aggression, and wandering. Problematic behaviors that occur during meals or bathing can be particularly challenging. It is important to recognize and realize that any new behavior could be a sign of an acute illness or an environmental influence. Unrecognized pain can cause disruptive behavior. The Progressively Lowered Stress Threshold (PLST) is a framework to optimize function, minimize disruption, and help the caregiver (M. Smith, Hall, Gerdner, & Buckwalter, 2006). The PLST model increases the positive appraisal and decreases the negative appraisal of the caregiving situation (Stolley, Reed, & Buckwalter, 2002) and helps the caregiver manage the aggressive behaviors demonstrated in AD (Cheung, Chien, & Lai, 2011; Lindsey & Buckwalter, 2009). By adapting the environment and routines, interventions are designed to help the patient with dementia use his or her functional skills and minimize potentially triggering reactions. There are six essential principles of care in the PLST:

1. Maximize safe function: Use familiar routines, limit choices, provide rest periods: reduce stimuli when stress occurs, and routinely identify and anticipate physical stressors (pain, urinary symptoms, hunger, or thirst).
2. Provide unconditional positive regard: Respectful conversation, simple and understandable language, and nonverbal expressions of touch.
3. Use behaviors to gauge activity and stimulation: Monitor for early signs of anxiety (pacing, facial grimacing) and intervene before behavior escalates.
4. Teach caregivers to "listen" to the behaviors: Monitor the language pattern (repetition, jargon) and behaviors (rummaging) that might be showing how the person reduces stress when needs are not being met.
5. Modify the environment: Assess the environment to assure safe mobility and promote way-finding and orientation through cues.
6. Provide ongoing assistance to the caregiver: Assess and address the need for education and support.

Advance Planning and EOL Care Interventions

Advance planning and providing directives for care are important in guiding the types of interventions used at the end of life and can decrease the caregiver stress in proxy decision making. Advance directives in cases of dementia have been a debated subject for although advance directives are considered valid, they are marginally effective. As many as 90% of Americans with dementia will be institutionalized before death (G. E. Smith, Kokmen, & O'Brien, 2000) making this environment in particular an important focus for EOL care. There is a lack of research published on EOL care in the nursing home and most of it is descriptive (Oliver, Porack, & Zewig, 2004). The end stage of AD may last for several years and frequently distressing signs and symptoms occur at this time. Nursing home patients and their families want physicians more involved in EOL care, to acknowledge the presence of the patient and caregiver, and provide guidance (Fosse, Schaufel, Reiths, & Malterud, 2014). See Chapter 39 "Advance Care Planning" for a fuller discussion.

Dementia itself or associated conditions can cause physical symptoms, such as poor nutrition, urinary incontinence, skin breakdown, pain, infection, shortness of breath, fatigue, difficulty in swallowing, choking, and gurgling, in addition to the behavioral symptoms mentioned earlier. There is no acceptable standard treatment for the consequences of advanced dementia and where guidelines do exist there is minimal palliative care content. Aggressive treatments, such as antibiotics, tube feedings, psychotropic drugs, and physical restrains to address problematic behaviors, appear to be prevalent although there is no substantial evidence that this approach is effective in end-stage dementia and that prognosis and life expectancy are improved by these strategies (Evers, Purohit, Perl, Khan, & Marin, 2002). Measuring quality of care at the end of life for those with dementia poses significant challenges because of the limitations in subjective reporting and therefore relies on the caregiver's analysis of cues to monitor the patient's condition and experience (Volicer, Hurley, & Blasi, 2001). In spite of the clear recognition that significant improvements in EOL care for those with dementia is needed (Scherder et al., 2005), there is a lack of systematic evidence on how to approach palliative care for this population (Sampson, Ritchie, Lai, Raven, & Blanchard, 2005).

CASE STUDY

Mrs. P is an 85-year-old Caucasian woman brought into the primary care clinic by her daughter for a geriatric consultation. She has a 4-year history of decline in cognitive impairment that began with memory loss and impaired judgment, which appears to be worsening; she is now experiencing some behavioral problems. Mrs. P is high school educated, widowed for 10 years, and is a retired short-order cook. She currently lives with her daughter, son-in-law (both work full time), and grandson.

Her primary care physician completed a dementia workup at the time the symptoms appeared 4 years ago and started her on donepezil, which was discontinued within a few days because of gastrointestinal side effects. The daughter reports she is allergic to it. Mrs. P recently had paranoid ideation in which she accused her 15-year-old grandson of listening in on her phone conversations and taking some money from her purse. Her daughter reports that Mrs. P has always had "a short fuse" and now gets agitated easily. "She called me a moron and even took a swing at me the other day when I told her she smelled bad and needed to take a shower."

Mrs. P performs her own personal hygiene though she needs reminders and cueing at times; she is continent. She does not perform any IADL (e.g., cooking, shopping) and it was unclear whether she truly was no longer capable of performing these functions or no longer had the opportunity or desire to do them. Mrs. P reports no desire to eat and had a weight loss resulting in a change in at least three clothing sizes that has occurred slowly over the past few years. She reports that she has always been overweight and is proud of this accomplishment. The daughter says she has tried to get her to eat by serving food that she likes but she just "plays with the food" pushing it around on her plate and has been seen sneaking it to the dog while at the table. When asked about her mood she becomes tearful and says, "I feel lonely; no one cares about me anymore." Mrs. P says she hates to be alone and that the family "just come and goes—they never talk with me." She used to take an evening walk in the neighborhood but now that she lives with her daughter she is unfamiliar with and fearful of her surroundings. Her MMSE score is 18/30 with deficits in memory, calculation, and ability to copy the intersecting pentagons. She scores 10/15 on the GDS.

Past medical history includes thyroidectomy, left cataract extraction, cholecystectomy, and hysterectomy for benign disease. Her daughter thinks that Mrs. P may have been on antihypertensives in the past. The only medication Mrs. P takes at present is for her thyroid but neither she nor her daughter know the name of the drug.

On physical examination Mrs. P is afebrile; blood pressure is 132/70, and she is about 10 pounds below her ideal body weight. Mrs. P is alert, cooperative,

(continued)

CASE STUDY *(continued)*

and smiles at intervals during the examination and has hearing loss bilaterally with clear canals; no thyromegaly. Cardiovascular examination reveals no murmur, edema, or discolorations of the extremities. Pulses are strong throughout. There are no focal neurological symptoms. Gait is slow but steady. She has full range of motion but her muscle tone and strength are diminished in both upper and lower extremities. Breasts are free of masses and abdomen is soft, nontender with no organ enlargement.

A diagnosis of depression and progressive dementia of the Alzheimer's type is made and she is started on the combination of donepezil and mementine, both to be titrated slowly. Additional information from Mrs. P's primary care physician will be consulted about potential lab work and diagnostic studies, including thyroid function. The need for a nutritional and hearing evaluation will be explored. Antidepressant therapy may be considered at a later date. Health teaching and additional resource information is provided to the family.

Discussion

Depression is not uncommon in those with a progressive dementia. Severe anxiety, agitation, and aggression can occur; tearfulness and decreased appetite with weight loss may also be present. Using the PLST model, the nurse focuses on teaching the daughter to recognize triggers and prodromal signs of increasing anxiety and intervene appropriately when anxiety and agitation occur. Strategies are emphasized in each of the PLST principles of care: maximize safe function, provide unconditional regard, use behaviors to gauge activity and stimulation, "listen" to the behaviors and modify the environment. Less confrontational language and behaviors are emphasized in approaches and interactions with Mrs. P. The daughter is also provided with specific contact information for the geriatrician's office as well as the local and national resources available through the Alzheimer's Association and the Alzheimer's Disease Education and Referral Center (ADEAR). Instructions include dietary strategies to increase nutritional density and an exploration of ways to increase social engagement and exercise while assuring safety. If available in the area, Meals on Wheels, Friendly Visitors, and Home Safety Assessment might be of benefit. Specific medication instructions with particular emphasis on how to use the titration packet are provided, with the recommendation to coadminister with food to reduce the likelihood of gastrointestinal side effects. It was explained that what Mrs. P experienced earlier was likely medication intolerance not an allergy and administering with food should help. The nurse plans a follow-up phone call for the next day and schedules a follow-up medical and health teaching appointment in 1 month to evaluate the effectiveness of the plan of care. The patient and family are instructed to call or return if new or changed behaviors or physical symptoms develop. Caregiving has its burdens and rewards and impacts the entire family. At the next visit the nurse plans to have the daughter, son-in-law, and grandson present to get their perspective and engage them in discussion on the development of a family-centered plan of care, including advance care planning.

SUMMARY

It is important that health care professionals identify cognitive impairments in older adults early and differentiate a progressive from a reversible etiology, such as delirium. Comprehensive assessment, monitoring, and pharmacological and nonpharmacological management of physical, functional, cognitive, and behavioral problems are important both in initial identification and in the ongoing care of the individual with progressive dementia. Education and support of the family and professional caregiver are essential. It is difficult to identify clearly what constitutes quality of life for the individual with progressive dementia, what interventions enhance this quality, and how this is accomplished. Overall, there is limited evidence in gerontological nursing to guide the care of older adults with dementia. It is imperative that geriatric nurses evaluate practice and generate new knowledge to assure best practice in the care of individuals with progressive dementia and their caregivers.

NURSING STANDARD OF PRACTICE

Protocol 16.1: Recognition and Management of Dementia: A Major Neurocognitive Disorder

I. GOALS

A. Early recognition of dementing illness
B. Appropriate management strategies in care of individuals with dementia and their families

II. OVERVIEW

The rapid growth of the aging population is associated with an increase in the prevalence of progressive dementias. It is imperative that a differential diagnosis be ascertained early in the course of cognitive impairment and that the patient is closely monitored for coexisting morbidities. Nurses have a central role in assessment and management of individuals with progressive dementia.

III. BACKGROUND

A. Definitions/distinctions
   1. Dementia (also referred to as a major neurocognitive disorder) is a clinical syndrome of disruptions in cognition.
   2. In addition to disruptions in cognition, dementias are commonly associated with changes in function, mood, and behavior.
   3. The most common forms of progressive dementia are AD, VaD, DLB, and FTD; the pathophysiology for each is poorly understood.
   4. Differential diagnosis of dementing conditions is complicated by the fact that concurrent disease states (i.e., comorbidities) often coexist.

B. Prevalence
   1. Dementia affects about 11% of individuals aged 65 years and older.
   2. Four to five million individuals in the United States have AD with a projected number of 13.8 million cases by 2050.
   3. Global prevalence of dementia is about 44.4 million with projections of 135.5 million by 2050.

C. Risk factors
   1. Advanced age
   2. MCI
   3. Cardiovascular disease
   4. Genetics: family history of dementia, PDD, cardiovascular disease, stroke, presence of ApoE4 allele on chromosome 19
   5. Environment: head injury, alcohol abuse

IV. PARAMETERS OF ASSESSMENT

No formal recommendations for cognitive screening are indicated in asymptomatic individuals. Clinicians are advised to be alert for cognitive and functional decline in older adults to detect dementia and dementia-like presentation in early stages. Assessment domains include cognitive, functional, behavioral, physical, caregiver, and environment.

A. Cognitive parameters
   1. Orientation: person, place, time
   2. Memory: ability to register, retain, recall information
   3. Attention: ability to attend and concentrate on stimuli
   4. Thinking: ability to organize and communicate ideas
   5. Language: ability to receive and express a message

(continued)

Protocol 16.1: Recognition and Management of Dementia: A Major Neurocognitive Disorder *(continued)*

6. Praxis: ability to direct and coordinate movements
7. Executive function: ability to abstract, plan, sequence, and use feedback to guide performance

B. Mental status screening tools
1. Folstein et al.'s MMSE is the most commonly used test to assess serial cognitive change. The MMSE is copyrighted and a comparable tool, SLUMS, is in the public domain.
2. CDT is a useful measure of cognitive function that correlates with executive control functions.
3. Mini-Cog combines the CDT with the three-word recall.

When the diagnosis remains unclear the patient may be referred for more extensive screening and neuropsychological testing, which might provide more direction and support for the patient and the caregivers.

C. Functional assessment
1. Tests that assess functional limitations, such as the FAQ and the FAST, can detect dementia. They are also useful in monitoring the progression of functional decline.
2. The severity of disease progression in dementia can be demonstrated by performance decline in ADL and IADL tasks and is closely correlated with mental status scores.

D. Behavioral assessment
1. Assess and monitor for behavioral changes, in particular the presence of agitation, aggression, anxiety, disinhibitions, delusions, hallucinations.
2. Evaluate for depression because it commonly coexists in individuals with dementia. The GDS is a good screening tool.

E. Physical assessment
1. A comprehensive physical examination with a focus on the neurological and cardiovascular system is indicated in individuals with dementia to identify the potential cause and/or the existence of a reversible form of cognitive impairment.
2. A thorough evaluation of all prescribed, over-the-counter, homeopathic, herbal, and nutritional products taken is done to determine the potential impact on cognitive status.
3. Laboratory tests are valuable in differentiating irreversible from reversible forms of dementia. Two laboratory tests specifically recommend in the initial evaluation are thyroid function and B_{12}. Structural neuroimaging with noncontrast CT or MRI scans are appropriate in the routine initial evaluation of patients with dementia.

F. Caregiver/environment
1. The caregiver of the patient with dementia often has as many needs as the patient with dementia so a detailed assessment of the caregiver and the caregiving environment is essential.
   a. Elicit the caregiver perspective of patient function and the level of support provided.
   b. Evaluate the impact that the patient's cognitive impairment and problem behaviors have on the caregiver (mastery, satisfaction, and burden). Two useful tools include the ZBI and the CSI tools.
   c. Evaluate the caregiver experience and patient/caregiver relationship.

V. NURSING CARE STRATEGIES

A. The PLST framework provides a framework for the nursing care of individuals with dementia.
1. Monitor the effectiveness and potential side effects of medications given to improve cognitive function or delay cognitive decline.
2. Provide appropriate cognitive-enhancement techniques and social engagement.
3. Assure adequate rest, sleep, fluid, nutrition, elimination, pain control, and comfort measures.
4. Avoid the use of physical and pharmacological restraints.
5. Maximize functional capacity: Maintain mobility and encourage independence as long as possible, provide graded assistance as needed with ADL and IADL, provide scheduled toileting and prompted voiding to reduce urinary incontinence, encourage an exercise routine that expends energy and promotes fatigue at bedtime, and establish bedtime routine and rituals.
6. Address behavioral issues: Identify environmental triggers, medical conditions, caregiver/patient conflict that may be causing the behavior; define the target symptom (i.e., agitation, aggression, wandering) and

(continued)

Protocol 16.1: Recognition and Management of Dementia: A Major Neurocognitive Disorder *(continued)*

pharmacological (psychotropics) and nonpharmacological (manage affect, limit stimuli, respect space, distract, redirect) approaches; provide reassurance; and refer to appropriate mental health care professionals as indicated.

7. Assure a therapeutic and safe environment: Provide an environment that is modestly stimulating avoiding overstimulation, which can cause agitation and increase confusion and understimulation, which can cause sensory deprivation and withdrawal. Use patient identifiers (name tags), medic-alert systems and bracelets, locks, wander guard. Eliminate any environmental hazards and modify the environment to enhance safety. Provide environmental cues or sensory aides that facilitate cognition, and maintain consistency in caregivers and approaches. Psychosocial interventions and cultural arts therapy in dementia may prove beneficial.
8. Encourage and support advance care planning: Explain the trajectory of progressive dementia, treatment options, and advance directives.
9. Provide appropriate EOL care in terminal phase: provide comfort measures, including adequate pain management; weigh the benefits/risks of the use of aggressive treatment (tube feeding, antibiotic therapy).
10. Provide caregiver education and support: Respect family systems/dynamics and avoid making judgments; encourage open dialogue, emphasize the patient's residual strengths; provide access to experienced professionals; and teach caregivers the skills of caregiving.
11. Integrate community resources into the plan of care to meet the needs for patient and caregiver information; identify and facilitate both formal (i.e., Alzheimer's Association, respite care, specialized long-term care) and informal (i.e., churches, neighbors, extended family/friends) support systems.

VI. EVALUATION/EXPECTED OUTCOMES

A. Patient outcomes: The patient remains as independent and functional in the environment of choice for as long as possible, the comorbid conditions the patient may experience are well managed, and the distressing symptoms that may occur at EOL are minimized or controlled adequately.
B. Caregiver outcomes (lay and professional): Caregivers demonstrate effective caregiving skills; verbalize satisfaction with caregiving; report minimal caregiver burden; are familiar with, have access to, and use available resources.
C. Institutional outcomes: The institution reflects a safe and enabling environment for delivering care to individuals with progressive dementia; the quality improvement plan addresses high-risk problem-prone areas for individuals with dementia such as falls and the use of restraints.

VII. FOLLOW-UP TO MONITOR CONDITION

A. Follow-up appointments are regularly scheduled; frequency depends on the patient's physical, mental, and emotional status and caregiver needs.
B. Determine the continued efficacy of pharmacological/nonpharmacological approaches to the care plan and modify as appropriate.
C. Identify and treat any underlying or contributing conditions.
D. Community resources for education and support are accessed and used by the patient and/or caregivers.

VIII. RELEVANT PRACTICE GUIDELINES/RESOURCES

A. American Academy of Neurology: Dementia: www.aan.com/guidelines
B. American Association of Geriatric Psychiatry: Position Statement: Principles of Care for Patients With Dementia Resulting From Alzheimer Disease: www.aagponline.org/index.php?src=news&submenu=Tools_Resources&srctype=detail&category=Position%20Statement&refno=35
C. Alzheimer's Foundation of America: Excellence in Care: www.alzfdn.org
D. American Medical Directors Association: www.amda.com/tools/guidelines.cfm#dementia
E. American Geriatrics Society: geriatricscareonline.org
F. Geriatric Advance Practice Nurse Association: www.gapna.org/resources/toolkit-gerontology-resources-advanced-practice-nurses
G. Hartford Institute for Geriatric Nursing: www.hartfordign.org

(continued)

Protocol 16.1: Recognition and Management of Dementia: A Major Neurocognitive Disorder *(continued)*

ABBREVIATIONS

AD	Alzheimer's disease
ADL	Activities of daily living
CDT	Clock Draw test
CSI	Caregiver Strain Index
DLB	Dementia with Lewy bodies
EOL	End of life
FAQ	Functional Activities Questionnaire
FAST	Functional Assessment Staging Test
FTD	Frontotemporal dementia
GDS	Geriatric Depression Scale
IADL	Instrumental activities of daily living
MCI	Mild cognitive impairment
Mini-COG	Mini-Cognitive
MMSE	Mini-Mental State Exam
PDD	Parkinson's disease
PLST	Progressively Lowered Stress Threshold
SLUMS	St. Louis University Mental Status Exam
VaD	Vascular dementia
ZBI	Zarit Burden Interview

RESOURCES

AARP
www.aarp.org/home-family/caregiving

Alzheimer's Association
www.alz.org/professionals_and_researchers_14899.asp

Alzheimer's Disease Education and Referral Center
https://www.nia.nih.gov/alzheimers

Caregiver Action Network (formerly National Family Caregiver's Association)
http://caregiveraction.org

ElderWeb
www.elderweb.com

Hartford Institute for Geriatric Nursing
www.hartfordign.org
www.consultgerirn.org/resources

Lewy Body Dementia Association
www.lbda.org

National Alliance for Caregiving
www.caregiving.org

National Council of Certified Dementia Practitioners
http://www.nccdp.org

National Hospice and Palliative Care Association
www.nhpco.org/resources-access-outreach/dementia-resources

REFERENCES

Ablitt, A., Jones, G. V., & Muers, J. (2009). Living with dementia: A systematic review of the influence of relationship factors. *Aging & Mental Health, 13*(4), 497–511. *Evidence Level I.*

Adelman, A. M., & Daly, M. P. (2005). Initial evaluation of the patient with suspected dementia. *American Family Physician, 71*(9), 1745–1750. *Evidence Level VI.*

Alzheimer's Association. (2015). *AD facts and figures, 10*(2). Retrieved from http://www.alz.org/facts. *Evidence Level IV.*

Alzheimer's Disease International. (2013). *The global voice of dementia: Dementia statistics.* Retrieved from www.alz.co.uk/research statistics. *Evidence Level IV.*

American Psychiatric Association. (2013). *Diagnostic and statistical manual of mental disorders* (5th ed.). Arlington, VA: American Psychiatric Publishing. *Evidence Level VI.*

Ariga, T., Miyatake, T., & Yu, R. K. (2010). Role of proteoglycans and glycosaminoglycans in the pathogenesis of Alzheimer's disease and related disorders: Amyloidogenesis and therapeutic strategies—A review. *Journal of Neuroscience Research, 88*(11), 2303–2315. *Evidence Level V.*

Atri, A., Molinuevo, J. L., Lemming, O., Wirth, Y., Pulte, I., & Wilkinson, D. (2013). Memantine in patients with Alzheimer's disease receiving donepezil: New analysis of efficacy and safety for combination therapy. *Alzheimer's Research and Therapy, 5*(1), 6. *Evidence Level I.*

Baird, A., & Samson, S. (2015). Music and dementia. *Progress in Brain Research, 217*, 207–235. *Evidence Level V.*

Bates, J., Boote, J., & Beverley, C. (2004). Psychosocial interventions for people with a milder dementing illness: A systematic review. *Journal of Advanced Nursing, 45*(6), 644–658. *Evidence Level I.*

Battaglini, E. (2013). *Dementia: Family support following diagnosis. Evidence summaries.* Retrieved from Joanna Briggs Institute EBP Resources website http://joannabriggslibrary.org. *Evidence Level V.*

Borson, S., Scanlan, J., Brush, M., Vitaliano, P., & Dokmak, A. (2000). The Mini-Cog: A cognitive "vital signs" measure for dementia screening in multi-lingual elderly. *International Journal of Geriatric Psychiatry, 15*(11), 1021–1027. *Evidence Level IV.*

Borson, S., Scanlan, J. M., Chen, P., & Ganguli, M. (2003). The Mini-Cog as a screen for dementia: Validation in a population based sample. *Journal of the American Geriatrics Society, 51*(10), 1451–1454. *Evidence Level IV.*

Borson, S., Scanlan, J. M., Watanabe, J., Tu, S. P., & Lessig, M. (2005). Simplifying detection of cognitive impairment: Comparison of the Mini-Cog and Mini-Mental State Examination in a multiethnic sample. *Journal of the American Geriatrics Society, 53*(5), 871–874. *Evidence Level IV.*

Brodaty, H., Low, L. F., Gibson, L., & Burns, K. (2006). What is the best dementia screening instrument for general practitioners to use? *American Journal of Geriatric Psychiatry, 14*(5), 391–400. *Evidence Level I.*

Brodaty, H., Pond, D., Kemp, N., Luscombe, G., Harding, L., Berman, K., & Huppert, F. (2002). The CPCOG: A new screening test for dementia designed for general practice. *Journal of the American Geriatrics Society, 50*(3), 530–534. *Evidence Level IV.*

Buschke, H., Kuslansky, G., Katz, M., Stewart, W. F., Sliwinski, J. J., Eckholdt, H. M., & Lipton, R. B. Screening for dementia with the memory impairment screen. *Neurology, 52*(2), 231–238. *Evidence Level IV.*

Carrion, C., Aymerich, M., Baillés, E., & López-Bermejo, A. (2013). Cognitive psychosocial intervention in dementia: A systematic review. *Dementia and Geriatric Cognitive Disorders, 36*(5–6), 363–375. *Evidence Level I.*

Castellani, R. J., Rolston, R. K., & Smith, M. A. (2010). Alzheimer disease. *Disease-a-Month, 56*(9), 484–546. *Evidence Level V.*

Cheung, D. S., Chien, W. T., & Lai, C. K. (2011). Conceptual framework for cognitive function enhancement in people with dementia. *Journal of Clinical Nursing, 20*(11–12), 1533–1541. *Evidence Level V.*

Cooper, C., Balamurali, T. B., & Livingston, G. (2007). A systematic review of the prevalence and covariates of anxiety in caregivers of people with dementia. *International Psychogeriatrics, 19*(2), 175–195. *Evidence Level I.*

Cummings, J. L., Mega, M., Rosenberg-Thompson, S., Carusi, D. I., & Gornbein, J. (1994). The neuropsychiatric inventory: Comprehensive assessment of psychopathology in dementia. *Neurology, 44*(12), 2308–2314. *Evidence Level IV.*

Declercq, T., Petrovic, M., Azermai, M., Vander Stichele, R., De Sutter, A. l., van Driel, M. L., & Christiaens, T. (2013). Withdrawal versus continuation of chronic antipsychotic drugs for behavioural and psychological symptoms in older people with dementia. *Cochrane Database of Systematic Reviews, 2013*(3), CD007726. *Evidence Level I.*

de la Torre, J. C. (2012). Cardiovascular risk factors promote brain hypoperfusion leading to cognitive decline and dementia. *Cardiovascular, Psychiatry, and Neurology, 2012,* 15. Article ID 367516. *Evidence Level V.*

de Medeiros, K., & Basting, A. (2014). "Shall I compare thee to a dose of donepezil?": Cultural arts interventions in dementia care research. *The Gerontologist, 54*(3), 344–353. *Evidence Level I.*

Evers, M. M., Purohit, D., Perl, D., Khan, K., & Marin, D.B. (2002). Palliative and aggressive end-of-life care for patients with dementia. *Psychiatric Services, 53*(5), 609–613. *Evidence Level IV.*

Ferreira, D., Rivero-Santana, A., Perestelo-Pérez, L., Westman, E., Wahlund, L. O., Sarría, A., & Serrano-Aguilar, P. (2014). Improving CSF biomarkers' performance for predicting progression from mild cognitive impairment to Alzheimer's disease by considering different confounding factors: A meta-analysis. *Frontiers in Aging Neuroscience, 6,* 287. *Evidence Level I.*

Ferrero-Arias, J., Goñi-Imízcoz, M., González-Bernal, J., Lara-Ortega, F., da Silva-González, A., & Díez-Lopez, M. (2011). The efficacy of nonpharmacological treatment for dementia-related apathy. *Alzheimer Disease and Associated Disorders, 25*(3), 213–219. *Evidence Level I.*

Folstein, M. F., Folstein, S. E., & McHugh, P. R. (1975). Mini-Mental State. *Journal of Psychiatric Research, 12*(3), 189–198. *Evidence Level IV.*

Forbes, D., Culum, I., Lischka, A., Morgan, D. G., Peacock, S., Forbes, J., & Forbes, S. (2009). Light therapy for managing cognitive, sleep, behavioural, or psychiatric disturbances in dementia. *Cochrane Database Systematic Reviews, 2009*(4), CD003946. *Evidence Level I.*

Fosse, A., Schaufel, M. A., Reiths, S., & Malterud, K. (2014). End of life expectations and experiences among nursing home patients and their relatives: A synthesis of qualitative studies. *Patient Education and Counseling, 97*(1), 3–9. *Evidence Level I.*

Freund, B., Gravenstein, S., Ferris, R., Burke, B. L., & Shaheen, E. (2005). Drawing clocks and driving cars. *Journal of General Internal Medicine, 20*(3), 240–244. *Evidence Level IV.*

Freund, B., Gravenstein, S., Ferris, R., & Shaheen, E. (2002). Evaluating driving performance of cognitively impaired and healthy older adults: A pilot study comparing on-road testing and driving simulation. *Journal of the American Geriatrics Society, 50*(7), 1309–1310. *Evidence Level IV.*

Futrell, M., & Melillo, K. D. (2002). Evidence-based protocol. Wandering. *Journal of Gerontological Nursing, 28*(11), 14–22. *Evidence Level V.*

Galasko, D., Bennett, D., Sano, M., Ernesto, C., Thomas, R., Grundman, M., & Ferris, S. (1997). An inventory to assess activities of daily living for clinical trials in Alzheimer's disease. The Alzheimer's Disease Cooperative Study. *Alzheimer Disease and Associated Disorders, 11*(Suppl. 2), S33–S39. *Evidence Level III.*

Gascon, E., & Gao, F. B. (2014). The emerging role of microRNA's with the pathogenesis of frontotemporal dementia-amyotropic lateral sclerosis spectrum disorders. *Journal of Neurogenetics, 28,* 30–40. *Evidence Level V.*

Geldmacher, D. S. (2003). Alzheimer's disease: Current pharmacotherapy in the context of patient and family needs. *Journal of the American Geriatrics Society, 51*(Suppl. 5), S289–S295. *Evidence Level V.*

Han, L., Cole, M., Bellavance, F., McCusker, J., & Primeau, F. (2000). Tracking cognitive decline in Alzheimer's disease using the Mini-Mental State Examination: A meta-analysis. *International Psychogeriatrics, 12*(2), 231–247. *Evidence Level I.*

Hanson, J. C., & Lippa, C. F. (2009). Lewy body dementia. *International Review Neurobiology, 84*, 215–228. *Evidence Level V.*

Hebert, L. E., Weuve, J., Scherr, P. A., & Evans, D. A. (2013). Alzheimer disease in the United States (2010–2050) estimated using the 2010 census. *Neurology, 80*(19), 1778–1783. *Evidence Level II.*

Higginson, I. J., Gao, W., Jackson, D., Murray, J., & Harding, R. (2010). Short-form Zarit Caregiver Burden Interviews were valid in advanced conditions. *Journal of Clinical Epidemiology, 63*(5), 535–542. *Evidence Level I.*

Howard, R., McShane, R., Lindesay, J., Ritchie, C., Baldwin, A., Barber, R., . . . Phillips, P. (2012). Donepezil and memantine for moderate-to-severe Alzheimer's disease. *New England Journal of Medicine, 366*(10), 893–903. *Evidence Level II.*

Ismail, Z., Rajji, T. K., & Shulman, K. J. (2010). Brief cognitive screening instruments: An update. *International Journal of Geriatric Psychiatry, 25*(2), 111–120. *Evidence Level I.*

Iverson, D. J., Gronseth, G. S., Reger, M. A., Classen, S., Dubinsky, R. M., Rizzo, M., & Quality Standards Subcomittee of the American Academy of Neurology. (2010). Practice parameter update: Evaluation and management of driving risk in dementia: Report of the Quality Standards Subcommittee of the American Academy of Neurology. *Neurology, 74*(16), 1316–1324. *Evidence Level I.*

Kane, R. L., Ouslander, J. G., Abrass, I. B., & Resnick, B. (2013). Delirium and dementia. In R. L. Kane, J. G. Ouslander, I. B. Abrass, & B. Resnick (Eds.), *Essentials of clinical geriatrics* (7th ed., Chap 6). Retrieved from http://accessmedicine.mhmedical.com.proxy.its.virginia.edu/content.aspx?bookid=678&Sectionid=44833884. *Evidence Level VI.*

Kilik, L. A., Hopkins, R., Day, D., Prince, C. R., Prince, P. N., & Rows, C. (2008). The progression of behavior in dementia: An in-office guide for clinicians. *American Journal of Alzheimer's Disease, 23*(3), 242–249. *Evidence Level IV.*

Kirshner, H. S. (2009). Vascular dementia: A review of recent evidence for prevention and treatment. *Current Neurology and Neuroscience Reports, 9*(6), 437–442. *Evidence Level V.*

Knopman, D. S., DeKosky, S. T., Cummings, J. L., Chui, H., Corey-Bloom, J., Relkin, N., . . . Stevens, J. C. (2001). Practice parameter: Diagnosis of dementia (an evidence-based review). Report of the Quality Standards Subcommittee of the American Academy of Neurology. *Neurology, 56*(9), 1143–1153. *Evidence Level V.*

Lai, C. K. (2014). The merits and problems of neuropsychiatric inventory as an assessment tool in people with dementia and other neurological disorders. *Clinical Interventions in Aging, 9*, 1051–1061. *Evidence Level I.*

Langa, K. M., Foster, N. L., & Larson, E. B. (2004). Mixed dementia: Emerging concepts and therapeutic implications. *Journal of the American Medical Association, 292*(23), 2901–2908. *Evidence Level V.*

Lee, H. B., & Lyketsos, C. G. (2003). Depression in Alzheimer's disease: Heterogeneity and related issues. *Biological Psychiatry, 54*(3), 353–362. *Evidence Level IV.*

Liefer, B. P. (2003). Early diagnosis of Alzheimer's disease: Clinical and economic benefits. *Journal of the American Geriatrics Society, 51*(5), S281–S288. *Evidence Level V.*

Lima-Silva, T. B., Bahia, V. S., Nitrini, R., & Yassuda, M. S. (2013). Functional status in behavioral variant frontotemporal dementia: A systematic review. *BioMed Research International, 2013*, 837120. *Evidence Level I.*

Lindsey, P. L., & Buckwalter, K. C. (2009). Psychotic events in Alzheimer's disease: Application of the PLST model. *Journal of Gerontological Nursing, 35*(8), 20–27; quiz 28. *Evidence Level V.*

Lonergan, E., Luxenberg, J., & Colford, J. (2002). Haloperidol for agitation in dementia. *Cochrane Database of Systematic Reviews, 2002*(2), CD002852. *Evidence Level I.*

Lowe, S. A., Rodríguez-Molinero, A., Glynn, L., Breen, P. P., Baker, P. M., Sanford, J., . . . Ólaighin, G. (2013). New technology-based functional assessment tools should avoid the weaknesses and proliferation of manual functional assessments. *Journal of Clinical Epidemiology, 66*(6), 619–632. *Evidence Level I.*

Luck, T., Luppa, M., Briel, S., & Riedel-Heller, S. G. (2010). Incidence of mild cognitive impairment: A systematic review. *Dementia and Geriatric Cognitive Disorders, 29*(2), 164–175. *Evidence Level I.*

Lyketsos, C. G., Toone, L., Tschanz, J., Rabins, P. V., Steinberg, M., Onyike, C. U., . . . Cache County Study Group. (2005). Population-based study of medical comorbidity in early dementia and "cognitive impairment, no dementia (CIND)": Association with functional and cognitive impairment: The Cache County Study. *American Journal of Geriatric Psychiatry, 13*(8), 656–664. *Evidence Level IV.*

Maher, A. R., Maglione, M., Bagley, S., Suttorp, M., Hu, J. H., Ewing, B., . . . Shekelle, P. G. (2011). Efficacy and comparative effectiveness of atypical antipsychotic medications for off-label uses in adults: A systematic review and meta-analysis. *Journal of the American Medical Association, 306*(12), 1359–1369. *Evidence Level I.*

Manly, J. J., & Espino, D. V. (2004). Cultural influences on dementia recognition and management. *Clinics in Geriatric Medicine, 20*(1), 93–119. *Evidence Level IV.*

Manning, C. (2004). Beyond memory: Neuropsychologic features in differential diagnosis of dementia. *Clinics in Geriatric Medicine, 20*(1), 45–58. *Evidence Level VI.*

Man-Son-Hing, M., Marshall, S. C., Molnar, F. J., & Wilson, K. G. (2007). Systematic review of driving risk and the efficacy of compensatory strategies in persons with dementia. *Journal of the American Geriatrics Society, 55*(6), 878–884. *Evidence Level I.*

Mayo, M. C., & Bordelon, Y. (2014). Dementia with Lewy bodies. *Seminars in Neurology, 34*(2), 182–188. *Evidence Level V.*

McKeith, I. G., Burn, D. J., Ballard, C. G., Collerton, D., Jaros, E., Morris, C. M., . . . O'Brien, J. T. (2003). Dementia with Lewy bodies. *Seminars in Clinical Neuropsychiatry, 8*(1), 46–57. *Evidence Level V.*

McShane, R., Areosa Sastre, A., & Minakaran, N. (2006). Memantine for dementia. *Cochrane Database of Systematic Reviews, 2006*(2), CD003154. *Evidence Level I.*

Milisen, K., Braes, T., Fick, D. M., & Foreman, M. D. (2006). Cognitive assessment and differentiating the 3 Ds (dementia, depression, delirium). *Nursing Clinics of North America, 41*(1), 1–22. *Evidence Level V.*

Miller, E. A., Schneider, L. S., & Rosenheck, R. A. (2011). Predictors of nursing home admission among Alzheimer's disease patients with psychosis and/or agitation. *International Psychogeriatrics, 23*(1), 44–53. *Evidence level II.*

Milne, A., Culverwell, A., Guss, R., Tuppen, J., & Whelton, R. (2008). Screening for dementia in primary care: A review of the use, efficacy and quality of measures. *International Psychogeriatrics, 20*(5), 911–926. *Evidence Level I.*

Mitchell, A. J. (2009). CSF phosphorylated tau in the diagnosis and prognosis of mild cognitive impairment and Alzheimer's disease: A meta-analysis of 51 studies. *Journal of Neurology, Neurosurgery & Psychiatry, 80*(9), 966–975. *Evidence Level I.*

Monastero, R., Mangialasche, F., Camarda, C., Ercolani, S., & Camarda, R. (2009). A systematic review of neuropsychiatric symptoms in mild cognitive impairment. *Journal of Alzheimer's Disease, 18*(1), 11–30. *Evidence Level I.*

Montine, R. J., Koroshetz, W. T., Babcock, D., Dickson, D. W., Galpern, W. R., Glymour, W. M.,... Corriveau, R. A. (2014). ADRD conference organizing committee: Recommendations of the Alzheimer's disease-related dementias conference. *Neurology, 83*, 851–860. *Evidence Level I.*

Morgan-Brown, M., Newton, R., & Ormerod, M. (2013). Engaging life in the Irish nursing home units for people with dementia: Qualitative comparison before and after implementing household environments. *Aging and Mental Health, 18*(1), 57–65. *Evidence Level IV.*

Nardell, M., & Tanjo, R. R. (2014). Pharmacological treatments for frontotemporal dementias: A systematic review of randomized control trials. *American Journal of Alzheimer's Disease and Other Dementias, 29*(2), 123–132. *Evidence Level I.*

Nasreddine, Z. S., Phillips, N. A., Bedirian, V., Charbonneau, S., Whitehead, V., ... Chertkow, F. F. (2005). The Montreal cognitive assessment: MoCA: A brief screening tool for mild cognitive impairment. *Journal of the American Geriatrics Society, 53*(4), 695–699. *Evidence Level III.*

Neal, M., & Barton Wright, P. (2003). Validation therapy for dementia. *Cochrane Database of Systematic Review, 2003*(3), CD001394. *Evidence Level I.*

O'Connor, D. W., Ames, D., Gardner, B., & King, M. (2009). Psychosocial treatments of psychological symptoms in dementia: A systematic review of reports meeting quality standards. *International Psychogeriatrics, 21*(2), 241–251. *Evidence Level I.*

Oliver, N. P., Porack, D., & Zewig, S. (2004). End of life care in U.S. nursing homes: A review of the evidence. *Journal of the American Medical Directors Association, 5*, 147–155. *Evidence Level I.*

Onega, L. L. (2006). Assessment of psychoemotional and behavioral status in patients with dementia. *Nursing Clinics of North America, 41*(1), 23–41. *Evidence Level VI.*

Onega, L. L. (2008). Helping those who help others: The Modified Caregiver Strain Index. *American Journal of Nursing, 108*(9), 62–69; quiz 69. *Evidence Level V.*

Parker, C., & Philp, I. (2004). Screening for cognitive impairment among older people in black and minority ethnic groups. *Age and Ageing, 33*(5), 447–452. *Evidence Level IV.*

Peters, R., & Pinto, E. M. (2008). Predictive value of the Clock Drawing Test. A review of the literature. *Dementia and Geriatric Cognitive Disorders, 26*(4), 351–355. *Evidence Level I.*

Potkin, S. G. (2002). The ABC of Alzheimer's disease: ADL and improving day-to-day functioning of patients. *International Psychogeriatrics, 14*(Suppl. 1), 7–26. *Evidence Level V.*

Quinn, T. J., Fearon, P., Noel-Storr, A. H., Young, C., McShane, R., & Stott, D. J. (2014). Informant Questionnaire on Cognitive Decline in the Elderly (IQCODE) for the diagnosis of dementia within community dwelling populations. *Cochrane Database of Systematic Reviews, 2014*(4), CD010079. *Evidence Level I.*

Reimer, M. A., Slaughter, S., Donaldson, C., Currie, G., & Eliasziw, M. (2004). Special care facility compared with traditional environments for dementia care: A longitudinal study of quality of life. *Journal of the American Geriatrics Society, 52*(7), 1085–1092. *Evidence Level IV.*

Riedl, L., MacKenzie, I. R., Forsti, H., Kurz, A., & Diehl-Schmid, J. (2014). Frontotemporal lobar degeneration: Current perspectives. *Neuropsychiatric Disease and Treatment, 10*, 297–310. *Evidence Level V.*

Riepe, M. W., Adler, G., Ibach, B., Weinkauf, B., Tracik, F., & Gunay, I. (2007). Domain-specific improvement of cognition on memantine in patients with Alzheimer's disease treated with rivastigmine. *Dementia and Geriatric Cognitive Disorders, 23*(5), 301–306. *Evidence Level III.*

Rikkert, M. G. M. O., Tona, K. D., Janssen, L., Burns, A., Lobo, A., Sartorius, N.,... Waldemar, G. (2011). Validity, reliability, and feasibility of clinical staging scales in dementia: A systematic review. *American Journal of Alzheimer's Disease and Other Dementias, 26*(5), 357–365. *Evidence Level I.*

Robinson, L., Hutchings, D., Dickinson, H. O., Corner, L., Beyer, F., Finch, T.... Bond, J. (2007). Effectiveness and acceptability of non-pharmacological interventions to reduce wandering in dementia: A systematic review. *International Journal of Geriatric Psychiatry, 22*(1), 9–22. *Evidence Level I.*

Román, G. C. (2003). Stroke, cognitive decline and vascular dementia: The silent epidemic of the 21st century. *Neuroepidemiology, 22*(3), 161–164. *Evidence Level VI.*

Ropacki, S. A., & Jeste, D. V. (2005). Epidemiology of and risk factors for psychosis of Alzheimer's disease: A review of 55 studies published from 1990 to 2003. *American Journal of Psychiatry, 162*(11), 2022–2030. *Evidence Level I.*

Sampson, E. L., Ritchie, C. W., Lai, R., Raven, P. W., & Blanchard, M. R. (2005). A systematic review of the scientific evidence for the efficacy of a palliative care approach in advanced dementia. *International Psychogeriatrics, 17*(1), 31–40. *Evidence Level I.*

Samson, S., Clement, S., Narme, P., Schiaratura, L., & Ehrle, N. (2015). Efficacy of musical interventions in dementia: Methodological requirements of nonpharmacological trials. *Annals of the New York Academy of Sciences, 1337*, 249–255. *Evidence Level II.*

Scherder, E., Oosterman, J., Swaab, D., Herr, K., Ooms, M., Ribbe, M.,... Benedetti, F. (2005). Recent developments in pain in dementia. *British Medical Journal, 330*(7489), 461–464. *Evidence Level V.*

Schoenmakers, B., Buntinx, F., & Delepeleire, J. (2010). Factors determining the impact of care-giving on caregivers of elderly patients with dementia. A systematic literature review. *Maturitas, 66*(2), 191–200. *Evidence Level I.*

Schwarz, S., Froelich, L., & Burns, A. (2012). Pharmacological treatment of dementia. *Current Opinion in Psychiatry, 25*(6), 542–550. *Evidence Level V.*

Seitz, D. P., Adunuri, N., Gill, S. S., Gruneir, A., Herrmann, N., & Rochon, P. (2011). Antidepressants for agitation and psychosis in dementia. *Cochrane Database of Systematic Reviews, 2011*(2), CD008191. *Evidence Level I.*

Shub, D., Ball, V., Abbas, A. A., Gottumukkala, A., & Kunik, M. E. (2010). The link between psychosis and aggression in persons with dementia: A systematic review. *Psychiatric Quarterly, 81*(2), 97–110. *Evidence Level I.*

Shulman, K. I. (2000). Clock-drawing is it the ideal screening test? *International Journal of Geriatric Psychiatry, 15*(6), 548–561. *Evidence Level I.*

Smith, G. E., Kokmen, E., & O'Brien, P. C. (2000). Risk factors for nursing home placement in a population-based dementia cohort. *Journal of the American Geriatrics Society, 48*(5), 519–525. *Evidence Level IV.*

Smith, M., Hall, G. R., Gerdner, L., & Buckwalter, K. C. (2006). Application of the Progressively Lowered Stress Threshold Model across the continuum of care. *Nursing Clinics of North America, 41*(1), 57–81, vi. *Evidence Level V.*

Stolley, J. M., Reed, D., & Buckwalter, K. C. (2002). Caregiving appraisal and interventions based on the progressively lowered stress threshold model. *American Journal of Alzheimer's Disease and Other Dementias, 17*(2), 110–120. *Evidence Level II.*

Tan, C. C., Yu, J. T., Wang, H. F., Tan, M. S., Meng, X. F., Wang, C., . . . Tan, L. (2014). Efficacy and safety of donepezil, galantamine, rivistagmine, and memantine for the treatment of Alzheimer's disease: A systematic review. *Journal of Alzheimer's Disease, 41*(2), 615–631. *Evidence Level I.*

Tariq, S. H., Tumosa, N., Chibnall, J. T., Perry, M. H., & Morley, J. E. (2006). Comparison of the Saint Louis University mental status examination and the Mini-Mental State Examination for detecting dementia and mild neurocognitive disorder—A pilot study. *American Journal of Geriatric Psychiatry, 14*(11), 900–910. *Evidence Level IV.*

Teng, E., Becker, B. W., Woo, E., Knopman, D. S., Cummings, J. L., & Lu, P. H. (2010). Utility of the functional activities questionnaire for distinguishing mild cognitive impairment from very mild Alzheimer disease. *Alzheimer Disease and Associated Disorders, 24*(4), 348–353. *Evidence Level III.*

Thorgrimsen, L., Spector, A., Wiles, A., & Orrell, M. (2003). Aroma therapy for dementia. *Cochrane Database of Systematic Reviews, 2003*(3), CD003150. *Evidence Level I.*

van der Lee, J., Bakker, T. J., Duivenvoorden, H. J., & Dröes, R. M. (2014). Multivariate models of subjective caregiver burden in dementia: A systematic review. *Ageing Research Reviews, 15*, 76–93. *Evidence Level I.*

Vann Jones, S. A., & O'Brien, J. T. (2014). The prevalence and incidence of dementia with Lewy bodies: A systematic review of population and clinical studies. *Psychological Medicine, 44*(4), 673–683. *Evidence Level I.*

Volicer, L., Hurley, A. C., & Blasi, Z. V. (2001). Scales for evaluation of end-of-life care in dementia. *Alzheimer Disease and Associated Disorders, 15*(4), 194–200. *Evidence Level IV.*

Wall, M., & Duffy, A. (2010). The effects of music therapy for older people with dementia. *British Journal of Nursing, 19*(2), 108–113. *Evidence Level I.*

Woods, B., Aguirre, E., Spector, A. E., & Orrell, M. (2012). Cognitive stimulation to improve cognitive functioning in people with dementia. *Cochrane Database of Systematic Reviews, 2012*(2), CD005562. *Evidence Level I.*

Yanhong, O., Chandra, M., & Venkatesh, D. (2013). Mild cognitive impairment in adult: A neuropsychological review. *Annals of Indian Academy of Neurology, 16*(3), 310–318. *Evidence Level V.*

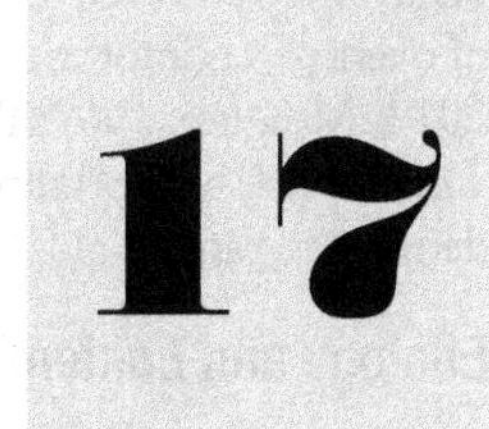

Delirium: Prevention, Early Recognition, and Treatment

Dorothy F. Tullmann, Cheri Blevins, and Kathleen Fletcher

EDUCATIONAL OBJECTIVES

On completion of this chapter, the reader should be able to:

1. Discuss risk factors of delirium in older hospitalized adults
2. Describe the negative sequelae of delirium in older adults during hospitalization
3. Discuss the importance of early recognition of delirium
4. List four nonpharmacological interventions to prevent and/or treat delirium
5. Identify long-term negative sequelae of delirium in older adults who have been hospitalized

OVERVIEW

Delirium is a common complication in hospitalized older adults and is one of the major contributors to poor outcomes of health care and institutionalization for older patients. The incidence and severity of delirium can be reduced by identifying modifiable risk factors, screening regularly for delirium, and implementing multicomponent interventions. If delirium does develop, early recognition is of paramount importance in order to treat the underlying pathology and minimize delirium's sequelae. Although many researchers are seeking to identify effective pharmacological agents to prevent and/or treat delirium, nonpharmacological, multicomponent interventions have the strongest evidence of accomplishing these goals. Nurses play a key role in the prevention, early recognition, and treatment of this potentially devastating condition in older hospitalized adults.

BACKGROUND AND STATEMENT OF PROBLEM

Definition

Delirium is a neurocognitive disorder that develops over a short period of time (hours to days), fluctuates in severity throughout the day, and is primarily a disturbance of attention. Delirium also manifests as a disturbance in cognition (memory defect, disorientation, etc.) that cannot be explained by a preexisting neurocognitive disorder; rather, delirium is a physiological consequence of substance intoxication or withdrawal, medication, another medical condition, or multiple etiologies (American Psychiatric Association, 2013). A patient may present with hyperactive, hypoactive, or mixed motoric subtypes of delirium (Hosie, Davidson, Agar, Sanderson, & Phillips, 2013; Meagher, 2009). Nurses typically associate delirium with hyperactivity and distressing, time-consuming, and harmful patient

For a description of evidence levels cited in this chapter, see Chapter 1, "Developing and Evaluating Clinical Practice Guidelines: A Systematic Approach."

behaviors. However, the hypoactive subtype, with its lack of overt psychomotor activity, is also common (Hosie et al., 2013; Meagher, 2009; Pandharipande et al., 2007) and has a higher risk of mortality, especially when superimposed on dementia (Yang et al., 2009).

Etiology and Epidemiology

Prevalence and Incidence

Among medical inpatients, delirium is present on admission to the hospital in 10% to 31% of older patients, and during hospitalization, 11% to 42% of older adults develop delirium (Siddiqi, House, & Holmes, 2006). Among hip surgery patients, the incidence of delirium is 4% to 53%. Those with hip fractures and preexisting cognitive impairment have the highest risk of delirium (Bruce, Ritchie, Blizard, Lai, & Raven, 2007). Older adults admitted to medical intensive care units (ICUs) have both prevalent and incident delirium of 31% (McNicoll et al., 2003; Salluh et al., 2010). In surgical ICUs (SICUs), the prevalence of delirium on admission is only 2.6%, but 28.3% develop delirium during their SICU stay (Balas et al., 2007). Up to 81.7% of mechanically ventilated patients in medical and SICUs experience delirium (Ely et al., 2004; Pisani, Murphy, Araujo, & Van Ness, 2010), and more than half of older patients in medical ICUs still have delirium when transferred (Pisani et al., 2010). From 13.3% to 42.3% of palliative care patients have delirium on admission, 26% to 62% during hospitalization, and 58.8% to 88% have delirium closer to death (Hosie et al., 2013). The incidence of delirium superimposed on dementia ranges from 22% to 89% (Fick, Agostini, & Inouye, 2002).

Pathophysiology

The pathogenesis of delirium is poorly understood and likely involves a complex interaction between neurotransmitter systems and psychoneuroimmunological pathways (AGS/NIA Delirium Conference Writing Group, Planning Committee and Faculty and AGS/NIA Delirium Conference Writing Group, 2015). More research is needed to determine the exact mechanisms and biomarkers to help identify different delirium pathways and whether or not there are differences between the biomarkers of risk, presence, and severity of delirium.

Risk Factors

The most common risk factors for delirium in acute hospital units are dementia, older age, comorbid illness, severity of medical illness, infection, "high risk" medication use, diminished activities of daily living, immobility, sensory impairment, urinary catheterization, urea and electrolyte imbalance, and malnutrition. Statistically significant risk factors are dementia, illness severity, urinary catheterization, low albumin level, and length of hospital stay (Ahmed, Leurent, & Sampson, 2014). In older patients admitted for hip surgery, early cognitive impairment, such as memory impairments, incoherence, disorientation, as well as an underlying physical illness and age, are especially strong predictors of delirium (de Jonghe et al., 2007; Kalisvaart et al., 2006). Other possible risk factors include sleep deprivation (Weinhouse et al., 2009), elevated blood urea nitrogen (BUN)/creatinine ratio, polypharmacy, physical restraints, and anemia (Inouye et al., 1990; Inouye, Viscoli, Horwitz, Hurst, & Tinetti, 1993; O'Keeffe & Lavan, 1996).

Outcomes

The outcomes of delirium in hospitalized older adults are grave. Those who develop delirium have an increased mortality rate (up to 22.7 months postdischarge [Witlox et al., 2010]), increased hospital length of stay, and transfer to long-term care facilities (Shi, Presutti, Selchen, & Saposnik, 2012; Witlox et al., 2013). Other sequelae of delirium are depression, decreased functional and cognitive status, and increased geriatric syndrome complications (Anderson, Ngo, & Marcantonio, 2012; Cole, McCusker, Ciampi, & Belzile, 2008; Witlox et al., 2010; Witlox et al., 2013). ICU patients who develop delirium have a higher mortality and complication rate, spend longer periods of time on mechanical ventilation, have increased ICU and hospital lengths of stay, and are more likely to be discharged to a long-term care facility (Ely et al., 2004; Shehabi et al., 2013; Zhang, Pan, & Ni, 2013). From 22% to 89% of older hospitalized adults with dementia also have delirium superimposed on the dementia (Fick et al., 2002), are at increased risk for developing delirium, and have worse outcomes when they do (Morandi et al., 2014; Yang et al., 2009).

ASSESSMENT OF THE PROBLEM

The first critically important step in the assessment of delirium is identifying the risk factors for delirium because eliminating or reducing these risk factors and intervening appropriately may prevent delirium or reduce its length or severity (Milisen, Lemiengre, Braes, & Foreman, 2005). Recognizing the features of delirium is important in order to further identify, eliminate, or reduce the precipitating factor(s) such as pain, infection, or other acute illnesses. This can best be done by routinely assessing patients at risk for delirium with a standardized screening tool for delirium although this is currently occurring only in 17% of hospitals (Neuman, Speck, Karlawish, Schwartz, & Shea, 2010) and nurses fail to recognize delirium 75% of the time (Rice et al., 2011).

The gold standard for diagnosing delirium is a full evaluation by a mental health expert using the criteria found in the most recent, fifth edition, of the *Diagnostic and Statistical Manual of Mental Disorders* (*DSM-5*; American Psychiatric Association [APA], 2013). However, given the rapid onset and typically fluctuating course of delirium, particularly in the hospital setting, a number of user-friendly and relatively rapid screening tools have been developed and utilized by nurses for over the past two decades.

The Confusion Assessment Method (CAM; Inouye et al., 1990) is the most widely used delirium screening instrument in hospitalized older adults, having been used in more than 5,000 original articles and translated into 13 languages (Inouye, 2015). The long CAM has 10 items and is preferred in research studies, whereas short CAM contains only the four items of the diagnostic algorithm. A version of the CAM for patients in ICUs (CAM-ICU; Ely, Gautam, et al., 2001) is recommended for use with critically ill older adults (Jacobi et al., 2002; Schuurmans, Deschamps, Markham, Shortridge-Baggett, & Duursma, 2003). The CAM instrument identifies the key features of delirium—acute onset and fluctuating course, inattention, disorganized thinking, and altered level of consciousness and is supported by the best evidence (Wong, Holroyd-Leduc, Simel, & Straus, 2010). Other robust and usable scales include the Delirium Rating Scale (DRS), the Memorial Delirium Assessment Scale (MDAS), and the NEECHAM Confusion Scale (Adamis, Sharma, Whelan, & Macdonald, 2010; Breitbart et al., 1997; Neelon, Champagne, Carlson, & Funk, 1996; Trzepacz et al., 2001).

Another delirium scale, growing in popularity, is the Nursing Delirium Screening Scale (Nu-DESC; Gaudreau, Gagnon, Harel, Tremblay, & Roy, 2005). The Nu-DESC is based on the Confusion Rating Scale (CRS; Gagnon, Allard, Masse, & DeSerres, 2000), the only delirium screening scale that does not require patient participation as it evaluates the presence of confusional symptoms. The CRS can be completed in less than 2 minutes during routine nursing care, and assesses four symptoms of delirium: disorientation, inappropriate behavior, inappropriate communication, and illusions or hallucinations. The CRS uses a score of 0 when there are no symptoms, 1 if there is one mild symptom, and 2 when a symptom is present and pronounced. A score of 2 or more is considered positive.

The NuDESC added a fifth symptom, psychomotor retardation, to account for the hypoactive variant of delirium (Gaudreau et al., 2005). When compared with blinded assessments of 59 patients with psychiatrists using the *Diagnostic and Statistical Manual of Mental Disorders* (4th ed.; *DSM–IV*; APA, 1994) criteria and research nurses using the CAM and MDAS assessments, the NuDESC showed 85.7% sensitivity and 86.8% specificity. When comparing the NuDESC to the CAM-ICU in ICU patients, the NuDESC had a sensitivity of 83% (compared to 81% for the CAM-ICU); however, the specificity of the NuDESC (81%) was significantly lower than that of CAM-ICU (96%; Luetz et al., 2010); so the CAM-ICU remains the preferred screening tool for delirium in critically ill patients.

Bedside nurses are in the best position to recognize delirium because they possess the skill and responsibility of ongoing patient assessment and are in key positions to recognize risk factors for delirium and the earliest cognitive changes heralding the onset of delirium. Early identification of risk factors and screening for the earliest onset of delirium are critical to implementing strategies to minimize the occurrence of this devastating pathology in hospitalized older adults.

Interventions

The Cochrane Review found that there are no strong-evidence randomized controlled trials (RCTs) from delirium prevention studies to guide clinical practice (Siddiqi, Stockdale, Britton, & Holmes, 2007). And although there is some preliminary evidence that some pharmacological agents may be effective in reducing delirium, it is not strong (Gosch & Nicholas, 2014). However, there is mounting evidence that multicomponent, nonpharmacological interventions are still the best practice for preventing and managing delirium as well as improving patient outcomes (Holroyd-Leduc, Khandwala, & Sink, 2010).

The American Geriatrics Society (AGS) views delirium as the most essential topic in the care of older hospitalized adults and strongly recommends nonpharmacological, multicomponent interventions (American Geriatrics Society Expert Panel, 2014). It is noteworthy that virtually all of the components of these recommended nonpharmacological interventions to prevent and manage delirium are basic nursing practices that should be part of every nurse's routine care of hospitalized patients. Supporting studies (Inouye et al., 1999; Lundstrom et al., 2005; Marcantonio, Flacker, Wright, & Resnick, 2001; Milisen et al., 2005; Rubin, Neal, Fenlon, Hassan, &

Inouye, 2011; Rubin et al., 2006; Zaubler et al., 2013) have included the following types of interventions:

1. Mobility
2. Reorientation
3. Cognitive stimulation
4. Maintenance of nutrition and hydration
5. Sleep enhancement
6. Vision and hearing adaptation
7. Nursing education
8. Geriatric consultation

CASE STUDY

Mr. Z is an 82-year-old patient admitted to your unit for prostate surgery. He is a retired accountant, lives with his wife, and is very active. He drives a car, plays golf, and regularly participates in activities at the senior center. His type 2 diabetes is well controlled on Actoplus Met (pioglitazone hydrochloride and metformin hydrochloride). Mr. Z reports that he has decreased his fluid intake so he can avoid waking several times during the night to urinate. He also has a history of hypertension, moderate hearing loss (hearing aids bilaterally), and previous surgery for inguinal hernia repair. He wears bifocal glasses for distance and reading. He is alert, oriented, and expresses a good understanding of his upcoming surgery. His preoperative laboratory values are within normal limits except for a low hematocrit and a slightly elevated BUN/creatinine (BUN/Cr) ratio. His medications include Actoplus Met (pioglitazone hydrochloride and metformin hydrochloride) for his diabetes and Calan (verapamil) for hypertension.

What Factors Present on Admission to the Hospital Put Mr. Z at Risk of Developing Delirium?

- *Age*: Older adults are at greater risk of delirium, particularly if they have underlying dementia or depression. Physiological changes that occur with aging can affect the ability of older adults to respond to physical and physiological stress and to maintain homeostasis.
- *Dehydration*: An elevated BUN/Cr ratio indicates dehydration (from decreased fluid intake), a frequent contributing factor (along with electrolyte imbalance) to delirium of hospitalized older adults.
- *Anemia*: Because of a low hematocrit, the body has diminished ability to deliver adequate oxygen to the brain, making delirium more likely.
- *Sensory deficits*: Those with vision and hearing loss are more likely to misinterpret sensory input, which places them at increased risk for delirium.

It is important to understand that it might not be one particular factor but the interplay of patient vulnerability (predisposing factors) and precipitating factors—common during hospitalization—that place the older adult at risk for delirium.

What Can You Do to Help Prevent Delirium in Mr. Z?

- Assist Mr. Z, as needed, to be as physically active as possible
  - Check his orientation regularly and reorient as needed
  - Encourage cognitive activities such as reading or crossword puzzles
- Make sure Mr. Z's glasses and hearing aids are on and functioning.
- Explore reasons for the low hematocrit and discuss correction preoperatively.
  - Assure correction of dehydration and adequate hydration preoperatively
  - Ensure adequate sleep and rest
  - Review Mr. Z's nutritional status and work with the interprofessional team to correct preoperatively
  - If possible, consult with a geriatric specialist (geriatrician or geriatric nurse practitioner) for a thorough geriatric assessment of Mr. Z

You provide care for Mr. Z again 2 days after surgery. He is confused and picking at the air and oriented to self only. An indwelling urinary catheter and peripheral intravenous line are in place. In his report, the day-shift nurse mentioned considering a physical restraint because Mr. Z was increasingly restless and impulsive. He was CAM positive, indicating that he may have delirium. The licensed independent practitioner was notified and confirmed delirium using the *DSM-5* criteria (APA, 2013).

What Are the Clinical Features of Delirium?

- *Disturbance of consciousness* characterized by reduced clarity and awareness of the environment: reduced ability to focus, sustain, and shift

(continued)

CASE STUDY *(continued)*

attention. Patients have trouble following instructions or making sense of their environment, even with cues. They may also get "stuck" on a particular concern or thought.

- *Cognitive changes*: Memory deficit, disorientation, language disturbance, and/or perceptual disturbance
- *Perceptual disturbances*: Hallucinations and delusions are common. Patients can be hyperactive and agitated or lethargic (hypoactive) and less active. The latter presentation is of particular concern because it is often not recognized by health care providers as delirium. The presentation may also be mixed, with the patient fluctuating from one to the other behavioral state.
- Delirium can be *characterized by* disturbances in the sleep–wake cycle and rapidly shifting emotional disturbances, with escalation of the disturbed behavior at night (sundowning).
- The clinical hallmarks of delirium are that the cited *changes occur rapidly* over several hours or days. There is a decreased attention span and a fluctuating course (waxing and waning of confusion).

It is also important to consider that delirium may occur concurrently with dementia or depression. In fact, these patients are at increased risk for developing delirium. Family and caregivers can be invaluable in helping to identify or distinguish cognitive changes in circumstances when the patient is not well known to you.

What Additional Factors May Now Be Contributing to Mr. Z's Delirium?

- *Anesthesia and other medications*: It takes several hours to days for the body to clear the effects of anesthesia. Inasmuch as older adults have a larger percentage of body fat than younger persons do, and many drugs are fat-soluble, drug effects will last longer. Also, older adults tend to have less cellular water; hence, water-soluble drugs will be more concentrated and have a more pronounced effect. Consider the possibility of alcohol withdrawal (often a hidden problem) as a contributing factor.
- *Pain*: What is Mr. Z's pain-control regimen and status? What is the dose and frequency of the pain medication? Is the dose appropriate?
- *Hypoxemia*: Mr. Z is at risk because of limited mobility and possible atelectasis after surgery. What is his oxygen saturation (SpO_2)? Does he have crackles or diminished breath sounds?
- *Infection, inflammation, or other medical illness*: Postoperative infections, intraoperative myocardial infarctions (MIs), or strokes are possible causes of delirium in this case. Could Mr. Z have a urinary tract infection (UTI) post prostate surgery, particularly because he has a Foley catheter? An inflammatory response to a new medical problem may be the cause of the delirium.
- *Unfamiliar surroundings*: Particularly for those with sensory deficits, unfamiliar environments can lead to misinterpretations of information, which may contribute to delirium.

What Steps Should Be Taken Now?

- *Avoid the use of restraints*, which could worsen Mr. Z's agitation.
- *Call the physician or nurse practitioner* immediately as postoperative delirium can be life threatening. Report your findings; request that the patient be evaluated to determine the underlying cause of the delirium. If the psychotic features of delirium worsen and the risk of harm to the patient or others is imminent, Mr. Z may also need medication to control his symptoms.
- *Frequent reality orientation*: Frequent orientation, reassurance, and helping Mr. Z interpret his environment and what is happening to him should be helpful. (Monitor the patient's reaction. If the patient becomes upset or angry, you will need to modify your approach to that of more reassurance and validating the patient's experience rather than reorienting.)
- Are Mr. Z's *hearing aids and glasses* in place; clean and functioning? Impaired sensory input contributes significantly to delirium. Also, he may seem more confused than he really is if he is not able to hear what you are saying.
- Invite *family/significant others* to stay as much as they are able to assist with his orientation, reassurance, and sense of well-being. Monitor the effect of family visitation. If the patient has increased agitation or anxiety, then limit the visitation of the individual who seems to be triggering Mr. Z's upset.
- *Mobilize the patient.* Mobility assists with orientation and helps prevent problems associated with immobility, such as atelectasis and deep venous thrombosis.
- *Judicious use of medications* for pain, sleep, or anxiety. Drugs used to address these issues can exacerbate the delirium. Try nonpharmacological approaches for sleep and anxiety first. If Mr. Z is having pain, are the drug and dose appropriate for

(continued)

CASE STUDY *(continued)*

him? A regular schedule of a smaller dose or non-narcotic pain medication almost always is better than as-needed dosing.

- Try to *provide for adequate sleep*: Reduce noise at night; play soft, relaxing music; offer warm milk or herbal tea, and massage; reschedule care in order not to interrupt sleep.
- Make sure the patient is well *hydrated and nourished.*
- Talk to the doctor or nurse practitioner about removing the indwelling urinary catheter. Because of his surgery, Mr. Z may need it immediately post-operation, but it should be removed as soon as possible. Additionally, recommend a urinalysis to rule out UTI.
- *Address safety concerns* (e.g., increase surveillance). Mr. Z is now also at greater risk for falls and other conditions and syndromes.

SUMMARY

Delirium is a common occurrence in hospitalized older adults and contributes to poor outcomes. Thus, it is important to promptly identify those patients at risk for delirium and implement preventive measures as well as promptly recognize delirium when it appears. Nursing assessments using validated delirium screening instruments must become routine. A standard-of-practice protocol provides concise information to guide nursing care of individuals at risk for or experiencing delirium.

NURSING STANDARD OF PRACTICE

PROTOCOL 17.1: Delirium Reduction

I. GOAL

Reduce the incidence of delirium in older hospitalized adults

II. OVERVIEW

A. Delirium is a common syndrome in hospitalized older adults and is associated with increased mortality, hospital costs, and long-term cognitive and functional impairment.
B. Delirium can sometimes be prevented or diminished with the recognition of high-risk patients and the implementation of a standardized multicomponent delirium-reduction protocol.
C. Recognition of risk factors and routine screening for delirium should be part of comprehensive nursing care for older adults.

III. BACKGROUND

A. Delirium is a neurocognitive disorder that develops over a short period of time (hours to days), fluctuates in severity throughout the day, and is primarily a disturbance of attention. Delirium is a physiological consequence of another underlying disorder (American Psychiatric Association, 2013).
B. Prevalence and incidence: In 10% to 31% of older medical patients, 31% of ICU patients, and 26% to 62% of palliative care patients delirium is *present on admission* (Siddiqi et al., 2006). Delirium *develops* in 11% to 42% of medical (Siddiqi et al., 2006), 4% to 53% of hip surgery (Bruce et al., 2007), 31% of medical ICU (McNicoll et al., 2003; Salluh et al., 2010), 28.3% of surgical ICU (Balas et al., 2007), up to 81.7% of mechanically ventilated (Ely et al., 2004; Pisani et al., 2010), and 26% to 62% of palliative care patients (Hosie et al., 2013).
C. Risk factors: The most common risk factors for delirium in acute hospital units are dementia, older age, comorbid illness, severity of medical illness, infection, "high risk" medication use, diminished activities of daily living, immobility, sensory impairment, urinary catheterization, urea and electrolyte imbalance and malnutrition (Ahmed et al., 2014). Other possible risk factors include sleep deprivation (Weinhouse et al., 2009), polypharmacy, physical restraints, and anemia (Inouye et al., 1990; Inouye et al., 1993; O'Keeffe & Lavan, 1996).

(continued)

Protocol 17.1: Delirium Reduction *(continued)*

D. Outcomes: The outcomes of delirium in hospitalized older adults are increased mortality (Witlox et al., 2010), hospital length of stay, transfer to long-term care facilities (Shi et al., 2012; Witlox et al., 2013), depression, decreased functional and cognitive status, increased geriatric syndrome complications, and dementia (Anderson et al., 2012; Cole et al., 2008; Witlox et al., 2010; Witlox et al., 2013). From 22% to 89% of older hospitalized adults with dementia also have delirium superimposed on the dementia (Fick et al., 2002), are at increased risk of developing delirium, and have worse outcomes when they do (Morandi et al., 2014; Yang et al., 2009).

IV. PARAMETERS OF ASSESSMENT

A. Assess for common and other risk factors (Ahmed et al., 2014).
   1. Cognitive dysfunction
   2. Illness severity
   3. Comorbidities
   4. Infection
   5. High-risk medication use (e.g., benzodiazepines)
   6. Immobility
   7. Decreased activities of daily living
   8. Urinary catheterization
   9. Urea and electrolyte imbalance and dehydration
   10. Malnutrition
   11. Physical restraints
   12. Anemia

B. Assess for delirium using a validated screening tool (see Resources)
   1. Key features of delirium (CAM, CAM-ICU)
      a. Acute onset and fluctuating course
      b. Inattention
      c. Disorganized thinking
      d. Altered level of consciousness
   2. Delirium symptoms (NuDESC)
      a. Disorientation
      b. Inappropriate behavior
      c. Inappropriate communication
      d. Illusions or hallucinations
      e. Psychomotor hypoactivity

V. NURSING CARE STRATEGIES

A. Eliminate or minimize risk factors
   1. Administer medications judiciously; avoid high-risk medications
   2. Prevent and/or promptly and appropriately treat infections
   3. Prevent and/or promptly treat dehydration and electrolyte disturbances
   4. Provide adequate pain control
   5. Maximize oxygen delivery (supplemental oxygen, blood, and BP support as needed).
   6. Use sensory aids as appropriate
   7. Regulate bowel/bladder function
   8. Provide adequate nutrition

B. Provide a therapeutic environment.
   1. Foster orientation: Frequently reassure and reorient patient (unless patient becomes agitated); use easily visible calendars, clocks, caregiver identification; carefully explain all activities; communicate clearly
   2. Provide appropriate sensory stimulation: quiet room, adequate light, pursue one task at a time, use noise-reduction strategies

(continued)

Protocol 17.1: Delirium Reduction *(continued)*

3. Facilitate sleep: Offer back massage, warm milk, or herbal tea at bedtime; play relaxation music/tapes; employ noise-reduction measures; avoid awaking patient
4. Foster familiarity: Encourage family/friends to stay at bedside, bring familiar objects from home, maintain consistency of caregivers, minimize relocations
5. Maximize mobility: Avoid restraints and urinary catheters; ambulate or active ROM exercises three times daily.
6. Communicate clearly, provide explanations
7. Reassure and educate family
8. Minimize invasive interventions
9. Consult with a geriatric specialist
10. Consider psychotropic medication as a last resort for agitation (Patel, Baldwin, Bunting, & Laha, 2014; Zaubler et al., 2014)

VI. EVALUATION/EXPECTED OUTCOMES

A. Patient
   1. Absence of delirium
   2. Cognitive status returned to baseline (before delirium)
   3. Functional status returned to baseline (before delirium)
   4. Discharged to same destination as prehospitalization

B. Health care provider
   1. Regular use of delirium screening tool
   2. Increased detection of delirium
   3. Implementation of appropriate interventions to prevent/treat delirium from standardized protocol
   4. Decreased use of physical restraints
   5. Decreased use of antipsychotic medications
   6. Increased satisfaction in care of hospitalized older adults

C. Institution
   1. Staff education and interprofessional care planning
   2. Implementation of standardized delirium screening protocol
   3. Decreased overall cost
   4. Decreased length of stay
   5. Decreased morbidity and mortality
   6. Increased referrals and consultation to earlier specified specialists
   7. Improved satisfaction of patients, families, and nursing staff

VII. FOLLOW-UP MONITORING OF CONDITION

A. Decreased delirium to become a measure of quality care
B. Incidence of delirium to decrease
C. Patient days with delirium to decrease
D. Staff competence in recognition and treatment of acute confusion/delirium
E. Documentation of a variety of interventions for acute confusion/delirium

ABBREVIATIONS

CAM	Confusion Assessment Method
CAM-ICU	CAM for patients in intensive care unit
NuDESC	Nursing Delirium Screening Scale
ROM	Range of motion

RESOURCES

Recommended Delirium Screening Instruments

Confusion Assessment Method (CAM)

http://www.hospitalelderlifeprogram.org/delirium-instruments/short-cam

Confusion Assessment Method for the Intensive Care Unit (CAM-ICU)

http://www.icudelirium.org/delirium/monitoring.html

Nursing Delirium Screening Scale (Nu-DESC)

http://www.jpsmjournal.com/article/S0885-3924(05)00053-9/abstract

Other Delirium Screening Instruments

Delirium Rating Scale (DRS)-revised-98

Memorial Delirium Assessment Scale (MDAS)

NEECHAM Confusion Scale

Additional Information About Delirium

Consult GeriRN: http://consultgerirn.org/resources: An online resource containing information regarding assessing and caring for older adults sponsored by the Hartford Institute for Geriatric Nursing at New York University College of Nursing.

REFERENCES

Adamis, D., Sharma, N., Whelan, P. J., & Macdonald, A. J. (2010). Delirium scales: A review of current evidence. *Aging & Mental Health, 14*(5), 543–555. doi:http://dx.doi.org/10.1080/13607860903421011. Retrieved from http://ovidsp.ovid.com/ovidweb.cgi?T=JS&CSC=Y&NEWS=N&PAGE=fulltext&D=med5&AN=20480420. *Evidence Level I.*

AGS/NIA Delirium Conference Writing Group, Planning Committee and Faculty, and AGS/NIA Delirium Conference Writing Group. (2015). The American Geriatrics Society/National Institute on Aging Bedside-to-Bench Conference: Research agenda on delirium in older adults. *Journal of the American Geriatrics Society, 63,* 843–852. doi:10.1111/jgs.13406. *Evidence Level VI.*

Ahmed, S., Leurent, B., & Sampson, E. L. (2014). Risk factors for incident delirium among older people in acute hospital medical units: A systematic review and meta-analysis. *Age & Ageing, 43*(3), 326–333. doi:http://dx.doi.org/10.1093/ageing/afu022. Retrieved from http://ovidsp.ovid.com/ovidweb.cgi?T=JS&CSC=Y&NEWS=N&PAGE=fulltext&D=medl&AN=24610863. *Evidence Level I.*

American Geriatrics Society Expert Panel. (2014). AGS Expert Panel on postoperative delirium in older adults. *Journal of the American Geriatrics Society, 63,* 142–150. *Evidence Level VI.*

American Psychiatric Association. (2004). *Diagnostic and statistical manual of mental disorders* (4th ed.). Arlington, VA: American Psychiatric Press. *Evidence Level I.*

American Psychiatric Association. (2013). *Desk reference to the diagnostic criteria from DSM-5.* Arlington, VA: American Psychiatric Press. *Evidence Level I.*

Anderson, C. P., Ngo, L. H., & Marcantonio, E. R. (2012). Complications in postacute care are associated with persistent delirium. *Journal of the American Geriatrics Society, 60*(6), 1122–1127. doi:http://dx.doi.org/10.1111/j.1532-5415.2012.03958.x. Retrieved from http://ovidsp.ovid.com/ovidweb.cgi?T=JS&CSC=Y&NEWS=N&PAGE=fulltext&D=medl&AN=22646692. *Evidence Level IV.*

Balas, M. C., Deutschman, C. S., Sullivan-Marx, E. M., Strumpf, N. E., Alston, R. P., & Richmond, T. S. (2007). Delirium in older patients in surgical intensive care units. *Journal of Nursing Scholarship, 39*(2), 147–154. *Evidence Level IV.*

Breitbart, W., Rosenfeld, B., Roth, A., Smith, M. J., Cohen, K., & Passik, S. (1997). The Memorial Delirium Assessment Scale. *Journal of Pain and Symptom Management, 13*(3), 128–137. *Evidence Level IV.*

Bruce, A. J., Ritchie, C. W., Blizard, R., Lai, R., & Raven, P. (2007). The incidence of delirium associated with orthopedic surgery: A meta-analytic review. *International Psychogeriatrics/IPA, 19*(2), 197–214. *Evidence Level I.*

Cole, M. G., McCusker, J., Ciampi, A., & Belzile, E. (2008). The 6- and 12-month outcomes of older medical inpatients who recover from subsyndromal delirium. *Journal of the American Geriatrics Society, 56*(11), 2093–2099. *Evidence Level II.*

de Jonghe, J. F., Kalisvaart, K. J., Dijkstra, M., van Dis, H., Vreeswijk, R., Kat, M. G., . . . van Gool, W. A. (2007). Early symptoms in the prodromal phase of delirium: A prospective cohort study in elderly patients undergoing hip surgery. *American Journal of Geriatric Psychiatry, 15*(2), 112–121. *Evidence Level IV.*

Ely, E. W., Gautam, S., Margolin, R., Francis, J., May, L., Speroff, T., . . . Inouye, S. K. (2001a). The impact of delirium in the intensive care unit on hospital length of stay. *Intensive Care Medicine, 27*(12), 1892–1900. *Evidence Level IV.*

Ely, E. W., Inouye, S. K., Bernard, G. R., Gordon, S., Francis, J., May, L., . . . Dittus, R. (2001b). Delirium in mechanically ventilated patients: Validity and reliability of the confusion assessment method for the intensive care unit (CAM-ICU). *Journal of the American Medical Association, 286*(21), 2703–2710. *Evidence Level IV.*

Ely, E. W., Shintani, A., Truman, B., Speroff, T., Gordon, S. M., Harrell, F. E., . . . Dittus, R. (2004). Delirium as a predictor of mortality in mechanically ventilated patients in the intensive care unit. *Journal of the American Medical Association, 291*(14), 1753–1762. doi:10.1001/jama.291.14.1753. *Evidence Level IV.*

Fick, D. M., Agostini, J. V., & Inouye, S. K. (2002). Delirium superimposed on dementia: A systematic review. *Journal of the American Geriatrics Society, 50*(10), 1723–1732. *Evidence Level I.*

Gagnon, P., Allard, P., Masse, B., & DeSerres, M. (2000). Delirium in terminal cancer: A prospective study using daily screening, early diagnosis, and continuous monitoring. *Journal of Pain and Symptom Management, 19*(6), 412–426. doi:S0885–3924(00)00143–3 [pii]. *Evidence Level II.*

Gaudreau, J. D., Gagnon, P., Harel, F., Tremblay, A., & Roy, M. A. (2005). Fast, systematic, and continuous delirium assessment in hospitalized patients: The Nursing Delirium Screening Scale. *Journal of Pain and Symptom Management, 29*(4), 368–375. doi:S0885–3924(05)00053–9 [pii]. *Evidence Level IV.*

Gosch, M., & Nicholas, J. A. (2014). Pharmacologic prevention of postoperative delirium. *Zeitschrift Fur Gerontologie und Geriatrie, 47*(2), 105–109. doi:http://dx.doi.org/10.1007/s00391–013-0598–1. Retrieved from http://ovidsp.ovid.com/ovidweb.cgi?T=JS&CSC=Y&NEWS=N&PAGE=fulltext&D=medl&AN=24619041. *Evidence Level I.*

Holroyd-Leduc, J., Khandwala, F., & Sink, K. M. (2010). How can delirium best be prevented and managed in older patients in hospital?" *Canadian Medical Association Journal, 182*(5), 465–470. doi:10.1503/cmaj.080519. *Evidence Level I.*

Hosie, A., Davidson, P. M., Agar, M., Sanderson, C. R., & Phillips, J. (2013). Delirium prevalence, incidence, and implications for screening in specialist palliative care inpatient settings: A systematic review. *Palliative Medicine, 27*(6), 486–498. doi:10.1177/0269216312457214. Retrieved from https://search.ebscohost.com/login.aspx?direct=true&AuthType=ip&db=cin20&AN=2012122082&site=ehost-live. *Evidence Level IV.*

Inouye, S. K. (2015). *Confusion Assessment Method (Long CAM).* Retrieved from http://www.hospitalelderlifeprogram.org/delirium-instruments/confusion-assessment-method-long-cam/. *Evidence Level VI.*

Inouye, S. K., Bogardus, S. T., Charpentier, P. A., Leo-Summers, L., Acampora, D., Holford, T. R., & Cooney, L. M. (1999). A multicomponent intervention to prevent delirium in hospitalized older patients. *New England Journal of Medicine, 340*(9), 669–676. *Evidence Level II.*

Inouye, S. K., van Dyck, C. H., Alessi, C. A., Balkin, S., Siegal, A. P., & Horwitz, R. I. (1990). Clarifying confusion: The Confusion Assessment Method (a new method for detection of delirium). *Annals of Internal Medicine, 113*(12), 941–948. *Evidence Level IV.*

Inouye, S. K., Viscoli, C. M., Horwitz, R. I., Hurst, L. D., & Tinetti, M. E. (1993). A predictive model for delirium in hospitalized elderly medical patients based on admission characteristics. *Annals of Internal Medicine, 119*(6), 474–481. *Evidence Level IV.*

Jacobi, J., Fraser, G. L., Coursin, D. B., Riker, R. R., Fontaine, D., Wittbrodt, E. T.,... American College of Chest Physicians. (2002). Clinical practice guidelines for the sustained use of sedatives and analgesics in the critically Ill adult. *Critical Care Medicine, 30*(1), 119–141. *Evidence Level VI.*

Kalisvaart, K. J., Vreeswijk, R., de Jonghe, J. F., van der Ploeg, T., van Gool, W. A., & Eikelenboom, P. (2006). Risk factors and prediction of postoperative delirium in elderly hip-surgery patients: Implementation and validation of a medical risk factor model. *Journal of the American Geriatrics Society, 54*(5), 817–822. *Evidence Level II.*

Luetz, A., Heymann, A., Radtke, F. M., Chenitir, C., Neuhaus, U., Nachtigall, I.,... Spies, C. D. (2010). Different assessment tools for intensive care unit delirium: Which score to use? *Critical Care Medicine, 38*(2), 409–418. doi:10.1097/CCM.0b013e3181cabb42. *Evidence Level IV.*

Lundstrom, M., Edlund, A., Karlsson, S., Brannstrom, B., Bucht, G., & Gustafson, Y. (2005). A multifactorial intervention program reduces the duration of delirium, length of hospitalization, and mortality in delirious patients. *Journal of the American Geriatrics Society, 53*(4), 622–628. doi:JGS53210 [pii]. *Evidence Level II.*

Marcantonio, E. R., Flacker, J. M., Wright, R. J., & Resnick, N. M. (2001). Reducing delirium after hip fracture: A randomized trial. *Journal of the American Geriatrics Society, 49*(5), 516–522. *Evidence Level II.*

McNicoll, L., Pisani, M. A., Zhang, Y., Ely, E. W., Siegel, M. D., & Inouye, S. K. (2003). Delirium in the intensive care unit: Occurrence and clinical course in older patients. *Journal of the American Geriatrics Society, 51*(5), 591–598. *Evidence Level IV.*

Meagher, D. (2009). Motor subtypes of delirium: Past, present and future. *International Review of Psychiatry, 21*(1), 59–73. *Evidence Level VI.*

Milisen, K., Lemiengre, J., Braes, T., & Foreman, M. D. (2005). Multicomponent intervention strategies for managing delirium in hospitalized older people: Systematic review. *Journal of Advanced Nursing, 52*(1), 79–90. *Evidence Level I.*

Morandi, A., Davis, D., Fick, D. M., Turco, R., Boustani, M., Lucchi, E.,... Bellelli, G. (2014). Delirium superimposed on dementia strongly predicts worse outcomes in older rehabilitation inpatients. *Journal of the American Medical Directors Association, 15*(5), 349–354. doi:10.1016/j.jamda.2013.12.084. *Evidence Level IV.*

Neelon, V. J., Champagne, M. T., Carlson, J. R., & Funk, S. G. (1996). The NEECHAM Confusion Scale: Construction, validation, and clinical testing. *Nursing Research, 45*(6), 324–330. *Evidence Level IV.*

Neuman, M. D., Speck, R. M., Karlawish, J. H., Schwartz, J. S., & Shea, J. A. (2010). Hospital protocols for the inpatient care of older adults: Results from a statewide survey. *Journal of the American Geriatrics Society, 58*(10), 1959–1964. *Evidence Level IV.*

O'Keeffe, S. T., & Lavan, J. N. (1996). Predicting delirium in elderly patients: Development and validation of a risk-stratification model. *Age and Ageing, 25*, 317–321. *Evidence Level IV.*

Pandharipande, P., Cotton, B. A., Shintani, A., Thompson, J., Costabile, S., Truman Pun, B.,... Ely, E. W. (2007). Motoric subtypes of delirium in mechanically ventilated surgical and trauma intensive care unit patients. *Intensive Care Medicine, 33*(10), 1726–1731. *Evidence Level II.*

Patel, J., Baldwin, J, Bunting, P., & Laha, S. (2014). The effect of a multicomponent multidisciplinary bundle of interventions on sleep and delirium in medical and surgical intensive care patients. *Anaesthesia, 69*(6), 540–549. *Evidence Level III.*

Pisani, M. A., Murphy, T. E., Araujo, K. L., & Van Ness, P. H. (2010). Factors associated with persistent delirium after intensive care unit admission in an older medical patient population. *Journal of Critical Care, 25*(3), 540.e1–540.e7. *Evidence Level IV.*

Rice, K. L., Bennett, M., Gomez, M., Theall, K. P., Knight, M., & Foreman, M. D. (2011). Nurses' recognition of delirium in the hospitalized older adult. *Clinical Nurse Specialist CNS, 25*(6), 299–311. doi:10.1097/NUR.0b013e318234897b. *Evidence Level IV.*

Rubin, F. H., Neal, K., Fenlon, K., Hassan, S., & Inouye, S. K. (2011). Sustainability and scalability of the hospital elder life program at a community hospital. *Journal of the American Geriatrics Society, 59*(2), 359–365. doi:10.1111/j.1532-5415.2010.03243.x. *Evidence Level V.*

Rubin, F. H., Williams, J. T., Lescisin, D. A., Mook, W. J., Hassan, S., & Inouye, S. K. (2006). Replicating the hospital elder life program in a community hospital and demonstrating effectiveness using quality improvement methodology. *Journal of the American Geriatrics Society, 54*(6), 969–974. doi:JGS744 [pii]. *Evidence Level II.*

Salluh, J. I., Soares, M., Teles, J. M., Ceraso, D., Raimondi, N., Nava, V. S., . . . Delirium Epidemiology in Critical Care Study Group. (2010). Delirium epidemiology in critical care (DECCA): An international study. *Critical Care, 14*(6), R210. doi:10.1186/cc9333. *Evidence Level IV.*

Schuurmans, M. J., Deschamps, P. I., Markham, S. W., Shortridge-Baggett, L. M., & Duursma, S. A. (2003). The measurement of delirium: Review of scales. *Research and Theory for Nursing Practice, 17*(3), 207–224. *Evidence Level V.*

Shehabi, Y., Bellomo, R., Reade, M. C., Bailey, M., Bass, F., Howe, B., . . . Australian and New Zealand Intensive Care Society Clinical Trials Group. (2013). Early goal-directed sedation versus standard sedation in mechanically ventilated critically ill patients: A pilot study. *Critical Care Medicine, 41*(8), 1983–1991. doi:http://dx.doi.org/10.1097/CCM.0b013e31828a437d. Retrieved from http://ovidsp.ovid.com/ovidweb.cgi?T=JS&CSC=Y&NEWS=N&PAGE=fulltext&D=medl&AN=23863230. *Evidence Level IV.*

Shi, Q., Presutti, R., Selchen, D., & Saposnik, G. (2012). Delirium in acute stroke: A systematic review and meta-analysis. *Stroke: A Journal of Cerebral Circulation, 43*(3), 645–649. doi:10.1161/STROKEAHA.111.643726. *Evidence Level I.*

Siddiqi, N., House, A. O., & Holmes, J. D. (2006). Occurrence and outcome of delirium in medical in-patients: A systematic literature review. *Age and Ageing, 35*(4), 350–364. *Evidence Level I.*

Siddiqi, N., Stockdale, R., Britton, A., & Holmes, J. (2007). Interventions for preventing delirium in hospitalised patients. *Cochrane Database of Systematic Reviews (Online), 2*(2): CD005563. *Evidence Level I.*

Trzepacz, P. T., Mittal, D., Torres, R., Kanary, K., Norton, J., & Jimerson, N. (2001). Validation of the delirium rating scale—revised-98: Comparison with the delirium rating scale and the cognitive test for delirium. *Journal of Neuropsychiatry and Clinical Neurosciences, 13*(2), 229–242. *Evidence Level IV.*

Weinhouse, G. L., Schwab, R. J., Watson, P. L., Patil, N., Vaccaro, B., Pandharipande, P., & Ely, E. W. (2009). Bench-to-bedside review: Delirium in ICU patients—Importance of sleep deprivation. *Critical Care, 13*(6), 234. doi:10.1186/cc8131. *Evidence Level VI.*

Witlox, J., Eurelings, L. S., de Jonghe, J. F., Kalisvaart, K. J., Eikelenboom, P., & van Gool, W. A. (2010). Delirium in elderly patients and the risk of postdischarge mortality, institutionalization, and dementia: A meta-analysis. *Journal of the American Medical Association, 304*(4), 443–451. *Evidence Level I.*

Witlox, J., Slor, C. J., Jansen, R. W. M. M., Kalisvaart, K. J., van Stijn, M. F. M., Houdijk, A. P. J., . . . de Jonghe, J. F. M. (2013). The neuropsychological sequelae of delirium in elderly patients with hip fracture three months after hospital discharge. *International Psychogeriatrics, 25*(9), 1521–1531. doi:10.1017/S1041610213000574. *Evidence Level IV.*

Wong, C. L., Holroyd-Leduc, J., Simel, D. L., & Straus, S. E. (2010). Does this patient have delirium?: Value of bedside instruments. *Journal of the American Medical Association, 304*(7), 779–786. doi:http://dx.doi.org/10.1001/jama.2010.1182. Retrieved from http://ovidsp.ovid.com/ovidweb.cgi?T=JS&CSC=Y&NEWS=N&PAGE=fulltext&D=med5&AN=20716741. *Evidence Level I.*

Yang, F. M., Marcantonio, E. R., Inouye, S. K., Kiely, D. K., Rudolph, J. L., Fearing, M. A., & Jones, R. N. (2009). Phenomenological subtypes of delirium in older persons: Patterns, prevalence, and prognosis. *Psychosomatics, 50*(3), 248–254. *Evidence Level IV.*

Zaubler, T., Murphy, K., Rizzuto, L., Santos, R., Skotzko, C., Giordano, J., . . . Inouye, S. (2013). Quality improvement and cost savings with multicomponent delirium interventions; replication of the hospital elder life program in a community hospital. *Psychosomatics, 54*(3), 219. *Evidence Level IV.*

Zhang, Z., Pan, L., & Ni, H. (2013). Impact of delirium on clinical outcome in critically ill patients: A meta-analysis. *General Hospital Psychiatry, 35*(2), 105–111. doi:http://dx.doi.org/10.1016/j.genhosppsych.2012.11.003. Retrieved from http://ovidsp.ovid.com/ovidweb.cgi?T=JS&CSC=Y&NEWS=N&PAGE=fulltext&D=medl&AN=23218845. *Evidence Level I.*

18

Pain Management

Ann L. Horgas, Mindy S. Grall, and Saunjoo L. Yoon

EDUCATIONAL OBJECTIVES

On completion of this chapter, the reader should be able to:

1. Discuss the importance of effective pain management for older adults
2. Describe the best methods of assessing pain
3. Discuss pharmacological and nonpharmacological strategies for managing pain
4. State at least two key points to include in education for patients and families

OVERVIEW

Pain is a common experience among older adults. The prevalence of persistent pain in older adults ranges from 25% to 76% among community-dwelling elders and from 83% to 93% among nursing home residents (Abdulla et al., 2013). Across all care settings and most specialty areas, nurses interact with older adults. By the year 2030, it is projected that there will be 72.1 million adults 65 years of age or older, representing 19% of the U.S. population, and those older than 85 years represent the fastest growing segment of the population (www.aoa.gov/Aging_Statistics). The Centers for Disease Control and Prevention reported that, in 2010, 13.6 million adults older than 65 years had been discharged from an acute care hospital and 298.4 million had at least one visit to an ambulatory care setting (Federal Interagency Forum on Aging-Related Statistics, 2012). Thus, care of older adults extends across many settings, and nurses in acute care settings also need to be knowledgeable about the most effective strategies for assessing and managing pain in this population (Herr, 2010).

There is a substantial body of literature that documents the high prevalence of pain in the U.S. older adult population (Institute of Medicine [IOM], 2011). Chronic diseases, including cardiovascular disease, diabetes mellitus, degenerative joint disease, osteoporosis, cancer, and peripheral neuropathies, are more prevalent in older adults and are often associated with persistent pain (Bruckenthal, 2010). In a study of a nationally representative sample of older adults with cancer receiving community-based hospice care, Herr et al. (2012) reported that pain was present in 83% of the population. These data highlight the need for increased knowledge of appropriate interventions to prevent and control pain in the elderly population.

Older adults commonly experience multiple causes and types of pain (Patel, Guralnik, Danise, & Turk, 2013). *Acute pain* is typically associated with surgery, fractures, or trauma (Herr, Bjoro, Steffensmeier, & Rakel, 2006). *Persistent pain* (i.e., pain that continues for more than 3–6 months) is most frequently associated with musculoskeletal conditions such as osteoarthritis (The American Geriatrics Society [AGS] Panel on the Pharmacological Management of Persistent Pain in Older Persons, 2009). In 2010, it was estimated that more than

For a description of evidence levels cited in this chapter, see Chapter 1, "Developing and Evaluating Clinical Practice Guidelines: A Systematic Approach."

19 million surgeries were performed on older adults, including 2.29 million musculoskeletal surgeries (including knee and hip replacements; Federal Interagency Forum on Aging-Related Statistics, 2012). In the acute care setting, older adults are therefore likely to have acute pain superimposed on persistent pain, particularly when admitted for a surgical procedure or acute illness.

Untreated or ineffectively treated moderate to severe persistent pain has major implications for older adults' health, functioning, and quality of life (Herr, 2011). Pain is associated with depression, social withdrawal, sleep disturbances, impaired mobility, decreased activity engagement, and increased health care use (AGS Panel on the Pharmacological Management of Persistent Pain in Older Persons, 2009). Other geriatric conditions that can be exacerbated by pain include falls, cognitive decline, deconditioning, malnutrition, gate disturbances, and slowed rehabilitation (AGS Panel on the Pharmacological Management of Persistent Pain in Older Persons, 2009). In the hospital setting, older adults suffering from acute pain have been reported to be at increased risk for thromboembolism, hospital-acquired pneumonia, and functional decline (Wells, Pasero, & McCaffery, 2008). Pain can also increase caregiving burdens for family members, who must often assist with treatments to alleviate pain at home (Herr, 2011). Pain also contributes to increased health care resource utilization and costs (IOM, 2011). Given the implications of unrelieved pain on the quality of life and health care use among older adults, it is not surprising that the IOM (2011) declared chronic pain a public health problem in the United States.

Over several recent decades, significant clinical and empirical efforts have been undertaken to improve the assessment and management of pain in older adults. Beginning in 2001, the Joint Commission on Accreditation of Healthcare Organizations (JCAHO) in the United States mandated pain assessment and management as part of the hospital survey and accreditation process (JCAHO, 2001). This accrediting body asserted that patients "have the right to appropriate assessment and management of pain" and declared pain as the fifth vital sign (JCAHO, 2001). This mandate exposed some of the challenges associated with assessing and managing pain in older adults in general, and in persons with dementia in particular. This, in part, spurred clinical and research activity to develop measures for assessing pain in older adults, particularly those with cognitive impairment. These behavioral measures have been reviewed in several published reports (Herr, Bursch, Ersek, Miller, & Swafford, 2010), including a comprehensive chapter focusing specifically on pain assessment tools in the classic reference by Pasero and McCaffery (2011). In addition, multiple clinical guidelines have been developed by leading scientific and clinical organizations, including the AGS (2009; Hadjistavropoulos et al., 2007), American Pain Society (Hadjistavropoulos et al., 2007), and the American Society for Pain Management Nursing (Herr, 2011). In 2011, the IOM convened a conference on pain care to evaluate the adequacy of pain assessment, treatment, and management, and to identify barriers to appropriate pain care in the United States. The ensuing report, *Relieving Pain in America: A Blueprint for Transforming Prevention, Care, Education, and Research*, comprehensively addresses the public health problem of chronic pain and the challenges of pain management (IOM, 2011). The report provided a blueprint for transforming the way pain is understood, assessed, treated, and prevented and delineated recommendations and objectives for researchers, practitioners, educators, and policy makers to facilitate the transformation of pain care. Among the key IOM recommendations are enabling self-management of pain, eliminating barriers to adequate pain care and disparities in assessment and treatment among high-risk groups, including older adults, and promoting interdisciplinary research and training for those who are conducting research on pain. Furthermore, the Affordable Care Act required a new focus on pain research at the National Institutes of Health (NIH) by directing it to continue and expand, through the Pain Consortium, an aggressive program of basic and clinical research on the causes of and potential treatments for pain. The NIH Pain Consortium enhances pain research and promotes collaboration among researchers across the many NIH institutes and centers that have programs and activities addressing pain. Most recent, the Gerontological Society of America (GSA), a major interdisciplinary organization promoting aging research, published a comprehensive monograph focusing on pain in the elderly population. The *From Policy to Practice* monograph, titled *An Interdisciplinary Look at the Potential of Policy to Improve the Health of an Aging America: Focus on Pain*, analyzes current policy initiatives aimed at improving pain care among older adults in America (GSA, 2014). Taken together, these initiatives highlight the attention that is being focused on improving pain care among older adults. Despite these efforts, there is persistent evidence that pain management for older adults in general, and specifically for those with dementia, remains suboptimal across care settings (Herr, 2011; Horgas, Elliott, & Marsiske, 2009, Titler et al., 2009). This chapter provides the best evidence on the assessment and treatment of pain in older adults, especially those with cognitive impairment. The goal is to provide information here that can be used to establish, implement, and evaluate protocols in the acute care setting that will improve pain management for older adults.

ASSESSMENT OF PAIN

Pain is defined as a complex, multidimensional subjective experience with sensory, cognitive, and emotional dimensions (AGS Panel on the Pharmacological Management of Persistent Pain in Older Persons, 2009; Melzack & Casey, 1968). For clinical practice, Margo McCaffery's classic definition of pain is perhaps the most relevant. She states, "Pain is whatever the experiencing person says it is, existing whenever he says it does" (McCaffery, 1968, p. 95). This definition serves as a reminder that pain is highly subjective and that patients' self-report and description of pain is paramount in the pain assessment process. This definition, however, also highlights the difficulty inherent in pain assessment. There is no objective measure of pain; the sensation and experience of pain are completely subjective. As such, there is a tendency for clinicians to doubt patients' reports of pain. Pasero and McCaffery (2011) provided a comprehensive chapter on biases, misconceptions, and misunderstandings that hampered clinicians' assessment and treatment of patients who reported pain. These issues apply to patients across the life span, and led the authors to conclude the following:

> A veritable mountain of literature published during the past three decades attests to the undertreatment of pain. Much of this literature is consistent with the hypothesis that human beings, including health care providers in all societies, have strong tendencies or motivations to deny or discount pain, especially severe pain, and to avoid relieving the pain. Certainly we should struggle to identify and correct personal tendencies that lean to inadequate pain management, but this may not be a battle that can be won. Perhaps it is best to assume that there are far too many biases to overcome and that the best strategy is to establish policies and procedures that protect patients and ourselves from being victims of these influences. (p. 48)

Among older adults, there is persistent evidence that pain is underdetected and poorly managed (Herr, 2011; Horgas et al., 2009). There are a number of factors that contribute to this situation, including individual-based, caregiver-based, and organizational-based factors. Individual-based factors that may impair pain assessment include the following: (a) belief that pain is a normal part of aging, (b) concern of being labeled a hypochondriac or complainer, (c) fear of the meaning of pain in relation to disease progression or prognosis, (d) fear of narcotic addiction and analgesics, (e) worry about health care costs, and (f) a belief that pain is not important to health care providers (AGS Panel on Persistent Pain in Older Persons, 2002). In addition, cognitive impairment is an important factor in reducing older adults' ability to report pain (Horgas et al., 2009; Lukas et al., 2013).

Pain detection and management are also influenced by provider-based factors. Health care providers have been found to share the mistaken belief that pain is a part of the normal aging process and to avoid using opioids because of fear about potential addiction and adverse side effects (Pasero & McCaffery, 2011). Similarly, cognitive status influences providers' assessment and treatment of pain. Several studies have documented that cognitively impaired older adults were prescribed and administered significantly less analgesic medication than were cognitively intact older adults (Horgas & Tsai, 1998; Morrison, Magaziner, Gilbert, et al., 2003). This finding may reflect cognitively impaired adults' inability to recall and report the presence of pain to their health care providers. It may also reflect caregivers' inability to detect pain, especially among frail older adults. Health care providers should face the challenge of pain assessment by first systematically examining their own biases, beliefs, and behaviors about pain, and eliciting and understanding the challenges and beliefs their patients bring to the situation as well (Pasero & McCaffery, 2011).

Self-Reported Pain

Patients' self-report is considered the gold standard for pain assessment (AGS Panel on the Pharmacological Management of Persistent Pain in Older Persons, 2009; Herr, 2011). There is no objective biological marker or laboratory test for the presence of pain. Diagnostic tests, however, often can reveal clinical problems, such as infection or inflammation, that may be associated with pain. The first principle of pain assessment is to *ask* about the presence of pain at regular and frequent intervals (Pasero & McCaffery, 2011). It is important to allow older adults sufficient time to process the questions and formulate answers, especially when working with cognitively impaired older adults. It is also important to explore different words that patients may use synonymously with pain, such as discomfort or aching. Use open-ended questions, such as "Tell me about your pain, aches, soreness, or discomfort," to elicit information about pain from older adults (Herr, 2011).

Pain intensity can be measured in various ways. Some commonly used tools include the numerical rating scale

(NRS), the verbal descriptor scale, and the Faces scale (Herr, 2011). The NRS is widely used in hospital settings. Patients are asked to rate the intensity of their pain on a 0 to 10 scale. The NRS requires the ability to discriminate differences in pain intensity and may be difficult for some older adults to complete. A recent study confirmed that the NRS was a reliable and valid tool for measuring pain and distress in community-residing elders (Wood et al., 2010). However, the authors reported a significantly higher failure rate in completing the NRS among those older than 81 years (11.1% failure rate) compared to those in the 61 to 70 (5.5% failure rate) or 71 to 80 (7.8% failure rate) age groups. This study also provides important information about the reliability of NRS ratings over time, a key factor in assessing treatment effectiveness and changes in pain ratings over time. Wood et al. (2010) reported that NRS current pain ratings has a reliability coefficient of .85, indicating high measurement reliability. There is evidence that older adults prefer a vertical orientation to the NRS when presented on paper (Herr, 2011).

The verbal descriptor scale, however, has been specifically recommended for use with older adults (Herr, 2011). This tool measures pain intensity by asking participants to select a word that best describes their present pain (e.g., no pain to worst pain imaginable). This measure has been found to be a reliable and valid measure of pain intensity and is reported to be the easiest to complete and the most preferred by older adults (Herr, 2011; Herr, Bjoro, & Decker, 2006). The Faces Pain Scale (FPS), initially developed to assess pain intensity in children, is often used to measure pain intensity, especially among cognitively impaired older adults. The FPS and the FPS–Revised (FPS-R) consists of facial expressions of pain, ranging from the least pain to the most pain possible (Herr, Bjoro, & Decker, 2006). Among adults, the FPS is considered more appropriate than other pictorial scales because the cartoon faces are not age, gender, or race specific. There is some evidence that cognitively impaired African American and Hispanic individuals prefer faces scales to numerical scales, possibly because of the impact of culture on pain expression (Herr, 2011). However, other studies suggest that the FPS has lower reliability and validity when used among older adults with cognitive impairment (Herr, 2011). See the Resources section for information on accessing these measurement tools.

Observed Pain Indicators

Dementia compromises older adults' ability to self-report pain. In patients with dementia, and other patients who cannot provide self-report, other assessment approaches must be used to identify the presence of pain. According to the American Society for Pain Management Nursing consensus statement on assessing pain in nonverbal patients, a hierarchical pain assessment approach is recommended (Herr, Coyne, et al., 2006). The four steps in the hierarchical process are as follows: (a) attempt to obtain a self-report of pain; (b) look for an underlying cause of pain, such as surgery or a procedure; (c) observe for pain behaviors; and (d) seek input from family and caregivers (Herr, Coyne, et al., 2006; Wells et al., 2008). If any of these steps are positive, the nurse should assume that pain is present and a trial of analgesics can be initiated. Pain behaviors should be observed before and after the analgesic trial in order to evaluate whether the analgesic was effective or if a stronger dose is needed.

Observational techniques for pain assessment focus on behavioral or nonverbal indicators of pain (Hadjistavropoulos et al., 2007; Herr, 2011; Herr, Coyne, et al., 2006; Horgas et al., 2009). Behaviors, such as guarded movement, bracing, rubbing the affected area, grimacing, painful noises or words, and restlessness, are often considered pain behaviors (AGS, 2006; Horgas et al., 2009). In the acute care setting, vital signs are often considered as physiological indicators of pain. It is important to note, however, that elevated vital signs are not considered a reliable indicator of pain, although they can be indicative of the need for pain assessment (Herr, Coyne, et al., 2006; Pasero & McCaffery, 2011).

Over the past few decades, approximately 20 different observational measurement tools have been developed to assess behavioral indicators of pain. These tools differ in their content, comprehensiveness, and scoring. Some have been tested empirically and show utility, but many require further psychometric testing of reliability and validity before they can be recommended for widespread use. (Herr, 2011). There is no perfect behavioral measure of pain that can be universally applied in all settings or with all nonverbal people. However, a recent team of experts developed a consensus statement for the use of pain behavior assessment tools in nursing homes (Herr, 2010). The panel recommended the Pain Assessment in Advanced Dementia (PAINAD) scale (Warden, Hurley, & Volicer, 2003) and the Pain Assessment Checklist for Seniors With Severe Dementia (PACSLAC; Fuchs-Lacelle & Hadjistavropoulos, 2004). A comprehensive review of these measures, as well as other similar tools, is available on the City of Hope website (see the Resources section). In addition, the Hartford Institute for Geriatric Nursing provides online resources for pain assessment in older adults with dementia that include information on the PAINAD tool, and an instructional video on how to use it (see the

Resources section for link). Several caveats about observational tools must be noted: (a) the presence of these behaviors is suggestive of pain but is not always a reliable indicator of pain and (b) the presence of pain behaviors does not provide information about the intensity of pain (Pasero & McCaffery, 2011). As such, pain behavior tools should be used as one part of a comprehensive pain assessment.

In summary, pain assessment is a clinical procedure that can be hampered by many factors. Systematic and thorough assessment, however, is a critical first step in appropriately managing pain in older adults. Assessment issues are summarized in the recommended pain management protocol. The use of a standardized pain assessment tool is important in measuring pain. It enables health care providers to document their assessment, measure change in pain, evaluate treatment effectiveness, and communicate to other health care providers, the patient, and the family. Comprehensive pain assessment includes measures of self-reported pain and pain behaviors. Information from family and caregivers should also be obtained, although these data should be considered supplemental rather than definitive.

INTERVENTIONS AND CARE STRATEGIES

Managing pain in older adults can be a challenging process. Many older adults suffer from comorbidity and frailty, which may complicate the management of their pain. Balancing the treatment for multiple comorbidities that can either cause or contribute to pain is especially challenging (Fine, 2012). As people age, the incidence and prevalence of illnesses that cause pain increase. These include rheumatological diseases, cancer, cardiac disease, postherpetic neuralgias, inflammatory diseases, and peripheral vascular diseases (Kaye, Baluch, & Scott, 2010). Additionally, it can be difficult to treat pain in older adults with an underlying dementia, as cognitively impaired adults often cannot self-report their pain.

The main goal in the management of pain in older adults is to maximize function and quality of life by minimizing pain to the extent possible (Herr, 2010; Wells et al., 2008). Pain relief is noted to be one of the most common goals of older adults (Makris, Abrams, Gurland, & Reid, 2014). There is a consensus supporting a multimodal approach to the management of pain, including pharmacological and nonpharmacological therapies (Makris et al., 2014). Pharmacological interventions are an integral component of pain management in older adults (Pasero & McCaffery, 2011). However, consideration must be given when devising a medication treatment plan given the physiological changes in older adults, which may both contribute to pain and be affected by pain treatments (Kaye et al., 2010). This means that the selection of pharmacological therapies must include a risk-and-benefit analysis taking into account the potential benefits versus the potential negative effects of pain medications on cognition and each organ system. It should be emphasized that pharmaceutical pain management is often more imperative in older adults with dementia because their ability to participate in nonpharmacological pain management strategies may be limited by their cognitive capacity (Buffum, Hutt, Chang, Craine, & Snow, 2007).

Barriers to pharmacological pain management should be noted. These can stem from both provider and patient perspectives. Patients often do not report pain for myriad reasons, including their expectation that pain is a normal part of aging, the desire to avoid testing, and not wanting to add medications to their regimens (Fine, 2012). Prescribers may also pose barriers, including the fear of stricter regulations surrounding the prescribing of opioids and potential concerns for diversion (Fine, 2012). Unfortunately, the result of these independent and/or combined barriers can lead to the undertreatment of pain in older persons, both with and without dementia.

When choosing pain strategies, consideration should be given to severity of pain because moderate and severe pain often require different modalities in order to provide adequate pain relief. In addition, nociceptive pain requires different pharmacological agents than neuropathic pain. It is also important to recognize the dangers in selecting potentially inappropriate medications (PIMs) for the treatment of pain in older adults. Medication-related problems can be costly and lead to poor outcomes (Campanelli, 2012). The AGS provides a list of PIMs, known as the Beers Criteria for PIMs, and updates this list regularly. Using an expert review panel, Beers et al. developed the original list of PIMs in 1991, which identified medications that had an "unfavorable balance of risk and benefits" (Campanelli, 2012, p. 2). This list has been updated and expanded several times, most recently in 2012. The intent of the Beers Criteria is to provide guidelines for the appropriate selection of medications while facilitating the education of clinicians and patients on proper drug use. Clinicians prescribing pain medications to persons aged 65 years and older should use the Beers Criteria to help identify medications that may have a greater risk-to-benefit ratio (Campanelli, 2012).

Several additional excellent pain management guidelines and protocols have been developed for use in the management of pain in older adults. For instance, the AGS updated their clinical practice guidelines for managing persistent pain in older adults (AGS Panel on the Pharmacological Management of Persistent Pain in Older Persons, 2009). The consensus statement by the World Health Organization (WHO) on the use of Step III opioids for chronic, severe pain in older adults provides detailed guidelines pertaining to the assessment of pain and use of opioids for cancer and non-cancer-related pain in 2008, and is due to be updated soon (Pergolizzi et al., 2008). In addition, there are other published guidelines for the assessment and management of pain in specific diseases, such as osteoarthritis (Hochberg et al., 2012). Pasero and McCaffery (2011) also provide one of the most comprehensive guides for pain management, including an updated edition that addresses pain management in older adults. Although there is a paucity of clinical practice guidelines for the management of pain in persons with dementia, there is strong support in the literature regarding the effects of untreated pain on persons with dementia (Corbett et al., 2014). In order to ensure that pain is treated in older persons with dementia, Corbett et al. (2014) provide guidance and recommendations for the treatment of pain in this population using multimodal approaches. See the Resources section for more information on accessing these items.

Pharmacological Pain Treatment

The management of pain in older adults can be optimized by using a multimodal approach. This includes the use of pharmacotherapy, psychological support, physical medicine, and interventional procedures as needed (Kaye et al., 2010). As noted, the use of pain medications involves decision making based on multiple considerations. Ideally, the treatment plan is a mutual process among health care providers, patients, and caregivers, with the goal of optimizing quality of life and functioning (Wells et al., 2008). An effective pain management strategy includes a careful discussion of risks versus benefits, and frequent reviews of drug regimens used by older adults. Guidelines from the AGS recommend the establishment of realistic goals with the acknowledgment that complete resolution of pain may not be achievable (Fine, 2012). Pain management is often a process of trial and error that aims to balance medication effectiveness with management of side effects, often in conjunction with the other treatment modalities mentioned.

Guiding principles for optimal pain management in older adults include the following components (Buffum et al., 2007; Gordon et al., 2005). First, the treatment of pain should be initiated immediately on the detection of pain. Second, regularly scheduled (rather than "as needed") dosing of pain medications should be employed. Additionally, multiple modalities for the evaluation of pain control should be used, including verbal, behavioral, and functional responses to pain medication, selected based on the patient's ability to communicate and interact. Pain medication should be titrated according to these responses, and a pain medication regimen should be chosen based on what is known about each individual patient. This includes the interaction of pain medications with other medications, and the knowledge of pain medication side effects, such as constipation. Titration must also take into account the severity of cognitive impairment and how this affects the patient's ability to express and report pain. For individuals with cancer-related pain, the WHO provides a three-step analgesic ladder that has been widely used as a guide for treating pain in this population. Choices are made from three drug categories based on pain severity: the nonopioids, opioids, and adjuvant agents. Combinations of drugs are used because two or more drugs can treat different underlying pain mechanisms, different types of pain, and allow for smaller doses of each analgesic to be used, thus minimizing side effects. In 2008, the WHO established guidelines for the use of Step III opioids (buprenorphine, fentanyl, hydromorphone, methadone, morphine, and oxycodone) in older adults with cancer and noncancer pain (Pergolizzi et al., 2008). Their criteria for the selection of analgesics in older adults with cancer are based on the type of pain, efficacy of the medication, side-effect profile, potential for abuse, and interactions with other medications (Pergolizzi et al., 2008). These guidelines make clear that Step III opioids are the gold standard of treatment for cancer pain and are also efficacious in noncancer diseases. The authors point out, however, a dearth of specific studies investigating the use of these drugs in older adults.

Special Considerations for Administering Analgesics

When considering the addition of pain medication to an older, and potentially frail person's medication regimen, several issues must be evaluated. Confounding factors for medication side effects include comorbidities, the use of multiple medications, and drug-to-drug interactions (Klotz, 2009). Advancing age is associated with physiological changes that can result in increased plasma levels of various medications (Fine, 2012). A reduction in renal and hepatic function, for example, can mean reduced efficacy in drug clearance and elimination. If not dosed accordingly, there is a higher risk for side effects and potential toxicity. These changes are the result of alterations in the pharmacodynamics (mechanisms of drug action in the body) and pharmacokinetics (processes of drug absorption, distribution, metabolism, and elimination in the body; Klotz, 2009) that occur with advancing age. It is important to take into account that adverse effects are not uncommon in older adults, regardless of whether a medication is new or used frequently (Makris et al., 2014). Adverse effects increase in the presence of comorbidities and the use of multiple medications. These effects are also a frequent cause for discontinuing pain medications. When starting a new medication, frequent follow-up is recommended to monitor for effect, side effects, and the need to titrate or change medications (Makris et al., 2014). Specific side effects to consider when prescribing and/or administering pain medications to the older adult include risks for sedation, mental status changes and cognition, balance, and gastrointestinal (GI) side effects—including bleeding and constipation (Buffum et al., 2007).

Recommendations for beginning pain medication treatment include starting at low doses and gradually titrating upward, while monitoring and managing side effects. The adage "start low and go slow" is often used. Titrate doses upward to desired effect using short-acting medications first, and consider using longer duration medications for long-lasting pain, once drug tolerability has been established. The use of short-acting medications can continue following the addition of long acting drugs in order to address breakthrough pain. If short-acting medications are being used regularly, then a reassessment of pain is essential to evaluate for the need to increase the long-acting medication (Fine, 2012). For most older adults, with mild to moderate pain, or those taking pain medications on an as-needed basis, choose a drug with a short half-life and the fewest side effects, if possible (Pasero & McCaffery, 2011; Wells et al., 2008).

The least invasive mode of drug delivery should be used. For most older adults, the oral route is the most convenient, provided their ability to swallow is intact. This route also provides steady plasma levels of medications. When a more rapid onset is needed, or when patients cannot take oral medications, intravenous, subcutaneous and intramuscular routes can be utilized. These modalities, however, tend to have a shorter duration, and require a skill set to administer; transdermal, rectal, and oral transmucosal routes can also be used (Fine, 2012). Intramuscular injections should generally be avoided in older adults because of the potential for tissue injury and unpredictable absorption, and because they produce pain. Overall, adopting a preventive approach to pain management, whenever possible, is recommended. By treating pain before it occurs, less medication is required than to relieve it (Wells et al., 2008). Examples of pain prevention are around-the-clock dosing and dosing before a painful treatment or event.

Types of Analgesic Medications

The AGS published updated guidelines for pain management in older adults in 2009 (AGS Panel on the Pharmacological Management of Persistent Pain in Older Persons, 2009). Information on accessing these guidelines is included in the Resources section at the end of this chapter. The guidelines provide comprehensive information about managing persistent pain, but the recommendations apply to acute pain management as well. Thus, the reader is referred to these guidelines for more comprehensive information.

Nonopioid Medications. Acetaminophen is recommended as the drug of first choice for the treatment of persistent pain in older adults (AGS Panel on the Pharmacological Management of Persistent Pain in Older Persons, 2009). It is considered the drug of choice for mild to moderate pain in older adults (Herr, Bjoro, Steffensmeier, et al., 2006). It is recommended that the total daily dose should not exceed 4 g/d (maximum 3 g/d in frail elders). A 50% to 75% reduction in the daily maximum dose should be made for older adults with hepatic insufficiency or a history of alcohol abuse (Food and Drug Administration [FDA] Announcement, 2011).

Nonsteroidal anti-inflammatory drugs (NSAIDs) are more effective than acetaminophen for patients with inflammatory pain, such as the pain associated with rheumatological diseases. Particular caution must be used when prescribing NSAIDs, to older adults, especially those with low creatinine clearance, gastropathy, cardiovascular disease or diseases that deplete vascular volume, such as congestive heart failure. In older adults, NSAID-induced side effects increase in frequency with advancing age. These side effects can include GI discomfort and bleeding. There are two types of NSAIDs: nonselective (e.g., ibuprofen, naproxen) and cyclooxygenase (COX)-2 selective inhibitors. The COX-2 drugs were introduced in the hopes of reducing the GI side effects seen with the nonselective NSAIDs. However, the GI protection provided by the COX-2 drugs is incomplete, and the side effects of both types of NSAIDs are otherwise unchanged. Two of the initial COX-2 drugs were withdrawn from the market because of their association with an increased risk for adverse cardiovascular events. All NSAIDs, including nonselective and COX-2 drugs, should be used with caution in older adults, especially in those with underlying cardiovascular diseases, renal disease, and history of gastropathy.

The concomitant use of gastro-protective agents, can reduce the risk of GI adverse events (AGS Panel on the Pharmacological Management of Persistent Pain in Older Persons, 2009).

Opioid Medications. Opioid drugs (e.g., codeine and morphine) are effective at treating moderate to severe pain from multiple causes. According to the AGS (AGS Panel on the Pharmacological Management of Persistent Pain in Older Persons, 2009), opioid analgesics can be used safely and effectively in older adults if they are properly selected and monitored. Patients with persistent uncontrolled pain requiring opioid therapy should receive around-the-clock, scheduled dosing, to ensure steady-state levels. As noted, the use of extended-release opioids can reduce the need for frequent dosing and provide better relief (Kaye et al., 2010). All providers caring for older patients should prescribe opioids based on clearly defined therapeutic goals. Prescribing should occur based on serial attempts to reach these goals, with the lowest doses chosen based on efficacy and side effects.

Many older adults and health care providers are reluctant to use opioids because of fears of addiction, side effects, and intolerance. Potential side effects include nausea, pruritus, constipation, drowsiness, cognitive effects, and respiratory depression. The most serious side effect, respiratory depression, is rare and can be mitigated by slow dose escalation and careful monitoring for signs of sedation (AGS Panel on the Pharmacological Management of Persistent Pain in Older Persons, 2009; Wells et al., 2008). To prevent constipation, preventive measures should be initiated when the opioid is started (e.g., stool softeners, adequate fluid intake, moderate activity; AGS Panel on Persistent Pain in Older Persons, 2002).

Adjuvant Drugs. Adjuvant drugs are those drugs administered in conjunction with analgesics to relieve pain. There are numerous drugs from various classes that provide pain relief beyond their intended indications. These primarily include antidepressants and antiepileptic medications. These adjuvant medications are often administered with nonopioids and opioids to achieve optimal pain control through additive analgesic effects, or to enhance response to analgesics. It is strongly recommended that patients with neuropathic pain be considered for adjuvant therapy (AGS Panel on the Pharmacological Management of Persistent Pain in Older Persons, 2009; Fine, 2012). Although tricyclic antidepressants (e.g., nortriptyline, desipramine) have shown dual effects on both pain and depression, they should be avoided because of their anticholinergic effects, which in the elderly increase the risk of side effects, including confusion, dry mouth and constipation among other risks associated with toxicity (Campanelli, 2012). Antidepressants that exert serotonin reuptake inhibition and mixed serotonin and norepinephrine uptake inhibition are safer to use in older adults as aduvant therapy for pain management because they are effective in the treatment of neuropathic pain and have a better side-effect profile (AGS Panel on the Pharmacological Management of Persistent Pain in Older Persons, 2009). Anticonvulsants (e.g., gabapentin) may be used as adjuvant drugs for neuropathic pain, such as trigeminal neuralgia and postherpetic neuralgia, and they have fewer side effects than tricyclic antidepressants (AGS Panel on the Pharmacological Management of Persistent Pain in Older Persons, 2009). They must, however, be titrated slowly and diligent monitoring is necessary to avoid side effects such as lethargy and confusion. Local anesthetics, such as lidocaine as a patch, gel, or cream, can be used as an additional treatment for the pain of postherpetic neuralgia.

Equianalgesia refers to equivalent analgesia effects. Understanding equianalgesic dosing (e.g., dose conversion chart, conversion ratio) improves prescribing practices for managing pain in older adults. Equianalgesic dosing charts provide lists of drugs and doses of commonly prescribed pain medications that are approximately equal in providing pain relief and can provide practical information for selecting appropriate starting doses when changing from one drug to another or finding optimal drug combinations (AGS Panel on the Pharmacological Management of Persistent Pain in Older Persons, 2009; Pasero & McCaffery, 2011; Pasero, Portenoy, & McCaffery, 1999).

Drugs to Avoid in Older Adults

Some medications should be generally avoided in older adults because they are either ineffective for them or cause higher risk of side effects. Per the updated Beers Criteria (2012), non-cox-selective NSAIDs—especially indomethacin, which has the most adverse effects of all of the NSAIDS—should be avoided. Additionally, certain opioids, such asmeperidine (Demerol) and pentazocine (Talwin), are considered to be inappropriate analgesic medications for older adults. Skeletal muscle relaxants should also be avoided because of adverse effects. These medications, like opioids, can cause central nervous system side effects, including confusion or hallucinations, and can increase the risk of falls. Because of the need to treat symptoms associated with pain syndromes, and often medication side effects, considerations to medication selection will be an imperative part of the treatment plan. When treating side effects using medications, such as sedatives, antihistamines, and antiemetics, consideration must be given to their long duration of action and side-effect profiles. These classes of drugs can increase risk of falls, hypotension, anticholinergic effects, and sedating effects (Gordon et al., 2005).

Nonpharmacological Pain Treatment

Older adults frequently experience multimorbidity with high prevalence of pain related to muscular skeletal conditions and depressive symptoms (Patel et al., 2013). Consequently, polypharmacy is common among older adults to relieve pain and other symptoms. And, therefore, special consideration should be paid to relieve multiple symptoms that they experience without adding further pharmacological regimen, if possible. Thus, nondrug strategies are a crucial component of pain management, which may be used alone or in combination with pharmacological therapies. The most commonly reported nonpharmacological strategies were exercise, nutritional supplements, ointments, massage, relaxation (e.g., breathing, meditation, imagery, music), activity modification, massage, and heat or cold application, although use of transcutaneous electrical nerve stimulation (TENS), chiropractics, vitamins, herbal remedies, magnets, and acupuncture was less prevalent in older adults (Stewart et al., 2012; Wells et al., 2008). Recently published pain management guidelines included the nonpharmacological therapies as recommendations (Abdulla et al., 2013; Zhang et al., 2008). Some of the recommended nonpharmacological therapies are acupuncture, mindfulness meditation, massage, TENS, and cognitive behavioral therapy (CBT), and supplements such as glucosamine and topical capsaicin cream (Abdulla et al., 2013; Zhang et al., 2008). Some of these nonpharmacological therapies demonstrated high levels of evidence (Makris et al., 2014). Older adult patients should be encouraged to use multimodal approaches, including nonpharmacological treatment, for more effective pain management (Makris et al., 2014).

Types of Nonpharmacological Treatment Strategies

Pain is strongly associated with biopsychosocial determinants such as anxiety and depression (Abdulla et al., 2013; Denise et al., 2014). Thus, multimodal approaches, including psychosocial interventions in combination with the pharmacological therapies for pain relief, are being increasingly encouraged (Abdulla et al., 2013; Keefe, Porter, Somers, Shelby, & Wren, 2013; Makris et al., 2014). Nonpharmacological pain treatment strategies, such as acupuncture, massage, mindfulness meditation, and yoga, may be beneficial to manage pain both physically and psychologically. Physical pain relief modalities include, but are not limited to, TENS, use of heat and cold, massage, physical activity, acupuncture, and exercise. Psychological pain relief modalities include guided imagery, mindfulness meditation, CBT, biofeedback, tai chi, and yoga (Abdulla et al., 2013; Makris et al., 2014). However, many physical and psychological nonpharmacological pain relief modalities are not often mutually exclusive and are rather beneficial for both aspects of pain treatment. Various types of dietary supplements are also commonly used nonpharmacological pain treatments among older adults. To date, many of these nonpharmacological strategies have been empirically evaluated for their effectiveness in pain management for older adults and reviewed for the level of evidence ratings (Makris et al., 2014). A brief explanation of some nonpharmacological pain treatments follows.

Acupuncture. Acupuncture is recommended mostly as an adjuctive therapy and considered an effective treatment with safety according to the reports of meta-analysis (Vickers et al., 2012), evidence-based review and guidelines (Abdulla et al., 2013; Makris et al., 2014; Park & Hughes, 2012), Osteoarthritis Research Society International (OARSI; Zhang et al., 2008) and AGS (2002), whereas a recent randomized clinical trial conducted in Australia (Hinman et al., 2014) does not support acupuncture as an effective treatment for chronic knee pain. Acupuncture demonstrates consistent evidence of effectiveness to manage various types of chronic pain, including back pain, shoulder pain, neck pain, and knee pain (Park & Hughes, 2012). Among the clinical trials, however, the frequency and duration of an acupuncture treatment varied from three times per week for 2 weeks to one time a week for 26 weeks.

Massage. Massage is considered to be an effective adjunctive therapy without serious adverse events (Abdulla et al., 2013; AGS, 2002; Makris et al., 2014; Zhang et al., 2008). Massage shows conflict findings and, based on the type of pain location, is more or less effective in managing chronic nonmalignant pain (Tsao, 2007). To be beneficial for pain, frequencies or duration of massage modalities have not been established in the studies.

Mindfulness Meditation. Meditation shows overall limited benefit to manage pain (Abdulla et al., 2013). One small clinical trial reported that 8 weeks of a meditation program was as effective as the education program to improve chronic low back pain (Morone, Rollman, Moore, Qin, & Weiner, 2009). Massage therapy may be effective in managing chronic low back pain and can be more beneficial when it is combined with education and exercise (Furlan, Imamura, Dryden, & Irvin, 2009).

TENS. TENS appears to be helful in managing pain particularly when it is combined with acupuncture (Abdulla et al., 2013; Park & Hughes, 2012). To obtain pain relief with TENS, adequate intensity and dosing should be established and applied (DeSantana, Walsh, Vance, Rakel, & Sluka, 2008).

Tai chi. Tai chi is a movement-based exercise regimen (Makris et al., 2014) that may be effective in managing pain and improving physical functioning without serious adverse events according to the findings of systematic review and meta-analysis (Kang, Lee, Posadzki, & Ernst, 2011); however, it may be considered as an option to manage pain if this movement-based approach can be delivered appropriately for an individual older adult (Abdulla et al., 2013). Despite many trials of tai chi, the effectiveness of this intervention for chronic pain in older adults is still inconclusive because of methodological issues in the studies (Hall, Maher, Latimer, & Ferreira, 2009) and, therefore, receives only limited support. Recommendations should be individualized based on the person's comorbidities, adherence, personal preference, and feasibility of exercise.

CBT. Cognitive behavioral treatments have also shown significant improvement in pain and mobility caused by osteoarthritis among older adults (Baird, Murawski, & Wu, 2010) and is recommended for pain relief if it is delivered by a professional therapist (Abdulla et al., 2013; AGS, 2002). One study (Green, Hadjistavropoulos, Hadjistavropoulos, Martin, & Sharpe, 2009) indicated that CBT intervention once a week for 10 weeks of provided maladapative pain behavior and higher level of relaxation, which is indicative of better coping.

Although these therapies are not an exhaustive list of nonpharmacological regimens, they demonstrate the levels of evidence to be used in older adults. Each of these nonpharmacological modalities has demonstrated mixed results, largely because of individual patient preferences and methodological differences in how the studies were conducted. Thus, there is no conclusive evidence that these modalities relieve pain. Among them, acupuncture seems to have the most consistently effective results for pain management. These nonpharmacolofical modalities should be considered on an individualized basis, depending on patient preference and response, physical function, psychological functioning, acceptability, and as an adjunct to pharmacological treatment.

In summary, nonpharmacological treatments are widely used comfort measures to help manage pain. These approaches are challenging to study because it is difficult to (a) find a convincing placebo and (b) establish optimal dose, frequency, and duration of an intervention. In addition, studies have contributed inconsistent findings because of differences in study designs, inconsistent measures, and mixed intervention durations. It may be also true that a specific type of nonpharmacolofical modality works for the specific type of chronic pain, which has not been fully investigated. Despite the lack of strong evidence and rigorous support for these nondrug approaches, they have received growing interest among the community of science and recently made a great advance. Thus, nurses and health care providers should consider all possible combinations and options for managing pain, and discuss these approaches with their older adult patients to identify the best options that are appropriate for each individual patient.

Special Considerations of Using Nonpharmacological Treatment for Older Adults

Individuals vary widely in their preferences for and ability to use nonpharmacological interventions to manage pain. Spiritual and/or religious coping strategies, for instance, must be consistent with individual values and beliefs. Other strategies, such as guided imagery, biofeedback, or relaxation, may not be feasible for cognitively impaired older adults. Tai chi or exercise should be customized based on functional ability and mental status of an individual adults. Therefore, it is important for health care providers to consider a broad array of nonpharmacological pain management strategies and to tailor selections to the individual. It is also important to gain individual and family input about the use of home and folk remedies because use of herbals or home remedies is often not disclosed to health care providers and may result in negative drug–herb interactions (Yoon & Horne, 2001; Yoon, Horne, & Adams, 2004; Yoon & Schaffer, 2006).

IMPROVING PAIN MANAGEMENT IN CARE SETTINGS

Nurses have a critical role in assessing and managing pain. The promotion of comfort and relief of pain is fundamental to nursing practice and, as integral members of interdisciplinary health care teams, nurses must work collaboratively to effectively assess and treat pain. Given the prevalence of pain in older adults and the burgeoning aging population seeking care in our health care systems, this nursing role is vitally important. In addition, nurses have the primary responsibility to teach the patient and family about pain and how to manage it, both pharmacologically and nonpharmacologically. As such, nurses must be knowledgeable about pain management in general, and about managing pain in older adults in particular. Moreover, nurses are responsible for basing their practice on the best evidence available, and helping to bridge the gap among evidence, recommendations, and clinical practice.

Nurses, however, must work within an organizational climate that supports and encourages efforts to improve pain management. These efforts must go beyond simply distributing guidelines and recommendations because this approach has not been effective (Dirks, 2010). Some quality-improvement processes that should be considered in promoting improved pain management include the following (Dirks, 2010):

1. Facilities/institutions demonstrate and maintain strong institutional commitment and leadership to improve pain management.
2. Facilities/institutions establish an internal pain team of committed and knowledgeable staff who can lead quality-improvement efforts to improve pain management practices.
3. Facilities/institutions establish evidence of documentation of pain assessment, intervention, and evaluation of treatment effectiveness. This includes adding pain assessment and reassessment questions to flow sheets and electronic forms.
4. Facilities/institutions provide evidence of using a multispecialty approach to pain management. This includes referral to specialists for specific therapies (e.g., psychiatry, psychology, physical therapy, interdisciplinary pain treatment specialists). Clinical pathways and decision support tools will be developed to improve referrals and multispecialty consultation.
5. Facilities/institutions provide evidence of pain management resources for staff (e.g., educational opportunities; print materials, access to web-based guidelines and information).

CASE STUDY

Mrs. B is a 93-year-old woman living with her daughter in the community. She has been diagnosed with anxiety disorder, hypertension, and diabetes, and has a severe hearing problem. Recently, Mrs. B fell in her bathroom and broke her right leg, which resulted in admission to the hospital. Before the fall, she typically walked around the neighborhood daily with her daughter. She now stays in her hospital bed with bruising, swelling, and pain in her right lower extremity. Her daughter has stayed with Mrs. B at the bedside and is worried about her anxiety and pain. Mrs. B is ordered oxycodone hydrochloride 5 to 10 mg every 6 hours orally or morphine sulfate 1 mg intravenously every 4 hours for pain as needed.

The nurse conducted an assessment of vital signs and completed a thorough pain assessment and mental status assessment, starting with self-report questions and asking the daughter for observations about her mother's response. The nurse explained the analgesic choices, including the types, routes, dosages, and potential side effects, to the patient and her daughter. When the nurse asked Mrs. B and her daughter about their perspective of pain medications and their acceptable level of pain (pain goal), both expressed fear of taking opioid medications. After further discussions with the nurse, Mrs. B and her daughter agreed to oxycodone 5 mg (instead of 10 mg) to manage Mrs. B's pain. They expressed that this was an informed decision—that Mrs. B's anxiety about pain medication was relieved, and that they felt relieved to be part of the pain treatment decision. Follow-up pain evaluation revealed that 5 mg of oxycodone did not relieve Mrs. B's pain. Another 5 mg of oxycodone was given to Mrs. B for pain. Afterward, Mrs. B rested comfortably. Her daughter was relieved to see her mother resting comfortably and felt more knowledgeable about her mother's pain experience and how to manage it.

SUMMARY

Pain is a significant problem for older adults, which has the potential to negatively impact independence, functioning, and quality of life. In the acute care setting, pain can negatively affect healing. In order for pain to be effectively managed, it must first be carefully and systematically assessed. Pain assessment in older adults should start with self-reported pain. It should also incorporate assessment of nonverbal pain behaviors and family input about usual pain responses and patterns, particularly in patients unable to communicate their pain. The use of established pain assessment/measurement tools is recommended. Pain treatment in older adults should be tailored to the type and severity of pain, with medications that can be safely used in older adults, or combined with nonpharmacological treatment for heightened effectiveness. Older adults, their families, and their care providers should be knowledgeable about pain and how to manage it. Thus, education is an important part of the process and should not be overlooked. Health care settings must emphasize the importance of effective pain management and empower their staff through resources, education, committed leadership, and organizational policies to provide high-quality pain management to older adults. Pain management is a critical nursing role that can improve the health care experience and quality of life for older adults.

NURSING STANDARD OF PRACTICE

Protocol 18.1: Pain Management in Older Adults

I. GOAL

All older adults will either be pain free or their pain will be controlled to a level that is acceptable to the patient and allows the person to maintain the highest level of functioning possible.

II. OVERVIEW

Pain, a common, subjective experience for many older adults, is associated with a number of acute (e.g., surgery, trauma) and chronic (e.g., osteoarthritis) conditions. Despite its prevalence, evidence suggests that pain is often poorly assessed and poorly managed, especially in older adults. Cognitive impairment resulting from dementia represents a particular challenge to pain management because older adults with these conditions may be unable to verbalize their pain. Nurses, an integral part of the interdisciplinary care team, need to understand the myths associated with pain management, including addiction and belief that pain is a normal result of aging, to provide optimal care and to educate patients and families about managing pain. Nurses must also examine their personal biases about pain and its management.

III. BACKGROUND

A. Definitions
   1. *Pain*: Pain is defined as "an unpleasant sensory and emotional experience" (AGS, 2002, 2009) and also as "whatever the experiencing person says it is, existing whenever he says it does" (McCaffery, 1968, p. 95). These definitions highlight the multidimensional and highly subjective nature of pain. Pain is usually characterized according to the duration of pain (e.g., acute vs. persistent) and the cause of pain (e.g., nociceptive vs. neuropathic). These definitions have implications for pain management strategies.
   2. *Acute pain*: Defines pain that results from injury, surgery, or trauma. It may be associated with autonomic activity such as tachycardia and diaphoresis. Acute pain is usually time limited and subsides with healing.
   3. *Persistent pain*: Defines pain that lasts for a prolonged period (usually more than 3–6 months) and is associated with chronic disease or injury (e.g., osteoarthritis; AGS, 2009). Persistent pain is not always time dependent, however, and can be characterized as pain that lasts longer than the anticipated healing time. Autonomic activity is usually absent, but persistent pain is often associated with functional loss, mood disruptions, behavior changes, and reduced quality of life.
   4. *Nociceptive pain*: This refers to pain caused by stimulation of specific peripheral or visceral pain receptors. This type of pain results from disease processes (e.g., osteoarthritis), soft-tissue injuries (e.g., falls), and medical treatment (e.g., surgery, venipuncture, and other procedures). It is usually localized and responsive to treatment.
   5. *Neuropathic pain*: Refers to pain caused by damage to the peripheral or central nervous system. This type of pain is associated with diabetic neuropathies, postherpetic and trigeminal neuralgias, stroke, and chemotherapy treatment for cancer. It is usually more diffuse and less responsive to analgesic medications.

B. Epidemiology
   1. Approximately 50% of community-dwelling older adults and 85% of nursing home residents experience persistent pain.
   2. More than one half of all inpatient hospital days are occupied by older adults, and more than 9 million surgeries are performed on older adults annually (Rosenthal & Kavic, 2004). Thus, pain is a common experience among older adults in the acute care setting (Herr, 2010).

C. Etiology
   1. More than 80% of older adults have chronic medical conditions that are typically associated with pain, such as osteoarthritis and peripheral vascular disease.
   2. Older adults often have multiple medical conditions, both chronic and/or acute, and may suffer from multiple types and sources of pain.

(continued)

Protocol 18.1: Pain Management in Older Adults *(continued)*

D. Significance
 1. Pain has major implications for older adults' health, functioning, and quality of life. If unrelieved, pain is associated with the following (Pasero & McCaffery, 2011; Wells et al., 2008):
  a. Impaired immune function and healing
  b. Impaired mobility
  c. Postoperative complications related to immobility (e.g., thrombosis, embolus, pneumonia)
  d. Sleep disturbances
  e. Mental health symptoms (e.g., depression, anxiety)
  f. Withdrawal and decreased socialization
  g. Functional loss and increased dependency
  h. Exacerbation of cognitive impairment
  i. Increased health care use and costs
 2. Nurses play a key role in pain management. The promotion of comfort and relief of pain is fundamental to nursing practice. Nurses need to be knowledgeable about pain in late life in order to provide optimal care, to educate patients and families, and to work effectively in interdisciplinary health care teams.
 3. The Joint Commission requires regular and systematic assessment of pain in all hospitalized patients. As older adults constitute a significant portion of the patient population in many acute care settings, nurses need to have the knowledge and skill to address specific pain needs of older adults.

IV. ASSESSMENT PARAMETERS

A. Assumptions (AGS, 2002, 2009; Herr, Coyne, et al., 2006; Pasero & McCaffery, 2011)
 1. Most hospitalized older patients suffer from both acute and persistent pain.
 2. Older adults with cognitive impairment experience pain but are often unable to verbalize it.
 3. Both patients and health care providers have personal beliefs, prior experiences, insufficient knowledge, and mistaken beliefs about pain and pain management that (a) influence the pain management process and (b) must be acknowledged before optimal pain relief can be achieved.
 4. Pain assessment must be regular, systematic, and documented in order to accurately evaluate treatment effectiveness.
 5. Self-report is the gold standard for pain assessment.
 6. Effective pain management requires an individualized approach.

B. Strategies for pain assessment
 1. Initial, quick pain assessment (Herr, Bjoro, Steffensmeier, et al., 2006)
  a. Assess older adults who present with acute pain of moderate to severe intensity or who appear to be in distress.
  b. Assess pain location, intensity, duration, quality, and onset.
  c. Assess vital signs. If changes in vital signs are absent, do not assume that pain is absent (Herr, Coyne, et al., 2006).
 2. Comprehensive pain assessment (AGS, 2009; Herr, Coyne, et al., 2006; Pasero & McCaffery, 2011)
  a. Review medical history, physical examination, and laboratory and diagnostic tests in order to understand sequence of events contributing to pain.
  b. Assess cognitive status (e.g., dementia, delirium), mental state (e.g., anxiety, agitation, depression), and functional status. If there is evidence of cognitive impairment, do not assume that the patient cannot provide a self-report of pain. Be prepared to augment self-report with observational measures and proxy report using the hierarchical approach.
  c. Assess present pain, including intensity, character, frequency, pattern, location, duration, and precipitating and relieving factors.
  d. Assess pain history, including prior injuries, illnesses, and surgeries; pain experiences; and pain interference with daily activities.
  e. Review medications, including current and previously used prescription drugs, over-the-counter drugs, and complementary therapies (including home remedies). Determine what pain control methods have

(continued)

Protocol 18.1: Pain Management in Older Adults *(continued)*

previously been effective for the patient. Assess patient's attitudes and beliefs about pain and the use of analgesics, adjuvant drugs, and nonpharmacological treatments. Assess history of medication or alcohol abuse.

f. Assess self-reported pain using a standardized measurement tool. Choose from published measurement tools and recall that older adults may have difficulty using 10-point NRSs. Vertical verbal descriptor scales or faces scales may be more useful with older adults.
g. Assess pain regularly and frequently; at least every 4 hours. Monitor pain intensity after giving medications to evaluate effectiveness.
h. Observe for nonverbal and behavioral signs of pain, such as facial grimacing, withdrawal, guarding, rubbing, limping, shifting of position, aggression, agitation, depression, vocalizations, and crying. Also watch for changes in behavior from the patient's usual patterns.
i. Gather information from family members about the patient's pain experiences. Ask about the patient's verbal and nonverbal/behavioral expressions of pain, particularly in older adults with dementia.
j. When pain is suspected but assessment instruments or observation is ambiguous, institute a clinical trial of pain treatment (i.e., in persons with dementia). If symptoms persist, assume that pain is unrelieved and treat accordingly.

V. NURSING CARE STRATEGIES

A. General approach
   1. Pain management requires an individualized approach.
   2. Older adults with pain require comprehensive, individualized plans that incorporate personal goals, specify treatments, and address strategies to minimize the pain and its consequences on functioning, sleep, mood, and behavior.

B. Pain prevention
   1. Develop a written pain treatment plan on admission to the hospital, or before surgery or treatments. Help the patient to set realistic pain treatment goals, and document the goals and plan.
   2. Assess pain regularly and frequently to facilitate appropriate treatment.
   3. Anticipate and aggressively treat for pain before, during, and after painful diagnostic and/or therapeutic treatments. Administer analgesics 30 minutes before activities.
   4. Educate patients, families, and other clinicians to use analgesic medications prophylactically before and after painful procedures.
   5. Educate patients and families about pain medications; their side effects; adverse effects; and issues of addiction, dependence, and tolerance.
   6. Educate patients to take medications for pain on a regular basis and to avoid allowing pain to escalate.
   7. Educate patients, families, and other clinicians to use nonpharmacological strategies to manage pain, such as relaxation, massage, and the use of heat and cold.

C. Treatment guidelines
   1. Pharmacological (AGS, 2009; Pasero & McCaffery, 2011)
      a. Administer pain drugs on a regular basis to maintain therapeutic levels. Use medications as needed for breakthrough pain.
      b. Document treatment plan to maintain consistency across shifts and with other care providers.
      c. Use equianalgesic dosing to obtain optimal pain relief and to minimize side effects.
      d. For postoperative pain, choose the least invasive route. Intravenous analgesics are the first choice after major surgery. Avoid intramuscular injections. Transition from parenteral medications to oral analgesics when the patient has oral intake.
      e. Choose the correct type of analgesic. Use opioids for treating moderate to severe pain and nonopioids for mild to moderate pain. Select the analgesic based on thorough medical history, comorbidities, other medications, and history of drug reactions.
      f. Among nonopioid medications, acetaminophen is the preferred drug for treating mild to moderate pain.

(continued)

Protocol 18.1: Pain Management in Older Adults *(continued)*

Guidelines recommend not exceeding 4 g/d (maximum 3 g/d in frail elders). The maximum dose should be reduced to 50% to 75% in adults with reduced hepatic function or history of alcohol abuse.

g. The other major class of nonopioid medications, NSAIDs, should be used with caution in older adults. Monitor for GI bleeding and consider giving with a proton pump inhibitor to reduce gastric irritation. Also monitor for bleeding, nephrotoxicity, and delirium.

h. Older adults are at increased risk for adverse drug reactions because of age- and disease-related changes in pharmacokinetics and pharmacodynamics. Monitor medication effects closely to avoid overmedication or undermedication and to detect adverse effects. Assess hepatic and renal functioning.

2. Nonpharmacological (Pasero & McCaffery, 2011; Wells et al., 2008)
   a. Investigate older patients' attitudes and beliefs about, preference for, and experience with nonpharmacological pain treatment strategies.
   b. Tailor nonpharmacological techniques to the individual.
   c. Cognitive behavioral strategies focus on changing the person's perception of pain (e.g., relaxation therapy, education, distraction) and may not be appropriate for cognitively impaired persons.
   d. Physical pain relief strategies focus on promoting comfort and altering physiological responses to pain (e.g., heat, cold, TENS units) and are generally safe and effective.

D. Follow-up assessment
   1. Monitor treatment effects within 1 hour of administration, and at least every 4 hours.
   2. Evaluate patient for pain relief and side effects of treatment.
   3. Document patient's response to treatment effects.
   4. Document treatment regimen in patient care plan to facilitate consistent implementation.

VI. EXPECTED OUTCOMES

A. Patient will
   1. Be either pain free or pain will be at a level that the patient judges as acceptable
   2. Maintain highest level of self-care, functional ability, and activity level possible
   3. Experience no iatrogenic complications, such as falls, GI upset/bleeding, or altered cognitive status

B. Nurse will
   1. Demonstrate evidence of ongoing and comprehensive pain assessment
   2. Document evidence of prompt and effective pain management interventions
   3. Document systematic evaluation of treatment effectiveness
   4. Demonstrate knowledge of pain management in older patients, including assessment strategies, pain medications, nonpharmacological interventions, and patient/family education

C. Institution/Facilities will (Dirks, 2010)
   1. Maintain strong institutional commitment and leadership to improve pain management. Evidence of institutional commitment includes:
      a. Providing adequate resources (including compensation for staff education and time; necessary materials)
      b. Clear communication of how better pain management is congruent with organizational goals
      c. Establishment of policies and standard operating procedures for the organization
      d. Requiring clear accountability for outcomes
   2. Establish an internal pain team of committed and knowledgeable staff who can lead quality-improvement efforts to improve pain management practices
   3. Require evidence of documentation of pain assessment, intervention, and evaluation of treatment effectiveness. This includes adding pain assessment and reassessment questions to flow sheets and electronic forms
   4. Provide evidence of using a multispecialty approach to pain management. This includes referral to specialists for specific therapies (e.g., psychiatry, psychology, physical therapy, interdisciplinary pain treatment specialists;

(continued)

Protocol 18.1: Pain Management in Older Adults *(continued)*

clinical pathways and decision support tools will be developed to improve referrals and multispecialty consultation

5. Provide evidence of pain management resources for staff (e.g., educational opportunities, print materials, access to web-based guidelines and information)

ABBREVIATIONS

AGS	American Geriatrics Society
GI	Gastrointestinal
NRS	Numerical rating scale
NSAIDs	Nonsteroidal anti-inflammatory drugs
TENS	Transcutaneous electrical nerve stimulation

RESOURCES

Agency for Healthcare Research and Quality National Clinical Guideline Clearinghouse
www.guideline.gov/content.aspx?id=10198

American Association of Pain Management Nurses (ASPMN). Geriatric Pain Assessment: Self-Directed Learning
www.commercecorner.com/aspmn/productlist1.aspx

American Association of Pain Management Nurses (ASPMN). Pain Assessment in the Non-Verbal Patient: Position Statement with Clinical Practice Recommendations
aspmn.org/Organization/position_papers.htm

American Geriatrics Society Guideline on the Management of Persistent Pain in Older Adults
www.americangeriatrics.org/files/documents/2009_Guideline.pdf

American Medical Directors Association (AMDA). Clinical Practice Guideline: Pain Management in the Long-Term Care Setting
http://amda.networkats.com/members_online/members/viewitem.asp?item=CPG11RE&catalog=CPGS&pn=1&af=AMDA

American Pain Society: Pain Guidelines and Online Resource Centers
http://americanpainsociety.org/education/guidelines/overview

City of Hope: State of the Art Review of Tools for Assessing Pain in Nonverbal Older Adults
prc.coh.org//elderly.asp

Gerontological Society of America
https://www.geron.org/publica-tions/from-policy-to-practice

Hartford Institute for Geriatric Nursing: Try This Series: Assessing Pain in Older Adults
www.consultgerirn.org/resources

Measurement Tools

See City of Hope website listed previously for comprehensive review of tools for persons with dementia.

REFERENCES

Abdulla, A., Adams, N., Bone, M., Elliott, A. M., Gaffin, J., Jones, D., . . . British Geriatric, S. (2013). Guidance on the management of pain in older people. *Age and Ageing, 42*(Suppl. 1), i1–i57. doi:10.1093/ageing/afs200. *Evidence Level I.*

American Geriatrics Society (AGS). (2009). Pharmacological management of persistent pain in older persons. *Journal of the American Geriatrics Society, 57*(8), 1331–1346. doi:JGS2376 [pii]10.1111/j.1532–5415.2009.02376.x. *Evidence Level I.*

American Geriatrics Society Panel on Persistent Pain in Older Persons. (2002). The management of persistent pain in older persons. *Journal of the American Geriatrics Society, 50*, S205–S224. *Evidence Level V.*

American Geriatrics Society Panel on the Pharmacological Management of Persistent Pain in Older Persons. (2009). Pharmacological management of persistent pain in older persons. *Journal of the American Geriatrics Society, 57*(8), 1331–1346. *Evidence Level I.*

Baird, C. L., Murawski, M. M., & Wu, J. (2010). Efficacy of guided imagery with relaxation for osteoarthritis symptoms and medication intake. *Pain Management Nursing, 11*(1), 56–65. *Evidence Level III.*

Bruckenthal, P. (2010). Integrating nonpharmacologic and alternative strategies into a comprehensive management approach for older adults with pain. *Pain Management Nursing, 11*(2), S23–S31. *Evidence Level VI.*

Buffum, M. D., Hutt, E., Chang, V. T., Craine, M. H., & Snow, A. L. (2007). Cognitive impairment and pain management: Review of issues and challenges. *Journal of Rehabilitation Research and Development, 44*(2), 315–330. *Evidence Level V.*

Campanelli, C. M. (2012). American Geriatrics Society updated Beers criteria for potentially inappropriate medication use in older adults: The American Geriatrics Society 2012 Beers criteria update expert panel. *Journal of the American Geriatrics Society, 60*(4), 616–631. *Evidence Level I.*

Corbett, A., Husebo, B., Achterberg, W. P., Aarsland, D., Erdal, A., & Flo, E. (2014). The importance of pain management in older people with dementia. *British Medical Bulletin, 111,* 139–148. *Evidence Level II.*

Denise, J. C., Hanssen, D. J. C., Naarding, P., Collard, R. M., Comijs, H. C., & Voshaar, R. C. O. (2014). Physical, lifestyle, psychological, and social determinants of pain intensity, pain disability, and the number of pain locations in depressed older adults. *Pain, 155,* 2088–2096. *Evidence Level IV.*

DeSantana, J. M., Walsh, D. M., Vance, C., Rakel, B. A., & Sluka, K. A. (2008). Effectiveness of transcutaneous electrical nerve stimulation for treatment of hyperalgesia and pain. *Current Rheumatology Reports, 10,* 492–499. *Evidence Level V.*

Dirks, F. (2010). A national framework for geriatric home care excellence. *American Journal of Nursing, 110*(8), 64. *Evidence Level VI.*

FDA Announcement Regarding Acetaminophen in Prescription Drugs. (2011). *Geriatric Pain.* Retrieved from http://www.geriatricpain.org/pages/acetaminophen.aspx. *Evidence Level I.*

Federal Interagency Forum on Aging-Related Statistics. (2012). *Older Americans 2012: Key indicators of well-being.* Washington, DC: Author. *Evidence Level IV.*

Fine, P. G. (2012). Treatment guidelines for the pharmacological management of pain in older persons. *Pain Medicine, 13*(S), S57–S66. *Evidence Level I.*

Fuchs-Lacelle, S., & Hadjistavropoulos, T. (2004). Development and preliminary validation of the pain assessment checklist for seniors with limited ability to communicate (PACSLAC). *Pain Management Nursing, 5*(1), 37–49. *Evidence Level IV.*

Furlan, A. D., Imamura, M., Dryden, T., & Irvin, E. (2009). Massage for low back pain: An updated systematic review within the framework of the Cochrane Back Review Group. *Spine, 34*(16), 1669–1684. *Evidence Level I.*

Gordon, D. B., Dahl, J. L., Miaskowski, C., McCarberg, B., Todd, K. H., Paice, J. A., . . . Carr, D. B. (2005). American pain society recommendations for improving the quality of acute and cancer pain management: American Pain Society Quality of Care Task Force. *Archives of Internal Medicine, 165*(14), 1574–1580. *Evidence Level I.*

Green, S. M., Hadjistavropoulos, T., Hadjistavropoulos, H., Martin, R., & Sharpe, D. (2009). A controlled investigation of a cognitive behavioral pain management program for older adults. *Behavioural and Cognitive Psychotherapy, 37,* 221–226. *Evidence Level II.*

Hadjistavropoulos, T., Herr, K., Turk, D. C., Fine, P. G., Dworkin, R. H., Helme, R., . . . Williams, J. (2007). An interdisciplinary expert consensus statement on assessment of pain in older persons. *Clinical Journal of Pain, 23*(Suppl. 1), S1–S43. *Evidence Level I.*

Hall, A., Maher, C., Latimer, J., & Ferreira, M. (2009). The effectiveness of tai chi for chronic musculoskeletal pain conditions: A systematic review and meta-analysis. *Arthritis and Rheumatism, 61*(6), 717–724. *Evidence Level I.*

Herr, K. (2010). Pain in the older adult: An imperative across all health care settings. *Pain Management Nursing, 11*(Suppl. 2), S1–S10. *Evidence Level VI.*

Herr, K. (2011). Pain assessment strategies in older patients. *Journal of Pain, 12*(3, Suppl. 1), S3–S13. *Evidence Level V.*

Herr, K., Bjoro, K., & Decker, S. (2006). Tools for assessment of pain in nonverbal older adults with dementia: A state-of-the-science review. *Journal of Pain and Symptom Management, 31*(2), 170–192. *Evidence Level I.*

Herr, K., Bjoro, K., Steffensmeier, J. J., & Rakel, B. (2006). *Acute pain management in older adults.* Iowa City, IA: University of Iowa Gerontological Nursing Interventions Research Center, Research Translation and Dissemination Core. *Evidence Level I.*

Herr, K., Bursch, H., Ersek, M., Miller, L. L., & Swafford, K. (2010). Use of pain-behavioral assessment tools in the nursing home: Expert consensus recommendations for practice. *Journal of Gerontological Nursing, 36*(3), 18–29; quiz 30–11. *Evidence Level VI.*

Herr, K., Coyne, P. J., Key, T., Manworren, R., McCaffery, M., Merkel, S., . . . Wild, L.; American Society for Pain Management Nursing. (2006). Pain assessment in the nonverbal patient: Position statement with clinical practice recommendations. *Pain Management Nursing, 7*(2), 44–52. *Evidence Level I.*

Herr, K., Titler, M., Fine, P. G., Sanders, S., Cavanaugh, J. E., Swegle, J., Tang, X., & Forcucci, C. (2012). The effect of a translating research into practice (TRIP)—cancer intervention on cancer pain management in older adults in hospice. *Pain Medicine, 13,* 1004–1017. *Evidence Level II.*

Hinman, R. S., McCrory, P., Pirotta, M., Forbes, A., Crossley, K. M., Williamson, E., . . . Bennell, K. L. (2014). Acupuncture for chronic knee pain: A randomized clinical trial. *Journal of the American Medical Association, 312,* 1313–1322. *Evidence Level II.*

Hochberg, M. C., Altman, R. D., April, K. T., Benkhalti, M., Guyatt, G., & McGowan, J. (2012). American College of Rheumatology 2012 recommendations for the use of nonpharmacologic and pharmacologic therapies in osteoarthritis of the hand, hip, and knee. *Arthritis Care & Research, 64*(4), 465–474. *Evidence Level I.*

Horgas, A. L., Elliott, A. F., & Marsiske, M. (2009). Pain assessment in persons with dementia: Relationship between self-report and behavioral observation. *Journal of the American Geriatrics Society, 57*(1), 126–132. *Evidence Level III.*

Horgas, A. L., & Tsai, P. F. (1998). Analgesic drug prescription and use in cognitively impaired nursing home residents. *Nursing Research, 47*(4), 235–242. *Evidence Level IV.*

Institute of Medicine (IOM). (2011). *Relieving pain in America: A blueprint for transforming prevention, care, education, and research.* Washington, DC: The National Academies Press. *Evidence Level VI.*

Joint Commission on Accreditation of Healthcare Organizations. (2001). *Accreditation manual for hospitals.* Oakbrook Terrace, IL: Author. *Evidence Level VI.*

Kang, J. W., Lee, M. S., Posadzki, P., & Ernst, E. (2011). Tai chi for the treatment of osteoarthritis: A systematic review and meta-analysis. *British Medical Journal, 1,* e000035. doi:10.1136/bmjopen-2010–000035. *Evidence Level I.*

Kaye, A. D., Baluch, A., & Scott, J. (2010). Pain management in the elderly population: A review. *Ochsner Journal, 10*(179), 187. *Evidence Level III.*

Keefe, F. J., Porter, L., Somers, T., Shelby, R., & Wren, A. V. (2013). Psychosocial interventions for managing pain in older adults: Outcomes and clinical implications. *British Journal of Anaesthesia, 111*(1), 89–94. doi:10.1093/bja/aet129. *Evidence Level III.*

Klotz, U. (2009). Pharmacokinetics and drug metabolism in the elderly. *Drug Metabolism Reviews, 41*(2), 67–76. *Evidence Level V.*

Lukas, A., Barber, J. B., Johnson, P., & Gibson, S. J. (2013). Observer-rated pain assessment instruments improve both the detection of pain and the evaluation of pain intensity in people with dementia. *European Journal of Pain, 17*(10), 1558–1568. *Evidence Level III.*

Makris, U. E., Abrams, R. C., Gurland, B., & Reid, M. C. (2014). Management of persistent pain in older patient: A clinical review. *Journal of the American Medical Association, 312,* 825–836. *Evidence Level II.*

McCaffery, M. (1968). *Nursing practice theories related to cognition, bodily pain, and man-environmental interaction.* Los Angeles, CA: UCLA Students Store. *Evidence Level V.*

Melzack, R., & Casey, K. L. (1968). Sensory, motivational, and central control determinants of pain: A new conceptual model. In D. R. Kenshalo (Ed.), *The skin senses* (pp. 423–443). Springfield, IL: Charles C. Thomas. *Evidence Level IV.*

Morone, N. E., Rollman, B. L., Moore, C. G., Qin, L., & Weiner, D. K. (2009). A mind-body program for older adults with chronic low back pain: Results of a pilot study. *Pain Medicine, 10,* 1395–1407. *Evidence Level II.*

Morrison, R. S., Magaziner, J., Gilbert, M., Koval, K. J., McLaughlin, M. A., Orosz, G.,...Siu, A. L. (2003). Relationship between pain and opioid analgesics on the development of delirium following hip fracture. *Journals of Gerontology. Series A, Biological Sciences and Medical Sciences, 58*(1), 76–81. *Evidence Level IV.*

Park, J., & Hughes, A. K. (2012). Nonpharmacological approaches to the management of chronic pain in community-dwelling older adults: A review of empirical evidence. *Journal of the American Geriatrics Society, 60,* 555–568. *Evidence Level V.*

Pasero, C., & McCaffery, M. (2011). *Pain assessment and pharmacologic management.* St. Louis, MO: Mosby Elsevier. *Evidence Level VI.*

Pasero, C., Portenoy, R. K., & McCaffery, M. (1999). Opioid analgesics. In M. McCaffery & C. Pasero (Eds.), *Pain clinical manual* (2nd ed., pp. 161–299). St. Louis, MO: Mosby. *Evidence Level V.*

Patel, K. V., Guralnik, J. M., Danise, E. J., & Turk, D. C. (2013). Prevalence and impact of pain among older adults in the United States: Findings from the 2011 National Health and Aging Trends Study. *Pain, 154,* 2649–2657.

Pergolizzi, J., Böger, R. H., Budd, K., Dahan, A., Erdine, S., Hans, G.,...Sacerdote, P. (2008). Opioids and the management of chronic severe pain in the elderly: Consensus statement of an International Expert Panel with focus on the six clinically most often used World Health Organization Step III opioids (buprenorphine, fentanyl, hydromorphone, methadone, morphine, oxycodone). *Pain Practice, 8*(4), 287–313. *Evidence Level I.*

Rosenthal, R. A., & Kavic, S. M. (2004). Assessment and management of the geriatric patient. *Critical Care Medicine, 32*(Suppl. 4), S92–S105. *Evidence Level V.*

Stewart, C., Leveille, S. G., Shmerling, R. H., Samelson, E. J., Bean, J. F., & Schofield, P. (2012). Management of persistent pain in older adults: The MOBILIZE Boston study. *Journal of Geriatrics Society, 60,* 2081–2086. *Evidence Level III.*

Titler, M. G., Herr, K., Brooks, J. M., Xie, X. J., Ardery, G., Schilling, M. L.,...Clarke W. R. (2009). Translating research into practice intervention improves management of acute pain in older hip fracture patients. *Health Services Research, 44*(1), 264–287. *Evidence Level V.*

Tsao, J. C. I. (2007). Effectiveness of massage therapy for chronic, non-malignant pain: A review. *Evidence-Based Complementary and Alternative Medicine, 4,* 165–179. *Evidence Level V.*

Vickers, A. J., Cronin, A. M., Maschino, A. C., Lewith, G., MacPherson, H., Foster, N. E.,...Linde, K. (2012). Acupuncture for chronic pain: Individual patient data meta-analysis. *Archives of Internal Medicine, 172,* 1444–1453. *Evidence Level I.*

Warden, V., Hurley, A. C., & Volicer, L. (2003). Development and psychometric evaluation of the Pain Assessment in Advanced Dementia (PAINAD) scale. *Journal of the American Medical Directors Association, 4*(1), 9–15. *Evidence Level IV.*

Wells, N., Pasero, C., & McCaffery, M. (2008). Improving the quality of care through pain assessment and management. In R. G. Hughes (Ed.), *Patient safety and quality: An evidence-based handbook for nurses* (Vol. 1, pp. 469–489). Rockville, MD: Agency for Healthcare Research and Quality. *Evidence Level VI.*

Wood, B. M., Nicholas, M. K., Blyth, F., Asghari, A., & Gibson, S. (2010). Assessing pain in older people with persistent pain: The NRS is valid but only provides part of the picture. *Journal of Pain, 11*(12), 1259–1266. *Evidence Level IV.*

Yoon, S. J., & Horne, C. H. (2001). Herbal products and conventional medicines used by community-residing older women. *Journal of Advanced Nursing, 33*(1), 51–59. *Evidence Level IV.*

Yoon, S. L., Horne, C. H., & Adams, C. (2004). Herbal product use by African American older women. *Clinical Nursing Research, 13*(4), 271–288. *Evidence Level IV.*

Yoon, S. L., & Schaffer, S. D. (2006). Herbal, prescribed, and over-the-counter drug use in older women: prevalence of drug interactions. *Geriatric Nursing, 27*(2), 118–129. *Evidence Level IV.*

Zhang, W., Moskowitz, R. W., Nuki, G., Abramson, S., Altman, R. D., Arden, N., . . . Tugwell, P. (2008). OARSI recommendations for the management of hip and knee osteoarthritis, Part II: OARSI evidence-based, expert consensus guidelines. *Osteoarthritis and Cartilage, 16,* 137–162. *Evidence Level VI.*

19

Preventing Falls in Acute Care

Deanna Gray-Miceli and Patricia A. Quigley

EDUCATIONAL OBJECTIVES

On completion of this chapter, the reader should be able to:

1. Evaluate the older adult patient who is unsafe and at risk for falls and injury, as well as corresponding nursing interventions to minimize risks for injury among fall-prone hospitalized older adults
2. Design nursing plans of care aimed at reducing serious injuries among older adults prone to falls based on the suspected fall type
3. Use findings from a comprehensive postfall assessment (PFA) to develop an individualized plan of nursing care for the secondary prevention of recurrent falls
4. Mobilize institutional resources to provide a collaborative interprofessional falls or safety team
5. Use the latest evidence innovations in practice to champion a nurse-led fall prevention intervention to prevent recurrent falls

OVERVIEW

Three specific aims of any effort in acute care institutions to reduce falls among older adults are (a) to reduce risk of injury from falls, including fatal falls; (b) reduction of injury; and (c) to champion an interprofessional fall-prevention program to prevent patient falls and fall-related injuries. These three aims seek to promote improvements in patient safety by reducing preventable falls through system-wide solutions whenever possible (The Joint Commission, 2006).

Overall, across *all* patient settings, evidence exists that fall-prevention programs are effective. The RAND report cites, from a meta-analysis of 20 randomized clinical trials (among all patient settings, but mostly long-term care), that fall-prevention programs reduced either the number of older adults who fell or the monthly rate of falling (U.S. Department of Health and Human Services, 2004). Hospital-based studies are emerging that provide solid scientific evidence of the effect of fall-prevention programs on fall rates and, more important, fall-related injuries.

Oliver et al. (2007; Oliver, Healy, & Haines, 2010) have produced a compilation of the best evidence of practice innovations used by hospitals across the United States and the United Kingdom, and their outcome effect on falls and injury reduction. After careful scrutiny (Oliver et al., 2007, 2010), they have identified the key components guiding multifactorial interventions used to prevent falls in hospitals (i.e., education, use of toileting schedules, and alarm devices). Oliver et al.'s (2007) approach has analyzed and weighed the individual intervention—within the multifactorial intervention—into its constituent parts, thereby minimizing any methodological design issues (Oliver et al., 2010). Many of these multifactorial interventions are

For a description of evidence levels cited in this chapter, see Chapter 1, "Developing and Evaluating Clinical Practice Guidelines: A Systematic Approach."

targeted on education initiatives and environmental issues, or they seek to improve equipment implicated in falls. Recent evidence from systematic reviews consistently suggest that, in acute hospitals, no single interventions are fully supported, rather multifactorial interventions in facilities may reduce falls by 18% to 31% (Oliver et al., 2010). To be most effective, action needs to be taken by both leaders and by frontline staff, to be championed by all members of the interprofessional team, including support workers, and tailored to the preferences and needs of individual patients (Degelau et al., 2012; Ganz et al., 2013; Oliver et al., 2010; Shekelle et al., 2013; Spoelstra, Given, & Given, 2012).

Before beginning any discussion on specific individual fall and injury prevention interventions, the acute care nurse must realize her or his role in championing a team effort in fall and injury prevention. Professional nurses are uniquely poised because they know the biopsychosocial and functional needs of their patients and situational contexts of how patients respond to the acute care environment. Such individual knowledge of each patient the nurse cares for positions the professional nurse, along with leadership skill, in a unique position to champion teamwork on their acute care unit.

BACKGROUND AND STATEMENT OF PROBLEM

The Importance of Fall and Injury Prevention in Acute Care

Many of the adverse health care outcomes resulting from falls, such as injury and/or functional decline, typically strike those patients older than 85 years *and* can be prevented. The most serious outcome is a *fatality*. The National Center for Injury Prevention and Control (NCIPC) ranks fatal falls as the number one cause of unintentional injury–fatality among older adults aged 65 to 85+ years between 1999 and 2010 (Centers for Disease Control and Prevention [CDC], NCIPC, 2015b). The fatal fall incidence increases with age—those older than 85 years being the most vulnerable.

Falls with injury populate our health care delivery system at alarming rates, resulting in more than 2.4 million injuries treated in emergency departments (EDs) annually, 772,000 hospitalizations, and more than 21,700 deaths (National Council on Aging, 2012). The CDC reports that every 29 minutes an older adult dies from a fall-related injury. Reported hospital in-patient falls vary according to the type of study conducted, that is, multi-site or single-site study, the type of unit (medical–surgical, telemetry, rehabilitation, or other), skill mix, and total number of nursing hours per patient day. The rate of falls in acute care hospitals, drawn from single-site studies, is estimated to range from 1.3 to 8.9 per 1,000 bed days, which translates into well more than 1,000 falls per year in a large facility (Oliver et al., 2010). The rate of falls, drawn from multisite studies, however, increases to three to five falls per 1,000 bed days (Oliver et al., 2010). In terms of unit type, recent evidence from a longitudinal study using National Database of Nursing Quality Indicators (NDNQI) data found the mean fall rates for most unit types are stable or are decreasing, whereas those for surgical units increased over time (He, Dunton, & Staggs, 2012). Changes in practice are cited as potential key drivers behind the increased rate of falls post-surgery. As early ambulation is encouraged, more patients on these units are out of bed. Fall rates have also been associated with registered nurse skill mix and total nursing hours per patient day. In He et al.'s study, lower fall rates were significantly associated ($p < .001$) with higher registered nurse skill mix and total number of nursing hours per patient day.

Serious injuries resulting from falls range from minor to severe types of injuries, such as hip fractures and traumatic brain injury (TBI), among others. And although we would like to believe that seemingly "minor" strikes to the head, spine, or limbs produce minor injury, evidence shows this simply is not true. We now know ground-level falls from a standing position among older adults older than 70 years cause more severe injuries, and those afflicted are less likely to survive compared with adults younger than 70 years (Spoelstra, Given, & Given, 2012). In fact, those 70 years and older are three times as likely to die from these low-level, ground falls compared with adults younger than age 70 years. Evidence suggests that seemingly minor strikes to the head can result in tears in cranial blood vessels and subdural matter (Weisberg, Garcia, & Strub, 2002). Given these findings, significant changes in clinical practice approaches are urgently needed for early identification of serious complications related to head trauma in older adults who appear to have "minimal head trauma, no obvious signs of head injury or concussion." New evidence supports a ramping up of the classic markers of head injury toward greater vigilance in recognition of other critical signs and symptoms of head trauma. Ergo, it is just not enough to assess older adults for risk of falls, but one must assess for risk for injury. Convential practice has always drilled into practitioners the need to assess for hip fracture injury or spinal fracture injury. Stepped up changes are warranted for heightened surveillance by health care professionals for all types of injury outcomes, most important, TBI as well as hip fracture. A brief overview of the evidence related to TBI and hip fracture incidence is presented.

Traumatic Brain Injury

About 1.7 million people sustain TBI annually (CDC, 2015a). Of all external causes implicated in TBI, such as assault, being struck, motor vehicle accident, falls account for 35%. The CDC reports falls as the leading cause of TBI for adults aged 75 years and older (CDC, 2015a). Of all the TBI-related ED visits in the United States during 2006 to 2010, the 65-years-and-older age group accounted for 81.8% of the TBI-related ED visits (CDC, 2015b). This age group also has the highest rates of TBI-related hospitalization and death. Because of limitations in study design, baseline health status, and inability to grade injury severity across studies, we have much less evidence of who, among the 75+-year-old cohort carries the greater risk for TBI. Is it the patient with type 2 diabetes, Parkinson's disease, or those patients on anticoagulation medication? One study that relied on a 15-state CDC TBI surveillance system found an increased incidence of depression, dementia, and Parkinson's disease in patients with fall-related TBI (Coronado, Thomas, Sattin, & Johnson, 2005).

The issue of increased comorbidity has been suggested as a likely contributing factor for the higher incidence of TBI in persons 65 years and older, owing to increased use of aspirin and anticoagulation in management of these chronic conditions (Thompson, McCormick, & Kagan, 2006).

Groups at risk for the development of TBI include men, who are twice as likely to sustain a TBI, adults aged 75 years or older, and African Americans who have the highest death rate from TBI (CDC, NCIPC, 2007). Older adult residents who experienced head injuries from a fall were more likely to live in assisted living (47.9%; $p < .04$) and to be walking at the time of their fall (69.0% versus 36.1%) compared with older adult fallers without a head injury (Gray-Miceli, Ratcliffe, & Thomasson, 2013). The link between ambulation and head injury when fall occurs from a standing position has clinical relevance across all settings of care.

Physiological changes in the brain matter itself, seen with aging, have also been suggested as contributing factors to the increased risk of TBI in older adults. It has been suggested that dura matter becomes more adherent to the skull with age (Thompson et al., 2006) giving way to the development of tears even with minor strikes or blows to the head. The field of cellular neuroscience has also isolated changes of the microglia, rendering them weaker against protection of the brain after an ischematic or traumatic insult (Lourbopoulos, Erturk, & Hellal, 2015). Although it is unknown, age-related changes among older adults' brain tissue and supporting structures may underlie accumulating evidence, which has shown that elderly patients with TBI have worse mortality and functional outcome than nonelderly patients who presented with head injury despite lower injury severity (Susman et al., 2002). Noted neurosurgical experts report that when the head hits a stationary object, such as the patient hitting his or her head on the floor, "lesions are produced in the white matter of the brain from these shearing forces... resulting in strain and stretching of axons and vessels." This damage is in addition to any bleeding or clot formation (Weisberg et al., 2002, p. 2).

Hip Fracture

The news headline, well known to older Americans, reads: "Death or Immobility Often Follows Hip Fractures in Nursing Homes." This common adverse outcome of a fall is realized not just in nursing homes, but also among those living independently in the community. The CDC estimates that more than 95% of hip fractures are caused by falling, often sideways, on the hip (CDC, 2015c). Annually, at least 258,000 hospital admissions for hip fracture among those 65 years and older occur nationwide (CDC, 2015c).

Women, especially White women, carry the greatest risk for hip fracture compared with men (National Hospital Discharge Survey), African American, or Asian women (Ellis & Trent, 2001). An underlying diagnosis of osteoporosis increases risk for fall-related hip fracture (National Osteoporosis Foundation, 2013). There are 54 million people with osteoporosis and/or low bone mass (43.4 million with low bone mass and 10.2 million with osteoporosis; National Osteoporosis Foundation, 2013). Classic risk factors for osteoporosis, pertinent to hospitalized patients, include immobility, insufficient calcium or vitamin D supplementation, and lack of weight-bearing exercises owing to the acute treatment of other diseases.

The U.S. Preventive Health Task Force recommends screening for osteoporosis in women aged 65 years and older and in younger women with other circumstances (U.S. Preventive Services Task Force, 2013). Health-promotion activities, including regular screening for osteoporosis, begin with a complete health history. Once detected, osteoporosis is treatable by medications that build bone, supplementation of calcium and vitamin D, coupled with regular walking and exercise. Although it would seem advantageous to recommend the use of hip pads to protect the hip bone from injury during a sideways fall, there is insufficient evidence to recommend hip protectors routinely for all persons at risk of a fall.

Falls with injury remain a major prioritized patient safety focus when considering that, in 2010, older adults who were aged 65+ years accounted for approximately 45% of the inpatient population. The repeat-fall age group is 75 years and older and compromised 28% of the inpatient population (CDC, 2015c).

Older adults in acute care hospitals are a vulnerable population at risk of falls and falls with injury, be it from age-related factors, disease-related factors, medications, functional declines or disabilities, or for all of these reasons taken together. Therefore, the nurse's antenna for suspicion for injury should be raised so that assessment for these serious types of injuries predominate our postfalls and fall risk analyses.

FALLS AND INJURY RISK ASSESSMENT

The older adult's risk potential of incurring a fall and or fall-related injury is contingent on several "real-time" underlying factors: (a) baseline pathophysiological changes at the time of the fall, such as presence of osteoporosis/osteopenia, sensory neuropathy, or prior falls and prior fracture history; (b) use of high-risk medications; (c) presence of fall risk factors, such as cognitive impairment (i.e., delirium and dementia) with impaired safety judgment; (d) situational factors; and (e) behavioral factors, such as the presence of agitation or overestimation of ability to function. Some of the more common issues seen in clinical practice are described in the following; a more complete discussion can be found elsewhere (Gray-Miceli, 2014).

Baseline Pathophysiological Changes

Pathophysiological changes of the sensory system, from age or from disease, can potentiate not only a fall but a fall with injury. Some of the more common age-related changes of the sensory system related to vision that predispose to falls include the presence of cataract formation or macular degeneration. With cataracts, the crystalline lens becomes yellowed and cloudy, thus creating a visual alteration and potential for blindness depending on the severity of the cataract. Age-related macular degeneration, however, causes loss of central vision, which can obfuscate ability to see objects directly in front of the patient. Assessment is geared at identifying unilateral visual loss and monocular vision. Seeing at night can become troublesome, therefore, higher levels of illumination are required. Consultation with an ophthalmologist for treatment of these disorders can prevent falls and falls with injury.

The contribution of vision to risk for falling has been summarized by fall experts (Lord, Smith, & Menant, 2010) substantiated by numerous studies of older persons' stance and balance. Evidence confirms significant increases in postural sway when loss of vision occurs, such as when older adults' eyes are closed (Lord, Clark, & Webster, 1991; Paulus, Straube, & Brandt, 1984).

A common sensory disorder affecting the peripheral nerves among older adults is peripheral neuropathy. Common among persons with B_{12} deficiency, disorder of the microvasculature, or type 2 diabetes, sensory neuropathy is a painful disorder that leads to loss of sensation typically affecting a stocking–glove distribution. Feeling one's feet on the floor can be a lost sensation altogether. Changes in gait are also evident with ambulation, as the foot is slapped against the floor surface in an attempt to secure foot placement. Referral to physiatry can be of help to find appropriate footwear and to discuss treatment options.

Age-related changes in the neurological system can also predispose to falls and falls with injury. The reduction in the righting reflex and an overall decrease in reflexes accompanying age cause not only slow movement but also potential for balance impairment resulting in a fall and/or injury, especially if ambulating on an uneven surface. With a slowed reflex, the ability of the older adult to reach out and stop the fall may be lost all together. In this situation, the person can fall flat on the face, shoulder, or back, resulting in serious cranial or extremity fractures. Although not considered normal aging, "frailty" is associated with a higher case incidence of falls. Frailty is defined according to clinical markers and, as suggested by Linda Fried, includes: gait speed slowness and slowness in movement, evidenced by an increased time to perform standard tests such as the Timed Get Up and Go test. It is estimated that frailty increases with age, and is highest among older adults aged 85 years and older and is more common among women.

Age-related changes in the musculoskeletal system are commonly encountered among older adults who fall and incur fall-related fractures. Normal aging results in some dimunition of muscle mass and strength and osteopenia (thinning of the bones). Older adults with diseases affecting the musculoskeletal system, such as osteoporosis, are at high risk of bone fracture as a result of underlying loss of trabeculated bone. In essence, the bone becomes porous and fragile and breaks with any impact.

Past Medical History of a Fall or Fracture Injury

Many studies have shown a prior fall to be the most potent predictor of another fall among older adults (Degelau et al., 2012; Gates, Smith, Fisher, Lamb, & Phil, 2008; Oliver et al., 2004). Therefore, careful fall-history screening is vital as a health-promotion measure and quality-of-care check for all newly admitted patients to the hospital or seen in the ED.

The presence of a current fracture injury, such as a hip fracture, could reoccur if care is not taken to protect such vulnerable patients. Older adult patients with a current hip fracture, and/or surgical repair, have muscular weakness, incisional and referred limb pain with potential loss of sensation, all of which contribute to their inability to maintain balance and prevent a fall from occurring should they become off balance. During ambulation or transferring, the patient puts less weight on the surgical limb, shifting it toward the unaffected limb, which bears the brunt of the patient's body weight. If osteoporosis exists and has been untreated, it is possible that the impact of walking can cause the "good" limb to fracture. In any event, the presence of pain or use of narcotic analgesia can also alter the patient's response to "avoid slips, spills, or obstacles" in her or his path.

An additional account of more of the common medical events and diseases associated with falls in older adults is described elsewhere (Gray-Miceli, Johnson, & Strumpf, 2005; Table 19.1).

High-Risk Medications Contributing to Falls and Injury Risk in Older Adults

"Culprit" drugs or medications implicated in increasing fall risk are those causing potentially dangerous side effects, including drowsiness, mental confusion, problems with balance or loss of urinary control, and sudden drops in blood pressure with standing (postural hypotension; Ensrud et al., 2002; Neutel, Perry, & Maxwell, 2002; Smith, 2003). Classifications of medications implicated in falls for older adults include psychotropic agents (benzodiazepines, sedatives/hypnotics, antidepressants, and neuroleptics), antiarrhythmics, digoxin, and diuretics (Leipzig, Cumming, & Tinetti, 1999). The risk of falls alone should not automatically disqualify a person from being treated with warfarin (Garwood & Corbett, 2008).

A recent review of medications and fall risks, taking into account a series of studies, finds strong evidence for benzodiazepines, antidepressants, and antipsychotics to increase risk of falls (Boyle, Naganathan, & Cumming, 2010; Bulat, Castle, Rutledge, & Quigley, 2008a, 2008b). Their analysis confirms that there is no evidence that very short or short half-life benzodiazepines, selective serotonin reuptake inhibitor (SSRI) antidepressants, or atypical antipsychotics are safer in terms of fall risks than earlier generations of drugs in the defined drug category. Furthermore, they conclude that antihypertensives, in particular diuretics, are associated with a modestly increased risk of falling (Bulat, Castle, Rutledge, & Quigley, 2008c).

In short, the use of medications in older adults is not without risks of fall or risks to injury. Reduction in medication use, whenever and wherever feasible, is the guiding light for practical management of older adults' health conditions. Constant attention to identifying risk versus benefits should be exercised by all practitioners caring for vulnerable populations of older adults at risk for falls and serious injuries.

TABLE 19.1

Medical Events and Diseases Associated With Falls in Older Adults

Age related
Dizziness with standing from physiological age-related changes
Dizziness with head rotation from physiological age-related changes
Accidental/environmental (Table 19.2)
Slipping or tripping on a wet/slippery surface
Trip/slip
Lack of support from equipment or assistive device
Acute (treatable) sudden symptoms
Mental confusion/delirium
Heart racing or skipping beats (arrhythmia)
Dizziness with standing up (orthostatic hypotension)
Dizziness with room spinning (vertigo)
Generalized weakness (infection, sepsis)
Involuntary movement of limbs accompanied by confusion, unresponsiveness, or absent facial features (seizure)
Lower extremity weakness (electrolyte imbalance)
Gait ataxia associated with acute alcohol ingestion
Feeling faint or dizzy or unable to sustain consciousness (hypoglycemia)
Blacking out or loss of recall of fall event (syncope)
Unilateral weakness, sudden speech change, and/or facial droop (TIA/CVA)
Postural hypotension/orthostatic hypotension
Chronic (manageable) gradual or recurrent symptoms
Lower extremity numbness (neuropathy, diabetes, PVD, B_{12} deficiency)
Lower extremity weakness (arthritis, CVA, thyroid disease)
Fatigue (anemia, CHF)
Dyspnea on exertion (emphysema, pneumonia)
Weakness (frailty, disuse, anemia)
Lightheadedness (carotid stenosis, cerebrovascular disease, emphysema)
Dizziness with standing (OH secondary to diabetes)
Dizziness with head rotation (carotid stenosis, hypersensitivity)
Dizziness with movement (labyrinthitis)
Forgetting the fall (dementia)
"I don't know" responses (depression)
Lower extremity joint pain (arthritis)
Unsteadiness with walking (dementia, CVA/MID)
Poor balance (Parkinson's disease)

CHF, congestive heart failure; CVA, cerebrovascular accident; OH, orthostatic hypotension; MID, multi-infarct dementia; PVD, peripheral vascular disease; TIA, transient ischemic attack.

Sources: Gray-Miceli et al. (2005); Rubenstein and Josephson (2006).

Why Do Older Adult Patients in an Acute Care Setting Fall and Who Is at Greatest Risk?

Evidence from systematic reviews of fall risk factors in hospital inpatients supports the following risk factors to be linked to falls: a recent fall, muscle weakness, behavioral disturbance, agitation or confusion, urinary incontinence or frequency, use of "culprit" medications (especially sedative/hypnotics), postural hypotension, syncope, and age greater than 85 years (Oliver et al., 2010).

The nursing assessment of the older adult patient who falls does not stop with administration of these assessment tools or other types of assessment. Rather, the assessment is a dynamic and continuous process of quality improvement, which extends to formulate an analysis of the information and situational context of the patient so that corrective plans of action can unfold.

The Value of Identifying Fall Type

Different types of falls exist. The three most commonly used types of falls are accidental fall (related to an unsafe environment or environmental risk factor), anticipated physiological fall (related to known intrinsic and extrinsic risk factors of the individual), and unanticipated physiological fall (resulting from an unexpected medical event) (Morse, 2009). Risk factors vary by the type of fall, and the interventions to reduce an accidental fall are different from the interventions used to reduce risk factors associated with anticipated physiological falls.

Reasons for patient falls and injuries are tied directly to impairments in consciousness, cognition, behavior, and acute and chronic types of medical conditions, in addition to the situational context of the fall. Some of these risks are caused by *intrinsic* factors, whereas others are the result of *extrinsic* factors. The standard of care calls for assessment of fall risk factors and then to develop an intervention plan targeted toward each of these factors. Not all fall risk factors are modifiable; those that are should be treated.

Accidental or environmental falls are potentially preventable because they encompass foreseeable events, such as spills or improper footwear, which is correctable (Connell, 1996). Important intrinsic risks that comprise anticipated physiological falls among older adults are summarized in Table 19.2; common extrinsic or environmental factors, which represent preventable falls, are highlighted in Table 19.3.

Fall risk is formally assessed through administration of fall risk tools (Table 19.4). The National Center for Patient Safety recommends the Morse Fall Scale, but *not* for long-term use (www.brighamandwomens.org/Patients_Visitors/pcs/nursing/nursinged/Medical/FALLS/Fall_TIPS_Toolkit_MFS%20Training%20Module.pdf). The Morse Fall Scale is a screening tool and should only be completed using the FACT acronym: after a fall, on admission of the patient, on change in patient status, and on transfer or discharge (National Center for Patient Safety [NCPS] Falls Toolkit, 2014). The St. Thomas Risk Assessment Tool in Falling Elderly Inpatients (STRATIFY) tool has also been widely used, but overall, researchers report that the use of any of the tools offers no added benefit over nursing staff's clinical judgment. Oliver et al. (2010) recommend the

TABLE 19.2
Intrinsic Risks to Falls

Lower extremity weakness
History of falls
Gait deficit
Balance deficit[a]
Use of an assistive device
Visual deficit
Arthritis
Impaired activity of daily living (ADL)
Dependency in transferring/mobility
Depression
Cognitive impairment
Delirium[a]
Agitated confusion
Older than 80 years[a]
Urinary incontinence/frequency
Diabetes[a]
Culprit medications: benzodiazepines, sedatives/hypnotics, alcohol, antidepressants, neuroleptics, antiarrhythmics, digoxin, and diuretics
Polypharmacy[a]

[a]Indicates independent predictor of falls with prolonged lengths of stay and increased nursing home placement (Corsinovi et al., 2009).

Sources: ECRI Institute (2006); Oliver et al. (2004); Papaioannou et al. (2004); Rubenstein and Josephson (2002).

TABLE 19.3
Extrinsic Risks to Falls

Medications
Floor surfaces that are slippery, wet, shiny or uneven or cracked
Equipment that is faulty, nonsupportive, or collapses when used, laden with debris
Intravenous (IV) poles, stretchers, or beds that are unsturdy or move away from the patient when used for support
Poor lighting or extraglaring "blinding" bright lights
Bathrooms lacking grab rails, bars, or nonskid appliqués or mats
Physical restraints
Inappropriate footwear

TABLE 19.4
Some Empirically Tested Fall-Assessment Tools

Name of Tool	Author	Setting	Training	Time to Administer	Sensitivity
Assessment of High Risk to Fall	Spellbring	IP	Y	17 minutes	UK
Berg Balance Test	Berg	OP	Y	15 minutes	77
Patient Fall Questionnaire	Rainville	IP	Y	UK	UK
STRATIFY	Oliver	IP	N	UK	93
Fall Prediction Index	Nyberg	IP-CVA	UK	UK	100
Resident Assessment Instrument	Morris	NH	Y	80 minutes	UK
Post-Fall Index	Gray-Miceli	NH	Y	22 minutes	UK
Morse Fall Scale	Morse	IP	Y	<1 minute	78
Fall Risk Assessment Tool	MacAvoy	IP	N	UK	93
Hendrich Fall Risk Model	Hendrich	IP	N	<1 minute	77
Timed Get Up and Go	Shumway-Cook	OP	Y	<1 minute	87
Tinetti Performance Oriented Mobility	Tinetti	IP	Y	20 minutes	80

CVA, cerebrovascular accident; IP, inpatient; N, no; NH, nursing home; OP, outpatient; UK, unknown; Y, yes.
Adapted from ECRI Institute (2006); Perell et al. (2001).

TABLE 19.5
Medical Factors Associated With Risk of Fall Caused by Impaired Safety Judgment

Summary of acute medical events, which can impair cognition, level of consciousness, or behavior predisposing to impaired patient judgment and safety

- Impaired level of consciousness
  - Volume-depletion disorders
  - Dehydration
  - Acute internal bleeding
  - Medication toxicity
- Infection/sepsis
  - Urinary tract infections
  - Pneumonia
- Intracranial mass/hemorrhage
  - Electrolyte imbalances
  - Diabetic ketoacidosis
  - Cerebral hypoxia
- Impaired cognition (memory, short-term attention span)
  - Dementia
  - Untreated depression
  - Medication toxicity
  - Mental illness/developmental disability/mental retardation
- Behavior agitation
  - Acute or chronic unmanaged pain
  - Medication toxicity
  - Depression

Morse Fall Scale and the STRATIFY tool as the two screening tools with best predictive properties, and the Morse Fall Scale was designed specifically to predict the probability of an anticipated physiological fall.

Some of the more commonly encountered risks of fall and injury observed in acute care are evident on many of the widely published and available risk-analysis tools. All of the tools include cognitive impairment (i.e., delirium and dementia).

It is very important to recognize cognitive impairment as studies have shown that early detection of acute mental status changes, that is, delirium, leads to early treatment and resolution. Moreover, early recognition of cognitive impairment caused by underlying chronic dementia is equally important. Acute care studies have shown that in patients with underlying dementia before hospitalization cognitive function typically worsens with hospitalization. Both acute delirum and chronic dementia are notorious conditions, potentiating impaired safety judgment. Impaired safety judgment is a nursing diagnosis that refers to the patients' inavailability to recognize whether their actions are safe or not. Therefore, when safety impairment exists in the acute care setting, it is incumbent on the registered nurse to protect the patient from harm. Table 19.5 illustrates some of the common medical problems, acute or chronic, that can result in impaired safety judgment.

TABLE 19.6

Matrix of the Patient Situation by Risk for Falls That Result in Injury

Situation of Patient	Fall While in Bed	Chair Fall	Fall While Transitioning	Ambulatory Fall
Acute delirium	✓	✓	✓	✓
Chronic cognitive impairment/ dementia	✓	✓	✓	✓
Visual impairment	✓	✓	✓	✓
Lower extremity weakness		✓	✓	✓
Gait or balance impairment		✓	✓	✓
Postural hypotension		✓	✓	✓

TABLE 19.7

Medical Conditions That Raise the Risk of Serious Injury/Internal Bleeding

Medical conditions
Underlying osteoporosis
Current hip or vertebral fracture
Thrombocytopenia
Acute lymphocytic leukemia
Acute anemia or loss of blood volume
Any state of alerted level of consciousness "delirium," lethargy, obtunded or comatose
Medications
Blood thinners
Thrombocytopenic agents

Table 19.6 lists some examples of age-related and associated conditions that cause falls. Positive predictive validity of falls has also been used as evidence by the patient's underlying history of falls, visual impairment, requiring toileting assistance, dependency in transfer/mobility, balance disturbance, and cognitive impairment (Blahak et al., 2009; Papaioannou et al., 2004; Tinetti, Williams, & Mayewski, 1986).

In addition, many medical conditions raise the risk for serious injury, as outlined in Table 19.7. An integral component of the nursing assessment is to evaluate patients who may possess these risk factors. If present, strategies must be integrated into the patient's individualized plan of care, which mitigate, reduce, or eliminate these risks altogether. Table 19.8 lists best practice interventions for patients suspected of injuries.

Diagnosis: Cognitive Dysfunction (Dementia/Delirium)

Important characteristics of level of alertness are the patients' ability to sustain attention, and determining whether the patient is awake or not. If impairment exists in level of consciousness, an assessment should be made to differentiate delirium from dementia. Cognitive impairment is a known fall risk factor, requiring clinical assessment to differentiate.

Delirium. Delirium has many synonyms, including acute confusional state, altered mental status, reversible dementia, and organic brain syndrome.

On admission, all patients older than the 65 years regardless of admitting diagnosis, should be assessed for both dementia and delirium. Assessment is usually completed with the Confusion Assessment Method (CAM; Degelau et al., 2012).

Dementia. Patients with dementia include those with a diagnosis of Alzheimer's disease, vascular dementia, Lewy-body dementia, frontotemporal lobe dementia, and those associated with other disorders. Such patients normally have slower reaction times and demonstrate impaired judgment. Individuals with dementia also possess varying degrees of alterations in visual–spatial orientation. Screening for dementia can be completed with the Mini-Cog, Mini-Mental State Exam (MMSE; Borson, Scanlan, Chen, & Ganguli, 2003; Folstein, Folstein, McHugh, 1975) and Kokmen Short Test of Mental Status Sources (Degelau et al., 2012; see Chapter 17). These patients are at risk of falls and injury, if injury-reduction practices are not implemented.

Additionally, any postoperative surgical patient is at great risk of injury from a fall owing to changes in the level of consciousness resulting from the sedative effects of medications. An important factor in determining a patient's safety within his or her environment will be whether he or she can process information and execute simple one-, two-, and/or three-stage commands. The ability to execute a command is contingent on the level of consciousness, behavior, and cognition.

Traditionally, the level of consciousness is assessed and written as alert and oriented times three, referring

TABLE 19.8

Best Practice Interventions for Patients Suspected of a Serious Injury

Notify the physician or health care professional immediately
Apply supplemental oxygen if indicated
Assess vital signs and pulse oximetry every 15 minutes
Prepare the patient for an x-ray of the extremity or CT scan of the head
Pad side rails if there is altered level of consciousness among the bedridden
Do not leave the patient alone; obtain a sitter or one-on-one assistance
Lower the height of the bed, use tab alarms or personal alarms
Maintain bed rest
Assess and maintain airway, breathing, and circulation
Assess and monitor pain (does it increase over time or is it unrelieved?)
Maintain an NPO status unless ordered otherwise
For suspected injury to soft tissue, apply ice for swelling, follow the RICE principle
Prepare the patient for laboratory data, frequently a serum blood count, type and cross match, bleeding time, and serum electrolytes are ordered
Observe and monitor the injured site: Does the swelling increase? Is there an open fracture? Does the tissue discolor? Is there loss of circulation?
Are there any coexisting symptoms, which worsen over time, such as headache, backache, pain in the extremity, or experiences of dizziness or shortness of breath?

NPO, nothing per mouth; RICE, rest, ice, compression, elevation.

to person, place, and time. The ability of the person to sustain attention can be gauged by observation of his or her ability (or not) to execute a command, for instance, following instructions. This type of assessment is typically routine when the nurse first greets the patient and is beyond a simple assessment of whether or not the patient is awake, "alert," and oriented and can say, "Hello." All of these determinations are critical factors in the nurse's judgment of patient safety. After the first assessment, the nurse should reassess the older patient frequently because the level of consciousness can change quickly. Thus, at first glance it appears to the nurse that the patient is awake and alert, but later in the shift, the patient may typify "delirium" and appear hyper-or hypoalert. Thus, patients require frequent monitoring of the level of consciousness.

Observation of a patient's behavior includes the patient's affect, demeanor, and ability to process stimuli in the environment. Agitated older adults are at risk of falls and injury because attention to the normal environmental cues is blunted or lost altogether. Depressed older adults may be at risk of impaired safety awareness and management because of blunted responses or apathy as well as centrally acting medications used to treat the depressants.

For each of these four factors—consciousness, affect, behavior, and cognition—nurses work with physicians to evaluate the underlying causes and find treatable solutions wherever possible. Note that the roots of many of the disturbances of *consciousness*, *behavior*, and *affect* are some classic acute medical events such as hypotension, infection, dehydration, profound blood loss, or toxicity from medications (Tables 19.5 and 19.7). If no identifiable solution exists, prudent and standard care (i.e., best practice) requires nurses to ensure the safety of patients by instituting interventions related to improved monitoring and assistance with activities. In the order of least to most restrictive, nurses employ various solutions until the patient is no longer judged by the nurse to be at risk of a safety issue or in danger of a serious fall-related injury (Table 19.8). Note that research on these best practices for fall prevention is slowly emerging, and the absence of research in this area does not justify not using the intervention, because it may be a best practice intervention accepted as standard care.

Critical-Thinking Points

How many times do nurses reassess their own judgment and make changes accordingly to their original impressions? Typically, in fall risk screening and clinical assessments, the reassessment is made during each shift and at the time of transition to another unit. Although a patient may "look to be safe" resting in bed, he or she may be totally unsafe if he or she sits up on the side of the bed or takes a step to walk. Therefore, it is very important to note the situational context.

Consider these points: while patients are safe in bed, are they also safe to be unsupervised alone? Are they safe to sit, transfer, or walk unassisted?

All of these nursing observations and ultimate clinical determination of patient safety hinge on the older patient's level of consciousness, level of alertness, as well as behavior and current cognitive capabilities.

The level of consciousness is formally measured by the use of standardized assessment tools such as the CAM and other such tools (see consultgerirn.org/resources).

Situational Context and Fall

When assessing the patient's risk of falls and risk of injury, it is imperative that the nurse consider the situational and environmental context as well as the medical stability of the patient (behavior, level of alertness, and cognition). So, although it may appear that the alert and oriented older patient with lower extremity weakness who is resting in a low-rise bed surrounded by floor mats is at a low risk of an injurious bed fall, his or her risk of injury increases as he or she walks, because of the lower extremity weakness. As the patient is out of bed and walking, with weakened limbs, risk of ambulatory falls occurs.

Thinking about the fall you are trying to prevent, whether it is a bed fall, an ambulatory fall, or a fall during transitioning from bed to chair, will further help in identifying risk fall and source of trauma for injury. With the older adult patient lying in bed or sitting on the chair, try to identify patient situations that place the older adult at a greater risk of falling or injury. Various circumstances of falls identified in the literature and commonly encountered in clinical practice include falls:

- From bed (patient rolls off the mattress or slips off the edge of the bed)
- From chair (patient slides from the chair, or falls getting into or out of the chair)
- While ambulating (patient falls while walking)
- While standing and/or transferring (patient falls getting on/off the toilet or when getting up to stand from a seated position)
- Found down, or unwitnessed activity resulting in falls

A risk-versus-benefit analysis should always be part of fall management decision making for patient safety and prevention of injury (Quigley & Goff, 2011), especially when patients move about on the hospital unit.

Given the patient's intrinsic and extrinsic risks of falls and risk of serious injury (based on the most recent nursing assessment), it can be helpful to use the matrix in Table 19.6 to envision the various risks of fall or injury with the patient in various types of positions.

Behavioral Factors

Older adults in the acute care setting enter hospitals for management of their conditions. They may have never encountered an illness or event that resulted in sudden changes in their bodies. When medically unstable or cognitively impaired, these factors pose a safety risk as physical capacity and physical independence in functioning are suddenly altered. These patients often cannot do the things they once could with ease and are admitted to an unfamiliar environment. As physical independence decreases, their autonomy and desire to do what they are accustomed to doing may remain. This creates a conflict. They wish to get up, but may not fully recognize it is really not safe for them to do so. Gender, degree of fraility or injury, cultural background, baseline personality, and prior hospitalization experience are all likely to influence how the patient is coping with this sudden illness (Agency for Healthcare Research and Quality [AHRQ], 2013). Assessment should include whether older adults perceive these changes as stressors; and, if so, do they believe they do not require help? Nurses caring for elderly patients must remember that they have many years of experience in coping, or not, with their chronic condition. How they have coped and managed day to day is likely to influence current reaction to the hospital experience and current behavior. Reminding the patient that he or she is ill and needs temporary help is one remedy through the use of teach-backs, but it is likely to be ignored or short lived by persons who refuse help and want to remain independent despite medical advice. Those with cognitive impairment, depending on the severity of impairment, may not have the current cognitive ability to recognize that they are overestimating their actual ability to perform.

Assess and Diagnose the Older Adult Patient's Risk of Serious Injury

Fractures

Nurses must ask a few commonsense questions when determining whether an elderly patient is at risk of serious injury (Tables 19.9 and 19.10). *Serious injury* is defined as injuries that result in loss of function and loss of life (Boushon et al., 2012). The National Quality Forum (NQF) defines moderate harm as the harm from falls resulting in suturing, Steri-Strips, fracture, or splinting; major harm as those falls that result in surgery, casting, or traction; then death (NQF, 2006). All of the items listed in Tables 19.1 to 19.3 are acute or chronic medical illnesses or conditions giving rise to the possibility that an acute injury could result. One of the most prevalent conditions increasing risk of serious injury in older patients, such as a fracture, is the presence of osteoporosis. For many reasons, the true incidence of osteoporosis is unknown in the older population, especially in men (Kaufman et al., 2000) who comprise a large percentage of the acute care hospital and long-term care beds. Therefore, it is entirely conceivable that the older adult will fracture an extremity or vertebrae with a fall, even though there is no documented diagnosis of osteopenia or osteoporosis. Depending on bone density and the severity of the trauma sustained during a fall, fracture risk must remain a consideration so that interventions to reduce harm can be implemented. Nurses must remember that osteopenia and osteoporosis can be present, even though they have not formally been diagnosed. Nurses must know risk factors for osteopenia and osteoporosis,

TABLE 19.9
Immediate Postfall Assessment

Actions taken by professional nurses and nursing staff:
If the older adult patient is found on the floor, remain with patient, summons additional help, proceed to:
Ask the older adult to explain what happened if possible.
Ask the older adult how he or she is feeling and whether there is pain.
Control any bleeding (follow unit protocol) from injured site.
Assess level of consciousness and perform neurological assessment, including pupillary checks (according to unit protocol).
Gather and document vital signs: Note the apical pulse rate and the supine blood pressure.
Examine for signs of external injury to the head, spine, neck, and extremities.
Determine oxygenation status.
Determine finger-stick glucose if hypoglycemia is suspected.
If stable, sit the patient up with support and assess sitting blood pressure.
Gather and review pertinent symptoms at the time of the fall.
Immobilize an extremity if fracture is suspected.
Reassure the older patient.
If stable, assist with transfer to an appropriate area for further evaluation.
Diagnosis and treatment

Reprinted with permission from ECRI Institute; (2006). Copyright © 2005 by Deanna Gray-Miceli.

TABLE 19.10
Critical Observations Made During the Immediate Postfall Assessment

Expressions or verbalizations of pain (facial grimacing, crying, screaming, agitation)
Changes in behavior or function, which may indicate pain
Swelling of an extremity (wrist, arm, leg) or head (hematoma, skull pain)
Unstable vital signs
Discolored cyanotic skin
Skin temperature (cold, clammy, diaphoretic)
Skin lacerations, contusions
LOC, no response to stimuli or significant change in LOC
Changed range of motion of extremities
Evidence of neck, head, or spinal cord injury
Abnormal or erratic neurological responses, such as absent pupil response, fixed or dilated pupils, seizures, or abnormal changes in posture

LOC, loss of consciousness.

Reprinted with permission from ECRI Institute (2006).

as not all older adults have received a dual-energy x-ray absorptiometry (DEXA) or bone densitometry scan. Most older individuals with hip fractures have osteoporosis; yet, findings from a retrospective analysis of records of patients receiving hip-fracture surgery show that the frequency of treating these high-risk older patients for osteoporosis is less than optimal; women are offered treatment more than men (Kamel, 2004).

If osteoporosis has been diagnosed, then certain protective interventions should be considered, such as the use of hip protectors (Applegarth et al., 2009; Bulat et al., 2008). As indicated for those older persons without safety judgment and who are unable to transfer and ambulate independently, the use of low-height beds and/or floor mats placed around the bedside will lessen the height of the fall, or padding a hard surface will reduce the chance of injury. Treatment for osteoporosis needs to be discussed, ranging from the use of medication agents to supplemental calcium and vitamin D, although research findings show a controversial association between vitamin D and physical performance improvements in gait and balance (Annweiler, Schott, Berrut, Fantino, & Beauchet, 2009). However, a recent meta-analysis found vitamin D to be the only intervention shown to be effective in reducing falls among female stroke survivors in an institutional setting (Batchelor, Hill, Mackintosh, & Said, 2010).

Other medical comorbidities that increase the risk of serious injury include bleeding disorders and use of blood-thinning medications to prevent stroke. A risk-versus-benefit analysis should always be part of fall management decision making for patient safety and prevention of injury (Quigley & Goff, 2011). Those with thrombocytopenia require monitoring of neurological status postfall in an effort to early identify a patient with a looming internal bleed or developing hematoma. These clinical conditions are very serious and can be fatal if not assessed early.

Best Practice Interventions for Suspected Serious Injury

Head Trauma

To detect the development of serious conditions, such as a subdural hematoma, frequent neurological checks are done for several days, depending on hospital clinical practice policies and guidelines, following head injury in older patients and those who are on blood thinners or who have coexisting medical conditions (Degelau et al., 2012; Ganz et al., 2013; Veterans Health Administration [VHA] Falls Toolkit, 2012). In addition, vital signs and assessing behavior, affect, cognition, and level of consciousness are all part of any assessment of a patient with head injury. Changes in speech, such as slurred speech, or subtle diminution in cognitive abilities (i.e., they no longer recognize you after recalling your name) are significant findings postfall head injury that require immediate attention. Recent evidence suggests that the major predictors of death in patients with ground-level falls were age greater than 70 years and a Glasgow Coma Scale score of less than 15 (Konstantinos et al., 2010). Older patients who have unwitnessed falls or do not recall falling despite evidence to the contrary should be monitored for head injury following the CDC guidelines for head injury (see Resources). TBI caused by head injuries is a condition that is preventable and, more important, readily recognizable. Subtle changes in cognition, level of consciousness, or behavior postfall indicate underlying head trauma. Table 19.8 details best practice interventions in cases in which a head injury is suspected postfall.

There is a strong clinical reason to suspect that older adults who are on anticoagulants are at higher risk of TBI, but empiric research in this age group is lacking. Still, best practice approaches to care of older adults must include a risk–benefit evaluation of medications, such as Coumadin, Plavix, and/or aspirin, among others, that place the older adult at an increased risk of bleeding following a fall. Additionally, use of helmets may be considered because they absorb trauma and reduce impact to the head (Quigley & Goff, 2011).

Postfall Management: Huddles and Assessment

Postfall Huddles

Many studies point out that a major determinant of a future fall is the history of previous falls (Degelau et al., 2012; Gates et al., 2008; Oliver et al., 2004). Finding the right intervention to prevent falls requires a multidisciplinary review to identify and intervene on modifiable risk factors (Ganz et al., 2013; Oliver et al., 2010). Because older adults continue to fall despite the implementation of evidence-based guidelines to prevent falls, identifying the causes of each fall is critical to preventing future falls. Within the inpatient settings, clinicians are able to act when a patient fall occurs, to quickly determine the event with the patient, using the postfall huddle (PFH) process. Implementing PFH shows promise for reducing repeat falls in individuals. Once a patient falls, the etiology and/or cause of the fall must be investigated to prevent future occurrences. Evidence reviews of PFAs are available (Cameron et al., 2012; Ganz et al., 2013).

PFHs are used in inpatient settings of care to determine the cause of the fall, and intervene appropriately (Anderson, Mokracek, & Lindy, 2009; Ganz et al., 2013; Quigley et al., 2009). The definition of *huddle* varies from study to study; but, a huddle is an immediate evaluation of each fall, by a team, preferably interprofessional, with the patient in the environment where the patient fell.

Postfall Assessment

Determination of why the fall occurred is of vital importance. The value of the PFA, if performed properly and comprehensively using appropriately empirically tested tools, is that underlying fall etiologies can be discerned so that appropriate plans of care can be instituted. To simply perform a fall risk assessment or perform a PFA and document the findings without linking the risk or actual fall cause to a strategy is *useless*. Once the type of fall is determined using a comprehensive postfall evaluation tool, the nurse can put into motion an appropriate plan of care.

Empirical research directed at determining the various types of falls occurring among older adults using a comprehensive PFA tool as the basis for determination has resulted in a broader classification scheme consisting of eight different fall types observed: falls caused by acute illness, chronic diseases, medications, behavior, unknown, environment, misjudgment, or poor patient safety awareness (Gray-Miceli, Ratcliffe, & Johnson, 2010). Fall risk screening tools identify the likelihood of an anticipated physiological fall with known intrinsic and extrinsic fall risk factors. These screening tools provide the first level of assessment data as the basis for comprehensive assessment. Only through comprehensive PFA can multifactorial, complex fall, and injury risk factors be defined (Quigley, Neily, Watson, Wright, & Strobel, 2007). Fall risk assessment and PFA are two very different and distinct approaches for fall prevention. Fall risk assessment tools offer limited types of inquiry, typically streamlined and focusing on five or six areas of inquiry, which are not a substitution or replacement for a comprehensive postfall inquiry or assessment. Critical information is missing in these streamlined fall risk assessment tools.

Therefore, the purpose of the PFA is to identify the clinical status of the older adult, verify and treat injuries, and to identify underlying causes of the fall whenever possible. Components of the PFA are typically routinely performed by professional nurses in all patient settings, although this evaluation may be skeletal or limited according to the completeness of questions and examination included in the tool used. Few empirically published tools for PFA exist, and previous research has shown that fall risk determination, using short forms, asking five to eight questions about risk, often replaced (inappropriately) PFA in institutionalized settings (Gray-Miceli,

Strumpf, Reinhard, Zanna, & Fritz, 2004; Ray et al., 1997; Rubenstein, Robbins, Josephson, Schulman, & Osterweil, 1990).

Evidence shows that comprehensive PFA tools are useful and available to assist professional registered nurses in performing a PFA, especially in institutionalized settings (Gray-Miceli, Strumpf, Johnson, Draganescu, & Ratcliffe, 2006). In institutional settings where teams are unavailable, comprehensive PFA may be carried out through consultation with specialty-trained providers.

The PFA is a comprehensive, yet fall-focused history and physical examination of the present problem (falling), coupled with a functional assessment, review of past medical problems, and medications. Clinical fall-prevention guidelines are very clear about all of the necessary components for inclusion of patients who have fallen, which include fall history; fall circumstance; medical problems; medication review; mobility assessment; vision assessment; neurological examination, including mental status; and cardiovascular assessment. In addition to this information, data are collected about the patient's physical status. Performing a comprehensive PFA allows the clinician to identify intrinsic risks and recent causes of a fall such as orthostatic hypotension and/or bradyarrhythmia or tachyarrhythmia associated with dizziness (Gray-Miceli et al., 2006). There are various stages of a postfall assessment, ranging from the immediate period following the fall (within 24 hours) to the interim period and then the longitudinal period where adverse outcomes such as pain from an injurious fall can occur. In the hospital setting, certain components of a PFA can be elicited immediately following a patient fall, with the decision to ask certain questions immediately depending on the medical stability of the patient and nursing judgment.

The Immediate PFA

As soon as possible, an assessment is made to determine the extent of any sustained injuries. Before any intervention is taken, any staff member should remain with the patient and call for help. During this time, the older adult patient is verbally reassured and kept warm (but not moved) until help arrives. There are many key observations to be noted about the fallen individual's medical and psychological condition, as well as condition of the environment. The medical stability of the patient determines the sequence of information gathered either immediately or in the interim period, according to current standards of practice followed by licensed professionals. For instance, if unconscious from a head injury sustained during the fall, neurological checks, vital signs with apical pulse rate, and pulse oxygenation are assessed first. Other assessments of gait or functional status are conducted after the patient has stabilized. While this is being performed, or if shoes or slippers are worn, other staff members can assess environmental spills. Information about the lighting and use of assistive devices can be gathered. Any verbalizations made by the patient should be noted about his or her condition. Critical observations made during the immediate PFA (Table 19.9) that should be communicated to the primary care provider include observation or verbalizations of pain, extremity swelling, unstable vital signs, discolored skin, temperature, laceration or contusions of the skin, loss of consciousness, decreased range of motion, evidence of head or neck injury and abnormal or erratic neurological responses, uncontrollable bleeding, and incontinence of bowel or bladder at the time of the fall.

Interim PFA

During the interim period of PFA and monitoring (anywhere from several hours to days), the nurses continue to review, determine, and communicate pertinent findings from this assessment and its progression or resolution. Once the patient is medically stable, fall risk assessment can be reassessed by the interprofessional team, revaluating intrinsic and extrinsic risks so that a plan of care can be determined. Developing a plan of care and requesting a change in physician orders for level of supervision required by nursing staff of the older patient or specific activity restrictions depend on the fall-assessment findings.

Longitudinal PFA

Following a patient fall, the presence of injury may not be apparent until days or even weeks later. When cognitive impairment exists, the accuracy of the historical accounts of pain obtained immediately after the fall may be questioned. Observations of functional status with attention to any subtle or blatant changes in mobility can signal an underlying fracture or a looming unstable joint that was not previously reported. Likewise, during a patient fall in which the older adult is cognitively intact, and then later develops an acute delirium, this should signal to the professional nurse the possibility of an injury. In these two instances, as part of the ongoing PFA, the standard of care warrants monitoring of vital signs and neurological status for a period of several days or more, as clinically indicated. Fall policy and procedures should reflect this provision because any change in patient condition warrants follow-through, documentation, and communication to senior level providers, other nursing staff, and family.

Overview of Effective Fall and Injury Prevention in Hospitals

Effective fall-prevention programs in acute care hospitals are championed by nurses using one or more approaches in collaboration with interprofessional teams. Moving beyond traditional measures of fall rates to assessing and measuring patient injury from falls provides more information and segmentation of vulnerable patients so that a new level of intervention is applied. This process advances the evidence related to falls into the quality-management program for fall prevention. Assessing risk for injury provides the evidence for nurses to provide specific interventions to reduce injury (e.g., hip protectors, floor mats, and helmets) based on using existing tools. The evidence is strong to support the benefit of multifactorial fall-prevention programs for injurious falls in acute care. System-level interventions with emerging evidence of effectiveness result from the work of innovation: nurse champions, safety huddles, teach-back strategies, PFHs, and interventions to reduce fall-related trauma.

Nurse Champions

Embracing nurse champions at the point of care, the Institute for Healthcare Improvement's (IHI) Transforming Care at the Bedside has partnered with the Veterans Integrated Service Network (VISN) 8 Patient Safety Center to focus on acute care fall and injury prevention for the past 5 years. Dedicated to building program capacity, infrastructure, and expertise, fall experts have mentored and coached nurses from across acute care settings to address vulnerable older adults who are at greatest risk of loss of function or loss of life if any type of fall occurs. This approach to nursing practice has been transformational (Boushon et al., 2012; Ganz et al., 2013).

Teach-Backs

Health literacy requires that providers evaluate the degree to which individuals learn by assessing their capacity to obtain information, process, and understand basic health information and services so that they can make informed health decisions (Institute of Medicine, 2004; Nielsen-Bohlman, Panzer, & Kindig, 2004). Teach-backs identify what the patient learned by a return demonstration or feedback, and, more important, what the patient had difficulty learning, so that the provider can fill that gap through ongoing education (Boushon et al., 2012). A more detailed discussion of teach-backs and patient education geared toward the older adult patient is available for practicing nurses (Gray-Miceli, 2014).

Comfort Care and Safety Rounds

Nursing staff complete routine and frequent comfort care and safety rounds as one of their tests of change. This intervention has emerging evidence of effectiveness for fall prevention based on the results of researchers Meade, Bursell, and Ketelsen (2006): hourly to 2-hour rounds in acute care reduced falls ($p = 0.01$), and by 60% 1 year later in the follow-up hospitals. There was a clinically significant reduction in falls by 23% but it was not of statistical significance. The fall rate declined from 3.37/1000 patient days to 2.6 or 0.77 falls per patient days. This intervention has been included in hospital fall-prevention toolkits (Boushon et al., 2012; Degelau et al., 2012; Ganz et al., 2013; National Center for Patient Safety Falls Toolkit, 2004, 2013). The IHI recommends implementing routine rounds that "combine frequent and regular toileting rounds with existing patient care tasks, such as patient turning, environmental safety assessments, and pain assessment. Address all patient needs (e.g., pain, position, toileting, and environment) in one effective encounter" (Boushon et al., 2012, p. 22).

Many hospital-based fall-prevention programs include toileting rounds. Toileting rounds use nurse's aides to regularly assess older adult patients for the need to urinate and to provide the patient with assistance. The purpose of toileting rounds is to prevent patients from incurring urinary accidents (and potential falls) by encouraging regular voiding. In many circumstances, urinary accidents can lead to falls. Scenarios include the older adult sensing a need to urinate, getting up out of bed unassisted, and incurring a fall by an unrecognized physiologic mechanism (e.g., orthostatic hypotension). Another scenario occurs on route to the bathroom; the older adult has a urinary accident on the floor and slips and falls on the wet floor. By offering toileting rounds on a regular basis, the potential for these occurrences is minimized, reducing fall rates as well as the iatrogenic complications (e.g., hip fracture). Toileting is a fundamental element of basic care that has an important place in the prevention of patient falls, but its importance is underrecognized. In a study by Brown et al. (2000), urge incontinence (and not stress), especially if occurring weekly or more often, increased the risk of falls and nonspinal, nontraumatic fractures in older White women living in the community.

Safety Huddle Postfall

Safety huddles were patterned after the military's "After Action Review" (AAR) process. Safety huddles provide a mechanism for immediate knowledge transfer for learning from errors and close calls. In a safety huddle, staff are instructed to immediately assess a situation or event to understand what happened, what should have happened, what accounted for the difference, and what corrective action could be implemented to prevent a similar event. This AAR mimics a modified root-cause analysis. All staff received a brochure explaining the AAR process and are instructed to perform a safety huddle as soon as possible after becoming aware of a fall. Nurse managers or advanced practice nurses coach staff in the safety-huddle process through role-playing and use of a brochure and presentation that describes the process. The nurse managers lead the initial huddles, and staff follow thereafter. Over time, staff begin to use safety huddles to examine other patient safety situations and to ensure that fall precautions are consistently applied in the shift-to-shift handoff process. Incorporation into the handoff process also provided the opportunity for staff to reassess a patient's status (Quigley et al., 2009).

Interventions to Reduce Trauma

Patients with risk factors for serious injury (osteoporosis or osteoporosis risk factors, anticoagulants, and postoperative patients) should be automatically placed on *high-risk* fall precautions and interventions to reduce risk for serious injury should be implemented (Boushon et al., 2012). Interventions to reduce the risk of trauma and to prevent injury include the following: place a bedside mat on floor at the side of the bed, unless contraindicated; use height-adjustable bed (low-bed position to reduce distance from bed to floor); helmet use for patients at risk of head injury (those on anticoagulants, patients with severe seizure disorder, and history of falling and hitting head); and dress with hip protectors for patients at risk of hip fracture (NCPS Falls Toolkit, 2014). These interventions, when combined, create protective bundles. For example, those patients at risk of hip fracture should be placed at high risk of falls and in height-adjustable beds, wear hip protectors, have floor mats at bedside when in bed, and receive comfort and safety rounds. Those patients at risk of hemorrhagic bleed should be placed at high risk of falls and in height-adjustable beds, have floor mats at bedside when in bed, and receive comfort and safety rounds. Helmets should be considered for patients with history of head injury and falls, and on anticoagulants. All patients should receive education about their fall and injury risks. Any patient at high risk of bleeding or other serious injury, residing in assisted living and who has a current diagnosis of cognitive impairment, should also be evaluated for safety to ambulate alone. When in doubt, err on the side of safety by making sure the cognitively impaired ambulatory patient has contact guarding or arm-in-arm assistance with a standby nurse's aide when walking. This nursing recommendation is in response to a recent single-site study that found that older adults at greatest risk of head injury (compared with older adults who fell without any head injury) were ambulating at the time of their fall (Gray-Miceli et al., 2013).

Program Evaluation

Many health systems use a specifically designed incident report form for falls that collects detailed literature-based data about fall occurrences (Elkins et al., 2004). For example, these data might include time of day, location, activity, orthostasis, and incontinence. From the analysis of the data, one can determine the type of fall, such as accidental, anticipated physiological, and unanticipated physiological fall, and severity of injury—minor, moderate, or major/severe (Donaldson, Brown, Aydin, Bolton, & Rutledge, 2005; Quigley et al., 2007). Analysis of data of this depth and scope enables clinicians, administrators, and risk managers to profile the level of fall risk of their patients along with actual factors contributing to the fall, as well as identifying overall patterns and trends surrounding fall occurrence.

Fall-Prevention Program

Fall prevention begins with an integrated/coordinated approach inclusive of fall risk determination and PFA to identify risk factors. Accurate documentation should be provided in the plan of care, nursing and interprofessional notes, and other aspects of the medical record, such as the problem-list, help to ensure communication and ongoing monitoring. A review of fall-related information collected about a fall event or a person deemed at risk of fall by the interprofessional team adds an important dimension to fall care. The team offers input from its unique perspective of the fall circumstance and how to best manage a fall or a patient at high risk of falls. The interpofessional team consists of the medical provider, nurse, physical or occupational therapist, risk manager, pharmacist, and other direct health care providers.

Hospital-based fall-prevention programs have been described in the literature, but few clinical trials have been conducted demonstrating their effectiveness because of methodological limitations associated with this complex fast-paced setting. One study examined the effect of a program of fall prevention that includes multifactorial components of fall risk assessment, a choice of interventions, patient education, and staff education, as well as labels or graphics alerting others to at-risk patients. Use of this model and its outcomes were examined prospectively for 5 years by Dempsey (2004), who reported a significant reduction in fall rates. However, over time, compliance deteriorated warranting further nursing inquiry considering use of a process approach to increase nurse autonomy in fall prevention.

Exemplary models of care also exist through the National Center for Patient Safety at the U.S.

Department of Veterans Affairs (http://www.ihi.org/resources/Pages/OtherWebsites/NationalCenterforPatientSafetyFallsToolkit.aspx). The Veterans Affairs, VISN 8 Patient Safety Center of Inquiry, under the direction of an advanced nurse practitioner–nurse scientist, spearheads an impressive program of fall prevention through its health care network of inpatient hospitals. Fall prevention through best practice approaches is evaluated and translated into standard practices among general fall prevention; interventions for high-risk patients; and education of staff, patients, and families.

Models of care, serving as exemplars of the geriatric nurse-centered approach, realize improvements in hospital lengths of stay and health outcomes as well as fewer iatrogenic geriatric syndromes such as inpatient falls. Use of the acute care of the elderly (ACE) units, Nurses Improving Care for Healthsystem Elders (NICHE) program, and the geriatric resource nurse (GRN) model, which use a system-level quality-improvement approach, including educational programs for staff, realized a decrease in fall rate by 5.8% (Smyth, Dubin, Restrepo, Nueva-Espana, & Capezuti, 2001).

INTERVENTIONS FOR FALL PREVENTION AND MANAGEMENT

Instituting General Safety Measures

Hospitals and their staff have a legal responsibility and due diligence to ensure freedom from environmental hazards and safety for all patients, staff, and visitors. Routine environmental assessment using a checklist should include the unit, corridors, entrance, and exits, as well as patient holding areas, patient rooms, and areas where patients are transported (radiology, nuclear imaging, and operating room). In each of these areas, an environmental assessment is performed focusing on floor surfaces; furniture; hallways; steps; device safety, such as stretchers, wheelchairs, and other types of chairs; presence or absence of clutter; bathrooms with appropriate grab rails; and routine assessment of equipment. Use of a checklist signed by the designated employee allows for audit review of compliance, serving as an internal benchmark of compliance.

As part of general safety, some facilities designate any older adult aged 65 years and older admitted to be on "safety precautions," which can include various other safety measures (presented in the following text). Clinically, it is important to recognize, in advance whenever possible, that if instructions are given to the patient for general safety precautions, that the older adult is actually able to hear, understand, and demonstrate that he or she can follow instructions. Simply "telling the older adult" to be careful or to not get up without assistance is insufficient in the face of an ongoing or new onset of delirium or cognitive impairment. Rather, other safety measures need to be immediately instituted, discussed with the team and the family caregiver, and incorporated as part of the plan of care. Immediate options always include (a) increasing surveillance by either staying with the patient continuously, (b) moving the patient to a closer location (provided there is staff constantly observing the patient), (c) considering need for a one-on-one type of sitter or surveillance technology service for continual surveillance, or (d) engaging the older patient in diversional activities or other forms of therapeutic recreation. Sitter-type services can be provided by hospital staff, volunteers, or through private-duty services. Discussion with family caregivers and the interprofessional team is essential in these cases. However, if a sitter program is to be used for fall prevention, specific criteria for use should be established, as effectiveness of sitters to prevent falls lacks empiric evidence (Feil & Wallace, 2014).

Early Mobility for Older Patients Who Fall

Early mobility, whenever older patients are medically stable, is a fundamental and basic aspect of care for all older adult patients to receive during their hospitalization. It is a step toward the prevention of deconditioning, reduced mobility and immobility, and other cascading problems that can result when less sedentary (for instance, orthostatic pneumonia or atelectasis). Early mobility as an intervention begins with the simple and conscious decision by nursing to assist the patient out of bed to walk to the bathroom whenever possible, rather than to use a bedpan or even a bedside commode that offers little opportunity for mobility. Wearing proper footwear, corrective lenses, and clearing a path that is free of clutter and spills are essential. Use of a walking aid, such as a standard cane or walker, may also be required; appropriate assistive devices can be ascertained through an occupational or physical therapist consultation (Quigley & Goff, 2011). For elderly patients who may have cognitive impairment and are at risk of serious injury, assistance with ambulation and their device is recommended, given findings that ambulatory elderly fallers in assisted living had greater risk of head injury than fallers residing in skilled nursing (Gray-Miceli, Ratcliffe, & Thomasson, 2013).

Another essential aspect for the older adult with comorbidities is for nurses to preemptively ask the older patient, who is transitioning with their assistance, from sitting to standing and then while walking, "How are you feeling?" Of concern is the detection of symptoms such as lightheadedness, vertigo with rotational movement, or muscular stiffness. These symptoms can be managed and monitored, if significant enough to prohibit mobility, once they are detected. Another concern exists for the older adult patient with orthostatic hypotension. In this instance, gradual upright incline with assistance while monitoring for symptoms of lightheadedness is important. Should an older adult experience symptoms or develop acute physiological evidence of a problem (for instance, near syncope, syncope, or changes in heart rate or blood pressure), slowly easing him or her back to a recumbent position and notifying the physician for further evaluation are warranted.

Mobility programs built on the positive feedback that the patient is feeling and objectively gaining strength each day are instituted. Checklists can monitor progress and serve to validate to the patient his or her clinical progression. Care must be taken, however, to remind persons who are restricted from independent mobility to always wait for assistance. Recommendations are to set a similar time each day and to use consistent staff. An integral component of any mobility program is the footwear of patients. A recent study found patients who wore their own footwear significantly improved participants' balance compared to being barefoot; in fact, the greatest benefit was seen in those individuals with the poorest balance (Horgan et al., 2009).

Specific Nursing Interventions

Personal alarms are routinely used to alert nursing staff about impending falls or changes in patient mobility status. Care should be taken when deciding to use these devices, because they do not prevent a fall from occurring (Oliver et al., 2010); rather, they heighten staff's awareness by sounding an alarm, indicating a change in position has occurred. There are many commercial products available, but generally, they are of two types: personal alarms clipped to the patient's gown or chair and bed–chair pressure sensors. Despite their widespread use, there is little evidence regarding their effectiveness in reducing falls in an acute care hospital setting. The use of a bed sensor alarm was studied in a geriatric rehabilitation unit with older adult patients, deemed by nurses to be at increased risk of falling (Kwok, Mok, Chien, & Tam, 2006). In this study, the availability of bed sensor devices neither reduced physical restraint use nor improved the clinical outcomes of older adults with perceived fall risk. In a nursing home–based study, however, use of the "NOC WATCH," a nonintrusive monitor used with older adults at high risk of falling (Kelly, Phillips, Cain, Polissar, & Kelly, 2002), reduced fall rate by 91%, thereby supporting other clinical trials using a randomized design. Effectiveness in the prevention of falls may best be gauged by the timeliness of the rescue (Quigley & Goff, 2011). Furthermore, greater nurse surveillance capacity was significantly associated with better quality care and fewer adverse events (Kutney-Lee, Lake, & Aiken, 2009).

Both floor mats and use of low-rise beds have an important place in the armamentarium of clinical interventions to prevent the occurrence of serious injury when a bed fall occurs. Floor mats are simply placed surrounding the bed and serve to cushion the impact of the fall. They vary in thickness, and, if portions of an area are uncovered, substantial injury could still occur if a patient attempts to get out of bed and a bed fall ensues. Little, if any, empirical research evidence exists regarding their effectiveness in preventing falls from bed causing fractures to the hip or TBI in acute care settings. However, one observational cluster randomized trial in 18 nursing homes found that both types of hip protectors (soft and hard), when worn correctly, had the potential to reduce the risk of a hip fracture in falls by nearly 60% (Bentzen, Bergland, & Forsen, 2008).

A recent meta-analysis, however, reported that hip protectors are an ineffective intervention for those living at home and that their effectiveness in the institutional setting is uncertain (Parker, Gillespie, & Gillespie, 2006).

Technological advances have occurred, offering staff and patients a greater variety of solutions to the problem of falling. Improvements are realized to have occurred with walking aides, such as canes that "talk" and provide feedback to the user, balance retraining that helps patients learn about where their body is in space and how to compensate for muscular impairments, and other types of equipment used at the bedside when transitioning patients. Although these devices are available, research is evolving and limited in terms of their effectiveness in fall prevention (Nelson et al., 2004).

An integral component of any fall-prevention educational intervention for hospitalized older adults or preparing for discharge home concerns their working knowledge of what caused their fall and what can be done about it. Exploring the older adults' beliefs and attitudes is important and can lead to dispelling myths they may hold about falling; for instance, they may believe it is a normal part of aging or that nothing can be done about it. An older person's view and conceptualization about falling is a starting point for a tailored educational intervention. A systematic review of the literature of many studies examining older adults' preferences, views, and experiences in relation to fall-prevention strategies reported several important findings (McInnes & Askie, 2004): (a) in clinical practice, it is important to consult with individuals to find out what they are willing to modify and (b) what changes they are prepared to make to reduce their risk of falling; otherwise they may not attend fall-prevention programs. Important aspects of patient education, as it relates to falls and injury prevention, and the use of teach-backs are recommended for practicing nurses in any setting (Gray-Miceli, 2014).

CASE STUDY

Mrs. S is an 80-year-old White female admitted to the step-down rehabilitation unit at the hospital following a 3-week admission for treatment of a community-acquired pneumonia. Mrs. S received intravenous antibiotics and fluids for management of the infiltrate and associated dehydration. Mrs. S.'s hospitalization was complicated by development of acute confusion, which escalated following the use of IV theophylline and the use of Ventolin nebulizers. Mrs. S also developed a deep vein thrombosis of the leg, which was treated with IV heparin, and she now receives Coumadin. Mrs. S's fall risk score was significant for visual impairment because of a cataract, delirium, focal lower extremity weakness resulting from osteoarthritis, chronic obstructive lung disease, osteoporosis, and forgetfulness with short-term memory loss.

Before this hospitalization, Mrs. S was functioning independently in her home, until her son and daughter found her on the floor, mildly confused and disoriented, complaining of dizziness. Mrs. S was transported to the emergency room for further evaluation. She was diagnosed with a right lung infiltrate via chest x-ray and moderate to severe dehydration. An IV line was started and she was treated with antibiotics and admitted for observation. A 12-lead electrocardiogram showed a sinus bradycardia at 54 beats per minute. A CT scan of the head was not performed; rather, Mrs. S was placed on observation and admitted to a medical–surgical unit.

After the 3-week long hospitalization, Mrs. S is transferred via wheelchair to the rehabilitation unit. During the admission assessment, you note Mrs. S's total fall risk score increased by 4 points as a result of increased confusion/disorientation, periods of restlessness, and reduced mobility. Mrs. S's vital signs are stable. You learn in the nursing report that Mrs. S needs constant supervision or she wanders off the unit. During the physical examination, you are paged overhead and respond by going to the nursing station. When you return to examine Mrs. S, she is gone. A second overhead page is called "stat" for assistance on your unit. Apparently, Mrs. S was found sitting on the floor outside of the elevator, complaining of pain in her right hip and right ankle.

The immediate PFA shows possible loss of consciousness as Mrs. S was observed unresponsive for a few seconds. There is evidence of a head injury with a laceration and hematoma to the scalp as well as right lower leg pain and swelling. Mrs. S's sitting blood pressure sitting is 80/50 mmHg, and her pulse rate is 60 bpm—regular, but weak. Ice is applied to her scalp and her leg is immobilized. The physician is notified immediately and a stat CT scan of the head is ordered, later confirming an acute intracranial bleed. Mrs. S is prepared for cranial surgery and then hip-fracture repair the following day.

Discussion

1. What nursing actions should have been taken to prevent the fall and serious injury?
   Mrs. S is at high risk of serious injury as indicated by her fall risk screen score and use of the anticoagulation medication Coumadin. The standard of practice for caring for an older adult hospitalized with increased risk of falls with serious injury requires the nurse to recognize that this patient is likely to have impaired judgment and inability to follow direction because of her disorientation, relocation to a new unit, and evidence of restlessness. Because she is ambulatory, but forgetful, this creates a situation in which the patient needs constant supervision. Mrs. S should be allowed to ambulate, but only with one-on-one supervision and/or physical assistance whenever possible. The nurse failed to recognize the importance of providing constant supervision to the patient. Actions that should have been undertaken include constant supervision by support staff, such as volunteers and/or a special assignment of a nurse's aide to stay with the patient. Family would need to be notified of this decision and to enlist their support for considering a private-duty nurse's assistant. Acute confusion or delirium renders Mrs. S unsafe to make the necessary decisions or judgments about her care.

   In terms of preventing serious injury, Mrs. S could be offered a hip protector as they are indicated for older adults who are deemed at high risk of fracture. Osteoporotic older adults who fall are likely to fracture an extremity or incur serious injury. A low-rise bed and floor mats should be used

(continued)

CASE STUDY ***(continued)***

because she is at high risk of falling from bed again. Her needs can be anticipated by regular rounds and by offering the use of the toilet, which can help prevent urinary accidents and/or falls walking toward the bathroom.

It is imperative that Mrs. S be allowed to continue to move freely and ambulate provided she is supervised and/or assisted because of her disorientation. Daily walking on the unit, in the patient's room, and whenever possible to increase mobility is essential.

2. How should the nursing assessment be focused?
   Further assessment for reversible causes of delirium is warranted. As Ventolin has precipitated acute confusion, this drug should be used sparingly and possibly substituted with less "anticholinergic agents." A pharmacy consultation, as part of the interprofessional assessment, would be appropriate. Alternative respiratory interventions for increased pulmonary secretions, such as clapping, postural drainage deep breathing, and the use of inspirometry, could be instituted.

   Further assessment of Mrs. S's falls (i.e., a fall evaluation) is clinically indicated. She has had two falls recently: one at home and one at the hospital. The etiology of these falls is not clear. The history of "being dazed" that occurred in both falls warrants additional workup. In the emergency room, the patient did not receive a CT scan of her head. The fall evaluation includes, among other tests, a 24-hour Holter monitor. A consultation with a geriatrician and/or neurologist is clinically warranted.

SUMMARY

Fall and serious injury prevention is a shared responsibility by all health care providers and professionals caring for older adult patients. National recommendations exist to guide practice and should be routinely incorporated into any fall-prevention program and practice policy. Some of the evidence-based research presented here can help clinicians make choices about which interventions may be the most efficacious or effective, bearing in mind that this choice changes with changes in the patient's condition. Therefore, selecting the most appropriate intervention will always depend on what the nursing and medical assessment determine the likely cause of the fall to be and the medical stability of the patient at that time. Among older adults with advanced years of age with complex illness and multiple comorbidities and geriatric syndromes, this determination becomes increasingly more challenging, but not impossible to make. The safety of older adults in the hospital and continuing on discharge home depends on continual assessment and reevaluation of their condition coupled with education, the use of the most effective and safest technology, and the older adults' knowledge and willingness to participate in evidence-based care.

Nursing staff and hospital organizations are fortunate to have resources of some best practice exemplars used by acute care hospitals in their efforts to reduce patient falls. Exemplars that have been reviewed by expert panels are available from the IHI and AHRQ's fall toolkits (NCPS, 2014; Ganz et al., 2013). Some best practice exemplars and compilation of evidence-based interventions are also addressed in the American Nurses Association publication (2014), *Five Easy Steps to Prevent Falls: The Comprehensive Guide for Nurses to Keeping Patients of All Ages Safe.* Framed around a public health model for fall prevention, content includes important steps for practicing professional nurses in fall history taking, fall-focused physical examination, environmental assessment, fall-focused nursing diagnosis and targeted interventions, and patient education through teach-backs (Gray-Miceli, 2014). These resources provide best practice examples to the nursing workforce, so that fall knowledge and falls and injury solutions can be implemented in practice.

Hospital organizations vary in their ability to successfully eradicate patient falls. Their success is contingent on many factors in addition to a trained, knowledgeable nursing and interprofessional team workforce. The Joint Commission has suggested that, to become a high-reliability hospital, a series of incremental changes should be undertaken. Leadership's commitment to zero falls, a fully functional culture of safety, along with widespread deployment of highly effective process improvement measures are required in their process approach for high-reliability health care (Chassin & Loeb, 2013). Quigley and White (2013) discuss components of patient safety culture and the integration of these components with fall prevention, the role of nurses, and high reliability.

NURSING STANDARD OF PRACTICE

Protocol 19.1: Fall Prevention

I. GOALS

A. Reduce preventable falls and serious injury in hospitalized older adults
B. Recognize multifactorial risks and causes of falls in older adults
C. Institute recommendations for fall prevention and management consistent with best available evidence, clinical practice guidelines, and standards of care that are age specific

II. OVERVIEW

Falls among older adults are not a normal consequence of aging; rather, they are considered a geriatric syndrome most often caused by discrete multifactorial and interacting, predisposing (intrinsic and extrinsic risks), and precipitating (dizziness and syncope) causes (Gray-Miceli et al., 2005; Rubenstein & Josephson, 2006). Fall epidemiology varies according to clinical setting. In acute care, fall incidence ranges from 2.3 to 7 falls per 1,000 patient-days depending on the unit. Nearly one third of older adults living in the community fall each year in their homes. The highest fall incidence occurs in the institutional long-term care setting (nursing home), where 50% to 75% of the 1.63 million nursing home residents experience a fall yearly. Falls rank as the eighth leading cause of unintentional injury for older Americans and were responsible for more than 16,000 deaths yearly (Oliver et al., 2010).

III. BACKGROUND/STATEMENT OF THE PROBLEM

A. Definition
   1. A *fall* is an unexpected event in which the participant comes to rest on the ground, floor, or lower level (Prevention of Falls Network Europe, 2006).
B. Fall etiology
   1. Fall *risk factors* include intrinsic risks of cognitive, vision, gait, or balance impairment, high-risk/contraindicated medications, and/or the extrinsic risks of assistive devices, inappropriate footwear, restraint, use of unsturdy furniture or equipment, poor lighting, uneven or slippery surfaces (Chang et al., 2004).
   2. Fall *causes* include, among others, orthostatic hypotension, arrhythmia, infection, generalized or focal muscular weakness, syncope, seizure, hypoglycemia, neuropathy, and medication.

IV. PARAMETERS OF ASSESSMENT

A. Assess and document all older adult patients for intrinsic risk factors to fall.
   1. Advancing age, especially if older than 75
   2. History of a recent fall, repeat falls, or fall-related injury (AGS/BGS, 2011)
   3. Specific comorbidities: dementia, hip fracture, type 2 diabetes, Parkinson's disease, arthritis, and depression
   4. Functional disability: use of assistive device
   5. Alteration in level of consciousness or cognitive impairment
   6. Gait, balance, or visual impairment
   7. Use of high-risk medications (Chang et al., 2004)
   8. Urge urinary incontinence (Brown et al., 2000)
   9. Physical restraint use (Capezuti, Maislin, Strumpf, & Evans, 2002)
   10. Bare feet or inappropriate footwear
   11. Identify risks for significant injury resulting from current use of anticoagulants, such as Coumadin, Plavix, or aspirin, and/or those with osteoporosis or risks for osteoporosis (John A. Hartford Foundation Institute for Geriatric Nursing, 2003).
B. Assess and document patient-care environment routinely for extrinsic risk factors for fall and institute corrective action:
   1. Floor surfaces for spills, wet areas, and unevenness
   2. Proper level of illumination and functioning of lights (night light works)

(continued)

Protocol 19.1: Fall Prevention *(continued)*

3. Table tops, furniture, and beds are sturdy and in good repair
4. Grab rails and bars are in place in the bathroom
5. Use of adaptive aids work properly and are in good repair
6. Bed rails do not collapse when used for transitioning or support
7. Patient gowns/clothing do not cause tripping
8. IV poles are sturdy if used during mobility and tubing does not pose a safety hazard for tripping

C. Perform PFH and a comprehensive PFA following a patient fall to identify possible fall causes (if possible, begin the identification of possible causes within 24 hours of a fall) as determined during the immediate, interim, and longitudinal postfall intervals. Because of known incidences of delayed complication of falls, including fractures, observe all patients for about 48 hours after an observed or suspected fall (ECRI Institute, 2006; Gray-Miceli et al., 2006; Panel on Prevention of Falls in Older Persons, 2011).

D. Perform a physical assessment of the patient at the time of the fall, including vital signs (which may include orthostatic blood pressure readings), neurological assessment, and evaluation for head, neck, spine, and/or extremity injuries.
1. Once the assessment rules out any significant injury:
   a. Obtain a history of the fall by the patient or witness description and document
   b. Note the circumstances of the fall, location, activity, time of day, and any significant symptoms
   c. Review underlying illness and problems
   d. Review medications
   e. Assess functional, sensory, and psychological status
   f. Evaluate environmental conditions
   g. Review risk factors for falling (American Medical Directors Association, 2003; ECRI Institute, 2006; John A. Hartford Foundation Institute for Geriatric Nursing, 2003; Panel on Prevention of Falls in Older Persons, 2011).

E. In the acute care setting, an integrated multidisciplinary team (comprised of the physician, nurse, health care provider, risk manager, physical therapist, and other designated staff) plans care for the older adult at risk of falls or who has fallen, hinged on findings from an individualized assessment (ECRI Institute, 2006; Joint Commission, 2006).

F. The process approach to an individualized PFA includes use of standardized measurement tools of patient risk in combination with a fall-focused history and physical examination, functional assessment, and review of medications (American Medical Directors Association, 2003; John A. Hartford Foundation Institute for Geriatric Nursing, 2003; Panel on Prevention of Falls in Older Persons, 2011). When plans of care are targeted to likely causes, individualized interventions are likely to be identified. If falling continues despite attempts at individualized interventions, the standard of care warrants a reexamination of the older adult and his or her fall.

V. NURSING CARE STRATEGIES

A. General safety precaution and fall-prevention measures that apply to all patients, especially older adults, include:
1. Assess the patient care environment routinely for extrinsic risk factors and institute appropriate corrective action.
   a. Use standardized environmental checklists to screen; document findings.
   b. Communicate findings to risk managers, housekeeping, maintenance department, all staff, and hospital administration if needed.
   c. Reevaluate environment for safety (ECRI Institute, 2006).
2. Assess/screen older adult patient for multifactorial risk factors for fall on admission, following a change in condition, on transfer to a new unit, and following a fall (ECRI Institute, 2006; NCPS Falls Toolkit, 2014):
   a. Use standardized or empirically tested fall risk tools in conjunction with other assessment tools to evaluate risk of falling (Panel on Prevention of Falls in Older Persons, 2011; Tinetti et al., 1986).
   b. Document findings in nursing notes, interprofessional progress notes, and the problem list.
   c. Communicate and discuss findings with interprofessional team members.
   d. In the interprofessional discussion, include review and reduction or elimination of high-risk medications associated with falling.

(continued)

Protocol 19.1: Fall Prevention *(continued)*

   e. As part of fall protocol in the facility, flag the chart or use graphic or color display of the patient's risk potential to fall.
   f. Communicate to the patient and the family caregiver the identified risk to fall, and specific interventions chosen to minimize the patient's risk.
   g. Include patient and family members in the interprofessional plan of care and discussion about fall-prevention measures.
   h. Promote early mobility and incorporate measures to increase mobility, such as daily walking, if medically stable and not otherwise contraindicated.
   i. On transfer to another unit, communicate the risk assessment and interventions chosen and their effectiveness in fall prevention.
   j. On discharge, review fall risk factors and measures to prevent falls in the home with the older patient and/or family caregiver. Provide patient literature/brochures, if available. If not readily available, refer to the Internet for appropriate websites/resources.
   k. Explore with the older patient and/or family caregiver avenues to maintain mobility and functional status; consider referral to home-based exercise or group exercises at community senior centers. If discharge is planned to a subacute or rehabilitation unit, label the older adult's mobility status at the time of discharge on the transfer or indicate other types of physical activity in the home to strengthen lower extremities or assist with gait/balance problems.
3. Institute general safety precautions according to the facility protocol, which may include:
   a. Referral to a fall-prevention program
   b. Use of a low-rise bed that measures 14 inches from the floor
   c. Use of floor mats if patient is at risk of serious injury such as osteoporosis
   d. Easy access to call light
   e. Minimization and/or avoidance of physical restraints
   f. Use of personal or pressure sensor alarms
   g. Increased observation/surveillance
   h. Use of rubber-soled/heeled shoes or nonskid slippers
   i. Regular toileting at set intervals and/or continence program; provide easy access to urinals and bedpans
   j. Observation during walking rounds or safety rounds
   k. Use of corrective glasses for walking
   l. Reduction of clutter in traffic areas
   m. Early mobility program (ECRI Institute, 2006)
4. Provide staff with clear, written procedures describing what to do when a patient fall occurs.

B. Identify specific patients requiring additional safety precautions and/or evaluation by a specialist or:
   1. Those with impaired judgment or thinking caused by acute or chronic illness (delirium and mental illness)
   2. Those with osteoporosis, at risk of fracture
   3. Those with current hip fracture
   4. Those with current head or brain injury (standard of care)

C. Review and discuss with the interprofessional team the findings from the individualized assessment and develop a multidisciplinary plan of care to prevent falls (Chang et al., 2004).
   1. Communicate to the physician significant PFA findings (ECRI Institute, 2006).
   2. Monitor the effectiveness of the fall-prevention interventions instituted.
   3. Following a patient fall, observe for serious injury resulting from a fall and follow facility protocols for management (standard of care).
   4. Following a patient fall, monitor vital signs, level of consciousness, neurological checks and functional status as per facility protocol. If significant changes in patient condition occur, consider further diagnostic tests, such as plain film x-rays, CT scan of the head/spine/extremity, provide a neurological consultation and/or transfer to a specialty unit for further evaluation (standard of care).

(continued)

Protocol 19.1: Fall Prevention *(continued)*

VII. EVALUATED/EXPECTED OUTCOMES

A. Patients will
   1. Maintain their safety
   2. Avoid preventable falls
   3. Not develop serious injury from a fall if it occurs
   4. Know their risks of falling
   5. Be prepared on discharge to prevent falls in their homes
   6. Continue prehospitalization level of mobility
   7. (Those who develop fall-related complications, such as injury or change in cognitive functive will) be promptly assessed and treated appropriately should fall related complications, injury or cognitive decline occur.
   8. Be fully engaged as a partner in the fall-prevention plan of care

B. Nursing staff will
   1. Accurately detect, refer, and manage older adults at risk of falling or who have experienced a fall
   2. Integrate into their practice comprehensive assessment and management approaches for fall prevention in the institution
   3. Gain appreciation for older adults' unique experience of falling and how it influences their daily living and functional, physical, and emotional status
   4. Educate older adult patients anticipating discharge about fall-prevention strategies
   5. Collaborate and coordinate fall prevention as members of interprofessional teams

C. Family caregivers will
   1. Benefit from added knowledge about fall prevention to become sensitized and more aware of simple strategies to prevent falls
   2. Be fully engaged in patient safety efforts

D. Health care organizations will
   1. Realize reduced fall and injurious fall rates
   2. Realize the benefits of fall-prevention programs that minimize liability
   3. Support budgetary lines for fall-prevention interventions directed to patients and health care staff

VIII. FOLLOW-UP MONITORING OF CONDITION

A. Monitor fall incidence and incidences of patient injury caused by a fall, comparing overall fall rates, rates by type of fall, root causes of fall events, within and across units over time.

B. Compare falls, falls with injury, percent age of falls with major injury per quarter against national benchmarks available in the National Database of Nursing Quality Indicators.

C. Incorporate continuous quality-improvement criteria into fall-prevention program

D. Identify fall team members and roles of clinical and nonclinical staff (ECRI Institute, 2006)

E. Educate patient and family caregivers about fall-prevention strategies so they are prepared for discharge

IX. RELEVANT PRACTICE GUIDELINES

A. Panel on Prevention of Falls in Older Persons (2011)

B. American Medical Directors Association (2003)

C. University of Iowa Gerontological Nursing Interventions Research Center (UIGN; 2004)

D. ECRI Institute (2006)

ABBREVIATIONS

PFA Postfall assessment

PFH Postfall huddle

RESOURCES

Barker, A., Brand, C., Haines, T., Hill, T., Brauer, S., Jolley, D.,... Kamar, J. (2011). The 6-PACK programme to decrease fall-related injuries in hospitals: Protocol for a cluster randomised controlled trial. *Injury Prevention, 17*, e5. doi:10.1136/injuryprev-2011–040074

Centers for Disease Control Guidelines for Head Injury
www.cdc.gov/concussion/pdf/TBI_Clinicians_Factsheet-a.pdf

Evidence-Based Clinical Practice Guidelines for Falls Prevention
www.americangeriatrics.org/files/documents/health_care_pros/Falls.Guidelines.pdf

Falls Prevention Strategies in Healthcare Settings
www.ecri.org

Gray-Miceli, D. (2014). *Five easy steps to prevent falls: The comprehensive guide for nurses to keeping patients of all ages safe.* Silver Spring, MD: American Nurses Association Publishers. Retrieved from www.nursesbooks.org/Homepage/Hot-off-the-Press/5-Easy-Steps-To-Prevent-Falls.aspx

National Center for Patient Safety, Department of Veterans Affairs, Fall Toolkit, 2014
www.patientsafety.va.gov

National Center for Patient Safety Falls Toolkit. Retrieved from http://www.ihi.org/resources/Pages/OtherWebsites/National-CenterforPatientSafetyFallsToolkit.aspx

VISN 8 Patient Safety Center of Inquiry/Fall
www.patientsafety.gov/SafetyTopics/fallstoolkit/index.html

REFERENCES

Agency for Healthcare Research and Quality (AHRQ). (2013). *Making health care safer II.* Rockville, MD: Agency for Healthcare Research and Quality. Retrieved from http://www.ahrq.gov/research/findings/evidence-based-reports/ptsafetyuptp.html. *Evidence Level II.*

American Geriatrics Society/British Geriatrics Society (AGS/BGS). (2011). Clinical practice guideline for prevention of falls in older persons. *Journal of the American Geriatrics Society, 59*, 148–157. *Evidence Level I.*

American Medical Directors Association. (2003). *Falls and fall risk.* Columbia, MD: Author. *Evidence Level II.*

American Nurses Association (ANA). (1996a). *Nursing quality indicators: Definitions and implications* Washington, DC: American Nurses Publishing. Retrieved from www.nursingworld.org/books/pdescr.cfm?cnum=11#NP-108. *Evidence Level II.*

American Nurses Association (ANA). (1996b). *Nursing quality indicators: Guide for implementation.* Washington, DC: American Nurses Publishing. *Evidence Level II.*

Anderson, J. J., Mokracek, M., & Lindy, C. N. (2009). A nursing quality program driven by evidence-based practice. *Nursing Clinics of North America, 44*(1), 83–91. *Evidence Level VI.*

Annweiler, C., Schott, A. M., Berrut, G., Fantino, B., & Beauchet, O. (2009). Vitamin D-related changes in physical performance: A systematic review. *Journal of Nutrition, Health & Aging, 13*(10), 893–898. *Evidence Level II.*

Applegarth, S. P., Bulat, T., Wilkinson, S., Fitzgerald, S. G., Ahmed, S., & Quigley, P. (2009). Durability and residual moisture effects on the mechanical properties of external hip protectors. *Gerontechnology, 8*(1), 26–34. *Evidence Level IV.*

Batchelor, F., Hill, K., Mackintosh, S., & Said, C. (2010). What works in falls prevention after stroke? A systematic review and meta-analysis. *Stroke, 41*(8), 1715–1722. *Evidence Level I.*

Bentzen, H., Bergland, A., & Forsen, L. (2008). Risk for hip fractures in soft protected, hard protected, and unprotected falls. *Injury Prevention: Journal of the International Society for Child and Adolescent Injury Prevention, 14*(5), 306–310. *Evidence Level II.*

Blahak, C., Baezner, H., Pantoni, L., Poggesi, A., Chabriat, H., Erkinjuntti, T.,... LADIS Study Group. (2009). Deep frontal and periventricular age related white matter changes but not basal ganglia and infratentorial hyperintensities are associated with falls: Cross sectional results from the LADIS study. *Journal of Neurology, Neurosurgery, and Psychiatry, 80*(6), 608–613. *Evidence Level III.*

Borson, S., Scanlan, J. M., Chen, P., & Ganguli, M. (2003). The Mini-Cog as a screen for dementia: Validation in a population-based sample. *Journal of the American Geriatrics Society, 51*(10), 1451–1454. *Evidence Level II.*

Boushon, B., Nielsen, G., Quigley, P., Rita, S., Rutherford, P., Taylor, J.,... Rita, S. (2012). *Transforming care at the bedside how-to guide: Reducing patient injuries from falls.* Cambridge, MA: Institute for Healthcare Improvement. *Evidence Level VI.*

Boyle, N., Naganathan, V., & Cumming, R. G. (2010). Medication and falls: Risk and optimization. *Clinical Geriatric Medicine, 26*, 583–605. doi:10.1016/j.cger.2010.06.007. *Evidence Level VI.*

Brown, J. S., Vittinghoff, E., Wyman, J. F., Stone, K. L., Nevitt, K. E., & Grady, D. (2000). Urinary incontinence: Does it increase risk for falls and fractures? Study of osteoporotic fractures research group. *Journal of the American Geriatrics Society, 48*(7), 721–725. *Evidence Level IV.*

Bulat, T., Applegarth, S., Wilkinson, S., Fitzgerald, S., Ahmed, S., & Quigley, P. (2008). Effect of multiple I impacts on protective properties of hip protectors. Original research. *Clinical Interventions in Aging, 3*(3), 1–5. *Evidence Level IV.*

Bulat, T., Castle, S., Rutledge, M., & Quigley, P. (2008a). Special Article. Clinical practice algorithm: Medication management to reduce fall risk in the elderly. Part 2. Summary algorithm. *Journal of the American Academy of Nurse Practitioners, 20*(1), 1–4. *Evidence Level VI.*

Bulat, T., Castle, S., Rutledge, M., & Quigley, P. (2008b). Special Article. Clinical practice algorithm: Medication management to reduce fall risk in the elderly. Part 3. Benzodiazepines, cardiovascular agents, and antidepressants. *Journal of the American Academy of Nurse Practitioners, 20*(2), 55–62. *Evidence Level VI.*

Bulat, T., Castle, S., Rutledge, M., & Quigley, P. (2008c). Special Article. Clinical practice algorithm: Medication management to reduce fall risk in the elderly. Part 4. Anticoagulants, and others. *Journal of the American Academy of Nurse Practitioners, 20*(4), 181–190. *Evidence Level VI.*

Cameron, I. D., Gillespie, L. D., Robertson, M. C., Murray, G. R., Hill, K. D., Cumming, R. G., & Kerse, N. (2012). Interventions for preventing falls in older people in care facilities and hospitals. *Cochrane Database of Systematic Reviews, 12,* CD005465. doi: 10.1002/14651858.CD005465.pub3. *Evidence Level I.*

Capezuti, E., Maislin, G., Strumpf, N., & Evans, L. K. (2002). Side rail use and bed-related fall outcomes among nursing home residents. *Journal of the American Geriatrics Society, 50*(1), 90–96. *Evidence Level III.*

Centers for Disease Control and Prevention, National Center for Injury Prevention and Control. (2007). *Preventing falls among older adults.* Retrieved from http://www.cdc.gov/ncipc/duip/preventadultfalls.htm. *Evidence Level VI.*

Centers for Disease Control and Prevention. (2015a). *Get the stats on traumatic brain injury in the United States.* Retrieved from http://www.cdc.gov/traumaticbraininjury/pdf/BlueBook_factsheet-a.pdf. *Evidence Level VI.*

Centers for Disease Control and Prevention. (2015b). *TBI data and statisitics.* Retrieved http://www.cdc.gov/traumaticbraininjury/data/index.html. *Evidence Level VI.*

Centers for Disease Control and Prevention. (2015c). *Hip fractures among older adults.* Retrieved from http:www.cdc.gov/Home-andRecreationalSafety/Falls/adulthipfx.html. *Evidence Level VI.*

Chang, J. T., Morton, S. C., Rubsenstein, L. Z., Mojica, W. A., Maglione, M., Suttorp, M. J., . . . Shekelle, P. G. (2004). Interventions for the prevention of falls in older adults: Systematic review and meta-analysis of randomized controlled trial. *British Medical Journal, 328*(7441), 680. *Evidence Level I.*

Chassin, M. R., & Loeb, J. M. (2013). High-reliability health care: Getting there from here. *Millbank Quarterly,* 91(3), 459–490. *Evidence Level VI.*

Connell, B. R. (1996). Role of the environment in falls prevention. *Clinics in Geriatric Medicine, 12*(4), 859–880. *Evidence Level VI.*

Coronado, V. G., Thomas, K. E., Sattin, R. W., & Johnson, R. L. (2005). The CDC traumatic brain injury surveillance system: Characteristics of persons aged 65 and older hospitalized with a TBI. *Journal of Head Trauma Rehabilitation, 20,* 215–228. *Evidence Level IV.*

Corsinovi, L., Bo, M., Aimonino, N. R.., Marinello, R., Gariglio, F., Marchetto, C., . . . Molaschi, M. (2009). Predictors of falls and hospitalization outcomes in elderly patients admitted to an acute geriatric unit. *Archives of Gerontology and Geriatrics, 49*(1), 142–145. *Evidence Level III.*

Degelau, J., Belz, M., Bungum, L., Flavin, P. L., Harper, C., Leys, K., . . . Institute for Clinical Systems Improvement. (2012). *Prevention of falls (acute care). Health care protocol.* Bloomington, MN: Institute for Clinical Systems Improvement (ICSI). *Evidence Level IV.*

Dempsey, J. (2004). Falls prevention revisited. A call for a new approach. *Journal of Clinical Nursing, 13*(4), 479–485. *Evidence Level IV.*

Donaldson, N., Brown, D. S., Aydin, C. E., Bolton, M. L., & Rutledge, D. N. (2005). Leveraging nurse-related dashboard benchmarks to expedite performance improvement and document excellence. *Journal of Nursing Administration, 35*(4), 163–172. *Evidence Level VI.*

Dube, A. H., & Mitchell, E. K. (1986). Accidental strangulation from vest restraints. *Journal of the American Medical Association, 256*(19), 2725–2726. *Evidence Level VI.*

ECRI Institute. (2006). *Falls prevention strategies in healthcare settings.* Plymouth Meeting, PA: ECRI Publishers. *Evidence Level VI.*

Elkins, J., Williams, L., Spehar, A., Marano-Perez, J., Gulley, T., & Quigley, P. (2004). Successful redesign: Fall incident report—A safety initiative. *Federal Practitioner, 21*(3), 29–44. *Evidence Level VI.*

Ellis, A. A., & Trent, R. B. (2001). Hospitalized fall injuries and reace in California. *Injury Prevention, 7,* 316–320. *Evidence Level II.*

Ensrud, K. E., Blackwell, T. L., Mangione, C. M., Bowman, P. J., Whooley, M. A., Bauer, D. C., . . . Study of Osteoporotic Fractures Research Group. (2002). Central nervous system-active medications and risk for falls in older women. *Journal of the American Geriatrics Society, 50*(10), 1629–1637. *Evidence Level II.*

Feil, M., & Wallace, S. C. (2014). The use of patient sitters to reduce falls: Best practices. *Pennsylvania Patient Safety Advisory, 11*(1) (March), 8–14.

Folstein, M. F., Folstein, S. E., McHugh, P. R. (1975). "Mini-mental state." A practical method for grading the cognitive state of patients for the clinician. *Journal of Psychiatric Research, 12*(3), 189–198. doi:10.1016/0022-3956(75)90026-6.PMID 1202204

Ganz, D. A., Huang, C., Saliba, D., Shier, V., Berlowitz, D., Lukas, C. V., . . . (2013). *Preventing falls in hospitals: A toolkit for improving quality of care.* Rockville, MD: Agency for Healthcare Research and Quality. *Evidence Level VI.*

Garwood, C. L., & Corbett, T. L. (2008). Use of anticoagulation in elderly patients with atrial fibrillation who are at risk for falls. *Annals of Pharmacotherapy, 42*(4), 523–532. *Evidence Level I.*

Gates, S., Smith, L. A., Fisher, J. D., Lamb, S. E., & Phil, D. (2008). Systematic review of accuracy of screening instruments for predicting fall risk among independently living older adults. *Journal of Rehabilitation Research & Development, 45*(8), 1105–1116. *Evidence Level I.*

Gray-Miceli, D. (2014). *Five easy steps to prevent falls: The comprehensive guide for nurses to keeping patients of all ages safe.* Silver Spring, MD: American Nurses Association. Retrieved from http://www.nursesbooks.org/Homepage/Hot-off-the-Press/5-Easy-Steps-To-Prevent-Falls.aspx. *Evidence Level VI.*

Gray-Miceli, D., Johnson, J. C., & Strumpf, N. E. (2005). A step-wise approach to a comprehensive postfall assessment. *Annals of Long-Term Care: Clinical Care and Aging, 13*(12), 16–24. *Evidence Level VI.*

Gray-Miceli, D., Ratcliffe, S. J., & Johnson, J. C. (2010). Use of a postfall assessment tool to prevent falls. *Western Journal of Nursing Research, 32*(7), 932–948. *Evidence Level III.*

Gray-Miceli, D., Ratcliffe, S. J., & Thomasson, A. (2013). Ambulatory assisted living elderly fallers at greatest risk for head injury. *Journal of the American Geriatrics Society, 61*(10), 1817–1819. doi:10.1111/jgs.12467. *Evidence Level III.*

Gray-Miceli, D., Strumpf, N. E., Johnson, J. C., Draganescu, M., & Ratcliffe, S. J. (2006). Psychometric properties of the Post-Fall Index. *Clinical Nursing Research, 15*(3), 157–176. *Evidence Level III.*

Gray-Miceli, D., Strumpf, N. E., Reinhard, S. C., Zanna, M. T., & Fritz, E. (2004). Current approaches to postfall assessment in nursing homes. *Journal of the American Medical Directors Association, 5*(6), 16–24. *Evidence Level IV.*

He, J., Dunton, N., & Staggs, V. (2012). Unit-level time trends in inpatient fall rates of US hospitals. *Medical Care, 50*(9), 801–807. *Evidence Level II.*

Horgan, N. F., Crehan, F., Bartlet, E., Keogan, F., O'Grady, A. M., Moore, A. R.,... Curran, M. (2009). The effects of usual footwear on balance amongst elderly women attending a day hospital. *Age & Aging, 38*(1), 62–67. *Evidence Level III.*

Institute of Medicine. (2004). *Health literacy: A prescription to end confusion.* Retrieved from http://www.ama-assn.org. *Evidence Level VI.*

John A. Hartford Foundation Institute for Geriatric Nursing. (2003). Preventing falls in acute care. In M. Mezey, T. Fulmer, I. Abraham, & D. Zwicker (Eds.), *Geriatric nursing protocols for best practice* (2nd ed., pp. 141–164). New York, NY: Springer Publishing Company. *Evidence Level VI.*

Kamel, H. K. (2004). Secondary prevention of hip fractures among hospitalized elderly: Are we doing enough? *Internet Journal of Geriatrics and Gerontology, 1*(1), 1–5. Retrieved from http://www.ispub.com/ostia/index.php?xmlFilePath=journals/ijgg/vol1n1/hip.xml. *Evidence Level IV.*

Kaufman, J. M., Johnell, O., Abadie, E., Adami, S., Audran, M., Avouac, B.,... Reginster, J. Y. (2000). Background for studies on the treatment of male osteoporosis: State of the art. *Annals of the Rheumatic Diseases*, 59(10), 765–772. *Evidence Level I.*

Kelly, K. E., Phillips, C. L., Cain, K. C., Polissar, N. L., & Kelly, P. B. (2002). Evaluation of a non-intrusive monitor to reduce falls in nursing home patients. *Journal of the American Medical Directors Association, 3*(6), 377–382. *Evidence Level IV.*

Konstantinos, S., Cheng, J. D., Gestring, M., Sangosanya, A., Stassen, N. A., & Bankey, P. E. (2010). Ground level falls are associated with significant mortality in elderly patients. *Journal of Trauma: Injury, Infection, and Critical Care, 69*(4), 821. doi:10.1097/TA.0b013e3181efc6c6. *Evidence Level II.*

Kutney-Lee, A., Lake, E. T., & Aiken, L. H. (2009). Development of the hospital nurse surveillance capacity profile. *Research in Nursing & Health, 32*(2), 217–228. *Evidence Level IV.*

Kwok, T., Mok, F., Chien, W. T., & Tam, E. (2006). Does access to bed-chair pressure sensors reduce physical restraint use in the rehabilitation setting. *Journal of Clinical Nursing, 15*(5), 581–587. *Evidence Level II.*

Leipzig, R. M., Cumming, R. G., & Tinetti, M. E. (1999). Drugs and falls in older people: A systematic review and meta-analysis: II. Cardiac and analgesic drugs. *Journal of the American Geriatrics Society, 47*(1), 40–50. *Evidence Level I.*

Lord, S. R., Clark, R. D., & Webster, I. W. (1991). Postural stability and associated physiological factors in a population of aged persons. *Journal of Gerontology, 46*(3), M69–M76. *Evidence Level IV.*

Lord, S. R., Smith, S. T., & Menant, J. C. (2010). Vision and falls in older people: Risk factors and intervention strategies. *Clinical Geriatric Medicine, 26*, 569–581. doi:10.1016/cger.2010.06.002. *Evidence Level VI.*

Lourbopoulos, A., Erturk, A., & Hellal, F. (2015). Microglia in action: How aging and injury can change the brain's guardians. *Frontiers in Cellular Neuroscience, 9*, 54. doi:10.3389/fnel.2015.00054.PCMID:PMC4337366. *Evidence Level VI.*

McInnes, E., & Askie, L. (2004). Evidence review on older people's views and experiences of falls prevention strategies. *Worldviews on Evidence-Based Nursing, 1*(1), 20–37. *Evidence Level I.*

Meade, C., Bursell, M., & Ketelsen, L. (2006). Effects of nursing rounds on patients' call light use, satisfaction and safety. *American Journal of Nursing, 106*(9), 58–70. *Evidence Level III.*

Morse, J. M., Morse, R. M., Tylko, S. J. (2009). *Preventing patient falls: Establishing a fall intervention program* (2nd ed.). New York, NY: Springer Publishing Company. *Evidence Level VI.*

National Center for Patient Safety Falls Toolkit. (2014). Retrieved from http://www.ihi.org/resources/Pages/OtherWebsites/National-CenterforPatient-SafetyFall-sToolkit.aspx. *Evidence Level VI.*

National Council on Aging. (2012). *Fall prevention fact sheet.* Retrieved from http:www.ncoa.org/press-room/fact-sheets/falls-prevention-fact-sheet. *Evidence Level VI.*

National Hospital Discharge Survey. (2010). 2007 Summary, National Health Statistics Report. Retrieved from http//205.207.175.93/hdi/ReportFolders.aspx?IF_ActivePath=p.18. *Evidence Level II.*

National Osteoporosis Foundation. (2013). *Clinician's guide to prevention and treatment of osteoporosis.* Retrieved from www.nof.org/files/nof/public/content/file/344/upload/159.pdf. *Evidence Level VI.*

National Quality Forum. (2006). Serious reportable events in healthcare 2006 update. Washington, DC: National Quality Forum. *Evidence Level II.*

Nelson, A., Powell-Cope, G., Gavin-Dreschnack, D., Quigley, P., Bulat, T., Baptiste, A. S.,... Friedman, Y. (2004). Technology to promote safe mobility in the elderly. *Nursing Clinics of North America, 39*(3), 649–671. *Evidence Level VI.*

Neutel, C. I., Perry, S., & Maxwell, C. (2002). Medication use and risk of falls. *Pharmacoepidemiological and Drug Safety, 11*(2), 97–104. *Evidence Level VI.*

Nielsen-Bohlman, L., Panzer, A. M., & Kindig, D. A. (Eds.). (2004). Committee on Health Literacy. *Health literacy: A prescription to end confusion.* Washington, DC: National Academies Press. Retrieved from http://www.nap.edu/catalog/10883.html. *Evidence Level VI.*

Oliver, D., Connelly, J. B., Victor, C. R., Shaw, F. E., Whitehead, A., Genc, Y.,... Gosney, M. A. (2007). Strategies to prevent falls and fractures in hospitals and care homes and effect of cognitive impairment: Systematic review and meta-analysis. *British Medical Journal, 334*(7584), 53–54. *Evidence Level I.*

Oliver, D., Daly, F., Martin, F. C., McMurdo, M. E. (2004). Risk factors and risk assessment tools for falls in hospital inpatients: A systematic review. *Age and Ageing, 33*(2), 122–130. *Evidence Level I.*

Oliver, D., Healy, F., & Haines, T. P. (2010). Preventing falls and fall-related injuries in hospitals. *Clinics in Geriatric Medicine, 26*(4), 645–692. *Evidence Level I.*

Panel on Prevention of Falls in Older Persons. (2011). Summary of the updated American Geriatrics Society/British Geriatrics Society Clinical Practice Guideline for prevention of falls in older persons. *Journal of the American Geriatrics Society, 59,* 148–157. doi:10.1111/j.1532–5415.2010.03234.x. *Evidence Level I.*

Papaioannou, A., Parkinson, W., Cook, R., Ferko, N., Coker, E., & Adachi, J. D. (2004). Prediction of falls using a risk assessment tool in the acute care setting. *BMC Medicine, 21*(2), 1. *Evidence Level III.*

Parker, M. J., Gillespie, W. J., & Gillespie, L. D. (2006). Effectiveness of hip protectors for preventing hip fractures in elderly people. *British Medical Journal, 332*(7541), 571–574. *Evidence Level I.*

Paulus, W. M., Straube, A., & Brandt, T. (1984). Visual stabilization of pursure. Physiological stimulus characteristics and clinical aspects. *Brain, 107,* 1143–1163. *Evidence Level III.*

Perell, K., Nelson, A., Goldman, R., Luther, S. L., Prieto-Lewis, N., & Rubenstein, L. Z. (2001). Fall risk assessment measures: An analytic review. *Journal of Gerontology, 56*(12), 761–766. *Evidence Level V.*

Prevention of Falls Network Europe. (2006). Retrieved from http://www.profane.eu.org. *Evidence Level VI.*

Quigley, P., & Goff, L. (2011, March). Current and emerging innovations to keep patients safe. Technological innovations play a leading role in fall-prevention programs. Special Report: Best practices for fall reduction. A practice guide. *American Nurse Today*, 14–17. *Evidence Level VI.*

Quigley, P., Hahm, B., Collazo, S., Gibson, W., Janzen, S., Powell-Cope, G.,... White, S. V. (2009). Reducing serious injury from falls in two veterans' acute medical-surgical units. *Journal of Nursing Care Quality, 24*(1), 33–41. *Evidence Level III.*

Quigley, P., Neily, J., Watson, M., Wright, M., & Strobel, K. (2007). Measuring fall program outcomes. *Online Journal of Issues in Nursing, 12*(2). doi:10.3912/OJIN.Vol12No02PPT01. *Evidence Level VI.*

Quigley, P., & White, S. V. (2013). Hospital-based fall program measurement and improvement in high reliability organizations. *Online Journal of Issues in Nursing, 18*(2). Manuscript 5. doi:10.3912/OJIN.Vol18No02Man05. *Evidence Level VI.*

Ray, W. A., Taylor, J. A., Meador, K. G., Thapa, P. B., Brown, A. K., Kajihara, H. K.,... Griffin, M. R. (1997). A randomized trial of a consultation service to reduce falls in nursing homes. *Journal of the American Medical Association, 278,* 557–562. *Evidence Level II.*

Rubenstein, L. Z., & Josephson, K. R. (2002). The epidemiology of falls and syncope. *Clinics of Geriatric Medicine, 18*(2), 141–158. *Evidence Level VI.*

Rubenstein, L. Z., & Josephson, K. R. (2006). Falls and their prevention in the elderly: What does the evidence show? *Medical Clinics of North American, 90*(5), 807–824. *Evidence Level I.*

Rubenstein, L. Z., Robbins, A. S., Josephson, K. R., Schulman, B. L., & Osterweil, D. (1990). The value of assessing falls in an elderly population: A randomized clinical trial. *Annals of Internal Medicine, 113*(4), 308–316. *Evidence Level II.*

Shekelle, P. G., Wachter, R. M., Pronovost, P. J., Schoelles, K., McDonald, K. M., Dy, S. M.,... Winters, B. D. (2013). Making health care safer II: An updated critical analysis of the evidence for patient safety practices. Comparative effectiveness review No. 211. (Prepared by the Southern California-RAND Evidence-based Practice Center under Contract No. 290–2007-10062-I. AHRQ Publication No. 13-E001-EF). Rockville, MD: Agency for Healthcare Research and Quality. Retrieved from www.ahrq.gov/research/findings/evidence-based-reports/ptsafetyuptp.html. *Evidence Level II.*

Smith, R. G. (2003). Fall-contributing adverse effects of the most frequently prescribed drugs. *Journal of the American Podiatric Medical Association; 93*(1), 42–50. *Evidence Level VI.*

Smyth, C., Dubin, S., Restrepo, A., Nueva-Espana, H., & Capezuti, E. (2001). Creating order out of chaos: Models of GNP practice with hospitalized older adults. *Clinical Excellence for Nurse Practitioners, 5*(2), 88–95. *Evidence Level IV.*

Spoelstra, S. L., Given, B. A., & Given, C. W. (2012). Fall prevention in hospitals: An integrative review. *Clinical Nursing Research, 21*(1), 92–112. *Evidence Level I.*

Susman, M., DiRusso, S. M., Sullivan, T., Risucci, D., Nealon, P., Cuff, S.,... Benzil, D. (2002). Traumatic brain injury in the elderly: Increased mortality and worse functional outcome at discharge despite lower injury severity. *Journal of Trauma, Injury, Infection and Critical Care, 53*(2), 219–224. doi:10.1097/01TA.0000024249.40070.BD. *Evidence Level II.*

The Joint Commission. (2006). *National patient safety goals.* Retrieved from http://www.jointcommission.org. *Evidence Level VI.*

Thompson, H. J., McCormick, W. C., & Kagan, S. H. (2006). Traumatic brain injury in older adults: Epidemiology, outcomes, and future implications. *Journal of the American Geriatrics Society, 54*(10), 1590–1595. doi:10.1111/j.1532–5415.2006.00894.x. *Evidence Level I.*

Tinetti, M. E., Williams, T. S., & Mayewski, R. (1986). Fall risk index for elderly patients based on number of chronic disabilities. *American Journal of Medicine, 80*(3), 429–434. *Evidence Level II.*

University of Iowa Gerontological Nursing Interventions Research Center (UIGN). (2004). *Fall prevention for older adults.* Iowa City, IA: University of Iowa Gerontological Nursing Interventions Research Center, Research Dissemination Core. *Evidence Level VI.*

U.S. Department of Health and Human Services Centers for Medicare and Medicaid Services. (2004). *Evidence report and evidenced-based recommendations: Fall prevention interventions in the medicare population* (RAND Contract No. 500–98-0281). *Evidence Level I.*

U.S. Preventive Services Task Force. (2013). *Osteoporosis screening.* Retrieved from http://www.uspreventiveservicestaskforce.org/Page/Topic/recommendations. *Evidence Level I.*

Veterans Health Administration (VHA). (2012). *Falls toolkit.* Retrieved from http://www.patientsafety.va.gov/professionals/onthejob/falls.asp

Weisberg, L. A., Garcia, C., & Strub, R. (2002). Head trauma. *In Essentials of clinical neurology* (4th ed.). St. Louis, MO: Mosby. *Evidence Level VI.*

20

Reducing Adverse Drug Events

DeAnne Zwicker and Terry Fulmer

EDUCATIONAL OBJECTIVES

On completion of this chapter, the reader should be able to:

1. Identify persons at high risk of adverse drug events (ADEs)
2. Conduct a comprehensive medication assessment
3. Specify four medications or medication classes having a high potential for toxicity in older adults
4. Describe five reasons that older adults experience adverse drug events
5. Delineate strategies to prevent common medication-related problems in older adults

OVERVIEW

One in seven Medicare beneficiaries experienced an adverse event while being hospitalized in 2008. Between 2007 and 2009, almost 100,000 emergency hospitalizations in the United States were caused by ADEs in adults 65 years of age or older. That is, nearly half of those were aged 80 years and older (Budnitz, Lovegrove, Shehab, & Richards, 2011). This number is likely much higher as ADEs often go unreported with only 50% being reported in U.S. hospitals. ADEs increase the costs to patients, length of hospital stay, and mortality, yet often go unreported and nearly half are likely preventable (Levinson, 2010; Salvi et al., 2012). Older adults are the largest consumers of prescription and over-the-counter (OTC) medications and the most at risk of ADEs (Hamilton, Gallagher, Ryan, Byrne, & Mahony, 2011; Qato et al., 2008; Sansgiry, Nadkarni, & Doan, 2011).

BACKGROUND AND STATEMENT OF PROBLEM

Adverse Drug Event

An ADE is "an untoward medical occurrence that may appear during treatment with a pharmaceutical product but which does not necessarily have a causal relationship with the treatment" (World Health Organization [WHO], 2002, p. 5). An ADE may occur during normal use of medication, inappropriate use, inappropriate or suboptimum prescribing, poor adherence, self-medication, or harm resuting from a medication error. An adverse drug reaction (ADR) is harm directly caused by a drug at normal doses (Nebeker et al., 2004; Table 20.1). Most ADRs are not ADEs. For example, if a patient experiences an expected ADR, as in the case of hypokalemia secondary to furosemide therapy, this would not be an ADE unless it is not identified as a clinically significant event. Likewise, medication errors are common but most do not result in actual patient harm. The use of prescription drugs has increased significantly over the past 25 years with a 90% increase and a consequent increase in ADEs reported to the Food and Drug Administration (FDA; National Center for Health Statistics [NCHS], 2012). Between 2004 and 2008, there was a 52% increase in the number of ADEs reported in U.S. hospitals (Lucado, Paez, & Elixhauser, 2008). Older adults are the greatest consumers of medications with on

---

For a description of evidence levels cited in this chapter, see Chapter 1, "Developing and Evaluating Clinical Practice Guidelines: A Systematic Approach."

TABLE 20.1
Summary of Definitions Relevant to Drug-Related Harm

Term	Definition	Example
Harm occurred		
Adverse event	Harm in a patient administered a drug but not necessarily caused by a drug	Traumatic death while taking lovastatin
Adverse drug reaction	Harm directly caused by a drug at normal doses *Unexpected adverse drug reaction:* *An adverse drug event whose nature or severity is not consistent with the product information*	Congestive heart failure from metoprolol
Adverse drug event	Harm caused by the use of drug *Effective definition in common practice:* *Harm caused by a drug or the inappropriate use of a drug*	Hematoma from tirofiban overdose
Harm may have occurred		
Medication error	Inappropriate use of a drug that may or may not result in harm	Failure to renew prednisone order on transfer to medical ward
Side effect	A usually predictable or dose-dependent effect of a drug that is not the principal effect for which the drug was chosen; the side effect may be desirable, undesirable, or inconsequential	(This term should be avoided when considering adverse events.)
Harm did not occur		
Potential adverse drug event	Circumstances that *could* result in harm by the use of a drug but *did* not harm the patient	Receipt of roommate's felodipine but no resulting hypotension

Source: Courtesy of John W. Devlin, PharmaD, Northeastern University (personal communication, March 2015).

average, older Americans taking three OTC medications and up to six or more prescription medications (Petrovic, van der Cammen, & Onder, 2012). Among older adults, up to 30% of all hospital admissions are secondary to an ADE—more than half could have been prevented (Figueiras, Herdeiro, Polónia, & Gestal-Otero, 2006; Steinman & Hanlon, 2010). Intrinsic factors, such as advanced age, frailty, and polypharmacy, place older adults at greater risk of adverse outcomes (Buck et al., 2009). Older adults are at high risk of further ADEs while in the hospital and often experience ADEs after discharge (Kanaan et al., 2013; Lucado et al., 2008; Salvi et al., 2012).

Persons older than 65 years experience medication-related events for five major reasons: (a) alteration in pharmacokinetics; a reduced ability to metabolize and excrete medications and pharmacodynamics, what the drug does in binding at the receptors (Ruscin & Linnebur, 2014; Steinman & Holmes, 2014); (b) polypharmacy, indicating multiple meds prescribed, which are often prescribed by multiple providers (Rogers et al., 2009); (c) therapeutic failures, for example, over or under therapeutic dosage (Marcum, Driessen, Thorpe, Gellad, & Donohue, 2014); (d) iatrogenic causes such as ADRs or inappropriate prescribing (Davies et al., 2009); medication errors (Hayes, Klein-Schwartz, & Gonzales, 2009); and using medication for treatment of symptoms that are not disease dependent or specific such as self-medication or prescribing cascades (Rochon, 2014; Rochon & Gurwitz, 1997); and (e) medication adherence (Steinman & Hanlon, 2010). Most ADRs are not ADEs. If a patient experiences an expected ADR (e.g., hypokalemia secondary to furosemide therapy), based on package insert information, this would not be an ADE unless it was not identified and a clinically significant event (e.g., cardiac arrest) occurred. Also, although medication errors are common, most do not result in actual patient harm.

Common OTC medications, such as aspirin and acetaminophen, often interact with prescription medications (Qato et al., 2008). Older adults often combine OTCs with prescription medications or herbal remedies yet do not report their use to health care providers. Likewise, providers often do not inquire about OTCs or herbal remedies. Underreporting may lead to ADEs, including unrecognized adverse drug–disease or drug–drug interactions (Lopez-Gonzalez, Herdeiro, & Figueiras, 2009). Patient safety in medication management is a major focus in older adults; however, current information on concurrent use of prescription medications, OTC medications, and dietary supplements is limited (Qato et al., 2008).

Iatrogenic Causes of ADE

The term *iatrogenic* may be defined as an ADR or complication induced by a nondrug medical intervention (Atiqi, van Bommel, Cleophas, & Zwinderman, 2010). An iatrogenic ADE is disease induced by a drug prescribed by a medical provider (WHO, 2002). An iatrogenic medication event is one that is preventable, such as the wrong dose of a medication given that resulted in an adverse outcome. ADRs, inappropriate prescribing of high-risk medications, and medication errors are all considered iatrogenic. An ADR is any noxious or unintended and undesired effect of a drug that occurs at normal human doses for prophylaxis, diagnosis, or therapy. Inappropriate prescribing of high-risk medication to older adults and medication errors are all considered iatrogenic (WHO, 1972).

Risk factors of iatrogenic complications in older adults include drug-induced iatrogenic disease, multiple medications and conditions, multiple physicians, hospitalizations, and medical or surgical procedures (Davies et al., 2009). Onder, van der Cammen, Petrovic, Somers, and Rajkumar (2013) developed and evaluated an ADR risk score based on prior evidence. The researchers reported that the number of drugs and history of a previous ADR were the strongest predictors of ADRs, followed by heart failure, liver disease, the presence of greater than or equal to four conditions, and renal failure. They determined that a GerontoNet ADR risk score of four out of 10 showed a good balance between specificity and sensitivity. In a sample of 513 acutely ill patients aged greater than or equal to 65 years, the GerontoNet ADR risk score missed almost 40% of those at risk of ADRs, although more research is needed to identify further risk factors (Onder et al., 2013). So far, this is the only tool available to determine potential ADR risk. Frail older adults with multiple medical problems, memory issues, and multiple prescribed and nonprescribed (OTC and herbal) medications are at highest risk of ADRs (Rochon, 2014).

Adverse Drug Reactions

It is important to differentiate an ADR from an ADE (Figure 20.1). An ADE may be an event caused by a number of different adverse outcomes and may be related to normal or inappropriate use of medications, suboptimum prescribing, poor adherence, self-medication, or harm resulting from a medication error (WHO, 2002). The WHO defines an ADR as "a response to a drug which is noxious and unintended, and which occurs at doses normally used in man for the prophylaxis, diagnosis, or therapy of disease, or for the modifications of physiological function" (p. 5). Thus, an ADR is attributable only to a drug, whereas an ADE includes many different types of adverse outcomes rather than just a drug reaction.

ADRs are the result of some action of a drug and may be classified as dose related (digoxin > 0.125 mg), nondose related (hypersensitivity), dose related and time related

FIGURE 20.1

Relationship between ADEs and ADRs.

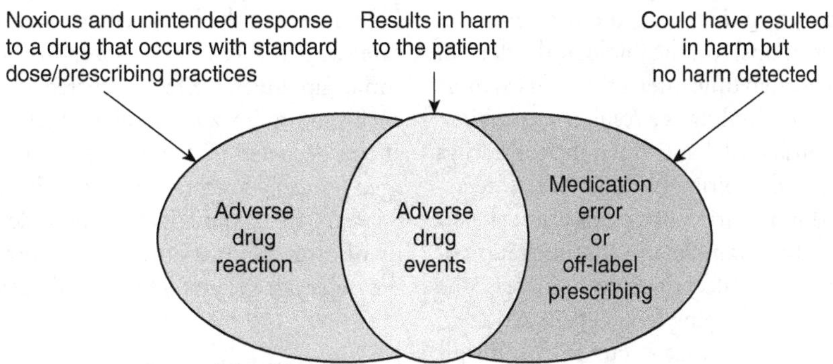

ADEs, adverse drug events; ADRs, adverse drug reactions.
Source: Nebeker et al. (2004).

(cumulative dose), time related, unexpected therapy failure, or the result of drug withdrawal (Salvi et al., 2012). In a systematic review, Kongkaew, Noyce, and Ashcroft (2008) reported a 10.7% prevalence rate of hospital admissions caused by ADRs in older adults; however, a confounding factor in the accuracy is that different methods and studies were employed to gather the data (Alomar, 2014). ADRs may occur because of drug interactions, duplication, additive effects, discontinuation of therapy, skipping medication, changing dose to costs, and physiologic antagonism (Alomar, 2014). Polypharmacy can also make it difficult for older adults to keep track of their multiple medications, particularly with added instructions such as taking meds with food, after meals, or at bedtime. Chronic side effects, such as fatigue, constipation, rashes, falls, and anxiety, can also lead to skipping medications. Finally, many process-related issues, such as lack of thorough medical reconciliation at each step of transition through the health care system, lead to error.

Frail older adults with multiple chronic medical problems requiring multiple medications are at high risk for ADRs (Hubbard, O'Mahony, & Woodhouse, 2013). Drug–drug and drug–disease interactions are the most common ADRs. Causes of drug interactions are multifaceted and include drug dosage, serum drug level, administration route, drug metabolism, therapy durations, and patient factors (Heuberger, 2012). Gray and Gardner (2009) reported that polypharmacy and multiple prescribers tend to be key factors in adverse reactions. Debate continues as to whether advancing age causes an increased ADR risk or if it is a marker for comorbid illness, change in pharmacokinetics, and polypharmacy. Many studies have shown that the key risk factors of adverse reactions are related to polypharmacy, multiple providers, and inappropriate use of medications (Gray & Gardner, 2009).

In hospitals, medications that are commonly associated with ADRs include diuretics, antihypertensives, anticoagulants, and antineoplastics. Drug–drug interactions occur when one therapeutic agent either alters the concentration (pharmacokinetic interactions) or the biological effect of another agent, a pharmacodynamic interaction. An example of drug–drug interaction is bleeding as a result of a combination of warfarin and nonsteroidal anti-inflammatory drugs (NSAIDs) or warfarin and aspirin. Drug–disease interactions occur when the administration of a medication alters a preexisting disease state. For example, the administration of aspirin to a patient with peptic ulcer disease will increase the risk for gastrointestinal (GI) bleeding (Salvi et al., 2012).

More than 80% of ADRs that occur in the hospital or cause admission are dose related, and therefore are predictable and potentially avoidable (Atiqi et al., 2010). Marcum et al. (2012) reported that inappropriate medications and therapeutic failures (a failure to accomplish treatment goals because of inadequate or inappropriate drug therapy) as well as adverse drug-withdrawal events (symptoms or signs related to removal of a drug) have not been studied as much as ADRs and often are a cause of hospitalizations (Z. A. Marcum et al., 2012).

Medication Errors

There is no international definition for *medication errors*; however, the most commonly used definition by the National Coordinating Council for Medication Error Reporting and Prevention (2015, p. 4) is "any preventable event that may cause or lead to inappropriate medication use or patient harm while the medication is in the control of the health care professional, patient, or consumer. Such events may be related to professional practice, health care products, procedures, and systems, including prescribing, order communication, product labeling, packaging, and nomenclature, compounding, dispensing, distribution, administration, education, monitoring, and use."

A large percentage of errors is caused by administration of the wrong medication or the correct medication with the wrong dose or at the wrong time interval between dosing. A medication error may be the result of negligence or prescribing errors. A reduction of these types of prescribing errors has been a high priority for health care policy in order to improve the safety profile of the health care delivery system (Aspden, Institute of Medicine [IOM], & Committee on Identifying and Preventing Medication, 2007).

In a retrospective review of 140,786 older adults, 49,320 experienced therapeutic errors resulting in adverse medical outcomes (Hayes et al., 2009). One example of therapeutic error may be taking twice the dose of prescribed medication, for example, which may or may not result in an adverse outcome. The majority of patients reporting ADEs (82%) were in the home environment or other non–health care facility (HCF). In those with a known adverse outcome, no adverse effect occurred in 62.9%, minor effects occurred in 25.2%, moderate effects in 10.7%, major effects occurred in 1.0%, and death in 0.2%. Older adults aged 65 to 74 years constituted 45% of major effects, 75 to 84 years 40%, and 85 years and older 14.5% of the majority of cases. Serious outcomes occurred more frequently in the older age groups (Hayes et al., 2009).

Medication Adherence

Costs of nonadherence are estimated at $100 billion annually (Ho, Bryson, & Rumsfeld, 2009). *Medication adherence* (or compliance) with a medication regimen is defined as "the extent to which a person's medication-taking behavior corresponds with agreed recommendations of a health care provider" (WHO, 2003, p. 3). A study by Marcumet al. (2014) revealed that older adults were nonadherent to treatment with chronic medications, such as 26% not taking calcium channel blockers. Those who used multiple pharmacies were more likely to be nonadherent to medications. There was no difference when demographics, health status, or access to care were considered. In a study providing elimination of copays for medications prescribed after a myocardial infarction, those with the usual coverage had an adherence rate from 35% to 49%; the full-coverage group was four to six points higher (Choudhry et al., 2011).

In a study of 7,108 patients enrolled in a pharmacy assistance program evaluating medication adherence, 40% to 50% adhered to their chronic medications with 80% of those patients reporting no income (Roberts et al., 2014). Older age and adherence to antihypertensive and statins (alone and combined) were significant predictors of adherence to medications. In patient admissions were much higher for the nonadherence population. Those who spoke English and those who took antihypertensives and oral hypoglycemic medication also had lower admission rates (Roberts et al., 2014).

Gellad, Grenard, and Marcum (2011) found the following barriers to medication adherence: health literacy, lack of knowledge of chronic disease, cognitive function, and adverse effects of drugs and polypharmacy; although they report there is a paucity of evidence on medication adherence in the literature and a need for using standardized measurements in research. Fried, Tinetti, Towle, Leary, and Iannone (2011) revealed that the presence of ADEs influenced the patient's decision whether to take a medication or not. Patients are often reluctant to admit nonadherence; however, pill counts and refill history can aid in determining this issue (Gearing, Townsend, Elkins, El-Bassel, & Osterberg, 2014; Steinman & Hanlon, 2010). Acute care nurses are ideally positioned to educate older adults and aid in evaluating reasons for nonadherence in hospitalized older adults.

EVALUATION OF THE PROBLEM

Assessment Tools

Geriatric assessment tools are used to evaluate an older adult's ability to self-administer medications, including physical and cognitive functional capacity (see Chapter 7, "Assessment of Physical Function" and Chapter 14, "Preventing Functional Decline in the Acute Care Setting;" review of the medication list for potentially inappropriate medications (PIMs; Campanelli, 2012), medications that are indicated but underused; medication reconciliation (MR), evaluation for potential drug–drug or drug–disease interactions; assessment of renal function; and encouraging the brown-bag method to augment reconciliation. Each of these methods should be patient/family centered and include collaboration with interprofessional team members. Common assessment tools include the following:

- **Beers Criteria**: American Geriatrics Society Beers Criteria for Potentially Inappropriate Medication Use in Older Adults (Campanelli, 2012)—This is used to assess the medication list for medications that should generally be avoided in older adults.
- **STOPP Criteria**: Screening Tool of Older Persons' Prescriptions—This tool identifies potentially inappropriate medications; identifies many more than the Beers Criteria and has identified greater number of older adults requiring hospitalization because of ADEs (Gallagher, O'Connor, & O'Mahony, 2011).
- **START Criteria:** Screening Tools to Alert Doctors to the Right Treatment—This is an evidence-based screening tool used to detect potential prescription omissions; recommends important medications for specific chronic conditions that are often omitted. This is intended to be used simultaneously with STOPP Criteria (Gallagher et al., 2011).
- **Drug–Drug Interactions:** Table 20.2 provides a list of *some* common medications known to interact with other medications. This is done using a computer order-entry program (COE) and computer decision support that includes drug–drug interaction alerts (Clyne, Bradley, Hughes, Fahey, & Lapane, 2012).
- **Cockroft–Gault Formula**—This is useful for estimating creatinine clearance based on age, weight, and serum creatinine levels (Terrell, Heard, & Miller, 2006). A creatinine clearance of less than 50 mL/min places older adults at risk of ADEs (Fouts, Hanlon, & Pieper, 1997) and virtually all people older than 70 years have a creatinine clearance of less than 50. An important point to note is that for older adults, particularly those of lower weight, this formula may estimate a creatinine clearance that is far higher than the actual glomerular filtration rate (GFR; Table 20.3).
- **Brown-Bag Method** (Nathan, Goodyer, Lovejoy, & Rashid, 1999)—This method is used to assess all medications an older adult has at home, including prescriptions from all providers, OTCs, and herbal remedies. All medications at home are placed in a bag and brought to hospital/other care setting. This should be used in conjunction with a complete medication history.

TABLE 20.2
Common Drug–Drug Interactions

Drug 1	Drug 2	Interaction	Effects
Warfarin	Diltiazem	Inhibits drug	↑ Anticoagulation
Warfarin	Verapamil	Metabolism	Potential bleeding
Warfarin	Metronidazole	Metabolism	Potential bleeding
Warfarin	NSAID	NSAID ↓ prostaglandins Increases GI erosion ↓ Platelet aggregation	GI bleeding
Warfarin	ASA	Same as NSAID	GI bleeding
Warfarin	Sulfa drugs	Unknown	↑ Warfarin effects
Warfarin	Acetaminophen—opiate combination Fluconazole Cipro Biaxin	↑ INR	Bleeding
Digoxin	Amiodorone	↓ Renal/nonrenal clearance of digoxin	Digoxin toxicity
Digoxin	Clarithromycin	↓ Renal clearance of digoxin	Digoxin toxicity
Digoxin toxicity	Verapamil	↓ Impulse conduction and muscle contraction	Potential bradycardia or heart block
Levothyroxine	Calcium carbonate	L-thyroxine (T_4) absorbs calcium carbonate	ACEIs absorption of L-thyroxine (T_4)
Glyburide	Co-trimoxazole	Potentiates effect of sulfonylureas	Hypoglycemia
ACEIs	Potassium sparing diuretics	Unknown	Life-threatening hyperkalemia
Diuretics	NSAIDs	ACEIs renal perfusion	Renal impairment
Phenytoin (Dilantin)	Cimetidine Erythromycin Fluconazole	Not specified	Increases levels of phenytoin within 1 week
Theophylline	Quinolones	↓ Liver metabolism of Theophylline	Theophylline toxicity
Acetylcholinesterase Inhibitor	Anticholinergics	↓ Ability to augment acetylcholine level	Therapy less effective

ACEIs, angiotensin-converting enzyme inhibitors; ASA, acetylsalicylic acid or aspirin; GI, gastrointestinal; INR, international normalized ratio; NSAIDs, nonsteroidal anti-inflammatory drugs.

Adapted from Ament, Bertolino, and Liszewski (2000); Cusak and Vestal (2000); Feldstein et al. (2006); Salvi et al. (2012).

TABLE 20.3
Cockroft–Gault Formula for Estimation of Creatinine Clearance (CrCl)

Formula for men:

$$\text{CrCl in milliliters per minute}^{a} = \frac{(140 - \text{age in years})\ (\text{weight in kilograms})}{72(\text{serum creatinine in milligrams per deciliter})}$$

Formula for women: Use formula for men and multiply by 0.85

[a]A creatinine clearance of less than 50 mL/min places older adults at risk of ADEs and virtually all people older than 70 years have a creatinine clearance of less than 50.

ADEs, adverse drug events.

Source: Fouts et al. (1997).

- **Drugs Regimen Unassisted Grading Scale (DRUGS) Tool**—This is a standardized method for assessing potential medication adherence problems. This requires a higher level of patient functioning, used at transfer to other levels of care (Edelberg, Shallenberger, & Wei, 1999; Hutchison, Jones, West, & Wei, 2006).
- **InterMed-Rx computer software**—This is new software that identifies cytochrome p-450 drug interactions. The cytochrome p-450 enzyme system is where drug–drug interactions often occur. It was evaluated in 100 patients with polypharmacy older than 82 years with a mean of 12 drugs prescribed. The software identified at least one drug–drug interaction and enabled the patients to have immediate pharmacist intervention, and 56% required further follow-up and medication adjustment. This software may aid in early identification of persons at risk of ADRs (Zakrzewski-Jakubiak et al., 2011).

ASSESSMENT STRATEGIES

Changes With Aging in Pharmacotherapy

Nurses and team members must first be aware of aging changes in pharmacokinetics and pharmacodynamics when assessing medications in older adults (Steinman & Holmes, 2014). New research is directed at pharmacogenetics and pharmacogenomics and has some application to ADRs. Interindividual variations of these genes may account for the differences observed in drug efficacy and the appearance of ADRs in elderly people (Cardelli, Marchegiani, Corsonello, Lattanzio, & Provinciali, 2012). The following describes aging changes.

- *Pharmacokinetics* is best defined as the time course of absorption, distribution across compartments, metabolism, and excretion of drugs in the body. As the body ages, the metabolism and excretion of many drugs declines and physiological changes require dosage adjustment for some drugs. The vast majority of drugs are cleared either through liver clearance or renal clearance (Steinman & Holmes, 2014).
- Changes in drug *absorption* (e.g., increased gastric pH and decreased GI motility in an absorptive surface) or underlying disease states such as diabetes. Older adult patients taking acid-suppressive agents, such as a proton pump inhibitors (e.g., Prilosec or Pepcid) or digoxin, may have decreased absorption (Steinman & Holmes, 2014).
- Drug *distribution* changes include decreased cardiac output, reduced total body water, decreased serum albumin (which is more likely to be related to malnutrition or acute illness than aging), and increased body fat. Changes in tissue or plasma binding can change the apparent volume of distribution (Vd) determined from plasma concentration measurements. Older people have a relative decrease in skeletal muscle mass and tend to have a smaller Vd, such as Vd of digoxin, which binds to muscle proteins. Reduced total body water creates a potential for higher serum drug levels because of a low Vd and occurs with water-soluble drugs (hydrophilic) such as alcohol or lithium. Decreased serum albumin results in higher unbound drug levels with protein-bound drugs, such as warfarin, phenytoin, digoxin, and theophylline. Drugs that distribute in fat (e.g., diazepam) may thus have a larger Vd. These lipophilic drugs (e.g., long-acting benzodiazepines [BZDs]) are stored in the body fat and slowly leech out, resulting in increased half-life and the drug staying around longer (Salvi et al., 2012; Steinman & Holmes, 2014).
- A significant change in *drug metabolism* is a reduction in the cytochrome p-450 system, which affects metabolism of many drugs cleared by this enzyme system. Drug metabolism includes the processes of absorption, distribution, metabolism, and elimination. These processes may change with aging; however, they are typically more influenced by genetic factors and by an individual's diseases, environment, and other medications (Steinman & Holmes, 2014). Many classes of drugs are cleared by the cytochrome p-450 enzyme system, including cardiovascular drugs, analgesics, NSAIDs, antibiotics, diuretics, psychoactive drugs, and others. Drugs, such as beta blockers, that go through the first-pass effect in the liver may be effective in lower doses in older adults (Steinman & Holmes, 2014). Drug metabolism may also be affected by alcohol abuse. Alcohol is metabolized and cleared slower in older adults thus stays around longer increasing the ADE risk. Metabolism may be affected by disease states common in older individuals (e.g., thyroid disease, congestive heart failure [CHF], and cancer) or drug-induced metabolic changes. Several drugs are cleared by multistage hepatic metabolism, which is more likely to be prolonged in older persons. Some drugs undergo hepatic metabolism and then renal clearance. BZDs have enormously longer half-lives in older adults because both systems are impaired, particularly with diazepam, clonezapam, and temazepam.
- *Elimination* or *renal clearance* of medications from the body may be slowed because of decline in GFR, renal tubular secretion, and renal blood flow that naturally

decreases with age (Steinman & Holmes, 2014). A decrease in clearance prolongs drug half-life and leads to increased plasma concentrations. A decrease in glomerular filtration is usually not accompanied by an increase in serum creatinine because of decreasing lean muscle mass with aging and a subsequent decline in creatinine production. Lack of dosage adjustment for renal insufficiency is a common reason for ADEs. Changes in renal function have the greatest impact on pharmacokinetics (Steinman & Holmes, 2014). Therefore, serum creatinine is not an accurate measure of renal function in the older adult. Instead, assessment of renal function using the Cockroft–Gault formula (see Table 20.3) should be made before initiation of renal clearing medications. Another instrument is the Modification of Diet in Renal Disease (MDRD) formula. This may be a more accurate reflection of renal function compared with the Cockroft–Gault equation; however, both are an estimate (Steinman & Holmes, 2014).

- *Pharmacodynamic* problems occur when two drugs act at the same or interrelated receptor sites, resulting in additive, synergistic (toxicity is greater than the sum of either agent used alone), or antagonistic effects (opposite effects). Many interactions of drugs are multifactorial, with a sequence of events that are both pharmacokinetic and pharmacodynamics (see Figure 20.2) (Steinman & Holmes, 2014).

Beers Criteria

The most recent Beers Criteria (Campanelli, 2012) were developed by experts in geriatrics and pharmacotherapy with a higher level of rigor using the IOM standards. The rigorous review includes the rating of quality and strength of the evidence. Medications included in this list should be avoided in older adults because of toxic effects; for example, avoidance of anticholinergic drugs or avoiding digoxin dosing greater than 0.125 mg. Other recommendations for specific problems, such as reducing doses for patients with a decline in kidney function or the potential of adverse effects from specific high-risk medications (BZD associated with falls). Avoiding PIMs is a very simple method to reduce inappropriate medications and thus ADEs in older adults.

Education and quality measures have been developed to inform and encourage all interprofessional providers to focus on PIMs to reduce the number of medications (Pugh et al., 2013). Although these criteria have been recommended as a standard by many regulatory and quality-improvement bodies for many years, PIMs

FIGURE 20.2

Multifactorial interactions leading to adverse drug events.

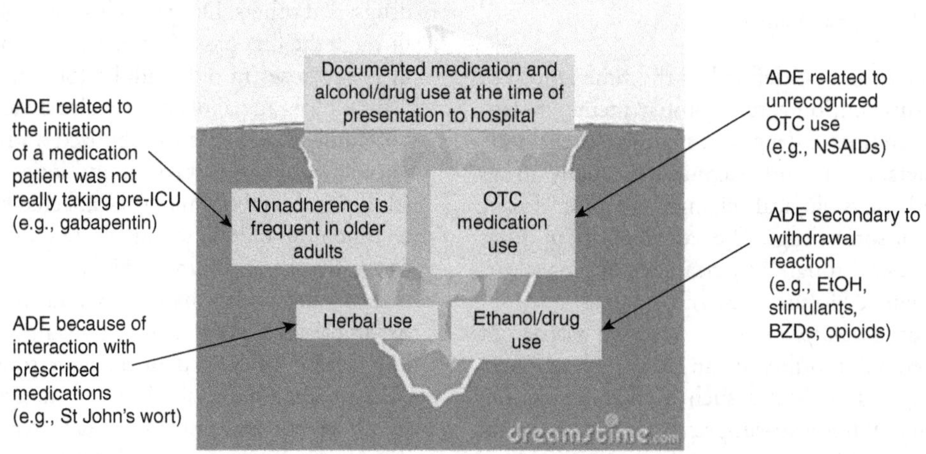

ADE, adverse drug event; BZDs, benxodiazepines; ICU, intensive care unit; NSAIDs, nonsteroidal anti-inflammatory drugs; OTC, over the counter.

Courtesy of John W. Devlin, PharmaD, Northeastern University (personal communication, March 2015).

continue to be prescribed in older adults. All members of the interprofessional team can aid in ensuring that PIMs are avoided.

STOPP and START Criteria

Like the Beers Criteria, the STOPP criteria are intended to identify potentially inappropriate prescriptions (PIPs vs. PIMs). These criteria include several more medications than the Beers Criteria. The prevalence of inappropriate medications in hospitalized older adults using these criteria was determined to be 77% (Lang et al., 2012). The START criteria identify omissions of medications that should be prescribed in hospitalized adults. According to the START criteria, 41.9% to 66% of hospitalized older adults experienced either undertreatment or omission of an appropriate medication (Lang et al., 2012). In a recent randomized controlled trial (RCT), the STOPP and START criteria were employed to identify PIPs and potentially omitted prescriptions (POPs) as determined by a pharmacist who made recommendations based on the criteria. Researchers reported a significant decrease in PIPs and POPs in the intervention group but not in the control group at the 6- to 12-month follow-up. The intervention group also showed a decline in falls (Frankenthal, Lerman, & Kalendaryev, 2014). This study indicates that pharmacist–physician collaboration in using the STOPP and START criteria in older adults may aid in decreasing ADEs.

Adverse Drug Reactions

ADRs are defined as any drug response that is noxious, unintended, and occurs at doses normally used for prophylaxis, diagnosis, or therapy of a disease (WHO, 2002). ADRs in older adults often go unidentified because of their atypical presentation in older adults or because the conventional symptoms of disease seen in younger persons are not evident (Steinman & Holmes, 2014) such as no pain with an acute abdomen. These changes are often a prodrome (symptom(s) indicative of an approaching disease) of an acute illness, especially in frail older adults. These symptoms may include a change in functional capacity, falls, vague cognitive changes, changes in behavior, decrease in appetite or anorexia, or new-onset incontinence (Steinman & Holmes, 2014). It is essential to take patients', families', and nonprofessional care providers' reports of subtle symptoms seriously so that they are not missed. Timely identification of acute illness with vague presentation enables early treatment of illness resulting in reduced morbidity and mortality and an enhanced quality of life in older adults. Atypical presentation makes ADRs difficult to accurately identify, thus nurses must be aware that ADRs may present atypically. One strategy for improving recognition of ADRs is to identify risk factors associated with ADRs. The most common risk factors include the following: increasing age (85 years or older), multiple medical conditions, polypharmacy or multiple medications, and physical or cognitive or functional impairment (Steinman & Holmes, 2014; Table 20.4).

Polypharmacy is common in older adults with multiple chronic conditions and multiple prescribed medications. The number of medications prescribed to older adults can be up to three OTC medications and up to six or more prescription medications (Petrovic et al., 2012). Research has shown that polypharmacy positively correlates with an increased risk for ADRs, such as drug–drug and drug–disease interactions, and increased risk for nonadherence to taking prescribed medications. Therefore, providers should perform regular reviews for unnecessary medications and consider whether any medication may be discontinued.

When a new symptom develops in a person taking multiple medications, it must always be considered to be an ADE first, particularly in the frail hospitalized patient. Providers should evaluate the relationship between the new symptom and the most recent medication given to identify the potential cause. Inappropriate treatment of a new symptom may result in a prescribing cascade of multiple drug treatment (see Figure 20.3) and possibly an ADR (Petrovic et al., 2012). In a systematic review conducted by Christensen and Lundh (2013), a medication review reduced emergency department visits in older adults. Although more research is needed on the efficacy of medication review, the authors suggest the review should be a part of regular geriatric care.

OTC Medications

Self-medication with OTC medications, herbal remedies, and dietary supplements may lead to adverse drug–drug or drug–disease interactions (Rochon, 2014; Tachjian, Maria, & Jahangir, 2010). Older adults are the largest consumer of OTC medications and dietary supplements. The seven top purchased herbal medicines include St. John's wort, ginseng, gingko biloba, echinacea, saw palmetto, and kava, all of which can interact with OTCs and prescription medications, warfarin being the drug that most commonly interacts with herbals and OTCs (Izzo & Ernst, 2009). In the United States, community-dwelling older adults take about as many OTC drugs as prescription drugs. In a study

TABLE 20.4

Risk Factors for Potential Adverse Drug Reaction in Older Adults

Medication-related factors	Patient characteristics
Class of medication	Polypharmacy
Anticoagulants and antiplatelets	Dementia/memory problems
Cardiovascular meds	Multiple chronic medical problems (> 4–6)
Hypoglycemics (oral and insulin)	Reduced homeostatic mechanisms
Benzodiazepines	Reduced lean body mass
Antipsychotics	Renal insufficiency (CrCl < 50 mL/min)
CNS agents/sedative/hypnotics	Recent hospitalization
Psychotropics	Advanced age (85 years of age)
Anticholinergics	Frailty
NSAIDs	Multiple prescribers
TCAs	Regular use of alcohol (~1 fl oz/d)
Opioid analgesics	Prior ADR
Corticosteroids	Nonadherence
	Alcohol misuse/abuse
Specific medication	
Warfarin	**Provider factors**
Digoxin	Prescribing potentially inappropriate medications
Diuretics	Individual clinical information for prescribing
Benadryl	Inadequate monitoring of adherence
Lithium salts	Adding medication for nonspecific indication
Chlorpropamide	Regular medication review
Theophylline	Monitoring: new medication, lab parameters, follow-up visit
Beta blockers	Identifying functional changes—self-administration ability; cognition
ACEIs/ARBs	
ASA	

ACEIs, angiotensin-converting enzyme inhibitors; ADR, adverse drug reaction; ARBs, angiotensin II receptor blockers; ASA, acetylsalicylic acid; CNS, central nervous system; CrCl, creatinine clearance; NSAIDs, nonsteroidal anti-inflammatory drugs; TCAs, tricyclic antidepressants;.

Sources: Buck et al. (2009); Chan, Hussain, Lawson, and Ormerod (2013); Kongkaew et al. (2013); Petrovic et al. (2012); Rochon (2014).

FIGURE 20.3

Prescribing cascade.

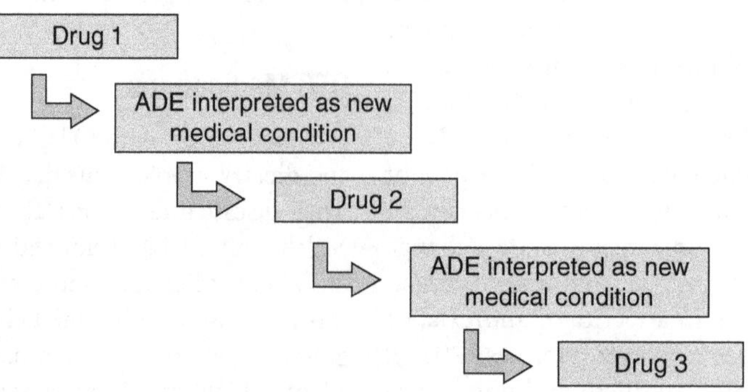

ADE, adverse drug event.

Reproduced from Rochon and Gurwitz (1997) with permission from BMJ Publishing Group Ltd.

of 6,887 patients, self-medication represented almost 4% of ADRs and prescribed and OTC drugs accounted for the rest of the ADRs (Schmiedl et al., 2014). ADRs related to self-medication occurred in women aged 70 to 79 years and in men aged 60 to 69 years. NSAIDs and acetylsalicylic acid (ASA or aspirin) were the most frequent ADRs, causing GI complaints. ADRs resulting from self-medication were caused by NSAIDs and OTC ASA most frequently.

According to the National Institute of Drug Abuse (NIDA, 2014), the combination of prescription medications and alcohol misuse is estimated to be 19% in older adults. The combination of alcohol and age-related renal insufficiency can worsen and result in chronic salicylate intoxication because of its water solubility. Cold remedies that include alcohol are a significant source of drug potentiation in aging adults. Indeed, alcohol consumption is frequently omitted from history taking of older adults, even though it interacts with OTC and prescription medications in frank and subtle ways to produce unintended drug harm (NIDA, 2014).

The OTCs most commonly implicated in hospital admissions are low-dose aspirin and NSAIDs (Schmiedl et al., 2014). In a study evaluating concomitant use of prescriptions, OTC, and herbal remedies (N = 1,000), more than half of major interactions involved the use of nonprescription therapies (Qato et al., 2008). Of those, almost half involved the use of anticoagulants (e.g., warfarin) or antiplatelet agents such as aspirin. Across all age groups, the concurrent use of aspirin and warfarin was significantly more common in men than women. Supplement use was typically nutritional products, including vitamins and minerals. Alternative treatments used for cardiovascular reasons included omega-3 fatty acids, garlic, coenzyme Q, and glucosamine-chondroitin (Qato et al., 2008). In this same study, major drug–drug interactions increased with age, with more than half of all major interactions caused by nonprescription medications. Half of the major interactions included warfarin and aspirin. The FDA has been evaluating OTC ingredients and encouraging active labeling of OTCs; although it has yet to be seen whether the FDA will be more specific on safety issues that relate to older adults. Health care providers need to specifically ask patients what OTC and herbal remedies they are taking and their frequency.

High-Risk Medications

Many studies have revealed common high-risk medications in older adults. Four medications or medication classes were implicated alone or in combination in 67% of hospitalizations: warfarin (33.3%), insulins (13.9%), oral antiplatelet agents (13.3%), and oral hypoglycemic agents (10.7%; Budnitz et al., 2011). Although warfarin is deemed high risk, it is often underprescribed because of provider fear of bleeding; however, older patients often gain a greater absolute reduction in risk of stroke (Steinman, Handler, Gurwitz, Schiff, & Covinsky, 2011). Purposeful monitoring and special attention given to these medications can significantly reduce the risk of serious adverse effects. Digoxin should also be closely monitored as one third of all emergency room visits are digoxin-related ADEs (Salvi et al., 2012; Steinman & Hanlon, 2010). According to a recent systematic review, monitoring of high-risk medications is more likely to reduce ADEs (vs. prescribing interventions) as providers can anticipate and address abnormal results immediately. Thus, proactive, appropriate monitoring is more likely than interventions to reduce ADEs. Other medications to monitor include BZDs, which are an independent risk factor for falls (Rochon, 2014). Prescription or OTC NSAIDs given with cardiac-dose ASA account for 30% of upper GI bleeding-related admissions. This may be prevented if NSAIDs were given with GI-protective agents such as a proton pump inhibitor or misoprostol. NSAIDs also lead to renal failure and heart failure (Salvi et al., 2012). Diphenhydramine (Benadryl) may lead to impaired cognition or urinary retention (in men) and antipsychotics may lead to falls, death, and are commonly associated with aspiration pneumonia (Steinman & Hanlon, 2010). These medications result in not only hospital admissions but also increased health care expenditures and morbidity (Bustacchini et al., 2009). Nurses should become familiar with high-risk medications prescribed for older adults and participate in monitoring and promptly reporting lab results to aid in reducing ADEs.

Hematological Agents

Anticoagulants and antiplatelet medications are commonly associated with ADEs resulting in hospital admissions in up to 42% of patients. Hemorrhage is the most common with GI bleeding causing around 85% of occurrences. Warfarin is more likely to cause bleeding than antiplatelet drugs, causing bleeding in 75% of all admissions (Salvi et al., 2012). However, RCTs have shown that some of the new anticoagulants are better than warfarin for prevention of stroke and systemic embolism, such as dabigatran (Salvi et al., 2012).

Warfarin has been identified throughout many research studies as among the highest risk medications, including prescription and herbal medications taken by older persons (Izzo & Ernst, 2009; Salvi et al., 2012). Warfarin is highly bound (approximately 97%) to plasma protein, mainly albumin. The high degree of protein binding is one of several mechanisms whereby other drugs interact with warfarin (Reine, Kongsgaard, Andersen, Thøgersen, & Olsen, 2010). Those with malnutrition and low albumin levels are at risk for unbound warfarin in the bloodstream and a higher risk of bleeding. Warfarin is metabolized by hepatic cytochrome p-450 isoenzymes predominantly to inactive metabolites excreted in the bile and by the kidneys. Warfarin metabolism may be altered in advanced age and in the presence of liver problems. Drug interactions with warfarin are extensive and include (a) drugs that inhibit warfarin metabolism and prolong prothrombin time (e.g., Cipro, phenytoin, amiodarone); (b) drugs that inhibit vitamin K activity (e.g., cephalosporins and high-dose penicillins); (c) additive effects with other anticoagulants such as aspirin, Lovenox, and others; and (d) drugs that reduce the effectiveness of warfarin such as phenytoin, barbiturates, cholestyramine, opioids, and others (Reine et al., 2010).

Warfarin must be monitored to evaluate the time it takes for blood to clot, using the international normalized ratio (INR), to ensure that the INR is within the target therapeutic range (2.0–3.0) although this range may vary depending on the reason for anticoagulation. This narrow therapeutic range is often difficult to achieve because of the many factors that can affect INR, including interactions with prescription and OTCs (Clarkesmith, Pattison, & Lane, 2013; Izzo & Ernst, 2009). In addition, the lab results must be acted on immediately as it will usually take 2 days to change the INR level; for example, if the level is too high the medication must be stopped to prevent bleeding. Evidence-based warfarin algorithms are available as is INR electronic monitoring. Older adults are at a significantly greater risk for bleeding on taking warfarin. Prescribing should be determined on accurate evaluation and the individual's benefit-versus-risk ratio. In some instances, the benefit of a higher risk medication may be deemed optimal and thus appropriate with close monitoring (Salvi et al., 2012). The safety literature recommends that all providers and nurses become educated in proficient warfarin management to improve safety for patients.

Fifty-eight percent of older persons do not report use of herbal supplements. Commonly used herbal remedies—ginkgo biloba, garlic, and St. John's wort—all interact with warfarin to increase its anticoagulant effect and may lead to serious bleeding problems (Clarkesmith et al., 2013; Izzo & Ernst, 2009; Tachjian et al., 2010). Many foods interact with warfarin, specifically those with high vitamin K content such as chickpeas, spinach, and green tea. It is imperative to identify older adults on warfarin who fall or are at risk of falling as their risk of serious injury increases. The risk of harm versus benefit must be weighed as a fall and head injury could lead to a serious outcome. The nurse should clarify the risk versus benefit with the primary prescriber when noting that a patient on warfarin is at high risk of a fall (Izzo & Ernst, 2009; Steinman & Hanlon, 2010).

Cardiovascular Drugs

Cardiovascular drug events represent up to 48% of all hospitalizations. Angiotensin-converting enzyme inhibitors (ACEIs), angiotensin II receptor blockers (ARBs), beta blockers, alpha blockers, calcium antagonists (all antihypertensive agents), as well as nitrates, digoxin, antiarrhythmics, and statins are of high risk for ADEs in older adults (Ho et al., 2009). In a systematic review, Salvi et al. (2012) reported that diuretics are involved in the larger number of hospital admissions across studies. Common diuretic interactions induce electrolyte disturbance, syncope, dehydration, hypotension, and falls. Hyponatremia and hyperkalemia caused ADEs related to loop and thiazide diuretics to be a significant problem in older adults and the risk increases if the person is also taking ACEIs and selective serotonin reuptake inhibitors (SSRIs; Salvi et al., 2012).

Digoxin is useful in treating CHF related to *systolic* dysfunction in the older adult but is not the recommended treatment for CHF from underlying *diastolic* dysfunction in older adults. Digoxin toxicity occurs more frequently in older adults, presents atypically, and may result in death. The dose of digoxin is often prescribed inappropriately (greater than 0.125 mg) in hospital patients, and toxic effects occur when digoxin is given in the presence of chronic kidney disease (Hamilton et al., 2011). Classic symptoms of digoxin toxicity (nausea, anorexia, and visual disturbance) may occur; however, symptomatic cardiac disturbance and arrhythmias are more common in the older adult. Older adults may experience toxicity symptoms even with normal plasma levels of digoxin (Hamilton et al., 2011).

Many older people will have some reduction in renal function with aging; therefore, monitoring for symptoms, especially atypical symptoms of digoxin toxicity, and monitoring renal function and potassium levels are key. Particular caution must be exercised when digoxin is prescribed with diuretics; this combination can cause hypokalemia and exacerbate renal impairment and potentiate digoxin toxicity. Because the therapeutic window for digoxin is narrow and it is water soluble, the drug has a smaller Vd, therefore, the plasma concentration is higher. Correct and safe dosing in older adults is challenging. The maximum recommended dose in older persons for treating systolic heart failure is 0.125 mg (Hamilton et al., 2011). Debilitated older adults who often have low serum albumin levels are at risk for elevated plasma levels resulting in digoxin toxicity.

Endocrine Agents

Antidiabetic medications and corticosteroids have been shown to be responsible for up to 28% of ADEs causing hospitalizations in older adults (Salvi et al., 2012). Older adults are at a higher risk of hypoglycemia because of age-related changes and changes in drug clearance and slowed hepatic metabolism (Lipska & Montori, 2013). Although diabetic complications have improved over the past 20 years, serious hypoglycemic events, which can result in rapid death, are on the rise and these events are more common than the adverse glycemic effects the tight control is treating; thus, the risk of harm may be considered greater than the benefit (Lipska et al., 2015).

Nearly 90% of all hospitalizations are caused by hypoglycemia with or without symptoms (Salvi et al., 2012). Older adults may present atypically with neurological symptoms, such as dizziness, confusion, delirium, and weakness, although seizures and loss of consciousness are also primary presentations in older adults. Falls, fractures, and cardiac events may also present as a hypoglycemic episode (Salvi et al., 2012). Hypoglycemic hospitalizations caused by insulin are more common than oral agents; yet sulfonylureas are commonly associated with hypoglycemia in older adults. In the hospital setting, many sulfonylureas prescribed with antibiotics have shown an increased risk of hypoglycemia, such as glipizide and glyburide. Antibiotics found to interact, including clarithromycin, levofloxacin, Bactrim, metronidazole, and ciprofloxacin, were associated with increased odds of severe hypoglycemia (Lipska et al., 2015).

Recently, sliding scale therapy was determined to be an ineffective treatment and it increased the risk of prolonged hypoglycemia, particularly in long-term care. Basal insulin, or basal plus rapid-acting insulin, with one or more meals (often called basal/bolus insulin therapy) is recommended as it most closely mimics normal physiologic insulin production. It also controls blood glucose more effectively. End-stage renal disease can be prevented or delayed with aggressive treatment in those at high risk; however, tight glycemic control must be assessed by closely evaluating the individual's risk of hypoglycemia. When the likelihood of benefit is examined in the context of limited life expectancy, the risk would be greater than the benefit. Intensive blood pressure control (less than or equal to 140/80 mmHg) is paramount to preserve renal function in diabetes mellitus (DM). Since the landmark United Kingdom Prospective Diabetes Study (UKPDS) in 2000, intensive blood pressure control has shown to preserve renal function and to reduce both diabetes-related morbidity and mortality, such as a significant reduction in microvascular and macrovascular complications, including strokes and heart failure, which were reduced in half with tight control. This also includes smoking cessation, glucose control, and lipid management (Steinman & Holmes, 2014). Again, limited life expectancy may make the risk of tighter blood pressure control greater than the benefit. ACEIs or ARBs are the primary choice for hypertensive treatment, although renal function must first be evaluated (Jarred & Kennedy, 2010; Steinman & Holmes, 2014).

Older adult diabetics are also susceptible to geriatric syndromes such as depression, cognitive impairment, urinary incontinence, chronic pain, polypharmacy, and injurious falls. The American Geriatrics Society (AGS) recommends that older adults be evaluated for atherosclerotic heart disease, functional status, and geriatric syndromes. Older adults should also be evaluated for their understanding of diabetes management, symptoms of hypoglycemia and, if they have any symptom, they should know the common presentation and treatment for them. Continual evaluation of this ability and support should be provided to older adults to avoid hypoglycemia. Diabetes management should be individualized. Annual self-management training is covered under Medicare Part B.

Factors contributing to polypharmacy in diabetes include tight glycemic control that often requires a multiple drug regimen. Likewise, the multiple comorbidities that tend to coexist with diabetes add to the number of medications and risk. Other co-occurring illnesses that may require more than one medication to control the disease include hypertension, coronary artery disease, early renal disease, glaucoma, and neuropathy. Polypharmacy, drug interactions (oral hypoglycemics with insulin or sulfonyureas), renal failure (decrease clearance of oral agents), and cognitive impairment (reduce ability to manage) increase the likelihood of hypoglycemia (Salvi et al., 2012). Multiple medications add to the cost for patients and may also lead to nonadherence.

Central Nervous System Agents

ADEs are often related to the following central nervous system (CNS) agents: BZDs; SSRIs and tricyclic antidepressants; antipsychotics; mood stabilizers such as lithium; and antiparkinson, antiseizure meds (especially Keppra), and dementia agents (Salvi et al., 2012). These drugs are responsible for up to 20% of all hospitalizations related to drugs. Change in mental status, syncope, falls, GI and respiratory disturbances, neuropsychiatric problems, and hyponatremia are often reported in older adults. Fall injuries are a leading injury related to psychotropic drug use, including hypnotics, antidepressants, and BZDs. Cholinesterase inhibitors and memantine, given for Alzheimer's disease, are associated with a high risk of bradycardia, syncope, and hip fractures. Treatment of behavioral problems is often inappropriately done with antipsychotics in patients with dementia. These medications have been associated with an increased risk of mortality, aspiration pneumonia, stroke, and sudden cardiac death secondary to arrhythmia. Psychotropic drugs have been associated with falls, including sedatives, hypnotics, and antidepressants. Recent literature suggests that SSRIs have a higher risk than tricyclics (Salvi et al., 2012).

INTERVENTIONS AND CARE STRATEGIES

Comprehensive Evaluation and Medication Management

Interventions to reduce ADEs in older adults include comprehensive geriatric assessment, evaluation of patient risk for ADEs; identifying high-risk drugs or classes of drugs to monitor closely; evaluating benefit versus risk of harm to prescribing; computerized decision-making support and prescribing systems with alerts for potential drug interactions; MR; comprehensive medication review with pharmacist support; geriatric medicine services and comprehensive geriatric evaluation and multidisciplinary team drug reviews; initiation of nonpharmacological interventions; multifaceted interventions to reduce polypharmacy (unnecessary medications and PIMs); and patient outreach and activation to be involved in education and self-management safety (Kongkaew et al., 2013; Salvi et al., 2012; Steinman et al., 2011; Topinková, Baeyens, Michel, & Lang, 2012).

Prevention of ADEs

It is prudent that health care team members are aware of the risk factors for ADEs in older adults and which medications put older adults at high risk of adverse events. In a prospective observational study, Kongkaew et al. (2013) reported that patient age, length of time since starting a new drug, total number of prescription drugs, and hospitalization were significantly associated with ADEs. The most common preventable ADEs were antiplatelet drugs, anticoagulants, diuretics (loop and thiazide diuretics), ACEIs, and antiepileptic drugs (Kongkaew et al., 2013). Knowing and recognizing these drug classes as being high risk for ADEs support the importance of regular INR monitoring and ongoing evaluation for anticoagulants or chemistry panels for diuretics to monitor electrolytes or potential orthostatic hypotension, particularly in frail older adults. In initiating ACEIs, serum potassium and increasing creatinine levels need to be monitored closely. It is important for nurses to identify that hypotension and/or hyponatremia can occur when a patient is dehydrated or volume depleted. Patients taking potassium-sparing diuretics may experience hypokalemia even in the presence of loop diuretics. These high-risk drugs should be on the radar for potential ADEs for all providers (Kongkaew et al., 2013).

Interventions for Reducing ADEs

In older adults with complex medical problems and needs, a global evaluation obtained through a comprehensive geriatric assessment (CGA) may be helpful in simplifying drug prescriptions. It will also aid in prioritizing pharmacological and health care needs, resulting in an improvement in quality of prescribing. Prescriptions should be evaluated for benefit versus harm choosing the safest and best medication for the individual. Before prescribing, providers should consider the individual's comorbidities, such as liver or kidney disease or a disease that may interact with a drug (Salvi et al., 2012). Likewise, consideration of life expectancy and health status should be evaluated in addition to the presence of frailty, which may increase the risk of ADEs and affect quality of life. Although many researchers have looked at reducing PIMs in research, the yield has been low. Computerized decision-support systems, pharmacist interventions, and CGA have shown more positive outcomes (Salvi et al., 2012). Nonpharmacological interventions and complementary and alternative medicine (CAM) therapies are underused in health care and should be considered before prescribing in many circumstances or used as an adjunctive therapy to prescribing.

Comprehensive Geriatric Assessment

An accurate medication history must be obtained from each patient and validate that the medication history is true. The amount and types of medication typically consumed, including OTCs and herbal remedies, should be examined as well as an estimate of how long each has been taken. The brown-bag method for medication review has shown to be a more accurate evaluation of a person's current medication regimen (Topinková et al., 2012). See the Assessment Tools section. Providers can also check the refill date and the number of medications remaining in the bottle or consult the pharmacy to aid in accuracy. FitzGerald (2009) recommends the following medication history:

- Currently prescribed drugs, doses, route of administration, frequency taken and duration of treatment
- OTC drugs and herbal remedies
- Drugs taken in the recent past
- Previous drug hypersensitivity reaction and the nature (rash or anaphylaxis)
- Previous ADRs and nature
- Adherence to therapy (are you taking your medication regularly? or how many pills did you miss this week/month?)
- Obtain up-to-date list from primary provider or pharmacy
- Check with pharmacy regarding prior ADRs and last order dates for each medication
- Inspect drugs and their container for name, dosage, and number of meds taken since dispensed

A CGA is a more global assessment that ensures a more specific plan for each single patient (Petrovic et al., 2012). An assessment should be conducted for each individual patient and repeated with a change in status when a new symptom develops. In a study of 746 patients receiving a CGA on admission, the following were reported as independent risk factors with in-hospital death: IADL dependence, malnutrition, acute kidney injury, and presence of pressure ulcers (Avelino-Silva et al., 2014) supporting the concept of CGA.

A comprehensive medication assessment must include a formal evaluation of the ability to manage medications on an individual basis. Of the 30 instruments developed to evaluate medication management ability, to date, none has shown sufficient validity and reliability. However, researchers report that the DRUGS tool and Medication Management Instrument for Deficiencies in Older Adults (Orwig, Brandt, & Gruber-Baldini, 2006) are the most promising. In a pilot study, patients were educated on and supervised administering their medication before discharge. This study reported improved medication management and adherence with postdischarge medications (Topinková et al., 2012). The Brief Medication Questionnaire (Svarstad, Chewning, Sleath, & Claesson, 1999) is a self-report tool that identifies persons at risk for nonadherence. It has been validated in a wide range of disease states (Rogers et al., 2009).

The Morisky Medication Adherence Questionnaire was developed to identify adherence to antihypertensive medications and has good concurrent and predicative validity in low-income and minority patients and it determines patient willingness and ability to take oral medications (Morisky, Ang, Krousel-Wood, & Ward, 2008). A thorough medication review should be performed and include patient adherence variations with attention to OTC drugs and herbal remedies. The review should include a previous history of ADRs as this is a harbinger for future ADRs (Steinman et al., 2011). Performing a systematic review of interventions using electronic reminders for patients to take medications, Vervloet et al. (2012) reported significant effects in patient adherence in seven of the eight studies reviewed. Of these, seven showed short-term effects in less than 6 months of follow-up. Adherence was improved using short message service (SMS) reminders, including four studies using an electronic recording device and one pager reminder (Vervloet et al., 2012).

Medication Reconciliation

The Institute of Healthcare Improvement (IHI; 2011) defines MR as "the process by which the most accurate patient medication list possible is obtained and compared to physician medication orders throughout the continuum of health care services" (p. 2). The IHI recommends including the drug name, dose, frequency, and administration route. It should include OTC medications, herbal remedies, vaccinations, supplements, and vitamins. MR should be performed and compared at each point during transitions in care, such as primary provider office, hospital, long-term care, rehabilitation or subacute facilities, surgery, or other levels of care transition or transfer (e.g., between hospital units). MR includes three steps, including verification, clarification, and reconciliation. Verification involves the collection of an accurate medication history from the patient, family, or other health care professionals involved in the patient's care. Clarification ensures that the medication name, dosage, route, and time of administration are accurate, and reconciliation includes the documentation of any changes made to the medication orders (Institute for Healthcare Improvement, 2011). Transmission is the final step, in which the updated list is communicated to the next care provider. MR reduced patient's ADEs caused by admission prescribing changes by 43%

(Boockvar et al., 2011). A recent study reported a reduction in emergency admissions with MR; however, two review articles reported difficulties in effective MR using HIT and reported there is insufficient evidence to support its value (McKibbon et al., 2011). See Resources: Medications at Transitions and Clinical Handoffs (MATCH).

Monitoring

Hospitalizations related to ADEs in U.S. older adults are more often related to drugs that require regular monitoring. Safety measures for monitoring high-risk medications, such as warfarin, anticonvulsants, and digoxin, have been endorsed by the National Quality Forum (Budnitz et al., 2011). Fifty-two percent of ADE-related hospitalizations can be attributed to monitoring problems. ADEs caused by errors in or lack of medication monitoring occur more frequently than precribing errors in older adults recently discharged from the hospital, as well as those in the community (Budnitz et al., 2011). Monitoring signs, symptoms, and laboratory parameters can determine whether an adverse event has only mild and short-term consequences or major long-term effects on morbidity and mortality (Steinman et al., 2011). Monitoring warfarin closely increases the benefit and decreases bleeding risk by increasing time in the therapeutic INR range. Ongoing monitoring with detection and mitigation of possible harms may improve the use of a very important medication often underprescribed in older adults (Steinman et al., 2011).

As an example, anticoagulants are most likely to cause harm to hospitalized patients because of a variety of factors, including complex dosing, the need for frequent monitoring, and transitions between parenterally and orally administered agents, such as in preparation for surgery or at the time of hospital discharge. Goals and strategies for improving anticoagulation management in inpatient settings have been identified and documented in the 2014 National Action Plan for Prevention of ADEs (2014; see Resources). The Joint Commission (TJC; 2010) identified the National Patient Safety Goal to reduce medication errors (omissions, duplications, dosing error, and drug interactions) by requiring MR at transitions from one level of care to another on admission and discharge.

Other strategies to improve monitoring include using health information technology (HIT) to link laboratory data with pharmacies, delineation of risk, and patient outreach using a multidisciplinary team–based approach to patient management and direct contact and follow-up with patients. Steinman et al. (2011) suggest that initial prescribing requires that benefits and harms of drugs are actively monitored, managed, and reassessed over time. They also recommend the use of risk-assessment tools. Those individuals predicted to be at risk should then be followed with more intensive monitoring of medication regimens. Likewise, patient outreach and activation for lab follow-up is recommended to improve monitoring. Medication management is led by pharmacists or nurses aiding in managing medications and contacting patients after a drug is started to inquire about side effects and target symptom assessment; they then can check in with the prescribing provider (Steinman et al. 2011).

Computerized Reminders

The Health Information Technology for Economic and Clinical Health Act (HITECH) was put into place in 2009 with the goals of improving patient care, decreasing errors and costs, and improving health (Beeuwkes Buntin, Burke, Hoaglin, & Blumenthal, 2011). Many criteria, including electronic health record use, had to be met before implementing computerized physician order entry (CPOE) and a Meaningful Use program. Many CPOE systems include drug safety alerts, which help to reduce prescribing errors and identify potential drug–drug interactions to improve patient safety; however, there are barriers to CPOE effectiveness. A recent systematic review reported a reduction in the number of medical errors with the implementation of CPOE (Charles, Cannon, Hall, & Coustasse, 2014). The review also showed a reduction in prescription orders and improved care coordination. One group found that the average time from physician order to when the patient received service decreased from 100 to 64 minutes. Another group found no difference in patient satisfaction form before to after CPOE was introduced, which was a concern of many providers (Charles et al., 2014). A consensus panel of physicians and pharmacists recommend increased use of CPOE systems (Steinman et al., 2011). Results of a systematic review performed by Steinman et al. recommend implementation of HIT tracking systems even in individual office practices. Topinková et al. (2012) reported that computerized decision-support systems significantly improved ADEs and inappropriate prescribing; other studies mentioned previously have shown the opposite outcome. One of the challenges reported is that alert fatigue can encourage busy providers to override alerts and compromise patient safety. Too many alerts with low credibility may cause providers to override important alerts along with unimportant ones (Steinman et al., 2011).

In addition to formal surveillance systems, including a clinical pharmacist in decision making and patient care within multidisciplinary geriatric teams, along with CPOE, is likely to minimize the occurrence of ADRs. In addition, a number of actions can be taken in hospitals to stimulate appropriate prescribing and to ensure adequate communication between primary and hospital care:

- Use a team-based approach to monitoring
- Create pharmacist-based outreach programs
- Use automated reminder calls to patients
- Send computer alerts to providers
- Establish collaborative agreements between physicians and pharmacists, in which
  - Physicians delegated test-ordering and prescribing authority to pharmacists
  - A legal mechanism for collaboration was provided
- Engage patients as active participants in monitoring
- Use systems that are acceptable to users
- Ensure MR at admission and discharge

Decision support in CPOE can be a good tool to improve patient safety but may encumber patient safety if poorly designed (Charles et al., 2014; Petrovic et al., 2012).

Medication Adherence

Evaluation for adherence is very challenging as there is no gold standard other than observing a person taking a medication, which is typically not feasible. Research includes the following six measures for evaluating adherence: pharmacy refills, pill counts, electronic medication event monitoring (MEM) caps, biologic measurements, self-report, and physician judgments. MEM devices contain a microprocessor inside a medication container that is activated when the container is opened indicating a pill has been taken (Jansen & Brouwers, 2012). This can then be downloaded at an office visit. However, it is not a perfect measure as a patient may remove more than one medication at a time, thus not accurately representing the adherence (Nieuwlaat et al., 2014).

In a systematic review, Viswanathan et al. (2012) reviewed medication adherence interventions in chronic disease. The study showed evidence for adherence improvement in diabetes using care coordination, behavioral support for hyperlipidemia, and a virtual clinic for osteoporosis. The study also reported improvement in health outcomes related to adherence in hypertension, depression, heart failure, and asthma. Blister packs helped improve adherence for hypertension, reminder calls and pharmacist-led interventions aided in improving heart failure adherence, case management and collaborative care enhanced antidepressant medication taking, and self-management and shared decision making improved asthma treatment adherence (Viswanathan et al., 2012). In another systematic review, financial incentives revealed an increase in adherence by a mean of 20% in 13 studies (Turner, Matthews, Linardatos, Tell, & Rosenthal, 2008). They also reported that the following interventions improved adherence: reduced out-of-pocket costs, case management, and patient education. Other methods of monitoring adherence included self-report, questionnaires, interview and/or logs and simply asking patient and family about the problems or difficulties they experience with taking medications. Topinková et al. (2012) also reported that patient behavioral interventions showed a significant impact on adherence versus educational interventions. Hubbard et al. (2013) reported that 92% of community pharmacies in the United States participated in electronic or e-prescribing in 2013 as did 73% of office practices. Although e-prescribing is still in its infancy, once it is fully functional it is expected that it can make a significant impact on medication adherence; for example, pharmacists follow up with patients when medications are not filled (Ryan et al., 2014).

Reducing Iatrogenic ADEs

Nurses must be vigilant in helping to prevent iatrogenic causes of ADEs, including identifying system issues to reduce medication errors (such as avoiding interruptions during medication passing), monitoring for inappropriate medications, and evaluating risk of nonadherence. Care should be focused on patient- and family-centered medication decisions (Dwamena et al., 2012) and culturally competent education on potential adverse effects of medicines. Nurses should also reinforce the need for drug monitoring with patients. Likewise, nurses must take a proactive role in ensuring patient safety through interprofessional collaboration with patient and family, doctors, advance practice nurses, pharmacists, and other team members to prevent adverse medication outcomes.

A systematic review (Spinewine, Fialová, & Byrne, 2012) reported that the involvement of a pharmacist with a geriatric evaluation and management (GEM) interprofessional team in patients older than 70 years showed appropriate use of medications during and after hospital stay using proactive review of medications and education of health care professionals. Other studies support involving pharmacists and multidisciplinary teams as well a geriatric medicine services (Topinková et al., 2012). The following outlines further interventions to reduce ADEs:

- Ask detailed questions about OTC and "recreational" drugs, alcohol use, and herbal or other folk remedies. Provide a list of herbal remedies and folk medicines to choose from (Tachjian et al., 2010). Be specific about the actual amount and under what circumstances these substances are used. Accurate information can help explain symptoms that otherwise may not make sense.
- Evaluate for duplicate medications or medication classes that occur because of unrecognized trade names versus generic names, and OTCs with the same active ingredients in them, especially acetaminophen.
- Consider medications as the underlying cause when falls or other new symptoms occur. Consider recently added medications that are high risk for causing falls such as BZDs, diuretics, and psychotropics.
- Collaborate with the interprofessional team to effect change in reducing the numbers of ADEs and ADRs, many of which are preventable (Topinková et al., 2012). Consider an interprofessional approach by including a medication care team (nurse, pharmacist, primary physician/nurse practitioner, and social worker) with specific functions assigned to review medications at admission and discharge utilizing evidence-based recommendations. Discharge interventions may be performed by various team members (Table 20.5).

Other recommendations to consider using an interprofessional approach include:

- *Reminder systems* may be instituted by pharmacists in collaboration with nurses, which have been reported to be effective, particularly in outreach to the patient at home for monitoring and follow-up of lab results (Steinman et al., 2011).
- *Pharmacist–physician or nurse collaboration* to review medication list at admission, when new medications are added, and before discharge for potential for drug–drug interactions, drug–disease interactions, and/or inappropriate medications. Monitoring and management of drug levels and medication changes in consultation with primary provider (preferably using a computer-based program). Collaboration in using the STOPP and START criteria (Frankenthal et al., 2014).
- *Computerized physician order-entry system* with decision support, including medication interaction alerts, has shown to prevent errors in dose, frequency, and route errors and reduces inappropriate medications. However, excess alerts with low credibility may cause physicians to override important alerts along with unimportant ones (Charles et al., 2014; Topinková et al., 2012).
- *Assess cognitive and affective status* to ensure that memory problems or vegetative symptoms associated with depression are not interfering with the safe use of prescription drugs (see Chapter 6, "Assessing Cognitive Function," and Chapter 15, "Late-Life Depression").
- *Assess abilities and limitations* such as functional ability, including the ability to read the medication label, to open the medication container, and consume or self-administer the prescribed medication as intended (Petrovic et al., 2012). (See Chapter 7, "Assessment of Physical Function" and Chapter 14, "Preventing Functional Decline in the Acute Care Setting."). The plan of care should address actual and potential problems and the need for reassessment at regular intervals and after major medical events (e.g., cerebrovascular accident or delirium).
- *Provide devices to accommodate impairments or barriers.* For example, tamperproof lids are often difficult for older adults to remove, particularly if there are arthritic changes. A simple request to the pharmacist to provide a nonchildproof lid may improve the safe and effective use of prescribed medication. Consult with occupational therapy for suggestions.
- *Assess health literacy.* Query whether the older person understands what the drug is to be used for, how often it is to be taken, circumstances of ingestion (e.g., with food), and other aspects of drug self-administration that signal intelligent drug use; use teach-back method to verify understanding. The Rapid Estimate of Adult Literacy in Medicine (REALM-SF instrument) is a common literacy assessment instrument that can be used to evaluate health literacy (Nutbeam, 2008).
- *Discuss the impact of medication expenses.* Many medications, particularly those that are new to the market, can be prohibitively expensive, particularly for persons on fixed incomes.

TABLE 20.5
Evidence-Based Interventions to Improve Adherence

Promising interventions to improve adherence and other key medicine-use outcomes, which require further investigation to be more certain of their effects, include:

- Simplified dosing regimens
- Interventions involving pharmacists in medicine management, for example, medicine reviews, pharmaceutical care services (consultation between pharmacist and patient to resolve medicines problems, develop a care plan, and provide follow-up)

Other strategies showed some positive effects, particularly relating to adherence and other outcomes, but their effects were less consistent overall and so need further study. These included:

- Delayed antibiotic prescriptions
- Practical strategies, such as reminders, cues, and/or organizers, reminder packaging, and material incentives
- Education delivered with self-management skills training, counselling, support, training or enhanced follow-up; information and counselling delivered together; or education/information as part of pharmacist-delivered packages of care
- Financial incentives

Several strategies also showed promise in promoting immunization uptake, but require further study to be more certain of their effects. These included:

- Organizational interventions, reminders and recall, financial incentives, home visits, free vaccination, lay health worker interventions, and facilitators working with physicians to promote immunizations. Education and/or information strategies also showed some positive, but even less consistent, effects on immunizations
- Positive effects on adherence
- Positive effects on adherence and knowledge
- Effective in decreasing antibiotic use but with mixed effects on clinical outcomes, adverse effects, and satisfaction
- Positive, although somewhat mixed effects on adherence
- Positive effects on adherence, use of medicines, clinical outcomes, and knowledge, but with mixed effects in some studies
- Positive, but mixed, effects on adherence
- Needs further assessment of effectiveness and investigation of heterogeneity

There are many different potential pathways through which consumers' use of medicines could be targeted to improve outcomes, and simple interventions may be as effective as complex strategies. However, no single intervention was effective in improving all medicine-use outcomes across all diseases, medicines, populations, or settings.

Note: Despite a doubling in the number of reviews included in this updated overview, uncertainty still exists about the effectiveness of many interventions, and the evidence on what works remains sparse for caregivers and people with multimorbidity.
Source: Ryan et al. (2014).

CASE STUDY

Mr. Johnson is a 75-year-old African American male who is re-admitted to the hospital for CHF for the fourth time in the past year. He was readmitted to the subacute unit for rehabilitation after another admission. He has a history of atrial fibrillation, type 2 diabetes with peripheral neuropathy. His other diagnoses include hypertension, low ejection fraction, hyperlipidemia, and a history of alcohol abuse. A year ago he had a suspected transient ischemic attack (TIA) with no recurrence. His wife of 56 years just died 6 months ago after a massive stroke. He has been living alone since then and his daughter stops by several times a week to check on him. Up until the last admission, he was able to make his own breakfast and lunch and received Meals on Wheels for dinner. He had a home care assistant once a week. Medications include warfarin, low-dose aspirin, Lasix 40 mg twice daily, Glyburide 5 mg every 12 hours, gabapentin 300 mg twice daily, Elavil 65 mg for a recent postherpetic neuralgia × 4 weeks, and atorvastatin 40 mg with a stable lipid panel over the past 2 years. What are your initial concerns with Mr. Johnson?

Your first concern is to ensure Mr. J's cardiovascular status is stable enough to remain in your cardiovascular unit. Is he hypotensive? Is he tachycardic? And how is his rhythm? How are his vital signs (V/S)? Is he tachypneic, unable to lie flat, or have a low O_2 saturation? If you answer is "yes" to any of these, he may need to be moved to intensive care.

His initial V/S are 160/100, heart rate is 110 irregular, and respiratory rate is 32. His O_2 saturation is 89%, but comes up to 91% with oxygen. He has bibasilar rales one third of the way up posteriorly,

(continued)

CASE STUDY *(continued)*

3+ edema up to knees. He is sitting up and increasingly short of breath transferring from gurney to bed; he is alert and oriented × 3 but anxious. He denies chest pain or other cardiovascuar symptoms. You provide O_2 and access a line and give him stat IV Lasix 80 mg as ordered, monitoring his urine output. Fortunately, he responds well to the stat dose and has excellent response with diuresis of a liter of fluid. His heart rate slows down to 86, O_2 sat is 93%, blood pressure is 150/82, and his symptoms start to improve. He will continue to receive Lasix every 12 hours and remain on telemetry × 24 hours.

Now you have time to sit down and evaluate his history and physical examination performed by the resident and see whether his lab results have returned. You recognize his story from his last admission when you helped care for Mr. Johnson with a CHF exacerbation 3 months ago. His admission weight shows he has gained 15 pounds since his last discharge and had digoxin 0.25 mg daily recently added by his cardiologist. You also learn about the loss of his wife who cared for him and made sure he ate "what he was supposed to." He also reported that he has had vague nausea over the past month.

What are your initial concerns about Mr. Johnson?

Now that he is stable you evaluate his pain, the fifth vital sign. Most important, we need to make sure he has adequate relief with his current regimen (gabapentin). In this case, evaluate whether his neuropathy is adequately controlled with gabapentin and whether he has pain anywhere else.

You decide to review and match each medicine with a corresponding diagnosis (recommended at your recent drug in-service) while you wait for the resident to arrive, and you do this in collaboration with the assigned admission RN.

Right away you question why he is on Elavil at 65 mg, which is a PIM (tricyclic). You look it up and discover that it may be given for postherpetic neuralgia but IF it is given it is maintained no longer than 3 weeks (the patient has been on it for 4 weeks). You note the patient is also on gabapentin for diabetic neuropathy and confirm with the pharmacist that this may also help postherpetic neuralgia pain, so, if the patient is still experiencing postherpetic neuralgia you may ask whether the Elavil can be tapered off and the Neurontin titrated up for neuralgia (one drug for two disorders) and reduce polypharmacy; the risk is likely greater than the benefit.

Next you notice his dose of digoxin is higher (0.25 mg/d) than the recommended digoxin dose of 0.125 mg/d for systolic heart failure; you make note of that as well. You remember Mr. Johnson is complaining of nausea and fatigue and wonder whether it may be an atypical presentation of digoxin toxicity (you note to check digoxin level) and see whether his electrolytes are off. You review his initial lab results: hemoglobin/hematocrit, electrolytes (chem panel) are normal except for a K^+ of 3.0, Na^+ of 124, and an albumin of 2.9. You notify the primary resident of the need for urgent K^+ replacement and tell him you will share other concerns when he arrives. You also note that in light of the low albumin he may be more likely to have an elevated digoxin level as the albumin is low, thus no place for the digoxin to bind to (noted). You will note this for the resident as well. Finally, you notice the patient is on warfarin, an anticoagulant, and aspirin, which also thins the blood (started after a suspected TIA). You remember a recent patient who had bleeding with this combination and will note it for the resident to evaluate risk versus benefit. Finally, you know that diuretics are one of the most common drugs to cause adverse events, but cannot sort out the underlying cause of the electrolyte imbalance, yet you know it needs to be addressed. You are also concerned about Mr. Johnson's risk for falls because he is fatigued and just received a diuretic that may cause syncope, dehydration, orthostatic hypotension, and falls in addition to the electrolyte imbalance.

You check Mr. Johnson for orthostatic hypotension and note he has a 15-mm Hg drop in blood pressure and instruct him about fall precautions, put the call light and bedside table in reach, and put a fall risk sign above his bed. You check his cognition and ask him to repeat his understanding of the fall prevention to ensure he is able to follow the safety plan. Finally, his random glucose and lipids are normal. However, you are already very concerned about whether Mr. Johnson is going to be safe at home when he is discharged this time. You ask the admission RN to notify the interprofessional team members about Mr. Johnson's challenges at home and his recent loss with both the case manager and social worker, who will follow up with his daughter when she gets off work today. Mr. Johnson's case will be reviewed in the interprofessional team meeting for a team-based discharge plan.

Finally, the resident arrives on the floor and you tell the resident what you have learned about Mr. Johnson thus far. Not surprising, the majority of the issues have been discussed/addressed through an ad hoc team of two nurses collaborating with other team members, including the pharmacist, case manager, social worker, and resident, to get Mr. Johnson off to a good start

(continued)

CASE STUDY ***(continued)***

of team-based care and avoidance of an ADE. Many nurses say, "but that is the doctors job" and other nurses say, "we make suggestions all the time" and "nurses are about the patients and keeping them safe." Although it may not be your job, it is incumbent on all nurses to be aware of the risks that face older adults, particularly in the high-risk hospital environment where older adults are at much higher risk for adverse events.

Here is a summary of medications and what might be considered by the geriatric team in collaborating with the patient and his daughter.

The patient should have a complete geriatric evaluation as outlined in the chapter along with a thorough history. A review of all his medications brought in with a brown bag is made and aligned with each diagnosis. In addition, alignment of drugs that may have drug–drug or drug–disease interactions is also done.

Discontinue/taper the Elavil and monitor the patient for increased pain (neuropathy or postherpetic neuralgia).

Check digoxin level, if toxic, need to hold the digoxin. If restarting digoxin, decrease dose to 0.125 mg/d in collaboration with the cardiologist who ordered it.

Warfarin and aspirin together may increase the risk of GI bleeding. Discontinuing the aspirin should be considered. The lipid panel is now within normal limits, this may likely allow Atorvostatin to be discontinued as there are likely few years to receive further benefit. Perhaps liberalizing his diet as well if that is an important issue for quality of life.

His likely prognosis will be discussed at the team meeting due to the recurrent hospitalizations, poor ejection fraction, CHF exacerbations, and progressing heart failure should be discussed by the team to arrive at his goals of care. Ensure that the team evaluates what he or his daughter understands about his diagnoses and recurrent hospitalizations. Ensure his wishes continue to be consistent with his current advance directive.

Continue to monitor diabetes.

It is likely diuretics will need to continue for the patient's comfort by improving pulmonary function. Monitoring of electrolytes will be very important if patient continues on diuretics; fall precautions are important. A discussion regarding risks associated with diuretics is key.

It is likely that the patient will need to be placed in an environment where he can be monitored for safety, but this decision will be based on the discussion of the patient's beliefs and wishes regarding quality of life. It is very important to ensure patient's/daughter's involvement in the decision making of medications to take or not to take along with the interprofessional team.

NURSING STANDARD OF PRACTICE

Protocol 20.1: Reducing Adverse Drug Events in Older Adults

I. GOAL

To proactively identify older adults at risk of ADEs

II. OVERVIEW

Around 31% of all adverse events in hospitals are caused by medication-related problems. The use of prescription drugs has increased 90% over the past 25 years with a consequent increase in ADEs reported to the FDA (NCHS, 2012). ADEs, whether from drug–drug or drug–disease interactions, inappropriate prescribing, poor adherence, or medication errors, lead to serious or potentially fatal outcomes for older adults. Between 2004 and 2008, there was a 52% increase in the number of ADEs reported in U.S. hospitals (Lucado et al., 2008). In U.S. hospitals, ADEs increase costs to patients, health care expenditures, length of hospital stay, and morbidity and mortality, yet nearly half are likely preventable. More than half of ADEs are potentially preventable (Kongkaew et al., 2013; Levinson, 2010; Rochon, 2014; Topinková et al., 2012).

III. BACKGROUND

A. Definitions
   1. *ADE*: An adverse outcome that occurs during normal use of medication, inappropriate use, inappropriate or suboptimum prescribing, poor adherence, self-medication, or harm caused by a medication error (WHO, 2002).

(continued)

Protocol 20.1: Reducing Adverse Drug Events in Older Adults *(continued)*

2. *Iatrogenic ADE*: This may be defined as ADRs or complications induced by nondrug medical interventions (Atiqi et al., 2010) and relates to medications induced by a drug prescribed by a medical provider (WHO, 2002).
3. *ADR*: Any noxious or unintended and undesired effect of a drug that occurs at normal human doses for prophylaxis, diagnosis, or therapy. Inappropriate prescribing of high-risk medication to older adults and medication errors are all considered iatrogenic (WHO, 1972).
4. *Drug–drug interactions*: These occur when one therapeutic agent alters either the concentration (pharmacokinetic interactions) or the biological effect of another agent or pharmacodynamic interactions (Levinson, 2010).
5. *Medication adherence*: This is defined as the extent to which a person's medication-taking behavior corresponds with agreed recommendations of a health care provider (WHO, 2003).
6. *Drug–disease interactions*: These are undesired drug effects (exacerbation of a disease or condition caused by a drug) that occur in patients with certain disease states. Common drug–disease interactions are aspirin given in peptic ulcer disease and beta blockers given in diabetes (Salvi et al., 2012).
7. *Pharmacokinetics*: This refers to the time course of absorption, distribution across compartments, metabolism, and excretion of drugs in the body. The metabolism and excretion of many drugs decrease and the physiological changes of aging require dose adjustment for some drugs (Levinson, 2010; Steinman & Holmes, 2014).
8. *Pharmacodynamics*: This is the response of the body to the drug that is affected by receptor binding, postreceptor effects, and chemical interactions. Pharmacodynamic problems occur when two drugs act at the same or interrelated receptor sites, resulting in additive, synergistic, or antagonistic effects. The effects of two or more drugs together can be either *additive* (combination of drugs "add up" to increase effect), *synergistic* (one agent magnifies the effect of the other), or *antagonistic* (one medication inhibits the effect of the other; Steinman & Holmes, 2014).
9. *Medication reconciliation*: Defined by TJC as "the process of comparing the medications a patient is taking (and should be taking) with newly ordered medications." It is a process of comparing the patient's current medication regimen against the physician's admission, transfer, and/or discharge orders to identify discrepancies (TJC, 2010).

B. Epidemiology
1. American older adults are the greatest consumers of medications, with this population taking, on average, three OTC medications and up to six or more prescription medications (Petrovic et al., 2012). Half of all prescriptions are prescribed to older adults; those in office practices take six or more medications. Medicare patients (older than 65 years) have the highest rates of ADEs, representing 75.3 per 10,000 discharges.
2. Older adults experience a 10.7% prevalence rate of hospital admissions caused by ADRs; however, a confounding factor in the accuracy is the different methods and studies employed to gather the data (Kongkaew et al., 2013).

C. Etiology

Older adults become increasingly susceptible to ADEs as they age, especially frail older adults (Hubbard et al., 2013). Physiological changes characteristic of aging predispose older adults to experience adverse events. ADEs increase the costs, length of hospital stay, and mortality, yet often go unreported, and nearly half are likely preventable (Levinson, 2010; Salvi et al., 2012). Persons older than age 65 years experience medication-related problems for five major reasons:
1. Age-related physiological changes that result in altered pharmacokinetics and pharmacodynamics (Levinson, 2010; Steinman & Holmes, 2014)
2. Polypharmacy (multiple medications); medications are often prescribed by multiple providers (Gray & Gardner, 2009; Rogers et al., 2009)
3. Therapeutic failures—over- or underdosing of medications (more than or less than a therapeutic dosage; Marcum et al., 2012)
4. Medication consumption for the treatment of symptoms that are not disease dependent or specific (self-medication and/or prescribing cascades; Rochon, 2014)

(continued)

Protocol 20.1: Reducing Adverse Drug Events in Older Adults *(continued)*

5. Iatrogenic causes such as:
   a. ADRs, including drug–drug or drug–disease interactions (Heuberger, 2012)
   b. Inappropriate prescribing for older adults (Hamilton et al., 2011)
   c. Problems with medication adherence (Marcum et al., 2014; Steinman & Hanlon, 2010)
   d. Medication errors (Charles et al., 2014; Steinman et al., 2011)

IV. ASSESSMENT TOOLS AND STRATEGIES

A. Assessment tools
   1. *Beers Criteria*—American Geriatrics Society Beers Criteria for Potentially Inappropriate Medication Use in Older Adults (2012)—used to assess medication list for medications that should generally be avoided in older adults
   2. *STOPP Criteria*—Screening Tool of Older Persons' Prescriptions—used to identify PIMs (Gallagher et al., 2011)
   3. *START Criteria*—Screening Tools to Alert Doctors to the Right Treatment—used to identify medications that are underused and potential prescription omissions (Gallagher et al., 2011).
   4. *Drug–Drug Interactions*—Table 20.2 gives a review list of common medications known to interact with other medications. This is done using computer decision-support and computer drug–drug interaction alerts (Clyne et al., 2012).
   5. *Cockroft–Gault Formula* (see Table 20.3)—This formula is useful for estimating creatinine clearance based on age, weight, and serum creatinine levels (Terrell et al., 2006). A creatinine clearance of less than 50 mL/min places older adults at risk for ADEs (Fouts et al., 1997).
   6. *Brown-Bag Method*—This method is used to assess all medications. Ask older adults to place all medications, OTCs, and herbal remedies in a bag and bring to hospital/other care setting to ensure med list is accurate (Nathan et al., 1999).
   7. *Drugs Regimen Unassisted Grading Scale (DRUGS) Tool*—This tool is used at transfer to other levels of care. A standardized method for assessing potential medication adherence problems. This requires a higher level of functioning (Edelberg et al., 1999; Hutchison et al., 2006).
   8. *Functional Capacity*—Evaluates ADL and IADL; Mini-Cog or MMSE can be used to evaluate the ability to self-administer medications (see Chapters 6 and 7).

B. Assessment strategies
   1. Identify aging changes in pharmacokinetics and pharmacodynamics when assessing medications in older adults (Levinson, 2010; Steinman & Holmes, 2014).
   2. Perform a CGA: Geriatric evaluation and management reduced inappropriate and unnecessary medications. A comprehensive assessment is important as it is a more global assessment that ensures a more specific plan for each single patient (Avelino-Silva et al., 2014; Petrovic et al., 2012).
   3. Perform a comprehensive medication history (FitzGerald, 2009):
      a. Currently prescribed drugs, doses, route of administration, frequency taken, and duration of treatment
      b. OTC drugs and herbal remedies
      c. Drugs taken in the recent past
      d. Previous drug hypersensitivity reaction and the nature of the reaction (rash or anaphylaxis)
      e. Previous ADRs and their nature
      f. Adherence to therapy (What medications are you having difficulty with? or How many pills have you missed this week/month?)
      g. Obtain an up-to-date medication list from primary provider or pharmacy.
      h. Check with pharmacy regarding prior ADRs and last order dates for each medication.
      i. Inspect drugs and their containers for name, dosage, and number taken since dispensed.

(continued)

Protocol 20.1: Reducing Adverse Drug Events in Older Adults *(continued)*

   j. The comprehensive medication assessment must include a formal evaluation of the ability to manage medications on an individual basis (Topinková et al., 2012); perform at discharge and intervals in between, including between units.
   k. Regular medication review to evaluate list for PIMs/PIPs (Beers Criteria and STOPP Criteria); consider drugs that may be discontinued (Campanelli, 2012; Gallagher et al., 2011)
4. Evaluate for patient-related and medication-related risk factors for ADRs (see Table 20.4).
5. Perform MR at admission, discharge, transfers, and transitions to other levels of care in consultation with a pharmacist, geriatric expert, or computer-based program (Frankenthal et al., 2014).
6. At discharge from hospital, use appropriate tools to assess individual's ability to self-administer medications (Ho et al., 2009).

V. INTERVENTIONS AND NURSING CARE STRATEGIES

A. Reducing ADEs (during and after hospitalization)
1. Patient/family-centered care and decision making include collaboration with interprofessional team members. Patients should be given the necessary information and the opportunity to exercise the degree of control they choose over health care decisions that affect them. Patients involved in decision making are less likely to make decisions that may lead to ADRs, such as abruptly discontinuing a medication that should be tapered off (Parchman, Zeber, & Palmer, 2010).
2. Comprehensive geriatric prescribing
   a. Evaluate prescriptions for benefit versus harm
   b. Choose the safest and best medication for the individual based on geriatric assessment and goals of care
   c. Before prescribing, consider the individual's comorbidities such as liver or kidney disease or a disease that may interact with a drug (Salvi et al., 2012).
   d. Prescribing principles. Although bedside nurses are not involved in prescribing, they are involved in reviewing and signing off medications, thus should be aware of prescribing principles.
      i. Monitoring for appropriate prescribing and alerting the prescriber to potential problem areas, monitoring for and reporting lab/drug levels to primary provider, monitoring for toxicity and medication effectiveness, and seeking consultation when necessary (Rochon, 2014).
      ii. Reduce the dose. "Start low and go slow" providing the lowest possible dose and slow upward titration to obtain clinical benefit; many ADEs are dose related (Rochon, 2014). Primary provider should be notified if the dosage ordered is higher than the recommended starting dose (e.g., digoxin maximum dose < 0.125 mg for treatment of systolic heart failure).
      iii. Discontinue unnecessary therapy. Prescribers are often reluctant to stop medications, especially if they did not initiate the treatment. This practice increases the risk for an adverse event (Rochon, 2014).
      iv. Attempt a trial of nonpharmacological interventions and treatments before requesting medication for new symptoms (e.g., therapeutic activity kit for agitation; Rochon, 2014).
      v. Recommend safer drugs. Avoid drugs that are likely to be associated with adverse outcomes (review Beers Criteria).
      vi. Assess renal function using the Cockroft–Gault formula (for renally cleared drugs) to determine accurate dosage before prescribing such as many routinely prescribed intravenous (IV) antibiotics. Dosage recommendations are available based on this formula and are presented in common prescribing resources.
      vii. Optimize drug regimen. When prescribing medications, focus on risk versus benefit in which the expected health benefit (e.g., relief of agitation in dementia with psychosis) exceeds the expected negative consequences (e.g., morbidity and mortality from falls that result in hip fracture).
      viii. Initiation of new medication. Assess risk factors for ADRs, potential drug–disease and drug–drug interactions, correct drug dosages, and follow-up to evaluate response to new medication.

(continued)

Protocol 20.1: Reducing Adverse Drug Events in Older Adults *(continued)*

h. Avoid the prescribing cascade. Avoid the prescribing cascade by first considering any new symptom as being an adverse effect of a current medication before adding a new medication (Rochon, 2014).
i. Avoid inappropriate medications. Review Beers and STOPP Criteria for potential inappropriate medications, drug–disease interactions, and potential drug–drug interactions.
j. Employ nonpharmacological approaches for primary symptom management or as adjunct to medication (e.g., therapeutic activity kit for agitation; Zwicker & Fletcher, 2009).
k. Evaluate for patient concern regarding difficulties in adherence to medication (Steinman & Hanlon, 2010).

B. Computerized order entry and decision-support systems
1. Monitor and attend to alerts for potential drug–drug interactions.
2. Pharmacist-based support of CPOE and electronic prescriptions direct to pharmacy
3. Reminder systems for monitoring (Charles et al., 2014)

C. Monitoring (Steinman et al., 2011)
1. Evaluate patients for adverse effects and efficacy after a new medication is started.
2. Educate patients about anticipated benefits and potential problem associated with a new drug. Partner with patient to actively engage to assess drug effectiveness, adherence, and adverse effects.
3. Monitor and inform primary care provider of lab results and/or drug levels particularly those with a narrow therapeutic range, such as digoxin, INR level, lithium levels.
4. Report questionable dosing amounts or schedule and medication allergy before medication administration.
5. Monitor for drug interactions and inform primary provider of new or recent medications that may be related to the negative interaction.
6. Use HIT to monitor labs where available, for example, lab tracing systems.
7. Use team-based approaches to monitor medications.
8. Risk assessment tools—individualize monitoring based on individual risk.
9. Generate a report when lab tests are not performed with follow-up mechanism.
10. Employ policy standards that mandate ability to track and report overdue lab tests easily.

VI. EXPECTED OUTCOMES

A. Patients will:
1. Experience fewer adverse outcomes from medication-related events
2. Demonstrate understanding of their medication regimens on discharge from the hospital and keep an updated medication list
3. Become an active member of medication decision making and monitoring

B. Health care providers will:
1. Use a range of interventions to prevent, alleviate, or ameliorate medication problems with older adults, including nonpharmacological and complementary therapies
2. Improve prescribing practices by documenting indication for initiation of new drug therapy, maintaining a current medication list, and documenting response to therapy as well as the need for ongoing treatment and follow-up monitoring
3. Evaluate nature and origins of medication-related problems in a timely manner
4. Increase knowledge about medication safety in older adults
5. Increase referrals to appropriate practitioners for collaboration and medication safety (e.g., pharmacist, geriatrician, geriatric/gerontological or psychiatric clinical nurse specialist, nurse practitioner, or consultation-liaison service, social worker, case manager, or interprofessional team)

C. Institution will:
1. Provide a culture of safety that encourages safe medication practices
2. Provide education to health care providers regarding prevention, identification, and reporting of ADRs
3. Make information on ADRs accessible to patients

(continued)

Protocol 20.1: Reducing Adverse Drug Events in Older Adults *(continued)*

4. Enhance surveillance and reporting of ADRs using a national surveillance system; consider use of computerized physician order entry system and drug interaction software
5. Track and report morbidity and mortality related to medication problems
6. Provide a system for MR and follow up its effectiveness regarding rehospitalization rates caused by ADRs
7. Review for careful documentation of iatrogenic medication and other iatrogenic events for CQI
8. Provide ongoing education related to safe medication management for physicians, other licensed independent providers, pharmacists, and nursing staff

VII. FOLLOW-UP

A. Health care providers will
   1. Provide consistent and appropriate care and follow-up in presence of a medication-related problem.
   2. Monitor and evaluate with physical examination and/or laboratory tests (as appropriate) on regular basis to ensure that the older adult is responding to therapy as expected.
   3. Review medication list, including OTC and herbal remedies, regularly and reconcile medications at transitions in care.
   4. Monitor high-risk medications more frequently for potential adverse events.

B. Institutions will
   1. Provide ongoing assessment of staff competence in assessing and intervening for prevention of ADEs.
   2. Embed reduction of ADEs in the institution's culture of safety.

VII. RELEVANT PRACTICE GUIDELINES

Noskin, M. D., & Gleason, K. (2012). Medications at Transitions and Clinical Handoffs (MATCH) Toolkit for Medication Reconciliation. AHRQ Publication No 11(12)-0059. Rockville, MD. Available at http://www.ahrq.gov/professionals/quality-patient-safety/patient-safety-resources/resources/match/match.pdf

ABBREVIATIONS

ADE	Adverse drug event
ADL	Activities of daily living
ADR	Adverse drug reaction
CGA	Comprehensive geriatric assessment
CQI	Continuous quality improvement
DRUGS	Drugs Regimen Unassisted Grading Scale
FDA	Food and Drug Administration
HIT	Health information technology
IADL	Independent activities of daily living
INR	International normalized ratio
MATCH	Medications at Transitions and Clinical Handoffs
MMSE	Mini-Mental State Exam
MR	Medication reconciliation
OTC	Over the counter
PIMs	Potentially inappropriate medications
PIPs	Potentially inappropriate prescriptions
TJC	The Joint Commission
WHO	World Health Organization

ACKNOWLEDGMENT

The authors wish to acknowledge the editorial review of Professor John W. Devlin, Northeastern University School of Pharmacy.

RESOURCES

ASHP Guidelines on Medication Errors: http://www.ashp.org/searchresults.aspx?q=medication%20error

CDC: Adverse Drug Events
http://www.cdc.gov/MedicationSafety/program_focus_activities.html

Cooper, J. A., Cadogan, C. A., Patterson, S. M., Kerse, N. Bradley, M. C., Ryan, C., & Hughes, C. M. (2015). Interventions to improve the appropriate use of polypharmacy in older people: A Cochrane Systematic Review. *British Medical Journal, 5*(12), e009235. doi: 10.1136/bmjopen-2015-009235

Dietary Supplement and Drug Interactions
http://www.merckmanuals.com/professional/special_subjects/dietary_supplements/overview_of_dietary_supplements.html#v1126015
Drugs with Potentially Serious Drug–Drug Interactions
http://www.merckmanuals.com/professional/clinical_pharmacology/factors_affecting_response_to_drugs/drug_interactions.html#v1108519 FDA: Medication Errors and Safety
http://www.fda.gov/Drugs/DrugSafety/MedicationErrors/default.htm

Gleason, K. M., McDaniel, M. R., Feinglass, J., Baker, D. W., Lindquist, L., Liss, D., & Noskin G. A. (2010). Results of the medications at transitions and clinical handoffs (MATCH) study: An analysis of medication reconciliation errors and risk factors at hospital admission. *Journal of General Internal Medicine, 25*(5), 441–447.

Institute for Safe Medication Practices
Offers webinars, lectures, and other programs related to safe medication practice, including reducing errors, identifying high-risk abbreviations:
www.ismp.org

Interventions to Improve Adherence. Systematic Review.
Medication Management Guideline. (2012). *Health Care Association of New Jersey (HCANJ). Medication management guideline.* Hamilton, NJ: Health Care Association of New Jersey (HCANJ). Retrieved from http://www.guideline.gov/content.aspx?id= 39268

Medications at Transitions and Clinical Handoffs (MATCH): Toolkit for Medication Reconciliation. Retrieved from http://psnet.ahrq.gov

Merck Manual, Professional Edition. Dietary supplement and drug interactions. Retrieved from http://www.merckmanuals.com/professional/special_subjects/dietary_supplements/overview_of_dietary_supplements.html#v1126015

U.S. Department of Health and Human Services, Office of Disease Prevention and Health Promotion. (2014). *National action plan for adverse drug event prevention.* Washington, DC: Author. Retrieved from http://health.gov/hcq/pdfs/ADE-Action-Plan-508c.pdf

U.S. Food and Drug Administration: http://www.fda.gov/

Youdim, A. (2013). Nutrient-drug interactions. *Merck Manual Professional Edition.* Kenilworth, NJ: Merck and Company. Retrieved from http://merckmanuals.com/professional/special_subjects/dietary_supplements/overview_of_dietary_supplements

REFERENCES

Alomar, M. (2014). Factors affecting the development of adverse drug reactions (review article) *Saudi Pharmacotherapy Journal, 22,* 83–94. *Evidence Level I.*

Ament, P. W., Bertolino, J. G., & Liszewski, J. L. (2000). Clinically significant drug interactions. *American Family Physician, 61*(6), 1745–1754. *Evidence Level V.*

Aspden, P., & Institute of Medicine. Committee on Identifying and Preventing Medication. (2007). *Preventing medication errors.* Washington, DC: National Academies Press. *Evidence Level VI.*

Atiqi, R., van Bommel, E., Cleophas, T., & Zwinderman, A. (2010). Prevalence of iatrogenic admissions to the departments of medicine/cardiology/pulmonology in a 1,250 bed general hospital. *International Journal of Clinical Pharmacology and Therapeutics, 48*(8), 517–524. *Evidence Level I.*

Avelino-Silva, T., Farfel, J., Curiati, J., Amaral, J., Campora, F., & Jacob, W. (2014). Comprehensive geriatric assessment predicts mortality and adverse outcomes in hospitalized older adults. *BMC Geriatrics, 3,* 14. doi:10.1186/1471–2318-14–129. *Evidence Level IV.*

Beeuwkes Buntin, M., Burke, M., Hoaglin, M., & Blumenthal, D. (2011). The benefits of health information technology: A review of the recent literature shows predominantly positive results. *Health Affairs, 30*(3), 464–471. *Evidence Level V.*

Boockvar, K. S., Blum, S., Kugler, A., Livote, E., Mergenhagen, K., Nebeker, J. R.,...Yeh, J. (2011). Effect of admission medication reconciliation on adverse drug events from admission medication changes. *Archives of Internal Medicine, 17*(9), 860–861. *Evidence Level V.*

Buck, M. D., Atreja, A., Brunker, C. P., Jain, A., Suh, T. T., Palmer, R. M.,...Wilcox, A. B. (2009). Potentially inappropriate medication prescribing in outpatient practices: Prevalence and patient characteristics based on electronic health records. *American Journal of Geriatric Pharmacotherapy, 7*(2), 84–92. *Evidence Level IV.*

Budnitz, D. S., Lovegrove, M. C., Shehab, N., & Richards, C. L. (2011). Emergency hospitalizations for adverse drug events in older Americans. *New England Journal of Medicine, 365*(21), 2002–2012. *Evidence Level IV.*

Bustacchini, S., Corsonello, A., Onder, G., Guffanti, E. E., Marchegiani, F., Abbatecola, A. M., & Lattanzio, F. (2009). Pharmacoeconomics and aging. *Drugs and Aging, 26*(Suppl. 1), 75–87. *Evidence Level VI.*

Campanelli, C. (2012). American Geriatrics Society updated Beers Criteria for potentially inappropriate medication use in older adults: The American Geriatrics Society 2012 Beers Criteria update expert panel. *Journal of the American Geriatrics Society, 60*(4), 616–631. *Evidence Level V.*

Cardelli, M., Marchegiani, F., Corsonello, A., Lattanzio, F., & Provinciali, M. (2012). A review of pharmacogenetics of adverse drug reactions in elderly people. *Management of Iatrogenic Risk in Older Patients, 35*(1), 3–20. doi: 10.1007/BF03319099. *Evidence Level IV.*

Chan, S. A., Hussain, F., Lawson, L. G., & Ormerod, A. D. (2013). Factors affecting adherence to treatment of psoriasis: comparing biologic therapy to other modalities. *Journal of Dermatological Treatment, 24*(1), 64–69. doi:10.3109/09546634.2011.607425. *Evidence Level IV.*

Charles, C., Cannon, M., Hall, R., & Coustasse, A. (2014). Can utilizing a computerized provider order entry (CPOE) system prevent hospital medical errors and adverse drug events? *Perspectives in health information management, 11,* 1b. *Evidence Level V.*

Choudhry, N., Avorn, J., Glynn, R., Antman, E., Schneeweiss, S., Toscano, M.,... Shrank, W. (2011). Full coverage for preventive medications after myocardial infarction. *New England Journal of Medicine, 365*(22), 2088–2097. *Evidence Level II.*

Christensen, M., & Lundh, A. (2013). Medication review in hospitalised patients to reduce morbidity and mortality. *Cochrane Database of Systematic Reviews. Evidence Level I.*

Clarkesmith, D. E., Pattison, H. M., & Lane, D. A. (2013). Educational and behavioural interventions for anticoagulant therapy in patients with atrial fibrillation. *Cochrane Database of Systematic Reviews, 6,* CD008600. doi:10.1002/14651858.CD008600.pub2. *Evidence Level I.*

Clyne, B., Bradley, M. C., Hughes, C., Fahey, T., & Lapane, K. L. (2012). Electronic prescribing and other forms of technology to reduce inappropriate medication use and polypharmacy in older people: A review of current evidence. *Clinics in Geriatric Medicine, 28*(2), 301–322. doi:10.1016/j.cger.2012.01.009. *Evidence Level I.*

Cusak, B., & Vestal, R. E. (2000). In M. H. Beers & R. Berkow (Eds.), *Clinical pharmacology.* Whitehouse Station, NJ: Merck Research Laboratories. *Evidence Level VI.*

Davies, E. C., Green, C. F., Taylor, S., Williamson, P. R., Mottram, D. R., & Pirmohamed, M. A. (2009). Adverse drug reactions in hospital in-patients: A prospective analysis of 3695 patient-episodes. *PLoS ONE, 4(2)* e4439. doi:10.1371/journal.pone.0004439. *Evidence Level V.*

Dwamena, F., Holmes-Rovner, M., Gaulden, C., Jorgenson, S., Sadigh, G., Sikorski, A., & Beasley, M. (2012). Interventions for providers to promote a patient-centered approach in clinical consultations. *Cochrane Database of Systematic Reviews, 12. Evidence Level I.*

Edelberg, H. K., Shallenberger, E., & Wei, J. Y. (1999). Medication management capacity in highly functioning community-living older adults: Detection of early deficits. *Journal of the American Geriatrics Society, 47*(5), 592–596. doi:10:1016/j.cger.2012.01.009. *Evidence Level I.*

Feldstein, A. C., Smith, D. H., Perrin, N., Yang, X., Simon, S. R., Krall, M., & Soumerai, S. B. (2006). Reducing warfarin medication interactions: An interrupted time series evaluation. *Archives of Internal Medicine, 166*(9), 10009–11015. *Evidence Level III.*

Figueiras, A., Herdeiro, M. T., Polónia, J., & Gestal-Otero, J. (2006). An educational intervention to improve physician reporting of adverse drug reactions: A cluster-randomized controlled trial. *Journal of the American Medical Association, 296*(9), 1086–1093. *Evidence Level II.*

FitzGerald, R. J. (2009). Medication errors: The importance of an accurate drug history. *British Journal of Clinical Pharmacology, 67*(6), 671–675. *Evidence Level V.*

Fouts, M., Hanlon, J., & Pieper, C. (1997). Identification of elderly nursing facility residents at high risk for drug related problems. *Consultant Pharmacist, 12,* 1103–1111. *Evidence Level VI.*

Frankenthal, D., Lerman, Y., & Kalendaryev, E. (2014). Intervention with the screening tool of older persons potentially inappropriate prescriptions/screening tool to alert doctors to right treatment criteria in elderly residents of a chronic geriatric facility: A randomized clinical trial. *Journal of American Geriatric Society, 62*(9), 1658–1665. *Evidence Level II.*

Fried, T., Tinetti, M. E., Towle, V., Leary, J. R., & Iannone, L. (2011). Effects of benefits and harms on older persons' willingness to take medication for primary cardiovascular prevention. *Archives of Internal Medicine, 171*(10), 923–928. *Evidence Level IV.*

Gallagher, P. F., O'Connor, M. N., & O'Mahony, D. (2011). Prevention of potentially inappropriate prescribing for elderly patients: A randomized controlled trial using STOPP/START criteria. *Clinical Pharmacology and Therapeutics, 89*(6), 845. *Evidence Level II.*

Gearing, R., Townsend, L., Elkins, J., El-Bassel, N., & Osterberg, L. (2014). Strategies to predict, measure, and improve psychosocial treatment adherence. *Harvard Review of Psychiatry, 22*(1), 31–45. *Evidence Level V.*

Gellad, W. F., Grenard, J. L., & Marcum, Z. A. (2011). A systematic review of barriers to medication adherence in the elderly: Looking beyond cost and regimen complexity. *American Journal of Geriatric Pharmacotherapy, 9*(1), 11–23. *Evidence Level I.*

Gray, C., & Gardner, C. (2009). Adverse drug events in the elderly: An ongoing problem. *Journal of Managed Care Pharmacy, 15*(7), 568–571. *Evidence Level V.*

Hamilton, H., Gallagher, P., Ryan, C., Byrne, S., & Mahony, D. (2011). Potentially inappropriate medications defined by STOPP criteria and the risk of adverse drug events in older hospitalized patients. *Archives of Internal Medicine, 171*(11), 1013–1019. *Evidence Level V.*

Hayes, B. D., Klein-Schwartz, W., & Gonzales, L. F. (2009). Causes of therapeutic errors in older adults: Evaluation of national poison center data. *Journal of the American Geriatric Society, 57*(4), 653–658. *Evidence Level IV.*

Heuberger, R. (2012). Polypharmacy and food–drug interactions among older persons: A review. *Journal of Nutrition in Gerontology and Geriatrics, 31*(4), 325–403. *Evidence Level V.*

Hines, L. E., & Murphy, J. E. (2011). Potentially harmful drug–drug interactions in elderly: A review. *American Journal of Geriatric Pharmacotherapy, 9*(6), 364–377. *Evidence Level V.*

Ho, P., Bryson, C., & Rumsfeld, J. (2009). Medication adherence its importance in cardiovascular outcomes. *Circulation, 119*(23), 3028–3035. *Evidence Level VI.*

Hubbard, R. E., O'Mahoney, M. S., & Woodhouse, K. W. (2013). Medication prescribing in frail older people. *European Journal of Clinical Pharmacology, 69*(3), 319–326. *Evidence Level VI.*

Hutchison, L. C., Jones, S. K., West, D. S., & Wei, J. Y. (2006). Assessment of medication management by community-living elderly persons with two standardized assessment tools: A cross-sectional study. *American Journal of Geriatric Pharmacotherapy, 4*(2), 144–153. *Evidence Level IV.*

Institute for Healthcare Improvement. (2011). *How-to guide: Prevent adverse drug events by implementing medication reconciliation.* (2011). Cambridge, MA: Author. *Evidence Level VI.*

Izzo, A. A., & Ernst, E. (2009). Interactions between herbal medicines and prescribed drugs: An updated systematic review (report). *Drugs, 69*(13), 1777. *Evidence Level I.*

Jansen, P. A. F., & Brouwers, J. R. B. J. (2012). Clinical pharmacology in old persons. *Scientifica,* Article ID: 723678. 17 pages. doi: 10.6064/2012/723678. *Evidence Level V.*

Jarred, G., & Kennedy, R. L. (2010). Therapeutic perspective: Starting an angiotensin-converting enzyme inhibitor or angiotensin II receptor blocker in a diabetic patient. *Therapeutic Advances in Endocrinology and Metabolism, 1*(1), 23–38. *Evidence Level VI.*

Kanaan, A. O., Donovan, J. L., Duchin, N. P., Field, T. S., Tjia, J., Cutrona, S. L.,... Gurwitz, J. H. (2013). Adverse drug events after hospital discharge in older adults: Types, severity, and involvement of Beers Criteria medications. *Journal of the American Geriatrics Society, 61*(11), 1894–1899. *Evidence Level IV.*

Kongkaew, C., Hann, M., Williams, S. D., Metcalfe, D., Noyce, P. R., & Ashcroft, D. M. (2013). Risk factors for hospital admissions associated with adverse drug events. *Pharmacotherapy, 33*(8), 827–837. *Evidence Level IV.*

Kongkaew, C., Noyce, P. R., & Ashcroft, D. M. (2008). Hospital admissions associated with adverse drug reactions: A systematic review of prospective observational studies. *Annals of Pharmacotherapy, 42,* 1017–1025. *Evidence Level I.*

Lang, P. O., Vogt-Ferrier, N., Hasso, Y., Le Saint, L., Drame, M., Zekry, D.,... Michel, J. P. (2012). Interdisciplinary geriatric and psychiatric care reduces potentially inappropriate prescribing in the hospital: Interventional study in 150 acutely ill elderly patients with mental and somatic comorbid conditions. *Journal of the American Medical Directors Association, 13*(4), 406. *Evidence Level IV.*

Levinson, D. (2010). *Adverse events in hospitals: National incidence among Medicare beneficiaries.* Department of Health & Human Services. Retrieved from http://oig.hhs.gov/oei/reports/oei-06-09-00090.pdf. *Evidence Level IV.*

Lipska, K. J., & Montori, V. M. (2013). Glucose control in older adults with diabetes mellitus—More harm than good? *Journal of the American Medical Association/Internal Medicine, 173*(14), 1–2. *Evidence Level VI.*

Lipska, K. J., Ross, J. S., Miao, Y., Shah, N. D., Lee, S. J., & Steinman, M. A. (2015). Potential overtreatment of diabetes mellitus in older adults with tight glycemic control. *Journal of the American Medical Association/Internal Medicine, 175*(3), 356–362. *Evidence Level IV.*

Lopez-Gonzalez, E., Herdeiro, M. T., & Figuerias, A. (2009). Determinants of under-reporting adverse drug reactions: A systematic review. *Drug Safety, 32*(1), 19–31. *Evidence Level I.*

Lucado, A., Paez, K., & Elixhauser, A. (2008). Medication-related adverse outcomes in U.S. hospitals and emergency departments (HCUP Statistical Brief #109). Agency for Healthcare Research and Quality, Rockville, MD. *Evidence Level IV.*

Marcum, A., Driessen, J., Thorpe, C. T., Gellad, W. F., & Donohue, J. M. (2014). Effect of multiple pharmacy use on medication adherence and drug–drug interactions in older adults with Medicare Part D. *Journal of the American Geriatrics Society, 62,* 244–252. *Evidence Level IV.*

Marcum, Z. A., Pugh, M. J., Amuan, M. E., Aspinall, S. L., Handler, S. M., Ruby, C. M.,... Hanlon, J. T. (2012). Prevalence of potentially preventable unplanned hospitalizations caused by therapeutic failures and adverse drug withdrawal events among older veterans. *Journals of Gerontology. Series A, Biological Sciences and Medical Sciences, 67*(8), 867–874. *Evidence Level VI.*

McKibbon, K. A., Lokker, C., Handler, S. M., Dolovich, L. R., Holbrook, A. M., O'Reilly, D.,... Raina, P. (2011). Enabling medication management through health information technology (AHRQ Publication No. 11-E008-EF). Rockville, MD: Agency for Healthcare Research and Quality. *Evidence Level IV.*

Morisky, D., Ang, A., Krousel-Wood, M., & Ward, H. (2008). Predictive validity of a medication adherence measure in an outpatient setting. *Journal of Clinical Hypertension, 10*(5), 348–354. *Evidence Level IV.*

Nathan, A., Goodyer, L., Lovejoy, A., & Rashid, A. (1999). "Brown bag" medication reviews as a means of optimizing patients' use of medication and of identifying potential clinical problems. *Family Practice, 16*(3), 278–282. *Evidence Level IV.*

National Center for Health Statistics. (2012). *Special feature on socioeconomic status and health.* Hyattsville, MD: Centers for Disease Control and Prevention. *Evidence Level VI.*

National Coordinating Council for Medication Error Reporting and Prevention. (2015). Two decades of coordinating medication safety efforts. *American Journal of Health-System Pharmacy, 66*(24), 2152. *Evidence Level VI.*

National Institute on Drug Abuse. (2014). *Specific population and prescription drug misuse and abuse.* Bethesda, MD: Author.

Nebeker, J. R., Barach, P., & Samore, M. H. (2004). Clarifying adverse drug events: A clinician's guide to terminology, documentation, and reporting. *Annals of Internal Medicine, 140*(10), 795–801. *Evidence Level V.*

Nieuwlaat, T., Wicznski, N., Navarro, T., Hobson, N., Jeffery, R., Kepanasseril, A., & Haynes, R. B. (2014). Interventions for enhancing med adhere. *Database of Systematic Reviews* (11). *Evidence Level I.*

Noskin, M. D., & Gleason, K. (2012). Medications at Transitions and Clinical Handoffs (MATCH) Toolkit for Reconciliation. AHRQ Publication No. 11(12)-0059. P 1. Retrieved from http://www.ahrq.gov/professionals/quality-patient-safety/patient-safety-resources/resources/match/match.pdf. *Evidence Level IV.*

Nutbeam, D. (2008). The evolving concept of health literacy. *Social Science & Medicine, 67*(12), 2072–2078. *Evidence Level VI.*

Onder, G., van der Cammen, T. J. M., Petrovic, M., Somers, A., & Rajkumar, C. (2013). Strategies to reduce the risk of iatrogenic illness in complex older adults. *Age and Ageing, 42*(3), 284–291. *Evidence Level V.*

Orwig, D., Brandt, N., & Gruber-Baldini, A. L. (2006). Medication management assessment for older adults in the community. *The Gerontologist, 46*(5), 661–668. *Evidence Level IV.*

Parchman, M. L., Zeber, J. E., & Palmer, R. (2010). Participatory decision making, patient activation, medication adherence, and intermediate clinical outcomes in type 2 diabetes: A STARNet study. *Annals of Family Medicine, 8*(5), 410–417. doi:10.1370/afm.1161. *Evidence Level V.*

Petrovic, M., van der Cammen, T., & Onder, G. (2012). Adverse drug reactions in older people: Detection and prevention. *Drugs & Aging, 29*(6), 453. *Evidence Level V.*

Pugh, M., Marcum, Z., Copeland, L., Mortensen, E., Zeber, J., Noel, P.,... Hanlon, J. (2013). The quality of quality measures: HEDISA (R) quality measures for medication management in the elderly and outcomes associated with new exposure. *Drugs & Aging, 30*(8), 645–654. doi:10.1007/s40266–013-0086–8. *Evidence Level IV.*

Qato, D. M., Alexander, G. C., Johnson, M., Conti, R. M., Schumm, P., & Lindau, S. T. (2008). Use of prescription and over-the-counter medications and dietary supplements among older adults in the United States (clinical report). *Journal of the American Medical Association, 300*(24), 2862–2878. *Evidence Level III.*

Reine, P. A., Kongsgaard, U. E., Andersen, A., Thøgersen, A. K., & Olsen, H. (2010). Infusions of albumin increase free fraction of naproxen in healthy volunteers: A randomized crossover study. *Acta Anaesthesiologica Scandinavica, 54*(4), 430–434. doi:10.1111/j.1399–6576.2009.02142. *Evidence Level II.*

Roberts, A. W., Crisp, G. D., Esserman, D. A., Roth, M. T., Weinberger, M., & Farley, J. F. (2014). Patterns of medication adherence and health care utilization among patients with chronic disease who were enrolled in a pharmacy assistance program. *North Carolina Medical Journal, 75*(5), 310. *Evidence Level IV.*

Rochon, P. (2014). *Drug prescribing in older adults.* Retrieved from http://www.uptodate.com/contents/drug-prescribing-for-older-adults. *Evidence Level V.*

Rochon, P. A., & Gurwitz, J. (1997). Optimising drug treatment for elderly people: The prescribing cascade. *British Medical Journal, 315*(7115), 1096–1099. *Evidence Level V.*

Rogers, S., Wilson, D., Wan, S., Griffin, M., Rai, G., & Farrell, J. (2009). Medication-related admissions in older people: A cross-sectional, observational study. *Drugs & Aging, 26*(11), 951–961. *Evidence Level IV.*

Ruscin, J. M., & Linnebur, S. A. (2014). *Drug-related problems in the elderly.* Whitehouse Station, NJ: Merck Research Laboratories. *Evidence Level VI.*

Ryan, R., Santesso, N., Lowe, D., Hill, S., Grimshaw, J., Prictor, M., . . . Taylor, M. (2014). Interventions to improve safe and effective medicines use by consumers: An overview of systematic reviews. *The Cochrane Database of Systematic Reviews, 4*, CD007768. doi: 10.1002/14651858.CD007768.pub3

Salvi, F., Marchetti, A., D'Angelo, F., Boemi, M., Lattanzio, F., & Cherubini, A. (2012). Adverse drug events as a cause of hospitalization in older adults. *Drugs & Aging, 35*(Suppl. 1), 29–45. *Evidence Level I.*

Sansgiry, S. S., Nadkarni, A., & Doan, T. (2011). Misuse of over-the-counter medications among community-dwelling older adults and associated adverse drug events. *Journal of Pharmaceutical Health Services Research, 1*(4), 175–179. doi:10.1111/j.1759–8893.2010.00032.x. *Evidence Level IV.*

Schmiedl, S., Rottenkolber, M., Hasford, J., Rottenkolber, D., Farker, K., Drewelow, B.,... Thürmann, P. (2014). Self-medication with over-the-counter and prescribed drugs causing adverse drug reaction-related hospital admissions: Results of a prospective, long-term multi-centre study. *Drug Safety, 37*(4), 225–235. doi:10.1007/s40264–014-0141–3. *Evidence Level IV.*

Spinewine, A., Fialová, D., & Byrne, S. (2012). The role of the pharmacist in optimizing pharmacotherapy in older people. *Drugs & Aging, 29*, 495–510. *Evidence Level I.*

Steinman, M. A., Handler, S. M., Gurwitz, J., Schiff, G., & Covinsky, K. E. (2011). Beyond the prescriptions: Medication monitoring and adverse drug events in older adults. *Journal of the American Geriatrics Society, 59*(8), 1513–1520. doi:10.1111/j.1532–5415.2011.03500.x. *Evidence Level IV.*

Steinman, M. A., & Hanlon, J. T. (2010). Managing medications in clinically complex elders: There's got to be a happy medium. *Journal of the American Medical Association, 304*(14), 1592–1601. *Evidence Level I.*

Steinman, M. A., & Holmes, H. M. (2014). Principles of prescribing in older adults. In B. A. Williams, A. Chang, C. Ahalt, H. Chen, R. Conant,... M. Yukawa (Eds.), *Current diagnosis & treatment: Geriatrics* (2nd ed.). Retrieved from http://accessmedicine.mhmedical.com/content.aspx?bookid=953§ionId=53375631. *Evidence Level VI.*

Svarstad, B. L., Chewning, B. A., Sleath, B. L., & Claesson, C. (1999). The brief medication questionnaire: A tool for screening patient adherence and barriers to adherence. *Patient Education and Counseling, 37*(2), 113–124. doi:10.1016/S0738–3991(98)00107–4. *Evidence Level IV.*

Tachjian, A., Maria, V., & Jahangir, A. (2010). Use of herbal products and potential interactions in patients with cardiovascular disease. *Journal of American Cardiology, 55*(6), 516–525. doi:10.1016/j.jacc.2009.07.074. *Evidence Level V.*

Terrell, K. M., Heard, K., & Miller, D. K. (2006). Prescribing to older ED patients. *American Journal of Emergency Medicine, 24*(4), 468–478. *Evidence Level V.*

The Joint Commission. (2010). *National patient safety goals*. Retrieved from http://www.jointcommission.org. *Evidence Level VI.*

Topinková, E., Baeyens, J., Michel, J.-P., & Lang, P.-O. (2012). Evidence based strategies for optimization of pharmacotherapy in older people. *Drugs & Aging, 29*(6), 477–494. *Evidence Level I.*

Turner, E. H., Matthews, A. M., Linardatos, E., Tell, R. A., & Rosenthal, R. (2008). Selective publication of antidepressant trials and its influence on apparent efficacy. *New England Journal of Medicine, 358*(3), 252–260. *Evidence Level I.*

Vervloet, M., Linn, A., van Weert, J., de Bakker, D., Bouvy, M., & van Dijk, L. (2012). The effectiveness of interventions using electronic reminders to improve adherence to chronic medication: A systematic review of the literature. *Journal of the American Medical Informatics Association, 19,* 696–704. *Evidence Level I.*

Viswanathan, M., Golin, C. E., Jones, C. D., Ashok, M., Blalock, S. J., Wines, R. C. M., . . . Lohr, K. N. (2012). Interventions to improve adherence to self-administered medications for chronic diseases in the United States: A systematic review (report; author abstract). *Annals of Internal Medicine, 157*(11), 785. *Evidence Level I.*

Volkow, N. D. (2010). National Institute on Drug Abuse National Institutes of Health Department of Health and Human Services. Retrieved from https://www.drugabuse.gov/about-nida/legislative-activities/testimony-to-congress/2010/09/prescription-drug-abuse. *Evidence Level VI.*

World Health Organization. (1972). International drug monitoring: The role of national centres. In T. S. Series (Ed.), *Report of a WHO meeting* (vol. 49, pp. 1–25). Geneva, Switzerland: Author. *Evidence Level V.*

World Health Organization. (2002). *Safety of medicines: A guide to detecting and reporting adverse drug reactions*. Geneva, Switzerland, Author. *Evidence Level VI.*

World Health Organization. (2003). *Adherence to long term therapies: Evidence for action*. Geneva, Switzerland: Author. *Evidence Level V.*

Zakrzewski-Jakubiak, H., Doan, J., Lamoureux, P., Singh, D., Turgeon, J., & Tannenbaum, C. (2011). Detection and prevention of drug–drug interactions in the hospitalized. *American Journal of Geriatric Pharmacotherapy, 9*(6), 461–470. *Evidence Level IV.*

Zwicker, D., & Fletcher, K. (2009). *Evidence based nonpharmacologic interventions for agitation*. Retrieved from http://www.consultgerirn.org. *Evidence Level V.*

21

Urinary Incontinence

Annemarie Dowling-Castronovo and Christine Bradway

EDUCATIONAL OBJECTIVES

On completion of this chapter, the reader should be able to:

1. Discuss transient and established etiologies of urinary incontinence (UI)
2. Describe the core components of a nursing assessment for UI in hospitalized older adults
3. Discuss the importance of nurse collaboration within the interprofessional team in an effort to best assess and document the type of UI
4. Develop an individualized plan of care for an older adult with UI

OVERVIEW

Despite evidence supporting UI management strategies (DuBeau, Kuchel, Johnson, Palmer, & Wagg, 2010; Fantl et al., 1996; Qaseem et al., 2014), nursing staff and laypersons often use containment strategies, such as adult briefs or other absorbent products, to manage UI. Individuals with UI believe that UI is a normal consequence of aging (Bush, Castellucci, & Phillips, 2001; Dowd, 1991; Kinchen et al., 2003; Milne, 2000; Mitteness, 1987a, 1987b), feel that UI is a difficult-to-discuss personal problem (Bush et al., 2001), and prefer self-help strategies, including containment, rather than seeking professional advice (Milne, 2000). Personal care strategies are often the result of information gained through lay media and personal contacts, not necessarily from health care professionals (Cochran, 2000; Miller, Brown, Smith, & Chiarelli, 2003; Milne, 2000). In comparison to nurses in other health care settings, nurses in hospitals view incontinent patients more negatively (Vinsnes, Harkless, Haltbakk, Bohm, & Hunskaar, 2001). Therefore, attitudes and beliefs regarding UI are important for the nurse to consider in an effort to best assess and manage UI.

BACKGROUND AND STATEMENT OF PROBLEM

UI affects more than 17 million adults in the United States and is most often defined as the involuntary loss of urine sufficient to be a problem (Fantl et al., 1996; National Association for Continence, 1998). Prevalence and incidence rates of UI are viewed cautiously because of inconsistencies with definitions and measurements of both these epidemiological statistics. In addition, variable or poorly articulated UI definitions (Abrams et al., 2003; Homma, 2008; Palmer, 1988) as well as underreporting and underassessment of UI (Schultz, Dickey, & Skoner, 1997) in the hospital setting can render data of questionable reliability.

For a description of evidence levels cited in this chapter, see Chapter 1, "Developing and Evaluating Clinical Practice Guidelines: A Systematic Approach."

Prevalence of UI in community-dwelling adult populations ranges from 8% to 46% (Du Moulin, Hamers, Ambergen, Janssen, & Halfens, 2008; Kwong et al., 2010; Lee, Cigolle, & Blaum, 2009; Sims, Browning, Lundgren-Lindquist, & Kendig, 2011). For individuals with dementia, UI prevalence rates range from 11% to 90%; higher prevalence rates reflect institutionalized cognitively impaired older adults (Brandeis, Baumann, Hossain, Morris, & Resnick, 1997; Skelly & Flint, 1995). Although the highest prevalence rate occurs in institutionalized older adults, 15% to 53% of homebound older adults and 10% to 42% of older adults admitted to acute care also suffer from UI (Dowd & Campbell, 1995; Fantl et al., 1996; McDowell et al., 1999; Palmer, Bone, Fahey, Mamon, & Steinwachs, 1992; Schultz et al., 1997). Twelve percent to 36% of older hospitalized adults develop acute UI (e.g., new-onset UI, meaning that these individuals were continent on hospital admission) (Kresevic, 1997; Sier, Ouslander, & Orzeck, 1987; Zisberg, 2011); for patients undergoing hip surgery, the incidence of acute UI ranges from 19% to 32% (Palmer, Baumgarten, Langenberg, & Carson, 2002; Palmer, Myers, & Fedenko, 1997).

In addition to being a common geriatric syndrome, UI significantly affects health-related quality of life (HRQOL; DuBeau, Simon, & Morris, 2006; Dugger, 2010; Kwong et al., 2010; Shumaker, Wyman, Uebersax, McClish, & Fantl, 1994). The consequences of UI may be characterized physically, psychosocially, and economically. For example, an episode of urge UI occurring once weekly, or more frequently, has been associated with falls or fracture (Brown, Sawaya, Thom, & Grady, 2000; Chiarelli, Mackenzie, & Osmotherly, 2009; Hasegawa, Kuzuya, & Iguchi, 2010). Other physical consequences associated with UI include skin irritations or infections, urinary tract infections (UTIs), bloodstream infections, pressure ulcers, and limitation of functional status (Fantl et al., 1996). UI is associated with psychological distress (Bogner et al., 2002; de Vries, Northington, & Bogner, 2012), including depression, poor self-rated health, and social isolation or condition-specific functional loss (Bogner et al., 2002; Fantl et al., 1996; Sims et al., 2011), and poststroke UI is a risk factor for poor outcomes (Pettersen, Saxby, & Wyller, 2007). Therefore, it is essential that nurses assess and treat UI when addressing other health problems such as depression or falls.

Although there is conflicting evidence regarding the role of UI as a predictor for nursing home placement, UI has been identified as a marker of frailty in community-dwelling older adults (Holroyd-Leduc, Mehta, & Covinsky, 2004) and a predictor of 1-year mortality among older adults hospitalized for an acute myocardial infarction (Krumholz, Chen, Chen, Wang, & Radford, 2001). The negative psychosocial impact of UI affects not only the individual but also family caregivers (CGs; Brittain & Shaw, 2007; Cassells & Watt, 2003; Gotoh et al., 2009; Jansen, McWilliam, Forbes, & Forchuk, 2013). Economically, the total direct cost for all incontinent individuals is estimated to be more than $16 billion annually in the United States (Landefeld et al., 2008; Wilson, Brown, Shin, Luc, & Subak, 2001).

Nurses are in a key position to identify and treat UI, a quality indicator (Donald et al., 2013; Wenger et al., 2011), in hospitalized older adults. This chapter reviews the etiologies and consequences of UI, with emphasis on the most common types of UI encountered in the acute care setting. Assessment parameters and care strategies for UI are highlighted and a nursing standard-of-practice protocol focused on comprehensive assessment and management of UI for hospitalized older adults is included.

ASSESSMENT OF THE PROBLEM

Adverse physiological consequences of UI commonly encountered in acute care settings include an increased potential for UTIs and indwelling urinary catheter use, dermatitis, skin infections, and pressure ulcers (Sier, Ouslander, & Orzeck, 1987). Moreover, UI that results in functional decline predisposes older individuals to complications associated with bed rest and immobility (Harper & Lyles, 1988).

Etiologies of UI

Continence is a complex, multidimensional phenomenon influenced by anatomical, physiological, psychological, and cultural factors (Gray, 2000). Thus, continence requires intact lower urinary tract function, as well as cognitive and functional ability to recognize voiding signals and use a toilet or commode, the motivation to maintain continence, and an environment that facilitates the process (Jirovec, Brink, & Wells, 1988). Physiologically, continence is a result of urethral pressure being equal to or greater than bladder pressure (Hodgkinson, 1965), of which angulation of the urethra, supported by pelvic muscles, plays a role (DeLancey, 1994, 2010). Continence also requires the ability to suppress autocontractility of the detrusor (Hodgkinson, 1965). Micturition (urination) involves voluntary as well as reflexive control of the bladder, urethra, detrusor muscle, and urethral sphincter. When the bladder volume reaches approximately 400 mL, stretch receptors in the bladder wall send a message to the brain and an impulse for voiding is sent back to the bladder. The detrusor muscle then contracts and the urethral sphincter relaxes to allow urination (Gray, Rayome, & Moore, 1995). Normally, the micturition reflex can be voluntarily inhibited (at least for a time) until an individual desires to void or finds an appropriate place for voiding. UI occurs as the result of a disruption at any point during this process. For a comprehensive review, Gray (2000) provided a detailed analysis of voiding physiology. Common age-associated changes, including a decrease in bladder capacity, benign prostatic hyperplasia (BPH) in men, and menopausal loss of estrogen in women, can affect lower urinary tract function and predispose older individuals to UI (Bradway & Yetman, 2002). Despite these aging changes, UI is not considered a normal consequence of aging.

The two major types of UI are transient (or acute/reversible) and established (or chronic/persistent; Ermer-Seltun, 2006; Newman & Wein, 2009). Transient UI is characterized by the sudden onset of potentially reversible symptoms that typically has a duration of less than 6 months (Specht, 2005). There may be cases of acute UI that do not resolve as in the case of acute UI caused by a spinal cord injury that then becomes an established UI. Causes of transient UI include delirium, infections (e.g., untreated UTI), atrophic vaginitis, urethritis, pharmaceuticals, depression, or other psychological disorders that affect motivation or function, excessive urine production, restricted mobility, and stool impaction or constipation (e.g., creates additional pressure on the bladder and can cause urinary urgency and frequency). Hospitalized older adults are at risk of developing transient UI. In the literature, these cases have been referred to as new-onset UI, hospital nosocomial, and hospital acquired (Ding & Jayaratnam, 1994; Kresevic, 1997; Paillard & Resnick, 1981; Palmer et al., 1997, 2002). Complicated by shorter hospital stays, older adults may also be at risk of being discharged without resolution of transient UI and, thus, urine leakage persists and may become established UI. However, transient UI is often preventable, or at least reversible (e.g., transient UI precipitated by a UTI that resolves with successful treatment, or acute UI related to diuretic therapy for heart failure exacerbation), if the underlying cause for the UI is identified and treated (Ding & Jayaratnam, 1994; Fantl et al., 1996; Palmer, 1996).

Kresevic (1997) reported that hospitalized older adults with new-onset UI were more likely to be on bed rest, restrained, depressed, dehydrated, malnourished, and dependent in ambulation when compared with their continent counterparts. Furthermore, the relative risk of developing new-onset UI was twofold for older adults with depression (odds ratio [OR] = 2.28), malnutrition (OR = 2.29), and dependent ambulation (OR = 2.55). Study participants identified that being able to walk, having use of a bedpan or commode, and nursing assistance fostered continence (Kresevic, 1997). Likewise, Palmer et al. (2002) determined that in addition to mobility dependency, other risk factors for new-onset UI, specific to a hip-fracture population, included institutionalization prior to hospitalization, the presence of confusion (identified by a retrospective chart review) preceding hip fracture, and being an African American woman. In addition to cognitive impairment, the use of indwelling urinary catheters and adult diapers statistically increased the odds of hospitalized older adults experiencing new-onset UI in a hospital in Israel (Zisberg, 2011).

Established UI has either a sudden or gradual onset and is often present prior to hospital admission; however, health care providers or family CGs may first identify UI during the course of an acute illness, hospitalization, or abrupt change in environment or daily routine (Palmer, 1996). Types of established UI include stress, urge, mixed, overflow, and functional UI.

Stress UI is defined as an involuntary loss of urine associated with activities that increase intra-abdominal pressure. Symptomatically, individuals with stress UI usually present with complaints of small amounts of daytime urine loss that occurs during physical effort or exertion (e.g., position change, coughing, sneezing) that result in increased intra-abdominal pressure. Stress UI is more common in women; however, stress UI may also occur in men postprostatectomy (Abrams et al., 2003; Fantl et al., 1996; Hunter, Moore, Cody, & Glazener, 2004; Jayasekara, 2009).

Urge UI is characterized by an involuntary urine loss associated with a strong desire to void (urgency). Individuals with urge UI often complain of being unable to hold the urge to urinate and leak on the way to the bathroom. This history is most helpful to the identification of urge UI (Holroyd-Leduc, Tannenbaum, Thorpe, & Straus, 2008). In addition to urinary urgency, signs and symptoms of urge UI most often include urinary frequency, nocturia and enuresis, and UI of moderate to large amounts. Bladder changes common in aging make older adults particularly prone to this type of UI (Abrams et al., 2003; Fantl et al., 1996; Jayasekara, 2009). Individuals with overactive bladder (OAB) may complain of urgency, with or without UI, as well as urinary frequency and nocturia. Assessment should focus on pathological or metabolic conditions that may explain these symptoms (Abrams et al., 2003).

Mixed UI is defined as involuntary urine loss as a result of both increased intra-abdominal pressure and detrusor instability (Fantl et al., 1996; Jayasekara, 2009). On history, individuals describe symptoms of stress UI in combination with symptoms of urge UI and OAB.

Overflow UI is an involuntary loss of urine associated with overdistention of the bladder, and may be caused by an underactive detrusor muscle or outlet obstruction leading to overdistention of the bladder and leakage of urine. Individuals with overflow UI often describe dribbling, urinary retention or hesitancy, urine loss without a recognizable urge, an uncomfortable sensation of fullness or pressure in the lower abdomen, and incomplete bladder emptying. Clinically, suprapubic palpation may reveal a distended or painful bladder as a result of urine retention, which may be acute or chronic. A common condition associated with this type of UI is BPH. Neurological conditions, such as multiple sclerosis and spinal cord injuries, or diabetes mellitus, which result in bladder muscle denervation, may also cause overflow UI (Abrams et al., 2003; Doughty, 2000; Fantl et al., 1996; Jayasekara, 2009).

Functional UI is caused by nongenitourinary factors, such as cognitive or physical impairments, that result in an inability for the individual to be independent in voiding. For example, acutely ill hospitalized individuals may be challenged by a combination of an acute illness and environmental changes. This, in turn, makes the voiding process even more complex, resulting in a functional type of UI (Fantl et al., 1996; Hodgkinson, Synnott, Josephs, Leira, & Hegney, 2008).

ASSESSMENT PARAMETERS

It is essential to ask patients about the presence of UI because they often will not offer this information or seek professional care (Qaseem et al., 2014). Nurse continence experts suggest that entry-level nurses demonstrate the ability to collect and organize data surrounding urine control and implement nursing interventions that promote continence (Jirovec, Wyman, & Wells, 1998). Nurses play a critical role in the basic assessment and management of UI in hospitalized older adults. Because UI is an interprofessional issue, collaboration with other members of the health care team is essential. It is not sufficient for nurses to only identify and document the presence of UI. Instead, the type of UI should be determined and documented based on a careful history and focused assessment; urodynamic tests are not required as part of the initial assessment of UI (DuBeau et al., 2010). Basic history and examination techniques are presented here to assist the nurse in identifying the type of UI along with a nursing standard of practice protocol (see Protocol 21.1 to guide UI assessment and management).

History

When a patient is admitted to the hospital, nursing history should include questions to determine whether the individual has preexisting UI or risk factors (Table 21.1) for UI. The nurse should be alert for the following UI-associated risk factors specific to the hospital setting: depression, malnourishment, dependent ambulation, being a resident of a long-term care institution, confusion, and being an African American woman (Kresevic, 1997; Palmer et al., 2002). Therefore, the nurse should screen for depression, determine body mass index (BMI), monitor albumin and total protein levels if available, consult with a dietitian, and perform a validated assessment of both cognitive and functional status.

The nurse should include screening questions for all older adult patients, such as Have you ever leaked urine? If yes, how much does it bother you? Although not validated in the hospital setting, examples of screening instruments used in other settings include the Urinary Distress Inventory-6 (UDI-6) and the Male Urinary Distress Inventory (MUDI). The UDI-6 is a self-report symptom inventory for UI that is reliable and valid for identifying the degree of bother and type of established UI in community-dwelling females (Lemack & Zimmern, 1999; Uebersax, Wyman, Shumaker, McClish, & Fantl, 1995). The MUDI is a valid and reliable measure of urinary symptoms in the male population (Robinson & Shea, 2002). Determining the degree of "bother" and the effect on HRQOL is important and should include the perspective of both the patient and CG or significant other. Various instruments for quantifying bother and HRQOL exist (Abrams et al., 2003; Bradway, 2003; Robinson & Shea, 2002; Shumaker et al., 1994).

Historical questions should focus on the characteristics of UI: time of onset, frequency, and severity of the problem. Questions also should review past health history and address possible precipitants of UI such as coughing, uncontrollable urinary urgency, functional decline, and acute illness (e.g., UTI, hip fracture). Nurses should inquire about lower urinary tract symptoms, such as nocturia, hematuria, and urinary hesitancy, as well as current management strategies for UI. The presence and rationale for an indwelling urinary catheter should be documented (see Chapter 22, "Prevention of Catheter-Associated Urinary Tract Infection").

A bladder diary or voiding record is recommended as a tool for obtaining objective information about the patient's voiding pattern, incontinent episodes, and UI severity (Lau, 2009). There are numerous voiding records

TABLE 21.1
Risk Factors Associated With Urinary Incontinence

Age (Hodgkinson et al., 2008; Holroyd-Leduc et al., 2004; Shamliyan, Wyman, Bliss, Kane, & Wilt, 2007)	Low fluid intake (Fantl et al., 1996)
Caffeine intake (Holroyd-Leduc et al., 2004)	Environmental barriers (Fantl et al., 1996; Offermans, Du Moulin, Hamers, Dassen, & Halfens, 2009)
Immobility/functional limitations (Fantl et al., 1996; Holroyd-Leduc & Straus, 2004; Kresevic, 1997; Offermans et al., 2009; Palmer, Baumgarten, Langenberg, & Carson, 2002; Shamliyan et al., 2007)	High-impact physical activities (Fantl et al., 1996)
Impaired cognition (Fantl et al., 1996; Palmer et al., 2002; Shamliyan et al., 2007)	Diabetes mellitus (Fantl et al., 1996; Holroyd-Leduc & Straus., 2004; Shamliyan et al., 2007)
Medications (Fantl et al., 1996; Newman & Wein, 2009; Offermans et al., 2009)	Parkinson's disease (Holroyd-Leduc & Straus, 2004; Vaughan et al., 2011)
Obesity (Fantl et al., 1996; Subak et al., 2005; Subak, Richter, & Hunskaar, 2009)	Stroke (Fantl et al., 1996; Holroyd-Leduc & Straus, 2004; Meijer et al., 2003; Shamliyan et al., 2007; Thomas et al., 2005)
Diuretics (Fantl et al., 1996)	Chronic obstructive pulmonary disease (Dowling-Castronovo, 2004; Holroyd-Leduc & Straus, 2004)
Smoking (Fantl et al., 1996)	Estrogen depletion (Fantl et al., 1996; Holroyd-Leduc & Straus, 2004)
Fecal impaction; fecal incontinence (Fantl et al., 1996; Offermans et al., 2009)	Pelvic organ prolapse (Shamliyan et al., 2007)
Malnutrition (Kresevic, 1997)	Pelvic muscle weakness (DeLancey, 1994; Fantl et al., 1996; Holroyd-Leduc & Straus, 2004; Kegel, 1956)
Depression (Kresevic, 1997)	Childhood nocturnal enuresis (Fantl et al., 1996)
Delirium (Fantl et al., 1996; Offermans et al., 2009)	Race (Fantl et al., 1996; Holroyd-Leduc et al., 2004; Palmer et al., 2002)
Pregnancy/vaginal delivery/episiotomy (DeLancey, 2010; Fantl et al., 1996; Holroyd-Leduc & Straus, 2004; Nygaard, 2006; Shamliyan et al., 2007)	Institutionalization prior to hospitalization (Palmer et al., 2002)
Treatment of prostate cancer, including radical prostatectomy and radiation therapy (Hunter et al., 2004; Shamliyan et al., 2007)	Arthritis and/or back problems (Holroyd-Leduc & Straus, 2004)
Hearing and/or visual impairment (Holroyd-Leduc & Straus, 2004)	

available; for example, visit consultgerirn.org/resources. Although the 7-day voiding record is the most evaluated and recommended tool used to quantify UI and identify activities associated with unwanted urine loss (Jeyaseelan, Roe, & Oldham, 2000), a 3-day voiding record has been recommended as more feasible in outpatient and long-term care settings (DuBeau et al., 2010; Fantl et al., 1996). A voiding record completed for even 1 day may help identify patients with bladder dysfunction or those requiring further referral. Advanced practice nurses or urologic/continence specialists can assist nursing staff with interpretation and offer suggestions regarding nursing interventions based on information from the voiding record.

Comprehensive Assessment

A wide variety of medications can adversely affect continence. Diuretics are the most commonly known class of medications that contribute to UI caused by polyuria, frequency, and urgency. Medications with anticholinergic and antispasmodic properties may cause mental status changes, urinary retention with or without overflow incontinence, and stool impaction. Various psychotropic medications (e.g., tricyclic antidepressants, antipsychotics, sedative-hypnotics) have anticholinergic effects, contribute to immobility, and cause sedation and possibly delirium—each of which negatively affects bladder control. Alpha-adrenergic blockers may cause urethral relaxation, whereas alpha-adrenergic agonists may cause urinary retention. Calcium channel blockers also may cause urinary retention (Newman & Wein, 2009).

Nurses should document all over-the-counter, herbal, and prescription medications on admission. In addition, nurses must closely scrutinize new medications as possible causes if UI suddenly develops during the patient's hospital stay. Medications that may contribute to iatrogenic (i.e., hospital caused) UI include diuretics and sedative-hypnotics. Essentially, when a hospitalized patient develops transient UI, the nurse must ask the question: Could a new medication be affecting this patient's bladder control? If the answer is yes, then the nurse reviews this finding with the prescribing practitioner to learn whether the contributing medication may be discontinued or modified. Although studies demonstrate that older women respond to pharmacological treatment for urgency UI and/or OAB, when these medications, specifically trospium, are included as part of a drug regimen of greater than seven total medications, there is a higher likelihood of adverse effects (Qaseem et al., 2014).

Important components of a comprehensive examination include abdominal, genital, rectal, and skin examinations. In particular, the abdominal examination should assess for suprapubic distention indicative of urinary retention. Inspection of male and female genitalia can be completed during bathing or as part of the skin assessment. Postmenopausal women are especially prone to atrophic vaginitis. Significant findings for atrophic vaginitis include perineal inflammation; tenderness (and, on occasion, trauma as a result of touch); and thin, pale genital tissues. During the genital examination, female patients should be instructed to cough or perform the Valsalva maneuver (sometimes referred to as a bladder stress test) to determine whether there is urine leakage caused by increased intra-abdominal pressure, which may be attributed to stress UI (Burns, 2000; Holroyd-Leduc et al., 2008).

Digital rectal and skin examinations are essential in identifying transient causes of UI such as constipation, fecal impaction, and the presence of fungal rashes. The "anal wink" (contraction of the external anal sphincter) indicates intact sacral nerve innervation and is assessed by lightly stroking the circumanal skin. Absence of the anal wink may suggest sphincter denervation (Burns, 2000) and risk of stress UI. In men, the prostate gland should be palpated during the rectal examination because BPH may contribute to urge or overflow UI. A normal prostate gland is symmetrically heart shaped, about the size of a large chestnut, and often described as "rubbery" or similar to the tip of the nose. When enlarged, as with BPH, the examiner may palpate symmetrical enlargement. Pain on palpation or asymmetrical borders may be indicative of prostatitis or prostate cancer, respectively (Gray & Haas, 2000).

TABLE 21.2
Postvoid Residual

Instruct the patient to void. Postvoid (ideally within 15 minutes or less), measure the residual urine remaining in the bladder by either:

- Bladder sonography (scan): Noninvasive ultrasound of the suprapubic area identifies the residual amount of urine
- Sterile catheterization

A PVR of greater than 100 mL or 20% of the voided volume is considered abnormal and requires further evaluation by a urology specialist.

PVR, postvoid residual.

Sources: Diokno, Laijness, and Griebling (2014); Dorsher and McIntosh (2012); Shinopulos (2000).

In some cases, diagnostic testing may provide additional information. The most common diagnostic tests include urinalysis, urine culture and sensitivity, and postvoid residual (PVR) urine (Dubeau et al., 2010). Urinalysis and urine cultures are used to identify the presence of a UTI and bacterial agent responsible, which may contribute to acute UI. A measurement of PVR may reveal incomplete bladder emptying. Two methods for accurately evaluating PVR are bladder sonography and sterile catheter insertion after the patient has voided (Table 21.2). In addition, in some patients, it may be useful to determine optimal bladder volume, which in one study was defined as the sum of the voided volume plus the PVR (Iwatsubo, Suzuki, Igawa, & Homma, 2014).

An additional diagnostic test, such as a simple bedside urodynamic test, which provides information regarding detrusor activity, may be warranted in some cases (Burns, 2000; Lenherr & Clemens, 2013; Newman & Wein, 2009). A simple bedside urodynamic test is most likely to be performed by an advanced practice nurse or physician. It is done after a PVR has been performed and measured via the sterile catheterization method. After the bladder is emptied, the catheter is maintained in the bladder, and a 50-mL syringe (without plunger) is connected to the catheter, with the center of the syringe in alignment with the symphysis pubis. Sterile water is then instilled to fill the bladder. The fluid level is monitored for evidence of bladder contractions, which are reflected in movement of the fluid level.

Functional, environmental, psychosocial, and mental status assessments are essential components of the UI evaluation in older adults. The nurse should observe the patient voiding, assess mobility, note any use of assistive devices, and identify any obstacles that interfere with appropriate use of toilets or toilet substitutes such as a bedside commode.

INTERVENTIONS AND CARE STRATEGIES

Evidence demonstrates that hospital nurses lack the knowledge necessary for evidence-based incontinence care (Coffey, McCarthy, McCormack, Wright, & Slater, 2007; Connor & Kooker, 1996; Cassells & Watt, 2003); therefore, adapting this UI protocol for the acute care environment includes staff education. A brief, unit-based in-service followed by patient rounds may be instrumental in identifying patients at risk for UI and those actually experiencing UI. The North American Nursing Diagnosis Association (NANDA), Nursing Interventions Classification (NIC), and Nursing Outcomes Classification (NOC) provide structure for planning and evaluating UI assessment and management (Johnson, Bulechek, McCloskey-Dochterman, Maas, & Moorhead, 2001). However, there is no structured guidance for the assessment and management of transient UI. Nurses are likely to be the first to identify, and perhaps prevent, transient UI; more research is needed to understand the role nurses play in preventing UI (Sampselle, Palmer, Boyington, O'Dell, & Wooldridge, 2004).

Treating Transient and Functional Causes of UI

First, transient causes of UI should be investigated, identified, and treated. Individuals with a history of established UI should have usual voiding routines and continence strategies immediately incorporated into the acute care plan, whenever possible. Nurses play an essential role in the initiation of discharge planning and patient or CG teaching regarding all aspects of UI. Teaching and discharge planning should begin at admission as appropriate, reviewed continually, and revised as necessary.

The environment is vital in managing UI, particularly functional UI. Incontinent older adults are often dependent on adaptive devices (e.g., walker), family CGs, and hospital staff for assistance with voiding, making them "dependently continent." Call bells should be identified and within easy reach. If limited mobility is anticipated, nursing staff should consider using an elevated toilet or commode seat, male or female urinal, or bedpan. Nurses should obtain referrals to physical and occupational therapy for ambulation aids, gait training, further assessment of activities of daily living associated with continence, and improved muscle strength. Physical and chemical restraints should be avoided, including side rails (see Case Study). Patients should be encouraged and assisted to void before leaving the unit for tests or therapy (Fantl et al., 1996; Jirovec, 2000; Jirovec et al., 1988; Palmer, 1996). Incorporation of an exercise program with support from physical therapists in nursing homes improved UI (Ouslander et al., 2005). In the hospital setting, patients describe worrying about having an "accident" in the therapy gym and request "diapers" for fear of being sent back to the nursing unit if they "wet themselves" or asking the therapists for assistance to use the bathroom during a therapy session (Dowling-Castronovo, 2014). A better understanding of the role of therapists, both occupational and physical, in an acute care continence promotion program is needed.

Toileting programs (e.g., individualized, scheduled toileting programs, including timed voiding; prompted voiding) have varied success rates (Colling, Ouslander, Hadley, Eisch, & Campbell, 1992; Eustice, Roe, & Paterson, 2000; Ostaszkiewicz, Johnston, & Roe, 2004; Rathnayake, 2009c). In contrast to hospitalized older adults, hospital nurses in one study reported preferring toileting programs over containment strategies, but this has not been explored further (Pfisterer, Johnson, Jenetzky, Hauer, & Oster, 2007). Timed voiding has been promoted as a strategy for managing UI in individuals who are not cognitively or physically able to participate in independent toileting (Rathnayake, 2009c). A voiding record is essential for developing an individualized, scheduled toileting or timed voiding program, which mimics the patient's normal voiding patterns and requires continual assessment and reevaluation for successful outcomes. For example, if the initial scheduled toileting time is set for 8:00 a.m., yet, at 6:30 a.m., the patient consistently attempts to independently void or is noted to be incontinent, then the toileting time should be adjusted to 6:00 a.m. Evidence is lacking regarding the effectiveness of timed voiding as a primary management strategy for UI; however, it may be used based on the nurse's judgment of the clinical situation (Rathnayake, 2009c).

Prompted voiding requires someone (nurse or the family CG) to ask whether the patient needs to void, offer assistance, and then offer praise for successful voiding (Eustice et al., 2000; Jirovec, 2000; Ostaszkiewicz et al., 2004). In nursing home residents with UI, prompted voiding may achieve short-term improvement in daytime UI and may be effective in reducing UI in cognitively intact older adults (Hodgkinson et al., 2008; Rathnayake, 2009b). Among hospitalized older adults in Japan, a prompted voiding program resulted in patients expressing a need to void, improvement in their ability to successfully void, and a decrease in the use of absorbent products (Iwatsubo et al., 2014).

The role of the family CG, such as spouses and children, needs to be explored in the acute care setting

(Dowling-Castronovo, 2014). In the home care setting, evidence suggests that these CGs may provide better consistency with the implementation of healthy bladder behavior skills (HBBS) than paid CGs (Egnatios, Dupree, & Williams, 2010). Moreover, a mutual learning process regarding management of UI (as well as other health problems) occurs when older adults with UI, their family CGs, nurses, and nursing aides interact (Jansen et al., 2013). In both home care and hospital settings, older adults attempt to build connections with nursing staff to meet their bladder needs (Dowling-Castronovo, 2014; Jansen et al., 2013). Therefore, from a practical and patient/family-centered approach, it is reasonable to suggest that both hospital nurses and therapists "coach" (Frampton et al., 2008) patients and their family CGs in the skills needed to manage UI.

Healthy Bladder Behavior Skills

Traditionally, nursing interventions for UI focus on containment strategies by means of receptacles (e.g., bedpan, urinal, commode, urinary catheters) or by various absorbent products (e.g., sanitary napkin, adult brief, incontinent pad; Harmer & Henderson, 1955; Henderson & Nite, 1978; Palese et al., 2007). Various treatments beyond containment strategies include dietary and fluid management (Vaughan et al., 2011), pelvic floor muscle exercises (PFMEs; Kegel, 1956; Qaseem et al., 2014; Vaughan et al., 2011), urge inhibition and bladder training (retraining) strategies, toileting programs (e.g., individualized, scheduled toileting programs/timed voiding; prompted voiding), pharmacological therapy, constipation management (Vaughan et al., 2011), and surgical options (Fantl et al., 1996; B. Hodgkinson et al., 2008; Qaseem et al., 2014). These treatments (excluding pharmacological and surgical options) are viewed as HBBS. Although the recommendation is to offer HBBS to all older adults with UI (Fantl et al., 1996; Teunissen, de Jonge, van Weel, & Lagro-Janseen, 2004), it is unclear how to best incorporate HBBS in the care of hospitalized older adults. Despite the fact that contemporary nursing practice textbooks list and describe HBBS as nursing interventions (Kozier, Erb, Berman, & Snyder, 2004; Newman & Wein, 2009; Taylor, Lillis, & LeMone, 2005), many of these interventions have not been adequately examined in the acute care setting, and nurses do not routinely implement these interventions in the acute care setting (Bayliss, Salter, & Locke, 2003; Schnelle et al., 2003; Watson, Brink, Zimmer, & Mayer, 2003). Underreporting and underassessment are barriers to optimally addressing UI in the hospital setting as reflected in the study by Schultz et al. (1997), which reported that only 0.1% of medical records captured the problem of UI present at the time of hospital admission. Accurate assessment and identification of type of UI are needed before care strategies are initiated.

Prior to instituting HBBS, the nurse needs to assess the motivation of the patient, family CG, and nursing staff because behavior modification is a premise of HBBS (Palmer, 2004). Examples of dietary management strategies include avoiding certain foods and beverages known to be bladder irritants such as caffeine, acidic foods or fluids, and aspartame (e.g., NutraSweet; Gray & Haas, 2000). Some individuals with a BMI greater than 27 may benefit from a weight-loss program. For example, in one study, a weight loss of 5% to 10% significantly decreased UI episodes for some obese women (Subak et al., 2005).

If not contraindicated, the nurse recommends adequate fluid intake, specifically water, and an increased intake of dietary fiber to maintain bowel regularity. It is important to work closely with older adults who fear that unwanted urine loss is a result of increased fluid intake. Education should focus on the adverse consequence of inadequate fluid intake, such as volume depletion or potential for dehydration, and that too little fluid intake may result in concentrated urine, which, in turn, may cause increased bladder contractions and increased feelings of urinary urgency. Finally, to manage and limit nocturia, patients may be advised to limit fluid intake a few hours before bedtime (Doughty, 2000; Fantl et al., 1996); however, this is questionable for older adults who do not have easy access to fluids or have diminished thirst sensation (DuBeau et al., 2010). In the hospital setting, the nurse must note the schedule of diuretics. For example, institutions may automatically schedule every-12-hour diuretic dose times at 10 a.m. and 10 p.m. For some patients, it will be extremely important that nurses navigate organizational processes to reschedule diuretic doses to an alternate time such as 6 a.m. and 6 p.m or even 4 p.m. This simple strategy may decrease nocturia, which, in turn, will likely decrease the risk of falls. Research that examines which UI interventions best modify fall risk is needed (Wolf, Riolo, & Ouslander, 2000).

For community-dwelling, cognitively intact older adults, PFMEs are at least as effective as pharmacological therapies in treating stress and urge UI (Hodgkinson et al., 2008). PFME holds promise for the primary prevention of UI, but requires additional research (Hay-Smith, Herbison, & Mørkved, 2002), particularly in the acute care setting. PFMEs were developed to augment the strength, endurance, and coordination of the pelvic muscles, which play a role in maintaining continence.

Integrating PFMEs into the plan of care requires an assessment of the patient's baseline understanding of PFMEs to identify knowledge deficits. Ideally, PFMEs are taught during a vaginal or rectal examination when the clinician manually assists the patient to identify the pelvic muscles by instructing the patient to squeeze around the gloved examination finger. This method allows for performance appraisal (Hay-Smith et al., 2002); and together with weekly phone consults and monthly performance appraisal, this method is known to improve UI outcomes for community-dwelling individuals (Tsai & Liu, 2009). Alternately, PFMEs may be verbally taught by instructing the patient to gently squeeze or contract the rectal or vaginal muscles. Either teaching method includes instructions to not squeeze the stomach, buttocks, or thigh muscles (because this only increases intra-abdominal pressure), but to isolate the contraction of the pelvic muscles.

Preferably, each exercise should consist of contracting for 10 seconds and relaxing for 10 seconds. Some patients may need to start with 3 or 5 seconds, and then increase as their muscle becomes stronger. There is no set "exercise dose" (Du Moulin, Hamers, Paulus, Berendsen, & Halfens, 2005); however, it is usual practice to recommend 15 PFMEs three times per day. For community-dwelling women with stress, urge, or mixed UI, PFMEs (at least 24 per day for at least 6 weeks) should be included in first-line conservative management programs (Choi, Palmer, & Park, 2007; Syah, 2010). Patients may notice improvement in 2 to 4 weeks, but not immediately. Nurses should reinforce compliance and other HBBS and initiate a referral for discharge follow-up with a continence specialist for PFME reinforcement via biofeedback, if available (Bradway & Hernly, 1998). In a study of community-dwelling adults, PFME instruction and reinforcement using biofeedback improved both UI outcomes and concurrent depressive symptoms (Tadic et al., 2007); therefore, hospitalized patients may benefit from a referral to a continence nurse or other provider specializing in care of individuals with UI (e.g., urologist, gynecologist, urogynecologist) for follow-up after discharge.

Urge inhibition is based on behavioral theory and is another recommended HBBS for treatment of urge UI (Teunissen et al., 2004), although the mechanism of how urge inhibition works is not well understood (Gray, 2005; Smith, 2000). Urge inhibition includes distraction techniques (e.g., reciting a favorite poem or song), relaxation techniques, and rapid pelvic floor muscle contractions with the goal being to suppress the urge to void until desirable (Smith, 2000).

Bladder training (retraining) is another behavioral technique used to treat urge UI (DuBeau et al., 2010; Teunissen et al., 2004) and OAB, is often used in conjunction with urge-inhibition techniques and functional incontinence training (FIT; DuBeau et al., 2010; Schnelle et al., 2003), and may be more effective if used in combination with PFMEs or anticholinergic drugs (Rathnayake, 2009a). Bladder training requires a baseline voiding record to determine the timing of voids and UI episodes. If urinary frequency is present, the patient is instructed to lengthen the time between voids in an effort to retrain the bladder. When a strong urge to void occurs, the patient is instructed to use urge-inhibition techniques to suppress urinary urgency. For example, if the patient is not in a position to empty the bladder in a socially appropriate manner, the nurse instructs the patient to quickly squeeze and relax pelvic floor muscles several times to suppress the urge to void. This technique is sometimes referred to as "quick flicks" (Gray, 2005). Relaxation and distraction and urge inhibition techniques are also beneficial during bladder training.

In some instances (e.g., for patients experiencing incomplete bladder emptying or overflow UI), patients and staff can use Crede's maneuvers (i.e., deep suprapubic palpation) to facilitate bladder emptying. The Crede's maneuver is used with caution and requires manual compression over the suprapubic area during bladder emptying. The Crede's maneuver should be avoided if vesicoureteral reflux (i.e., abnormal flow of urine from the bladder back up the ureters) or overactive sphincter mechanisms are suspected because it may dangerously elevate pressure within the bladder (Doughty, 2000). Therefore, if the nurse suspects that UI is related to neurologic impairments, a urologic specialist should be consulted before implementing this specific HBBS. In some cases, instructing patients to double void (i.e., after an initial void, instruct patients to stand or reposition for a second void) also facilitates bladder emptying.

Additional Nursing Interventions

Maintaining skin integrity is a goal of nursing care. Decomposition of urinary urea by microorganisms releases ammonia and forms ammonium hydroxide, an alkali. This alkali makes the protective "acid mantle" of the skin vulnerable and jeopardizes skin integrity. If UI episodes persist despite management strategies, perineal skin care interventions should focus on maintaining the integrity of the protective acid mantle of the skin (Ersser, Getliffe, Voegeli, & Regan, 2005; see Chapter 24, "Preventing Pressure Ulcers and Skin Tears").

Although absorbent products are commonly used for UI containment, there is little evidence available to guide product selection and no evidence of how absorbent products may interact with the acid mantle (Fader, Cottenden, & Getliffe, 2008). Community-dwelling women with light UI reported important characteristics of absorbent pads, including the ability to hold and hide UI and ease of use (Getliffe, Fader, Cottenden, Jamieson, & Green, 2007). In hospitals, nursing staff reported problems with quality and availability of absorbent products

(Clayman, Thompson, & Forth, 2005). Pertaining to reusable versus disposable absorbent products, there is no demonstrable risk of cross-infection with reusable absorbent products when appropriate laundering protocols are followed, and there are no clear cost savings with using one over the other. Reusable products have limited acceptability among users (Fader et al., 2008), and use of adult briefs is significantly associated with an increased risk of infection (Zimakoff, Stickler, Pontoppidan, & Larsen, 1996). Although bed pads absorb urine, consumer satisfaction is questionable, and there are no studies on the use of chair pads. In the hospital, patients fear "wetting the bed." Some gain a sense of control when able to contain and conceal UI with adult diapers; however, in one study, patients described a preference for brand name over the generic absorbent products provided by the hospital (Dowling-Castronovo, 2014). Although limited evidence suggesting that disposable insert pads may be more effective for women with UI than other absorbent products exists (Rathnayake, 2009d), there is no clear evidence to suggest one absorbent product is superior to another, particularly in the acute care setting. Evidence does support pilot testing of absorbent products according to individual circumstances, including patient, family, and institutional preferences, and offering a choice of products to women with UI (Dunn, Kowanko, Paterson, & Pretty, 2002; Fader et al., 2008; Rathnayake, 2009d).

CASE STUDY

A student nurse received a report on Mr. G, an 86-year-old man with a history of Alzheimer's dementia, who is hospitalized for delirium. The nurse was told that Mr. G was "pleasantly confused," required full assistance with personal care, and spent most of the day in a Geri-chair. The student nurse performed an assessment that revealed the following:

Patient sleeping in bed with all side rails up, call bell within reach, no urinal in sight
Past medical history: coronary artery disease, mild hypertension, mild osteoarthritis, AD
Past surgical history: none
Medications: diphenhydramine (Benadryl) 25 mg as needed for sleep, enalapril (Vasotec) 5 mg by mouth every day for hypertension, multivitamin 1 tablet by mouth daily, donepezil (Aricept) 10 mg by mouth every day for Alzheimer's dementia
Vital signs: 114/60, 72, 14, 98.0°F
Alert and oriented to self; sleepy; no focal deficits
Heart rate: regular
Breath sounds clear, slightly decreased at the bases
Abdomen: +BS (bowel sounds) in all quadrants, soft, nontender, no suprapubic tenderness; left quadrant slightly dull to percussion; no palpable masses
Dry adult brief in place

The student nurse learns from the patient's wife (i.e., the primary CG at home) that the patient has experienced occasional urinary leaking in the past, but not to the extent of needing "diapers." He has a history of chronic constipation. With the nursing instructor's guidance, the student nurse assisted Mr. G to a dangling position at the side of the bed. After assessing and evaluating that the patient's muscular strength was strong, ambulation was attempted. The patient ambulated to the bathroom, the adult brief was removed, and Mr. G was prompted to void. He successfully voided and had a bowel movement. He proceeded to wash his hands and returned to the bedside chair. The adult brief was left off during the time the student nurse was there to assist him. During this time, Mr. G made one attempt to initiate voiding and was successfully assisted by the student nurse.

Discussion

The importance of ongoing nursing assessment was stressed as being vital to quality of care. Had the student nurse just transferred the patient to the chair, he may not have effectively emptied his bowel and bladder. Mr. G's constipation was addressed by providing appropriate fluid and fiber intake and by continuing with an individualized toilet schedule as tolerated. The avoidance of diphenhydramine for the older adults was also discussed because it is known to cause anticholinergic effects, including urinary retention. Diphenhydramine raises concerns about sedation as well, which may alter Mr. G's response to the need to void.

Evidence suggests that prompted voiding and individualized toileting schedules reduce the number of UI episodes (Eustice et al., 2000; Fink, Taylor, Tacklind, Rutks, & Wilt, 2008; Ostaszkiewicz et al., 2004). In addition, prompted voiding in cognitively impaired long-term care residents has demonstrated an increase in self-initiative toileting activities (Holroyd-Leduc & Straus, 2004). These strategies have not been extensively studied in the hospital setting; however, this case study demonstrates that nursing interventions used in other settings may also be beneficial for acutely hospitalized older adults. For example, one published case report highlights the importance of nurses working with older adults and their CGs to address UI during the transitional period from hospital to home (Bradway, Bixby, Hirschman, McCauley, & Naylor, 2013).

SUMMARY

Although acute care stays are generally short, UI is a significant health problem that should not be overlooked. Behavioral and supportive therapies and patient education should be initiated by nurses if the patient is cognitively, physically, and emotionally able to participate. Evidence from long-term care and community settings suggests that nurse continence experts play an essential role in improving the quality of continence care (Du Moulin et al., 2005; McDowell et al., 1999; Watson, 2004). Therefore, if patients remain incontinent at discharge, hospital nurses have the responsibility to design a plan that includes referral to a continence nurse specialist or other continence expert for follow-up.

Other than identifying UI as a risk for falls, there are no requirements specific to UI from The Joint Commission (www.jointcommission.org). Nevertheless, it is recommended that a continuous quality-improvement (CQI) criterion should encompass critical elements in an effective and successful urinary continence program. For example, quality indicators for UI in the vulnerable older adult population that may be used in the hospital setting include documentation of (a) the presence of UI, (b) the bothersome nature for the older adult and significant other, (c) focused history and physical examination, (d) documentation of urinalysis and/or culture, (e) PVR and, if elevated to more than 100 mL, consider referral for further evaluation; (f) type of UI; (g) discussion of HBBS; (h) interprofessional evaluation for urodynamic evaluation and pharmacological/surgical treatments; and (i) response to treatment (Fung, Spencer, Eslami, & Crandall, 2007). Hospital quality-improvement teams may use an if–then approach (Schnelle & Smith, 2001). For example, if a hospitalized older adult experiences transient UI, then a focused assessment is performed to identify etiology.

Nurses have a significant role in improving the assessment and treatment of UI in hospitalized older adults. It is recommended that nurses are particularly vigilant for patients who are "admitted dry and become wet" during a hospitalization. These patients will particularly benefit from evidence-based assessment and management. Moreover, nurses can help to promote changes in attitudes toward UI and provide education on individual, facility-wide, community, and national levels.

NURSING STANDARD OF PRACTICE

Protocol 21.1: Urinary Incontinence in Older Adults Admitted to Acute Care

I. GOAL

A. Nursing staff will utilize comprehensive assessments and implement evidence-based management strategies for patients identified with UI.
B. Nursing staff will collaborate with interprofessional team members to identify and document type of UI.
C. Patients with UI will not have UI-associated complications.

II. OVERVIEW

UI affects approximately 17 million Americans (Fantl et al., 1996; Landefeld et al., 2008; National Association for Continence, 1998; Resnick & Ouslander, 1990). More than 35% of older adults admitted to the hospital develop UI (Kresevic, 1997). In addition to medications, constipation/fecal impaction, low fluid intake, environmental barriers, diabetes mellitus, and stroke (Fantl et al., 1996; Holroyd-Leduc & Straus, 2004; Meijer et al., 2003; Offermans, Du Moulin, Hamers, Dassen, & Halfens, 2009; Shamliyan, Wyman, Bliss, Kane, & Wilt, 2007; Thomas et al., 2005), immobility, impaired cognition, malnutrition, and depression are additional factors specific to identifying older adults at risk of UI in the hospital setting (Kresevic, 1997). Complications of UI include falls, skin irritation leading to pressure ulcers, social isolation, and depression (Bogner et al., 2002; Brown et al., 2000; Fantl et al., 1996; Morris & Wagg, 2007). Nurses play a key role in the assessment and management of UI.

III. BACKGROUND

A. Definitions
   1. *UI* is the involuntary loss of urine sufficient to be a problem (Fantl et al., 1996). UI may be transient (acute) or established (chronic).

(continued)

Protocol 21.1: Urinary Incontinence in Older Adults Admitted to Acute Care *(continued)*

a. *Transient UI* is characterized by the sudden onset of potentially reversible symptoms that typically has a duration of less than 6 months (Specht, 2005).

B. Types of established UI include the following:
   1. *Stress UI* is defined as an involuntary loss of urine associated with activities that increase intra-abdominal pressure (Abrams et al., 2003; Fantl et al., 1996; Hunter et al., 2004).
   2. *Urge UI* is characterized by an involuntary urine loss associated with a strong desire to void (urgency; Abrams et al., 2003; Fantl et al., 1996). An individual with OAB may complain of urinary urgency, with or without UI (Abrams et al., 2003).
   3. *Mixed UI* is defined as a combination of stress UI and urge UI (Jayasekara, 2009).
   4. *Overflow UI* is an involuntary loss of urine associated with overdistention of the bladder, and may be caused by an underactive detrusor muscle or outlet obstruction leading to overdistention of the bladder and overflow of urine (Abrams et al., 2003; Doughty, 2000; Fantl et al., 1996; Jayasekara, 2009).
   5. *Functional UI* is caused by nongenitourinary factors, such as cognitive or physical impairments that result in an inability for the individual to be independent in voiding (Fantl et al., 1996; Hodgkinson et al., 2008).

C. Epidemiology
   1. UI affects approximately 17 million Americans (Fantl et al., 1996; Landefeld et al., 2008; National Association for Continence, 1998; Resnick & Ouslander, 1990).
   2. UI studies specific to the hospital setting demonstrate that UI is present in 10% to 42% of older adults (Dowd & Campbell, 1995; Fantl et al., 1996; Kresevic, 1997; Palmer et al., 1992; Schultz et al., 1997); therefore, assessment and implementation of an evidence-based protocol are essential.

IV. PARAMETERS OF ASSESSMENT

A. Document the presence or absence of UI for all patients on admission (DuBeau et al., 2010).

B. Document the presence or absence of an indwelling urinary catheter.

C. For patients with UI, the nurse collaborates with interprofessional team members to
   1. Determine whether the UI is transient, established (stress/urge/mixed/overflow/functional), or both and document (DuBeau et al., 2010; Fantl et al., 1996; Jayasekara, 2009; Johnson et al., 2001; Qaseem et al., 2014).
   2. Identify and document the possible etiologies of the UI (DuBeau et al., 2010; Fantl et al., 1996).

V. NURSING CARE STRATEGIES

A. General principles that apply to prevention and management of all forms of UI
   1. Identify and treat causes of transient UI (DuBeau et al., 2010).
   2. Identify and continue successful prehospital management strategies for established UI.
   3. Develop an individualized plan of care using data obtained from the history and physical examination, and in collaboration with other team members. Implement toileting programs as needed (Ostaszkiewicz et al., 2004; Rathnayake, 2009c).
   4. Avoid medications that may contribute to UI (Newman & Wein, 2009).
   5. Avoid indwelling urinary catheters whenever possible to avoid the risk of CAUTI (Bouza, San Juan, Muñoz, Voss, &Kluytmans, 2001; Dowd & Campbell, 1995; Gould et al., 2009; Zimakoff et al., 1996).
   6. Monitor fluid intake and maintain an appropriate hydration schedule.
   7. Limit dietary bladder irritants (Gray & Haas, 2000).
   8. Consider adding weight loss as a long-term goal in discharge planning for those with a BMI greater than 27 (Subak et al., 2005; Qaseem et al., 2014).
   9. Modify the environment to facilitate continence (Fantl et al., 1996; Jirovec, 2000; Palmer, 1996).
   10. Provide patients with usual undergarments in expectation of continence, if possible.
   11. Prevent skin breakdown by providing immediate cleansing after an incontinent episode and utilizing barrier ointments (Ersser et al., 2005).

(continued)

Protocol 21.1: Urinary Incontinence in Older Adults Admitted to Acute Care *(continued)*

12. Pilot test absorbent products to best meet patient, staff, and institutional preferences (Dunn et al., 2002), bearing in mind adult briefs have been associated with UTIs (Zimakoff et al., 1996).

B. Strategies for specific problems:
   1. Stress UI
      a. Teach PFMEs (DuBeau et al., 2010; Hodgkinson et al., 2008; Qaseem et al., 2014).
      b. Provide toileting assistance and bladder training as needed (whenever necessary; DuBeau et al., 2010; Qaseem et al., 2014).
      c. Consider referral to other team members if pharmacological or surgical therapies are warranted.
   2. Urge UI and OAB
      a. Implement bladder training (retraining; DuBeau et al., 2010; Qaseem et al., 2014; Teunissen et al., 2004).
      b. If patient is cognitively intact and is motivated, provide information on urge inhibition (Gray, 2005; Smith, 2000).
      c. Teach PFMEs to be used in conjunction with bladder training, and instruct in urge inhibition strategies (Flynn, Cell, & Luisi, 1994; Rathnayake, 2009a; Teunissen et al., 2004).
      d. Collaborate with prescribing team members if pharmacological therapy is warranted.
      e. Initiate referrals for those patients who do not respond to the aforementioned strategies.
   3. Overflow UI
      a. Allow sufficient time for voiding.
      b. Discuss with interprofessional team the need for determining a PVR (Newman & Wein, 2009; Shinopulos, 2000; see Table 21.2).
      c. Instruct patients in double voiding and Crede's maneuver (Doughty, 2000).
      d. If catheterization is necessary, sterile intermittent catheterization is preferred over indwelling catheterization (Saint et al., 2006; Terpenning, Allada, & Kauffman, 1989; Warren, 1997).
      e. Initiate referrals to other team members for patients requiring pharmacological or surgical intervention.
   4. Functional UI
      a. Provide individualized scheduled toileting, timed voiding, or prompted voiding (Eustice et al., 2000; Jirovec, 2000; Lee et al., 2009; Ostaszkiewicz et al., 2004).
      b. Provide adequate fluid intake.
      c. Refer for physical and occupational therapy as needed.
      d. Modify environment to maximize independence with continence (Fantl et al., 1996; Jirovec, 2000; Jirovec et al., 1988; Palmer, 1996).

VI. EVALUATION OF EXPECTED OUTCOMES

A. Patients will
   1. Have fewer or no episodes of UI or complications associated with UI

B. Nurses will
   1. Document assessment of continence status at admission and throughout hospital stay. If UI is identified, document and determine type of UI
   2. Use interprofessional expertise and interventions to assess and manage UI during hospitalization
   3. Include UI in discharge planning needs and refer as needed

C. Institutions will
   1. Make sure incidence and prevalence of transient UI will decrease
   2. Require assessment and documentation policies for continence status (Fung et al., 2007; Schnelle & Smith, 2001)
   3. Provide access to evidence-based guidelines for evaluation and management of UI
   4. Instruct staff to receive administrative support and ongoing education regarding assessment and management of UI

(continued)

Protocol 21.1: Urinary Incontinence in Older Adults Admitted to Acute Care *(continued)*

VII. FOLLOW-UP MONITORING OF CONDITION

A. Provide patient/CG discharge teaching regarding outpatient referral and management.
B. Incorporate CQI criteria into existing program ("Assessing Care," 2007; Fung et al., 2007), and measure quality indicators using an if–then approach (Schnelle & Smith, 2001).
C. Identify areas for improvement and enlist multidisciplinary assistance in devising strategies for improvement.

VIII. RELEVANT PRACTICE GUIDELINES

National Guideline Clearinghouse: Guideline Synthesis
www.guideline.gov/syntheses
Agency for Healthcare Research and Quality
http://www.guideline.gov/content.aspx?id=43941

ABBREVIATIONS

BMI	Body mass index
CAUTI	Catheter-associated urinary tract infection
CG	Caregiver
CQI	Continuous quality improvement
OAB	Overactive bladder
PFME	Pelvic floor muscle exercises
PVR	Postvoid residual
UI	Urinary incontinence
UTI	Urinary tract infection

RESOURCES

GeroNurseOnline
Geriatric Resources and tools
consultgerirn.org

Hartford Institute for Geriatric Nursing
Click resources tab in urinary incontinence topic
This website will bring the reader to the "Try This" series to share with hospital staff.
www.hartfordign.org

International Continence Society
A registered charity improving the quality of life for people across the globe affected by urinary incontinence.
www.ics.org

National Association for Continence (NAFC)
A not-for-profit organization dedicated to improving the lives of individuals with incontinence
www.nafc.org

Society of Urologic Nurse and Associates (SUNA)
An international organization dedicated to nursing care of individuals with urologic disorders
www.suna.org

Wound, Ostomy Continence Nurses Society
An international society providing a source of networking and research for nurses specializing in enterostomal and continence care
www.wocn.org

REFERENCES

Abrams, P., Cardozo, L., Fall, M., Griffiths, D., Rosier, P., Ulmsten, U., . . . Wein, A.; Standardisation Sub-Committee of the International Continence Society. (2003). The standardisation of terminology in lower urinary tract function: Report from the standardisation sub-committee of the International Continence Society. *Urology, 61*(1), 37–49. *Evidence Level I.*

Bayliss, V., Salter, L., & Locke, R. (2003). Pathways for continence care: An audit to assess how they are used. *British Journal of Nursing, 12*(14), 857–863. *Evidence Level IV.*

Bogner, H. R., Gallo, J. J., Sammel, M. D., Ford, D. E., Armenian, H. K., & Eaton, W. W. (2002). Urinary incontinence and psychological distress in community-dwelling older adults. *Journal of the American Geriatrics Society, 50*(3), 489–495. *Evidence Level IV.*

Bouza, E., San Juan, R., Muñoz, P., Voss, A., & Kluytmans, J.; Cooperative Group of the European Study Group on Nosocomial Infections. (2001). A European perspective on nosocomial urinary tract infections II. Report on incidence, clinical characteristics and outcome (ESGNI-004 study). European Study Group on Nosocomial Infection. *Clinical Microbiology and Infection: The Official Publication of the European Society of Clinical Microbiology and Infectious Diseases, 7*(10), 532–542. *Evidence Level IV.*

Bradway, C. (2003). Urinary incontinence among older women. Measurement of the effect on health-related quality of life. *Journal of Gerontological Nursing, 29*(7), 13–19. *Evidence Level VI.*

Bradway, C., Bixby, M. B., Hirschman, K. B., McCauley, K., & Naylor, M. D. (2013). Case study: Transitional care for a patient with benign prostatic hyperplasia and recurrent urinary tract infections. *Urologic Nursing, 33*(4), 177–9, 200. *Evidence Level V.*

Bradway, C., & Hernly, S. (1998). Urinary incontinence in older adults admitted to acute care. The NICHE Faculty. *Geriatric Nursing (New York, N.Y.), 19*(2), 98–102. *Evidence Level VI.*

Bradway, C. W., & Yetman, G. (2002). Genitourinary problems. In V. T. Cotter & N. E. Strumpf (Eds.), *Advanced practice nursing with older adults: Clinical guidelines* (pp. 83–102). New York, NY: McGraw-Hill. *Evidence Level VI.*

Brandeis, G. H., Baumann, M. M., Hossain, M., Morris, J. N., & Resnick, N. M. (1997). The prevalence of potentially remediable urinary incontinence in frail older people: A study using the Minimum Data Set. *Journal of the American Geriatrics Society, 45*(2), 179–184. *Evidence Level IV.*

Brittain, K. R., & Shaw, C. (2007). The social consequences of living with and dealing with incontinence—A carers perspective. *Social Science & Medicine (1982), 65*(6), 1274–1283. *Evidence Level IV.*

Brown, J. S., Sawaya, G., Thom, D. H., & Grady, D. (2000). Hysterectomy and urinary incontinence: A systematic review. *Lancet, 356*(9229), 535–539. *Evidence Level I.*

Burns, P. A. (2000). Stress urinary incontinence. In D. B. Doughty (Ed.), *Urinary & fecal incontinence nursing management* (2nd ed., pp. 63–89). St. Louis, MO: Mosby. *Evidence Level VI.*

Bush, T. A., Castellucci, D. T., & Phillips, C. (2001). Exploring women's beliefs regarding urinary incontinence. *Urologic Nursing, 21*(3), 211–218. *Evidence Level IV.*

Cassells, C., & Watt, E. (2003). The impact of incontinence on older spousal caregivers. *Journal of Advanced Nursing, 42*, 607–616. *Evidence Level IV.*

Chiarelli, P. E., Mackenzie, L. A., & Osmotherly, P. G. (2009). Urinary incontinence is associated with an increase in falls: A systematic review. *Australian Journal of Physiotherapy, 55*(2), 89–95. *Evidence Level I.*

Choi, H., Palmer, M. H., & Park, J. (2007). Meta-analysis of pelvic floor muscle training: Randomized controlled trials in incontinent women. *Nursing Research, 56*(4), 226–234. *Evidence Level I.*

Clayman, C., Thompson, V., & Forth, H. (2005). Development of a continence assessment pathway in acute care. *Nursing Times, 101*(18), 46–48. *Evidence Level IV.*

Cochran, A. (2000). Don't ask, don't tell: The incontinence conspiracy. *Managed Care Quarterly, 8*(1), 44–52. *Evidence Level VI.*

Coffey, A., McCarthy, G., McCormack, B., Wright, J., & Slater, P. (2007). Incontinence: Assessment, diagnosis, and management in two rehabilitation units for older people. *Worldviews on Evidence-Based Nursing/Sigma Theta Tau International, Honor Society of Nursing, 4*(4), 179–186. *Evidence Level IV.*

Colling, J., Ouslander, J., Hadley, B. J., Eisch, J., & Campbell, E. (1992). The effects of patterned urge-response toileting (PURT) on urinary incontinence among nursing home residents. *Journal of the American Geriatrics Society, 40*(2), 135–141. *Evidence Level II.*

Connor, P. A., & Kooker, B. M. (1996). Nurses' knowledge, attitudes, and practices in managing urinary incontinence in the acute care setting. *Medsurg Nursing: Official Journal of the Academy of Medical-Surgical Nurses, 5*(2), 87–92, 117. *Evidence Level IV.*

DeLancey, J. O. (1994). Structural support of the urethra as it relates to stress urinary incontinence: The hammock hypothesis. *American Journal of Obstetrics and Gynecology, 170*(6), 1713–20; discussion 1720. *Evidence Level IV.*

Delancey, J. O. (2010). Why do women have stress urinary incontinence? *Neurourology and Urodynamics, 29*(Suppl. 1), S13–S17. *Evidence Level VI.*

de Vries, H. F., Northington, G. M., & Bogner, H. R. (2012). Urinary incontinence (UI) and new psychological distress among community dwelling older adults. *Archives of Gerontology and Geriatrics, 55*(1), 49–54. *Evidence Level IV.*

Ding, Y. Y., & Jayaratnam, F. J. (1994). Urinary incontinence in the hospitalised elderly—A largely reversible disorder. *Singapore Medical Journal, 35*(2), 167–170. *Evidence Level VI.*

Diokno, A. C., Laijness, M. J., & Griebling, T. L. (2014). Urinary incontinence: Evaluation and diagnosis. In T. L. Griebling (Ed.), *Geriatric urology* (pp. 127-140). New York, NY: Springer Publishing Company. *Evidence Level V.*

Donald, F., Martin-Misener, R., Carter, N., Donald, E. E., Kaasalainen, S., Wickson-Griffiths, A., ... DiCenso, A. (2013). A systematic review of the effectiveness of advanced practice nurses in long-term care. *Journal of Advanced Nursing, 69*(10), 2148–2161. *Evidence Level I.*

Dorsher, P. T., & McIntosh, P. M. (2012). Neurogenic bladder. *Advances in Urology, 2012*, 816274. *Evidence Level V.*

Doughty, D. B. (2000). Retention with overflow. In D. B. Doughty (Ed.), *Urinary & fecal incontinence nursing management* (2nd ed., pp. 159–180). St. Louis, MO: Mosby. *Evidence Level VI.*

Dowd, T. T. (1991). Discovering older women's experience of urinary incontinence. *Research in Nursing & Health, 14*(3), 179–186. *Evidence Level IV.*

Dowd, T. T., & Campbell, J. M. (1995). Urinary incontinence in an acute care setting. *Urologic Nursing, 15*(3), 82–85. *Evidence Level IV.*

Dowling-Castronovo, A. (2004). Urinary incontinence: An exploration of the relationship between age, COPD, and obesity. Unpublished. *Evidence Level VI.*

Dowling-Castronovo, A. (2014). *Regaining control* (Doctoral disseration). Retrieved from http://dx.doi.org/doi:10.7282/T3057D5P *Evidence Level IV.*

DuBeau, C. E., Kuchel, G. A., Johnson, T., Palmer, M. H., & Wagg, A.; Fourth International Consultation on Incontinence. (2010). Incontinence in the frail elderly: Report from the 4th International Consultation on Incontinence. *Neurourology and Urodynamics, 29*(1), 165–178. *Evidence Level I.*

Dubeau, C. E., Simon, S. E., & Morris, J. N. (2006). The effect of urinary incontinence on quality of life in older nursing home residents. *Journal of the American Geriatrics Society, 54*(9), 1325–1333. *Evidence Level IV.*

Dugger, B. R. (2010). Concept analysis of health-related quality of life in nursing home residents with urinary incontinence. *Urologic Nursing, 30*(2), 112–118; quiz 119. *Evidence Level I.*

Du Moulin, M. F., Hamers, J. P., Ambergen, A. W., Janssen, M. A., & Halfens, R. J. (2008). Prevalence of urinary incontinence among community-dwelling adults receiving home care. *Research in Nursing & Health, 31*(6), 604–612. *Evidence Level IV.*

Du Moulin, M. F., Hamers, J. P., Paulus, A., Berendsen, C., & Halfens, R. (2005). The role of the nurse in community continence care: A systematic review. *International Journal of Nursing Studies, 42*(4), 479–492. *Evidence Level I.*

Dunn, S., Kowanko, I., Paterson, J., & Pretty, L. (2002). Systematic review of the effectiveness of urinary continence products. *Journal of Wound, Ostomy, and Continence Nursing: Official Publication of the Wound, Ostomy and Continence Nurses Society/WOCN, 29*(3), 129–142. *Evidence Level I.*

Egnatios, D., Dupree, L., & Williams, C. (2010). Performance improvement in practice: Managing urinary incontinence in home health patients with the use of an evidence-based guideline. *Home Healthcare Nurse, 28*(10), 620–628; quiz 629. doi:10.1097/NHH.0b013e3181f85d44. *Evidence Level IV.*

Ermer-Seltun, J. (2006). Assessment and management of acute or transient urinary incontinence. In D. B. Doughty (Ed.), *Urinary & fecal incontinence: Current management concepts* (3rd ed., pp. 55–76). St. Louis, MO: Mosby Elsevier. *Evidence Level: VI.*

Ersser, S. J., Getliffe, K., Voegeli, D., & Regan, S. (2005). A critical review of the inter-relationship between skin vulnerability and urinary incontinence and related nursing intervention. *International Journal of Nursing Studies, 42*(7), 823–835. *Evidence Level I.*

Eustice, S., Roe, B., & Paterson, J. (2000). Prompted voiding for the management of urinary incontinence in adults. *Cochrane Database of Systematic Reviews, 2000*(2), CD002113. *Evidence Level I.*

Fader, M., Cottenden, A. M., & Getliffe, K. (2008). Absorbent products for moderate-heavy urinary and/or faecal incontinence in women and men. *Cochrane Database of Systematic Reviews, 2008*(4), CD007408. *Evidence Level I.*

Fantl, A., Newman, D. K., Colling, J., DeLancey, J. O., Keeys, C., & Loughery, R. (1996). *Urinary incontinence in adults: Acute and chronic management* (Report No. Publication No. 92–0047). Rockville, MD: Agency for Health Care Policy and Research. *Evidence Level I.*

Fink, H. A., Taylor, B. C., Tacklind, J. W., Rutks, I. R., & Wilt, T. J. (2008). Treatment interventions in nursing home residents with urinary incontinence: A systematic review of randomized trials. *Mayo Clinic Proceedings, 83*(12), 1332–1343. *Evidence Level I.*

Flynn, L., Cell, P., & Luisi, E. (1994). Effectiveness of pelvic muscle exercises in reducing urge incontinence among community residing elders. *Journal of Gerontological Nursing, 20*(5), 23–27. *Evidence Level IV.*

Frampton, S., Guastello, S., Brady, C., Hale, M., Horowitz, S., Bennett Smith, S., & Stone, S. (2008). *Patient-centered care improvement guide.* Derby, CT: Plantree. Retrieved from http://www.ihi.org/knowledge/Pages/Tools/PatientCentered-CareImprovementGuide.aspx. *Evidence Level V.*

Fung, C. H., Spencer, B., Eslami, M., & Crandall, C. (2007). Quality indicators for the screening and care of urinary incontinence in vulnerable elders. *Journal of the American Geriatrics Society, 55*(Suppl. 2), S443–S449. *Evidence Level I.*

Getliffe, K., Fader, M., Cottenden, A., Jamieson, K., & Green, N. (2007). Absorbent products for incontinence: "Treatment effects" and impact on quality of life. *Journal of Clinical Nursing, 16*(10), 1936–1945. *Evidence Level IV.*

Gotoh, M., Matsukawa, Y., Yoshikawa, Y., Funahashi, Y., Kato, M., & Hattori, R. (2009). Impact of urinary incontinence on the psychological burden of family caregivers. *Neurourology and Urodynamics, 28*(6), 492–496. *Evidence Level IV.*

Gould, C. V., Umscheid, C. A., Agarwal, R. K., Kuntz, G., Pegues, D. A., & the Healthcare Infection Control Practices Advisory Committee. (2009). *Guideline for prevention of catheter-associated urinary tract infections.* Retrieved from http://www.cdc.gov/hicpac/cauti/001_cauti.html. *Evidence Level I.*

Gray, M. (2005). Assessment and management of urinary incontinence. *Nurse Practitioner, 30*(7), 32–33, 36. *Evidence Level VI.*

Gray, M., Rayome, R., & Moore, K. (1995). The urethral sphincter: An update. *Urologic Nursing, 15*(2), 40–53; quiz 54. *Evidence Level VI.*

Gray, M. (2000). Physiology of voiding. In D. B. Doughty (Ed.), *Urinary & fecal incontinence: Nursing management* (2nd ed., pp. 1–27). St. Louis, MO: Mosby. *Evidence Level V.*

Gray, M. L., & Haas, J. (2000). Assessment of the patient with urinary incontinence. In D. B. Doughty (Ed.), *Urinary & fecal incontinence: Nursing management* (2nd ed., pp. 209–284). St. Louis, MO: Mosby. *Evidence Level VI.*

Harmer, B., & Henderson, V. (1955). *Textbook of the principles and practice of nursing* (5th ed.). New York, NY: MacMillan. *Evidence Level VI.*

Harper, C. M., & Lyles, Y. M. (1988). Physiology and complications of bed rest. *Journal of the American Geriatrics Society, 36*(11), 1047–1054. *Evidence Level V.*

Hasegawa, J., Kuzuya, M., & Iguchi, A. (2010). Urinary incontinence and behavioral symptoms are independent risk factors for recurrent and injurious falls, respectively, among residents in long-term care facilities. *Archives of Gerontology and Geriatrics, 50*(1), 77–81. *Evidence* Level IV.

Hay-Smith, J., Herbison, P., & Mørkved, S. (2002). Physical therapies for prevention of urinary and faecal incontinence in adults. *Cochrane Database of Systematic Reviews, 2002*(2), CD003191. *Evidence Level I.*

Henderson, V., & Nite, G. (1978). *Principles and practice of nursing* (6th ed.). New York, NY: MacMillan. *Evidence Level VI.*

Hodgkinson, B., Synnott, R., Josephs, K., Leira, E., & Hegney, D. (2008). A systematic review of the effect of educational interventions for urinary and faecal incontinence by health care staff/carers/clients in the aged care, on level knowledge, frequency of incontinence episodes and hours spent on the management of incontinence episodes. *JBI Library of Systematic Review, 6*(1), 1–66. Publication 318. *Evidence Level I.*

Hodgkinson, C. P. (1965). Stress urinary incontinence in the female. *Surgery, Gynecology & Obstetrics, 120*, 595–613. *Evidence Level V.*

Holroyd-Leduc, J. M., Mehta, K. M., & Covinsky, K. E. (2004). Urinary incontinence and its association with death, nursing home admission, and functional decline. *Journal of the American Geriatrics Society, 52*(5), 712–718. *Evidence Level I.*

Holroyd-Leduc, J. M., & Straus, S. E. (2004). Management of urinary incontinence in women: Scientific review. *Journal of the American Medical Association, 291*(8), 986–995. *Evidence Level I.*

Holroyd-Leduc, J. M., Tannenbaum, C., Thorpe, K. E., & Straus, S. E. (2008). What type of urinary incontinence does this woman have? *Journal of the American Medical Association, 299*(12), 1446–1456. *Evidence Level I.*

Homma, Y. (2008). Lower urinary tract symptomatology: Its definition and confusion. *International Journal of Urology: Official Journal of the Japanese Urological Association, 15*(1), 35–43. *Evidence Level V.*

Hunter, K. F., Moore, K. N., Cody, D. J., & Glazener, C. M. (2004). Conservative management for postprostatectomy urinary incontinence. *Cochrane Database of Systematic Reviews, 2004*(2), CD001843. *Evidence Level I.*

Iwatsubo, E., Suzuki, M., Igawa, Y., & Homma, Y. (2014). Individually tailored ultrasound-assisted prompted voiding for institutionalized older adults with urinary incontinence. *International Journal of Urology: Official Journal of the Japanese Urological Association, 21*(12), 1253–1257. *Evidence Level III.*

Jansen, L., McWilliam, C. L., Forbes, D., & Forchuk, C. (2013). Social-interaction knowledge translation for in-home management of urinary incontinence and chronic care. *Canadian Journal on Aging = La Revue Canadienne Du Vieillissement, 32*(4), 392–404. *Evidence Level IV.*

Jayasekara, R. (2009). Urinary incontinence: Evaluation. *JBI Database Evid Summaries*, Publication ES0610. *Evidence Level I.*

Jeyaseelan, S. M., Roe, B. H., & Oldham, J. A. (2000). The use of frequency/volume charts to assess urinary incontinence. *Physical Therapy Reviews, 5*(3), 141–146. *Evidence Level I.*

Jirovec, M. M. (2000). Functional incontinence. In D. B. Doughty (Ed.), *Urinary and fecal incontinence nursing management* (2nd ed., pp. 145–157). St. Louis, MO: Mosby. *Evidence Level VI.*

Jirovec, M. M., Brink, C. A., & Wells, T. J. (1988). Nursing assessments in the inpatient geriatric population. *Nursing Clinics of North America, 23*(1), 219–230. *Evidence Level VI.*

Jirovec, M. M., Wyman, J. F., & Wells, T. J. (1998). Addressing urinary incontinence with educational continence-care competencies. *Image—The Journal of Nursing Scholarship, 30*(4), 375–378. *Evidence Level VI.*

Johnson, M., Bulechek, G., McCloskey-Dochterman, J., Maas, M., & Moorhead, S. (2001). *Nursing diagnoses, outcomes, and interventions: NANDA, NOC and NIC linkages*. St. Louis, MO: Mosby. *Evidence Level VI.*

Kegel, A. H. (1956). Stress incontinence of urine in women; physiologic treatment. *Journal of the International College of Surgeons, 25*(4 Pt 1), 487–499. *Evidence Level VI.*

Kinchen, K. S., Burgio, K., Diokno, A. C., Fultz, N. H., Bump, R., & Obenchain, R. (2003). Factors associated with women's decisions to seek treatment for urinary incontinence. *Journal of Women's Health (2002), 12*(7), 687–698. *Evidence Level IV.*

Kozier, B., Erb, G., Berman, A., & Snyder, S. (2004). *Fundamentals of nursing concepts, process, and practice* (7th ed.). Upper Saddle River, NJ: Prentice Hall. *Evidence Level VI.*

Kresevic, D. M. (1997). *New-onset urinary incontinence among hospitalized elders* (Doctoral dissertation). Case Western Reserve University. (UMI No. 9810934). *Evidence Level IV.*

Krumholz, H. M., Chen, J., Chen, Y. T., Wang, Y., & Radford, M. J. (2001). Predicting one-year mortality among elderly survivors of hospitalization for an acute myocardial infarction: Results from the Cooperative Cardiovascular Project. *Journal of the American College of Cardiology, 38*(2), 453–459. *Evidence Level IV.*

Kwong, P. W., Cumming, R. G., Chan, L., Seibel, M. J., Naganathan, V., Creasey, H., . . . Handelsman, D. (2010). Urinary incontinence and quality of life among older community-dwelling Australian men: The CHAMP study. *Age and Ageing, 39*(3), 349–354. *Evidence Level IV.*

Landefeld, C. S., Bowers, B. J., Feld, A. D., Hartmann, K. E., Hoffman, E., Ingber, M. J., . . . Trock, B. J. (2008). National Institutes of Health state-of-the-science conference statement: Prevention of fecal and urinary incontinence in adults. *Annals of Internal Medicine, 148*(6), 449–458. *Evidence Level I.*

Lau, J. B. C. (2009). Urinary incontinence: Clinical assessment. *JBI Database Evid Summary*, Publication ES0599. *Evidence Level I.*

Lee, P. G., Cigolle, C., & Blaum, C. (2009). The co-occurrence of chronic diseases and geriatric syndromes: The health and retirement study. *Journal of the American Geriatrics Society, 57*(3), 511–516. *Evidence Level IV.*

Lemack, G. E., & Zimmern, P. E. (1999). Predictability of urodynamic findings based on the Urogenital Distress Inventory-6 questionnaire. *Urology, 54*(3), 461–466. *Evidence Level IV.*

Lenherr, S. M., & Clemens, J. Q. (2013). Urodynamics: With a focus on appropriate indications. *Urologic Clinics of North America, 40*, 545–557. *Evidence Level V.*

McDowell, B. J., Engberg, S., Sereika, S., Donovan, N., Jubeck, M. E., Weber, E., & Engberg, R. (1999). Effectiveness of behavioral therapy to treat incontinence in homebound older adults. *Journal of the American Geriatrics Society, 47*(3), 309–318. *Evidence Level II.*

Meijer, R., Ihnenfeldt, D. S., de Groot, I. J., van Limbeek, J., Vermeulen, M., & de Haan, R. J. (2003). Prognostic factors for ambulation and activities of daily living in the subacute phase after stroke. A systematic review of the literature. *Clinical Rehabilitation, 17*(2), 119–129. *Evidence Level I.*

Miller, Y. D., Brown, W. J., Smith, N., & Chiarelli, P. (2003). Managing urinary incontinence across the lifespan. *International Journal of Behavioral Medicine, 10*(2), 143–161. *Evidence Level IV.*

Milne, J. (2000). The impact of information on health behaviors of older adults with urinary incontinence. *Clinical Nursing Research, 9*(2), 161–176. *Evidence Level IV.*

Mitteness, L. S. (1987a). The management of urinary incontinence by community-living elderly. *The Gerontologist, 27*(2), 185–193. *Evidence Level IV.*

Mitteness, L. S. (1987b). So what do you expect when you're 85? Urinary incontinence in late life. In J. A. Roth & P. Conrad (Eds.), *Research in the sociology of health care* (pp. 177–219). Greenwich, CT: JAI Press. *Evidence Level IV.*

Morris, V., & Wagg, A. (2007). Lower urinary tract symptoms, incontinence and falls in elderly people: Time for an intervention study. *International Journal of Clinical Practice, 61*(2), 320–323. *Evidence Level VI.*

National Association for Continence. (1998, December). *Release of findings from consumer survey on urinary incontinence: Dissatisfaction with treatment continues to rise.* Spartansburg, SC: Author. *Evidence Level IV.*

Newman, D. K., & Wein, A. J. (2009). *Managing and treating urinary incontinence* (2nd ed.). Baltimore, MD: Health Professions Press. *Evidence Level VI.*

Nygaard, I. (2006). Urinary incontinence: Is cesarean delivery protective? *Seminars in Perinatology, 30*(5), 267–271. *Evidence Level VI.*

Offermans, M. P., Du Moulin, M. F., Hamers, J. P., Dassen, T., & Halfens, R. J. (2009). Prevalence of urinary incontinence and associated risk factors in nursing home residents: A systematic review. *Neurourology and Urodynamics, 28*(4), 288–294. *Evidence Level I.*

Ostaszkiewicz, J., Johnston, L., & Roe, B. (2004). Timed voiding for the management of urinary incontinence in adults. *Cochrane Database of Systematic Reviews, 4*(1), 1-21. CD002802. *Evidence Level I.*

Ouslander, J. G., Griffiths, P., McConnell, E., Riolo, L., & Schnelle, J. (2005). Functional incidental training: Applicability and feasibility in the Veterans Affairs nursing home patient population. *Journal of the American Medical Directors Association, 6*(2), 121–127. *Evidence Level II.*

Paillard, M., & Resnick, N. (1981). Natural history of nosocomial urinary incontinence. *The Gerontologist, 24,* 212. *Evidence Level IV.*

Palese, A., Regattin, L., Venuti, F., Innocenti, A., Benaglio, C., Cunico, L., & Saiani, L. (2007). Incontinence pad use in patients admitted to medical wards: An Italian multicenter prospective cohort study. *Journal of Wound, Ostomy, and Continence Nursing: Official Publication of the Wound, Ostomy and Continence Nurses Society/WOCN, 34*(6), 649–654. *Evidence Level IV.*

Palmer, M. H. (1988). Incontinence. The magnitude of the problem. *Nursing Clinics of North America, 23*(1), 139–157. *Evidence Level V.*

Palmer, M. H. (1996). *Urinary continence: Assessment and promotion.* Gaithersburg, MD: Aspen. *Evidence Level VI.*

Palmer, M. H. (2004). Use of health behavior change theories to guide urinary incontinence research. *Nursing Research, 53*(Suppl. 6), S49–S55. *Evidence Level VI.*

Palmer, M. H., Baumgarten, M., Langenberg, P., & Carson, J. L. (2002). Risk factors for hospital-acquired incontinence in elderly female hip fracture patients. *Journals of Gerontology. Series A, Biological Sciences and Medical Sciences, 57*(10), M672–M677. *Evidence Level IV.*

Palmer, M. H., Bone, L. R., Fahey, M., Mamon, J., & Steinwachs, D. (1992). Detecting urinary continence in older adults during hospitalization. *Applied Nursing Research, 5,* 174–180. *Evidence Level IV.*

Palmer, M. H., Myers, A. H., & Fedenko, K. M. (1997). Urinary continence changes after hip-fracture repair. *Clinical Nursing Research, 6*(1), 8–21; discussion 21. *Evidence Level IV.*

Pettersen, R., Saxby, B. K., & Wyller, T. B. (2007). Poststroke urinary incontinence: One-year outcome and relationships with measures of attentiveness. *Journal of the American Geriatrics Society, 55*(10), 1571–1577. *Evidence Level IV.*

Pfisterer, M. H., Johnson, T. M., Jenetzky, E., Hauer, K., & Oster, P. (2007). Geriatric patients' preferences for treatment of urinary incontinence: A study of hospitalized, cognitively competent adults aged 80 and older. *Journal of the American Geriatrics Society, 55*(12), 2016–2022. *Evidence Level IV.*

Qaseem, A., Dallas, P., Forciea, M. A., Starkey, M., Denberg, T. D., & Shekelle, P.; Clinical Guidelines Committee of the American College of Physicians. (2014). Nonsurgical management of urinary incontinence in women: A clinical practice guideline from the American College of Physicians. *Annals of Internal Medicine, 161*(6), 429–440. *Evidence Level I.*

Rathnayake, T. (2009a). Urinary incontinence: Bladder training. *JBI Database of Evidence Summaries,* Publication ES5237. *Evidence Level I.*

Rathnayake, T. (2009b). Urinary incontinence: Prompted voiding. *JBI Database of Evidence Summaries,* Publication ES5396. *Evidence Level I.*

Rathnayake, T. (2009c). Urinary incontinence: Timed voiding. *JBI Database of Evidence Summaries,* Publication ES5330. *Evidence Level I.*

Rathnayake, T. (2009d). Urinary incontinence: Treatments. *JBI Database of Evidence Summaries,* Publication ES6918. *Evidence Level I.*

Resnick, N. M., & Ouslander, J. G. (1990). National Institutes of Health consensus development conference on urinary incontinence. *Journal of the American Geriatrics Society, 38,* 263–386. *Evidence Level IV.*

Robinson, J. P., & Shea, J. A. (2002). Development and testing of a measure of health-related quality of life for men with urinary incontinence. *Journal of the American Geriatrics Society, 50*(5), 935–945. *Evidence Level IV.*

Saint, S., Kaufman, S. R., Rogers, M. A., Baker, P. D., Ossenkop, K., & Lipsky, B. A. (2006). Condom versus indwelling urinary catheters: a randomized trial. *Journal of the American Geriatrics Society, 54*(7), 1055–1061. *Evidence Level II.*

Sampselle, C. M., Palmer, M. H., Boyington, A. R., O'Dell, K. K., & Wooldridge, L. (2004). Prevention of urinary incontinence in adults: Population-based strategies. *Nursing Research, 53*(Suppl. 6), S61–S67. *Evidence Level VI.*

Schnelle, J. F., Cadogan, M. P., Grbic, D., Bates-Jensen, B. M., Osterweil, D., Yoshii, J., & Simmons, S. F. (2003). A standardized quality assessment system to evaluate incontinence care in the nursing home. *Journal of the American Geriatrics Society, 51*(12), 1754–1761. *Evidence Level IV.*

Schnelle, J. F., & Smith, R. L. (2001). Quality indicators for the management of urinary incontinence in vulnerable community-dwelling elders. *Annals of Internal Medicine, 135*(8 Pt 2), 752–758. *Evidence Level V.*

Schultz, A., Dickey, G., & Skoner, M. (1997). Self-report of incontinence in acute care. *Urologic Nursing, 17*(1), 23–28. *Evidence Level IV.*

Shamliyan, T., Wyman, J., Bliss, D. Z., Kane, R. L., & Wilt, T. J. (2007). Prevention of urinary and fecal incontinence in adults. *Evidence Report/Technology Assessment,* (161), 1–379. *Evidence Level I.*

Shinopulos, N. (2000). Bedside urodynamic studies: Simple testing for urinary incontinence. *Nurse Practitioner, 25*(6 Pt 1), 19–22, 25. *Evidence Level VI.*

Shumaker, S. A., Wyman, J. F., Uebersax, J. S., McClish, D., & Fantl, J. A. (1994). Health-related quality of life measures for women with urinary incontinence: The Incontinence Impact Questionnaire and the Urogenital Distress Inventory. Continence Program in Women (CPW) Research Group. *Quality of Life Research: An International Journal of Quality of Life Aspects of Treatment, Care and Rehabilitation, 3*(5), 291–306. *Evidence Level IV.*

Sier, H., Ouslander, J., & Orzeck, S. (1987). Urinary incontinence among geriatric patients in an acute-care hospital. *Journal of American Medical Association, 257*(13), 1767–1771. *Evidence Level IV.*

Sims, J., Browning, C., Lundgren-Lindquist, B., & Kendig, H. (2011). Urinary incontinence in a community sample of older adults: Prevalence and impact on quality of life. *Disability and Rehabilitation, 33*(15–16), 1389–1398. *Evidence Level IV.*

Skelly, J., & Flint, A. J. (1995). Urinary incontinence associated with dementia. *Journal of the American Geriatrics Society, 43*(3), 286–294. *Evidence Level V.*

Smith, D. A. (2000). Urge incontinence. In D. B. Doughty (Ed.), *Urinary & fecal incontinence: Nursing management* (2nd ed., pp. 91–104). St. Louis, MO: Mosby. *Evidence Level VI.*

Specht, J. K. (2005). 9 Myths of incontinence in older adults: Both clinicians and the over-65 set need to know more. *American Journal of Nursing, 105*(6), 58–68; quiz 69. *Evidence Level V.*

Subak, L. L., Richter, H. E., & Hunskaar, S. (2009). Obesity and urinary incontinence: Epidemiology and clinical research update. *Journal of Urology, 182*(Suppl. 6), S2–S7. *Evidence Level I.*

Subak, L. L., Whitcomb, E., Shen, H., Saxton, J., Vittinghoff, E., & Brown, J. S. (2005). Weight loss: A novel and effective treatment for urinary incontinence. *Journal of Urology, 174*(1), 190–195. *Evidence Level II.*

Syah, N. A. (2010). Urinary (incontinence) management. *JBI Database of Evidence Summaries,* Publication ES6985. *Evidence Level I.*

Tadic, S. D., Zdaniuk, B., Griffiths, D., Rosenberg, L., Schäfer, W., & Resnick, N. M. (2007). Effect of biofeedback on psychological burden and symptoms in older women with urge urinary incontinence. *Journal of the American Geriatrics Society, 55*(12), 2010–2015. *Evidence Level IV.*

Taylor, C., Lillis, C., & LeMone, P. (2005). *Fundamental of nursing: The art and science of nursing care* (5th ed.). New York, NY: Lippincott, Williams, & Wilkins. *Evidence Level VI.*

Terpenning, M. S., Allada, R., & Kauffman, C. A. (1989). Intermittent urethral catheterization in the elderly. *Journal of the American Geriatrics Society, 37*(5), 411–416. *Evidence Level IV.*

Teunissen, T. A., de Jonge, A., van Weel, C., & Lagro-Janssen, A. L. (2004). Treating urinary incontinence in the elderly—Conservative therapies that work: A systematic review. *Journal of Family Practice, 53*(1), 25–30, 32. *Evidence Level I.*

Thomas, L. H., Barrett, J., Cross, S., French, B., Leathley, M., Sutton, C., & Watkins, C. (2005). Prevention and treatment of urinary incontinence after stroke in adults. *Cochrane Database of Systematic Reviews, 2005*(3), CD004462. *Evidence Level I.*

Tsai, Y. C., & Liu, C. H. (2009). The effectiveness of pelvic floor exercises, digital vaginal palpation and interpersonal support on stress urinary incontinence: An experimental study. *International Journal of Nursing Studies, 46*(9), 1181–1186. *Evidence Level II.*

Uebersax, J. S., Wyman, J. F., Shumaker, S. A., McClish, D. K., & Fantl, J. A. (1995). Short forms to assess life quality and symptom distress for urinary incontinence in women: The Incontinence Impact Questionnaire and the Urogenital Distress Inventory. Continence Program for Women Research Group. *Neurourology and Urodynamics, 14*(2), 131–139. *Evidence Level IV.*

Vaughan, C., Juncos, J., Burgio, K., Goode, P., Wolf, R., & Johnson, T. (2011). Behavioral therapy to treat urinary incontinence in Parkinson disease. *Neurology, 76*(19), 1631–1634. *Evidence Level III.*

Vinsnes, A. G., Harkless, G. E., Haltbakk, J., Bohm, J., & Hunskaar, S. (2001). Healthcare personnel's attitudes towards patients with urinary incontinence. *Journal of Clinical Nursing, 10*(4), 455–462. *Evidence Level IV.*

Warren, J. W. (1997). Catheter-associated urinary tract infections. *Infectious Disease Clinics of North America, 11*(3), 609–622. *Evidence Level VI.*

Watson, N. M. (2004). Advancing quality of urinary incontinence evaluation and treatment in nursing homes through translational research. *Worldviews on Evidence-Based Nursing/Sigma Theta Tau International, Honor Society of Nursing, 1*(Suppl. 1), S21–S25. *Evidence Level VI.*

Watson, N. M., Brink, C. A., Zimmer, J. G., & Mayer, R. D. (2003). Use of the Agency for Health Care Policy and Research Urinary Incontinence Guideline in nursing homes. *Journal of the American Geriatrics Society, 51*(12), 1779–1786. *Evidence Level VI.*

Wenger, N. S., Roth, C. P., Martin, D., Nickels, L., Beckman, R., Kamberg, C., . . . Ganz, D. A. (2011). Quality of care provided in a special needs plan using a nurse care manager model. *Journal of the American Geriatrics Society, 59*(10), 1810–1822. *Evidence Level IV.*

Wilson, L., Brown, J. S., Shin, G. P., Luc, K. O., & Subak, L. L. (2001). Annual direct cost of urinary incontinence. *Obstetrics and gynecology, 98*(3), 398–406. *Evidence Level IV.*

Wolf, S. L., Riolo, L., & Ouslander, J. G. (2000). Urge incontinence and the risk of falling in older women. *Journal of the American Geriatrics Society, 48*(7), 847–848. *Evidence Level VI.*

Zimakoff, J., Stickler, D. J., Pontoppidan, B., & Larsen, S. O. (1996). Bladder management and urinary tract infections in Danish hospitals, nursing homes, and home care: A national prevalence study. *Infection Control and Hospital Epidemiology, 17*(4), 215–221. *Evidence Level IV.*

Zisberg, A. (2011). Incontinence brief use in acute hospitalized patients with no prior incontinence. *Journal of Wound, Ostomy, and Continence Nursing: Official Publication of the Wound, Ostomy and Continence Nurses Society/WOCN, 38*(5), 559–564. *Evidence Level IV.*

22

Prevention of Catheter-Associated Urinary Tract Infection

Heidi L. Wald, Regina M. Fink,
Mary Beth Flynn Makic, and Kathleen S. Oman

EDUCATIONAL OBJECTIVES

On completion of this chapter, the reader should be able to:

1. Define catheter-associated urinary tract infection (CAUTI)
2. Describe the epidemiology of CAUTI
3. Define indications for indwelling urinary catheters (IUC)
4. Identify evidence-based strategies and interventions for the prevention of CAUTI
5. Describe key components of a nurse-driven protocol for IUC removal
6. Understand how to engage an interdisciplinary team in the prevention and management of CAUTIs

OVERVIEW

Health care–associated infections (HAIs) have received increasing scrutiny over the past decade. It is now widely recognized that HAIs are often preventable adverse events related to medical care. CAUTIs are among the most common HAIs, occurring at a rate of 0.2 to 4.8 infections per 1,000 catheter days for adult inpatient units (Centers for Disease Control and Prevention [CDC], 2013), CAUTIs are associated with significant morbidity and excess health care costs (Klevens et al., 2007; Tambyah, 2002). Catheter use and CAUTIs are disproportionately reported among older adults (Fakih et al., 2010; Vincitorio et al., 2014). Although once largely overlooked as part of the price of doing business in hospitals, a significantly changed regulatory environment has emerged that has brought increased scrutiny to HAIs in general, and CAUTIs in particular. Examples of this oversight include process and outcome measurement and reporting and financial incentives to improve these measures. Since 2008, the Centers for Medicare & Medicaid Services (CMS) no longer reimburses for additional costs required to treat hospital-acquired urinary tract infections (UTIs; CMS, 2007). Long-term care facilities also follow CMS regulatory guidance and their federal regulations (F-315 Tag) mandate that IUC use must be medically justified and care rendered to reduce infection risk in all residents with or without an IUC (CMS, 2005). Enhanced public reporting and financial incentives figure prominently in the Patient Protection and Affordable Care Act of 2010; HAIs were singled out for inclusion in both of these initiatives (Patient Protection and Affordable Care Act, 2010). In related rulemaking, CAUTI is included as a measure in the new HAI reduction program and the value-based purchasing composite measure (PSI 90) for acute care hospitals (Agency for Healthcare Research and Quality,

For a description of evidence levels cited in this chapter, see Chapter 1, "Developing and Evaluating Clinical Practice Guidelines: A Systematic Approach."

2013a; CMS, 2007, 2008). Therefore, it is imperative that health care professionals in all settings develop strategies and interventions to reduce IUC duration and prevent CAUTIs, thus benefitting both clinical and financial outcomes.

This focus on reducing harm occurs even as the evidence base for the prevention of CAUTI continues to evolve. Between 2008 and 2014, multiple stakeholder organizations, including the CDC, and several major professional societies critically examined the literature on CAUTI prevention (Cottenden et al., 2005; Gould et al., 2010; Greene et al., 2008; Hooten et al., 2010; Joanna Briggs Institute, 2010; Lo, Nicolle, & Classen, 2008; Lo et al., 2014; Society of Urologic Nurses, 2006; see Resources section). Also, the CDC's National Healthcare Safety Network (NHSN) significantly revised the surveillance definition for CAUTI several times since 2009, including a major revision in January 2015, with the cumulative effect of focusing surveillance efforts on only the most clinically important events (CDC, 2015). Despite this attention, CAUTI rates have been stable. A 2012 data report showed an overall 3% increase in CAUTIs reported to the CDC nationwide, even as rates of other HAIs decline (CDC, 2013). However, a large national collaborative reported preliminary success in CAUTI reduction by pairing a technical bundle with a socio-adaptive change model (Agency for Healthcare Research and Quality, 2013b).

In light of these rapid changes in the field and the regulatory focus on CAUTI, the regular review of policies, procedures, practices, and products is imperative for all health care facilities. In this chapter, we review the rationale for CAUTI prevention strategies, suggest an approach to implementing a comprehensive CAUTI prevention program, and catalog the most important CAUTI prevention strategies.

BACKGROUND AND STATEMENT OF PROBLEM

Health care–associated UTIs are frequent and costly, resulting in increased morbidity and possible mortality in hospitalized elders. There are estimated to be more than 400,000 hospital-acquired UTIs in the United States annually (Klevens et al., 2007; Scott, 2009; Tambyah et al., 2002). At a mean cost of $589 per episode, this epidemic results in $250 million of excess health care costs each year (Tambyah et al., 2002). In a multihospital study in Quebec, 21% of bacteremias were from a urinary source, with 71% associated with IUCs. Thus, CAUTI is an important cause of hospital-acquired bacteremia (Fortin, Rocher, Frenette, Tremblay, & Quach, 2012).

The majority of UTIs are associated with the ubiquitous IUC, also known as a Foley catheter, after urologist Frederick Foley who developed the modern device. Urinary catheters are among the most widely used medical devices. Despite their utility in acutely ill patients, they have many downsides, including the CAUTI. Other complications include delirium (Inouye, 2006), accidental removal, gross hematuria, leakage, urethral injury, and restriction of mobility. Taken together, these complications of IUCs occur as frequently as CAUTI (Hollingsworth et al., 2013; Saint, Lipsky, & Goold, 2002). Therefore, the benefits of managing urinary output with an IUC must be weighed against the many risks.

Unfortunately, the indiscriminate use of IUCs is widespread. IUCs are used in up to 16% of adult hospital inpatients and are more commonly used in the older patient (Vincitorio et al., 2014). Older age and female sex are risk factors for catheterization, and older women are more likely to have no clear indication for catheterization than other patients (Vincitorio et al., 2014). Of Medicare patients undergoing elective surgery, 86% have an IUC (Wald, Ma, Bratzler, & Kramer, 2008). According to the Infectious Diseases Society of America, 21% to 54% of all IUCs are inappropriately placed and are not medically indicated (Fakih et al., 2010; Gokula, Murthy, Hickner, & Smith, 2004; Hooten et al., 2010). Thus, interventions aimed at evidence-based use of catheters are needed to reduce unnecessary catheter days, and to prevent CAUTIs. To better understand the potential approaches to prevention of CAUTIs, an understanding of CAUTI pathogenesis is essential.

CAUTI Pathogenesis

The urinary tract is normally a sterile body site, therefore, any positive urine culture can be considered abnormal. Asymptomatic bacteriuria is of questionable clinical significance, however, and should not be treated except in pregnant patients or those undergoing urologic surgery (Nicolle et al., 2005). The CDC's surveillance definition therefore only focuses on symptomatic or bacteremic infections, which occur in the presence of an IUC (CDC, 2015).

When a patient has an IUC, microorganisms can gain access to the urinary tract on either the extraluminal surface of the IUC or intraluminal surface through breaks in the catheter system (Figure 22.1). Extraluminal infection can occur early if bacteria are introduced during insertion, but more commonly, extraluminal infection occurs later (Tillekeratne et al., 2014). Once they gain access to the urinary tract, microorganisms can thrive in a "biofilm" layer on either the extra- or intraluminal surface of the IUC. The biofilm, made up of bacteria, host proteins, and bacterial slime, is thought to be important in the development of late CAUTIs. Because the formation of a biofilm and colonization with bacteria takes time, most CAUTI occurs after 48 hours of catheterization and increases approximately 5% per day (Schaeffer, 1986; Stamm, 1975).

The mechanisms described earlier provide the rationale for evidence-based care of IUCs and highlights four potential opportunities for intervention during the use of IUCs (Figure 22.2). The first opportunity is avoidance of catheters at the time of the decision for insertion, the second is evidence-based product selection and care practices regarding IUCs (including insertion and maintenance), and the third is minimizing duration through timely removal. A fourth set of additional strategies for CAUTI prevention includes education of providers, surveillance of processes, and reporting practice outcomes and CAUTI rates. This set of strategies can be applied at any of the opportunities for intervention. A comprehensive program to eliminate CAUTIs includes elements of each of the aforementioned strategies.

FIGURE 22.1

Routes of entry of uropathogens to catheterized urinary tract.

Extraluminal
• *Early*, at insertion
• *Late*, by capillary action
Intraluminal
• Break in closed drainage
• Contamination of collection bag urine

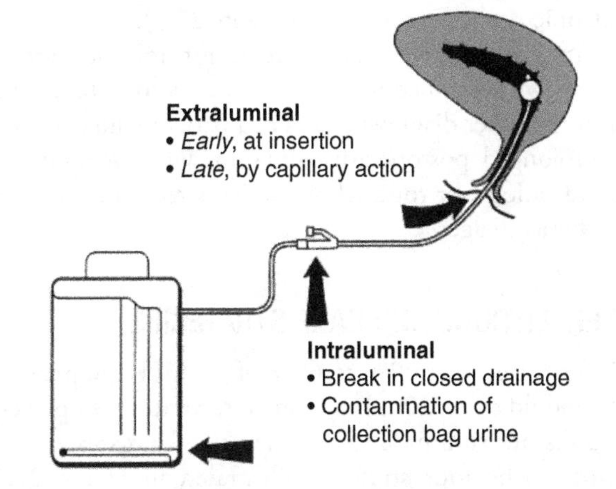

Source: Maki and Tambyah (2001).

ASSESSMENT OF THE PROBLEM

Surveillance Definition of CAUTI

Although clinical diagnosis of CAUTI allows for clinical judgment, the CDC has developed explicit surveillance criteria for CAUTI in acute care for use by infection control practitioners (CDC, 2015). In brief, the patient must have:

1. An IUC for at least 2 days, which is either still in place or removed within 1 day before the date of the event.
2. One of the following: fever more than 38°C, suprapubic tenderness, costovertebral angle pain, or tenderness, (additional symptoms may include urinary urgency, frequency, or dysuria if the catheter has already been

FIGURE 22.2

Stages of catheter use and potential intervention strategies.

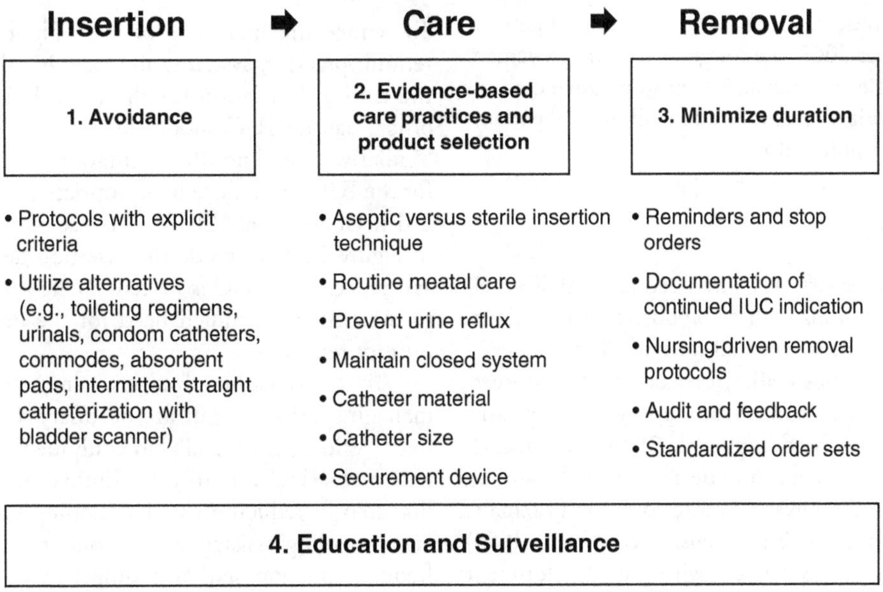

Insertion
Care
Removal
1. Avoidance
2. Evidence-based care practices and product selection
3. Minimize duration
• Protocols with explicit criteria
• Utilize alternatives (e.g., toileting regimens, urinals, condom catheters, commodes, absorbent pads, intermittent straight catheterization with bladder scanner)
• Aseptic versus sterile insertion technique
• Routine meatal care
• Prevent urine reflux
• Maintain closed system
• Catheter material
• Catheter size
• Securement device
• Reminders and stop orders
• Documentation of continued IUC indication
• Nursing-driven removal protocols
• Audit and feedback
• Standardized order sets
4. Education and Surveillance

removed); or a positive blood culture with the same organism as in the urine.

3. A positive urine culture sent more than 48 hours after admission to the health care facility. A positive urine culture is defined as having no more than two species of microorganism, at least one of which is a bacteria of greater than or equal to 10 colony-forming units/mL of urine (CMS, 2005).

All elements of the definition must occur within a 7-day window. A CAUTI diagnosed within 48 hours of arrival to a health care facility or unit is attributed to the previous location.

In nonbacteremic cases, this surveillance definition requires that the patient have symptoms referable to the urinary tract or a fever without another cause. For the purposes of infection-control surveillance in acute care, new alterations in mental status do not meet the diagnostic criteria for CAUTI. Of note, the CDC's surveillance definition for UTI in long-term care facilities differs substantially from the acute care definition. Practitioners in long-term care facilities should acquaint themselves with that definition (Stone et al., 2012).

CAUTIs are generally reported as infections per 1,000 catheter days on a given patient care unit. More than half of all states require public reporting of HAIs, among them many specify reporting of CAUTIs. Hospitals participating in the Medicare program must report all CAUTIs to the CDC's NHSN for the purposes of surveillance, public reporting on Hospital Compare, and incentive programs.

Additional important process measurement includes the catheter usage ratio reported as catheter days per patient-days. Since October 2009, the Surgical Care Improvement Project (SCIP) collects a measure of postoperative catheter removal on catheterization day 1 or 2 for all surgical patients (The Joint Commission, n.d.).

Indications for IUC

Avoidance of unnecessary IUCs may reduce CAUTI incidence and complications such as bloodstream infections. A decrease in IUC use is expected to result in decreases in length of stay, cost of hospitalization associated with treatment of CAUTI and bloodstream infections (Apisarnthanarak et al., 2007b; Meddings et al., 2014). Elpern et al. (2009) evaluated the inappropriate use of IUCs among inpatients and found them to be more common in female, nonambulatory, and medical intensive care unit (ICU) patients. Risk factors associated with the development of CAUTI in hospitalized patients include older age, not maintaining a closed drainage system, neutropenia, renal disease, and male gender (Greene et al., 2012; Lo et al., 2014). Explicit criteria for appropriate insertion may result in significant reductions in catheter duration and CAUTI prevalence. The University of Colorado Health System developed criteria for appropriate insertion of IUCs in hospitalized patients based on evidence (Chenoweth et al., 2014; Fuchs, Sexton, Thronlow, & Champagne, 2011; Lo et al., 2014; Mori, 2014) and disseminated this information to nursing and physician staff through the integration of a nurse-driven protocol for IUC removal within the electronic health record (EHR; Figure 22.3).

An IUC should not be used for routine care of patients who are incontinent, as a means to obtain urine culture or other diagnostic tests in a patient who can void, for prolonged postoperative duration without appropriate indications, or routinely in patients receiving epidural anesthesia/analgesia.

INTERVENTIONS AND CARE STRATEGIES

It is estimated that 20% to 69% of CAUTIs are preventable (Gould et al., 2009). Specific interventions to prevent CAUTIs are summarized as follows and organized with regard to the four strategies illustrated in Figure 22.2. Many of these recommendations are supported by low-quality evidence and expert opinion. Further study may impact these recommendations. A proposed approach to a comprehensive CAUTI intervention follows.

Strategy 1: Avoidance

To reduce the incidence of CAUTI, it is important to rethink practice, systems, and examine the "why" behind the clinical indication for the IUC. Elimination options other than an IUC should be explored before insertion. Similarly, providing documentation of a clear indication for the IUC can reduce inappropriate device use (Lo et al., 2014; Uberoi et al., 2013). The use of explicit criteria (as in Figure 22.3) to guide the insertion decision may be of assistance. If an IUC is placed, an algorithm may be used to determine continued need for the device or promote prompt removal.

To avoid catheterizations, alternative strategies for managing urine output are necessary. Completing a systems evaluation of available equipment to provide alternatives to IUC for urinary elimination is an important first step in reducing use. Developing toileting schedules and providing assistance with toileting incorporated into frequent nursing staff rounding is another strategy that can be used to reduce urgency and incontinence episodes

FIGURE 22.3

University of Colorado Health System nurse-driven indwelling urinary catheter removal protocol.

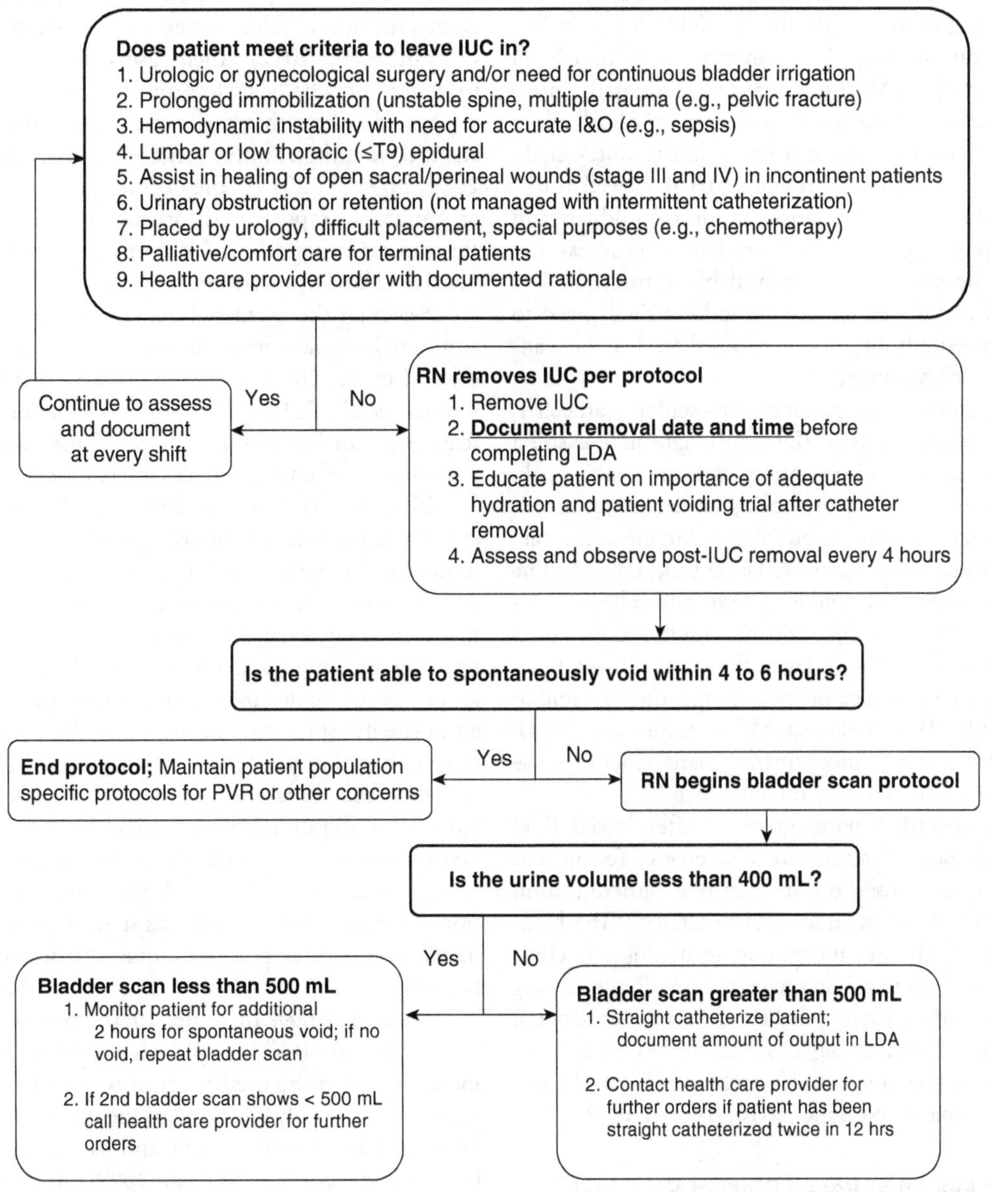

I&O, input and output; IUC, indwelling urinary catheter; LDA, lines, drains, airways; PVR, postvoid residual.

(Uberoi et al., 2013). If the patient is mobile or has limited mobility, alternatives to an IUC include the use of a bedside commode with a toileting schedule (Gray, 2010; Uberoi et al., 2013), condom catheters for male patients (Dowling-Castronovo & Bradway, 2008; Saint et al., 2013), moisture-wicking incontinence pads (Covidien Maxicare Underpad; Medline Ultrasorb Underpad), intermittent straight catheterization with the use of a bladder scanner to determine bladder urine volume (Hooten et al., 2010; Parry et al., 2013; Saint et al., 2013), as well as urinals and bedpans. Careful consideration of products and how and where they are stocked is essential to success. For instance, commodes need to be available in multiple sizes and need to include bariatric commodes; urinals need to fit snugly on bedrails; bladder ultrasound needs to be readily available for assessment.

For less mobile male patients, the condom catheter is an effective alternative to an IUC, although there is still a small risk of infection with condom catheters (Saint et al., 2013). Moisture-absorbing or wicking underpads for incontinence management are an alternative for the acute care environment (Covidien Maxicare Underpad, n.d.; Medline Ultrasorb Underpad n.d.) and long-term care or home environments (NAFC.org). Incontinence underpad products pull effluent moisture/urine away from the skin and can absorb up to 2 L of fluid before becoming saturated (Junkin & Selekof, 2008; Padula Manish, Makic, & Sullivan, 2011). For a full discussion of incontinence management, please refer to Chapter 21, "Urinary Incontinence."

Urinary retention postsurgery or after initial IUC removal may pose clinical care challenges. To prevent IUC insertion or reinsertion, intermittent catheterization should be considered as an avoidance strategy. The bladder scanner, which uses ultrasound technology, is clinically beneficial in determining urinary retention, reducing unnecessary intermittent catheterizations, enhancing patient comfort, and saving costs associated with inappropriate catheterizations, and possible CAUTIs (Palese, Buchini, Deroma, & Barbone, 2010; Saint et al., 2013).

Strategy 2: Evidence-Based Product Selection, Insertion, and Routine Care

If an IUC is determined to be clinically indicated, selection of the right catheter, proper technique during insertion of the device, and evidence-based ongoing care management are needed to reduce infection.

Catheter material remains an area of ongoing debate. Although antimicrobial catheter materials have been shown to reduce catheter-associated bacteriuria (Lo et al., 2014; Pickard et al., 2012), the impact of antimicrobial catheters on symptomatic CAUTIs remains unproven. Research syntheses have failed to conclusively demonstrate effectiveness of silver-coated or antibiotic impregnated catheters on prevention of CAUTIs for short-term catheterization of adult patients versus standard materials (Pickard et al., 2012). There also is insufficient evidence to determine whether selection of a latex catheter, hydrogel-coated latex catheter, silicone-coated latex catheter, or all-silicone catheter influences CAUTI risk (Hooten et al., 2010; Lo et al., 2014). The decision to use a silver-coated or antibiotic impregnated catheter should be made with the understanding that it does not substitute for a comprehensive CAUTI prevention program.

Selecting the smallest IUC size, when possible, is an additional consideration to reduce the risk of infection (Gould et al., 2009; L. Greene, Marx, & Oriola, 2008; Hooten et al., 2010). The selection of a smaller catheter (e.g., less than 18 French) reduces irritation and inflammation of the urethra and reduces infection risk (Gray, 2010).

Placing an IUC is a fundamental skill for nurses; however, current evidence supporting sterile versus aseptic technique for the procedure is inconclusive (Lo et al., 2014). A strict sterile technique involves using a sterile gown, mask, prolonged hand washing (greater than 4 minutes), opening and using a sterile insertion kit, donning sterile gloves, cleansing the urethral meatus and perineal area with an antiseptic solution, and inserting the catheter using a no-touch technique (Gray, 2010). Wilson et al. (2009) reviewed the literature and found that most clinicians employ an aseptic technique, which was most frequently defined as the use of sterile gloves, sterile barriers, perineal washing using an antiseptic cleanser, and no-touch insertion. Current recommendations suggest an IUC insertion be placed under aseptic technique with sterile equipment (Gould et al., 2009; Greene et al., 2008; Hooten et al., 2010; Joanna Briggs Institute, 2010; Lo et al., 2014).

Once an IUC is placed, optimal management includes care of the urethral meatus according to "routine hygiene" (e.g., daily cleansing of the meatal surface during bathing with soap and water and as needed following a bowel movement; Gould et al., 2009; Greene et al., 2008; Hooten et al., 2010; Joanna Briggs Institute, 2010). Metal cleansing with antiseptics, creams, lotions, or ointment has been found to irritate the meatus, possibly increasing the risk of infection (Jeong et al., 2010; Joanna Briggs Institute, 2010; Lo et al., 2014).

Securing the IUC after placement to reduce friction from movement is an important element of catheter management supported by current guidelines, researchers, and expert opinion panels (Clarke et al., 2013; Darouiche et al., 2006; Gould et al., 2009; Hooten et al., 2010; Joanna

Briggs Institute, 2010). Maintaining a closed catheter system is also supported by current guidelines (Gould et al., 2009; Greene et al., 2008; Hooten et al., 2010; Joanna Briggs Institute, 2010; Lo et al., 2014) to eliminate the introduction of microbes that occurs when breaking the prepackaged seals on the IUC. A systems analysis should be conducted to purchase and stock the most commonly needed IUC insertion and drainage-bag kits to optimize the maintenance of a closed system. Similarly, maintaining the urine-collection bag below the level of the bladder minimizes reflux into the catheter itself preventing retrograde flow of urine (Clarke et al., 2013; Gould et al., 2009; Greene et al., 2008; Hooten et al., 2010; Joanna Briggs Institute, 2010). Establishing workflow protocols to routinely empty the drainage bag frequently and before transport are important in reducing urine reflux and opportunities for CAUTI.

Strategy 3: Timely Removal

Developing systems that prompt health care providers to review the need for the IUC and encourage early removal have been found to reduce IUC use and CAUTI rates (Alessandri, Mistrangelo, Lijoi, Ferrero, & Ragni, 2006; Alexaitis et al., 2014; American Nurses Association CAUTI Prevention Tool, 2015; Andreessen, Wilde, & Herendeen, 2012; Carter, Reitmeier, & Goodloe, 2014; Fakih et al., 2012; Fuchs et al., 2011; Knoll et al., 2011; Marigliano et al., 2012; Meddings et al., 2014; Mori, 2014; Parry, Grant, & Sestovic, 2013; Purvis et al., 2014; Rosenthal et al., 2012; Saint et al., 2013; Titsworth et al., 2012). Meddings et al. (2014) updated an earlier systematic review and meta-analysis and found that urinary catheter removal reminders and stop orders appeared to reduce CAUTI rates. Implementation of systems that provide physicians and nurses with routine reminders to evaluate the need for the IUC or automatic stop orders were found to reduce the CAUTI rate by 53% ($p \leq .0001$). In this study, automatic stop orders were more effective than reminders in reducing catheter duration ($p < .0001$ and $p = .071$, respectively).

Other approaches to reducing catheter days include audit and feedback and reminders to recommend reevaluation of the need for the IUC (Marigliano et al., 2012; Meddings et al., 2014; Parry et al., 2013; Purvis et al., 2014; Saint et al., 2013) and early removal (Alexaitis et al., 2014; American Nurses Association CAUTI Prevention Tool, 2015; Fuchs et al., 2011; Meddings et al., 2014; Mori, 2014; Parry et al., 2013; Saint et al., 2013; Titsworth et al., 2012). EHR icons (Purvis et al., 2014) or flags that calculate the number of days the IUC has been placed are effective forms of electronic reminders that can easily be incorporated into the EHR. Automatic stop orders or IUC orders that expire in a defined time frame have shown to reduce both catheter usage and CAUTI (Fuchs et al., 2011; Knoll et al., 2011; Saint et al., 2013). Daily nursing rounds (Alexaitis et al., 2014; Fakih et al., 2012; Purvis et al., 2014), and the use of checklists (Andreessen et al., 2012; Fuchs et al., 2011) have also been shown to reduce catheter usage and CAUTI.

Nurse-driven catheter removal protocols are being developed and implemented successfully in many acute care settings (Andreessen et al., 2012; Carter et al., 2014; Fakih et al., 2012; Knoll et al., 2011; Purvis et al., 2014; Saint et al., 2013; Titsworth et al., 2012). Protocols range in degree of nurse autonomy in catheter removal decision making; some require a physician order, most allow the nurse to remove the catheter when there is no evidence-based indication for continuation. Protocols also differ in complexity, with some only addressing the IUC removal aspect of the protocol and others that address follow-up bladder management strategies with bladder scanning guidelines (Alexaitis et al., 2014; American Nurses Association CAUTI Prevention Tool 2015; Carter et al., 2014; Mori, 2014; Purvis et al., 2014; Saint et al., 2013). Figure 22.3 is an example of a nurse-driven IUC removal protocol developed and implemented by the University of Colorado Hospital.

If premature, early removal of IUCs poses the risk of unnecessary recatheterization. It is important to monitor the need for recatheterization to avoid unintended harm. In the meta-analysis conducted by Meddings et al. (2014), low recatheterization rates were noted in studies using reminders and automatic stop orders.

Most of the implementation and quality-improvement research employs multiple interventions (or bundles), as CAUTI prevention is a multifaceted issue. These bundled approaches are also effective and are providing explicit criteria for catheter usage and structured approaches to CAUTI reduction (Andreessen et al., 2012; Fakih et al., 2012; Knoll et al., 2011; Purvis et al., 2014; Rosenthal et al., 2012; Titsworth et al., 2012).

It is well established that duration of IUC increases CAUTI risk. The SCIP is a national quality partnership of organizations interested in improving surgical care by significantly reducing surgical complications (The Joint Commission, n.d.). One of the key performance measures in this program is CAUTI prevention; specifically that IUCs be removed by postoperation day 2, also known as SCIP-inf-9. This SCIP performance measure has had significant impact on decreasing catheter usage in surgical patients (CMS, 2015).

Keeping the IUC as long as thoracic epidural analgesia is maintained (higher than T9) may result in a higher incidence of CAUTI and increased hospital stay. IUC removal on the morning after surgery while the thoracic epidural catheter is still in place does not lead to increased incidence of urinary retention, infection, or higher rates of recatheterizations (Basse, Werner, & Kehlet, 2000; Chia, Wei, Chang, & Liu, 2009; Stubbs et al., 2013; Zaouter, Kanera, & Carli, 2009; Zaouter, Wuethrich, Miccoli, & Carli, 2012).

Strategy 4: Surveillance and Education

Ensuring that leadership of organizations and systems are in place to effectively evaluate and sustain practice change is essential to improving patient outcomes (Kabcenell, Nolan, Martin, & Gill, 2010; Reinertsen, Bisognano, & Pugh, 2008). In particular, surveillance is a cornerstone of CAUTI prevention but is resource intensive, typically relying on manual surveillance by trained infection prevention personnel (Wald, Bandle, & Richard, 2014). There is emerging evidence that electronic surveillance, using EHR algorithms, are effective in increasing the efficiency of CAUTI identification (Shepard et al., 2014; Wald et al., 2014). Catheter usage data and CAUTI rates are key data elements to collect and trend. IUC usage is determined by the number of catheter days divided by the number of patient days and is expressed as a ratio. CAUTI rate is determined by the number of CAUTIs divided by 1,000 catheter days. Both data elements can then be benchmarked against the NHSN pooled means to assess unit level performance. However, the use of a catheter days denominator can produce unstable CAUTI rates when catheter usage is low (Wright, Kharasch, Beaumont, Peterson, & Robicsek, 2011).

Measurement must be accompanied by provision of knowledge and skills to frontline providers through appropriate education and training, which may be central to a multicomponent CAUTI intervention. Multiple studies and quality-improvement projects found that multifaceted educational interventions bundled with the use of algorithms/checklists, automated stop orders, physician EHR reminder prompts, and/or nurse-driven removal protocols are effective in decreasing CAUTIs and catheter usage (Alexaitis & Broome, 2014; Andreessen et al., 2012; Apisarnthanarak, 2007a; Carter et al., 2014; Knoll et al., 2011; Marigliano et al., 2012; Mori, 2014; Purvis et al., 2014; Roser et al., 2012). Ongoing system evaluation, nursing reeducation, practice reminders, and public reporting of unit-based CAUTI rate data are strategies to inform the health care team of current practice outcomes and effectiveness of CAUTI prevention strategies. Implementing systems that encompass the whole health care team to question the need for the IUC and, when indicated, ensuring proper care and early removal can be pivotal in reducing CAUTI rates (Wenger, 2010).

Approach to a Comprehensive CAUTI Intervention

Evidence-based practice (EBP) guidelines derived from valid, current research and other evidence sources can successfully improve patient outcomes and quality care. However, simply disseminating scientific evidence is often ineffective in changing clinical practice. Learning how to implement findings is critically important to promoting high-quality, safe care. How EBPs are adopted in practice depend on the type, complexity, and strength of the evidence and how the knowledge is communicated to clinicians (Titler, 2011). There are a number of models that can guide the implementation of EBP (Rycroft-Malone & Bucknall, 2010) but there is not a single way to implement new findings into practice. What works in one setting may need modification to be successful in another context (Titler, 2011). Understanding health care provider decisions, experiences, practice processes, and barriers is considered essential. These elements must be explored to successfully implement practice change based on best evidence (Melnyk & Fineout-Overholt, 2011).

The explicit use of a socio-adaptive model has been employed in large-scale HAI prevention activities, including the Agency for Healthcare Research and Quality's On the Comprehensive Unit-based Safety Program (CUSP): STOP CAUTI initiative. Here, the technical interventions for CAUTI reduction were paired with the CUSP developed by Pronovost et al., which provides tools for improving safety climate on clinical units (Pronovost et al., 2005). The preliminary results of this work are promising for a decrease in CAUTI, but show no change in IUC usage (Agency for Healthcare Research and Quality, 2013a).

At a minimum, the development of an interdisciplinary champion team and the creation of a multifaceted intervention to implement evidence-based procedures for IUC insertion and maintenance must be a priority in all practice settings. The ultimate goals are to reduce routine catheter insertions, provide evidence-based catheter care, and prompt early removal when possible, thus decreasing the risk of and prevention of CAUTI.

Steps used for protocol development at the University of Colorado Hospital are highlighted as follows. Improved patient outcomes (decreased catheter days, decreased CAUTIs) and decreased costs have been realized.

Protocol Development

1. Recruit an interdisciplinary champion team to include nurses (clinical, educators, operating room [OR] RNs, emergency department [ED] RNs); physicians [hospitalists, infectious disease, ED MDs, surgeons, anesthesiologists]); rehabilitation therapists and transport

personnel; infection control preventionists; and quality-improvement, central supply, and clinical informatics representatives.

2. Examine and synthesize the evidence (search, review, critique, and hold journal clubs in various care areas to present the evidence).
3. Identify and understand product use, availability, and costs in your health care setting. Refine product use based on the best evidence and cost analysis. Examine:
   - Urinary catheter materials, sizes, kits, drainage bags
   - Catheter securement device
   - Urinal and bedpan availability
   - Commodes (availability and size)
   - Bladder scanners
   - Alternatives (incontinence pads, condom catheters, etc.)
4. Identify barriers to optimal IUC care practices by surveying staff or holding focus groups throughout your health care setting.
5. Update your policy and procedures related to IUC insertion and care based on the evidence.
6. Consider dividing the project into manageable phases. Avoidance strategies may require a different approach than care or removal strategies. For instance, avoidance starts in the ED and OR; removal occurs on inpatient floors.
7. Develop and use algorithms, decision aids, and factoid posters displaying evidence-based caveats.
8. Development of a nurse-driven IUC removal protocol.
   - Recruit an interdisciplinary team to include nurses (clinical educators, physicians [hospitalists, infectious disease physicians, surgeons, anesthesiologists]) and clinical informatics representatives.
   - Examine and synthesize the evidence (search, review, critique) and protocol examples.
   - Develop protocol with interdisciplinary and key stakeholder (clinical nurses, charge nurses, educators, physicians [all specialties], midlevel providers, regulatory personnel) input and feedback
   - Incorporate protocol into hospital policy/procedure.
   - Develop EHR interface.
   - Plan education and implementation procedures.
     a. Identify champions to assist with implementation: infection control champions, nurse educators, clinical nurse educators, and specialists.
     b. Journal club presentations, RN tip sheets, provider tip sheets, EHR screenshot tip sheets, nursing unit posters/clings, PowerPoint presentations.
   - Plan evaluation strategies
     a. Verbal feedback from clinicians
     b. EHR reports on protocol usage/documentation
     c. Audits
9. Update patient and family educational materials on the importance of prompt and early removal of IUCs.
10. Educate staff (including radiology, transport, rehabilitation therapy staff [physical therapy, occupational therapy]) focusing on policy and procedure revision, insertion indication guidelines, insertion procedures, maintenance and care, catheter-bag placement, removal prompts or removal protocols, and bladder scanner use and procedures.
11. Work with infection control and clinical informatics staff to audit and measure outcomes. Provide feedback to staff. Potential measurable outcomes include:
    - CAUTIs/1,000 catheter days
    - Catheter days/hospital days
    - Postoperative catheter days/patient
    - Proportion of catheterized/admitted patients from ED or OR
12. Continually evaluate and update practice changes based on new evidence.

CASE STUDY

CASE 1

Mrs. F is an 87-year-old female with a history of Alzheimer's dementia, incontinence, and a recent fall at home. She presents to your hospital with failure to thrive, increased pain on movement, and a Stage II pressure ulcer on her coccyx. Mrs. F lives at home alone; her daughter frequently checks on her condition.

Mrs. F arrives to your medical unit with an IUC that was placed in the ED. Given the patient's incontinence, fall risk, pain, and concern about pressure ulcer progression, the IUC is left in place. After stabilization of her pain (no fractures are present), Mrs. F is able to ambulate with assistance. Three days after admission while awaiting placement in a skilled nursing facility (SNF), Mrs. F develops fever and delirium and is diagnosed with a UTI. This delays her transfer to the SNF.

Questions to Consider

1. Was the IUC placement medically indicated? If so, what were the indications?

(continued)

CASE STUDY *(continued)*

2. What could have been used as alternatives to IUC placement?
3. Discuss various strategies that may have been used to remind the nursing team to remove the patient's IUC in a timely manner.

Discussion

As incontinence, fall risk, pain, and a Stage II pressure ulcer are not medically appropriate indications for an IUC, it should have been avoided in the ED or removed as soon as the patient arrived to the floor. Alternatives to indwelling catheterization in this patient would include a bedside commode with nursing assistance and/or moisture-wicking incontinence pads. Attentiveness to the appropriate medical indications for catheter use, familiarity with catheter alternatives, and recognition of the clinical and economic impacts may have prevented the infection and eased the placement of this patient. The use of a nurse-driven IUC removal protocol, automatic stop orders in the EHR, and daily nursing rounds on patients with IUCs may call attention to the unnecessary use of the IUC and encourage timely removal.

CASE 2

Mr. B is a 69-year-old alert male with a diagnosis of nonsmall cell lung cancer admitted for a thoracotomy. The patient is transferred from the postanesthesia care unit to the surgical ICU with an IUC that was placed in the OR and a thoracic epidural for pain management with morphine and bupivicaine infusion. Mr. B is doing well 48 hours postoperatively, experiencing little pain and is able to cough and breathe deeply. He is transferred out of the ICU to the surgical floor with the urinary catheter and thoracic epidural still in place. When prompted by nursing staff to write an order for urinary catheter removal, the surgeon says he is waiting for the anesthesiology team to pull the epidural catheter before removing the urinary catheter.

Questions to Consider

1. Was the IUC placement surgically indicated?
2. When should the IUC be removed?
3. When the IUC is removed what can be used as alternatives?
4. If the patient does not void after the IUC is removed, when is a bladder scanner indicated? What are the indications for recatheterization?

Discussion

The IUC was probably indicated because of the length of surgery (greater than 2 hours) and need for accurate monitoring for intake and output. The misconception that the IUC needs to be in place as long as the thoracic epidural remains for pain management purposes needs clarification. Multiple studies have supported IUC removal on the morning after surgery to decrease CAUTI risk in the setting of a thoracic epidural higher than the T9 level (Stubbs et al., 2013; Zaouter et al., 2012). Early removal typically does not lead to urinary retention or higher rates of recatheterization. After IUC removal, toileting with assistance, use of a bedpan or urinal, placement of an incontinence pad, or use of a bladder scanner for postvoid residual volume assessment and use of straight catheterization if indicated are alternatives.

If the patient is unable to spontaneously void 4 to 6 hours post-IUC removal, a bladder scanning protocol should be instituted to determine the amount of urine in the bladder. If the bladder scan indicates less than 400 mL of urine, then Mr. B should be monitored for 2 additional hours postvoid. If he is still unable to void, the bladder scan is repeated. If the second bladder scan shows greater than 400 mL postvoid, the nurse needs to straight catheterize the patient, documenting the amount of output in the EHR. Additional orders will be necessary if Mr. B has been straight catheterized twice or more within 12 hours.

SUMMARY

A rapidly changing evidence base and regulatory environment necessitates a continued focus on the prevention of CAUTI, which is informed by an understanding of CAUTI pathogenesis and rational IUC use. Critical elements of a CAUTI prevention program include maximizing catheter avoidance, ensuring EBP and product use, and timely catheter removal. Additional strategies include staff education, continuing monitoring of CAUTI incidence, and catheter use. Multicomponent technical interventions have been used successfully in the prevention of CAUTIs when paired with a socio-adaptive change strategy.

NURSING STANDARD OF PRACTICE

Protocol 22.1: Prevention of Catheter-Associated Urinary Tract Infection

I. GOALS

To ensure that nurses in acute care are able to

A. Define CAUTI
B. Describe the epidemiology of CAUTI
C. Define indications for IUC
D. Identify evidence-based strategies and interventions for the prevention of CAUTI
E. Describe key components of a nurse-driven protocol for IUC removal
F. Understand how to engage an interdisciplinary team in the prevention and management of CAUTIs in the setting

II. OVERVIEW

A. CAUTIs are the single most common HAI, accounting for 34% of all HAIs and associated with significant morbidity and excess health care costs.
B. Since 2008, the CMS no longer reimburses for additional costs required to treat nosocomial UTIs.
C. Multiple EBP strategies, recommendations, and/or guidelines for preventing CAUTI in hospitals and long-term care have been published.
D. In light of these rapid changes in the field, the review of policies, procedures, practices, and products is imperative for all health care facilities.

III. BACKGROUND/STATEMENT OF PROBLEM

A. Introduction
   1. It is suggested that there are more than 449,000 health care–associated CAUTIs annually. At an approximate cost of $749 to $1,007 per hospital admission, this epidemic results in $452 million of excess health care costs each year.
   2. The vast majority of UTIs are associated with the ubiquitous IUC, also known as a Foley catheter.
   3. According to the Infectious Diseases Society of America 21% to 54% of all IUCs are inappropriately placed and are not medically indicated.
B. Definitions
   1. *Symptomatic UTI*: A patient has at least one of the following signs or symptoms with no other recognized cause: Fever (more than 38°C), urgency, frequency, dysuria, or suprapubic tenderness and a positive urine culture; may or may not be catheter associated.
   2. *Asymptomatic bacteriuria*: A positive urine culture in a patient who does not have fever or symptoms referable to the urinary tract; may or may not be catheter associated.
   3. *CAUTI*: A symptomatic UTI that occurs while a patient has an IUC inserted for at least 2 days or within 24 hours of its removal.
C. Essential elements
   1. The urinary tract is normally a sterile body site. In the presence of an IUC, microorganisms can gain access to the urinary tract on either the extraluminal surface of the IUC or intraluminal surface through breaks in the catheter system.
   2. Once bacteria gain access to the urinary tract, microorganisms can thrive in a "biofilm" layer on either the extra- or intraluminal surface of the IUC.
   3. Because the formation of a biofilm and colonization with bacteria takes time, most CAUTI occurs after 48 hours of catheterization and increases approximately 5% per day.
   4. The mechanisms described earlier provide the rationale for evidence-based care of IUCs. Four potential opportunities for intervention include:
      a. Avoid the use of catheters
      b. Evidence-based care practices and product selection

(continued)

Protocol 22.1: Prevention of Catheter-Associated Urinary Tract Infection *(continued)*

c. Timely removal
d. Education and surveillance

IV. ASSESSMENT OF CAUTI

A. The CDC has developed explicit surveillance criteria for CAUTI. In brief, the patient must have:
   1. A positive urine culture sent more than 48 hours after admission to the health care facility
   2. An IUC at the time of or within 24 hours before the culture
   3. One of the following: suprapubic tenderness, costovertebral angle pain or tenderness, or a fever more than 38°C without another recognized cause; or a positive blood culture with the same organism as in the urine
B. Measures
   1. Outcomes
      a. CAUTIs/1,000 catheter days
   2. Processes
      a. Catheter days/hospital days
      b. Patients with catheter removed on postoperative day 1 or 2 eligible surgical patients
C. Indications for IUCs can be operationalized using algorithms or protocols.

V. NURSING CARE STRATEGIES

Twenty percent to 69% of CAUTIs are preventable through the application of evidence-based care strategies.

A. Catheter avoidance
   1. Established insertion guidelines
   2. Alternative strategies to manage urine output available:
      a. Bedside commodes
      b. Condom catheters
      c. Moisture-wicking incontinence pads
      d. Intermittent straight catheterization
      e. Bladder scanner for monitoring and assessment
      f. Bedpans and urinals that are functional
   3. Toileting schedules and frequent nursing rounds
B. Product selection and routine care
   1. Catheter material:
      a. Antimicrobial catheter materials have been shown to reduce catheter-associated bacteriuria (colonization), but impact on prevention of symptomatic CAUTIs during short-term insertions is unproven.
      b. There is insufficient evidence to determine whether selection of a latex catheter, hydrogel-coated latex catheter, silicone-coated latex catheter, or all-silicone catheter influences CAUTI risk.
   2. Select the smallest size possible (less than 18 French).
   3. Use aseptic technique and sterile product during catheter insertion.
   4. Routine urethral meatus cleansing with soap and water during bath and after bowel movement.
   5. Secure catheter to leg using a catheter securement device.
   6. Maintain a closed system at all times.
   7. Keep drainage bag below level of bladder.
   8. Empty the bag when two thirds full and before transport.
C. Timely removal
   1. Systems that prompt providers to review need for the catheter and encourage early removal. Examples include stop orders and reminder systems; audit/feedback, nurse-prompted reminders, nurse-driven removal protocols.
   2. Measure of removal: SCIP, SCIP-inf-9 measure; catheter removal on postoperative day 1 or 2.

(continued)

Protocol 22.1: Prevention of Catheter-Associated Urinary Tract Infection *(continued)*

D. Surveillance and education
   1. Measurement of processes and outcomes
   2. Ongoing system evaluation, nursing reeducation, practice reminders, and public reporting of unit-based CAUTI-rate data are strategies to inform the health care team of current practice outcomes and effectiveness of CAUTI prevention strategies.

VI. EVALUATION/EXPECTED OUTCOMES

A. Plan of care
   1. Assessment that patient meets established insertion criteria
   2. Adherence to prompts for early catheter removal
   3. Standardized catheter care guidelines followed
B. Documentation
   1. Dates of insertion and removal
   2. Type of catheter (new indwelling, chronic indwelling, reinsertion, change of device)
   3. Reason for catheter insertion
   4. Justification that catheter is still necessary
   5. Postvoid residual catheter removal if patient is unable to void in 4 to 6 hours; bladder volume; intervention
C. Catheter usage
   1. Monitor unit-specific CAUTI rates.
   2. Monitor average catheter duration (catheter days).
   3. Monitor SCIP postoperative catheter removal on catheterization day 1 or 2.
   4. Trend unit-specific IUC usage.

ABBREVIATIONS

CAUTI	Catheter-associated urinary tract infection
CMS	Centers for Medicare & Medicaid Services
EBP	Evidence-based practice
HAI	Health care–associated infection
IUC	Indwelling urinary catheters
SCIP	Surgical Care Improvement Project
IUC	Indwelling urinary catheter

ACKNOWLEDGMENTS

We thank Lilian Hoffecker, MLS, Research Librarian, Health Sciences Library at the University of Colorado Anschutz Medical Campus for her evidence-based search and Cynthia Drake, MA, for assistance with the formatting of this chapter.

RESOURCES

American Nurses Association: CAUTI Prevention Tool Kit. (2015).
www.nursingworld.org/MainMenuCategories/ThePracticeofProfessionalNursing/Improving-Your-Practice/ANA-CAUTI-Prevention-Tool

Association for Professionals in Infection Control and Epidemiology (APIC). (2014). *APIC Implementation Guide. Guide to Prevention Catheter-Associated Urinary Tract Infections.*
apic.org/Resource_/EliminationGuideForm/6473ab9b-e75c-457a-8d0f-d57d32bc242b/File/APIC_CAUTI_web_0603.pdf

Centers for Disease Control and Prevention. (2015). *Catheter-Associated Urinary Tract Infections (CAUTI).*
www.cdc.gov/HAI/ca_uti/uti.html

Centers for Disease Control and Prevention. (2015). *Urinary Tract Infection (Catheter-Associated Urinary Tract Infection [CAUTI] and Non-Catheter-Associated Urinary Tract Infection [UTI]) and Other Urinary System Infection [USI]) Events.*
www.cdc.gov/nhsn/PDFs/pscManual/7pscCAUTIcurrent.pdf

Drekonja, D. M., Kuskowski, M. A., & Johnson, J. R. (2010). Internet survey of Foley catheter practices and knowledge among Minnesota nurses. *American Journal of Infection Control, 38*(1), 31–37.

Dunn, T. S., Shlay, J., & Forshner, D. (2003). Are in-dwelling catheters necessary for 24 hours after hysterectomy? *American Journal of Obstetrics and Gynecology, 189*(2), 435–437.

Goetz, A. M., Kedzuf, S., Wagener, M., & Muder, R. R. (1999). Feedback to nursing staff as an intervention to reduce catheter-associated urinary tract infections. *American Journal of Infection Control, 27*, 402–424.

Huang, W. C., Wann, S. R., Lin, S. L., Kunin, C. M., Kung, M. H., Lin, C. H., . . . Lin, T. W. (2004). Catheter-associated urinary tract infections in intensive care units can be reduced by prompting physicians to remove unnecessary catheters. *Infection Control & Hospital Epidemiology, 25*(11), 974–978.

ICS fact sheets
www.ics.org/Documents/Documents.aspx?DocumentID=2172

IDSA Diagnosis, Prevention, &Treatment of CAUTI in Adults: 2009 International Clinical Practice Guideline
www.guideline.gov/content.aspx?id=24060

IDSA Guidelines: Catheter-Associated Bacteriuria
eguideline.guidelinecentral.com/i/53990-catheter-associated-bacteriuria (available as an electronic app)

International Continence Society (International Consultation on Incontinence Committee [an international group of continence researchers])
www.ics.org

Johnson, J. R., Kuskowski, M. A., & Wilt, T. J. (2006). Systematic review: Antimicrobial urinary catheters to prevent catheter-associated urinary tract infections in hospitalized patients. *Annals of Internal Medicine, 144*(2), 116–126.

Ladak, S. S., Katznelson, R., Muscat, M., Sawhney, M., Beattie, W. S., & O'Leary, G. (2009). Incidence of urinary retention in patients with thoracic patient controlled epidural analgesia (TCPEA) undergoing thoracotomy. *Pain Management Nursing, 10*(2), 94–98.

Lee, Y. Y., Tsay, W. L., Lou, M. F., & Dai, Y.-T. (2006). The effectiveness of implementing a bladder ultrasound programme in neurosurgical units. *Journal of Advanced Nursing, 57*(2), 192–200.

Loeb, M., Hunt, D., O'Halloran, K., Carusone, S. C., Dafoe, N., & Walter, S. D. (2008). Stop orders to reduce inappropriate urinary catheterization in hospitalized patients: A randomized controlled trial. *Journal of General Internal Medicine, 23*(6), 816–820.

Meddings, J., Rogers, M. A., Macy, M., & Saint, S. (2010). Systematic review and meta-analysis: Reminder systems to reduce catheter-associated urinary tract infections and urinary catheter use in hospitalized patients. *Clinical Infectious Diseases, 51*(5), 550–560.

Parker, D., Callan, L., Harwood, J., Thompson, D. L., Wilde, M., & Gray, M. (2009). Nursing interventions to reduce the risk of catheter-associated urinary tract infection: Part 1: Catheter selection. *Journal of Wound Ostomy & Continence Nursing, 36*(1), 23–34.

Saint, S. (2000). Clinical and economic consequence of nosocomial catheter-related bacteruria. *American Journal of Infection Control, 28*(1), 68–75.

Saint, S., Kaufman, S. R., Robers, M. A. M., Baker, P. D., Ossenkop, K., & Lipsky, B. A. (2006). Condom versus indwelling urinary catheters: A randomized trial. *Journal of the American Geriatrics Society, 54*(7), 1055–1061.

Saint, S., Kowalski, C. P., Kaufman, S. R., Hofer, T. P., Kauffman, C. A., Olmsted, R. N., . . . Krein, S. L. (2008). Preventing hospital-acquired urinary tract infection in the United States: A national study. *Clinical Infectious Diseases, 46*(2), 243–250.

Saint, S., Olmsted, R. N., Fakih, M. G., Kowalski, C. P., Watson, S. R., Sales, A. E., & Krein, S. L. (2009). Translating health care-associated urinary tract infection prevention research into practice via the bladder bundle. *Joint Commission Journal on Quality Patient Safety, 35*(9), 449–455.

Saint, S., Wiese, J., Amory, J., Bernstein, M. L., Patel, U. D., Zemencuk, J. K., . . . Hofer, T. P. (2000). Are physicians aware of which of their patients have indwelling urinary catheters? *American Journal of Medicine, 109*(6), 476–480.

Society for Healthcare Epidemiology of America and the Infectious Diseases Society of America (SHEA-IDSA). (2014). *Compendium of Strategies to Prevent HAIs in Acute Care Hospitals.*
www.shea-online.org/PriorityTopics/CompendiumofStrategiesto-PreventHAIs.aspx

Sparks, A., Boyer, D., Gambrel, A., Lovett, M., Johnson, J., Grimm, E., . . . Palermo, D. (2004). The clinical benefits of the bladder scanner: A research synthesis. *Journal of Nursing Care Quality, 19*(3), 188–192.

Wound, Ostomy, and Continence Nurses Society
c.ymcdn.com/sites/www.wocn.org/resource/resmgr/Publications/Catheter_Associated_Urinary_.pdf

REFERENCES

Agency for Healthcare Research and Quality. (2013a). *Eliminating CAUTI: Interim data report: A national patient safety imperative.* Rockville, MD: Author. Retrieved from http://www.ahrq.gov/professionals/quality-patient-safety/cusp/cauti-interim/index.html. *Evidence Level III.*

Agency for Healthcare Research and Quality. (2013b). *Patient safety for selected indicators technical specifications, patient safety indicators #90 (PSI #90) Version 4.5.* Retrieved from http://qualityindicators.ahrq.gov/Downloads/Modules/PSI/V45/TechSpecs/PSI%2090%20Patient%20Safety%20for%20Selected%20Indicators.pdf. *Evidence Level III.*

Alessandri, F., Mistrangelo, E., Lijoi, D., Ferrero, S., & Ragni, N. (2006). A prospective, randomized trial comparing immediate versus delayed catheter removal following hysterectomy. *Acta Obstetricia et Gynecologica Scandinavica, 85*(6), 716–720. *Evidence Level II.*

Alexaitis, I., & Broome, B. (2014). Implementation of a nurse-driven protocol to prevent catheter-associated urinary tract infections.

Journal of Nursing Care Quality, 29(3), 245–252. *Evidence Level V.*

American Nurses Association. (2015). CAUTI prevention tool. *Nursingworld.org.* Retrieved from http://nursingworld.org/ANA-CAUTI-Prevention-Tool. *Evidence Level VI.*

Andreessen, L., Wilde, M. H., & Herendeen, P. (2012). Preventing catheter-associated urinary tract infections in acute care: The bundle approach. *Journal of Nursing Care Quality, 27*(3), 209–217. *Evidence Level V.*

Apisarnthanarak, A., Rutjanawech, S., Wichansawakun, S., Ratanabunjerdkul, H., Patthranitima, P., Thongphubeth, K., . . . Fraser, V. J. (2007b). Initial inappropriate urinary catheters use in a tertiary-care center: Incidence, risk factors, and outcomes. *American Journal of Infection Control, 35*(9), 594–599. *Evidence Level V.*

Apisarnthanarak, A., Thongphubeth, K., Sirinvaravong, S., Kitkangvan, D., Yuekyen, C., Warachan, B., . . . Fraser, V. J. (2007a). Effectiveness of multifaceted hospitalwide quality improvement programs featuring an intervention to remove unnecessary urinary catheters at a tertiary care center in Thailand. *Infection Control & Hospital Epidemiology, 28*(7), 791–798. *Evidence Level IV.*

Basse, L., Werner, H., & Kehlet, H. (2000). Is urinary drainage necessary during continuous epidural analgesia after colonic resection? *Regional Anesthesia and Pain Medicine, 25*(5), 498–501. *Evidence Level II.*

Carter, N. M., Reitmeier, L., & Goodloe, L. R. (2014). An evidence-based approach to the prevention of catheter-associated urinary tract infections. *Urologic Nursing, 34*(5), 238–245. *Evidence Level V.*

Centers for Disease Control and Prevention. (2013). *2011 National and state healthcare—Associated infections standardized infection ratio report.* Atlanta, GA: Author. Retrieved from http://www.cdc.gov/hai/pdfs/SIR/SIR-Report_02_07_2013.pdf. *Evidence Level VI.*

Centers for Disease Control and Prevention. (2015). *Urinary tract infection (catheter-associated urinary tract infection [CAUTI] and non-catheter-associated urinary tract infection [UTI]) and other urinary system infection [USI]) events.* Retrieved from http://www.cdc.gov/nhsn/PDFs/pscManual/7pscCAUTIcurrent.pdf. *Evidence Level VI.*

Centers for Disease Control and Prevention, CDC's National Healthcare Safety Network. (2015). *Urinary tract infection (catheter-associated urinary tract infection [CAUTI] and non-catheter-associated urinary tract infection [UTI]) and other urinary system infection [USI]*). Retrieved, from http://www.cdc.gov/nhsn/pdfs/pscManual/7pscCAUTI current.pdf/. *Evidence Level VI.*

Centers for Medicare & Medicaid Services. (2005). *Manual system DHHS and CMS urinary incontinence Tag F-315.* Retrieved from https://www.cms.gov/transmittals/downloads/R8SOM.pdf. *Evidence Level VI.*

Centers for Medicare & Medicaid Services. (2008). *Inpatient prospective payment system (IPPS) fiscal year (Fy) 2009 final rule.* CMS-1390. Retrieved from http://www.cms.gov/Medicare/Medicare-Fee-for-Service-Payment/AcuteInpatientPPS/IPPS-Regulations-and-Notices-Items/CMS1227598.html. *Evidence Level VI.*

Centers for Medicare & Medicaid Services. (2015). *Hospital compare.* Retrieved from http://www.hospitalcompare.hhs.gov. *Evidence Level VI.*

Centers for Medicare & Medicaid Services, Department of Health and Human Services. Medicare Program. (2007). *Changes to the hospital inpatient prospective payment systems and fiscal year 2008 rates.* CMS-1390-F. 8-1-2007. Retrieved from http://www.cms.gov/Medicare/Medicare-Fee-for-Service-Payment/AcuteInpatientPPS/IPPS-Regulations-and-Notices-Items/CMS1228401.html. *Evidence Level VI.*

Chia, Y., Wei, R. J., Chang, H. C., & Liu, K. (2009). Optimal duration of urinary catheterization after thoracotomy in patients under post operative patient controlled epidural analgesia. *Acta Anaesthesiologica Taiwanica, 47*(4), 173–179. *Evidence Level II.*

Chenoweth, C., Gould, C., & Saint, S. (2014). Diagnosis, management, and prevention of catheter-associated urinary tract infections. *Infectious Disease Clinics of North America, 28*(1), 105–119. doi:10.1016/j.idc.2013.09.002. *Evidence Level VI.*

Clarke, K., Tong, D., Pan, Y., Easley, K. A., Norrick, B., Ko, C., . . . Stein, J. (2013). Reduction in catheter-associated urinary tract infections by bundling interventions. *International Journal for Quality Health Care, 25*(1), 43–49. *Evidence Level IV.*

Cottenden, A., Bliss, D., Fader, M., Getliffe, K., Herrera, H., Paterson, J., . . . Wilde, M. (2005). Management with continence products. In P. Abrams, L. Cardozo, S. Khoury, & A. Wein (Eds.), *Incontinence: Basics & evaluation* (pp. 149–253). Paris, France: Health Publications. *Evidence Level VI.*

Darouiche, R. O., Goetz, L., Kaldis, T., Cerra-Stewart, C., AlSharif, A., & Priebe, M. (2006). Impact of StatLock securing device on symptomatic catheter-related urinary tract infection: A prospective, randomized, multicenter clinical trial. *American Journal of Infection Control, 34*(9), 555–560. *Evidence Level II.*

Dowling-Castronovo, A., & Bradway, C. (2008). *Urinary incontinence: Nursing standard of practice protocol in older adults admitted to acute care.* Retrieved from http://consultgerirn.org/resources. *Evidence Level V.*

Elpern, E. H., Killeen, K., Ketchem, A., Wiley, A., Patel, G., & Lateef, O. (2009). Reducing use of indwelling urinary catheters and associated urinary tract infections. *American Journal of Critical Care, 18*(6), 535–542. *Evidence Level IV.*

Fakih, M. G., Shemes, S. P., Pena, M. E., Dye, N., Rey, J. E., Szpunar, S. M., & Saravolatz, L. D. (2010). Urinary catheters in the emergency department: Very elderly women are at high risk for unnecessary utilization. *American Journal of Infection Control, 38*(9), 683–688. *Evidence Level IV.*

Fakih, M. G., Watson, S. R., Greene, T., Kennedy, E. H., Olmsted, R. N., Krein, S., & Saint S. (2012). Reducing inappropriate urinary catheter use: A statewide effort. *Archives of Internal Medicine, 172*(3), 255–260. *Evidence Level IV.*

Fortin, E., Rocher, I., Frenette, C., Tremblay, C., & Quach, C. (2012). Healthcare-associated bloodstream infections secondary to a urinary focus: The Quebec provincial surveillance results. *Infection Control & Hospital Epidemiology, 33*(5), 456–462. *Evidence Level III.*

Fuchs, M. A., Sexton, D. J., Thronlow, D. K., & Champagne, M. T. (2011). Evaluation of an evidence-based, nurse driven checklist to prevent hospital-acquired catheter-associated urinary tract infections in intensive care units. *Journal of Nursing Care Quality, 26*(1), 101–109. *Evidence Level V.*

Gokula, R., Hickner, J. A., & Smith, M. A. (2004). Inappropriate use of urinary catheters in elderly patients at a midwestern community teaching hospital. *American Journal of Infection Control, 32*(4), 196–199. *Evidence Level III.*

Gould, C. V., Umscheid, C. A., Agarwal, R. K., Kuntz, G., Pegues, D. A., & Healthcare Infection Control Practices Advisory Committee. (2010). Guideline for prevention of catheter-associated urinary tract infections 2009. *Infect Control Hosp Epidemiol, 31*(4), 319–326. doi:10.1086/651091. *Evidence Level VI.*

Gray, M. (2010). Reducing catheter-associated urinary tract infection in the critical care unit. *AACN Advanced Critical Care, 21*(2), 247–257. *Evidence Level V.*

Greene, L., Marx, J., & Oriola, S. (2008). *Guide to the elimination of catheter-associated urinary tract infections (CAUTIs).* Washington, DC: Association for Professionals in Infection Control and Epidemiology (APIC). Retrieved from http://www.apic.org/Resource_/EliminationGuideForm/c0790db8-2aca-4179-a7ae-676c27592de2/File/APIC-CAUTI-Guide.pdf. *Evidence Level VI.*

Greene, M. T., Chang, R., Kuhn, L., Rogers, M. A., Chenoweth, C. E., Shuman, E., & Saint, S. (2012). Predictors of hospital-acquired urinary tract-elated bloodstream infection. *Infection Control & Hospital Epidemiology, 33*, 1001–1007. *Evidence Level III.*

Hollingsworth, J. M., Rogers, M. A., Krein, S. L., Hickner, K. A. L., Cheng, A., Chang, R., & Saint, S. (2013). Determining the noninfectious complications of indwelling urethral catheters: A systematic review and meta-analysis. *Annals of Internal Medicine, 159*(6), 401–410. *Evidence Level I.*

Hooten, T. M., Bradley, S. F., Cardenas, D. D., Colgan, R., Geerlings, S. E., Rice, J. C., . . . Nicolle, L. E. (2010). Diagnosis, prevention, and treatment of catheter-associated urinary tract infection in adults: 2009 International clinical practice guidelines from the Infectious Diseases Society of America. *Clinical Infectious Diseases, 50*, 625–663. *Evidence Level VI.*

Inouye, S. K. (2006). Delirium in older persons. *New England Journal of Medicine, 354*, 1157–1165. *Evidence Level IV.*

Jeong, I., Park, S., Joeng, J., Sun Kim, D., Choi, Y. S., Lee, Y. S., & Park, Y. M. (2010). Comparison of catheter-associated urinary tract infection rates by perineal care agents in intensive care units. *Asian Nursing Research, 4*(3), 142–150. *Evidence Level II.*

Joanna Briggs Institute. (2010). *Management of short term indwelling urethral catheter to prevent urinary tract infections.* Retrieved from http://connect.jbiconnectplus.org/ViewSourceFile.aspx?0=5381. *Evidence Level I.*

Junkin, J., & Selekof, J. L. (2008). Beyond "diaper rash": Incontinence-associated dermatitis: Does it have you seeing RED? *Nursing, 38*(Suppl. 11), 56hn1–56hn10. *Evidence Level VI.*

Kabcenell, A., Nolan, T. W., Martin, L. A., & Gill, Y. (2010). *The pursuing perfection initiative: Lessons on transforming health care.* IHI Innovation Series white paper. Cambridge, MA: Institute for Healthcare Improvement. Retrieved from http://www.ihi.org/resources/Pages/IHIWhitePapers/PursuingPerfectionInitiativeWhitePaper.aspx. *Evidence Level VI.*

Klevens, R. M., Edwards, J. R., Richards, C. L., Jr, Horan, T. C., Gaynes, R. P., Pollock, D. A., & Cardo, D. M. (2007). Estimating health care-associated infections and deaths in US hospitals, 2002. *Public Health Report, 122*(2), 160–166. *Evidence Level V.*

Knoll, B. M., Wright, D., Ellingson, L. A., Kraemer, L., Patire, R., Kuskowski, M. A., & Johnson, J. R. (2011). Reduction of inappropriate urinary catheter use at a veterans affairs hospital through a multifaceted quality improvement project. *Clinical Infectious Disease, 52*(11), 1283–1290. *Evidence Level V.*

Lo, E., Nicolle, L., & Classen, D. (2008). Strategies to prevent catheter-associated urinary tract infections in acute care hospitals. *Infection Control and Hospital Epidemiology, 29*(Suppl. 1), S41–S50. *Evidence Level VI.*

Lo, E., Nicolle, L. E., Coffin, S. E., Gould, C., Maragakis, L. L., Meddings, J., . . . Yokoe, D. S. (2014). Strategies to prevent catheter-associated urinary tract infections in acute care hospitals: 2014 Update. *Infection Control and Hospital Epidemiology, 35*(Suppl. 2), S32–S47. *Evidence Level V.*

Maki, D. G., & Tambyah, P. A. (2001). Engineering out the risk of infection with urinary catheters. *Emerging Infectious Diseases, 7*(2), 342–347. Retrieved from http://www.cdc.gov/ncidod/eid/vol7no2/makiG1.htm. *Evidence Level VI.*

Marigliano, A., Barbadoro, P., Pennacchietti, L., D'Errico, M. M., Prospero, E., & CAUTI Working Collaborative Group. (2012). Active training and surveillance: 2 Good friends to reduce urinary catheterization rate. *American Journal of Infection Control, 40*(8), 692–695. *Evidence Level V.*

Meddings, J., Rogers, M. A. M., Krein, S., Fakih, M. G., Olmsted, R. N., & Saint, S. (2014). Reducing unnecessary urinary catheter use and other strategies to prevent catheter-associated urinary tract infection: An integrative review. *British Medical Journal Quality and Safety, 23*(4), 277–289. *Evidence Level I.*

Melnyk, B. M., & Fineout-Overholt, E. (2011). Creating a vision and motivating a change to evidence-based practice in individual, teams, and organizations. In B. M. Melnyk & E. Fineout-Overholt (Eds.), *Evidence-based practice in nursing & healthcare: A guide to best practice* (2nd ed., pp. 276–290). Philadelphia, PA: Lippincott, Williams, & Wilkins. *Evidence Level V.*

Mori, C. (2014). A-voiding catastrophe: Implementing a nurse-driven protocol. *MedSurg Nursing, 23*(1), 15–28. *Evidence Level V.*

National Association for Continence. (2015). Retrieved from http://www.nafc.org/tools. *Evidence Level VI.*

Nicolle, L., Bradley, S., Colgan, R., Rice, J. C., Schaeffer, A., & Hooten, T. M. (2005). Infectious Diseases Society of America guidelines for the diagnosis and treatment of asymptomatic bacteriuria in adults. *Clinical Infectious Diseases, 40*(5), 643–654. *Evidence Level VI.*

Padula, W. V., Manish, K. M., Makic, M. B. F., & Sullivan, P. W. (2011). Improving the quality of pressure ulcer care with prevention: A cost-effectiveness analysis. *Medical Care, 49*(4), 385–392. *Evidence Level V.*

Palese, A., Buchini, S., Deroma, L., & Barbone, F. (2010). The effectiveness of the ultrasound bladder scanner in reducing urinary tract infections: A meta-analysis. *Journal of Clinical Nursing, 19*(21–22), 2970–2979. *Evidence Level I.*

Parry, M. F., Grant, B., & Sestovic, M. (2013). Successful reduction in catheter-associated urinary tract infections: Focus on nurse-directed catheter removal. *American Journal of Infection Control, 41*(12), 1178–1181. *Evidence Level III.*

Patient Protection and Affordable Care Act, 42 U.S.C. § 18001 (2010). Retrieved from https://democrats.senate.gov/pdfs/reform/patient-protection-affordable-care-act-as-passed.pdf. *Evidence Level VI.*

Pickard, R., Lam, T., MacLennan, G., Starr, K., Kilonzo, M., McPherson, G.,... N'dow, J. (2012). Types of urethral catheters for reducing symptomatic urinary tract infections in hospitalized adults requiring short-term catheterization: Multicenter randomized controlled trail and economic evaluation of antimicrobial and antiseptic impregnated ureteral catheters. *Health Technology Assessment, 16*(47), 47. *Evidence Level II.*

Pronovost, P., Weast, B., Rosenstein, B., Sexton, J. B. P., Holzmueller, C. G. B., Paine, L. M.,... Rubin, H. R. (2005). Implementing and validating a comprehensive unit-based safety program. *Journal of Patient Safety, 1*(1), 33–40. *Evidence Level VI.*

Purvis, S., Gion, T., Kennedy, G., Rees, S., Safdar, N., VanDne-Bergh, S., & Weber, J. (2014). Catheter-associated urinary tract infection: A successful prevention effort employing a multipronged initiative at an academic medical center. *Journal of Nursing Care Quality, 29*(2), 141–148. *Evidence Level V.*

Reinertsen, J. L., Bisognano, M., & Pugh, M. D. (2008). *Seven leadership leverage points for organization-level improvement in health care* (2nd ed.). IHI Innovation Series white paper. Cambridge, MA: Institute for Healthcare Improvement. Retrieved from http://www.IHI.org. *Evidence Level VI.*

Rosenthal, V. D., Ramachandran, B., Duenas, L., Alvarez-Moreno, C., Navoa-Ng, J. A., Armas-Ruiz, A.,.... Dursun, O. (2012). Findings of the international nosocomial infection control consortium (INICC), Part I: Effectiveness of a multidimensional infection control approach on catheter-associated urinary tract infection rates in pediatric intensive care units of 6 developing countries. *Infection Control and Hospital Epidemiology, 33*(7), 696–703. *Evidence Level IV.*

Roser, L., Altpeter, T., Anderson, D., Dougherty, M., Walton, J. E., & Merritt, S. (2012). A nurse driven foley catheter removal protocol proves clinically effective to reduce the incidents of catheter related urinary tract infections. *American Journal of Infection Control, 40*(5), e92–e93. *Evidence Level V.*

Rycroft-Malone, J., & Bucknall, T. (2010). *Models and frameworks for implementing evidence-based practice: Linking evidence to action.* West Sussex, UK: John Wiley. *Evidence Level VI.*

Saint, S., Greene, T., Kowalski, C. P., Watson, S. R., Hofer, T. P., & Krein, S. L. (2013). Preventing catheter-associated urinary tract infection in the United States. *JAMA Internal Medicine, 173*(10), 874–879. *Evidence Level IV.*

Saint, S., Lipsky, B. A., & Goold, S. D. (2002). Indwelling urinary catheters: A one-point restraint? *Annals of Intern Medicine, 137*(2), 125–127. *Evidence Level VI.*

Schaeffer, A. J. (1986). Catheter-associated bacteriuria. *Urologic Clinics of North America, 13*(4), 735–747. *Evidence Level V.*

Scott, R. (2009). *The direct medical costs of healthcare-associated infections in US hospitals and the benefits of prevention.* Atlanta, GA: Centers for Disease Control and Prevention. Retrieved from http://www.cdc.gov/hai/pdfs/hai/scott_costpaper.pdf. *Evidence Level V.*

Shepard, J., Hadhazy, E., Frederick, J., Nicol, S., Gade, P., & Cardon, A. (2014). Using electronic medical records to increase the efficiency of catheter-associated urinary tract infection surveillance for National Health and Safety Network reporting. *American Journal of Infection Control, 42*(3), e33–e36. *Evidence Level IV.*

Society of Urologic Nurses and Associates: Clinical Practice Guidelines Task Forces. (2006). Care of the patient with an indwelling catheter. *Urologic Nursing Journal, 26*(1), 80–81. *Evidence Level VI.*

Stamm, W. E. (1975). Guidelines for prevention of catheter-associated urinary tract infections. *Annals of Intern Medicine, 82*(3), 386–390. *Evidence Level VI.*

Stone, N. D., Ashraf, M. S., Calder, J., Crnich, C. J., Crossley, K., Drinka, P. J.,... Group Society for Healthcare Epidemiology Long-Term Care Special Interest. (2012). Surveillance definitions of infections in long-term care facilities: Revisiting the Mcgeer Criteria. *Infection Control & Hospital Epidemiology, 33*(10), 965–977. *Evidence Level I.*

Stubbs, B. M., Bakcock, K. J., Hayams, C., Rizal, F. E., Warren, S., & Francis, D. (2013). A prospective study of early removal of the urethral catheter after colorectal surgery in patients having epidural analgesia as part to the enhanced recovery after surgery programme. *Colorectal Disease, 15*(6), 733–736. *Evidence Level IV.*

Tambyah, P. H., Knasinski, V., & Maki, D. G. (2002). The direct costs of nosocomial catheter-associated urinary tract infection in the era of managed care. *Infection Control & Hospital Epidemiology, 23*(1), 27–31. *Evidence Level IV.*

The Joint Commission. (n.d.). Surgical Care Improvement Project. Retrieved from http://www.jointcommission.org/assets/1/6/Surgical%20Care%20Improvement%20Project.pdf. *Evidence Level VI.*

Tillekeratne, L. G., Linkin, D. R., Obino, M., Omar, A., Wanjiku, M., Holtzman, D., & Cohn, J. (2014). A multifaceted intervention to reduce rates of catheter-associated urinary tract infections in a resource-limited setting. *American Journal of Infection Control, 42*(1), 12–16. *Evidence Level IV.*

Titler, M. G. (2011). Nursing science and evidence-based practice. *Western Journal of Nursing Research, 33*(3), 291–295. *Evidence Level VI.*

Titsworth, W. L., Hester, J., Correia, T., Reed, R., Williams, M., Guin, P.,... Mocco, J. (2012). Reduction of catheter-associated urinary tract infections among patients in a neurological intensive care unit: A single institution's success. *Journal of Neurosurgery, 116*(4), 911–920. *Evidence Level V.*

Uberoi, V., Calixte, N., Coronel, V. R., Furlong, D. J., Orlando, R. P., & Lerner, L. B. (2013). Reducing urinary catheter days. *Nursing, 43*(1), 16–20. *Evidence Level IV.*

Vincitorio, D., Barbadoro, P., Pennacchietti, L., Pellegrini, I., David, S., Ponzio, E., & Prospero, E. (2014). Risk factors for catheter-associated urinary tract infection in Italian elderly. *American Journal of Infection Control, 42*(8), 898–901. *Evidence Level III.*

Wald, H. L., Bandle, B., & Richard, A. (2014). Accuracy of electronic surveillance of catheter-associated urinary tract infection at an academic medical center. *Infection Control & Hospital Epidemiology, 35*(6), 685–691. *Evidence Level IV.*

Wald, H. L., Ma, A., Bratzler, D. W., & Kramer, A. M. (2008). Indwelling urinary catheter use in the postoperative period: Analysis of the national surgical infection prevention project data. *Archives of Surgery, 143*(6), 551–557. *Evidence Level VI.*

Wenger, J. E. (2010). Reducing rates of catheter-associated urinary tract infection. *American Journal of Nursing, 110*(8), 40–45. *Evidence Level V.*

Wilson, M., Wilde, M., Webb, M. L., Thompson, D. L., Parker, D., Harwood, J.,... Gray, M. (2009). Nursing interventions to deduce the risk of catheter-associated urinary tract infection: Part 2: Staff education, monitoring, and care techniques *Journal of Wound, Ostomy, and Continence Nursing, 36*(2), 137–154. *Evidence Level V.*

Wright, M. O., Kharasch, M., Beaumont, J. L., Peterson, L. R., & Robicsek, A. (2011). Reporting catheter-associated urinary tract infections: Denominator matters. *Infection Control & Hospital Epidemiology, 32*(7), 635–640. *Evidence Level IV.*

Zaouter, C., Kanera, P., & Carli, F. (2009). Less urinary tract infection by earlier removal of bladder catheter in surgical patients receiving thoracic epidural analgesia. *Regional Anesthesia and Pain Medicine, 34*(6), 542–548. *Evidence Level II.*

Zaouter, C., Wuethrich, P., Miccoli, V., & Carli, F. (2012). Early removal of urinary catheter leads to greater post-void residuals in patients with thoracic epidural. *Acta Anaesthesiologica Scandinavica, 56*(8), 1020–1025. *Evidence Level II.*

Zhan, C., Elixhauser, A., Richards, C., Wang, Y., Baine, W., Pineau, M.,... Hunt, D. (2009). Identification of hospital-acquired catheter-associated urinary tract infections from medicare claims: Sensitivity and positive predictive value. *Medical Care, 47*(3), 364–369. *Evidence Level IV.*

23

Physical Restraints and Side Rails in Acute and Critical Care Settings

Cheryl M. Bradas, Satinderpal K. Sandhu, and Lorraine C. Mion

EDUCATIONAL OBJECTIVES

On completion of this chapter, the reader should be able to:

1. Describe the consequences of physical restraint use, including side rails, on older adults
2. Describe the characteristics of an effective restraint reduction program
3. Develop individualized care plan strategies that promote alternatives to restraint use through evidence-based care for falls, delirium, nutrition, medications, sleep, pain, and function
4. Evaluate educational needs of patients and families related to restraint reduction
5. Facilitate interprofessional team collaboration to ensure all aspects of restraint reduction program are addressed

OVERVIEW

The Centers for Medicare & Medicaid Services (CMS) defines *physical restraint* as "any manual method, physical or mechanical device, material, or equipment that immobilizes or reduces the ability of the patient to move his or her arms, legs, body or head freely" (U.S. Department of Health and Human Services [USHHS], 2007). Examples include wrist or leg restraints, Geri-chairs, and, in certain situations, full side rails and reclining chairs. Many consider hand mitts a restraint only when wrist ties are used, but this is not universally agreed on; others consider hand mitts a type of restraint because they involuntarily limit the individual's ability to feed and groom himself or herself. Despite the federal regulations placed on hospitals since 1999, eliminating the use of physical restraints for the management of patients in acute nonpsychiatric settings has remained challenging. It is typical for health care professionals to use physical restraints and/or side rails to protect the patient or others (Evans & FitzGerald, 2002). However, the use of physical restraints or side rails for the involuntary immobilization of the patient may not only be an infringement of the patient's rights, but can also result in patient harm, including soft tissue injury, fractures, delirium, and even death (Bower, McCullough, & Timmons, 2003; Evans, Wood, & Lambert, 2003; Krexi, Georgiou, Krexi, & Sheppard, 2015; McPherson et al., 2013; Miles, 1993).

The standards from The Joint Commission (TJC) and regulations from CMS have raised concerns among hospital professionals about the feasibility and safety of eliminating use of physical restraints and side rails in hospitals. The almost nonexistent use of physical restraint in the United Kingdom in comparable settings provides evidence that this can be achieved (O'Keeffe, Jack, & Lye, 1996; Williams & Finch, 1997). This chapter focuses on the issues of physical restraint in acute, nonpsychiatric hospital settings with particular attention to older adult patients.

For a description of evidence levels cited in this chapter, see Chapter 1, "Developing and Evaluating Clinical Practice Guidelines: A Systematic Approach."

BACKGROUND AND LEGAL ISSUES

U.S. Regulations and Accrediting Standards

In 1992, the U.S. Food and Drug Administration (FDA) issued a medical alert on the potential hazards of restraint devices (U.S. FDA, 2006a). Any harm that arises from the use of a restraining device, which now includes bedside rails, must be reported to the FDA. TJC hospital standards began to address the use of physical restraints in the early 1990s. In the ensuing years, the standards have become increasingly prescriptive.

In 1999, CMS established an interim rule for hospitals and, in December 2006, finalized the Patients' Rights Condition of Participation (USDHHS, 2007). These conditions establish the minimum protections of patients' rights and safety and may be superseded by state regulations or accrediting agencies. In brief, the use of physical restraint should be used as a last resort, only used when less restrictive mechanisms have been determined to be ineffective, the use of restraint must be in accordance with a written modification to the patient's plan of care, used in accordance with the order of a physician or licensed independent practitioner (LIP), and must never be written as an "as needed" order. Each order must be renewed every 24 hours for nonviolent behavior and every 4 hours for violent or self-destructive behavior. Orders must be renewed in accordance with hospital policy. Last, restraint must be discontinued at the earliest possible time.

Risks of Liability

A major obstacle in reducing clinicians' use of physical restraint or side rails is the fear of liability if restraints are not used. Case law has been mixed; hospitals have been found liable both for the use of physical restraints and for not using physical restraints (Kapp, 1994, 1996). Although hospitals have a clear duty to protect patients from harm, they do not have a duty to restrain patients. As the practice in hospitals becomes one of reduced restraints because of changing legal and accrediting standards, it will become easier for hospitals to justify nonuse of restraints in instances of patient injury in which use of nonrestraint interventions was clearly demonstrated (Kapp, 1999).

Professional Standards of Care

A number of organizations have established guidelines for the use of physical restraints, including the American Nurses Association and the Society for Critical Care Medicine (American Nurses Association, 2001; Maccioli et al., 2003). The National Quality Forum has designated physical restraint as a nursing-sensitive measure to be monitored in hospitals and nursing facilities. Last, as part of the condition for participation as a *Magnet™ facility*, hospitals must examine the use of physical restraint in relation to nursing skill mix and hours. These guidelines have become the standard for customary practice and are used as an appropriate legal standard that defines the parameters of liability. Furthermore, these guidelines, in combination with TJC and CMS requirements, are used to establish hospital-based policies and procedures and quality of performance activities.

PREVALENCE AND RATIONALE OF STAFF

Extent of Use

These standards and guidelines have led to an overall decrease in physical restraint use in acute care and a change in practice patterns. In the 1980s, the overall prevalence rate of physical restraint use on general floors ranged from 6% to 13%, with higher rates (18%–22%) among older adult patients (Frengley & Mion, 1998). In the late 1990s, the overall hospital restraint prevalence decreased but varied as much as threefold, with rates ranging from 39 restraint days/1,000 patient days to 82 restraint days/1,000 patient days (Minnick, Mion, Leipzig, Lamb, & Palmer, 1998; Mion et al., 2001). For the first time, restraint use was examined in critical care units and was noted to be as high as 500 restraint days/1,000 patient days. Intensive care unit (ICU) rates varied markedly, among units in the same hospital setting as well as matched units among hospitals.

A U.S. national prevalence study involving 434 units in 40 acute care hospitals selected at random from five geographical areas was completed in 2005 (Minnick, Mion, Johnson, Catrambone, & Leipzig, 2007). Findings from this study revealed overall hospital prevalence of 50 restraint days/1,000 patient days but with a ten-fold variation among hospitals from a rate of 9 to 94 restraint days/1,000 patient days. The majority of use was accounted for in the ICUs. The pattern of differences by type of unit was again present (e.g., medical vs. surgical and adult vs. pediatric). However, even when controlling by type of unit, more than ten-fold variation existed among similar settings. For example, overall prevalence among the 41 general ICUs was 202.6 restraint days/1,000 patient days with a range of 9 to 351/1,000 patient days. Further, analyses revealed that variation in practice persisted even when controlling for size of hospital, academic or nonacademic status, geographical region, type of hospital (e.g., nonprofit, profit, and government), staffing ratios, and nursing skill mix. Clearly, there are major practice differences *even when controlling for patient population.*

Similarly, a recent Canadian study involving 51 ICUs revealed that (a) more than half of the patients were in restraints and (b) patient and hospital characteristics were *not* associated with restraint use of duration (Luk et al., 2014). Rather, treatment characteristics, such as use of sedative, analgesic, and antipsychotic drugs, were predictive of restraint use and duration.

Decision to Use Physical Restraint

Today's hospital nurses cite prevention of patient therapy disruption as the primary reason for restraint use (reported for 75% of restraint days), presence of "confusion" (25.4% of the restraint days), and fall prevention (17.6% of the restraint days; Minnick et al., 2007). Other less commonly voiced reasons included management of agitation or violent behavior, wandering, and positioning. Although most nurses cite patient care issues as the rationale to use physical restraint, a small proportion of nurses have cited insufficient staffing or legal concerns (Diercks de Casterle, Goethals, & Gastmans, 2014; Evans & FitzGerald, 2002; Minnick et al., 1998).

The CMS regulations mandate that physicians or LIPs must order physical restraint. Similar to nurses, physicians vary in their decisions to order physical restraint (Mion et al., 2010; Sandhu et al., 2010). Factors associated with physicians' decisions to order restraint include (a) lack of knowledge of physical restraint and hospital policy, (b) higher appraisal of patient harm, (c) specialty (family practice or general surgery), (d) trusting the nurse; (e) patient behavior; and (f) presence of dementia. Given the variation in actual use of restraint, it appears that the decision to use physical restraint continues to be one based on individual judgment and beliefs rather than on scientifically validated guidelines or protocols.

ETHICAL ISSUES IN THE USE OF PHYSICAL RESTRAINT

The primary ethical dilemma resulting from physical restraint is the clinician's value or emphasis of beneficence versus the patient's autonomy (Schafer, 1985; Slomka, Agich, Stagno, & Smith, 1998). Clinicians believe that physical restraint prevents patient falls and patient disruption of therapy (Frengley & Mion, 1998; Lamb, Minnick, Mion, Palmer, & Leipzig, 1999). The presence of a physical restraint, by its very nature, is applied against a patient's wishes and inevitably compromises the individual's dignity and diminishes respect for the person. Beneficence requires that at least no harm should arise from the use of physical restraint and that, optimally, a good outcome would result from use. The lack of beneficial results from the use of physical restraints has been well documented in many health care settings. Little is known, however, of the risk-to-benefit ratio of use or nonuse of physical restraint in patients who are critically ill (Maccioli et al., 2003).

The discussion of physical restraints from an ethical viewpoint must also incorporate the sociocultural and political contexts. For example, clinicians have reported on low to nonexistent use of physical restraint in the United Kingdom, stemming perhaps from a legal mandate existing since the 1800s prohibiting their use. It has been suggested that in the United States, the domination of risk in geriatric assessment (e.g., prevent harm, prevent falls) shapes much of clinicians' understanding of old age (Kaufman, 1994). If one's primary focus is on the likelihood of patient risk resulting in harm, one is less likely to see self-esteem or dignity as the more important value or model to guide clinical decisions (Slomka et al., 1998). Interestingly, Slomka and associates point out the contradictory nature of the frequent use of physical restraint in the United States—that is, a society that places a high value on autonomy yet is so willing to violate that autonomy in the interest of perceived patient benefit (Slomka et al., 1998).

The discussion of ethics in clinical practice must also acknowledge the realities of reduced resources and escalating costs (Minnick et al., 2007; Slomka et al., 1998). Decisions and protocols about the use of physical restraints and methods to reduce and/or eliminate restraints will be impacted by cost-containment efforts, and clinicians and administrators alike may be reluctant to minimize or eliminate restraints. If alternatives to physical restraints in acute care settings can be shown to contribute to quality outcomes (e.g., patient safety, patient dignity, or satisfaction) and within existing cost-containment efforts, then there is an increased likelihood of successfully implementing and maintaining practice guidelines. There is a chance, however, that if restraint reduction efforts are seen as too expensive (e.g., use of "sitters"), then the emphasis on cost constraint may trump other considerations (Slomka et al., 1998).

ADMINISTRATIVE RESPONSIBILITIES

Changing established practices and philosophies of care can be a daunting task. Although education and training are important, the single most important factor in affecting a major shift in the present paradigm of care to one that is restraint-free care is the commitment by administrators and key clinical leaders (Mion et al., 2001; Williams & Finch, 1997). Indeed, the huge variation seen in the rates among 40 hospitals that cannot be explained by size of hospital, type of hospital, or geographical location lends support to this observation. Administrators, including nurse managers, set the tone for the practice on the unit. Reducing health care providers' reliance on physical restraint in managing confused or agitated patients, especially in the critical care units, is a major shift that leaves many staff uneasy. Clinical staff, especially the frontline care providers, must feel supported during the transition period. The goal set and supported by administration of a restraint-free environment would establish the presence of a physical restraint as an outlier that requires a full analysis as for a sentinel event. The outcome of such analyses may well lead to the recognition of system problems and organizational arrangements that can be improved, which, in turn, lead to even fewer restraints in use.

INTERVENTIONS AND CARE STRATEGIES

The studies of the prevalence of the use of physical restraints for nonpsychiatric purposes in hospitals have shown that there is great discrepancy among general medical and surgical units and ICUs in terms of the extent of use and rationale for it. Therefore, the use of physical restraints and approaches to possible alternatives can be considered separately for general hospital units and critical care units.

General Medical and Surgical Units

Although rates of physical restraint use on general medical and surgical units have declined in the past 20 years, wide variation exists: from 3 to 123 restraint days/1,000 patient days on medical units and from 0 to 65 restraint days/1,000 patient days on surgical units (Minnick et al., 2007). It is apparent that there are units that demonstrate best practices, but also that further efforts are needed to eliminate this practice as a national standard. Otherwise, significant numbers of patients will continue to be restrained.

Many hospitals provide care for acutely ill, frail older adults in settings that are not designed environmentally for the care of such older people (Catrambone, Johnson, Mion, & Minnick, 2009; Mion et al., 2006; Palmer, Landefeld, Kresevic, & Kowal, 1994). Environmental structure can either facilitate or inhibit monitoring and surveillance, noise control, appropriate lighting, socialization, cognition, and function (Catrambone et al., 2009; Diercks de Casterle et al., 2014; Palmer et al., 1994). Studies in long-term care settings have demonstrated that the use of environmental strategies can enhance function among those suffering from dementia; similar strategies need to be considered in acute care settings.

Besides environmental strategies, organizational factors, such as systems to determine staffing numbers and mix, models of care delivery, and transmission or communication of the plan of care among multiple disciplines and departments, are gaining increased recognition in the patient safety movement (Leape & Berwick, 2005). Many health care providers lack the knowledge, skills, and sensitivity in providing appropriate care to older adults. TJC standard to ensure age-specific education and training is a step in the right direction, but further efforts are required.

No single approach to eliminating physical restraints on general medical and surgical units can be successful. Studies in a variety of settings have shown that the use of advanced practice nurses, comprehensive interprofessional approaches to enhance cognitive and physical function, staff education, organizational strategies, and environmental interventions can eliminate or reduce physical restraints in a cost-effective manner while promoting other patient outcomes such as reduced fall rates (Amato, Salter, & Mion, 2006; Enns, Rhemtulla, Ewa, Fruetel, & Holroyd-Leduc, 2014; Inouye et al., 1999; Landefeld, Palmer, Kresevic, Fortinsky, & Kowal, 1995; Mion et al., 2001).

Critical Care Units

The use of physical restraints now predominantly occurs within the ICUs to maintain needed life-sustaining therapies or life-maintaining therapies (Luk et al., 2014; Minnick et al., 2007). Strategies that have been used with success in long-term care settings, rehabilitation settings, and general hospital units are not as successful in critical care environments (Mion et al., 2001). The severity of illness of patients, the intensity and delivery of care, the pace of activity, and the consequences of interruptions, delays, or disruptions of therapeutic devices differ significantly between non-ICUs and ICUs. The thought of delirious patients dislodging external ventricular drains with subsequent brain damage, pulling out central lines with threat of hemorrhage, or self-extubation from mechanical ventilation with subsequent respiratory arrest is one that heavily influences critical care nurses' decisions to use physical restraints (Frengley & Mion, 1998; Happ, 2000; Luk et al., 2014).

Efforts to limit physical restraint use in the ICU are hampered by lack of information regarding the extent of therapy disruption in these units or the resulting immediate and subsequent harm to patients (Maccioli et al., 2003). A number of studies, mostly single site, have examined self-extubation from mechanical ventilation (Frengley & Mion, 1998). Rates have ranged from 0.3% to 14.3%, with higher rates in medical ICUs. Reintubation after self-extubation ranged from 11% to 76%. *It is important to note that 33% to 91% of those who self-extubated did so while physically restrained.* As part of the national prevalence study described earlier, the authors also examined the prevalence of patient-initiated device removal, patient contexts, patient risk-adjusted factors, and consequences (Mion, Minnick, Leipzig, Catrambone, & Johnson, 2007). In 49 ICUs in 39 hospitals, the authors collected data on 49,482 patient days. Patients removed 1,623 devices on 1,097 occasions for an overall rate of 22.1 episodes/1,000 patient days. Similar to results on physical restraint prevalence, wide variation in rates was noted: from none to 102.4 episodes/1,000 patient days. Approximately half the episodes occurred on day shift, and 44% were in physical restraint at the time of the episode. Patient harm occurred in 250 (23%) events, mostly minor in nature. In 10 (0.9%) episodes, patients incurred major harm. No deaths occurred. The authors examined rates of reinsertion and found these varied by type of device. Devices that are easily applied, such as monitor lead or oxygen masks, had much higher reinsertion rates than devices that are more complex and difficult to insert (such as endotracheal tubes or surgical drains). It may be that devices are used too long, which could contribute to prolonged use of physical restraint. In turn, physical restraint may contribute to agitation and delirium (Inouye & Charpentier, 1996). Additional hospital resources (e.g., x-rays, laboratory tests) were used in slightly more than half the episodes; thus posing a potentially costly problem (Fraser, Riker, Prato, & Wilkins, 2001).

Information gathered on staffing levels and mix showed little variation among these ICUs; hence, there was no association between staffing ratios and therapy disruptions. Of the three studies on self-extubation that examined relationship to staffing levels, two also showed no association (Boulain, 1998; Chevron et al., 1998; Marcin et al., 2005). The authors found *no* association between a unit's restraint rate and rate of therapy disruption, a finding similar to some studies (Kapadia, Bajan, & Raje, 2000; Mion et al., 2001) but not others (Carrión et al., 2000; Tominaga, Rudzwick, Scannell, & Waxman, 1995).

Finally, the pattern of sedation and analgesia in these units was unclear, and 30% of the patients had received no analgesia or sedation in the 24 hours before the episode. Others have reported on inconsistent sedation and analgesia practices in ICUs (Bair et al., 2000; Egerod, Christensen, & Johansen, 2006; Mehta et al., 2006). In an earlier cohort study, the authors examined medical intensive care unit (MICU) patient outcomes after implementing sedation and analgesia guidelines and found that those cared for with the guidelines had less self-extubation events and less use of physical restraints (Bair et al., 2000). Examining appropriate strategies for sedation and analgesia in critically ill patients may well result in improved clinical outcomes while providing care in a more humane fashion.

Attention to the environment of the ICU is as important as any other setting. Indeed, the environment can affect more strongly persons whose personal competence is low and who are unable to exert control over the environment. Inouye and Charpentier (1996) exquisitely demonstrated the inverse relationship of the individual's level of vulnerability with that of environmental or process insults on subsequent development of delirium among hospitalized older adults. Environmental features, such as noise, light, and unit design, have been shown to be associated with agitation, anxiety, and disorientation of ICU patients (Frengley & Mion, 1998).

Lack of communication with ICU patients by care providers has been documented and results in distress, anxiety, and confusion (Fontaine, 1994). Attention to the physical environment, use of communication techniques with seemingly noncommunicative patients; encouragement of collaborative practice among ICU disciplines; and nonpharmacological approaches to relieve patient distress, anxiety, and agitation have been suggested but largely untested (Maccioli et al., 2003). Nevertheless, a multipronged approach to optimize physical and cognitive function, address onset, as well as manage delirium and appropriate and adequate pain control is likely to affect nurses' and physicians' reliance on physical restraint.

ALTERNATIVES TO PHYSICAL RESTRAINTS

This book has provided the reader with a number of protocols addressing care issues such as falls, delirium, sleep, nutrition, medications, and function. The reader is encouraged to review these protocols closely. Implementing best practices aimed at these areas in itself will reduce the use of physical restraints. A brief overview of an approach that the authors have found successful is presented herein.

Addressing the two major reasons for using physical restraints, to prevent therapy disruption and falls, requires comprehensive yet targeted approaches. The act of self-terminating therapy among hospitalized, acutely ill older adults is most likely a manifestation of delirium and less likely a desire to enact a clinical decision, as with advance directives. Both falls and delirium are well-known syndromes with significant morbidity and mortality among older adults. Both are complex syndromes with multiple underlying etiologies that require a combination of individual-, environmental-, and organization-specific strategies (Tinetti, Inouye, Gill, & Doucette, 1995). Inouye et al. (1999) have demonstrated a multicomponent approach to preventing delirium in a randomized controlled trial subsequently implemented in a number of hospitals (Bradley, Webster, Schlesinger, Baker, & Inouye, 2006). Fall prevention also requires a multicomponent approach (Hempel et al., 2013; Oliver, Healey, & Haines, 2010). Given the complexity of falls and delirium, it is unlikely that any single intervention will suffice as an alternative to physical restraint. Rather, attention to the environment and organization of the unit, as described in the two previous sections, combined with patient-specific approaches, provides the most successful way to eliminate restraint use (Amato et al., 2006; Enns et al., 2014; Mion et al., 2001).

Fall Prevention

Falls are common, serious events in hospitalized older patients. Although nurses perceive that physical restraint prevents falls from occurring, the reality is that physical restraints have not been shown to prevent falls and can actually contribute to fall injury (Frengley & Mion, 1998). The goal is to minimize the risk or probability of falling without compromising the older individual's mobility and functional independence. Using a systematic or standardized approach, the nurse and physician assess the patient for intrinsic (personal), extrinsic (environment), and situational (activity) factors. Common intrinsic risk factors include impaired gait or balance, sedating medications, vision and hearing impairments, and cognitive impairment, including impaired memory, impulsiveness, or poor judgment. Given the multiple potential causes of falls, no single intervention or combination of interventions has been found effective in preventing falls in hospital settings (Cameron, Murray, & Gillespie, 2010; Hempel et al., 2013). A number of fall risk assessment guidelines are available (Oliver et al., 2010). The reader is referred to Chapter 19, "Preventing Falls in Acute Care," for a more in-depth discussion. What is important to note is that the evaluation for intrinsic factors need not be complex or time consuming. For instance, the nurse can do a simple evaluation of gait and balance by simply observing the person's ability to transfer in and out of bed or chair and ability to walk to and from the bathroom. The nurse can quickly note any difficulty with steadiness, ability to stand up independently without using a rocking motion or use of upper extremities, ability to sit down without "plopping" onto the surface of the chair, and the ability to walk steadily to the bathroom without holding onto objects or the wall. At this time, notation can be made of lightheadedness or dizziness, presence of orthostatic hypotension, and use of sedating medications.

Extrinsic factors include clothing and footwear. Shoes or slippers should be nonskid, but rubber-soled footwear is not recommended because this material can "grip" the floor causing the person to pitch forward. Furniture design, such as beds at a proper height and chairs with extended armrests for easier leverage, can facilitate mobility. Reclining chairs are helpful for those with poor trunk control and who slide out of chairs with a 90° seating angle. On the other hand, reclining chairs can act as a type of restraint if used for patients with general deconditioning or weakened states who subsequent struggle to rise out of the chair. Beds low to the floor assist with preventing fall injury because the distance from bed to floor is reduced (Bower, Lloyd, Lee, Powell-Cope, & Baptiste, 2008). Padded floor mats may be used in combination with the very low beds. However, caution must be taken in determining which patients receive very low beds with or without the floor mats. There have been case reports of patient falls and injury from very low beds or floor mats (Bower, et al., 2008; Doig & Morse, 2010). Falls can occur either because of difficulty rising to a standing position from a very low height and/or tripping on the mat. Thus, care must be taken in determining those patients most likely to benefit from these beds. We suggest use of these beds for patients who are identified at moderate to high risk for falls, unable to stand without assistance, and who forget or refuse to call for help (B. Bower, et al., 2008; Capezuti et al., 2008; Doig & Morse, 2010; Tzeng & Yin, 2008). Use of these beds is no guarantee that falls or fall injuries will be reduced. Haines, Bell, and Varghese (2010) conducted a cluster randomized trial and found no effect on either falls or fall injury with the use of these beds. Similarly, we found that bed and chair alarms have no effect on overall fall rates on general medical and surgical floors (Shorr et al., 2010). Last, hospital equipment can contribute to falls, such as legs collapsing on bedside commodes, wheelchairs tipping when a patient leans forward, or tubing from lower extremity intermittent-compression devices that may be left on when a patient stands up from bed. In determining equipment use, the nurse must weigh each patient's risk factors for the most effective and appropriate use.

The findings of either intrinsic or extrinsic factors should lead to targeted interventions. There are some fall-prevention strategies that one can consider "universal,"—that is, to be implemented for all patients regardless of the risk level. For instance, all patients should have beds at appropriate heights for ease of exiting and entering, have call bells within reach, and have clear pathways. Depending on the type of unit, some units may elect to incorporate universal interventions that other floors would consider a targeted intervention. For example, an acute stroke unit may elect to automatically place all patients on a toileting schedule at time of admission and reevaluate continually whether this intervention is required, whereas the other units in the hospital would elect to use this as a targeted intervention only for those patients with cognitive impairment and incontinence. An important fall-prevention strategy in any setting is mobilization and exercise. Even in critical care settings, there is a growing body of literature that demonstrates the physiological and physical benefits of early mobilization and rehabilitation (Truong, Fan, Brower, & Needham, 2009).

Protection of Medical Devices

Disruption of therapy or self-termination of devices can be dealt with by first identifying the underlying reason for the patient's attempts to terminate therapies. In many cases, the nurse will identify "confusion" as the underlying cause. As discussed in earlier chapters, the nurse needs to differentiate dementia, delirium, or delirium superimposed on dementia. Additionally, the interprofessional team must discern the underlying causes of delirium, including pain. A systematic approach to determine the cause of the behavior is necessary for treatment. For example, if an older adult is suffering from alcohol withdrawal, it is unlikely that interventions, such as increased surveillance or pain relief, will have much impact on the person's agitation and delirium. Refer to Chapter 6, "Assessing Cognitive Function,"; Chapter 16, "Dementia: A Neurocognitive Disorder"; and Chapter 17, "Delirium: Prevention, Early Recognition, and Treatment" for further protocols to identify cognitive impairments and to prevent and manage delirium.

In the past, the options for managing agitation in the critical care unit have been sedation and/or physical restraint. The type and amount of sedation, however, may actually contribute to delirium and agitation (Wunsch & Kress, 2009). Multiple studies suggest that limiting the use of benzodiazepines and use of an alternative medication, dexmedetomidine, can decrease ventilator time, length of stay, and long-term brain dysfunction (Wunsch & Kress, 2009). The use of physical restraint in critical care settings has been associated with delirium as well as posttraumatic stress disorder (Jones et al., 2007; McPherson et al., 2013; Micek, Anand, Laible, Shannon, & Kollef, 2005; Nirmalan, Dark, Nightingale, & Harris, 2004; Wallen, Chaboyer, Thalib, & Creedy, 2008).

As the health care team works to address the patient's behavior, nonpharmacological approaches to protecting the device from self-termination can be made. First, evaluate daily whether the device is absolutely necessary. Since the CMS designation of nonpayment of nosocomial catheter infections (e.g., urinary tract infections from indwelling catheters, ventilator-related pneumonia), many ICUs have implemented multidisciplinary daily mandatory checklists that incorporate assessment for compliance to infection control and timely discontinuation of devices (Byrnes et al., 2009; DuBose et al., 2010). Even in the critical care environment, major therapy devices may not be reinserted once a patient pulls it out. Thus, always question whether the device is absolutely necessary or whether a less noxious device or approach may be used instead. For example, if a nasogastric tube is used for nutrition, request the assessment of other disciplines, such as speech or occupational therapists (OTs), to determine whether oral feeding could be introduced. If long-term enteral feeding is required, an interprofessional team plan with the patient and family is warranted given the known deleterious effects of tube feedings with certain conditions.

Some therapeutic devices cannot be altered or discontinued, for example, use of endotracheal tubes, nasal cannula, or oxygen masks. A second approach is to use anchoring techniques to secure the device against the patient's attempts to dislodge the device or to use camouflage to "hide" the device from the patient. Proper anchoring addresses comfort as well as stabilization of the device(s). For example, it is not unusual for pressure ulcers to develop on nares or behind ears and neck because of undue pressure from the device; clearly a source of discomfort for the patient. Proper stabilization of the tube or device with secure anchoring can minimize accidental dislodgment as well as deter more purposeful removal. For instance, a nasogastric tube can be placed so as to not interfere with or interrupt the person's visual field. Seeing the tube dangling in front of one's eyes or pulling on one's nares is an obvious irritant. If a gastrostomy tube is determined to be appropriate in the person's plan of care, abdominal binders can aid in reducing the person's ability to pull it out. There are a number of commercial products available to secure various tubes, including nasogastric tubes, endotracheal tubes, IV lines, and indwelling bladder catheters. Although none of these devices is likely to prevent a determined person from pulling out a device, they do provide anchoring and stability of the device that is probably more secure than taping methods.

Side Rails

A discussion on physical restraints in hospitals would not be complete without mentioning side rails. Side rails, in and of themselves, are not considered a restraining device by either TJC or CMS. It is the nurse's intent of their use that determines whether side rails are a restraining device or a protective device. This has led to some confusion by nurses. Full side rails to transfer patients in carts, during procedures (e.g., conscious sedation), or protect a sedated or lethargic patient from rolling out of the bed can be considered as protective devices. A number of specialty beds, such as ICU pulmonary beds or bariatric beds, require full side rails in use. Many bed manufacturers have bed controls and call systems embedded in the side rail frames, resulting in patients requesting the side rails be kept raised for ease of control. Hospital patients have also been observed to request partial to full side rails to be raised because of the narrowness of the beds or to facilitate movement (e.g., transfers, repositioning).

In ICU settings, full side rails are used predominantly because of bed equipment specification (e.g., pulmonary beds) or because of procedural considerations (e.g., sedation protocols; Minnick, Mion, Johnson, Catrambone, & Leipzig, 2008). In non-ICUs, nurses use full side rails primarily for fall prevention (46%), especially for older patients (Minnick et al., 2008). Full side rails used to keep patients in bed who *desire* to leave the bed are restraints. It does not matter what the cognitive level of the person is. If a severely demented patient wishes to leave the bed, full side rails are considered a restraint, even if the nurse believes that the side rails are for "patient safety." Side rails have been shown to increase fall injuries because patients either try to squeeze through rails or climb over the foot of the bed; hence they are not recommended as a fall prevention strategy for conscious patients, even in the presence of cognitive impairment (Braun & Capezuti, 2000). Rather, side rails should be limited for use with patients who may inadvertently roll off the bed because of impaired levels of consciousness from sedation, anesthesia, or medical conditions. Indeed, the FDA has received reports of more than 400 deaths as a direct result of side rail entrapment from a variety of health care settings, including hospitals (U.S. FDA, 2006b). The reader is referred to Braun and Capezuti (2000) for an excellent review of the legal and medical aspects of side rail use.

SUMMARY

The pattern and rationale for physical restraint use has changed over the past two decades. Focusing on assessment and prevention of delirium and falls will likely minimize their use. Further work is needed in the ICU setting for best strategies to identify, prevent, and manage delirium that would include nonpharmacological as well as pharmacological approaches. To avoid the use of physical restraints, practical and cost-effective strategies need to be devised and tested. This would best be done in an interprofessional patient-centered fashion.

NURSING STANDARD OF PRACTICE

Protocol 23.1: Physical Restraints and Side Rails in Acute and Critical Care Settings

I. GOAL

To eliminate the use of physical restraints and side rails in acute and critical care settings

II. OVERVIEW

A. The use of physical restraints or side rails for the involuntary immobilization of the patient may not only be an infringement of the patient's rights, but can also result in patient harm, including soft tissue injury, fractures, delirium, and even death (F. L. Bower et al., 2003; Evans et al., 2003; Miles, 1993).
B. The primary ethical dilemma resulting from physical restraint is the clinician's value or emphasis of beneficence versus the patient's autonomy.
C. Use of physical restraint should be used as a last resort; only used when less restrictive mechanisms have been determined to be ineffective; the use of restraint must be in accordance with a written modification to the patient's plan of care; used in accordance with the order of a physician or LIP and must never be written as an "as needed" order. Each order must be renewed every 24 hours for nonviolent behavior and every 4 hours for violent or self-destructive behavior. Orders must be renewed in accordance with hospital policy. Last, restraint must be discontinued at the earliest possible time (USDHHS, 2007).

(continued)

Protocol 23.1: Physical Restraints and Side Rails in Acute and Critical Care Settings *(continued)*

III. BACKGROUND AND STATEMENT OF PROBLEM

A. Definition: The CMS defines physical restraint as "any manual method, physical or mechanical device, material, or equipment that immobilizes or reduces the ability of the patient to move his or her arms, legs, body or head freely" (USDHHS, 2007). Examples include wrist or leg restraints, Geri-chairs, and, in certain situations, mitts, full side rails and reclining chairs.

B. Etiology: Hospital nurses' reasons for use of physical restraint are prevention of patient disruption of medical devices and therapy (75%), confusion (25%), and fall prevention (18%; Minnick et al., 2007).

C. Epidemiology
   1. Prevalence of physical restraint use on individual non-ICU rates range from 0 to 123 restraint-days/1,000 patient days, with overall rates ranging among types of units from 3.6 (pediatric units) to 49.2 (neuroscience units; Minnick et al., 2007).
   2. Individual ICU rates range from 0 to 267.9 restraint-days/1,000 patient-days with overall rates ranging by types from 50.6 (pediatric ICUs) to 267 (neurology and neurosurgery ICUs; Minnick et al., 2007).

IV. PARAMETERS OF ASSESSMENT

A. Assess for underlying cause(s) of agitation and cognitive impairment leading to patient-initiated device removal (refer to Chapter 6; Chapter 15, "Late-Life Depression"; Chapter 16; and Chapter 17).
   1. If abrupt change in perception, attention, or level of consciousness:
      a. Assess for life-threatening physiological impairments
      b. Respiratory, neurological, fever and sepsis, hypoglycemia and hyperglycemia, alcohol or substance withdrawal, and fluid and electrolyte imbalance
      c. Notify physician of change in mental status and compromised physiological status
   2. Differential assessment (interprofessional)
      a. Obtain baseline or premorbid cognitive function from family and caregivers
      b. Establish whether the patient has history of dementia or depression
      c. Review medications to identify drug–drug interactions, adverse effects
      d. Review current laboratory values

B. Assess fall risk: intrinsic, extrinsic, and situational factors (refer to Chapter 19)

C. Assess for medications that may cause drug–drug interactions and adverse drug effects (refer to Chapter 20, "Reducing Adverse Drug Events").

V. NURSING CARE STRATEGIES

A. Interventions to minimize or reduce patient-initiated device removal
   1. Disruption of any device
      a. Reassess daily to determine whether it is medically possible to discontinue device; try alternative mode of therapy (DuBose et al., 2010; Mion et al., 2001; Nirmalan et al., 2004).
      b. For mild to moderate cognitive impairment, explain device and allow patient to understand nurse's guidance.
   2. Attempted or actual disruption: ventilator
      a. Determine underlying cause of behavior for appropriate medical and/or pharmacological approach
      b. More secure anchoring
      c. Appropriate sedation and analgesia protocol
      d. Start with less restrictive means: mitts, elbow extenders
   3. Attempted or actual disruption: nasogastric tube
      a. If for feeding purposes, consult with nutritionist and speech or OT for swallow evaluation
      b. Consider gastrostomy tube for feeding as appropriate if other measures are ineffective
      c. Anchoring of tube, either by taping techniques or commercial tube holder
      d. If restraints are needed, start with least restrictive: mitts, elbow extenders

(continued)

Protocol 23.1: Physical Restraints and Side Rails in Acute and Critical Care Settings *(continued)*

4. Attempted or actual disruption: IV lines
   a. Commercial tube holder for anchoring
   b. Long-sleeved robes, commercial sleeves for arms
   c. Consider Hep-Lock and cover with skin sleeve. White gauze may also be used, but case reports exist in which patients focus on the white gauze and unravel it.
   d. Taping, securement of IV line under gown, sleeves
   e. Keep IV bag out of visual field
   f. Consider alternative therapy: oral fluids, drugs
5. Treatment (interprofessional)
   a. Treat underlying disorder(s)
   b. Judicious, low-dose use of medication if warranted for agitation
   c. Communication techniques: low voice, simple commands, reorientation
   d. Frequent reassurance and orientation
   e. Surveillance and observation: Determine whether family member(s) is willing to stay with patient, move patient closer to nurses' station, perform safety checks more frequently, redeploy staff to provide one-on-one observation if other measure is ineffective
6. Attempted or actual disruption: bladder catheter
   a. Consider intermittent catheterization if appropriate
   b. Proper securement, anchoring to leg; commercial tube holders available

B. Interventions to reduce fall risk
1. Patient-centered interventions
   a. Supervised, progressive ambulation even in ICUs (Inouye et al., 1999; Truong et al., 2009)
   b. PT/OT consultation: weakened or unsteady gait, trunk weakness, upper arm weakness
   c. Provide physical aids in hearing, vision, walking
   d. Modify clothing: skidproof slippers, slipper socks, robes no longer than ankle length
   e. Bedside commode if impaired or weakened gait
   f. Postural hypotension: behavioral recommendations such as ankle pumps, hand clenching, reviewing medications, elevating head of bed
2. Organizational interventions (Mion et al., 2001)
   a. Examine pattern of falls on unit (e.g., time of day, day of week)
   b. Examine unit factors that can contribute to falls that can be ameliorated (e.g., report in staff room vs. walking rounds to improve surveillance during shift change)
   c. Restructure staff routines to increase number of available staff throughout the day
   d. Set and maintain toilet schedules
   e. Install electronic alarms for wanderers
   f. Consider bed and chair alarms (note: no to little evidence on effectiveness; Shorr et al., 2012)
   g. Move patient closer to nurse station
   h. Increase checks on high-risk patients
3. Environmental interventions (Amato et al., 2006; Landefeld et al., 1995)
   a. Keep bed in low, locked position
   b. Ensure safety features, such as grab bars, call bells, bed alarms, are in good working order
   c. Ensure bedside tables and dressers are in easy reach
   d. Clear pathways of hazards
   c. Bolster cushions to assist with posture, maintain seat in chair
   d. Ensure adequate lighting, especially in bathroom at night
   e. Choose furniture to facilitate seating: reclining chairs (note: may be considered restraint in some instances), extended arm rests, high back

C. Review medications using Beers Criteria for potentially inappropriate medications

(continued)

Protocol 23.1: Physical Restraints and Side Rails in Acute and Critical Care Settings *(continued)*

VI. EVALUATION AND EXPECTED OUTCOMES

A. Patient will
   1. Remain free of restraints
   2. Be put in physical restraints only as a last resort
B. Nursing staff will
   1. Be able to accurately assess patients who are at risk for use of physical restraint
   2. Only use physical restraints when less restrictive mechanisms have been determined to be ineffective
   3. Have an increased use of nonrestraint, safety alternatives
C. Organization will
   1. Have a decrease in incidence and/or prevalence of restraints
   2. Not have an increase of falls, agitated behavior, and patient-initiated removal of medical devices

VII. FOLLOW-UP MONITORING OF CONDITION

A. Monitor restraint incidence comparing benchmark rates over time by unit
B. Document prevalence rate of restraint use on an ongoing basis
C. Focus education on assessment and prevention of delirium and falls
D. Consult with interprofessional members to identify additional safety alternatives

VIII. RELEVANT PRACTICE GUIDELINES

A. American Nurses Association (2012)
B. Maccioli et al. (2003)

ABBREVIATIONS

CMS	Centers for Medicare & Medicaid Services
ICU	Intensive care unit
LIP	Licensed independent practitioner
OTs	Occupational therapists
PT	Physical therapist
USDHHS	U.S. Department of Health and Human Services

RESOURCES

Additional Information About Restraints

Consult GeriRN
An online resources containing information regarding assessing and caring for older adults sponsored by the Hartford Institute for Geriatric Nursing at New York University College of Nursing.
consultgerirn.org/resources

The Joint Commission (TJC): Sentinel Event Alert
www.jointcommission.org/sentinel_event_alert_issue_8_preventing_restraint_deaths

REFERENCES

Amato, S., Salter, J. P., & Mion, L. C. (2006). Physical restraint reduction in the acute rehabilitation setting: A quality improvement study. *Rehabilitation Nursing, 31*(6), 235–241. *Evidence Level III.*

ANA (American Nurses Association) Board of Directors. ANA Position Statement. Reduction of Patient Restraint and Seclusion in Health Care Settings. (2012). Retrieved from http://www.nursingworld.org/MainMenuCategories/EthicsStandards/Ethics-Position-Statements/Reduction-of-Patient-Restraint-and-Seclusion-in-Health-Care-Settings.pdf. *Evidence Level VI.*

Bair, N., Bobek, M., Hoffman-Hogg, L., Mion, L. C., Slomka, J., & Arroliga, A. C. (2000). Introduction of sedative, analgesic, and neuromuscular blocking agent guidelines in a medical intensive care unit: Physician and nurse adherence. *Critical Care Medicine, 28*(3), 707–713. *Evidence Level III.*

Boulain, T. (1998). Unplanned extubations in the adult intensive care unit: A prospective multicenter study. Association des Réanimateurs du Centre-Ouest. *American Journal Respiratory and Critical Care Medicine, 157*(4 Pt. 1), 1131–1137. *Evidence Level IV.*

Bower, B., Lloyd, J., Lee, W., Powell-Cope, G., & Baptiste, A. (2008). Biomechanical evaluation of injury associated with patient falls from bed. *Rehabilitation Nursing, 33*, 253–259. *Evidence Level III.*

Bower, F. L., McCullough, C. S., & Timmons, M. E. (2003). A synthesis of what we know about the use of physical restraints and seclusion with patients in psychiatric and acute care settings: 2003 update. *Online Journal of Knowledge Sysnthesis for Nursing, 10*, 1. *Evidence Level V.*

Bradley, E. H., Webster, T. R., Schlesinger, M., Baker, D., & Inouye, S. K. (2006). Patterns of diffusion of evidence-based clinical programmes: A case study of the Hospital Elder Life Program. *Quality & Safety in Health Care, 15*(5), 334–338. *Evidence Level IV.*

Braun, J. A., & Capezuti, E. (2000). The legal and medical aspects of physical restraints and bed siderails and their relationship to falls and fall-related injuries in nursing homes. *DePaul Journal of Healthcare Law, 3*(1), 1–72. *Evidence Level I.*

Byrnes, M. C., Schuerer, D. J., Schallom, M. E., Sona, C. S., Mazuski, J. E., Taylor, B. E.,... Coopersmith, C. M. (2009). Implementation of a mandatory checklist of protocols and objectives improves compliance with a wide range of evidence-based intensive care unit practices. *Critical Care Medicine, 37*(10), 2775–2781. *Evidence Level III.*

Cameron, I., Murray, G. L., & Gillespie, L. (2010). Interventions for preventing falls in older people in nursing care facilities and hospitals. *Cochrane Database of Systematic Reviews, 2010*(1), CD005465. *Evidence Level I.*

Capezuti, E., Wagner, L., Brush, B., Boltz, M., Renz, S., & Secic, M. (2008). Bed and toilet height as potential environmental risk factors. *Clinical Nursing Research, 17*(1), 50–66. *Evidence Level IV.*

Carrión, M. I., Ayuso, D., Marcos, M., Paz Robles, M., de la Cal, M. A., Alía, I., & Esteban, A. (2000). Accidental removal of endotracheal and nasogastric tubes and intravascular catheters. *Critical Care Medicine, 28*(1), 63–66. *Evidence Level III.*

Catrambone, C., Johnson, M. E., Mion, L. C., & Minnick, A. F. (2009). The design of adult acute care units in U.S. hospitals. *Journal of Nursing Scholarship, 41*(1), 79–86. *Evidence Level IV.*

Chevron, V., Ménard, J. F., Richard, J. C., Girault, C., Leroy, J., & Bonmarchand, G. (1998). Unplanned extubation: Risk factors of development and predictive criteria for reintubation. *Critical Care Medicine, 26*(6), 1049–1053. *Evidence Level IV.*

Diercks de Casterle, B., Goethals, S., & Gastmans, C. (2015). Contextual influences on nurses' decision-making in cases of physical restraint. *Nursing Ethics, 22*, 642–651. *Evidence Level V.*

Doig, A., & Morse, J. (2010). The hazards of using floor mats as a fall protection device at the bedside. *Journal of Patient Safety, 6*(2), 68–75. *Evidence Level V.*

DuBose, J., Teixeira, P. G., Inaba, K., Lam, L., Talving, P., Putty, B.,... Belzberg, H. (2010). Measurable outcomes of quality improvement using a daily quality rounds checklist: One-year analysis in a trauma intensive care unit with sustained ventilator-associated pneumonia reduction. *Journal of Trauma, 69*(4), 855–860. *Evidence Level III.*

Egerod, I., Christensen, B. V., & Johansen, L. (2006). Trends in sedation practices in Danish intensive care units in 2003: A national survey. *Intensive Care Medicine, 32*(1), 60–66. *Evidence Level IV.*

Enns, E., Rhemtulla, R., Ewa, V., Fruetel, K., & Holroyd-Leduc, J. M. (2014). A controlled quality improvement trial to reduce the use of physical restraints in older hospitalized adults. *Journal of the American Geriatrics Society, 62*(3), 541–545. *Evidence Level III.*

Evans, D., & FitzGerald, M. (2002). Reasons for physically restraining patients and residents: A systematic review and content analysis. *International Journal of Nursing Studies, 39*(7), 735–743. *Evidence Level I.*

Evans, D., Wood, J., & Lambert, L. (2003). Patient injury and physical restraint devices: A systematic review. *Journal of Advanced Nursing, 41*(3), 274–282. *Evidence Level I.*

Fontaine, D. K. (1994). Nonpharmacologic management of patient distress during mechanical ventilation. *Critical Care Clinics, 10*(4), 695–708. *Evidence Level VI.*

Fraser, G. L., Riker, R. R., Prato, B. S., & Wilkins, M. L. (2001). The frequency and cost of patient-initiated device removal in the ICU. *Pharmacotherapy, 21*(1), 1–6. *Evidence Level IV.*

Frengley, J. D., & Mion, L. C. (1998). Physical restraints in the acute care setting: Issues and future direction. *Clinics in Geriatric Medicine, 14*(4), 727–743. *Evidence Level V.*

Haines, T., Bell, R., & Varghese, P. (2010). Pragmatic, cluster randomized trial of a policy to introduce low-low beds to hospital wards for the prevention of falls and fall injuries. *Journal of the American Geriatrics Society, 58*(3), 435–441. *Evidence Level II.*

Happ, M. B. (2000). Preventing treatment interference: The nurse's role in maintaining technologic devices. *Heart & Lung: The Journal of Critical Care, 29*(1), 60–69. *Evidence Level IV.*

Hempel, S., Newberry, S., Wang, Z., Booth, M., Shanman, R., Johnsen, B., . . . Ganz, D. A. (2013). Hospital fall prevention: A systematic review of implementation, components, adherence, and effectiveness. *Journal of the American Geriatrics Society, 61*(4), 483–494. *Evidence Level I.*

Inouye, S. K., Bogardus, S. T., Jr., Charpentier, P. A., Leo-Summers, L., Acampora, D., Holford, T. R., & Cooney, L. M., Jr. (1999). A multicomponent intervention to prevent delirium in hospitalized older patients. *New England Journal of Medicine, 340*(9), 669–676. *Evidence Level II.*

Inouye, S. K., & Charpentier, P. A. (1996). Precipitating factors for delirium in hospitalized elderly persons. Predictive model and interrelationship with baseline vulnerability. *Journal of the American Medical Association, 275*(11), 852–857. *Evidence Level IV.*

Jones, C., Bäckman, C., Capuzzo, M., Flaaten, H., Rylander, C., & Griffiths, R. D. (2007). Precipitants of post-traumatic stress disorder following intensive care: A hypothesis generating study of diversity of care. *Intensive Care Medicine, 33*(6), 978–985. *Evidence Level IV.*

Kapadia, F. N., Bajan, K. B., & Raje, K. V. (2000). Airway accidents in intubated intensive care unit patients: An epidemiological study. *Critical Care Medicine, 28*(3), 659–664. *Evidence Level IV.*

Kapp, M. B. (1994). Physical restraints in hospitals: Risk management's reduction role. *Journal of Healthcare Risk Management, 14*(1), 3–8. *Evidence Level VI.*

Kapp, M. B. (1996). Physical restraint use in critical care: Legal issues. *AACN Clinical Issues, 7*(4), 579–584. *Evidence Level VI.*

Kapp, M. B. (1999). Physical restraint use in acute care hospitals: Legal liability issues. *Elder's Advisor, 1*(1), 1–10. *Evidence Level VI.*

Kaufman, S. R. (1994). Old age, disease, and the discourse on risk: Geriatric assessment in U.S. health care. *Medical Anthropology Quarterly, 8*(4), 430–447. *Evidence Level VI.*

Krexi, L., Georgiou, R., Krexi, D., & Sheppard, M. N. (2015). Sudden cardiac death with stress and restraint: The association with sudden adult death syndrome, cardiomyopathy and coronary artery disease. *Medicine Science Law*, January 26, 2015. Pii:002802414568483. [Epub ahead of print]. *Evidence Level V.*

Lamb, K. V., Minnick, A., Mion, L. C., Palmer, R., & Leipzig, R. (1999). Help the health care team release its hold on restraint. *Nursing Management, 30*(12), 19–23. *Evidence Level IV.*

Landefeld, C. S., Palmer, R. M., Kresevic, D. M., Fortinsky, R. H., & Kowal, J. (1995). A randomized trial of care in a hospital medical unit especially designed to improve the functional outcomes of acutely ill older patients. *New England Journal of Medicine, 332*(20), 1338–1344. *Evidence Level II.*

Leape, L. L., & Berwick, D. M. (2005). Five years after to err is human: What have we learned? *Journal of the American Medical Association, 293*(19), 2384–2390. *Evidence Level VI.*

Luk, E., Sneyers, B., Rose, L., Perreault, M. M., Williamson, D. R., Mehta, S.,... Burry, L. (2014). Predictors of physical restraint use in Canadian intensive care units. *Critical Care, 18*, R:46. Retrieved from http://ccforum.com/content/18/2/R46. *Evidence Level IV.*

Maccioli, G. A., Dorman, T., Brown, B. R., Mazuski, J. E., McLean, B. A., Kuszaj, J. M.,... Society of Critical Care Medicine. (2003). Clinical practice guidelines for the maintenance of patient physical safety in the intensive care unit: Use of restraining therapies—American College of Critical Care Medicine Task Force 2001–2002. *Critical Care Medicine, 31*(11), 2665–2676. *Evidence Level VI.*

Marcin, J. P., Rutan, E., Rapetti, P. M., Brown, J. P., Rahnamayi, R., & Pretzlaff, R. K. (2005). Nurse staffing and unplanned extubation in the pediatric intensive care unit. *Pediatric Critical Care Medicine, 6*(3), 254–257. *Evidence Level IV.*

McPherson, J. A., Wagner, C. E., Boehm, L. M., Hall, J. D., Johnson, D. C., Miller, L. R.,... Pandharipande, P. P. (2013). Delirium in the cardiovascular intensive care unit: Exploring modifiable risk factors. *Critical Care Medicine, 41*(2), 405–413. *Evidence Level IV.*

Mehta, S., Burry, L., Fischer, S., Martinez-Motta, J. C., Hallett, D., Bowman, D.,... Canadian Critical Care Trials Group. (2006). Canadian survey of the use of sedatives, analgesics, and neuromuscular blocking agents in critically ill patients. *Critical Care Medicine, 34*(2), 374–380. *Evidence Level IV.*

Micek, S. T., Anand, N. J., Laible, B. R., Shannon, W. D., & Kollef, M. H. (2005). Delirium as detected by the CAM-ICU predicts restraint use among mechanically ventilated medical patients. *Critical Care Medicine, 33*(6), 1260–1265. *Evidence Level IV.*

Miles, S. H. (1993). Restraints and sudden death. *Journal of the American Geriatrics Society, 41*(9), 1013. *Evidence Level V.*

Minnick, A. F., Mion, L. C., Johnson, M. E., Catrambone, C., & Leipzig, R. (2007). Prevalence and variation of physical restraint use in acute care settings in the US. *Journal of Nursing Scholarship, 39*(1), 30–37. *Evidence Level IV.*

Minnick, A. F., Mion, L. C., Johnson, M. E., Catrambone, C., & Leipzig, R. (2008). The who and why's of side rail use. *Nursing Management, 39*(5), 36–44. *Evidence Level IV.*

Minnick, A. F., Mion, L. C., Leipzig, R., Lamb, K., & Palmer, R. M. (1998). Prevalence and patterns of physical restraint use in the acute care setting. *Journal of Nursing Administration, 28*(11), 19–24. *Evidence Level IV.*

Mion, L. C., Fogel, J., Sandhu, S., Palmer, R. M., Minnick, A. F., Cranston, T.,... Leipzig, R. (2001). Outcomes following physical restraint reduction programs in two acute care hospitals. *Joint Commission Journal on Quality Improvement, 27*(11), 605–618. *Evidence Level III.*

Mion, L. C., Hazel, C., Cap, M., Fusilero, J., Podmore, M. L., & Szweda, C. (2006). Retaining and recruiting mature experienced nurses: A multicomponent organizational strategy. *Journal of Nursing Administration, 36*(3), 148–154. *Evidence Level IV.*

Mion, L. C., Minnick, A. F., Leipzig, R., Catrambone, C. D., & Johnson, M. E. (2007). Patient-initiated device removal in intensive care units: A national prevalence study. *Critical Care Medicine, 35*(12), 2714–2720. *Evidence Level IV.*

Mion, L. C., Sandhu, S. K., Khan, R. H., Ludwick, R., Claridge, J. A., Pile, J.,... Winchell, J. (2010). Effect of situational and clinical variables on the likelihood of physicians ordering physical restraint. *Journal of the American Geriatrics Society, 58*(7), 1279–1288. *Evidence Level III.*

Nirmalan, M., Dark, P. M., Nightingale, P., & Harris, J. (2004). Editorial IV: Physical and pharmacological restraint of critically ill patients: Clinical facts and ethical considerations. *British Journal of Anesthesia, 92*(6), 789–792. *Evidence Level V.*

O'Keeffe, S., Jack, C. L., & Lye, M. (1996). Use of restraints and bedrails in a British hospital. *Journal of the American Geriatrics Society, 44*(9), 1086–1088. *Evidence Level IV.*

Oliver, D., Healey, F., & Haines, T. P. (2010). Preventing falls and fall-related injuries in hospitals. *Clinics in Geriatric Medicine, 26*(4), 645–692. *Evidence Level I.*

Palmer, R. M., Landefeld, C. S., Kresevic, D., & Kowal, J. (1994). A medical unit for the acute care of the elderly. *Journal of the American Geriatrics Society, 42*(5), 545–552. *Evidence Level VI.*

Sandhu, S. K., Mion, L., Khan, R. H., Ludwick, R., Claridge, J., Pile, J. C.,... Dietrich, M. S. (2010). Likelihood of ordering physical restraints: Influence of physician characteristics. *Journal of the American Geriatrics Society, 58*(7), 1272–1278. *Evidence Level III.*

Schafer, A. (1985). Restraints and the elderly: When safety and autonomy conflict. *Canadian Medical Association Journal, 132*(11), 1257–1260. *Evidence Level VI.*

Shorr, R. I., Chandler, A. M., Mion, L. C., Waters, T. M., Liu, M., Daniels, M. J., … Miller, S. T. (2010). Effects of an intervention to increase bed alarm use to prevent falls in hospitalized patients: A cluster randomized trial. *Annals of Internal Medicine, 157*(10), 692–699. *Evidence Level III.*

Shorr, R. I., Chandler, A. M., Mion, L. C., Waters, T. M., Liu, M., Daniels, M. J., … Miller, S. T. (2012). Increasing bed alarm use to prevent falls in hospitalized patients: A cluster-randomized trial. *Annals of Internal Medicine, 157*(10), 692–699. *Evidence Level II.*

Slomka, J., Agich, G. J., Stagno, S. J., & Smith, M. L. (1998). Physical restraint elimination in the acute care setting: Ethical considerations. *HEC Forum, 10*(3–4), 244–262. *Evidence Level VI.*

Tinetti, M. E., Inouye, S. K., Gill, T. M., & Doucette, J. T. (1995). Shared risk factors for falls, incontinence, and functional dependence. Unifying the approach to geriatric syndromes. *Journal of the American Medical Association, 273*(17), 1348–1353. *Evidence Level VI.*

Tominaga, G. T., Rudzwick, H., Scannell, G., & Waxman, K. (1995). Decreasing unplanned extubations in the surgical intensive care unit. *American Journal of Surgery, 170*(6), 586–590. *Evidence Level III.*

Truong, A. D., Fan, E., Brower, R. G., & Needham, D. M. (2009). Bench-to-bedside review: Mobilizing patients in the intensive care unit—From pathophysiology to clinical trials. *Critical Care, 13*(4), 216. *Evidence Level I.*

Tzeng, H. M., & Yin, C. Y. (2008). Heights of occupied patient beds: A possible risk factor for inpatient falls. *Journal of Clinical Nursing, 17*(11), 1503–1509. *Evidence Level IV.*

U.S. Department of Health and Human Services. (2006). *Medicare and Medicaid Programs; hospital conditions of participation: Patients' rights.* Retrieved from https://federalregister.gov/a/06-9559.

U.S. Department of Health and Human Services. (2007). Medicare program; proposed changes to the hospital inpatient prospective payment systems and fiscal year 2008 rates; correction. *Federal Register, 72*(109), 31507–31540.

U.S. Food and Drug Administration (FDA). (2006a). *A guide for modifying bed systems and using accessories to reduce the risk of entrapment.* Retrieved from http://www.fda.gov/MedicalDevices/ProductsandMedicalProcedures/GeneralHospitalDevicesandSupplies/HospitalBeds/ucm123673.htm

U.S. Food and Drug Adminstration. (2006b). FDA news: FDA issues guidance on hospital bed design to reduce patient entrapment. 2006; *P0–36:FDA News.* Retrieved from http://www.fda.gov/bbs/topics/NEWS/2006/NEW01331.html

Wallen, K., Chaboyer, W., Thalib, L., & Creedy, D. K. (2008). Symptoms of acute posttraumatic stress disorder after intensive care. *American Journal of Critical Care, 17*(6), 534–544. *Evidence Level IV.*

Williams, C. C., & Finch, C. E. (1997). Physical restraint: Not fit for woman, man, or beast. *Journal of the American Geriatrics Society, 45*(6), 773–775. *Evidence Level VI.*

Wunsch, H., & Kress, J. P. (2009). A new era for sedation in ICU patients. *Journal of the American Medical Association, 301*(5), 542–544. *Evidence Level VI.*

24

Preventing Pressure Ulcers and Skin Tears

Elizabeth A. Ayello and R. Gary Sibbald

EDUCATIONAL OBJECTIVES

On completion of this chapter, the reader should be able to:

1. Complete a comprehensive pressure ulcer risk assessment
2. Classify pressure ulcers using the correct staging definitions (check for applicability in your clinical care setting or country)
3. Develop a comprehensive, holistic plan to prevent pressure ulcers in individuals at risk
4. Identify older adults at risk of skin tears
5. Classify skin tears using the International Skin Tear Advisory Panel (ISTAP) classification system
6. Develop a plan to prevent and treat skin tears

OVERVIEW

The skin is the largest external organ; so preserving its integrity is an important aspect of nursing care. Performing a risk assessment and implementing a consistent prevention protocol may avoid disruption of the skin integrity, including pressure ulcers or skin tears. Although, pressure ulcers and skin tears may look similar, they are different types of skin injury; skin tears are acute traumatic wounds, whereas pressure ulcers are chronic wounds. It is important, therefore, to assess the wound and to determine the correct etiology so that the proper individualized treatment plan can be implemented.

BACKGROUND AND STATEMENT OF PROBLEM

Pressure Ulcers

Pressure ulcers are a significant health care problem worldwide (Bolton, 2010). They have a significant impact on health-related quality of life (HRQL; Gorecki et al., 2009). The word friction was first eliminated from the definition of a pressure ulcer in the 2009 joint pressure ulcer clinical guideline written by the National Pressure Ulcer Advisory Panel and the European Pressure Ulcer Advisory Panel (NPUAP, EPUAP, 2009). In the most recent international pressure ulcer clinical guideline by the NPUAP, EPUAP and now joined by the Pan Pacific Pressure Injury Alliance the word friction has been eliminated (NPUAP, EPUAP, PPPIA, 2014; Table 24.1). The NPUAP has upheld its position that friction is a superficial force that is not an important etiological factor for pressure ulcers (Brienza et al., 2015). Pressure ulcers are believed to develop as a result of the tissues' internal mechanical deformation in response to external mechanical loading (EPUAP, NPUAP, & PPPIA, 2014). A case series by Berke (2015) can help clinicians differentiate friction injuries from pressure ulcers, moisture-associated skin damage such as incontinence-associated dermatitis, and other skin problems or injuries.

For a description of evidence levels cited in this chapter, see Chapter 1, "Developing and Evaluating Clinical Practice Guidelines: A Systematic Approach."

TABLE 24.1

2014 International NPUAP–EPUAP–PPPIA Pressure Ulcer Definition and Classification System

Pressure ulcer definition

A pressure ulcer is localized injury to the skin and/or underlying tissue, usually over a bony prominence, as a result of pressure, or pressure in combination with shear. A number of contributing or confounding factors are also associated with pressure ulcers; the significance of these factors is yet to be elucidated.

NPUAP/EPUAP/PPPIA pressure ulcer classification system

Category/Stage I: Nonblanchable erythema

Intact skin with nonblanchable redness of a localized area, usually over a bony prominence. Darkly pigmented skin may not have visible blanching; its color may differ from the surrounding area.

The area may be more painful, firm, soft, warmer, or cooler as compared to adjacent tissue. Category/Stage I may be difficult to detect in individuals with dark skin tones. May indicate "at-risk" individuals (a heralding sign of risk).

Category/Stage II: Partial-thickness skin loss

Partial-thickness loss of dermis, presenting as a shallow open ulcer with a red or pink wound bed, without slough. May also be present as an intact or open/ruptured serum-filled blister.

Presents as a shiny or dry shallow ulcer without slough or bruising.[a] This category/stage should not be used to describe skin tears, tape burns, perineal dermatitis, maceration, or excoriation.

Category/Stage III: Full-thickness skin loss

Full-thickness tissue loss. Subcutaneous fat may be visible but bone, tendon, or muscle are not exposed. Slough may be present, but does not obscure the depth of tissue loss. May include undermining and tunneling.

The depth of a category/Stage III pressure ulcer varies by anatomical location. The bridge of the nose, ear, occiput, and malleolus do not have subcutaneous tissue and category/Stage III ulcers can be shallow. In contrast, areas of significant adiposity can develop extremely deep category/Stage III pressure ulcers. Bone or tendon is not visible or directly palpable.

Category/Stage IV: Full-thickness tissue loss

Full-thickness tissue loss with exposed bone, tendon, or muscle. Slough or eschar may be present. Often includes undermining and tunneling.

The depth of a category/Stage IV pressure ulcer varies by anatomical location. The bridge of the nose, ear, occiput, and malleolus do not have subcutaneous tissue and these ulcers can be shallow. Category/Stage IV ulcers can extend into muscle and/or supporting structures (e.g., fascia, tendon, or joint capsule) making osteomyelitis possible. Exposed bone/tendon is visible or directly palpable.

Unstageable: Depth unknown

Full-thickness tissue loss in which the base of the ulcer is covered by slough (yellow, tan, gray, green, or brown) and/or eschar (tan, brown, or black) in the wound bed.

Until enough slough and/or eschar is removed to expose the base of the wound, the true depth and therefore category/stage, cannot be determined. Stable (dry, adherent, intact, without erythema, or fluctuance) eschar on the heels serves as "the body's natural (biological) cover" and should not be removed.

Suspected deep tissue injury—depth unknown

Purple or maroon localized area of discolored, intact skin or blood-filled blister resulting from damage of underlying soft tissue from pressure and/or shear. The area may be preceded by tissue that is painful, firm, mushy, boggy, warmer, or cooler as compared to adjacent tissue.

Deep tissue injury may be difficult to detect in individuals with dark skin tones. Evolution may include a thin blister over a dark wound bed. The wound may further evolve and become covered by thin eschar. Evolution may be rapid exposing additional layers of tissue even with optimal treatment.

[a]Bruising indicates suspected deep tissue injury.

Reprinted with permission from the National Pressure Ulcer Advisory Panel (NPUAP), European Pressure Ulcer Advisory Panel (EPUAP), and Pan Pacific Pressure Injury Alliance (PPPIA, 2014).

The exact combination of pressure, ischemia, muscle deformation, and reperfusion injury that leads to a pressure ulcer remains unclear (NPUAP, EPUAP, & PPPIA, 2014). Most pressure ulcers on adults are found on the sacrum, with heels being the second most common site (VanGilder, Amlung, Harrison, & Meyer, 2009). In a study of hospitalized adults, a hospital-acquired pressure ulcer (HAPU) rate of 4.5% was identified, with the majority of HAPUs on the coccyx or sacrum (41%) with heels and hip/buttock region both being at 23% (Lyder et al., 2012). Data in 2009 from 92,408 U.S. facilities reported an overall prevalence rate of 12.3%, with a facility-acquired rate of 5.0%, which lowers to 3.2% rate when Stage I ulcers are excluded (VanGilder et al., 2009). This same study of 86,932 U.S. acute care facilities reported an overall prevalence rate of 11.9%, with a facility-acquired rate of 5.0%, which reduced to 3.1% when Stage I ulcers were excluded (VanGilder et al., 2009).

Table 24.2 summarizes the number of pressure ulcers by stages from this study (VanGilder et al., 2009). The distribution of pressure ulcers has changed over the years, with the number of Stage I ulcers decreasing and the number of unstageable pressure ulcers increasing to 15%, and suspected deep tissue injury (sDTI) to 9% (VanGilder, MacFarlane, Harrison, Lachenbruch, & Meyer, 2010). The most common site for deep tissue injury (DTI) is the heel (41%) followed by the sacrum (19%) and buttocks (13%; VanGilder et al., 2010).

In hospice patients, in addition to the usual sites on the sacrum and heels, elbows are a common site for ulcers with most ulcers occurring within 2 weeks before death (Hanson et al., 1991). In one hospital's 10-bed palliative care unit, 5% of their patients developed a Kennedy terminal pressure ulcer (shaped like a pear, over the sacrum, bruise-like discoloration that is yellow and brown-black; Brennan & Trombley, 2010).

TABLE 24.2

2009 Pressure Ulcer Prevalence by Stages in Acute Care

Type of Pressure Ulcer	Number of Pressure Ulcers
Stage I or II	4,985
Stage III or IV, eschar or unable to stage	876
DTI	642
Stage unspecified	86
Device-related	1,631

DTI, deep tissue injury.
Adapted from VanGilder, Amlung, Harrison, and Meyer (2009).

TABLE 24.3

Location of Device-Related Pressure Ulcers

Location	Percentage
Ears	20
Sacral/coccyx	17
Heel	12
Buttocks	10

Adapted from VanGilder, Amlung, Harrison, and Meyer (2009).

Device-Related Pressure Ulcers

Device-related pressure ulcers account for 9.1% of ulcers, with ears being the most common location (Table 24.3; VanGilder et al., 2009). The NPUAP has a position paper specifically on medical device–related pressure ulcers; a one-page educational resource (often referred to as an enabler for practice by educators), to raise awareness of the prevention and treatment of these pressure ulcers that can be downloaded for free from their website (www.npuap.org). Device-related pressure ulcers on the mucosa are not staged using the NPUAP classification system, as mucosa does not keratinalize and therefore the staging definitions cannot be applied (NPUAP position paper on device-related pressure ulcers; NPUAP, EPUAP, & PPPIA, 2014). Because of this ruling, in the United States, the Centers for Medicare & Medicaid Services (CMS) has directed long-term care (LTC) facilities and long-term acute care hospitals (LTCHs) that mucosal device-related pressure ulcers should not be recorded on the resident assessment instrument (RAI) under the pressure ulcer section.

Pressure Ulcer Risk Factors

No single factor puts a patient at risk of pressure ulcer skin breakdown. The 2014 NPUAP EPUAP PPPIA pressure ulcer clinical guideline confirms what the CMS has required in LTC facilities, LTCHs, and inpatient rehabilitation units, which is that pressure ulcer risk assessment should be comprehensive and should include assessment of all patient risk factors. Clinicians need to go beyond just relaying on validated pressure ulcer risk assessment tools (e.g., the Braden Scale, Norton Scale, and so forth; NPUAP, EPUAP, & PPPIA, 2014).

Nonnemacher et al. (2009) addressed the question of what combination of factors increase the pressure ulcer risk by exploring 12 factors that seem to have the most impact on predicting pressure ulcer risk. Historically, pressure ulcers occur from a combination of intensity and duration of pressure as well as from tissue tolerance

(Bergstrom, Braden, Laguzza, & Holman, 1987; Braden & Bergstrom, 1987, 1989). Immobility as seen in bedbound or chair-bound patients and those unable to change body positions can lead to shear, undernourishment or malnutrition, incontinence, friable skin, impaired cognitive ability, and decreased ability to respond to one's environment, which are some of the important identified risk factors for pressure ulcers (Braden, 1998).

True pressure ulcers need to be distinguished from moisture-associated dermatitis or surface injury in the buttocks region caused by the contact irritation of local friction (Berke, 2015) and moisture factors (Gray et al., 2011). In a large study by Bergquist-Beringer and Gajewski (2011), immobility and incontinence were the two predictors of pressure ulcer development in older persons receiving home care.

A study of 20 hospitals of patients waiting for surgery determined a higher incidence of pressure ulcers for longer surgery waiting times or time in an intensive care unit (ICU; Baumgarten et al., 2003). Most pressure ulcers, in one study of 84 surgical patients, occurred within the first three postoperative days (Karadag & Gümüskaya, 2006). A large study of more than 50,000 hospitalized Medicare beneficiaries reported that 4.5% developed at least one new pressure ulcer during their hospital stay, had higher mortality rates during their hospitalization as well as within 30 days of discharge, and had longer hospital stays (Lyder et al., 2012). The following patient characteristics were found in those who developed HAPUs: a diagnosis of congestive heart failure (CHF), chronic obstructive pulmonary disease (COPD), cardiovascular disease (CVD), or diabetes mellitus, and presence of obesity (Lyder et al., 2012). A 2015 study found that in hospitalized patients, immobility, a diagnosis of diabetes mellitus, peripheral vascular disease, and a Braden Scale score of 18 or below were independent predictors for hospital-acquired heel pressure ulcers (Delmore, Lebovits, Suggs, Rolnitzky, & Ayello, 2015).

Patients With Hip Fracture and Pressure Ulcer Risk

In a study of nine hospitals, the cumulative incidence of Stage II or higher pressure ulcer in older adults with hip fractures was 36.1% (Baumgarten et al., 2009). The less time patients waited to go to the operating room (OR) for repair of the hip fracture, the fewer the number of associated Stage IV pressure ulcers (Hommel, Ulander, & Thorngren, 2003). The length of time on the OR table also increased the risk of pressure ulcers in patients with hip fracture (Houwing et al., 2004). Campbell, Woodbury, and Houghton (2010b) found that one third of their sample of patients with hip fracture developed Stage II or higher pressure ulcers. Implementation of a Heel Pressure Ulcer Prevention Program (HPUPP) for orthopedic patients in Canada resulted in complete elimination of heel pressure ulcers compared to the preimplementation level of 13.8% (Baumgarten et al., 2008).

Critically Ill, Intensive Care Unit Patients and Pressure Ulcer Risk

In a case–control study of medical patients in two hospitals, Baumgarten et al. (2008) found that the odds of developing a pressure ulcer were twice as high for those having an ICU stay. In contrast, Shahin, Dassen, and Halfens (2009) found a low incidence of pressure ulcers in their 121 ICU patients as a result of prevention measures, including foam and alternating air-pressure reducing mattresses. Acute Physiology and Chronic Health Evaluation II (APACHE II) scores, physiological criteria, and Glasgow Coma Scale scores are used to predict ICU outcomes, with higher scores indicating poorer outcome; scores were higher in patients who developed pressure ulcers. In contrast, other researchers found no relationship between pressure ulcer development and APACHE II scores (Kaitani, Tokunaga, Matsui, & Sanada, 2010). Shanks, Kleinhelter, and Baker (2008) found that despite the consistent implementation of pressure ulcer prevention protocols in their critically ill patients, the patients who developed more hypotensive episodes were more likely to develop pressure ulcers.

Several authors have published case series that provide emerging support that when polyurethane foam dressings are applied prophylactically on the sacrum of critically ill, emergency department (ED), or medical–surgical (med–surg) patients, there is a reduction in incidence of pressure ulcers (Brindle & Wegelin, 2012; Brindle, 2010; Chaiken, 2012; Cubit, NcNally, & Lopez, 2013; Keily, 2012; Ohura, Takahaski, & Ohura, 2008; Park, 2014; Philbin, Shaw, Walker, & Bishop, 2013; Santamaria et al., 2013; Torrabou et al., 2009; Walsh et al., 2012). Based on their review of the evidence, the 2014 NPUAP, EPUAP, PPPIA Pressure Ulcer Clinical Guideline has provided a recommendation at the B level of evidence to consider using polyurethane foam dressing prophylactically to prevent pressure ulcers on bony prominences such as the heels or sacrum (NPUAP, EPUAP, & PPPIA, 2014, p. 18).

Regulatory and Government Initiatives

Regulatory and government initiatives continuously support the importance of pressure ulcer prevention. Beginning October 1, 2008, CMS no longer reimbursed hospitals at a higher rate for pressure ulcers acquired during hospitalization (CMS Hospital Acquired Conditions, 2011). Recording of location and stage of any Stage III and IV pressure ulcers present on admission (POA) now holds clinicians who are legally responsible for establishing the medical diagnosis accountable for documenting this information in the patient's medical record; otherwise, the hospital is not reimbursed for the pressure ulcer diagnosis (Russo, Steiner, & Spector, 2006). Data from the Healthcare Cost and Utilization Project (HCUP) statistical review reveal that, over the past years, pressure ulcers have increased in hospitalized patients by 80%, even though the number of hospitalizations during this period of 1993 to 2006 only increased by 15% (CMS Hospital Acquired Conditions, 2011). In the state of New Jersey, Stage III and IV pressure ulcers are now reportable in acute care (New Jersey Department of Health and Senior Services, 2004). Pressure ulcers are one of the 12 targeted areas to reduce harm to hospitalized patients in the United States as part of the Institute for Healthcare Improvement's (IHI) "5 Million Lives Campaign" launched in December 2006 (IHI, 2006). Therefore, at the beginning of the 21st century, appropriate risk assessment and preventative care take on even more important meanings.

Several successful initiatives to decrease pressure ulcer incidence are reported in the literature (Anderson et al., 2015; Lyder & Ayello, 2009; McInerney, 2008; Pancorbo-Hidalgo, Garcia-Fernandez, Lopez-Medina, & Alvarez-Nieto, 2006). Nurses will find the Agency for Healthcare Research and Quality (AHRQ) toolkit available at www.ahrq.gov/professionals/systems/hospital/pressureulcertoolkit helpful in developing quality initiatives to decrease pressure ulcer incidence (AHRQ, 2012). A summary of successful characteristics of pressure ulcer reduction initiatives can be found in the literature (Niederhauser et al., 2012; Padula, Valuck, Makic, & Wald, 2015).

ASSESSMENT OF THE PROBLEM

When to Do an Assessment

The assessment of the relative pressure ulcer risk is the first step of any individual patient or health care system plan for prevention. Some pressure ulcer clinical guidelines recommend that patients are assessed for pressure ulcer development on admission to a care facility, on discharge, whenever the patient's condition changes, and then reassessed based on the person's acuity (NPUAP, EPUAP, & PPPIA, 2014).

Pressure Ulcer Risk-Assessment Tools

Guidelines recommend that a comprehensive assessment for pressure ulcer risk be structured and include evaluation of all relevant risk factors and avoid reliance on just one risk factor or assessment tool total score (NPUAP, EPUAP, & PPPIA, 2014). The assessment should include a history (comorbidities, previous pressure ulcer, medications, and so forth) and physical examination, including skin inspection for skin status, and a pressure ulcer risk assessment using a valid and reliable assessment tool, including subscale scores. Both the Braden (Braden & Bergstrom, 1989) and the Norton Scales (Norton, McLaren, & Exton-Smith, 1962; Norton, McLaren, & Exton-Smith, 1975) are considered reliable and valid. A study of 429 patients in acute care found the modified Braden Scale to be a better predictor than the Norton Scale (Kwong et al., 2005). Although Kottner and Dassen (2010) found that the Braden Scale was more valid and reliable than the Waterlow Scale, they do not recommend either of these scales for ICU patients. Research to create new scales specific to ICU patients continues (Suriadi, Sanada, Sugama, Thigpen, & Subuh, 2008).

The Braden Scale was created in 1987 (Bergstrom et al., 1987) as part of a research study. The scale has six factors and is the most widely used scale in the United States. The first three subscales, sensory/perception, mobility, and activity, address clinical situations that predispose the patient to intense and prolonged pressure. The last three subscales, moisture, nutrition, and friction/shear, address factors that alter tissue tolerance for pressure. Each of the six categories is ranked with a numerical score, with 1 representing the lowest possible subscore and indicating the greatest risk. The sum of the six subscores and the greatest risk is the final Braden Scale score, which can range from 6 to 23.

A low Braden Scale score indicates that a patient is at risk for pressure ulcers. The original onset-of-risk score on the Braden Scale was 16 or less (Braden & Bergstrom, 1987). Further research on older adults (Bergstrom & Braden, 1992) and on persons with darkly pigmented skin (Lyder et al., 1998, 1999) supports a score of 18 or less. Research by Chan, Tan, Lee, and Lee (2005) also determined that the total Braden Scale score was the only significant predictor of pressure ulcers in hospitalized patients. In 2009, Chan, Pang, and Kwong (2009) applied a modified Braden Scale and calculated a cutoff score of 19 in a 107-bed orthopedic department of an acute care hospital in Hong Kong, with 9.1% of patients developing a pressure ulcer. In a retrospective study of intensive care patients in Korea using a cutoff score of 13, the Braden Scale (without a more comprehensive approach to patient-risk assessment) had low to moderate positive predictive performance (Cho & Noh, 2010). Risk was associated with pressure ulcer development in ICU patients who had low Braden Scale scores on the first day of hospitalization and low Glasgow Scale scores (Fernances & Caliri, 2008).

The NPUAP, EPUAP, and PPPIA 2014 clinical guidelines recommend that clinicians not only consider total Braden Scale scores but also address any low subscale scores (these indicate a higher risk) in planning pressure ulcer prevention care. Once high risk is identified, either for overall score or in *any* low subscales (CMS, 2004), prevention interventions need to be implemented. However, one study determined that in a sample of 792 hospitalized patients with a high risk of pressure ulcer development, only 51% of patients 65 years and older had a preventive device in place (Rich, Shardell, Margolis, & Baumgarten, 2009).

DOES RACE MAKE A DIFFERENCE?

When it comes to severity of pressure ulcers, race may make a difference. Ayello and Lyder (2001) analyzed and summarized the existing data about pressure ulcers across the skin pigmentation spectrum. Blacks have the lowest incidence (19%) of superficial tissue damage classified as Stage I pressure ulcers, and Whites have the highest incidence at 46% (Barczak, Barnett, Childs, & Bosley, 2007). Despite the lower Stage I rate, the more severe tissue injury detected in Stages II to IV pressure ulcers is higher in persons with darkly pigmented skin (Barczak et al., 2007; Meehan, 1990, 1994). Three national surveys identified that Blacks had 39% (Barczak et al., 2007), 16% (Meehan, 1990), and 41% (Meehan, 1994) higher incidence of Stage II pressure ulcers compared to Caucasians. Subsequent studies by Lyder et al. (1998, 1999) continue to support a higher incidence of pressure ulcers in persons with darkly pigmented skin. Fogerty, Guy, Barbul, Nanney, and Abumrad (2009) determined that not only was there a higher prevalence of pressure ulcers, but also that they occurred at a younger age in African Americans as compared to Caucasians.

Inadequate detection of Stage I pressure ulcers in persons with darkly pigmented skin may be a result of clinicians erroneously believing that dark skin tolerates pressure better than light skin (Bergstrom, Braden, Kemp, Champagne, & Ruby, 1996), or that only color changes indicate an ulcer (Bennett, 1995; Henderson et al., 1997; Lyder, 1996; Lyder et al., 1998, 1999; Rich et al., 2009). Research has begun to validate these assessment characteristics in the Stage I definition. In 2001, Lyder et al. (2001) reported a higher diagnostic accuracy rate of 78% using the revised definition compared with 58% with the original definition. Sprigle, Linden, McKenna, Davis, and Riordan (2001) evaluated changes in skin temperature; in particular, that warmth followed by coolness accompanied most Stage I pressure ulcers.

Clinicians should pay careful attention to a variety of factors when assessing a patient with darkly pigmented skin for Stage I pressure ulcers. Differences in skin over bony prominences (e.g., the sacrum and the heels) as compared with surrounding skin may be indicators of a Stage I pressure ulcer. The skin should be assessed for alterations in pain or local sensation. In addition, a change of skin color should be noted; doctors need to be familiar with the range of skin pigmentation that is normal for a particular patient (Bennett, 1995; Henderson et al., 1997).

INTERVENTIONS AND CARE STRATEGIES

Determining a patient's risk for developing a pressure ulcer is only the first step in providing best practice care. Once risk is identified, implementing a consistent protocol to prevent the development of a pressure ulcer is essential. A nursing standard-of-practice protocol for pressure ulcer prevention is presented later in the chapter to facilitate proactive interventions to prevent pressure ulcers. A change in attitudes of health care professionals may be required to facilitate prevention (Buss, Halfens, Abu-Saad, & Kok, 2004). Educating nursing students (Holst et al., 2010) and nurses in an ICU unit resulted in decrease in pressure ulcers (Uzun, Aylaz, & Karadag, 2009). Several clinical guidelines exist detailing pressure ulcer prevention (NPUAP, EPUAP, & PPPIA, 2014; Wound, Ostomy, and Continence Nurses Society, 2010). Components of a pressure ulcer prevention protocol should minimally include interventions targeting the following: skin care (including addressing moisture and friction), pressure redistribution, repositioning, and nutrition.

Skin Care

Skin that is too dry or too wet has been associated with pressure ulcers. Although there is limited research, dry skin is believed to predispose ulcer formation (Allman, Goode, Patrick, Burst, & Bartolucci, 1995; Reddy, Gill, & Rochon, 2006). The type of cream used on the skin for different parts of the body may make a difference as evidenced by a study of 79 patients treated with dimethyl sulfoxide cream, with an increase in pressure ulcers when this cream was used on the heels as compared to the buttocks (Houwing, Van der Zwet, van Asbeck, Halfens, & Arends, 2008). Other researchers (Stratton et al., 2005) found that a silicone-based dermal nourishing cream reduced the proportion of HAPUs to 0 after 8 months. Each of these creams are lubricating, adding an external ointment layer preventing insensible losses. The stratum corneum has 10% moisture content maintained by a complex structure of a number of chemicals referred to as the natural moisturizing factor (NMF). When the NMF decreases to below a critical level, the skin integrity is lost, with defects occurring between the keratin layers (dry skin, winter itch, eczema craquelé). The second way to moisturize the skin is with humectants (urea, lactic acid, glycerin, ceramides), which actually bind water to the stratum corneum. These substances will sting or burn when applied to open skin because of their hydroscopic properties but this does not indicate an allergy. Skin can also be too wet, causing a macerated stratum corneum, decreasing the cutaneous barrier and subjecting affected individuals to an increased risk of yeast and bacterial infections.

Use of a soft silicone dressing on the sacrum of critically ill patients resulted in zero pressure ulcers in one ICU (Brindle, 2010). Other researchers have reported similar pressure ulcer occurrence reduction when polyurethane foam dressings are placed prophylactically on heels or sacrum (Brindle & Wegelin, 2012; Chaiken, 2012; Cubit et al., 2013; Keily, 2012; Park, 2014; Philbin et al., 2013; Santamaria et al., 2013; Torrabou et al., 2008; Walsh et al., 2012). Hydrocolloid dressings decreased pressure ulcers from nasotracheal intubation (Huang, Tseng, Lee, Yeh, & Lai, 2009). When hydrocolloid or film dressings were applied to the skin under facemasks, there were fewer device-related pressure ulcers (Weng, 2008).

Repositioning and Pressure Redistribution

Because hospitalized patient immobility is a risk factor for the development of pressure ulcers (Lindgren, Unosson, Fredrikson, & Ek, 2004), efforts must be implemented to address pressure. Although repositioning patients is a key intervention to redistribute the pressure and prevent pressure ulcers, the best frequency for turning and repositioning, as well as which support surface to use, remains a challenge (Defloor, De Bacquer, & Grypdonck, 2005; Norton et al., 1975; Young, 2004). Patients on a particular support surface may not have to be repositioned every 2 hours, depending on their tolerance to pressure. There is no one repositioning timetable for all, the timing needs to be individualized (EPUAP & NPUAP, 2009). The use of a wedge-shaped cushion rather than a pillow may be more effective in decreasing pressure ulcers in some patients (Heyneman, Vanderwee, Grypdonck, & Defloor, 2009).

Redistributing pressure is a key pressure ulcer prevention component. When compared to alternating pressure overlays, alternating pressure mattresses reduced length of stay for hospitalized patients, thus decreasing costs as well as having the added benefit of delaying the time at which a pressure ulcer appeared (Iglesias et al., 2006; Nixon et al., 2006).

The incidence of heel pressure ulcers decreased when the appropriate heel-suspending device was used to relieve pressure (Gilcreast et al., 2005). In 2010, a prospective 150-patient, 6-month study by Campbell, Woodbury, and Houghton (2010a), indicated pressure ulcer incidence was being lowered significantly, by 16%, (p = .016) for those who received help with pressure relief interventions. No new pressure ulcers developed in a single study of persons with a body mass index (BMI) greater than 35 who were placed on appropriately sized low air-loss equipment (Pemberton, Turner, & VanGilder, 2009). Clinicians may find the Wound, Ostomy, and Continence Nursing Society (WOCN) evidence-based algorithm for selecting a support surface to be a helpful tool in practice (McNichol, Watts, Mackey, Beitz, & Gray, 2015).

In Australia, where medical grade sheepskin (animal source, not synthetic) is available, one study with some questionable methodology demonstrated that hospitalized patients randomly assigned to the animal-source sheepskin mattress overlay had a 9.6% lower incidence of risk of pressure ulcers compared to the control group, which had a risk of 16.6% (Jolley et al., 2004). The results were that 58 patients developed pressure ulcers (sheepskin group, 21; referent group, 37). The cumulative incidence risk was 9.6% in the sheepskin group (95% CI, 6.1%–14.3%) versus 16.6% in the referent group (95% CI, 12.0%–22.1%). Patients in the sheepskin group developed new pressure ulcers at a rate less than half that of referent patients (rate ratio, 0.42; 95% CI, 0.26–0.67).

Nutrition

There is lack of consensus about the best way to assess nutritional impairment but, generally, consultation by a dietitian for nutritional status, determination of any unintended weight loss, and evaluation of laboratory values, including serum albumin or prealbumin, should be considered. Cordeiro et al. (2005) found that the concentrations of ascorbic acid and alpha-tocopherol were significantly decreased in patients with pressure ulcers or active infection. In a randomized double-blind study on the effect of a daily supplement with protein, arginine, zinc, and antioxidants versus a water-based placebo supplement in patients with hip fractures, there was a 9% difference in the incidence of Stage II pressure ulcers between the nutritionally supplemented group and the placebo group (Houwing et al., 2003). The Cochrane Database reviewed the role of nutrition in pressure ulcer prevention and treatment. The analysis of the database was inconclusive because of the lack of high-quality trials (Langer, Schloemer, Knerr, Kuss, & Behrens, 2003). When and how patients should be nutritionally supplemented to prevent pressure ulcers remains unclear (Houwing et al., 2003; Reddy et al., 2006; Stratton et al.,

2005), with contradictions in the literature. The NPUAP nutritional recommendations (NPUAP, EPUAP, & PPPIA, 2014; Posthauer, Banks, Dorner, & Schols, 2015) for pressure ulcer prevention are included in Protocol 24.1.

SKIN TEARS

Skin tears were originally conceptualized as traumatic wounds caused by shear and friction (O'Regan, 2002) when the epidermis is separated from the dermis (Malone, Rozario, Gavinski, & Goodwin, 1991). Extensive work of the ISTAP has provided the following new skin tear definition: "a wound caused by shear, friction, and/or blunt force resulting in separation of skin layers. A skin tear can be partial-thickness (separation of the epidermis form the dermis) or full-thickness (separation of both the epidermis and dermis from underlying structures)" (LeBlanc et al., 2013, p. 460). Because aging skin has a thinner epidermis, a flatter dermal–epidermal junction, and decreased dermal collagen, older persons are more prone to skin injury from mechanical trauma (Baranoski, 2000; Payne & Martin, 1993; White, Karam, & Cowell, 1994). Therefore, skin tears are common in older adults, with more than 1.5 million occurring annually in institutionalized adults in the United States (Thomas, Goode, LaMaster, Tennyson, & Parnell, 1999), although the incidence in acute care is unknown. Skin tears are frequently located at areas of age-related purpura (Malone et al., 1991; White et al., 1994).

Assessment of Skin Tears

The following areas should be assessed for skin tears: shins, face, dorsal aspect of hands, and plantar aspect of the foot (Malone et al., 1991). Besides older adults, others with thinning skin who are at risk of skin tears are patients on long-term steroid therapy, women with decreased hormone levels, persons with peripheral vascular disease or neuropathy (the decreased sensation making them more susceptible to injury), and those with inadequate nutritional intake (O'Regan, 2002).

The three-group risk assessment tool was developed during a research study by White et al. (1994). Because of its length, and awkward format, it is not often used clinically to assess for risk of skin tears (White et al., 1994). Within the tool, there are three groups delineated by the level of risk: Groups 1, 2, and 3 (Table 24.4). Summarizing the components of this tool, the clinician should assess patients for five criteria:

TABLE 24.4
Enabler for Skin-Tear Risk Assessment

Criteria for High Risk of Skin Tears	Group 1: Either Criteria	Group 2: Any 4 of 6 Criteria	Group 3: Any 5 of 13 Criteria
Skin tears	■ Currently present ■ Seen in the past 90 days		
Challenged mentation		■ Decision-making skills are either impaired or slightly impaired, or extensive assistance and total dependence for ADL is noted	■ Physically abusive ■ Resists ADL care ■ Agitation
Mobility impaired		■ Wheelchair assistance needed ■ Loss of balance ■ Confined to bed or chair ■ Unsteady gait	■ Wheels self ■ Manually or mechanically lifted ■ Hemiplegia and hemiparesis ■ Trunk, partial, or total inability to balance or turn body
Skin changes		■ Bruises	■ Pitting edema of legs ■ Open lesions on extremities ■ Three or four discrete senile purpura lesions on extremities ■ Dry, scaly skin
Physical impediments			■ Hearing impaired ■ Decreased tactile stimulation ■ Contractures of arms, legs, shoulders, and/or hands

ADL, activities of daily living.

Adapted from White, Karam, and Cowell (1994). Copyright © Sibbald and Ayello (unpublished).

- Skin tears present or within the past 90 days
- Impaired mentation or resistance to treatment or activities of daily living (ADL)
- Mobility challenged—there are several criteria for persons who cannot walk normally with a steady gait (we would add a falls history or susceptibility as an additional risk)
- Skin changes—bruising of the extremities, pitting edema of the lower legs and dry scaly skin
- Physical limitations, including hearing loss, decreased tactile sensation, along with contractures

Any of these criteria should alert clinicians to institute a skin tear prevention program, especially the presence of skin tears or history in the past 90 days, along with mobility challenges with impaired mentation, skin changes, and physical limitations further increasing the risk.

The recent work of ISTAP affirms the importance of reviewing both intrinsic and extrinsic factors to assess skin tear risk (LeBlanc et al., 2013).

Several authors have suggested protocols to prevent skin tears (Baranoski, 2000; Battersby, 1990; LeBlanc et al., 2013; Mason, 1997; O'Regan, 2002; White et al., 1994). Lacking research in acute care, some nursing home research supports the value of skin ulcer care protocols to reduce the incidence of skin tears (Bank, 2005; Birch & Coggins, 2003; Hanson, Anderson, Thompson, & Langemo, 2005). After changing from soap and water to a no-rinse, one-step bed product, skin tears declined from 23.5% to 3.5% in one nursing home (Birch & Coggins, 2003). Hanson et al. (2005) also found that skin tears could be reduced in two different nursing homes when staff were educated in appropriate skin cleaning and protection strategies. A reduction in monthly average of skin tears from 18 to 11 after using longer lasting moisturizer lotion, sleeves to protect the arms, and padded side rails was reported in yet another nursing home study (Bank, 2005). One study claims a decrease in skin tears when skin is treated with cream (Groom, Shannon, Chakravarthy, & Fleck, 2010).

Interventions for Skin Tears

If a skin tear does occur, it is important to correctly identify it and begin an appropriate plan of care. ISTAP (LeBlanc et al., 2013) has suggested replacing the original three-category Payne–Martin classification system (Payne & Martin, 1993) with their newer and more simplified classification system of three types, as follows:

- Type 1: A skin tear with no skin loss
- Type 2: A skin tear with partial flap loss
- Type 3: A skin tear with total flap loss

The usual healing time for skin tears is 3 to 10 days (Krasner, 1991). Although skin tears are prevalent in the older adult patient, there is no consistent approach to managing these skin injuries (Baranoski, 2000; O'Regan, 2002). The extensive work of ISTAP has attempted to provide a research base for consistent care to prevent and treat skin tears worldwide (LeBlanc et al., 2013).

Research is just beginning to provide evidence on the best dressings for skin tears. One study (Edwards, Gaskill, & Nash, 1998) compared the use of four different types of dressings in treating skin tears in a nursing home: three occlusive (transparent film, hydrocolloid, and polyurethane foam) and one nonocclusive dressing of Steri-strips covered by a nonadhesive cellulose-polyester material. The nonocclusive dressing facilitated healing at a faster rate than the occlusive dressings. Another study by Thomas et al. (1999) studied older adult skin tears in three nursing homes and identified that there was a higher rate of complete healing with foam dressings compared to transparent films. ISTAP has published a skin tear product selection guide that directs clinicians to avoid adhesives, hydrocolloids, transparent films and closure strips, and instead consider using lipocolloid mesh, silicone mesh, foam, impregnated gauze, hydrogel, calcium alginate, hydrofibers, or acrylic dressings (LeBlanc et al., 2013).

Goals of care for skin tears include retaining the skin flap if present, providing a moist, nonadherent dressing, and protecting the site from further injury (LeBlanc et al., 2013; O'Regan, 2002). A consensus protocol for treating skin tears based on suggested plans of care has been developed by several authors (Baranoski, 2000; Baranoski & Ayello, 2008; Edwards et al., 1998; LeBlanc et al., 2013; O'Regan, 2002) as well as ISTAP, and can be found in Protocol 24.2.

CASE STUDY 1

Mr. Randy Gonnagetawound, 70 years old, has diabetes mellitus with several microvascular and macrovascular complications. He was admitted to the hospital after a right-sided cerebral vascular accident. Past history includes retinal hemorrhages, a previous myocardial infarction, peripheral vascular disease, and a neuroischemic foot ulcer (healed after a left femoral popliteal bypass, intravenous antibiotics, and plantar pressure redistribution with deep-toed shoe and orthotic). He is incontinent of feces and urine, and responds by nodding to verbal commands. His left arm and leg are paralyzed. He has a gag reflex but cannot swallow. His Braden Score is 10.

(continued)

CASE STUDY 1 *(continued)*

Current Data

Physical examination: There is an area of persistent erythema with bruising on the left buttock along with a number of superficial nonpalpable purpuric lesions on the arms and legs.

Physical Assessment and Pertinent Admission History

General: Responds to verbal questioning but he cannot move his left side. Over the past 3 days, he has been increasingly fatigued, completely bedridden. He can change position only with movement of the right side.

Vital signs

- Temperature: 39.2°C
- Respiration: 10 breaths per minute and regular
- Pulse: 88 and irregular
- Blood pressure: 162/94 mmHg
- Weight: 195 pounds
- Height: 5 feet, 9 inches
- Abdominal: Intake has been limited to half bowl of cereal twice a day and piece of toast and tea for lunch for the past 3 days. Last bowel movement was 3 days ago; + bowel sounds.
- Cardiovascular: Irregular heartbeat, no S_3S_4 at apex, +1 pedal edema, faintly palpable pedal pulses; capillary refill prolonged at 8 seconds.
- Respiratory: Crackles over right lower lobe, coughing periodically, nonproductive of mucus
- Renal: Episodes of urinary incontinence for the past 3 days before admission
- Integumentary: Skin is warm, dry, and translucent; tenting noted

Laboratory data: hemoglobin 10, hematocrit 28, red bood cells: 3.2, white blood cells: 11,000 shift to the left. Albumin 3.0 g/dL, potassium: 3.1, blood urea nitrogen (BUN): 32 mg/100 mL, glucose and/or HbA_{1c} not available

Medical Orders

Dextrose 5% in water with equal parts normal saline and 10 mEq KCl at 100 cc/hr

Colace 100 mg by mouth, three times a day
Pulse oximetry monitoring continuously
Metamucil one package every day
Bed rest
Multivitamin one tablet every day
Daily weights
Soft diet as tolerated

Discussion

Mr. Gonnagetawound is a prime candidate for developing a pressure ulcer. His low numerical score on the Braden Scale (10), comorbidities, lack of movement, and other risk factors put him at high risk. Immediate strategies to prevent the occurrence of an ulcer are needed. Immobility is a leading risk factor for pressure ulcer development, so a major part of his plan of care needs to first be directed to initiate moving as much as possible. A physiotherapy consult is needed to evaluate and recommend a plan of progressive exercise and activity. The plan should be to get him out of bed and moving within the constraints of his limitations from the stroke, as well as being in the chair rather than the bed. When in the chair, he should have a gel cushion for pressure redistribution. He will need to be repositioned every hour when in the chair. A Group 2, alternating low-air-loss mattress needs to be placed on his bed. For the limited time when he is in bed, he needs to be turned and positioned. His skin should be assessed every shift to evaluate signs for early skin injury.

A consult with a speech therapist is essential. A swallowing study is warranted to determine his ability to safely take an oral diet. A nutritional consult with a dietitian will address his needs for appropriate calories, protein, and vitamins or minerals. A toileting regimen needs to be implemented to address the fecal and urinary incontinence. A discussion with the prescribing health care provider can explore whether he should continue on the Colace and Metamucil. His skin needs cleansing after each episode of incontinence. Use of a no-rinse bathing system is preferred here rather than soap and water. This vulnerable skin needs protection through use of one of the many skin barriers available on the market.

Both Mr. Gonnagetawound and his family need instruction on why it is so important to get him moving and why nutrition, skin care, turning, and repositioning are so critical to his skin health.

Considering his general health, low hemoglobin, possibility of sepsis, and increase in capillary refill must also be monitored and addressed. It would be beneficial to know the HbA_{1c} to determine blood sugar control and prevent long-term complications.

CASE STUDY 2

Mrs. Keri Sight, 88 years old, is admitted to the hospital from an LTC facility with a primary diagnosis of pneumonia, and secondary diagnosis of senile dementia of the Alzheimer's type with impaired communication skills. She has a history of congestive heart failure and osteoporosis. She spends most of the day in a wheelchair and needs two-person assistance for ambulation. Her skin is thin and dry, resembling an onion; each arm and leg has a purpura area. She weighs 15 pounds less than her ideal body weight and has difficulty swallowing. Laboratory values are as follows: total protein, 5.5 g/dL; albumin, 2.6 g/dL; and BUN, 28. She is verbally aggressive to the staff on which she depends for assistance for her ADL.

Assessment of Mrs. Sight on admission for skin integrity as well as pressure ulcer risk needs to be done. Because she has four of the criteria from Group 2 of the skin tear risk assessment tool developed by White et al. (1994; impaired decision-making skills caused by senile dementia, dependence for ADL, wheelchair or bed confined, unsteady gait), she is at risk of developing skin tears. Other factors that would put her at risk are her thin, dry skin with four purpura present and poor nutritional status (LeBlanc et al., 2013). Her dependence on staff for ADL and assistance, coupled with her dementia, predispose her to skin injury during bathing and other ADL. A comprehensive pressure ulcer risk assessment, including her skin assessment, comorbidities, and Braden Scale score, puts her at very high risk for developing pressure ulcers. A pressure ulcer prevention protocol, such as in Protocol 24.1 is implemented. The rest of this case discussion focuses on her skin tear risk needs.

Discussion

A skin tear prevention protocol needs to be implemented for Mrs. Sight immediately. In order to achieve a safe environment for her, the staff must know how to approach her with her dementia. To address her nutrition and hydration risk factors, a dietary consultation should be performed. Her ability to safely swallow needs to be evaluated by a speech therapist. After the swallowing evaluation, a plan to encourage frequent fluids and assistance with eating should be implemented. To protect Mrs. Sight's skin from additional injury, avoid using hot water to bathe her and, instead, use one of the nonrinse, soapless bathing products. Her family can be asked to bring in a soft fleece jogging suit for her to wear. The purpura areas on her arms and legs should be covered with stockinet or some other soft nonadherent dressing or skin-protective barrier product to further protect these areas. Her bed rails, and the arms and legs of her wheelchair, should be padded. Staff should use the palms of their hands and a turn sheet when repositioning Mrs. Sight in bed. A moisturizer can be applied twice a day to her dry skin. Daily assessment of her skin, including the five minimal characteristics proposed by CMS, should be performed (Rich et al., 2009).

SUMMARY

The skin is the body's largest organ, so pay attention to it. Although the research into prevention strategies is limited, there is support for following the appropriate risk assessment and practice guidelines for these two types of skin injuries: pressure ulcers (NPUAP, EPUAP, & PPPIA, 2014) and skin tears (LeBlanc et al., 2013). Make sure you correctly identify the type of skin injury so the proper plan of care can be implemented.

General skin assessment is important for early breakdown, protecting the skin by using appropriate bathing techniques, using products to minimize the effects of friction and shear on the skin, and paying attention to nutritional status. In the case of pressure ulcers, redistributing the pressure by turning and repositioning and appropriate use of support surfaces are also critical. Immediate initiation of prevention protocols after risk identification is key with correctiion of each major abnormal risk factor part of the treatment protocol. Following these suggestions can prevent and treat skin integrity problems such as skin tears and pressure ulcers.

NURSING STANDARD OF PRACTICE

Protocol 24.1: Pressure Ulcer Prevention

I. GOALS

A. Prevention of PU
B. Early recognition of PU development and skin changes

II. BACKGROUND AND STATEMENT OF PROBLEM

A. Pressure ulcer 2009: Occurrence data reported for 2009 (VanGilder et al., 2009)
  1. All U.S. facilities
    a. Overall prevalence: 12.3%
    b. FA prevalence: 5.0 %
    c. Prevalence excluding Stage I: 9.0%
    d. FA prevalence excluding Stage I: 3.2%
  2. Acute care
B. Etiology and/or epidemiology
  1. Risk factors (immobility, undernutrition or malnutrition, incontinence, friable skin, impaired cognitive ability)
  2. Higher incidence of Stage II and higher in persons with darkly pigmented skin

III. PARAMETERS OF ASSESSMENT

A. Perform a structured pressure ulcer risk assessment that includes complete skin assessment, consideration of all risk factors, and inclusion of subscores as well as total score when using a valid risk assessment tool (NPUAP, EPUAP, & PPPIA, 2014).
  1. Inspect skin regularly for color changes such as redness in lightly pigmented persons and discoloration in darkly pigmented persons (EPUAP & NPUAP, 2009).
  2. Look at the skin located under any medical device (e.g., catheters, oxygen, airway or ventilator tubing, face masks, braces, collars at least twice daily and more frequently in persons with fluid shifts or localized or generalized edema [NPUAP, EPUAP, & PPPIA, 2014]).
  3. Palpate skin for changes in temperature (warmth), edema, or hardness.
  4. Ask the patient whether he or she has any areas of pain or discomfort over bony prominences.
B. Assess for intrinsic and extrinsic risk factors
C. Braden Scale risk score—18 or less for older adults and persons with darkly pigmented skin; pay attention to low subscale scores also

IV. NURSING CARE STRATEGIES AND INTERVENTIONS

A. Risk-assessment documentation
  1. On admission to acute care
  2. Reassess at intervals taking into account the patient's acuity, any change in condition, and based on patient care setting:
    a. Based on patient acuity every 24 to 48 hours on general units
    b. Assess critically ill patients every 12 hours
  3. Use a reliable and standardized tool as part of a risk assessment, such as the Braden Scale, as part of a comprehensive risk assessment (available at www.bradenscale.com/braden.PDF). Do not rely only on a standardized tool for risk assessment!
  4. Document risk-assessment scores and implement prevention protocols based on overall scores, low subscores, and the comprehensive assessment of other risk factors.
  5. Assess risk of surgical patients for increased risk of PU, including the following factors: length of operation, number of hypotensive episodes, and/or low-core temperatures intraoperatively, reduced mobility on first day postoperatively.

(continued)

Protocol 24.1: Pressure Ulcer Prevention *(continued)*

B. General care issues and interventions
  1. Culturally sensitive early assessment for Stage I PU in patients with darkly pigmented skin
     a. Use a halogen light to look for skin color changes—may be purple hues or other discoloration based on patient's skin tone.
     b. Compare skin over bony prominences to surrounding skin—may be boggy or stiff, warmer or cooler.
  2. Prevention recommendations:
     a. Skin care (NPUAP, EPUAP, & PPPIA, 2014)
        i. Assess skin regularly.
        ii. Clean skin at time of soiling—avoid hot water and irritating cleaning agents.
        iii. Use emollients on dry skin.
        iv. Do not massage bony prominences as a pressure ulcer prevention strategy; do not vigorously rub skin at risk for PU.
        v. Protect skin from moisture-associated damage (e.g., urinary and/or fecal incontinence, perspiration, wound exudates) by using barrier products.
        vi. Use lubricants, protective dressings, and proper lifting techniques to avoid skin injury from friction and shear during transferring and turning of patients. Avoid drying out the patient's skin; use lotion after bathing.
        vii. Avoid hot water and soaps that are drying when bathing older adults. Use body wash and skin protectant (Hunter et al., 2003).
        viii. Teach patient, caregivers, and staff the prevention protocol.
        ix. Manage moisture by determining the cause; use absorbent pad that wicks moisture away from the skin.
        x. Consider protecting high-risk areas, such as elbows, heels, sacrum, prophylactically from friction injury using foam dressing (NPUAP, EPUAP, & PPPIA, 2014).
     b. Repositioning and support surfaces
        i. Assess skin and other patient characteristics, pressure ulcer risk, and consider using the WOCN evidence and consensus based support surface algorithm (McNichol et al., 2015).
        ii. Keep patients off the reddened areas of skin.
        iii. Repositioning schedules should be individualized based on the patient's condition, care goals, vulnerable skin areas, and type of support surface being used (NPUAP, EPUAP, & PPPIA, 2014).
        iv. Communicate the repositioning schedule to all the patient's caregivers.
        v. Raise heels of bedbound patients off the bed using either pillows or heel-protection devices; do not use donut-type devices (Gilcreast et al., 2005).
        vi. Use a 30° tilted, side-lying position; do not place patients directly in a 90° side-lying position on their trochanter.
        vii. Keep head of the bed at lowest height possible.
        viii. Use transfer and lifting devices (trapeze, bed linen) to move patients rather than dragging them in bed during transfers and position changes.
        ix. Use pressure-reducing devices (static air, alternating air, gel, or water mattresses; Hampton & Collins, 2005; Iglesias et al., 2006). Use higher specification foam mattresses rather than standard hospital mattress for patients at risk for PU. If the patient cannot be frequently repositioned manually, use an active support surface (overlay or mattress).
        x. Use high-specification reactive or alternating pressure support surfaces on the operating table for patients identified at risk for developing PU. Additional support surfaces, such as facial pads, are needed for patients in the prone position (NPUAP, EPUAP, & PPPIA, 2014).
        xi. Reposition chair-bound or wheelchair-bound patients every hour. In addition, if patient is capable, have him or her do small weight shifts every 15 minutes.
        xii. Use a pressure-reducing device (not a donut) for chair-bound patients.
        xiii. Keep the patient as active as possible; encourage mobilization.

(continued)

Protocol 24.1: Pressure Ulcer Prevention *(continued)*

xiv. Avoid positioning the patient directly on his or her trochanter.
xv. Avoid using donut-shaped devices.
xvi. Offer a bedpan or urinal in conjunction with turning schedules.
xvii. Keep heels off the bed using heel suspension devices or other equipment that also avoids placing pressure on the Achilles tendon (NPUAP, EPUAP, & PPPIA, 2014).
xviii. Manage friction and shear:
a) Elevate the head of the bed no more than 30°.
b) Have the patient use a trapeze or other transfer devices to lift self up in bed.
c) Staff should use transfer devices, a lift sheet, or mechanical lifting device to move patient.

c. Nutrition
i. Assess nutritional status of patients at risk for PU.
ii. Assess and monitor weight status (NPUAP, EPUAP, & PPPIA, 2014).
iii. For at-risk patient, follow nutritional guidelines for hydration (1 mL/kcal of fluid per day), calories (30–35 kcal/kg of body weight per day), and protein 1.25 to 1.5 g/kg/d). Give high-protein supplements or tube feedings in addition to the usual diet in persons at nutritional and pressure ulcer risk (NPUAP, EPUAP, & PPPIA, 2014; Posthauer et al., 2015).
iv. Manage nutrition
v. Consult a dietitian and correct nutritional deficiencies by increasing protein and calorie intake and A, C, or E vitamin supplements as needed (CMS, 2004; Houwing et al., 2003).
vi. Offer a glass of water with turning schedules to keep patient hydrated.

C. Interventions linked to Braden risk scores (Ayello & Braden, 2001)
Prevention protocols linked to Braden risk scores are as follows:
1. At risk: score of 15 to 18
   a. Frequent repositioning, turning; use a written schedule
   b. Maximize patient's mobility.
   c. Protect patient's heels.
   d. Use a pressure-reducing support surface if patient is bedbound or chair bound.
2. Moderate risk: score of 13 to 14
   a. Same as cited, but provide foam wedges for 30° lateral position.
3. High risk: score of 10 to 12
   a. Same as cited, but add the following (b and c).
   b. Increase the turning frequency.
   c. Do small shifts of position.
4. Very high risk: score of 9 or less
   a. Same as cited but use a pressure-relieving surface.
   b. Manage moisture, nutrition, and friction and shear.

V. EVALUATION AND EXPECTED OUTCOMES

A. Patient
1. Skin will remain intact
2. Pressure ulcer will heal

B. Provider or nurse will
1. Accurately perform PU risk assessment using standardized tool
2. Implement PU prevention protocols for patients interpreted as at risk for PU
3. Perform a skin assessment for early detection of PU

C. Institution will
1. Reduce development of new PU

(continued)

Protocol 24.1: Pressure Ulcer Prevention *(continued)*

2. Increase number of risk assessments performed
3. Develop cost-effective prevention protocols

VI. FOLLOW-UP MONITORING OF CONDITION

A. Monitor effectiveness of prevention interventions.
B. Monitor healing of any existing PU.

ABBREVIATIONS

EPUAP	European Pressure Ulcer Advisory Panel
FA	Facility acquired
NPUAP	National Pressure Ulcer Advisory Panel
PPPIA	Pan Pacific Pressure Injury Alliance
PU	Pressure ulcer

NURSING STANDARD OF PRACTICE

Protocol 24.2: Skin Tear Prevention

I. GOALS

A. Prevent skin tears in older adult patients.
B. Identify patients at risk for skin tears (Mason, 1997; LeBlanc et al., 2013).
C. Foster healing of skin tears by:
   1. Retaining skin flap
   2. Providing a moist, nonadherent dressing (Edwards et al., 1998; LeBlanc et al., 2013; Thomas et al., 1999)
   3. Protecting the site from further injury

II. BACKGROUND AND STATEMENT OF THE PROBLEM

A. Traumatic wounds from mechanical injury of skin
B. Need to clearly differentiate etiology of skin tears from PU
C. Common in the older adult, especially over the areas of age-related purpura

III. PARAMETERS OF ASSESSMENT

A. Use either the three-group risk assessment tool (White et al., 1994) or the ISTAP (LeBlanc et al., 2013) recommendations to assess for skin tear risk.
B. Use ISTAP-validated simplified classification system to classify skin tears (LeBlanc et al., 2013).
   1. Type 1: a skin tear with no skin loss
   2. Type 2: a skin tear with partial flap loss
   3. Type 3: a skin tear with total flap loss

IV. NURSING CARE STRATEGIES AND INTERVENTIONS

A. Preventing skin tears (Baranoski, 2000; Baranoski & Ayello, 2012; LeBlanc et al., 2013)
   1. Provide a safe environment:
      a. Do a risk assessment of older adult patients on admission.
      b. Implement prevention protocol for patients identified as at risk for skin tears.

(continued)

Protocol 24.2: Skin Tear Prevention *(continued)*

c. Have patients wear long sleeves or pants to protect their extremities (Bank, 2005).
d. Have adequate light to reduce the risk of bumping into furniture or equipment.
e. Provide a safe area for wandering.

2. Educate staff or family caregivers in the correct way to handle patients to prevent skin tears. Maintain nutrition and hydration:
   a. Offer fluids between meals.
   b. Use lotion, especially on dry skin on arms and legs, twice daily (Hanson et al., 1991).
   c. Obtain a dietary consultation.
3. Protect from self-injury or injury during routine care:
   a. Use a lift sheet to move and turn patients.
   b. Use transfer techniques that prevent friction or shear.
   c. Pad bed rails, wheelchair arms, and leg supports (Bank, 2005).
   d. Support dangling arms and legs with pillows or blankets.
   e. Use nonadherent dressings on frail skin.
      i. Apply skin-protective products (creams, ointments, liquid sealants, and so forth) or a nonadherent wound dressing, such as hydrogel dressing with gauze as a secondary dressing, silicone, or Telfa-type dressings.
   f. Use gauze wraps, stockinettes, flexible netting, or other wraps to secure dressings rather than tape.
   g. Use no-rinse, soapless bathing products (Birch & Coggins, 2003; Mason, 1997).
   h. Keep skin from becoming dry; apply moisturizer (Bank, 2005; Hanson et al., 1991).

B. Treating skin tears (Baranoski & Ayello, 2012; LeBlanc et al., 2013)
   1. Gently clean the skin tear with normal saline.
   2. Let the area air dry or pat dry carefully.
   3. Approximate the skin tear flap.
   4. Use caution when removing dressings as skin damage can occur when removing dressings.
   5. Consider adding an arrow on the dressing to indicate the direction of the skin tear to minimize any further skin injury during dressing removal.
      a. Skin sealants, petroleum-based products, and other water-resistant products, such as protective barrier ointments or liquid barriers, may be used to protect the surrounding skin from wound drainage or dressing, or tape-removal trauma.
      b. Always assess the size of the skin tear; consider doing a wound tracing.
      c. Document assessment and treatment findings.

V. EVALUATION AND EXPECTED OUTCOMES

A. No skin tears will occur in at-risk patients.
B. Skin tears that do occur will heal.

VI. FOLLOW-UP MONITORING OF CONDITION

A. Continue to reassess for any new skin tears in older adults.

ABBREVIATIONS

CMS	Centers for Medicare & Medicaid Services
EPUAP	European Pressure Ulcer Advisory Panel
ISTAP	International Skin Tear Advisory Panel
NMF	Natural moisturizing factor
NPUAP	National Pressure Ulcer Advisory Panel
PPPIA	Pan Pacific Pressure Injury Alliance
PU	Pressure ulcers

RESOURCES

Tools

Agency for Healthcare Research and Quality (AHRQ). (2011). *Preventing pressure ulcers in hospitals: A toolkit for improving quality of care.* Retrieved from http://www.ahrq.gov/research/ltc/pressureulcertoolkit

Anderson, M., Guthrie, P. F., Kraft, W., Reicks, P., Skay, C., & Beal, A. L. (2015). Universal pressure ulcer prevention bundle with WOCN nurse support. *Journal of Wound, Ostomy, and Continence Nursing, 42*(3), 217–275.

Ayello, E. A. (2007). *Try this: Best practices in nursing care to older adults. Predicting pressure ulcer risk.* Retrieved from http://www.consultgerirn.org/resources

Braden, B., & Bergstrom, N. (1988). *Braden Scale for predicting pressure sore risk.* Retrieved from http://www.bradenscale.com/braden.PDF

Authoritative Sites

Agency for Healthcare Research and Quality (AHRQ). (2011). *USDHHS supported clinical guidelines: Pressure ulcers.* Retrieved from http://www.guideline.gov

International Skin Tear Advisory Panel (ISTAP)
http:www.skintears.org

National Pressure Ulcer Advisory Panel (NPUAP)
Pressure ulcer prevention and treatment, research, and policy information
http://www.npuap.org

Wound, Ostomy, and Continence Nursing Society (WOCN)
Guidelines, position statements, best practices, and much more
http://www.wocn.org

Other Related Professional Organizations

American Professional Wound Care Association (APWCA)
http://www.apwca.org

European Pressure Ulcer Advisory Panel (EPUAP)
http://www.epuap.org

World Council of Enterostomal Therapists (WCET)
http://www.wcetn.org

World Union of Wound Healing Societies (WUWHS)
http://www.wuwhs.org

Wound Healing Society (WHS)
http://www.woundheal.org

REFERENCES

Agency for Healthcare Research and Quality (AHRQ). (2015). *Preventing pressure ulcers in hospitals: A toolkit for improving quality of care.* Retrieved from http://www.ahrq.gov/professionals/systems/hospital/pressureulcertoolkit. *Evidence Level I.*

Allman, R. M., Goode, P. S., Patrick, M. M., Burst, N., & Bartolucci, A. A. (1995). Pressure ulcer risk factors among hospitalized patients with activity limitations. *Journal of the American Medical Association, 273*(11), 865–870. *Evidence Level IV.*

Anderson, M., Guthrie, P. F., Kraft, W., Reicks, P., Skay, C., & Beal, A. L. (2015). Universal pressure ulcer prevention bundle with WOCN nurse support. *Journal of Wound, Ostomy, and Continence Nursing, 42*(3), 217–275. *Evidence Level III.*

Ayello, E. A., & Braden, B. (2001). Why is pressure ulcer risk so important? *Nursing, 31*(11), 74–79. *Evidence Level V.*

Ayello, E. A., & Lyder, C. H. (2001). Pressure ulcers in persons of color: Race and ethnicity. In J. G. Cuddigan, E. A. Ayello, & C. Sussman (Eds.), *Pressure ulcers in America: Prevalence, incidence, and implications for the future* (pp. 153–162). Reston, VA: National Pressure Ulcer Advisory Panel. *Evidence Level V.*

Bank, D. (2005). Decreasing the incidence of skin tears in a nursing and rehabilitation center. *Advances in Skin and Wound Care, 18*, 74–75. *Evidence Level IV.*

Baranoski, S. (2000). Skin tears: The enemy of frail skin. *Advances in Skin and Wound Care, 13*(3 Pt. 1), 123–126. *Evidence Level V.*

Baranoski, S., & Ayello, E. A. (2012). *Wound care essentials: Practice principles* (3rd ed.). Springhouse, PA: Lippincott, Williams, & Wilkins. *Evidence Level V.*

Barczak, C. A., Barnett, R. I., Childs, E. J., & Bosley, L. M. (1997). Fourth national pressure ulcer prevalence survey. *Advances in Wound Care, 10*(4), 18–26. *Evidence Level IV.*

Battersby, L. (1990). Exploring best practice in the management of skin tears in older people. *Nursing Times, 105*(16), 22–26. *Evidence Level V.*

Baumgarten, M., Margolis, D. J., Berlin, J. A., Strom, B. L., Garino, J., Kagan, S. H., . . . Carson, J. L. (2003). Risk factors for pressure ulcers among older hip fracture patients. *Wound Repair and Regeneration, 11*(2), 96–103. *Evidence Level IV.*

Baumgarten, M., Margolis, D. J., Localio, A. R., Kagan, S. H., Lowe, R. A., Kinosian, B., . . . Mehari, T. (2008). Extrinsic risk factors for pressure ulcers early in the hospital stay: A nested case-control study. *Journals of Gerontology. Series A, Biological Sciences and Medical Sciences, 63*(4), 408–413. *Evidence Level IV.*

Baumgarten, M., Margolis, D. J., Orwig, D. L., Shardell, M. D., Hawkes, W. G., Langenberg, P., . . . Magaziner, J. (2009). Pressure ulcers in elderly patients with hip fracture across the continuum of care. *Journal of the American Geriatrics Society, 57*(5), 863–870. *Evidence Level V.*

Bennett, M. A. (1995). Report of the task force on the implications for darkly pigmented intact skin in the prediction and prevention of pressure ulcers. *Advances in Wound Care, 8*(6), 34–35. *Evidence Level V.*

Bergquist-Beringer, S., & Gajewski, B. J. (2011). Outcome and assessment information set data that predict pressure ulcer development in older adult home health patients. *Advances in Skin and Wound Care, 24*(9), 404–414. *Evidence Level IV.*

Bergstrom, N., & Braden, B. J. (1992). A prospective study of pressure sore risk among institutionalized elderly. *Journal of the American Geriatrics Society, 40*(8), 747–758. *Evidence Level III.*

Bergstrom, N., Braden, B. J., Kemp, M., Champagne, M., & Ruby, E. (1996). Multi-site study of incidence of pressure ulcers and the relationship between risk level, demographic characteristics, diagnoses, and prescription of preventive interventions. *Journal of the American Geriatrics Society, 44*(1), 22–30. *Evidence Level IV.*

Bergstrom, N., Braden, B. J., Laguzza, A., & Holman, V. (1987). The Braden Scale for predicting pressure sore risk. *Nursing Research, 36*(4), 205–210. *Evidence Level III.*

Berke, C. T. (2015). Pathology and clinical presentation of friction injuries. Case series and literature review. *Journal of Wound, Ostomy, and Continence Nursing, 42*(1), 47–61. *Evidence Level V.*

Birch, S., & Coggins, T. (2003). No-rinse, one-step bed bath: The effects on the occurrence of skin tears in a long-term care setting. *Ostomy/Wound Management, 49*(1), 64–67. *Evidence Level IV.*

Bolton, L. (2010). Pressure ulcers. In J. M. Macdonald & M. J. Geyer (Eds.), *Wound and lymphedema management* (pp. 95–101). Geneva, Switzerland: World Health Organization. *Evidence Level V.*

Braden, B. J. (1998). The relationship between stress and pressure sore formation. *Ostomy/Wound Management, 44*(Suppl. 3A), 26S–36S. *Evidence Level IV.*

Braden, B. J., & Bergstrom, N. (1987). A conceptual schema for the study of the etiology of pressure sores. *Rehabilitation Nursing, 12*(1), 8–12. *Evidence Level II.*

Braden, B. J., & Bergstrom, N. (1989). Clinical utility of the Braden Scale for predicting pressure sore risk. *Decubitus, 2*(3), 44–51. *Evidence Level III.*

Brennan, M. R., & Trombley, K. (2010). Kennedy terminal ulcers—A palliative care unit's experience over a 12 month period of time. *World Council of Enterostomal Therapists Journal, 30*(3), 20–22. *Evidence Level IV.*

Brienza, D., Antokal, S., Herbe, L., Maguire, J., Van Ranst, J., & Siddiqui, A. (2015). Friction-induced skin injuries- are they pressure ulcers? An updated NPUAP white paper. *Journal of Wound, Ostomy, and Continence Nursing, 41*(1), 62–64. *Evidence Level I.*

Brindle, C. T. (2010). Outliers to the Braden Scale: Identifying high-risk ICU patients and the results of prophylactic dressing use. *World Council of Enterostomal Therapists Journal, 30*(1), 11–18. *Evidence Level IV.*

Brindle, C. T., & Wegelin, J. A. (2012). Prophylactic dressing application to reduce pressure ulcer formation in cardiac surgery patients. *Journal of Wound, Ostomy, and Continence Nursing, 39*, 133–142. *Evidence Level III.*

Buss, I. C., Halfens, R. J., Abu-Saad, H. H., & Kok, G. (2004). Pressure ulcer prevention in nursing homes: Views and beliefs of enrolled nurses and other health care workers. *Journal of Clinical Nursing, 13*(6), 668–676. *Evidence Level III.*

Campbell, K. E., Woodbury, M. G., & Houghton, P. E. (2010a). Heel pressure ulcers in orthopedic patients: A prospective study of incidence and risk factors in an acute care hospital. *Ostomy/Wound Management, 56*(2), 44–54. *Evidence Level V.*

Campbell, K. E., Woodbury, M. G., & Houghton, P. E. (2010b). Implementation of best practice in the prevention of heel pressure ulcers in the acute orthopedic populations. *International Wound Journal, 7*(1), 28–40. *Evidence Level V.*

Centers for Medicare & Medicaid Services (CMS). (2004). *Guidance for surveyors in long term care. Tag F 314. Pressure ulcers.* Retrieved from http://www.cms.hhs.gov/manuals/downloads/som107ap_pp_guidelines_ltcf.pdf. *Evidence Level V.*

Centers for Medicare & Medicaid Services (CMS) Hospital Acquired Conditions. (2011). *Present on admission indicator.* Retrieved from https://www.cms.gov/hospitalacqcond/06_hospital-acquired_conditions.asp

Chaiken, N. (2012). Reduction of sacral pressure ulcers in the intensive care unit using a silicone border foam dressing. *Journal of Wound, Ostomy, and Continence Nursing, 39*, 143–145. *Evidence Level III.*

Chan, E. Y., Tan, S. L., Lee, C. K., & Lee, J. Y. (2005). Prevalence, incidence and predictors of pressure ulcers in a tertiary hospital in Singapore. *Journal of Wound Care, 14*(8), 383–384, 386–388. *Evidence Level IV.*

Chan, W. S., Pang, S. M., & Kwong, E. W. (2009). Assessing predictive validity of the modified Braden scale for prediction of pressure ulcer risk of orthopaedic patients in an acute care setting. *Journal of Clinical Nursing, 18*(11), 1565–1573. *Evidence Level IV.*

Cho, I., & Noh, M. (2010). Braden Scale: Evaluation of clinical usefulness in an intensive care unit. *Journal of Advanced Nursing, 66*(2), 293–302. *Evidence Level III.*

Cordeiro, M. B., Antonelli, E. J., da Cunha, D. F., Júnior, A. A., Júnior, V. R., & Vannucchi, H. (2005). Oxidative stress and acute-phase response in patients with pressure sores. *Nutrition, 21*(9), 901–907. *Evidence Level IV.*

Cubit, K., NcNally, B., & Lopez, V. (2013). Taking the pressure off in the emergency department: Evaluation of the prophylactic application of a low shear soft silicon sacral dressing on high risk medical patients. *International Wound Journal, 10*(5), 579–584. *Evidence Level III.*

Defloor, T., De Bacquer, D., & Grypdonck, M. (2005). The effect of various combinations of turning and pressure reducing devices on the incidence of pressure ulcers. *International Journal of Nursing Studies, 42*(1), 37–46. *Evidence Level III.*

Delmore, B., Lebovits, S., Suggs, B., Rolnitzky, L., & Ayello, E. A. (2015). Risk factors associated with heel pressure ulcers in hospitalized patients. *Journal of Wound, Ostomy, and Continence Nursing, 42*(3), 242–248. *Evidence Level IV.*

Edwards, H., Gaskill, D., & Nash, R. (1998). Treating skin tears in nursing home residents: A pilot study comparing four types of dressings. *International Journal of Nursing Practice, 4*(1), 25–32. *Evidence Level III.*

European Pressure Ulcer Advisory Panel (EPUAP) and National Pressure Ulcer Advisory Panel (NPUAP). (2009). *Treatment of pressure ulcers: Quick reference guide.* Washington, DC: National Pressure Ulcer Advisory Panel. *Evidence Level I.*

Fernances, L. M., & Caliri, M. H. (2008). Using the Braden and Glasgow scales to predict pressure ulcer risk in patients hospitalized at intensive care units. *Revista Latino-Americana De Enfermagem, 16*(6), 973–978. *Evidence Level V.*

Fogerty, M., Guy, J., Barbul, A., Nanney, L. B., & Abumrad, N. N. (2009). African Americans show increased risk for pressure ulcers: A retrospective analysis of acute care hospitals in America. *Wound Repair and Regeneration, 17*(5), 678–684. *Evidence Level IV.*

Gilcreast, D. M., Warren, J. B., Yoder, L. H., Clark, J. J., Wilson, J. A., & Mays, M. Z. (2005). Research comparing three heel ulcer-prevention devices. *Journal of Wound, Ostomy, and Continence Nursing, 32*(2), 112–120. *Evidence Level II.*

Gorecki, C., Brown, J. M., Nelson, E. A., Briggs, M., Schoonhoven, L., Dealey, C.,…Nixon, J; European Quality of Life Pressure Ulcer Project Group. (2009). Impact of pressure ulcers on quality of life in older patients: A systematic review. *Journal of the American Geriatrics Society, 57*(7), 1175–1183. *Evidence Level I.*

Gray, M., Black, J. M., Baharestani, M. M., Bliss, D., Colwell, J. C., Goldberg, M.,…Ratliff, C. R. (2011). Moisture-associated skin damage, overview and pathophysiology. *Journal of Wound, Ostomy, and Continence Nursing, 38*(3), 233–241. *Evidence Level V.*

Groom, M., Shannon, R. J., Chakravarthy, D., & Fleck, C. A. (2010). An evaluation of costs and effects of a nutrient-based skin care program as a component of prevention of skin tears in an extended convalescent center. *Journal of Wound, Ostomy, and Continence Nursing, 37*(1), 46–51. *Evidence Level V.*

Hampton, S., & Collins, F. (2005). Reducing pressure ulcer incidence in a long-term setting. *British Journal of Nursing, 14*(15 Suppl.), S6–S12. *Evidence Level II.*

Hanson, D. H., Anderson, J., Thompson, P., & Langemo, D. (2005). Skin tears in long term care: Effectiveness on skin care protocols on prevalence. *Advances in Skin and Wound Care, 18*, 74. *Evidence Level III.*

Hanson, D., Langemo, D. K., Olson, B., Hunter, S., Sauvage, T. R., Burd, C., & Cathcart-Silberberg, T. (1991). The prevalence and incidence of pressure ulcers in the hospice setting: Analysis of two methodologies. *American Journal of Hospice & Palliative Care, 8*(5), 18–22. *Evidence Level IV.*

Henderson, C. T., Ayello, E. A., Sussman, C., Leiby, D. M., Bennett, M. A., Dungog, E. F.,…Woodruff, L. (1997). Draft definition of stage I pressure ulcers: Inclusion of persons with darkly pigmented skin. NPUAP Task Force on Stage I Definition and Darkly Pigmented Skin. *Advances in Wound Care, 10*(5), 16–19. *Evidence Level IV.*

Heyneman, A., Vanderwee, K., Grypdonck, M., & Defloor, T. (2009). Effectiveness of two cushions in the prevention of heel pressure ulcers. *Worldviews on Evidenced-base Nursing/ Sigma Theta Tau International, Honor Society of Nursing, 6*(2), 114–120. *Evidence Level III.*

Holst, G., Willman, A., Fagerström, C., Borg, C., Hellström, Y., & Borglin, G. (2010). Quality of care: Prevention of pressure ulcers—Nursing students as facilitators of evidence-based practice. *Vård i Norden, 30*(1), 40–42. *Evidence Level V.*

Hommel, A., Ulander, K., & Thorngren, K. (2003). Improvements in pain relief, handling time and pressure ulcers through internal audits of hip fracture patients. *Scandinavian Journal of Caring Sciences, 17*(1), 78–83. *Evidence Level IV.*

Houwing, R. H., Rozendaal, M., Wouters-Wesseling, W., Beulens, J. W., Buskens, E., & Haalboom, J. R. (2003). A randomised, double-bind assessment of the effect of nutritional supplementation on the prevention of pressure ulcers in hip-fracture patients. *Clinical Nutrition, 22*(4), 401–405. *Evidence Level II.*

Houwing, R. H., Rozendaal, M., Wouters-Wesseling, W., Buskens, E., Keller, P., & Haalboom, J. (2004). Pressure ulcer risk in hip fracture patients. *Acta Orthopaedica Scandinavica, 75*(4), 390–393. *Evidence Level IV.*

Houwing, R., van der Zwet, W., van Asbeck, S., Halfens, R., & Arends, J. W. (2008). An unexpected detrimental effect on the incidence of heel pressure ulcers after local 5% DMSO cream application: A randomized, double-blind study in patients at risk for pressure ulcers. *Wounds: A Compendium of Clinical Research and Practice, 20*(4), 84–88. *Evidence Level II.*

Huang, T. T., Tseng, C. E., Lee, T. M., Yeh, J. Y., & Lai, Y. Y. (2009). Preventing pressure sores of the nasal ala after nasotracheal tube intubation: From animal model to clinical application. *Journal of Oral and Maxillofacial Surgery, 67*(3), 543–551. *Evidence Level III.*

Hunter, S., Anderson, J., Hanson, D., Thompson, P., Langemo, D., & Klug, M. G. (2003). Clinical trial of a prevention and treatment protocol for skin breakdown in two nursing homes. *Journal of Wound, Ostomy, and Continence Nursing, 30*(5), 250–258. *Evidence Level III.*

Iglesias, C., Nixon, J., Cranny, G., Nelson, E. A., Hawkins, K., Phillips, A.,…Cullum, N.; PRESSURE Trial Group. (2006). Pressure relieving support surfaces (PRESSURE) trial: Cost effectiveness analysis. *British Medical Journal, 332*(7555), 1416. *Evidence Level II.*

Institute for Healthcare Improvement (IHI). (2006). *5 million lives saved campaign: Pressure ulcers.* Retrieved from http://www.ihi.org/IHI/Programs/Campaign. *Evidence Level V.*

Jolley, D. J., Wright, R., McGowan, S., Hickey, M. B., Campbell, D. A., Sinclair, R. D., & Montgomery K. C. (2004). Preventing pressure ulcers with the Australian Medical Sheepskin: An open-label randomized controlled trial. *Medical Journal of Australia, 180*(7), 324–327. *Evidence Level II.*

Kaitani, T., Tokunaga, K., Matsui, N., & Sanada, H. (2010). Risk factors related to the development of pressure ulcers in the critical care settings. *Journal of Clinical Nursing, 19*(3–4), 414–421. *Evidence Level IV.*

Karadag, M., & Gümüskaya, N. (2006). The incidence of pressure ulcers in surgical patients: A sample hospital in Turkey. *Journal of Clinical Nursing, 15*(4), 413–421. *Evidence Level IV.*

Keily, C. (2012). Cultural transformation I pressure ulcer prevention and care. *Journal of Wound, Ostomy, and Continence Nursing, 39*, 443–446. *Evidence Level V.*

Kottner, J., & Dassen, T. (2010). Pressure ulcer risk assessment in critical care: Interrater reliability and validity studies of the Braden and Waterlow scales and subjective rating in two intensive care units. *International Journal of Nursing Studies, 47*(6), 671–677. *Evidence Level III.*

Krasner, D. (1991). An approach to treating skin tears. *Ostomy/ Wound Management, 32*, 56–58. *Evidence Level VI.*

Kwong, E., Pang, S., Wong, T., Ho, J., Shao-ling, X., & Li-jun, T. (2005). Predicting pressure ulcer risk with the modified Braden, Braden, and Norton scales in acute care hospitals in Mainland China. *Applied Nursing Research, 18*(2), 122–128. *Evidence Level IV.*

Langer, G., Schloemer, G., Knerr, A., Kuss, O., & Behrens, J. (2003). Nutritional interventions for preventing and treating pressure ulcers. *Cochrane Database of Systematic Reviews, 2003*(4), CD003216. *Evidence Level I.*

LeBlanc, K., Baranoski, S., Christensen, D., Langemo, D., Sammon, M. A., Edwars, K., . . . Regan, M. (2013). International Skin Tear Advisory Panel: A tool kit to aid in the prevention, assessment, and treatment of skin tears using a Simplified Classification System ©. *Advances in Skin and Wound Care, 26*(10), 459–476. *Evidence Level VI.*

Lindgren, M., Unosson, M., Fredrikson, M., & Ek, A. C. (2004). Immobility—A major risk factor for development of pressure ulcers among adult hospitalized patients: A prospective study. *Scandinavian Journal of Caring Sciences, 18*(1), 57–64. *Evidence Level VI.*

Lyder, C. H. (1996). Examining the inclusion of ethnic minorities in pressure ulcer prediction studies. *Journal of Wound, Ostomy, and Continence Nursing, 23*(5), 257–260. *Evidence Level IV.*

Lyder, C. H., & Ayello, E. A. (2009). Annual checkup: The CMS pressure ulcer present-on-admission indicator. *Advances in Skin & Wound Care, 22*(10), 476–484. *Evidence Level V.*

Lyder, C. H., Preston, J., Grady, J. N., Scinto, J., Allman, R., Bergstrom, N., & Rodeheaver, G. (2001). Quality of care for hospitalized Medicare patients at risk for pressure ulcers. *Archives of Internal Medicine, 161*(12), 1549–1554. *Evidence Level III.*

Lyder, C. H., Yu, C., Emerling, J., Mangat, R., Stevenson, D., Empleo-Frazier, O., & McKay, J. (1999). The Braden Scale for pressure ulcer risk: Evaluating the predictive validity in Black and Latino/Hispanic elders. *Applied Nursing Research, 12*(2), 60–68. *Evidence Level IV.*

Lyder, C. H., Yu, C., Stevenson, D., Mangat, R., Empleo-Frazier, O., Emerling, J., & McKay, J. (1998). Validating the Braden Scale for the prediction of pressure ulcer risk in Blacks and Latino/Hispanic elders: A pilot study. *Ostomy/Wound Management, 44*(Suppl. 3A), 42S–49S. *Evidence Level IV.*

Lyder, C. H., Wang, Y., Metersky, M., Curry, M., Kliman, R., Verzier, N. R., & Hunt, D. R. (2012). Hospital-acquired pressure ulcers: Results from the National Medicare patient safety monitoring system study. *Journal of the American Geriatrics Society, 60*(9), 1603–1608. *Evidence Level IV.*

Malone, M. L., Rozario, N., Gavinski, M., & Goodwin, J. (1991). The epidemiology of skin tears in the institutionalized elderly. *Journal of the American Geriatrics Society, 39*(6), 591–595. *Evidence Level IV.*

Mason, S. R. (1997). Type of soap and the incidence of skin tears among residents of a long-term care facility. *Ostomy/Wound Management, 43*(8), 26–30. *Evidence Level IV.*

McInerney, J. A. (2008). Reducing hospital-acquired pressure ulcer prevalence through a focused prevention program. *Advances in Skin & Wound Care, 21*(2), 75–78. *Evidence Level V.*

McNichol, L., Watts, C., Mackey, D., Beitz, J. M., & Gray, M. (2015). Identifying the right surface for the right patient at the right time: Generation and content validation of an algorithm for support surface selection. *Journal of Wound, Ostomy, and Continence Nursing, 42*(1), 19–37. *Evidence Level IV.*

Meehan, M. (1990). Multisite pressure ulcer prevalence survey. *Decubitus, 3*(4), 14–17. *Evidence Level IV.*

Meehan, M. (1994). National pressure ulcer prevalence survey. *Advances in Wound Care, 7*(3), 27–30, 34. *Evidence Level IV.*

National Pressure Ulcer Advisory Panel (NPUAP), European Pressure Ulcer Advisory Panel (EPUAP), and Pan Pacific Pressure Injury Alliance (PPPIA). (2014). *Prevention and treatment of pressure ulcers: Quick reference guide.* Emily Haesler (Ed.). Osborne Park, Western Australia: Cambridge Media. Retrieved from www.npuap.org. *Evidence Level VI.*

National Pressure Ulcer Advisory Panel (NPUAP). (1989). Pressure ulcers prevalence, cost, and risk assessment: Consensus development conference statement. *Decubitus, 2*(2), 24–28. *Evidence Level I.*

National Pressure Ulcer Advisory Panel (NPUAP). (2008). *Mucosal press ulcers: An NPUAP position Statement.* Retrieved from http://www.npuap.org/wp-content/uploads/2012/01/Mucosal_Pressure_Ulcer_Position_Statement_final.pdf. *Evidence Level VI.*

National Pressure Ulcer Advisory Panel (NPUAP). (2015). *Best practices for prevention of medical device related pressure ulcers.* Retrieved from http://www.npuap.org/resources/educational-and-clinical-resources/best-practices-for-prevention-of-medical-device-related-pressure-ulcers. *Evidence Level VI.*

New Jersey Department of Health and Senior Services. (2004). *Interim mandatory patient safety reporting requirements for general hospitals. Patient safety reporting initiative.* Retrieved from http://www.state.nj.us/health/ps/documents/irr.pdf. *Evidence Level VI.*

Niederhauser, A., VanDeusen Lukas, C., Parker, V., Ayello, E. A., Zulkowski, K., & Berlowitz, D. (2012). Comprehensive programs for preventing pressure ulcers: A review of the literature. *Advances in Skin and Wound Care, 25*(4), 167–188. *Evidence Level V.*

Nixon, J., Cranny, G., Iglesias, C., Nelson, E. A., Hawkins, K., Phillips, A., . . . Cullum, N. (2006). Randomized, controlled trial of alternating pressure mattresses compared with alternating pressure overlays for the prevention of pressure ulcers: PRESSURE (pressure relieving support surfaces) trial. *British Medical Journal, 332*(7555), 1413. *Evidence Level II.*

Nonnemacher, M., Stausberg, J., Bartoszek, G., Lottko, B., Neuhaeuser, M., & Maier, I. (2009). Predicting pressure ulcer risk: A multifactorial approach to assess risk factors in a large university hospital population. *Journal of Clinical Nursing, 18*(1), 99–107. *Evidence Level V.*

Norton, D., McLaren, R., & Exton-Smith, A. N. (1962). *An investigation of geriatric nursing problems in hospitals.* London, UK: Corporation for the Care of Old People. *Evidence Level IV.*

Norton, D., McLaren, R., & Exton-Smith, A. N. (1975). *An investigation of geriatric nurse problems in hospitals.* Edinburgh, UK: Churchill Livingstone. *Evidence Level IV.*

Ohura, T., Takahaski, M., Ohura, N., Jr. (2008). Influence of external forces (pressure and shear force) on superficial layer and subcutis of porcine skin and effects of dressing materials: Are dressing materials beneficial for reducing pressure and shear force in tissues. *Wound Repair and Regeneration, 16*, 102–107. *Evidence Level IV.*

O'Regan, A. (2002). Skin tears: A review of the literature. *Journal of Wound, Ostomy, and Continence Nursing, 39*(2), 26–31. *Evidence Level V.*

Padula, W. V., Valuck, R. J., Makic, M. B. F., & Wald, H. L. (2015). Factors influencing adoption of hospital-acquired pressure ulcer prevention programs in US academic Medical Centers. *Journal of Wound, Ostomy, and Continence Nursing, 42*(4), 327–330. *Evidence Level IV.*

Pancorbo-Hidalgo, P. L., Garcia-Fernandez, F. P., Lopez-Medina, I. M., & Alvarez-Nieto, C. (2006). Risk assessment scales for pressure ulcer prevention: A systematic review. *Journal of Advanced Nursing, 54*(1), 94–110. *Evidence Level I.*

Park, K. H. (2014). The effect of silicone border foam dressing for prevention of pressure ulcers an incontinence-associate dermatitis in intensive care unit patients. *Journal of Wound, Ostomy, and Continence Nursing, 41*, 424–429. *Evidence Level III.*

Payne, R. L., & Martin, M. L. (1993). Defining and classifying skin tears: Need for common language. *Ostomy/Wound Management, 39*(5), 16–26. *Evidence Level IV.*

Pemberton, V., Turner, V., & VanGilder, C. (2009). The effect of using a low-air-loss surface on the skin integrity of obese patients: Results of a pilot study. *Ostomy/Wound Management, 55*(2), 44–48. *Evidence Level IV.*

Philbin, S., Shaw, H., Walker, M., & Bishop, S. (2013). The role of new foam dressing technology in prevention of skin breakdown. *Ostomy Wound Management, 59*(4), 8, 10. *Evidence Level V.*

Posthauer, M. E., Banks, M., Dorner, B., & Schols, J. M. (2015). The role of nutrition for pressure ulcer management: National Pressure Ulcer Advisory Panel, European Pressure Ulcer Advisory Panel, and Pan Pacific Pressure Injury Alliance White Paper. *Advances in Skin and Wound Care, 28*(4), 175–188. *Evidence Level VI.*

Reddy, M., Gill, S. S., & Rochon, P. A. (2006). Preventing pressure ulcers: A systematic review. *Journal of the American Medical Association, 296*(8), 974–984. *Evidence Level I.*

Rich, S. E., Shardell, M., Margolis, D., & Baumgarten, M. (2009). Pressure ulcer preventive device use among elderly patients early in the hospital stay. *Nursing Research, 58*(2), 95–104. *Evidence Level IV.*

Russo, C. A., Steiner, C., & Spector, W. (2006). *Hospitalizations related to pressure ulcers among adults 18 years and older, 2006.* Retrieved from http://www.hcup-us.ahrq.gov/reports/statbriefs/sb64.jsp. *Evidence Level IV.*

Santamaria, N., Gerdtz, M., Sage, S., McCann, J., Freeman, A., Vassiliou, T., . . . Knott, J. (2015). A randomized controlled trial of the effectiveness of soft silicone multi-layered foam dressings in the prevention of sacral and heel pressure ulcers in trauma and critically ill patients: The border trial. *International Wound Journal, 12*(3), 302–308. *Evidence Level II.*

Shahin, E. S., Dassen, T., & Halfens, R. (2009). Incidence, prevention and treatment of pressure ulcers in intensive care patients: A longitudinal study. *International Journal of Nursing Studies, 46*(4), 413–421. *Evidence Level III.*

Shanks, H. T., Kleinhelter, P., & Baker, J. (2008). Skin failure: A retrospective review of patients with hospital-acquired pressure ulcers. *World Council of Enterostomal Therapists Journal, 29*(1), 6–10. *Evidence Level IV.*

Sprigle, S., Linden, M., McKenna, D., Davis, K., & Riordan, B. (2001). Clinical skin temperature measurement to predict incipient pressure ulcers. *Advances in Skin & Wound Care, 14*(3), 133–137. *Evidence Level IV.*

Stratton, R. J., Ek, A. C., Engfer, M., Moore, Z., Rigby, P., Wolfe, R., & Elia, M. (2005). Enteral nutritional support in prevention and treatment of pressure ulcers: A systematic review and meta-analysis. *Ageing Research Reviews, 4*(3), 422–450. *Evidence Level I.*

Suriadi, Sanada, H., Sugama, J., Thigpen, B., & Subuh, M. (2008). Development of a new risk assessment scale for predicting pressure ulcers in an intensive care unit. *Nursing in Critical Care, 13*(1), 34–43. *Evidence Level IV.*

Thomas, D. R., Goode, P. S., LaMaster, K., Tennyson, T., & Parnell, L. K. (1999). A comparison of an opaque foam dressing versus a transparent film dressing in the management of skin tears in institutionalized subjects. *Ostomy/Wound Management, 45*(6), 22–28. *Evidence Level III.*

Torra I Bou, J. E., Rueda López, J., Camañes, G., Herrero Narváez, E., Blanco Blanco, J., Ballesté Torralba, J., . . . Soriano, J. V. (2009). Preventing pressure ulcers on the heel: A Canadian cost study. A cost study. *Dermatology Nursing/Dermatology Nurses' Association, 21*(5), 268–272. *Evidence Level V.*

Uzun, O., Aylaz, R., & Karadağ, E. (2009). Prospective study: Reducing pressure ulcers in intensive care units at a Turkish medical center. *Journal of Wound, Ostomy, & Continence Nursing, 36*(4), 404–411. *Evidence Level V.*

VanGilder, C., Amlung, S., Harrison, P., & Meyer, S. (2009). Results of the 2008–2009 International Pressure Ulcer Prevalence Survey and a 3-year, acute care, unit-specific analysis. *Ostomy/Wound Management, 55*(11), 39–45. *Evidence Level IV.*

VanGilder, C., MacFarlane, G. D., Harrison, P., Lachenbruch, C., & Meyer, S. (2010). The demographics of suspected deep tissue injury in the United States: An analysis of the International Pressure Ulcer Prevalence Survey 2006–2009. *Advances in Skin & Wound Care, 23*(6), 254–261. *Evidence Level IV.*

Walsh, N. S., Blanck, A. W., Smith, L., Cross, M., Andersson, L., & Polito, C. (2012). Use of sacral silicone border foam dressing as one component of a pressure ulcer prevention program in an intensive care unit setting. *Journal of Wound, Ostomy, and Continence Nursing, 39*(2), 146–149. *Evidence Level IV.*

Weng, M. H. (2008). The effect of protective treatment in reducing pressure ulcers for non-invasive ventilation patients. *Intensive & Critical Care Nursing, 24*(5), 295–299. *Evidence Level III.*

White, M. W., Karam, S., & Cowell, B. (1994). Skin tears in frail elders: A practical approach to prevention. *Geriatric Nursing, 15*(2), 95–98. *Evidence Level IV.*

Wound, Ostomy, and Continence Nurses Society. (2010). *Guideline for prevention and management of pressure ulcers.* Mt. Laurel, NJ: Author. *Evidence Level I.*

Young, T. (2004). The 30 degree tilt position vs the 90 degree lateral and supine positions in reducing the incidence of non-blanching erythema in a hospital inpatient population: A randomized controlled trial. *Journal of Tissue Viability, 14*(3), 88–96. *Evidence Level IV.*

25

Mealtime Difficulties in Dementia

Melissa Batchelor-Murphy and Sarah Crowgey

EDUCATIONAL OBJECTIVES

On completion of this chapter, the reader should be able to:

1. Assess the person with dementia for issues related to performance at mealtimes, including cognitive/affective status, functional ability, feeding behaviors, and environmental factors
2. Use a problem-solving framework to determine the most effective intervention strategies, the C3P Model: change the person, change the people, and/or change the place
3. Educate staff and caregivers on hand-feeding techniques for individualized assistance at mealtimes while preserving the dignity and independence of the person being assisted

OVERVIEW

Florence Nightingale's first textbook articulated the importance of providing nutritional support for any person requiring nursing care. Her chapters, "Taking Food" and "What Food" provided critical information for improving health outcomes that is still applicable today (Nightingale, 1859a, 1859b). Since the inception of the nursing profession, life expectancy has increased dramatically. As life spans increase, so does the risk for developing cognitive impairment (dementia). Dementia is the fifth leading cause of death for persons older than 65 years, and one third of people 85 years and older have some form of cognitive impairment (Alzheimer's Association, 2014). By the year 2050, the number of persons with dementia is expected to triple to nearly 14 million, and most of the care needed will be provided by family caregivers (Alzheimer's Association, 2014). When caregiving demands increase to the point that families can no longer bear the tremendous burden, many persons with dementia will be placed in the nursing home setting. In 2014, 64% of residents in our nation's nursing homes had some form of dementia (Alzheimer's Association, 2014).

Malnutrition is a hidden epidemic among older Americans across weight categories (underweight, normal, and obese/overweight) and across care settings (home, health care systems, and long-term care institutions). In the nursing home setting, malnutrition is more prevalent than falls or pressure ulcers (Centers for Medicare & Medicaid Services, 2015); and in hospitals, malnutrition is the biggest risk factor associated with readmission and mortality (Gerontological Society of America, 2014). Interventions to combat this problem fall into five major categories: nutritional supplements, training/education, environment/routine modification, feeding assistance, and mixed interventions (Wen, Jooyoung, & Thomas, 2014). The majority of interdisciplinary studies to date are descriptive and correlational studies, pointing to the

For a description of evidence levels cited in this chapter, see Chapter 1, "Developing and Evaluating Clinical Practice Guidelines: A Systematic Approach."

need for research in the areas of eating ability, cognitive and behavioral function, and tailoring interventions according to the level of dependence (Aselage, Amella, & Watson, 2011; Wen et al., 2014). Randomized controlled clinical trials are predominant in the category of nutritional supplements and training/education (Aselage et al., 2011; Hanson, Ersek, Gilliam, & Carey, 2011; Wen et al., 2014). In spite of all efforts, current evidence demonstrates that specialized feeding interventions may not impact how long a person with dementia lives or improve function (Hanson et al., 2011). The goals of care should be discussed with patients and families from the time dementia is diagnosed, and throughout the disease trajectory. The reality is that dementia is terminal; and the issue of mealtime difficulties will be a major factor at end of life. Early in the disease process, advance-directive discussions should include information related to hand feeding or tube feeding until death. This allows the caregivers who will eventually be responsible for making the decisions at the end of life to be guided by the person with dementia's expressed wishes, and these can be clearly communicated to health care providers and documented (Hickman, Keevern, & Hammes, 2015).

Mealtime difficulties include a wide range of issues. In institutions, restrictive diets are sometimes barely palatable and no longer appropriate in the most advanced stages of dementia (Sekerak & Stewart, 2014). The eating environment ranges from a cluttered hospital room to a large, noisy dining room. Staff treat the meal as a task to complete rather than a process to enjoy. As the demographic projections for rates of dementia increase exponentially, formal and informal caregivers alike will continue to need adequate training and support to effectively battle the epidemic of malnutrition (Alzheimer's Association, 2014). Intervening with supportive nursing care that is evidence based will be integral to reduce costs associated with tube-feeding placement in end-stage dementia. There are financial costs for our health care system, but also costs to the person with dementia related to quality of life, dignity, and discomfort when feeding tubes are used (Finucane, Christmas, & Leff, 2007; Mitchell, Buchanan, Littlehale, & Hamel, 2003). The goals of care should be to promote quality of life until the end of life in this vulnerable population.

BACKGROUND AND STATEMENT OF PROBLEM

There have been several reviews which demonstrate that, even with increased use of feeding tubes in dementia, outcomes, such as aspiration pneumonia and pressure ulcer development, do not improve (Finucane, Christmas, & Travis, 1999; Mitchell, Buchanan, Littlehale, & Hamel, 2004). Hand feeding is the current recommendation (DiBartolo, 2006; Palecek et al., 2010). One feasibility study has been undertaken to prospectively compare hand feeding to tube feeding. It was met with significant challenges at the institutional and individual caregiver levels (Zapka et al., 2014). This study reiterates the emotional difficulties a legally authorized representative faces when presented with the "decision" to tube feed or continue care with hand feeding. The reality with dementia is that it is a terminal diagnosis; the person will die from dementia, not from "starving to death." Unfortunately, this reality is not well understood by the public. Skillful and educated clinicians must be available to provide the necessary emotional support for family caregivers as the disease reaches the end stage. Although there is no cure for dementia, there are care options—and hand feeding until death is the preferred care option (American Geriatrics Society, 2014; Palecek et al., 2010; Sekerak & Stewart, 2014; Sherman, 2003; Zapka et al., 2014). This chapter details the care options nursing has in its repertoire to provide nutritional support to this vulnerable population across the disease trajectory.

Over the past decade, hand feeding has emerged as the recommendation for persons with dementia (American Geriatrics Society, 2014; Chernoff, 2006; DeLegge, 2009; DiBartolo, 2006; Palmer & Metheny, 2008). Hand feeding is a significant part of managing mealtime difficulties in dementia; yet there is no evidence to support how and when to use any particular hand-feeding technique, and very few practicing clinicians realize that there are three different techniques to choose from. There are three practice-driven hand-feeding techniques—direct hand, hand-over-hand, and hand-under-hand feeding, and evidence is emerging that each of them has its place in daily care (Batchelor-Aselage, Bales, Amella, & Rose, 2014; Batchelor-Murphy, 2015; Batchelor-Murphy, Amella, Zapka, Mueller, & Beck, 2015). Although evidence is forthcoming, patient safety is the ultimate priority and using individual judgment when providing any feeding assistance to a person with dementia should be exercised (Aselage, 2012; Batchelor-Murphy, 2014). How and when each technique should be used depends on the response of the individual person with dementia, his or her functional ability, and individual preferences; and these preferences are typically communicated through nonverbal behaviors (Batchelor-Aselage et al., 2014; Batchelor-Murphy et al., 2015). For an event that occurs at least three times daily, how and when to use any hand-feeding technique is usually based on individual knowledge, beliefs, and perceptions (Pelletier, 2004, 2005). In the literature, only one scientific study has been identified reporting use of a specific hand-feeding technique, hand-over-hand feeding. The hand-feeding technique was not the focus of the study, but when used to provide feeding assistance, meal intake improved (Simmons & Schnelle, 2006).

More emphasis is being placed on preparing staff in nursing homes to safely assist with meals; this has not occurred with equal vigor in acute care or in the community setting where older adults may be the most vulnerable and the most support is needed (Aselage et al., 2011). Only two studies have been identified to teach nursing home staff to improve feeding strategies, and both demonstrated increased time spent providing feeding assistance and increased meal intake after training in research studies (Batchelor-Murphy et al., 2015; Chang & Lin, 2005). Even with training the nursing home staff, the feeding behaviors (e.g., clamping mouth shut, turning head away) demonstrated by persons with dementia increased in both the control and intervention groups in both studies—the trained staff responded differently and meal intake increased in the intervention groups (Batchelor-Murphy et al., 2015; Chang & Lin, 2005; Chang, Wykle, & Madigan, 2006).

When originally studied in the mid-1990s, feeding behaviors, such as turning the head away and clamping the mouth shut, were framed in the literature as "aversive" behaviors, and the typical response by caregivers has been to interpret these behaviors as "resistive," and the response was to cease feeding attempts (Pelletier, 2004, 2005; Watson, 1993; Watson & Green, 2006). The goals of research have been to decrease these "aversive" or "resistant" types of feeding behaviors. During the same time frame that the primary clinical measurement instrument was developed for "aversive" feeding behaviors, the Edinburgh Feeding Evaluation in Dementia (EdFED) Scale, the movement toward understanding behaviors in dementia as "unmet" needs was also emerging (Algase et al., 1996; Aselage, 2010; Watson & Deary, 1994). Evidence that these behaviors are more likely a *form of communication*, and the *only form of control* a person with dementia has over a feeding interaction has emerged with tremendous implications for clinical care (Batchelor-Murphy et al., 2015). For example, if a person with dementia clamps his or her mouth shut, he or she may be trying to communicate the need for a sip of his or her drink. Once the drink is offered, the meal can resume, increasing meal intake. Viewing aversive feeding behaviors as communication of an "unmet" need is a clinical practice and research paradigm shift, and creates the opportunity for caregivers and researchers to respond differently to the behaviors to improve nutritional outcomes (Algase et al., 1996; Batchelor-Murphy et al., 2015).

C3P MODEL FOR ASSESSMENT AND CARE STRATEGIES

The C3P Model is a problem-solving strategy that frames how licensed nurses can think through an identified mealtime difficulty: **c**hange the **p**erson, **c**hange the **p**eople, and/or **c**hange the **p**lace (Amella & Batchelor-Aselage, 2014). The assessment and interventions for this chapter are framed around this model. The recommendations for assessment of mealtime difficulties and nutritional assessment will vary depending on the person with dementia's place of residence (community, long-term care, or acute care). Assessment is not a static event, especially when an older adult experiences the downward spiral of a life-limiting cognitive or physical illness. As an individual ages, the likelihood of functional impairment increases. With increased frailty, loss of function follows a predictable pattern, with the ability to feed oneself the last activity of daily living (ADL) to be lost (Katz, Downs, Cash, & Grotz, 1970; Katz, Ford, Moskowitz, Jackson, & Jaffe, 1963).

Quite often, mealtime difficulties are first noticed by caregivers when the person with dementia has lost weight. In the nursing home setting, weight loss is quantified as a "5% loss in one month, or 10% loss in past six months" (Centers for Medicare & Medicaid Services, 2013). These parameters are a good "rule of thumb" for community-dwelling elders also. In early dementia, weight loss may be a sign of forgetting to prepare and eat meals. In moderate to advanced dementia, there may be issues more related to functional ability and/or deficits related to the disease process with apraxia, agnosia, and aphasia. As the disease progresses, if meal intake is affected, the general "rules" for dietary restrictions should be carefully weighed for risk versus benefit. Liberalizing diets may increase intake, especially when the goals of care are comfort, quality of life, and dignity (Sekerak & Stewart, 2014).

Change the Person

Physical Assessment and Daily Care Record Review

A head-to-toe physical assessment by a licensed nurse is vital. Investigation should focus on identifying any reversible, physical cause for weight loss. Potential factors at the individual level include but are not limited to pain, infection, medication interaction, abnormal lab values, food preferences, and/or sociocultural considerations. Along with the physical assessment, review any daily care documents available in the medical record. Looking back over several days (or weeks, if available) for patterns of daily intake through the meal intake record may provide information related to the onset of a reversible problem (e.g., urinary tract infection, constipation, new medication cause decrease in meal intake). Additionally, these patterns may provide insight in to the best time of day to target meal intake. For example, if a person consumes 100% of breakfast, and less over the course of the day, one strategy would be to double the breakfast portions to increase the caloric intake at that time of day. Review of lab values for any abnormalities that may be easily remedied, and/or new or unnecessary medications that could be eliminated are important components of a comprehensive geriatric assessment.

In addition to the physical examination and meal intake records, output records for "regular" bowel movements should be reviewed for regularity or changes in bowel habits. Teaching staff to correctly quantify bowel movement size is also a little known but critical assessment skill. Small bowel movements should be quantified as the size of a closed fist, medium bowel movements quantified as half the length of the forearm, and large bowel movements quantified as the full length of the forearm. The rationale for quantifying in this manner is that the full forearm is the same length as the colon. If a person is only outputting a series of small bowel movements every few days, he or she is not emptying the colon—increasing risk for a major constipation episode or fecal impaction, which will impact any person's appetite.

Change the People

Successful completion of the meal is dependent on who assists or feeds the patient and the interpersonal process that the person uses to interact with the patient (Altus, Engelman, & Mathews, 2002; Amella, 2002). Caregivers who are able to let the patient set the tempo of the meal and allow others to make choices will be more effectual in increasing intake. These studies point to a need for patient-centered approaches that individualize mealtimes for patients and indicate that the responsibility for ensuring this occurs rests with a sensitive and well-trained staff.

Several patient-centered factors have been identified as critical to older adults: Each mealtime was seen as a unique process, and patients are central to the process through their actions not only at meals but also during the time surrounding meals, such as socializing while waiting (Evans, Crogan, & Shultz, 2005; Gibbs-Ward & Keller, 2005). Encouraging the family to eat with the patient can be beneficial; this has been shown to be an effective strategy in nursing homes, increasing body weight and fine motor function in a randomized controlled trial (Altus et al., 2002; Nijs et al., 2006).

Paradigm Shift for Resistive/Aversive Feeding Behaviors

The EdFED instrument was developed around the same time frame that the person-centered care approach was emerging, and the Need-Driven Dementia-Compromised Behavior Model developed to support the notion that "resistive" behaviors were attempts by persons with dementia to communicate an "unmet" need (Algase et al., 1996). When caregivers respond appropriately to these needs, the "resistive" behaviors diminish and care outcomes are achieved more easily (Conti, Voelkl, & McGuire, 2008; Kolanowski, Litaker, Buettner, Moeller, & Costa, 2011; Penrod et al., 2007).

This emerging problem-solving framework is the C3P Model: **c**hange the **p**erson, **c**hange the **p**eople, and/or **c**hange the **p**lace (Amella & Batchelor-Aselage, 2014). This framework is an adaptation of the Social Ecology Model and is used to guide assessment and interventions related to mealtime difficulties. More recent work used the C3P Model, combined with the Need-Driven Dementia-Compromised Behavior Model, and the evidence-based protocol for managing mealtime difficulties. Information was also provided on the practice-based hand-feeding techniques. In this feasibility study, the dementia feeding skills training program taught nursing home staff that these behaviors may be the only form of communication and control a person with dementia has over a meal interaction, and should be responded to as such to increase meal intake (Algase et al., 1996; Amella & Batchelor-Aselage, 2014; Aselage, 2012, 2013; Batchelor-Aselage et al., 2014; Batchelor-Murphy et al., 2015).

Meal Observation of Feeding Behaviors

Assessment of the entire process of eating and mealtimes was divided into the following components: *eating behavior* assessed by the Level of Eating Independence Scale (LEIS) and the Eating Behavior Scale (EBS); *feeding behavior* assessed by the EdFED, Feeding Abilities Assessment (FAA), Self-Feeding Assessment Tool of Osborn and Marshall, the McGill Ingestive Skills Assessment (MISA), Feeding Behavior Inventory, the Feeding Traceline Technique (FTLT), Feeding Dependency Scale (FDS), and the Aversive Feeding Inventory; and *meal behavior* assessed by the Meal Assistance Screening Tool (MAST) and Structured Meal Observation (Aselage, 2010). This critical appraisal of instruments determined that most are primarily used in research, and most are setting specific, with an emphasis on either long-term care or rehabilitation settings—few have been used in the community; these are often lengthy instruments to administer and may not be practical in a clinical setting.

Only the EdFED has been used across acute and long-term care settings and in the community, has strong psychometrics, and appears to be the most practical across domains (Watson & Deary, 1994; Watson, Green, & Legg, 2001). It was designed to evaluate individuals with dementia—clearly not all older persons having difficulties with meals, but in all likelihood a significant portion. The EdFED focuses on six feeding behaviors that are often interpreted as "resistance" by formal and informal caregivers (e.g., clamping mouth shut, turning head away, refusing to open mouth, letting food fall from mouth, spillage, and spitting food; Watson, 1993, 1994a, 1994b).

Change the Place

Because of the strong social and cultural components of eating, where one dines is sometimes as important as what one eats. Nurses should simply ask themselves, "Would I want to eat my next meal where this person is eating?" If the answer is no, then steps should be taken to improve the dining environment. Small changes in the dining environment may make large improvements in a patient's capacity and motivation to eat or be fed. It is unfortunate that, in institutions, the mealtime experience is often not focused on individual needs (Sydner & Fjellström, 2005). External factors, such as decreased noise, increased lighting, and playing relaxing music, at meals positively influenced appetite (Hicks-Moore, 2005; McDaniel, Hunt, Hackes, & Pope, 2001). Using contrasting colors (foreground/background) in tableware and tablecloth, and always placing dishes in similar positions may help persons with low vision be more independent (Ellexson, 2004). Proper positioning using the appropriate, supportive chair (instead of eating in bed or sitting on the bedside) promotes good eating posture (Rappl & Jones, 2000). Meals eaten in small groups—much like family dining—are considered an ideal method; however, this intervention had more effect on staff's perception of meals and willingness to spend time in the process of attending to meals (Kofod & Birkemose, 2004).

Hand-Feeding Assistance

For a video demonstration depicting the three feeding techniques, please visit the website: youtube/NYzH_B7XfjY; or go to YouTube and search "Hand Feeding Techniques in Dementia." Photographs of the differences are also available (Batchelor-Aselage et al., 2014).

Fine motor ability declines with aging, and one area that specifically relates to the ability to feed oneself is grip strength and the ability to coordinate motor movements. Although motor decline is a normal part of aging, older adults with dementia do experience more severe decline when compared to an unaffected age group (Rogers & Jarrott, 2008; Scherder, Dekker, & Eggermont, 2008). As cognitive impairment progresses, older adults lose fine motor ability before they lose gross motor ability (Bottiggi & Harrison, 2008). Assessing gross and fine motor functional ability is a critical need when making decisions about how much assistance to provide to a person with dementia and which hand-feeding technique may be more appropriate. Formal and informal caregivers should promote self-feeding as much as possible, for as long as possible, and only offer the least amount of support necessary to maximize meal intake.

The hand-feeding techniques are labeled according to where the caregiver (feeding assistant) places his or her hand in relation to the person he or she is assisting. When first learning about these techniques, it is helpful to do a "role play" with a partner. Each person can alternate being in the role of the feeding assistant and the person with dementia. Kinesthetically experiencing each technique oneself provides insight for the feeding assistant as to how the person with dementia may perceive that feeding assistance—these hand-feeding techniques feel differently in the areas of feeling as though you have control over the movement and/or if someone is forcing your hand toward your face. The hand-feeding techniques may be used interchangeably during a mealtime. Decisions on which technique to use should consider the upper extremity range of motion the person with dementia has, whether or not the person has contractures of the hands, and/or which technique appears to be the most comfortable to the person with dementia. Every person with dementia is an individual, and clinical judgment should be exercised to promote safety, comfort, dignity, and quality of life during every meal interaction.

For the hand-over-hand and hand-under-hand techniques, the feeding assistant should first assess which hand is the dominant hand of the person with dementia. The feeding assistant should sit on the person with dementia's dominant side, and use the same hand to provide assistance (e.g., if the person with dementia is right-handed, the feeding assistant should sit on the right side and use his or her right hand to provide assistance). These two techniques are more challenging if attempting to provide feeding assistance while the person with dementia is in bed. It is recommended that the person with dementia be in a chair during mealtimes as often as possible.

Hand-Over-Hand Feeding

For the hand-over-hand feeding technique, the feeding assistant places his or her hand over the hand of the person being assisted with the meals. The person with dementia must still possess the fine motor ability to hold the utensil, and have the upper extremity range of motion and strength to move the utensil with food from the plate to the mouth. This technique may also be used to stabilize any hand tremor that results in spillage of food off the utensil. The feeding assistant may need to keep his or her hand over the person with dementia's hand all the way through the feeding cycle, or just long enough to initiate the movement of the utensil to the mouth. If the person with dementia pushes away the feeding assistance, this behavior may be because he or she is capable of performing the movement on his or her own and/or he or she feels as though you are forcing the movement.

Hand-Under-Hand Feeding

In the hand-under-hand feeding technique, the caregiver (feeding assistant) holds the utensil, and places his or her hand under the hand of the person with dementia (Batchelor-Aselage, Bales, Amella, & Rose, 2014; Snow, 2015). This technique is most likely to be effective if the person with dementia is losing the fine motor ability of being able to hold the utensil on his or her own. From the perspective of the person with dementia, this will likely feel as though he or she has control over the movement and that he or she initiated the movement. In addition to the verbal and visual cues that should be provided, the hand-under-hand technique may serve as a motor cue. This motor cue may allow a person who has lost language ability to understand that the feeding assistant is "really" that person feeding himself or herself. The person with dementia may actively engage in this technique by pulling the feeding assistant's hand and/or the feeding assistant's forearm.

Direct Hand Feeding

This technique should be reserved for a person who has progressed in the disease process of dementia to the point that he or she is totally dependent on care. Rather than being the first line of assistance, direct hand feeding makes the experience of eating a completely passive event for the person with dementia. The feeding assistant using this technique does all of the work, with no active engagement of the person he or she is assisting.

Role of Nutritional Supplements

Nutritional supplements include high-calorie supplements and appetite stimulants (Hanson et al., 2011). Although there is evidence that nutritional supplements improve body weight by 1 to 4 pounds in persons with dementia, there is less evidence that these supplements reduce risk of infections or promote wound healing (Hanson et al., 2011). In addition, these supplements have not demonstrated improvement in function or improved life expectancy (Hanson et al., 2011). Nutritional supplements are expensive, and between 55% and 65% of the time are not actually consumed by the person with dementia (Allen, Methven, & Gosney, 2014; Kayser-Jones et al., 1998). A recent randomized controlled clinical trial indicated that when offered the supplement in a glass or beaker rather than inserting a straw into a container, persons with dementia did increase the amount of the supplements consumed (Allen et al., 2014). Even with this delivery modification, supplement consumption averaged 65%. Nutritional supplements given midmorning have also been associated with decreasing lunch intake (Young, Greenwood, van Reekum, & Binns, 2004).

The interdisciplinary team may have neglected to perform a thorough assessment of underlying issues prior to using nutritional supplements. Potentially reversible conditions, such as adequate staffing and lack of supervision, poor oral health, or identifying other factors requiring intervention such as dysphagia, should be investigated (Kayser-Jones et al., 1998). This in-depth assessment into the etiology of a mealtime difficulty should occur, and results documented prior to using a nutritional supplement. Real food should be offered first, with deliberate attention paid to providing adequate support in order to achieve meal intake, based on individual preferences and functional ability, as outlined in this chapter.

CASE STUDY

Mr. Robertson is an 80-year-old male who has been admitted to the acute care medical unit after experiencing general debilitation subsequent to an influenza diagnosis. Previously functioning independently at home with a private caregiver, he has a diagnosis of Alzheimer's dementia. He has been taking Aricept for the previous year. Mr. Robertson was found in his home disoriented, dehydrated, and incontinent 3 days ago. Throughout hospitalization, he has exhibited behaviors consistent with decompensation of cognitive and functional status. His son, who lives locally, has become concerned with his deterioration in functioning, and has decided it will be best if he is transferred to a long-term care facility for rehabilitation prior to returning home.

Since arriving to the skilled nursing facility, Mr. Robertson has been monitored closely, and has required total care. On one particular midmorning round, the certified nursing assistant (CNA) enters Mr. Robertson's room by first calling his name (auditory cue), and entering his visual field (visual cue) before finally coming to

(continued)

CASE STUDY *(continued)*

touch his shoulder (tactile cue). This sequence of cueing prompts the most positive response from Mr. Robertson. The CNA is directly hand feeding Mr. Robertson, and during his mealtimes, he will occasionally clamp his mouth shut and turn his head away when offered food. After several failed attempts to encourage eating, she consults the nurse about his "refusal" to eat.

The nurse uses the C3P Model and begins with *change the person:* She conducts a head-to-toe physical examination, medication reconciliation, meal intake review, and bowel review. The physical assessment is negative; no new medications have been added and all have a supporting diagnosis; his meal intake has been steady around 50% to 75% for all three meals; and he has been having regular, large bowel movements. In addition to this assessment information, the nurse also consults the interdisciplinary team to decide what options would be available for improving Mr. Robertson's issue. To assess his swallowing abilities, a speech and language pathologist conducts a videofluoroscopic swallowing study. The study revealed a slight deterioration in physiological swallowing function, and recommends changing to a mechanically altered diet. The occupational therapist recommends using adaptive equipment to help him independently hold his utensils because of his limited dexterity and loss of fine motor control. The dietary manager reviews food preferences with Mr. Robertson's son, and adjustments are made to foods served to him. *Change the people:* Next, the nurse uses the EdFED Scale and observes several mealtimes over the course of the day. The nurse also observes the behaviors of clamping his mouth shut and turning his head away when offered some food items. When some staff members offer him a sip of water when this behavior occurs, the meal resumes; when other staff interpret these behaviors as "refusing," the meal assistance ceases. *Change the place:* During the meal observations, the nurse notes that several staff members enter and exit the room frequently. When a staff member catches Mr. Robertson's attention, it takes additional time to get him refocused on his meal. The tables are set with contrasting placemats, and the noise level is kept to a minimum.

With the *change the person* interventions recommended by the therapy departments in place (modified food texture, adaptive equipment, food preferences), the nurse and CNA work collaboratively to provide meal assistance. *Change the people:* After initial attempts to verbally encourage independent feeding are not successful, the nurse and CNA begin a trial of the three hand-feeding techniques to determine which would be most appropriate for Mr. Robertson, given his current ability. The CNA provides Mr. Robertson with his adaptive utensil, which he is able to hold. Using the hand-over-hand technique, she begins to guide the utensil toward his face. While using this technique, Mr. Robertson begins to push the assistance away, but he is unable to complete the feeding cycle and eat his food. In the second attempt to provide assistance, the CNA holds his utensil and uses the hand-under-hand feeding technique. Mr. Robertson does not push this type of assistance away and consumes his food. After a few cycles of hand under hand, Mr. Robertson again clamps his mouth shut and turns his head away. The nurse encourages the CNA to offer a sip of water at this point. Mr. Robertson takes several sips of water. The CNA then resumes using the hand-under-hand feeding technique, responds to his feeding behaviors by offering fluids, and Mr. Robertson consumes 100% of his meal and fluids. *Change the place:* A brief in-service is held with staff to praise the use of contrasting placemats in the dining room and minimizing the noise. Staff are encouraged to try to limit the traffic in and out of the dining room, as it is a distraction for the residents with dementia.

The approaches from the C3P Model assessment are added to his care plan. Over the next several weeks, Mr. Robertson improves his meal intake to 75% to 100% consistently and the staff are able to transition from hand-under-hand assistance to hand-over-hand assistance. As his nutritional status improves, he makes gains with his rehabilitation therapy, and regains the ability to feed himself independently. His functional and cognitive status return to baseline prior to the hospitalization for influenza. The social worker collaborates with the son and prior community support is available. Mr. Robertson's son agrees and Mr. Robertson is able to be discharged to his home with his private caregiver.

SUMMARY

Solving a mealtime problem for a person with dementia is very challenging. Formal and informal caregivers must be prepared to conduct a thorough investigation into potentially reversible causes of weight loss, and to provide an adequate amount of support as dependence increases over time. Examining whether a problem exists for the person with dementia, the approach used by his or her caregivers, or an environmental etiology allows for a comprehensive assessment that will provide insight into the most effective care strategies. Hand feeding is the recommended course of care, until death, in this devastating illness.

NURSING STANDARD OF PRACTICE

Protocol 25.1: Assessment and Management of Mealtime Difficulties in Dementia

I. GOAL

To maintain or improve nutritional intake during mealtimes and provide a quality mealtime experience that fosters dignity and maximum independence in eating, while respecting personal preferences and cultural/social aspects, for as long as possible

II. OVERVIEW

A. Guiding principles
   1. Adequate intake of nutrients is necessary to maintain physical and emotional health.
   2. Mealtimes are critical to socialization as well as maximizing nutritional intake; therefore, mealtime rituals, cultural norms, and food preferences will be observed to the extent possible.
   3. Persons will be encouraged to self-feed as long as possible, and support provided with hand feeding/hand-feeding technique(s), as necessary.
   4. As persons require more assistance with eating, dignity will be maintained.
   5. The quality of mealtime interactions is an indicator of quality of life and quality of care provided to individuals.

III. BACKGROUND

A. Basic definitions
   1. *Feeding* is "the process of getting the food from the plate to the mouth. It is a primitive sense without concern for social niceties" (Katz et al., 1970, p. 23).
   2. *Eating* is "the ability to transfer food from plate to stomach through the mouth" (Katz et al., 1970, p. 23). Eating involves the ability to recognize food, the ability to transfer food to the mouth, and the phases of swallowing.
   3. *Dysphagia* is "an abnormality in the transfer of a bolus from the mouth to the stomach" (Groher, 1997, p. 2).

B. Impact of dementia on independent meal management
   4. *Apraxia* is an inability to carry out voluntary muscular activities related to neuromuscular damage. As it relates to eating and feeding, it involves loss of the voluntary stages of swallowing or the manipulation of eating utensils.
   5. *Agnosia* is the inability to recognize familiar items when sensory cueing is limited. As it relates to feeding, a utensil (e.g., spoon or fork) is not recognized as an object for moving food from the plate to the mouth.
   6. *Aphasia* is the inability to communicate effectively, this may be receptive or expressive. As it relates to feeding, spoken language may not be spoken or understood.

C. Hand-feeding techniques
   1. *Direct hand feeding* is when the caregiver holds the fork or spoon, and moves food from plate to mouth; the person being assisted is passive in the interaction (Batchelor-Aselage et al., 2014).
   2. *Hand-over-hand feeding* is when the person with dementia still possesses the fine motor skill needed to hold the utensil. The caregiver puts his or her hand over the hand of the person with dementia and guides it toward the mouth. The person being assisted is active in the process, but may misinterpret the assistant as controlling and push assistance away (Batchelor-Aselage et al., 2014).
   3. *Hand-under-hand feeding* is when the caregiver holds the fork or spoon, and places his or her hand under the hand of the person with dementia. From the perspective of the person with dementia, this type of assistance may convey a feeling of control over the movement and provides fine motor assistance when it no longer exists (Batchelor-Aselage et al., 2014; Snow, 2015).

For a video demonstration depicting the three techniques, please visit the website youtu.be/NYzH_B7XfjY or go to YouTube and search "Hand Feeding Techniques in Dementia." Photographs of the differences are also available (Batchelor-Aselage et al., 2014).

(continued)

Protocol 25.1: Assessment and Management of Mealtime Difficulties in Dementia *(continued)*

D. Etiology
Mealtime difficulties can have multiple causes of both physiological and psychological origins. Health professionals need to consider multiple etiologies and not assume that difficulties are related only to increased confusion from a cognitive decline.
1. Cognitive/neurological: Parkinson's disease; amyotrophic lateral sclerosis; dementia, especially Alzheimer's disease; stroke
2. Psychological: depression
3. Iatrogenic: lack of adaptive equipment; use of physical restraints that limit the ability to move, position, or self-feed; improper chair or table surface or discrepancy of chair to table height; use of wheelchair in lieu of table and chair; and use of disposable dinnerware, especially for patients with cognitive or neuromuscular impairments

IV. PARAMETERS OF ASSESSMENT

A. Meal observation
1. EdFED Scale: observe a few mealtimes at different times of the day using the EdFED Scale to examine the present feeding behaviors and possible meaning of behavior (Watson, 1996):
   a. Turning head away, clamping mouth shut: Are these behaviors indicating a dislike of food offered, or desire for fluids at that moment? When choice honored, does meal intake continue?
   b. Refusing to open mouth/not swallowing/allowing food to drop out of mouth: Does speech therapy need to evaluate swallowing problem? Dental consult?
   c. Spillage of food: Does person need stabilization of utensils with hand-feeding technique?

B. Care record review
1. Meal intake record for patterns of intake, or reduction in meal intake; clinical investigation should occur to determine underlying cause, as these patterns may indicate:
   a. Acute illness/infection onset (e.g., meal intake decreased few days prior)
   b. Daily patterns of meal intake (e.g., breakfast always 100%, dinner 25%)
2. Review of bowel movement records; auscultate for bowel sounds: look for patterns of 3 days without equivalent of a large bowel movement
   a. Chronic constipation will affect appetite.

V. NURSING INTERVENTIONS

A. **C**hange the **p**erson
1. Allow time for rituals before meals (e.g., handwashing and toilet use); dressing for dinner; saying blessing of food or grace, if appropriate.
2. Observe religious rites or prohibitions observed in preparation of food or before meal begins (e.g., Muslim, Jewish, Seventh-Day Adventist; consult pastoral counselor or family as needed).
3. Acknowledge cultural or special cues: family history, special holiday occasions, especially rituals surrounding meals.
4. Follow preferences about end-of-life decisions regarding withdrawal or administration of food/fluids in the face of incapacity; request of designated health care proxy; ethicist or social worker may facilitate process.
5. Develop interdisciplinary care plan for any chronic, treatable conditions, such as constipation, depression, anxiety, that may impact meal intake.

B. **C**hange the **p**eople
1. Provide an adequate number of well-trained staff.
2. Deliver an individualized approach to meals, including choice of food, tempo of assistance.
3. If meal patterns indicate one meal eaten better than an other (100% breakfast intake, 25% dinner), provide double meal portions for the associated meal.
4. Position of caregiver relative to older adult: caregiver seated beside older adult, on the older adult's dominant side; eye contact; older adult able to see facial expressions and feeding behaviors emulated by the caregiver with visual cueing.
5. Cueing: Caregiver provides verbal and visual cues whenever possible with short statements of simple commands to direct meal behavior (e.g., here is your corn, open your mouth, swallow the food).

(continued)

Protocol 25.1: Assessment and Management of Mealtime Difficulties in Dementia *(continued)*

6. Self-feeding: Encourage to self-feed with multiple methods based on functional ability; allow time for person to complete task, rather than provide assistance to minimize time.
7. Mealtime rounds: Interdisciplinary team to examine multifaceted process of meal service, environment, and individual food preferences.

C. **C**hange the **p**lace
1. Dining or patient room: Encourage the older adult to eat in the dining room to increase food intake, personalize the dining room; no treatments or other activities to occur during the mealtime; no distractions.
2. Tableware: Use standard dinnerware (e.g., glasses, cups, saucer, flatware) versus disposable tableware and bibs.
3. Contrasting background/foreground: Use contrasting background and foreground colors with minimal design to aid person with decreased vision.
4. Furniture: Seat older adult in stable armchair rather than in a wheelchair or in bed; place table at appropriate height.
5. Noise level: Environmental noise from music, caregivers, and television is minimal; personal conversation between person and caregiver is encouraged.
6. Music: pleasant, preferred by patient
7. Light: adequate and nonglaring versus dark, shadowy, or glaring
8. Odor: Prepare food in area adjacent to or in dining area to stimulate appetite.
9. Adaptive equipment: available, appropriate, and clean; caregivers and/or older adult knowledgeable in use; occupational therapist assists in evaluation

VI. EVALUATION/EXPECTED OUTCOMES

A. Change the person
1. Corrective and supportive strategies reflected in plan of care
2. Quality-of-life issues emphasized in maintaining social aspects of dining
3. Culture, personal preferences, and end-of-life decisions regarding nutrition respected

B. Change the people
1. System disruptions at mealtimes minimized
2. Family and staff informed and educated to patient's special needs to promote safe and effective meals
3. Maintenance of normal meals and adequate intake for the patient reflected in care plan
4. Competence in diet assessment; knowledge of and sensitivity to cultural norms and preferences for mealtimes reflected in care plan

C. Change the place
1. Documentation of nutritional status and eating and feeding behavior meets expected standard
2. Alterations in nutritional status; eating and feeding behaviors assessed and addressed in a timely manner
3. Involvement of interdisciplinary team (geriatrician, advanced practice nurse, dietitian, speech therapist, dentist, occupational therapist, social worker, pastoral counselor, ethicist) is appropriate and timely
4. Nutritional, eating, and/or feeding problems modified to respect individual preferences and cultural norms
5. Adequate number of well-trained staff who are committed to delivering knowledgeable and individualized care

VII. FOLLOW-UP MONITORING

A. Providers' competency to monitor eating and feeding behaviors
B. Documentation of eating and feeding behaviors
C. Documentation of care strategies and follow-up of alterations in nutritional status and eating and feeding behaviors
D. Documentation of staffing and staff education; availability of supportive interdisciplinary team

ABBREVIATION

EdFED Edinburgh Feeding Evaluation in Dementia

ACKNOWLEDGMENTS

The first author would like to acknowledge the generous support of the National Center for Gerontological Nursing Excellence (NHCGNE) Claire M. Fagin Fellowship program; the Robert Wood Johnson Nurse Faculty Scholars Program; the National Institute of Nursing Research (NIH P30NR014139); and R.A. Anderson and S. Docherty, principal investigators, Duke University School of Nursing, in completion of this chapter.

REFERENCES

Algase, D. L., Beck, C., Kolanowski, A., Whall, A., Berent, S., Richards, K., & Beattie, E. (1996). Need-driven dementia-compromised behavior: An alternative view of disruptive behavior. *American Journal of Alzheimer's Disease, 11*(6), 10–19. *Evidence Level V.*

Allen, V. J., Methven, L., & Gosney, M. (2014). Impact of serving method on the consumption of nutritional supplement drinks: Randomized trial in older adults with cognitive impairment. *Journal of Advanced Nursing, 70*(6), 1323–1333. doi:10.1111/jan.12293. *Evidence Level II.*

Altus, D. E., Engelman, K. K., & Mathews, R. M. (2002). Using family-style meals to increase participation and communication in persons with dementia. *Journal of Gerontological Nursing, 28*(9), 47–53. *Evidence Level III.*

Alzheimer's Association. (2014). 2014 Alzheimer's disease facts and figures. *Alzheimer's & Dementia, 10*(2). *Evidence Level V.*

Amella, E. J. (2002). Resistance at mealtimes for persons with dementia. *Journal of Nutrition, Health & Aging, 6*(2), 117–122. *Evidence Level IV.*

Amella, E. J., & Batchelor-Aselage, M. B. (2014). Facilitating ADLs by caregivers of persons with dementia: The C3P model. *Occupational Therapy in Health Care, 28*(1), 51–61. doi:10.3109/07380577.2013.867388. *Evidence Level V.*

American Geriatrics Society. (2014). Feeding tubes in advanced dementia position statement. *Journal of the American Geriatrics Society, 62*(8), 1590–1593. doi:10.1111/jgs.12924. *Evidence Level VI.*

Aselage, M. (2010). Measuring mealtime difficulties: Eating, feeding and meal behaviours in older adults with dementia. *Journal of Clinical Nursing, 19*(5–6), 621–631. doi:10.1111/j.1365-2702.2009.03129.x. *Evidence Level V.*

Aselage, M. (2012). *Comparison of careful hand feeding techniques for persons with dementia in the nursing home.* Duke University School of Nursing: National Centers for Gerontological Nursing Excellence, Claire M. Fagin Fellowship. *Evidence Level II.*

Aselage, M. (2013). Eating and feeding behaviors: Problems in dementia. In E. Capezuti (Ed.), *Encyclopedia of elder care* (3rd ed., pp. 247–249). New York, NY: Springer Publishing Company. *Evidence Level VI.*

Aselage, M., Amella, E. J., & Watson, R. (2011). State of the science: Alleviating mealtime difficulties in nursing home residents with dementia. *Nursing Outlook, 59*(4), 210–214. doi:10.1016/j.outlook.2011.05.009. *Evidence Level VI.*

Batchelor-Aselage, M., Bales, C., Amella, E., & Rose, S. (2014). Dementia-related mealtime difficulties: Assessment and management in the long-term-care setting. In C. Bales, J. Locher, & E. Salzman (Eds.), *Handbook of clinical nutrition and aging* (3rd ed., pp. 287–301). New York, NY: Springer Publishing Company. *Evidence Level V.*

Batchelor-Murphy, M. (2014). *Adaptive approaches for effectively managing mealtimes in dementia.* Duke University School of Nursing, Robert Wood Johnson Foundation Nurse Faculty Scholars Program. *Evidence Level IV.*

Batchelor-Murphy, M. (Producer). (2015, March). *Hand feeding techniques for assisting persons with dementia.* [Video] Retrieved from https://youtu.be/NYzH_B7XfjY. *Evidence Level VI.*

Batchelor-Murphy, M., Amella, E. J., Zapka, J., Mueller, M., & Beck, C. (2015). Feasibility of a web-based dementia feeding skills training program for nursing home staff. *Geriatric Nursing, 36*(3), 212–218. *Evidence Level III.*

Bottiggi, K., & Harrison, A. L. (2008). The association between change in motor function and cognition in older adults: A descriptive review. *Physical Therapy Reviews, 13*(2), 91–101. *Evidence Level V.*

Centers for Medicare & Medicaid Services. (2010). *Minimum Data Set (MDS) Version 3.0: Resident assessment and care screening, nursing home comprehensive (NC) item set.* Retrieved from http://www.ltcombudsman.org/sites/default/files/ombudsmen-support/training/MDS-3.0-Item-set.pdf. *Evidence Level V.*

Centers for Medicare & Medicaid Services. (2013). *Section K: Swallowing/Nutritional StatusCMS's RAI Version 3.0 Manual (Vol. 2015, pp. K–4).* Retrieved from http://www.aanac.org/docs/mds-3.0-rai-users-manual/11126_mds_3-0_chapter_3_-_section_k_v1-12.pdf?sfvrsn=6. *Evidence Level V.*

Centers for Medicare & Medicaid Services. (2015). *Nursing home compare.* Retrieved from http://www.medicare.gov/NHCompare. *Evidence Level V.*

Chang, C. C., & Lin, L. C. (2005). Effects of a feeding skills training programme on nursing assistants and dementia patients. *Journal of Clinical Nursing, 14*(10), 1185–1192. doi:10.1111/j.1365–2702.2005.01240.x. *Evidence Level IV.*

Chang, C. C., Wykle, M. L., & Madigan, E. A. (2006). The effect of a feeding skills training program for nursing assistants who feed dementia patients in Taiwanese nursing homes. *Geriatric Nursing 27*(4), 229–237. *Evidence Level IV.*

Chernoff, R. (2006). Tube feeding patients with dementia. *Nutrition in Clinical Practice: Official Publication of the American Society for Parenteral and Enteral Nutrition, 21*(2), 142–146. *Evidence Level V.*

Conti, A., Voelkl, J. E., & McGuire, F. A. (2008). Efficacy of meaningful activities in recreation therapy on passive behaviors of older adults with dementia. *Annual in Therapeutic Recreation, 16,* 91–104. *Evidence Level IV.*

DeLegge, M. H. (2009). Tube feeding in patients with dementia: Where are we? *Nutrition in Clinical Practice: Official Publication of the American Society for Parenteral and Enteral Nutrition, 24*(2), 214–216. doi:10.1177/0884533609332006. *Evidence Level V.*

DiBartolo, M. C. (2006). Careful hand feeding: A reasonable alternative to PEG tube placement in individuals with dementia. *Journal of Gerontological Nursing, 32*(5), 25–33; quiz 34. *Evidence Level V.*

Ellexson, M. T. (2004). Access to participation: Occupational therapy and low vision. *Topics in Geriatric Rehabilitation, 20*(3), 154–172. *Evidence Level IV.*

Evans, B. C., Crogan, N. L., & Shultz, J. A. (2005). The meaning of mealtimes: Connection to the social world of the nursing home. *Journal of Gerontological Nursing, 31*(2), 11–17. *Evidence Level IV.*

Finucane, T. E., Christmas, C., & Leff, B. A. (2007). Tube feeding in dementia: How incentives undermine health care quality and patient safety. *Journal of the American Medical Directors Association, 8*(4), 205–208. *Evidence Level IV.*

Finucane, T. E., Christmas, C., & Travis, K. (1999). Tube feeding in patients with advanced dementia: A review of the evidence. *Journal of the American Medical Association, 282*(14), 1365–1370. *Evidence Level V.*

Gerontological Society of America. (2014, December 18). Malnutrition: A hidden epidemic among elders. *Science Daily.* Retrieved from www.sciencedaily.com/releases/2014/12/141218120846.htm. *Evidence Level V.*

Gibbs-Ward, A. J., & Keller, H. H. (2005). Mealtimes as active processes in long-term care facilities. *Canadian Journal of Dietetic Practice and Research: A Publication of Dietitians of Canada = Revue Canadienne de La Pratique Et de La Recherche En Diététique: Une Publication Des Diététistes Du Canada, 66*(1), 5–11. *Evidence Level IV.*

Groher, M. (1997). *Dysphagia: Diagnosis and management.* Boston, MA: Butterworth-Heinemann. *Evidence Level V.*

Hanson, L. C., Ersek, M., Gilliam, R., & Carey, T. S. (2011). Oral feeding options for people with dementia: A systematic review. *Journal of the American Geriatrics Society, 59*(3), 463–472. doi:10.1111/j.1532-5415.2011.03320.x. *Evidence Level I.*

Hickman, S. E., Keevern, E., & Hammes, B. J. (2015). Use of the physician orders for life-sustaining treatment program in the clinical setting: A systematic review of the literature. *Journal of the American Geriatrics Society, 63*(2), 341–350. doi:10.1111/jgs.13248. *Evidence Level I.*

Hicks-Moore, S. L. (2005). Relaxing music at mealtime in nursing homes: Effect on agitated patients with dementia. *Journal of Gerontological Nursing, 31*(12), 26–32. *Evidence Level III.*

Katz, S., Downs, T., Cash, H., & Grotz, R. (1970). Progress in the development of the index of ADL. *The Gerontologist, 10*(1), 20–30. *Evidence Level IV.*

Katz, S., Ford, A., Moskowitz, R., Jackson, B., & Jaffe, M. (1963). Studies of illness in the aged. The index of ADL: A standardized measure of biological and psychological function. *Journal of the American Medical Association, 185,* 914–919. *Evidence Level IV.*

Kayser-Jones, J., Schell, E. S., Porter, C., Barbaccia, J. C., Steinbach, C., Bird, W. F., . . . Pengilly, K. (1998). A prospective study of the use of liquid oral dietary supplements in nursing homes. *Journal of the American Geriatrics Society, 46*(11), 1378–1386. *Evidence Level IV.*

Kofod, J., & Birkemose, A. (2004). Meals in nursing homes. *Scandinavian Journal of Caring Sciences, 18*(2), 128–134. *Evidence Level IV.*

Kolanowski, A., Litaker, M., Buettner, L., Moeller, J., & Costa, J. P. T. (2011). A randomized clinical trial of theory-based activities for the behavioral symptoms of dementia in nursing home residents. *Journal of the American Geriatrics Society, 59*(6), 1032–1041. doi:10.1111/j.1532-5415.2011.03449.x. *Evidence Level II.*

McDaniel, J. H., Hunt, A., Hackes, B., & Pope, J. F. (2001). Impact of dining room environment on nutritional intake of Alzheimer's residents: A case study. *American Journal of Alzheimer's Disease & Other Dementias, 16*(5), 297–302. *Evidence Level III.*

Mitchell, S. L., Buchanan, J. L., Littlehale, S., & Hamel, M. B. (2003). Tube-feeding versus hand-feeding nursing home residents with advanced dementia: A cost comparison. *Journal of the American Medical Directors Association, 4*(1), 27–33. *Evidence Level IV.*

Mitchell, S. L., Buchanan, J. L., Littlehale, S., & Hamel, M. B. (2004). Tube-feeding versus hand-feeding nursing home residents with advanced dementia: A cost comparison. *Journal of the American Medical Directors Association, 5*(Suppl. 2), S22–S29. doi:10.1097/01.jam.0000043421.46230.0e. *Evidence Level IV.*

Nightingale, F. (1859a). Taking food. *Notes on Nursing* (pp. 45–50). New York, NY: Barnes & Noble. *Evidence Level VI.*

Nightingale, F. (1859b). What food? *Notes on Nursing* (pp. 51–58). New York, NY: Barnes & Noble. *Evidence Level VI.*

Nijs, K. A., de Graaf, C., Sebelink, E., Blauw, Y. H., Vanneste, V., Kok, F. J., & van Staveren, W. A. (2006). Effect of family-style meals on energy intake and risk of malnutrition in Dutch nursing home residents: A randomized controlled trial. *Journals of Gerontology. Series A, Biological Sciences & Medical Sciences, 61A*(9), 935–942. *Evidence Level II.*

Palecek, E. J., Teno, J. M., Casarett, D. J., Hanson, L. C., Rhodes, R. L., & Mitchell, S. L. (2010). Comfort feeding only: A proposal to bring clarity to decision-making regarding difficulty with eating for persons with advanced dementia. *Journal of the American Geriatrics Society, 58*(3), 580–584. doi:10.1111/j.1532-5415.2010.02740.x. *Evidence Level VI.*

Palmer, J. L., & Metheny, N. A. (2008). Preventing aspiration in older adults with dysphagia: Aspiration can lead to aspiration pneumonia, a serious health problem for older adults. *American Journal of Nursing, 108*(2), 40. *Evidence Level V.*

Pelletier, C. A. (2004). What do certified nurse assistants actually know about dysphagia and feeding nursing home residents? *American Journal of Speech-Language Pathology, 13*(2), 99–113. *Evidence Level IV.*

Pelletier, C. A. (2005). Innovations in long-term care. Feeding beliefs of certified nurse assistants in the nursing home: A factor influencing practice. *Journal of Gerontological Nursing, 31*(7), 5–10. *Evidence Level IV.*

Penrod, J., Yu, F., Kolanowski, A., Fick, D. M., Loeb, S. J., & Hupcey, J. E. (2007). Reframing person-centered nursing care for persons with dementia. *Research & Theory for Nursing Practice, 21*(1), 57–72. *Evidence Level V.*

Rappl, L., & Jones, D. A. (2000). Seating evaluation: Special problems and interventions for older adults. *Topics in Geriatric Rehabilitation, 16*(2), 63–72. *Evidence Level V.*

Rogers, S. D., & Jarrott, S. E. (2008). Cognitive impairment and effects on upper body strength of adults with dementia. *Journal of Aging & Physical Activity, 16*(1), 61–68. *Evidence Level IV.*

Scherder, E., Dekker, W., & Eggermont, L. (2008). Higher-level hand motor function in aging and (preclinical) dementia: Its relationship with (instrumental) activities of daily life—A mini-review. *Gerontology, 54*(6), 333–341. *Evidence Level V.*

Sekerak, R. J., & Stewart, J. T. (2014). Caring for the patient with end-stage dementia. *Annals of Long Term Care, 22*(12), 36–43. *Evidence Level V.*

Sherman, F. T. (2003). Nutrition in advanced dementia. Tube-feeding or hand-feeding until death? *Geriatrics, 58*(11), 10, 12. *Evidence Level VI.*

Simmons, S. F., & Schnelle, J. F. (2004). Individualized feeding assistance care for nursing home residents: Staffing requirements to implement two interventions. *Journals of Gerontology. Series A, Biological Sciences & Medical Sciences, 59A*(9), 966–973. *Evidence Level III.*

Simmons, S. F., & Schnelle, J. (2006). Feeding assistant needs of long-stay nursing home residents and staff time to provide care. *Journal of the American Geriatrics Society, 54*, 919–924. *Evidence Level IV.*

Snow, T. (2015). *Positive approach to brain change*. Retrieved from http://teepasnow.com. *Evidence Level VI.*

Sydner, Y. M., & Fjellström, C. (2005). Food provision and the meal situation in elderly care—Outcomes in different social contexts. *Journal of Human Nutrition & Dietetics, 18*(1), 45–52. *Evidence Level IV.*

Watson, R. (1993). Measuring feeding difficulty in patients with dementia: Perspectives and problems. *Journal of Advanced Nursing, 18*(1), 25–31. doi:10.1046/j.1365-2648.1993.18010025.x. *Evidence Level V.*

Watson, R. (1994a). Measuring feeding difficulty in patients with dementia: Developing a scale. *Journal of Advanced Nursing, 19*(2), 257–263. doi:10.1111/j.1365-2648.1994.tb01079.x. *Evidence Level IV.*

Watson, R. (1994b). Measuring feeding difficulty in patients with dementia: Replication and validation of the EdFED Scale #1. *Journal of Advanced Nursing, 19*(5), 850–855. doi:10.1111/j.1365-2648.1994.tb01160.x. *Evidence Level III.*

Watson, R. (1996). The Mokken scaling procedure (MSP) applied to the measurement of feeding difficulty in elderly people with dementia. *International Journal of Nursing Studies, 33*(4), 385–393. *Evidence Level III.*

Watson, R., & Deary, I. J. (1994). Measuring feeding difficulty in patients with dementia: Multivariate analysis of feeding problems, nursing intervention and indicators of feeding difficulty. *Journal of Advanced Nursing, 20*(2), 283–287. doi:10.1046/j.1365-2648.1994.20020283.x. *Evidence Level III.*

Watson, R., & Green, S. M. (2006). Feeding and dementia: A systematic literature review. *Journal of Advanced Nursing, 54*(1), 86–93. doi:10.1111/j.1365-2648.2006.03793.x. *Evidence Level I.*

Watson, R., Green, S. M., & Legg, L. (2001). The Edinburgh Feeding Evaluation in Dementia Scale #2 (EdFED #2): Convergent and discriminant validity. *Clinical Effectiveness in Nursing, 5*(1), 44–46. doi:10.1111/j.1365-2702.2012.04250.x. *Evidence Level III.*

Wen, L., Jooyoung, C., & Thomas, S. A. (2014). Interventions on mealtime difficulties in older adults with dementia: A systematic review. *International Journal of Nursing Studies, 51*(1), 14–27. doi:10.1016/j.ijnurstu.2012.12.021. *Evidence Level I.*

Young, K. W. H., Greenwood, C. E., van Reekum, R., & Binns, M. A. (2004). Providing nutrition supplements to institutionalized seniors with probable Alzheimer's disease is least beneficial to those with low body weight status. *Journal of the American Geriatrics Society, 52*(8), 1305–1312. doi:10.1111/j.1532-5415.2004.52360.x. *Evidence Level II.*

Zapka, J., Amella, E., Magwood, G., Madisetti, M., Garrow, D., & Batchelor-Aselage, M. (2014). Challenges in efficacy research: The case of feeding alternatives in patients with dementia. *Journal of Advanced Nursing, 70*(9), 2072–2085. doi:10.1111/jan.12365. *Evidence Level II.*

26

Excessive Sleepiness

Grace E. Dean, Michelle L. Klimpt, Jonna Lee Morris, and Eileen R. Chasens

EDUCATIONAL OBJECTIVES

On completion of this chapter, the reader should be able to:

1. Identify the signs and symptoms of excessive sleepiness and quantify them using a standardized scale
2. Describe the signs, symptoms, and usual treatments for the most primary sleep disorders causing excessive sleepiness in older adults: obstructive sleep apnea (OSA), restless legs syndrome (RLS), insomnia, and short sleep duration
3. Discuss the implications of chronic illness, medications, and acute hospitalization on sleep
4. Provide nursing care that incorporates sleep hygiene measures and provide consistent ongoing treatment for existing sleep disorders
5. Educate patients and families about sleep disorders and sleep hygiene measures

OVERVIEW

Excessive sleepiness, sometimes called *excessive daytime sleepiness*, is common in older adults. Fatigue manifests as difficulty in sustaining a high level of physical performance; *excessive sleepiness* refers to the inability to maintain alertness or vigilance because of hypersomnolence. Many factors can affect nighttime sleep and result in daytime sleepiness in older adults. These include psychological disorders, symptoms of chronic illnesses (e.g., pain), medication side effects, environmental factors, and lifestyle preferences. Increases in sleepiness can result from age-related changes in chronobiology and sleep disorders. In older adults, the most common primary sleep disorders are OSA, RLS, and insomnia. The extent to which changes in sleep patterns experienced by older adults are caused by normal physiological alterations, pathological events, sleep disorders, or poor sleep hygiene remains unclear. Hospitalization and institutionalization can also interfere with sleep quality or quantity. There are many effective treatments for sleep disorders, but the first step is to identify the cause of excessive daytime sleepiness and then to quantify and aggressively treat this condition in the older adult. This chapter outlines an overview of sleep disorders common in older adults, describes how to assess sleep, and provides interventions to improve sleep in older adults.

BACKGROUND AND STATEMENT OF PROBLEM

The Institute of Medicine (Colten & Altevogt, 2006) reports that 50 to 70 million Americans are affected by chronic disorders of sleep and wakefulness. Recent data

For a description of evidence levels cited in this chapter, see Chapter 1, “Developing and Evaluating Clinical Practice Guidelines: A Systematic Approach.”

from the Behavioral Risk Factor Surveillance System (BRFSS) conducted by the Centers for Disease Control and Prevention (CDC) found that among community-dwelling persons older than 65 years (n = 23,167), nearly a quarter (24.5%) reported sleeping, on average, less than 7 hours in a 24-hour period and more than half (50.5%) of these older adults reported snoring (CDC, 2011b). Data from the 2005 to 2008 National Health and Nutrition Examination Survey (NHANES) show that 32% of persons older than 60 years (n = 3,716) slept less than 7 hours per night on weekdays or workdays (CDC, 2011a). Likewise, the Cardiovascular Health Study documented excessive sleepiness in 20% of subjects older than 65 years (n = 4,578; Whitney et al., 1998). Further, some sleep disorders are more common in patients in acute and chronic care settings. Ancoli-Israel et al. (1991) and Ancoli-Israel, Kripke, and Mason (1987) studied only persons older than 65 years and found undiagnosed sleep apnea in 24% of those living independently in the community, in 33% of those in acute care settings, and in 42% of older adults in nursing home settings.

CONSEQUENCES OF EXCESSIVE SLEEPINESS

The primary consequences of sleepiness are decreased alertness, delayed reaction time, and reduced cognitive performance (Ohayon & Vecchierini, 2002). The BRFSS found that nearly half (44%) of subjects in this telephone survey reported that they unintentionally fell asleep during the day at least once in the preceding month and that one out of 50 older adults had fallen asleep while driving in the preceding month (CDC, 2011a). The 2005 to 2008 NHANES data also show that older adults reported difficulty concentrating (18%) and remembering (14.7%) because of sleep-related problems (CDC, 2011a). Recent studies show that daytime sleepiness is significantly associated with declining cognitive function (Cohen-Zion et al., 2001), falls (Brassington, King, & Bliwise, 2000), cardiovascular events (Whitney et al., 1998) and higher levels of disability and depressive symptomatology (Anderson et al., 2014).

In the Cardiovascular Health Study, daytime sleepiness was the only sleep symptom associated with mortality, incident cardiovascular disease morbidity and mortality, myocardial infarction, and congestive heart failure, particularly among women (Newman et al., 2000). More recent, the risk for developing depression was examined in older women with few or no depressive symptoms at baseline, reports found poor sleep and objectively fragmented sleep at baseline indicated greater odds of worsening depressive symptoms 5 years later (Maglione et al., 2014). This link between sleep and medical conditions is consistent with the 2005 to 2008 NHANES results that demonstrated a greater rate of sleep-related problems with concentration, memory, and activities of daily living among women (CDC, 2011a).

Sleep problems, such as changes in sleep architecture and an increased incidence of OSA, are prevalent among persons with Alzheimer's disease (Harper, 2010). Persons with Alzheimer's disease demonstrate a pattern of decreased slow-wave sleep similar to older adults with normal aging. However, patients with Alzheimer's disease also exhibit greatly reduced rapid eye movement (REM) sleep and decreased stability of their circadian sleep–wake cycle that is not part of normal aging. Frequently, before the diagnosis of a permanent neurocognitive disorder, an evaluation of sleep is performed to rule out impaired cognitive functioning resulting from a potentially treatable sleep disorder. Research suggests that improved sleep consolidation may be neuroprotective. According to Lim, Kowgier, Yu, Buchman, and Bennett (2013), better sleep consolidation, sleep that is uninterrupted by repeated awakenings, reduces the effect of apolipoprotein E (APOE) ε4 allele, the most well established genetic risk factor for Alzheimer disease. Nearly 700 community-dwelling older adults without dementia participating in the Rush Memory and Aging Project were monitored with up to 10 days of actigraphy to quantify sleep consolidation and ascertain APOE genotype over 6 years. Better sleep consolidation substantially reduced the negative impact of the ε4 allele on incidence of Alzheimer's disease risk, leading the investigators to conclude that interventions to enhance sleep consolidation should be studied as potential means to reduce the risk of Alzheimer's disease in APOE ε4+ individuals (Lim, Kowgier, Yu, Buchman, & Bennett, 2013).

PHYSIOLOGICAL CHANGES IN SLEEP THAT ACCOMPANY AGING

Normal changes in sleep that occur as part of human development and lifestyle choices must be differentiated from pathological sleep conditions, which are common among older adults. Although older adults require as much sleep as younger adults, older adults may divide their sleep between nighttime slumber and daytime naps, rather than a single consolidated period. The endogenous circadian pacemaker, located in the suprachiasmatic nucleus, along with exogenous environmental cues and a homeostatic need for sleep, mediate the normal wake and sleep pattern. With aging, the circadian pattern for sleep–wake decreases in amplitude, possibly in association with less robust changes in core body temperature (Richardson,

Carskadon, Orav, & Dement, 1982). Compared with younger adults, healthy older adults have a more pronounced biphasic pattern of sleepiness during the afternoon hours (about 2–6 p.m.) and a phase advancement of nighttime sleepiness earlier in the evening (Roehrs, Turner, & Roth, 2000).

Changes in sleep architecture associated with normal aging include increased difficulty in falling asleep, poorer sleep quality with decreased sleep efficiency (SE), more time awake after sleep onset, increased "light" sleep (stages 1 and 2 sleep), and decreased quantity and amplitude of restorative "deep" slow-wave sleep (stages 3 and 4). Although older women report more sleep disturbances than older men, studies indicate that their sleep is less disturbed than that of men (Rediehs, Reis, & Creason, 1990). Gender partially accounts for differences in the outcomes of poor sleep quality in older adults. Women report more difficulty then men sleeping at night but studies indicate that their sleep is objectively less disturbed. When women and men both sleep less than 7 hours at night, men report better next-day function the following day (Krishnan & Collup, 2006). A cross-sectional study of community-dwelling older adults examined the independent association between nighttime sleep and daytime napping for all-cause mortality for 19 years from baseline. Increased mortality was associated in women sleeping more than 9 hours per night and in men napping 30 minutes or more during the day (Jung, Song, Ancoli-Israel, & Barrett-Connor, 2013).

PRIMARY CAUSES OF EXCESSIVE DAYTIME SLEEPINESS

Obstructive Sleep Apnea

OSA is a condition in which intermittent pharyngeal obstruction causes cessation of respiratory airflow (apneas) or reductions of airflow (hypopneas) that last for at least 10 seconds. This results in a microarousal that restores upper airway patency, permitting breathing and airflow to resume. According to the American Academy of Sleep Medicine (AASM, 2005) Task Force, OSA is diagnosed when these events occur at a rate of greater than 5 per hour of sleep and is accompanied by daytime sleepiness and impaired daytime functioning. It is common for patients with severe symptoms to experience multiple arousals during the night. These multiple arousals severely fragment sleep, preventing the deep sleep (stages 3 and 4) and REM sleep necessary for healthy mental and physical functioning.

OSA is both an age-related and an age-dependent condition, with an overlap in both distributions in the 60- to 70-year-old age range (Bliwise, King, & Harris, 1994). Age-related risk factors for OSA in older adults include an increased prevalence of overweight and obesity. Conversely, age-dependent risk factors include increased collapsibility of the upper airway, decreased lung capacity, altered ventilatory control, decreased muscular endurance, and altered sleep architecture (Brassington et al., 2000; Edwards et al., 2014). Treatments for OSA depend on the contributing pathology and patient preference and include nocturnal positive airway pressure, surgical procedures designed to increase the posterior pharyngeal area, oral appliances, and weight reduction when obesity is a contributing factor. Nasal continuous positive airway pressure (CPAP) therapy, which is highly effective when individually titrated to eliminate apneas and hypopneas, is currently the gold standard for treating OSA (Morgenthaler et al., 2006). Older adults tolerate CPAP therapy, with patterns of compliance similar to that of middle-aged adults (Weaver & Chasens, 2007). Although oral appliances offer a low-tech treatment option, they require a stable dentition that may be problematic for persons with extensive tooth loss or dentures.

Insomnia

Insomnia can be defined as delayed sleep onset, difficulty in maintaining sleep, premature waking, and/or very early arousals that result in insufficient sleep (American Psychiatric Association, 2013; Ancoli-Israel & Martin, 2006). Insomnia can be transient or chronic, and the perception of sleep loss may not correspond to objective assessment. The frequent awakenings suggestive of insomnia may be a conditioned arousal response because of environmental (e.g., noise or extremes of temperature) or behavioral cues. Anxiety associated with emotional conflict, stress, recent loss, feeling insecure at night, or significant changes in living arrangements can also produce insomnia (Ancoli-Israel & Martin, 2006). Chronic insomnia can result in a conditioned response of anxiety and arousal at bedtime in anticipation of difficulty falling asleep; this may prompt the use of hypnotic medications, over-the-counter (OTC) drugs, or alcohol. Although the use of hypnotics may produce short-term relief, they also affect sleep architecture and consequently lead to deterioration of sleep quality. The cycle of dependency and substance abuse is a potential problem in this age group (see Chapter 20 , "Reducing Adverse Drug Events"). At this time, the general recommendation is, when hypnotics are indicated, the most short-acting drug should be selected and, optimally, used in conjunction with an appropriate behavioral intervention (Ancoli-Israel, 2000).

Risk factors for insomnia include older age, being female, comorbidities, shift work, and possibly lower socioeconomic status (Schutte-Rodin, Broch, Buysse, Dorsey, & Sateia, 2008). Both the cause and duration of insomnia should inform the choice of treatment. For example, insomnia associated with a psychological origin, such as depression or anxiety, is best treated from that perspective. If pain is affecting sleep, pain management should be addressed first and strategies to promote sleep onset should be added secondarily. Short-term pharmacotherapy may be appropriate if insomnia is situational and of recent onset. When insomnia has been "learned" and the behavior becomes chronic, behavioral interventions are most appropriate. Behavioral treatments for insomnia include stimulus control, progressive muscle relaxation, paradoxical intention, sleep restriction, biofeedback, and multifaceted cognitive behavioral therapy (CBT; Morin et al., 1999). Data show that 70% to 80% of patients benefit from behavioral therapies and that improvement in sleep is often sustained for a minimum of 6 months after treatment. Recently, a brief, 4-week, group-based CBT program in adults (mean age = 64 years) with sleep-maintenance insomnia produced robust and durable improvements in sleep quality and daytime functioning that was maintained at 3-month follow-up compared to the waitlist group (Lovato, Lack, Wright, & Kennaway, 2014).

Restless Legs Syndrome

RLS is a neurological condition that is characterized by the irresistible urge to move the legs. It is usually associated with disagreeable leg sensations that become worse during inactivity and often interferes with initiating and maintaining sleep. As a secondary condition, this movement disorder can be caused by iron deficiency anemia, uremia, neurological lesions, diabetes, Parkinson's disease, rheumatoid arthritis, or it can be a side effect of certain drugs (e.g., tricyclic antidepressants, serotonin reuptake inhibitors, lithium, dopamine blockers, xanthines). Periodic leg movement disorder (PLMD) is a similar condition, but it is characterized by involuntary flexion of the leg and foot that produces microarousals or full arousals from sleep that interfere with achieving and maintaining restorative slow-wave sleep (stages 3 and 4). Although the etiology and associated mechanism of this specific movement disorder are not well defined, this condition has been linked to metabolic, vascular, and neurologic causes (Claman et al., 2013). Dopaminergic drugs are the most effective agents for treating RLS and PLMD as well as opioids, benzodiazepines, anticonvulsants, adrenergics, and iron supplements. However, their efficacy for long-term treatment in older adults has not been sufficiently evaluated (Ancoli-Israel & Martin, 2006; Gamaldo & Earley, 2006).

SECONDARY CAUSES OF EXCESSIVE DAYTIME SLEEPINESS

Medical and psychiatric illness can interfere with sleep quality and disturb sleep. For example, depression or anxiety appear to have a bidirectional relationship with insomnia (Buysse, 2004). Painful chronic conditions, such as arthritis, reduce SE, or simply changing body position may be painful enough to cause awakenings. Nighttime voiding, or nocturia, worsens sleep in older individuals with insomnia. However, it is unclear whether the urge for urination causes the awakenings or whether some other cause of awakening led to the need for urination (Zeitzer, Bliwise, Hernandez, Friedman, & Yesavage, 2013).

Because older adults frequently have multiple medical conditions, they are also more likely to take OTC and prescription medications for symptom relief. However, many medications and nonprescription drugs (e.g., pseudoephedrine, alcohol, caffeine, and nicotine) interfere with sleep. Thus, health care providers must be acutely aware of which OTC medications and beverages can cause sleep problems. Symptom management must be balanced against preventing polypharmacy in older adults to maintain sleep quality (Ancoli-Israel, 2005).

Sleep Disturbance During Hospitalization

Studies have shown that as many as 22% to 61% of hospitalized patients experience impaired sleep (Redeker, 2000). Many older adults have primary sleep disorders (OSA, insomnia, RLS) and these conditions can become more pronounced or acute during acute illness and hospitalization. Sleep disorders may go unrecognized in acute care settings, thus patients may experience acute sleep deprivation concurrently with a medical crisis or surgical intervention.

Protecting sleep and monitoring sleep quality should be routine elements of care in hospital settings (Young, Bourgeois, Hilty, & Hardin, 2008). There are three common causes for sleep disruption in hospitals that are often overlooked by nursing staff: noise, light, and patient-care activities (Redeker, 2000). Further, anesthesia, cardiopulmonary disorders, and pain medications can reduce the respiratory drive and lead to hypopnea and apnea. Medications typically administered postoperatively can affect alertness by causing excessive sedation, changes in sleep architecture, decreased REM sleep, nightmares, or

TABLE 26.1
Sleep History

Basic Sleep History Questions	Follow-Up Questions	Sleep Disorders to Consider
■ Do you have any difficulty falling asleep? ■ Are you having any difficulty sleeping until morning? ■ Are you having difficulty sleeping throughout the night? ■ Have you or anyone else ever noticed that you snore loudly or stop breathing in your sleep? ■ Do you find yourself falling asleep during the day when you do not want to?	■ What time do you usually go to bed? ■ What time do you fall asleep? ■ What prevents you from falling asleep? ■ Review intake of alcohol, nicotine, caffeine, all medications. ■ Review of depressive symptoms: weight loss, sadness, or recent losses ■ How often do you waken? ■ How long are you awake? ■ Do you have any pain, discomfort, or shortness of breath during the night? ■ How many times do you void during the night? ■ What prevents you from falling back to sleep? ■ Are you sleepy or tired during the day? ■ Review risk factors (e.g., obesity, arthritis, poorly controlled illnesses). ■ Do your legs kick or jump around while you sleep? ■ Do you stay outdoors in natural daylight on most days?	■ Shift work/sleep schedule disorders ■ Psychophysiological insomnia ■ Restless legs syndrome ■ Psychiatric disorders ■ Substance/medications related disorders ■ Depression ■ Insomnia ■ Medical causes of sleep disturbance ■ Obstructive sleep apnea ■ Functional impairment resulting from sleep disorder ■ Periodic leg movement disorders

Adapted from Avidan (2005); Bloom et al. (2009).

insomnia. Pain and anxiety may also cause older patients to have insomnia. Inadequate sleep impedes healing and recovery and may be associated with acute mental confusion in older adults (Young, Bourgeois, Hilty, & Hardin, 2009).

Additionally, a significant association between sleep disturbances and falls in older adults exists, especially in individuals who have trouble staying asleep (Helbig et al., 2013). It is unfortunate that the two common fall risk assessment scales used in hospitals do not include questions on sleep disturbances (Hendrich, Bender, & Nyhuis, 2003; Morse, Black, Oberle, & Donahue, 1989). Many acute care patients fall in the evenings or at night. Half of these falls may be attributable to the need for elimination (Hitcho et al., 2004). Therefore, nocturia may contribute to the problem of falls in older adults.

In summary, older adults in acute care settings are exposed to many conditions that can negatively affect sleep and result in excessive daytime sleepiness. The sleep environment and the quality of patients' sleep can be improved in hospital settings if caregivers recognize the essential importance of sleep in illness and health. The American Academy of Nursing (2014) recommends that nurses should not wake patients for routine care unless the patient's condition necessitates it. As a standard practice, nurses should include a thorough sleep history (Table 26.1) during admission to determine usual sleep patterns and/or symptoms of sleep disorders. Patients with OSA who use CPAP at home should be instructed to bring their machines with them to the hospital. Sleep-hygiene measures should be incorporated into nursing care routines during evening and night hours and also incorporated into care plans on every nursing unit. This includes simple practices, such as reducing light intensity, maintaining a quiet environment, and efficient delivery of patient care, to minimize sleep disruption among patients. Anticipatory and preventive pain management is also an important element of care to promote adequate sleep in the hospital setting (Young et al., 2009).

ASSESSMENT OF THE PROBLEM

There are valid and reliable measures to assess subjective and objective sleep disorders in adults, however, not all have been evaluated in older persons (Luyster et al., 2015). The Insomnia in the Elderly Scale (IES) has been validated in persons aged 65 years and older. With only nine questions to be scored, it can easily be completed in less than 5 minutes and takes only a minute or 2 to assess (Navarro et al., 2013). Although OSA can only be diagnosed with a sleep study, the risk of OSA is frequently evaluated in adults using the Berlin Questionnaire (Netzer, Stoohs, Netzer, Clark, & Strohl, 1999) or the Snore, Tired, Observed, Pressure, Body Mass Index, Age, Neck, Gender (STOP-Bang) Questionnaire (Chung et al., 2008). However, a study of older adults (n = 643; mean age of 65.6 years), found that the Berlin questionnaire was not able to accurately identify OSA in older adults (Sforza et al., 2011). The STOP-Bang, first developed to screen for OSA in persons scheduled for anesthesia, consists of eight questions and has sensitivity from 76% to 96%. Although men have a higher risk for OSA compared to women, the ratio of men to women in the general population is not as high as in early studies or in clinic populations. This results in women being frequently underdiagnosed (Young et al., 1996). One of the questions on the STOP-Bang is "gender" with women automatically having a lower score, therefore the STOP-Bang may underestimate OSA in older women.

The Functional Outcomes of Sleep Questionnaire (Weaver et al., 1997b) is used to evaluate the impact of sleepiness on functional status, and the Pittsburgh Sleep Quality Index (PSQI; Buysse, Reynolds, Monk, Berman, & Kupfer, 1989) quantifies sleep quality over the past month. Many sleep clinicians use the Epworth Sleepiness Scale (ESS) to screen for sleepiness and track symptoms over the previous week during common activities such as sitting and reading, watching TV, or riding in a car. It is easy to administer and includes a scoring parameter to indicate the need for a medical evaluation (Johns, 1991). Recent research questions the validity of the ESS in older adults (Onen et al., 2013). Results of a study of independently living older adults (n = 104; age > 65 years) who answered affirmatively to the question, "Do you feel excessively sleepy during the day recently?" found that over half the participants could not answer at least one of the questions on the ESS and that only 25% had an abnormal ESS score.

Therefore, although subjective questionnaires should be used to assist in the evaluation of sleep disorders in the older adult, the nurse needs to recognize that older adults may not be as aware of impaired sleep. The diagnosis of sleep disorders requires both an in-depth history and an objective sleep evaluation in both younger and older adults. A brief sleep history can be obtained by using the questionnaire in Table 26.1. In a sleep-laboratory setting, a completed evaluation of sleep is conducted using polysomnography that includes EEG, electromyogram (EMG), electro-oculogram (EOG), respiratory effort, oxygen saturation, and electrophysiological cardiac aspects of sleep. Additional electrophysiological tests, such as the Multiple Sleep Latency Test, are also used to quantify daytime sleepiness. Most important in the assessment of sleepiness is an evaluation of the patient's knowledge and application of sleep-hygiene measures (Table 26.2) that are also effective behavioral strategies to maximize, promote, and protect sleep.

TABLE 26.2
Sleep-Hygiene Measures

- Use the bed only for sleeping or sex.
- Develop consistent and rest-promoting bedtime routines.
- Maintain the same bedtime and waking time every day.
- Exposure to bright sunlight is desirable on awakening.
- On awakening, get out of bed slowly, no matter what time it is, to prevent postural hypotension.
- If awakened during the night, avoid looking at the clock; frequent time checks may heighten anxiety and hinder sleep onset.
- Avoid naps if they negatively affect nighttime sleep. Limit naps to 15 to 30 minutes' duration.
- Sleep in a cool, quiet environment.
- If you cannot fall asleep after 15 or 20 minutes in bed, get up and go into another room, read, or do a quiet activity, using dim lighting, until you are sleepy again.
- Before bedtime, avoid the following:
  - caffeine and nicotine after noon
  - alcohol intake (more than three drinks)
  - large meals or exercise 3 to 4 hours before bedtime
  - emotional upset or emotionally charged activities, including television programs that are troubling

INTERVENTIONS AND CARE STRATEGIES

The first line of defense against excessive sleepiness is a lifestyle that promotes and ensures adequate sleep and rest. By maintaining a daily routine, daytime sleepiness can be minimized. Characteristics of a routine that have been found to be helpful are timing, frequency, and duration of activities (Zisberg, Gur-Yaish, & Shochat, 2010). Although humans have a natural drive to sleep, environment and habituation play an important behavioral role in sleep. Sleep hygiene, those practices that permit and promote sleep onset and sleep maintenance, has many aspects and requires regular reinforcement. Regardless of health status, sleep-hygiene practices and routines are as important for older adults as they are for children, adolescents, and other adults.

CASE STUDY

Ms. K stopped attending her weekly bingo night with her girlfriends, saying, "I just don't have the energy." Usually the ringleader, she had become more withdrawn from her friends and family. Work had also become a struggle for Ms. K, but she blamed it on poor sleep. Her daughter suggested that she may need professional help and encouraged her to make an appointment with her primary care provider.

Ms. K is a 67-year-old African American woman who is overweight (height, 62 inches; weight, 140 lbs; body mass index [BMI] 25.6). She is a lung cancer survivor. She is hypertensive and takes a variety of medications. She has a 53-pack-year history of smoking and currently smokes approximately three to 12 cigarettes per day because she is bored and lonely. She lives alone in a second-story apartment with a cat, although she states that she is a dog person. She reports that she stopped going to bingo night at the local fire station about 2 months ago. She said that she loved hanging out with her girlfriends but feels like it is such an effort now. She is a self-employed aide working in the home care setting.

Fatigue, irritability, and the inability to get going in the morning are her major complaints because they interfere with her ability to work and socialize. Ms. K worries when she goes out whether she will make it back home under her own power. She would like to stop smoking, but because of her poor energy level she stays home and smokes. She can only work 4 hours per day and must take frequent rest periods because she becomes short of breath easily. She takes long naps and then cannot fall asleep at night. Her cat wakes her up frequently, too. She also becomes short of breath when climbing the stairs to her apartment.

Ms. K has severe fatigue and worries about her lack of nighttime sleep, which may be the result of comorbid insomnia related to her diagnosis of lung cancer and poor sleep hygiene. Ms. K often falls asleep watching TV with the cat and then the cat wakes her up in the middle of the night and she cannot get back to sleep, tossing and turning, worrying about her poor sleep. She then will have a cigarette because she is bored. Although Ms. K has no bed partner, her daughter has stayed overnight and never reported to Ms. K about any loud snoring, gasping for breath, or breath holding. She also denies the occurrence of morning headaches. Because her sleep problem is interfering with her daytime functioning (e.g., ability to work), Ms. K warrants a referral to a sleep specialist. The self-limiting of her socialization and reports of boredom and loneliness suggest a need for depression screening.

The sleep specialist ordered an overnight portable screening for sleep apnea (e.g., ApneaLink) to rule out OSA, which is a common cause for daytime sleepiness. The results demonstrated that Ms. K does not have OSA (Table 26.3). A 14-day sleep diary screening for insomnia revealed the following: SE = 62% (slept 240 minutes; in bed 390 minutes); sleep latency (SL) = 33 minutes; wake after sleep onset (WASO) = 117 minutes; naps = 84 minutes; ESS = 9.

Normal Sleep Values

SE > 85%; SL < 30; WASO < 30; ESS < 11; naps < 30

Ms. K was also referred for CBT for her insomnia. CBT for insomnia (CBT-I) is now accepted as the standard of care for patients with insomnia regardless of etiology. CBT-I consists of sleep restriction, stimulus control, relaxation, sleep-hygiene education and cognitive therapy that focuses on dysfunctional sleep-related thoughts and unhelpful sleep behaviors that may exacerbate insomnia.

TABLE 26.3

Results of Overnight Apnea Link to Rule Out OSA

Total recording time	274 minutes	Apnea/ Hypopnea Index	1.9/ hours of sleep
Lowest O_2 saturation	88%	Saturation less than or equal to 90%	10 minutes

Ms. K returned to her primary care provider who diagnosed her as having a major depressive episode and discussed further treatment options. Her insomnia is being managed with CBT-I, is improving, but not yet resolved. Therefore, an antidepressant medication with sedating side effects was indicated. Celexa, Lexapro, Paxil, and Zoloft were considered. Zoloft was eventually chosen, but knowing that there were other alternatives was appealing to Ms. K.

Diagnosis

Comorbid insomnia with major depressive episode

Treatment

CBT-I—individual therapy

(continued)

CASE STUDY *(continued)*

6-Month Follow-Up

While working with the CBT-I therapist, who just happened to be a nurse practitioner, Ms. K's 14-day sleep-diary data improved: SE = 86% (slept 360 minutes; in bed 420 minutes); SL = 15 minutes; WASO = 45; naps = 36 minutes; ESS = 8. Although she is still taking naps, she is not taking them every day and she is taking them earlier so that they do not interfere with her ability to fall asleep at bedtime. The cat is out of the bedroom and she has started to volunteer at her local library as well as rejoining her friends at bingo. She is still smoking, but is now down to only three to five cigarettes per day. The nurse practitioner discussed how smoking is a stimulant that may increase insomnia and the importance of smoking-cessation programs. Ms. K declines to stop smoking completely at this time, she states she is "working at it on her own," but agrees to give up her bedtime cigarette. The nurse practitioner plans to continue to encourage sleep hygiene and smoking cessation on follow-up visits.

SUMMARY

Nurses must be able to identify, screen, and refer patients with excessive daytime sleepiness and symptoms of sleep disorders. No other group of health care providers watch more people sleep than nurses, and sleep disorders can affect all aspects of health and illness. Sleep medicine is a relatively new specialty, and many health care providers have had no preparation in the science of sleep. Nurses also must incorporate sleep-hygiene measures and actively address existing sleep disorders in care plans of older adults to ensure adequate sleep in all settings: acute care, primary care, and at home. Failing to identify, diagnose, or treat excessive sleepiness and its underlying cause(s) can adversely affect the health and longevity of older adults.

NURSING STANDARD OF PRACTICE

Protocol 26.1: Excessive Sleepiness

I. GOAL

Older adults will maintain an optimal state of alertness while awake and optimal quality and quantity of sleep during their preferred sleep period

II. OVERVIEW

Although normal aging is accompanied by decreased "deep sleep," sleep efficiency, and increased time awake after sleep onset, these changes should not result in excessive daytime sleepiness. Daytime sleepiness is not only a symptom of sleep disorders but also results in decreased health and functional outcomes in the older adult.

III. BACKGROUND

A. Definition

Excessive sleepiness: somnolence, hypersomnia, excessive daytime sleepiness, subjective sleepiness. Sleepiness is a ubiquitous phenomenon, experienced not only as a symptom in a number of medical, psychiatric, and primary sleep disorders, but also as a normal physiological state in most individuals over any given 24-hour period. Sleepiness can be considered abnormal when it occurs at inappropriate times, or does not occur when desired (Shen, Barbera, & Shapiro, 2006).

B. Etiology and epidemiology

1. Excessive sleepiness may be caused by difficulty initiating sleep, impaired sleep maintenance, waking prematurely, sleep disorders, or sleep fragmentation.
2. There are many types of sleep diagnoses and the most common disorders reported by older adults are OSA, insomnia, and RLS.

(continued)

Protocol 26.1: Excessive Sleepiness *(continued)*

3. Many sleep disorders share excessive sleepiness as a common symptom, but this symptom is often not evaluated or treated because health care providers are uninformed about the nature of sleep disorders, the symptoms of these disorders, and the many effective treatments available for these conditions.

IV. PARAMETERS OF ASSESSMENT

A. A sleep history (see Table 26.1) should include information from both the patient and family members. People who share living and sleeping spaces can provide important information about sleep behavior that the patient may not be able to convey.
B. The Epworth Sleepiness Scale (Johns, 1991) is a brief instrument to screen for severity of daytime sleepiness in the community setting. It can also be found under "Resources" at consultgerirn.org/resources.
C. The Pittsburgh Sleep Quality Index (Buysse et al., 1989) is useful to screen for sleep problems in the home environment and to monitor changes in sleep quality. This instrument can be found under "Resources" at consultgerirn.org/resources.

V. NURSING CARE STRATEGIES

A. Vigilance by nursing staff in observing patients for snoring, apneas during sleep, excessive leg movements during sleep, and difficulty staying awake during normal daytime activities (Ancoli-Israel & Martin, 2006; Avidan, 2005)
B. Management of medical conditions, psychological disorders, and symptoms that interfere with sleep, such as depression, pain, hot flashes, anemia, or uremia (Ancoli-Israel & Martin, 2006; Avidan, 2005)
C. For patients with a current diagnosis of a sleep disorder, ongoing treatments, such as continuous positive airway pressure should be documented, maintained, and reinforced through patient and family education (Avidan, 2005). Nursing staff should reinforce patient instruction in cleaning and maintaining positive airway pressure equipment and masks.
D. Instruction for patients and families regarding sleep-hygiene techniques to protect and promote sleep among all family members (see Table 26.2; Avidan, 2005)
E. Review and, if necessary, adjust medications that interact with one another or whose side effects include drowsiness or sleep impairment (Ancoli-Israel & Martin, 2006).
F. Referral to a sleep specialist for moderate or severe sleepiness or a clinical profile consistent with major sleep disorders such as OSA or RLS (Avidan, 2005)
G. Aggressive planning, monitoring, and management of patients with OSA when sedative medications or anesthesia are given (Avidan, 2005)
H. Ongoing assessment of adherence to prescriptions for sleep hygiene, medications, and devices to support respiration during sleep (Avidan, 2005)
I. Hospital staff should avoid waking a patient for routine care, such as baths, vitals signs, and routine blood tests (American Academy of Nursing, 2014).

VI. EVALUATION AND EXPECTED OUTCOMES

A. Quality-assurance actions
    1. Provide staff education on the major causes of excessive sleepiness (i.e., OSA, insomnia, RLS).
    2. Provide staff with in-services on how to use and monitor CPAP equipment.
    3. Have individual nursing units conduct environmental surveys regarding noise level during the night hours and then develop strategies to reduce sleep disruption caused by noise and care patterns.
    4. Add sleep as a parameter of the admission assessment for patients and provide written instructions for patients using CPAP at home to always bring the equipment with them to the hospital. Include sleep quality (e.g., see PSQI tool; www.hartfordign.org) in the assessment
    5. Use posthospital surveys of patient satisfaction with sleep while in the hospital and provide feedback for nursing staff (see www.hartfordign.org, Sleep topic).
B. Quality outcomes
    Improved quality and/or quantity of sleep during normal sleep intervals as reported by patients and staff

(continued)

Protocol 26.1: Excessive Sleepiness *(continued)*

VII. FOLLOW-UP MONITORING

A. Depending on the diagnosis, follow-up may include long-term reinforcement of the original interventions along with support for adhering to treatments prescribed by a sleep specialist. For example, patient compliance with CPAP therapy for OSA is critical to its efficacy and should be assessed during the first week of treatment (Weaver et al., 1997a). All patients benefit from positive reinforcement while trying to acclimate to nightly use of a positive airway pressure device.
B. CPAP masks may require minor adjustments or refitting to find the most comfortable fit. Most such changes are needed during the acclimation period, but patients should be encouraged to seek assistance if mask problems develop (Weaver et al., 1997a). In the acute care setting, respiratory care technicians are valuable in-house resources when staff from a sleep center are not readily available.
C. During the initial treatment phase of insomnia, sleep deprivation may cause rebound sleepiness, which should subside over time. Follow-up should include ongoing assessment of napping habits and sleepiness to track treatment effectiveness (Avidan, 2005).
D. If obesity has been a complicating health factor, weight loss is a desirable long-term goal. With reduction in daytime sleepiness, the timing is ripe for increasing the activity level. Treatment of sleep disorders should include planning for strategic changes in lifestyle that include regular exercise, which is also consistent with cardiovascular health and long-term diabetes control (Ancoli-Israel & Ayalon, 2006).

ABBREVIATIONS

CPAP Continuous positive airway pressure
OSA Obstructive sleep apnea
PSQI Pittsburgh Sleep Quality Index
RLS Restless legs syndrome

RESOURCES

American Academy of Sleep Medicine (AASM)
This organization for sleep professionals is also a great source of information for the public and for practice guidelines for professionals.
http://www.aasmnet.org

Basics of Sleep Guide
This Sleep Research Society publication is designed for students, sleep researchers, and nonsleep professionals interested in studying sleep across the life cycle, sleep deprivation or restriction, and sleep physiology. Information about this publication and how to order it can be found on the Sleep Research Society website.
http://www.sleepresearchsociety.org/Products.aspx

National Institutes of Health, National Center on Sleep Disorders Research
This site includes brochures that may be downloaded or printed for distribution to patients or for the education of other health care providers.
For health care professionals: http://www.nhlbi.nih.gov/health/prof/sleep/index.htm
For patients and the general public: http://www.nhlbi.nih.gov/health/resources/sleep

Sleep Research Society
This professional organization fosters scientific investigation, professional education, and career development in sleep research and academic sleep medicine. It is an excellent resource for nurses who are interested in studying issues of sleep and circadian processes.
http://www.sleepresearchsociety.org

Willis-Ekbom Disease Foundation (formerly Restless Legs Syndrome Foundation)
This organization is dedicated to improving the lives of those living with this often devastating disease. The organization's goals are to increase awareness of WED/RLS, to improve treatments, and to find a cure through research.
http://www.rls.org

REFERENCES

American Academy of Nursing. (2014). *Choosing wisely: Sleep*. Retrieved from http://www.choosingwisely.org/clinician-lists/

american-academy-nursing-avoid-waking-patients-for-routine-care. *Evidence Level VII.*

American Academy of Sleep Medicine. (2005). *International classification of sleep disorders: Diagnostic and coding manual* (2nd ed.). Westchester, MN: Author. *Evidence Level I.*

American Psychiatric Association. (2013). *Diagnostic and statistical manual of mental disorders* (5th ed.). Arlington, VA: American Psychiatric Press. *Evidence Level I.*

Ancoli-Israel, S. (2000). Insomnia in the elderly: A review for the primary care practitioner. *Sleep, 23*(Suppl. 1), S23–S30; discussion S36–S38. *Evidence Level I.*

Ancoli-Israel, S. (2005). Sleep and aging: Prevalence of disturbed sleep and treatment considerations in older adults. *Journal of Clinical Psychiatry, 66*(Suppl. 9), 24–30; quiz 42–43. *Evidence Level I.*

Ancoli-Israel, S., & Ayalon, L. (2006). Diagnosis and treatment of sleep disorders in older adults. *American Journal of Geriatric Psychiatry, 14*(2), 95–103. *Evidence Level I.*

Ancoli-Israel, S., Kripke, D. F., Klauber, M. R., Mason, W. J., Fell, R., & Kaplan, O. (1991). Sleep-disordered breathing in community-dwelling elderly. *Sleep, 14*(6), 486–495. *Evidence Level IV.*

Ancoli-Israel, S., Kripke, D. F., & Mason, W. (1987). Characteristics of obstructive and central sleep apnea in the elderly: An interim report. *Biological Psychiatry, 22*(6), 741–750. *Evidence Level IV.*

Ancoli-Israel, S., & Martin, J. L. (2006). Insomnia and daytime napping in older adults. *Journal of Clinical Sleep Medicine, 2*(3), 333–342. *Evidence Level VI.*

Anderson, K. N., Catt, M., Collerton, J., Davies, K., von Zglinicki, T., Kirwood, T. B. L., & Jagger, C. (2014). Assessment of sleep and circadian rhythm disorders in the very old: The Newcastle 85+ cohort study. *Age and Ageing, 43*, 57–63. *Evidence level IV.*

Avidan, A. Y. (2005). Sleep in the geriatric patient population. *Seminars in Neurology, 25*(1), 52–63. *Evidence Level I.*

Bliwise, D. L., King, A. C., & Harris, R. B. (1994). Habitual sleep durations and health in a 50–65 year old population. *Journal of Clinical Epidemiology, 47*(1), 35–41. *Evidence Level IV.*

Bloom, H. G., Ahmed, I., Alessi, C. A., Ancoli-Israel, S., Buysse, D. J., Kryger, M. H., . . . Zee, P. C. (2009). Evidence-based recommendations for the assessment and management of sleep disorders in older persons. *Journal of the American Geriatrics Society, 57*(5), 761–789. *Evidence Level I.*

Brassington, G. S., King, A. C., & Bliwise, D. L. (2000). Sleep problems as a risk factor for falls in a sample of community-dwelling adults aged 64–99 years. *Journal of the American Geriatrics Society, 48*(10), 1234–1240. *Evidence Level III.*

Buysse, D. J. (2004). Insomnia, depression and aging. Assessing sleep and mood interactions in older adults. *Geriatrics, 59*(2), 47–51. *Evidence Level VI.*

Buysse, D. J., Reynolds, C. F., III, Monk, T. H., Berman, S. R., & Kupfer, D. J. (1989). The Pittsburgh Sleep Quality Index: A new instrument for psychiatric practice and research. *Psychiatry Research, 28*(2), 193–213. *Eveidence Level IV.*

Centers for Disease Control and Prevention (CDC). (2011a). Effect of short sleep duration on daily activities—United States, 2005–2008. *Morbidity and Mortality Weekly Report, 60*(8), 239–242. *Evidence Level IV.*

Centers for Disease Control and Prevention. (2011b). Unhealthy sleep-related behaviors—12 States, 2009. *Morbidity and Mortality Weekly Report, 60*(8), 233–238. *Evidence Level IV.*

Chung, F., Yegneswaran, B., Liao, P., Chung, S. A., Vairavanathan, S., Islam, S., . . . Shapiro, C. M. (2008). STOP questionnaire: A tool to screen patients for obstructive sleep apnea. *Anesthesiology, 108*(5), 812–821. *Evidence Level IV.*

Claman, D. M., Ewing, S. K., Redine, S., Ancoli-Israel, S., Cauley, J. A., & Stone, K. L. (2013). Periodic leg movements are associated with reduced sleep quality in older men: The MrOS sleep study. *Journal of Clinical Sleep Medicine, 9*(11), 1109–1117. *Evidence Level IV.*

Cohen-Zion, M., Stepnowsky, C., Marler, Shochat, T., Kripke, D. F., & Ancoli-Israel, S. (2001). Changes in cognitive function associated with sleep disordered breathing in older people. *Journal of the American Geriatrics Society, 49*(12), 1622–1627. *Evidence Level III.*

Colten, H. R., & Altevogt, B. M. (Eds.). (2006). *Sleep disorders and sleep deprivation: An unmet public health problem.* Washington, DC: National Academies Press. *Evidence Level I.*

Edwards, B. A., Wellman, A., Sands, S. A., Owens, R. L., Eckert, D. J., White, D. P., & Malhotra, A. (2014). Obstructive sleep apnea in older adults is a distinctly different physiological phenotype. *Sleep, 37*(7), 1227–1236. *Evidence Level IV.*

Gamaldo, C. E., & Earley, C. J. (2006). Restless legs syndrome: A clinical update. *Chest, 130*(5), 1596–1604. *Evidence Level I.*

Harper, D. G. (2010). Sleep and circadian disturbances in Alzheimer's disease. In S. R. Randi-Permual, J. M. Monti, & A. A. Monjan (Eds.), *Principles and practice of geriatric sleep medicine* (pp. 214–226). New York, NY: Cambridge University Press. *Evidence Level V.*

Helbig, A. K., Doring, A., Heier, M., Emeny, R. T., Zimmermann, A. K., Autenrieth, C. S., . . . Meisinger, C. (2013). Association between sleep disturbances and falls among the elderly: Results from the German Cooperative Health Research in the region of Augsburg-Age study. *Sleep Medicine, 14*, 1356–1363. *Evidence Level IV.*

Hendrich, A. L., Bender, P. S., & Nyhuis, A. (2003). Validation of the Hendrich II Fall Risk Model: A large concurrent case/control study of hospitalized patients. *Applied Nursing Research, 16*(1), 9–21. [Context Link] *Evidence Level II.*

Hitcho, E. B., Krauss, M. J., Birge, S., Dunagan, W. C., Fischer, I., Johnson, S., . . . Fraser, V. J. (2004). Characteristics and circumstances of falls in a hospital setting: A prospective analysis. *Journal of General Internal Medicine, 19*(7), 732–739. *Evidence Level IV.*

Johns, M. W. (1991). A new method for measuring daytime sleepiness: The Epworth sleepiness scale. *Sleep, 14*(6), 540–545. *Evidence Level VI.*

Jung, K. I., Song, C. H., Ancoli-Israel, S., & Barrett-Connor, E. (2013). Gender differences in nighttime sleep and daytime napping as predictors of mortality in older adults: The Rancho Bernardo study. *Sleep Medicine, 14*(1), 12–19. *Evidence Level IV.*

Krishnan, V., & Collup, N. (2006). Gender differences in sleep disorders. *Current Opinion in Pulmonary Medicine, 12*(6), 383–389. *Evidence Level V.*

Lim, A. S., Kowgier, M., Yu, L., Buchman, A. S., & Bennett, D. A. (2013). Sleep fragmentation and the risk of incident Alzheimer's disease and cognitive decline in older persons. *Sleep, 36*(7), 1027–1032. *Evidence Level IV.*

Lovato, N., Lack, L., Wright, H., Kennaway, D. J. (2014). Evaluation of a brief treatment program of cognitive behavior therapy for insomnia in older adults. *Sleep, 37*(1), 117–126. *Evidence Level II.*

Luyster, F. S., Choi, J. Y., Yeh, C. H., Imes, C. C., Johannson, A., & Chasens, E. R. (2015). Screening and evaluation tools for sleep disorders in older adults. *Applied Nursing Research, 28*(4), 334–340. doi:10.1016/j.apnr.2014.12.007. *Evidence Level V.*

Maglione, J. E., Ancoli-Israel, S., Peters, K. W., Paudel, M. L., Yaffe, K., Ensrud, K. E., & Stone, K. L. (2014). Depressive symptoms and subjective and objective sleep in community-dwelling older women. *Journal of the American Geriatrics Society, 60*(4), 635–643. *Evidence Level VI.*

Morgenthaler, T. I., Kapen, S., Lee-Chiong, T., Alessi, C., Boehlecke, B., Brown, T., . . . Swick, T. (2006). Practice parameters for the medical therapy of obstructive sleep apnea. *Sleep, 29*(8), 1031–1035. *Evidence Level I.*

Morin, C. M., Hauri, P. J., Espie, C. A., Spielman, A. J., Buysse, D. J., & Bootzin, R. R. (1999). Nonpharmacologic treatment of chronic insomnia. An American Academy of Sleep Medicine review. *Sleep, 22*(8), 1134–1156. *Evidence Level I.*

Morse, J. M., Black, C., Oberle, K., & Donahue, P. (1989). A prospective study to identify the fall-prone patient. *Social Sciences & Medicine, 28*, 81–86. Level IV.

Navarro, B., Lopez-Torres, J., Andres, F., Latorre, J. M., Montes, M. J., & Parraga, I. (2013). Validation of the Insomnia in the Elderly Scale for the detection of insomnia in older adults. *Geriatrics & Gerontology International, 13*, 646–653. *Evidence Level VI.*

Netzer, N. C., Stoohs, R. A., Netzer, C. M., Clark, K., & Strohl, K. P. (1999). Using the Berlin Questionnaire to identify patients at risk for the sleep apnea syndrome. *Annals of Internal Medicine, 131*(7), 485–491. *Evidence Level VI.*

Newman, A. B., Spiekerman, C. F., Enright, P., Lefkowitz, D., Manolio, T., Reynolds, C. F., & Robbins, J. (2000). Daytime sleepiness predicts mortality and cardiovascular disease in older adults. The Cardiovascular Health Study Research Group. *Journal of the American Geriatrics Society, 48*(2), 115–123. *Evidence Level III.*

Ohayon, M. M., & Vecchierini, M. F. (2002). Daytime sleepiness and cognitive impairment in the elderly population. *Archives of Internal Medicine, 162*(2), 201–208. *Evidence Level IV.*

Onen, F., Moreau, T., Gooneratne, N. S., Petit, C., Falissard, B. & Onen, S. H. (2013). Limits of the Epworth Sleepiness Scale in older adults. *Sleep and Breathing, 17*, 343–350. *Evidence Level IV.*

Redeker, N. S. (2000). Sleep in acute care settings: An integrative review. *Journal of Nursing Scholarship, 32*(1), 31–38. *Evidence Level I.*

Rediehs, M. H., Reis, J. S., & Creason, N. S. (1990). Sleep in old age: Focus on gender differences. *Sleep, 13*(5), 410–424. *Evidence Level I.*

Richardson, G. S., Carskadon, M. A., Orav, E. J., & Dement, W. C. (1982). Circadian variation of sleep tendency in elderly and young adult subjects. *Sleep, 5*(Suppl. 2), S82–S94. *Evidence Level VI.*

Roehrs, T., Turner, L., & Roth, T. (2000). Effects of sleep loss on waking actigraphy. *Sleep, 23*(6), 793–797. *Evidence Level IV.*

Schutte-Rodin, S., Broch, L., Buysse, D., Dorsey, C., & Sateia, M. (2008). Clinical guideline for the evaluation and management of chronic insomnia in adults. *Journal of Clinical Sleep Medicine, 4*(5), 487–504. *Evidence Level I.*

Sforza, E., Chouchou, F., Pichot, V., Herrmann, F., Barthelemy, J. C., & Roche, F. (2011). Is the Berlin questionnaire a useful tool to diagnose obstructive sleep apnea in the elderly? *Sleeep Medicine, 12*, 142–146. *Evidence Level IV.*

Shen, J., Barbera, J., & Shapiro, C. M. (2006). Distinguishing sleepiness and fatigue: Focus on definition and measurement. *Sleep Medicine Reviews, 10*(1), 63–76. *Evidence Level VI.*

Weaver, T. E., & Chasens, E. R. (2007). Continuous positive airway pressure treatment for sleep apnea in older adults. *Sleep Medicine Reviews, 11*(2), 99–111. *Evidence Level I.*

Weaver, T. E., Kribbs, N. B., Pack, A. I., Kline, L. R., Chugh, D. K., Maislin, G., . . . Dinges, D. F. (1997a). Night-to-night variability in CPAP use over the first three months of treatment. *Sleep, 20*(4), 278–283. *Evidence Level II.*

Weaver, T. E., Laizner, A. M., Evans, L. K., Maislin, G., Chugh, D. K., Lyon, K., . . . Dinges, D. F. (1997b). An instrument to measure functional status outcomes for disorders of excessive sleepiness. *Sleep, 20*(10), 835–843. *Evidence Level VI.*

Whitney, C. W., Enright, P. L., Newman, A. B., Bonekat, W., Foley, D., & Quan, S. F. (1998). Correlates of daytime sleepiness in 4578 elderly persons: The Cardiovascular Health Study. *Sleep, 21*(1), 27–36. *Evidence Level III.*

Young, J. S., Bourgeois, J. A., Hilty, D. M., & Hardin, K. A. (2008). Sleep in hospitalized medical patients, part 1: Factors affecting sleep. *Journal of Hospital Medicine, 3*(6), 473–482. *Evidence Level VI.*

Young, J. S., Bourgeois, J. A., Hilty, D. M., & Hardin, K. A. (2009). Sleep in hospitalized medical patients, part 2: Behavioral and pharmacological management of sleep disturbances. *Journal of Hospital Medicine, 4*(1), 50–59. *Evidence Level VI.*

Young, T., Hulton, R., Finn, L., Badr, S., & Palta, M. (1996). The gender bias in sleep apnea diagnosis. Are women missed because they have different symptoms? *Archives of Internal Medicine, 156*(21), 2445–2451. *Evidence Level VI.*

Zeitzer, J. M., Bliwise, D. L., Hernandez, B., Friedman, L., & Yesavage, J. A. (2013). Nocturia compounds nocturnal wakefulness in older individuals with insomnia. *Journal of Clinical Sleep Medicine, 9*(3), 259–262. *Evidence Level V.*

Zisberg, A., Gur-Yaish, N., & Shochat, T. (2010). Contribution of routine sleep quality in community elderly. *Sleep, 33*(4), 509–514. *Evidence Level IV.*

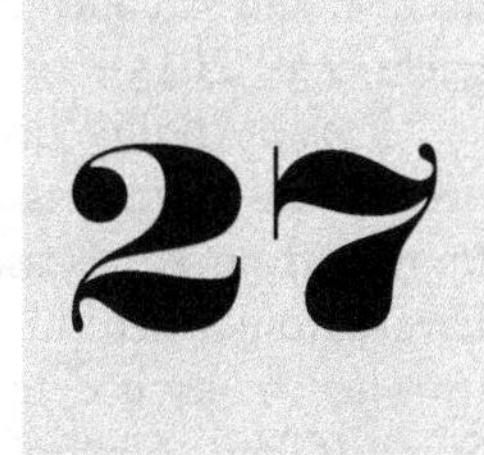

The Frail Hospitalized Older Adult

Stewart M. Bond, Rebecca Bolton, and Marie Boltz

EDUCATIONAL OBJECTIVES

On completion of this chapter, the reader should be able to:

1. Describe frailty in hospitalized older adults
2. List complications associated with frailty in hospitalized older adults
3. Discuss the importance of early recognition of frailty
4. Develop a patient-centered plan for frail hospitalized older adults

OVERVIEW

Frailty is a multidimensional geriatric syndrome characterized by multisystem dysregulation and decreased physiological reserve. The interaction of these biological abnormalities (including inflammation) results in an increased vulnerability to stressors and adverse health outcomes (Clegg, Young, Iliffe, Rikkert, & Rockwood, 2013; Song, Mitnitski, & Rockwood, 2010). Frailty is characterized by diminished strength, endurance, and reduced physiological function that increases an individual's risk for dependence on caregivers and/or death. A longitudinal study conducted among community-dwelling older adults found that the course of disability closely mirrored the prevalence of hospital admission, indicating that aggressive measures are needed to prevent complications in frail older adults during hospitalization (Gill, Gahbauer, Han, & Allore, 2015). Nurses play a central role in the detection of frailty and in providing timely interventions to prevent complications in those who are frail, both during hospitalization and the transition to the postacute setting.

BACKGROUND AND STATEMENT OF PROBLEM

Presentation and Prevalence

Frail older adults exhibit three or more of the following characteristics: low physical activity, muscle weakness, slowed performance, fatigue or poor endurance, and unintentional weight loss (Fried et al., 2001). Between 25% and 50% of people older than 85 years are estimated to be frail (Song et al., 2010) with prevalence estimates of 7% to 16% reported in noninstitutionalized, community-dwelling older adults (Fried et al., 2001). Declines in physiological reserves and resilience are the essence of being frail (Fedarko, 2011). The development of frailty involves declines in energy production, energy usage, and repair systems in the body, resulting in declines in the function of many different physiological systems (Bandeen-Roche et al., 2006). This decline in multiple systems affects the normal, complex adaptive behavior that is essential to health (Fried et al., 2009). Frail individuals are significantly more likely to have cognitive decline, memory

For a description of evidence levels cited in this chapter, see Chapter 1, "Developing and Evaluating Clinical Practice Guidelines: A Systematic Approach."

decline, and sarcopenia than nonfrail older adults (Nishiguchi et al., 2014).

Primary frailty occurs in the absence of significant overt disease, whereas *secondary* frailty is associated with known advanced disease. Although many frail older adults have chronic medical conditions and may have disability when frailty is detected, in the Cardiovascular Health Study (CHS), 63% of frail patients had no impairment in activities of daily living (ADL) and 32% had none or only one of nine chronic diseases (Fried et al., 2001). Persons with secondary frailty may have worse prognoses than those with primary frailty, as suggested by a study in which patients with diabetes, cancer, heart failure, and lung disease showed worse 4-year survival independent of features such as low weight and decreased walking (Lee, Lindquist, Segal, & Covinsky, 2006). Frailty can potentially be prevented or treated with specific modalities, such as exercise, protein-calorie supplementation, vitamin D, and reduction of polypharmacy (Morley et al., 2013). In the hospitalized older adult, the clinical presentation of frailty often includes nonspecific symptoms (e.g., extreme fatigue, unexplained weight loss, and frequent infections), and gait and balance impairment with potential falls, delirium, and functional abilities that vary day to day (Parker, Fadayevatan, & Lee, 2006).

Etiology and Epidemiology

A number of risk factors have been identified for frailty, including (a) chronic diseases, such as cardiovascular disease, diabetes, chronic kidney disease, depression, and cognitive impairment (Fried, Ferrucci, Darer, Williamson, & Anderson, 2004); (b) physiological impairments, such as activation of inflammation and coagulation systems (Walston et al., 2002); (c) anemia (Chaves et al., 2005; Roy, 2011); (d) atherosclerosis (Chaves et al., 2008); (e) autonomic dysfunction, (Varadhan et al., 2009); (f) hormonal abnormalities (Cappola, Xue, & Fried, 2009); (g) obesity (Blaum, Xue, Michelon, Semba, & Fried, 2005); (h) hypovitaminosis D in men (Shardell et al., 2009); and (i) environmental factors within the living space and the neighborhood (Xue, Fried, Glass, Laffan, & Chaves, 2008). The occurrence of frailty increases incrementally with advancing age, and is more common in older women than men and among those of lower socioeconomic status (Fried et al., 2004).

Pathophysiology

The pathophysiology of frailty is multifaceted. In addition to sarcopenia (Ferrucci, Penninx, & Volpato, 2002), a proinflammatory state that is present in cardiovascular disease, diabetes mellitus, renal insufficiency, and other diseases (Walston et al., 2002) are believed to contribute to frailty. Anemia (Chaves et al., 2005; Roy, 2011), deficiencies in anabolic hormones (e.g., androgens and growth hormone; Cappola et al., 2009), excess exposure to cortisol (Varadhan et al., 2008), insulin resistance (Barzilay et al., 2007), compromised altered immune function (Wang et al., 2010; Yao, Li, & Leng, 2011), micronutrient deficiencies, and oxidative stress (Semba et al., 2007) are also each individually associated with a higher likelihood of frailty. Thus, frailty is a consequence of cumulative decline in many physiological systems during a lifetime rather than the presence of a measurable disease state.

Outcomes Associated With Frailty

Frail older adults are at high risk of major adverse health outcomes, including disability, falls, institutionalization, hospitalization, and mortality (Fried et al., 2001; Lahousse et al., 2014). Frailty, cognitive impairment, and functional status were markers of perceived risk for negative outcomes (e.g., institutionalization, hospitalization, and death) in frail older adults (O'Caoimh et al., 2014). In older surgical patients, frailty independently predicts postoperative complications, length of stay, discharge to a skilled or assisted-living facility, and mortality (Afilalo et al., 2010; Lee, Buth, Martin, Yip, & Hirsch, 2010; Makary et al., 2010; Sundermann et al., 2011). A systematic review conducted by Sepehri et al. (2014) examined the relationship between objective frailty assessments and postoperative outcomes. Frailty, defined using multiple criteria, had a strong positive relationship with the risk of major adverse cardiac and cerebrovascular events (MACCE; odds ratio, 4.89; 95% CI [1.64, 14.60]). The authors concluded that further study is needed to determine which components of frailty are most predictive of negative postoperative outcomes before integration in risk prediction scores (Sepehri et al., 2014). In a study of older adults admitted to a Geriatric Evaluation and Management Unit (GEMU) in Australia, Dent, Chapman, Howell, Piantadosi, and Visvanathan (2014) found that psychosocial factors modify the association of frailty with adverse outcomes. Frail patients had an increased likelihood of 12-month mortality, discharge to a higher level of care, longer length of stay, and 1-month emergency rehospitalization. Psychosocial factors that increased the likelihood of adverse outcomes included anxiety, and low ratings for well-being, sense of control, social activities, and home/neighborhood satisfaction.

TABLE 27.1

The Phenotype Model: Indicators of Frailty and Measures

Indicators	Measures
Unintentional weight loss	Self-reported weight loss of 10 lbs or recorded weight loss greater than or equal to 5% per year
Exhaustion	Self-reported exhaustion on U.S. Center for Epidemiological Studies Depression Scale (3–4 days per week or most of the time)
Slow gait speed	Standardized cutoff times to walk 15 feet, stratified by sex and height
Muscle weakness	Grip strength, stratified by sex and body mass index
Low activity levels	Energy expenditure less than 383 kcal/wk (men) or less than 270 kcal/wk (women)

Frailty Models

Frailty models are underpinned by biological principles of causality and are offered to predict the clinical course and response to treatment (Bell, 2010). The two main emerging models of frailty are the phenotype model (Fried et al., 2001) and the cumulative deficit model (Rockwood et al., 2005).

The frailty phenotype proposed by Fried et al. (2001) includes five dimensions: unintentional weight loss, exhaustion, muscle weakness, slowness while walking, and low levels of activity (Table 27.1). A criticism of this model is that cognitive impairment, a highly prevalent condition associated with functional decline and disability, is not included as part of the phenotype (Rothman, Leo-Summers, & Gill, 2008). In addition, it may be difficult to use this model in hospitalized older adults whose clinical presentation may be altered by the acute illness or injury.

The cumulative deficit model views frailty as the combined effect of individual symptoms (e.g., low mood), signs (e.g., tremor), abnormal laboratory values, disease states, and disabilities (collectively referred to as deficits). This model supports the idea of reduced homoeostatic reserve, as no one deficit causes frailty but it is the accumulation of deficits that contribute to risk. Frailty, then, is viewed as a gradable syndrome (Rockwood & Mitnitski, Skoog, 2008).

ASSESSMENT OF THE PROBLEM

The International Frailty Consensus Group recommends that all individuals with significant weight loss (greater than or equal to 5%) resulting from chronic disease should be screened for frailty (Morley et al., 2013). Although many methods have been proposed in academic trials, a universally accepted screening tool for frailty in acute admissions does not exist.

Single Markers of Frailty

Grip strength and walking speed are commonly used single measures of frailty. Grip strength is evaluated as the maximum of three attempts of the dominant hand using a handheld dynamometer: low grip strength is less than 18 kg in women and less than 30 kg in men (Fairhall et al., 2008). Walking speed is measured over 6 m, with or without the use of a walking aid. Slow walking speed is defined as an inability to walk 6 m in less than or equal to 30 seconds (Smith, 1994).

Phenotypic Frailty Indices

The frailty phenotype (Fried et al., 2001), with its five indicators described earlier, is commonly used to identify frailty. Older adults with three or more of the five factors are considered to be frail, those with one or two factors as prefrail, and those without any factors as robust or not frail. Table 27.1 describes the measures associated with each indicator.

The SOF (Study of Osteoporotic Fractures) Index defines frailty as two or more of the following: weight loss (5% loss either intentional or unintentional over the past year), self-report of low energy and low mobility (unable to rise from a chair five times; Ensrud et al., 2008). The CHS Index defines frailty as three or more of the following: shrinking (unintentional weight loss of more than or equal to 4.5 kg in the past year), weakness (low grip strength), exhaustion (self-report), slowness, and low physical activity (low walking speed, defined as unable to walk 6 m in 30 seconds; Fried et al., 2001).

Multidimensional Indices

Frailty, conceptualized as an accumulation of deficits, can be assessed using a frailty index (Rockwood & Mitnitski, 2007). A frailty index allows one to quantify frailty or vulnerability resulting from multiple, interacting health-related problems (i.e., individuals with more accumulated deficits are more likely to be frail). A frailty index demonstrated greater discriminatory ability for people with moderate and severe frailty than that shown by the categorical phenotype model—a finding that has been validated independently (Kulminski et al., 2008).

A frailty index can be constructed using different numbers and types of health deficits (Searle, Mitnitski, Gahbauer, Gill, & Rockwood, 2008). It is recommended that a frailty index include at least 30 to 40 deficits to enhance its precision. Typically, the index includes information that is gathered in routine health assessments or health surveys. To score the frailty index, the deficits that are present are summed and divided by the total number of deficits on the index. Kulminski et al. (2008) created a Cumulative Deficit Index (DI) based on a set of 48 deficits, including multiple chronic medical conditions, health attitudes, symptoms, functional impairments, ADL, depression and other mental health problems, eyesight/hearing difficulties, and social support. Hubbard et al. (2011) used a frailty index based on a comprehensive geriatric assessment (FI-CGA) in conjunction with balance and mobility to assess illness and recovery in older hospitalized patients. The FI-CGA comprised 52 items covering the following: cognition, mood, motivation, health attitude, communication, strength, mobility, continence, nutrition, instrumental and basic ADL, sleep, medical problems, and medications. Similarly, Dent et al. (2014) developed and used the Frailty Index of Cumulative Deficits (FI-CD) to predict outcomes in patients admitted to a geriatric evaluation and management unit. The FI-CD included 50 multidimensional health-related deficits that were largely obtained from patients' CGAs.

SHERPA (Score Hospitalier d'Evaluation du Risque de Perte d'Autonomie) dimensions include age, falls in the previous year before hospitalization, Mini-Mental State Exam (first 21 questions), perception of health, and instrumental activities of daily living (IADL). Scores are summed and frailty is defined as scores greater than 6 out of 11.5, consistent with the category of high risk for functional decline during hospitalization (Cornette et al., 2006).

The Multidimensional Prognostic Index (MPI) is based on a CGA and includes the following components: ADL, IADL, mental status, comorbidity, nutrition, pressure ulcer risk assessment, medication number, and living status. Problems for each component are classified as: major (1 point), minor (0.5 point), and none (0 point). Scores were summed, divided by eight, and scores greater than 0.66 are graded as frailty (Pilotto et al., 2008).

Two tools are efficient for use in the busy acute care setting. The nine-point Clinical Frailty Scale is easy to use and classifies frailty status on a range from very fit to terminally ill (Dalhouse University, n.d.). The scale has shown to be valid and reliable, and highly correlated (r = 0.80) with the Frailty Index (Rockwood et al., 2005). The five-item FRAIL scale (Fatigue, Resistance, Ambulation, Illnesses, & Loss of Weight) is another tool used to screen for frailty and the risk for disability (Abellan van Kan et al., 2008). The tool inquires about whether patients are fatigued, are unable to climb a flight of stairs or walk one block, have more than five illnesses, and lost more than 5% of body weight in the past year. Three or more positive items indicate frailty.

Care of the Hospitalized Frail Older Adult

The older adult who demonstrates characteristics of frailty requires a multifaceted approach to address the potential for or actual presence of the hazards of hospitalizations. In addition to the increased predisposition to deep vein thrombosis and adverse medication effects, frail individuals are at increased risk for worsening functional status, delirium, falls, nosocomial infections, malnutrition, dehydration, immobilization, and decubitus ulcers while in the hospital (Boockvar & Meier, 2006).

Nutritional supplements, including fortified foods and essential vitamins and minerals, may be necessary (Torpy, Lynm, & Glass, 2006). Randomized controlled trials showed oral nutritional supplements during acute illness and recovery was associated with reduced non-elective hospital readmissions (Bergstrom, 2007) and in patients recovering from hip fracture, a decreased hospital length of stay (Myint et al., 2013). Ongoing oral assessment and adequate oral hygiene are standard care. Exercise and promotion of physical activity has demonstrated a decrease in length of stay and an increased likelihood of being discharged to home (de Morton, Keating, & Jeffs, 2007). Strategies to mitigate fall risk should be implemented without restricting physical activity. Nursing processes that emphasize promotion of physical and cognitive activity, nonpharmacological approaches to behavioral manifestations of distress, the avoidance of both physical restraint and the use of indwelling urinary catheters are key elements of care and may potentially benefit frail older people, particularly those with dementia or at high risk of delirium (Parker et al., 2006).

It is critical to mobilize these interventions in tandem to address the clinical complexity of the frail older adult. Multidisciplinary collaboration with physicians, dietitians, rehabilitation therapists, and social workers will facilitate these interventions. Evidence-based approaches to prevent, detect, and manage the syndromes associated with frailty are described in detail in various chapters throughout this book.

Discussions of goals of care and advance care planning are routinely indicated when the frail older person is hospitalized (Boockvar & Meier, 2006). For patients with advanced frailty, palliative care focused on relief of discomfort and enhancement of quality of life is highly appropriate. Studies suggest that patients with serious end-stage conditions, such as cancer, end-stage kidney disease, or neurodegenerative disease, have the following priorities for treatment: symptom management, measures to optimize quality of life, sense of control, minimized burden on family, and promoting relationships with loved ones (Singer, Martin, & Kelner, 1999; Steinhauser et al., 2000).

Current evidence indicates that hospital discharge planning for frail older people can be improved if interventions address family inclusion and education, communication between health care workers and family, interdisciplinary communication and ongoing support after discharge (Bauer, Fitzgerald, Haesler, & Manfrin, 2009). Interventions that combine discharge planning and discharge support (i.e., postacute health monitoring and teaching) tend to have the greatest effects (Mistiaen, Francke, & Poot, 2007). In addition to the traditional approaches that include coordination and teaching related to the management and follow-up of the acute admitting problem, discharge planning of the frail older adult requires attention to preventing future disability (Clegg et al., 2013; Parker et al., 2006). Transitional planning requires additional foci: (a) exercise, including resistance, strength, physical movement (gait and balance) training, and lingual exercise; (b) nutritional maintenance and/or supplementation; (c) maintenance of oral health; (d) environmental modifications and; (e) family and professional caregiver education (Benefield & Higbee, 2013)

Referral to postacute services is warranted to address rehabilitative needs, dental care, assistive support, and social engagement. Alerting the postacute provider to the degree and nature of the older adult's frailty status is critical to promote a smooth transition and prepare for care in the postacute setting. An important priority is modifying the living environment to enhance opportunities for independence and self-reliance. These interventions include grab bars; walk-in showers with shower seats; counter and cabinet height adjustments; wide doors and hallways; contrasting colors of counters, floors, walls, and dishes; nonslip surfaces; ramps; proper lighting; and emergency call systems (Crews & Zavotka, 2006). Physical therapy should include both resistance and aerobic exercise training (Carr, Flood, Steger-May, Schechtman, & Binder, 2006). Resistance training involves weight-lifting or weight-bearing exercises of the large skeletal muscle groups to increase lean body mass and improve strength, exercise tolerance, and walking speed (Fiatarone et al., 1994). After the older adult's condition stabilizes, a recommendation for tai chi may be considered. Tai chi is a slow and gentle exercise regimen that involves both physical movement and meditation to improve balance and gait (Adler & Roberts, 2006). Additionally, lingual exercises (i.e., isometric exercises compressing an air-filled bulb between the tongue and hard palate) may help to enhance swallowing (Robbins et al., 2005).

When a frail older adult is transferred to the nursing home, details of the treatment of the acute problem as well as supportive measures to promote functional recovery need to be communicated. Family and caregiver education are needed to address the need for use of medications, nutritional approaches, oral health, promotion of socialization, and engagement in physical activity.

CASE STUDY

Ms. T is an 88-year-old woman who was admitted to the medical unit after being brought to the emergency room from the assisted-living facility where she resides. Her admitting diagnosis is acute change in mental status. Her other medical problems include Alzheimer's disease, a history of falls, and atrial fibrillation. The emergency department reports that Ms. T has a low-grade fever and an area of consolidation in the right lower lobe. Her lab values indicate dehydration and an elevated international normalized ratio (INR). Her medications before admission included donepezil hydrochloride/Aricept, Coumadin, and Risperdal. After spending 6 hours in the emergency department because of high patient volume and demands there, Ms. T is restless and irritable on transfer to the medical unit. Her daughter, who has her power of attorney, reports that Ms. T was admitted to the assisted-living facility 6 months ago after she lost 20 pounds over several months and began to require assistance with medications, bathing, and dressing.

Ms. T's physical examination reveals a small, disheveled woman with an anxious appearance. An intravenous (IV) line is running; she is receiving hydration and antibiotics. The IV site is "camouflaged" and secured for comfort. Her oral mucosa is dry and dentition is fair (a few missing teeth). Ms. T is oriented to person and place but has difficulty with the Clock Draw test and can recall only one of three words. She is able to respond to a two-step verbal command. Her heart rate is 80 with an irregularly, irregular rhythm. She is able to rise from the chair very slowly with maximum help and states she is "too tired" and "too weak" to walk. Ms. T's balance is poor, as she sways back onto the bed, when assisted to stand. Her motor strength is diminished in all extremities; range of motion is intact. Her body mass index is 18. Ms. T's unintended weight loss,

(continued)

CASE STUDY ***(continued)***

exhaustion, muscle weakness, and low activity levels are consistent with a frailty state.

The initial plan of care developed with the input of Ms. T and her daughter includes:

- Evaluation with the geriatric consultation service with a plan to secure physical therapy consultation, nutritional evaluation, and discussion of treatment goals and advance directives
- A fall-prevention plan, including an adjustable height low bed and a room close to the nurses' station
- Careful monitoring of her INR is warranted especially with the addition of new medications
- Diligent oral care
- Careful monitoring of food and fluid intake; follow-up with the dietitian to provide dietary supplements and address food preferences
- Ongoing monitoring for delirium and implementation of nonpharmacological delirium prevention strategies
- Avoiding physical and chemical restraints
- Encouraging her daughter to bring in a few familiar items from home
- A plan for family visits/frequent presence at the bedside
- Assistance to a chair for meals and a commode for elimination. Range of motion and self-care during bathing are encouraged. Follow-up needed with physical therapy to develop a plan for ambulation, including the assistive device, as soon as possible.
- Discuss with the assisted-living facility staff the supports and resources available at discharge, including the need for postacute rehabilitation, nutritional support and monitoring, and therapeutic activities that provide social engagement, cognitive stimulation, and physical activity.

SUMMARY

Frailty has been conceptualized as a diminished capacity to withstand stress that places individuals at risk for adverse health outcomes (Boockvar & Meier, 2006). The acute care stay creates further risk for disability and other complications for the frail older adult. A multifaceted, nurse-led approach provided by a multidisciplinary team that engages family caregivers is warranted to prevent hospital-acquired complications. Hospitalization also provides an opportunity to initiate measures to promote maximum function, health, and quality of life while acknowledging the patient's unique circumstances and preferences.

NURSING STANDARD OF PRACTICE

Protocol 27.1: Frailty in the Hospitalized Older Adult

I. GOALS

To ensure that nurses in acute care are able to

A. Describe frailty in hospitalized older adults
B. List complications associated with frailty in hospitalized older adults
C. Discuss the importance of early recognition of frailty
D. Develop a patient-centered plan for frail hospitalized older adults

II. OVERVIEW

A. Frailty is a multidimensional geriatric syndrome characterized by multisystem dysregulation and decreased physiological reserve.
B. Frailty is associated with increased vulnerability to stressors.
C. Frailty is characterized by diminished strength, endurance, and reduced physiological function that increases an individual's vulnerability for developing increased dependency and/or death.
D. Hospitalization increases the risk of disability in frail older adults.
E. Nurses play a central role in the detection of frailty, timely interventions to both prevent frailty and prevent complications in those who are frail, both during hospitalization as well as the transition to the postacute setting.

(continued)

Protocol 27.1: Frailty in the Hospitalized Older Adult *(continued)*

III. BACKGROUND/STATEMENT OF PROBLEM

A. Presentation and prevalence
   1. To be considered frail, a person must have three or more of these characteristics: low physical activity, muscle weakness, slowed performance, fatigue or poor endurance, and unintentional weight loss.
   2. Between 25% and 50% of people older than 85 years are estimated to be frail with estimates of 7% to 16% reported in noninstitutionalized, community-dwelling older adults.
   3. Decline in multiple systems affects the normal complex adaptive behavior that is essential to health.
   4. *Primary* frailty occurs in the absence of significant overt disease, whereas *secondary* frailty is associated with known advanced disease.
   5. Frailty can potentially be prevented or treated with specific modalities, such as exercise, protein-calorie supplementation, vitamin D, and reduction of polypharmacy.
   6. In the hospitalized older adult, the clinical presentation of frailty often includes nonspecific symptoms, and gait and balance impairment with potential falls, delirium, and functional abilities that vary day to day.

B. Etiology and epidemiology
   1. Risk factors include (a) chronic diseases; (b) physiological impairments, such as activation of inflammation and coagulation systems; (c) anemia; (d) atherosclerosis; (e) autonomic dysfunction; (f) hormonal abnormalities; (g) obesity; (h) hypovitaminosis D in men; and (i) environmental characteristics.
   2. The occurrence of frailty increases incrementally with advancing age, and is more common in older women than men and among those of lower socioeconomic status.

C. Pathophysiology
   1. The pathophysiology of frailty is considered to be multifaceted, and it reflects a consequence of cumulative decline in many physiological systems during a lifetime.
   2. Contributors to frailty include: sarcopenia, a proinflammatory state, anemia, deficiencies in anabolic hormones, excess exposure to cortisol, insulin resistance, compromised or altered immune function, micronutrient deficiencies, and oxidative stress.

D. Outcomes of frailty
   1. Frail older adults are at high risk of disability, falls, institutionalization, hospitalization, and mortality.
   2. Frailty increases risk of MACCE.
   3. Frailty independently predicts postoperative complications, length of stay, discharge to a skilled or assisted-living facility in older surgical patients, and mortality.
   4. Psychosocial factors that increase the likelihood of adverse outcomes include anxiety, and low sense of well-being, sense of control, social activities, and home/neighborhood satisfaction.

E. Frailty models
   1. The frailty phenotype proposed by Fried et al. includes five dimensions: unintentional weight loss, exhaustion, muscle weakness, slowness while walking, and low levels of activity.
   2. The cumulative deficit model views frailty as the combined effect of individual symptoms (e.g., low mood); signs (e.g., tremor); and abnormal laboratory values, disease states, and disabilities (collectively referred to as deficits

IV. ASSESSMENT OF FRAILTY

A. Single markers of frailty
   1. Grip strength is evaluated as the maximum of three attempts of the dominant hand using a hand-held dynamometer: low grip strength less than 18 kg (women), less than 30 kg (men).
   2. Walking speed is measured over 6 m, with or without the use of a walking aid. Slow walking speed is defined as unable to walk 6 m in 30 seconds.

B. Phenotypic frailty indices
   1. The frailty phenotype, with its five indicators, is commonly used to identify frailty. Those with three or more of the five factors are considered to be frail, those with one or two factors as prefrail, and those with no factors as not frail or robust older adults.

(continued)

Protocol 27.1: Frailty in the Hospitalized Older Adult *(continued)*

2. The SOF Index (Study of Osteoporotic Fractures frailty scale) defines frailty as two or more of: weight loss (5% loss either intentional or unintentional over the past year) and self-report of low energy and low mobility (unable to rise from a chair five times).
3. The FRAIL Index classifies frailty as three or more of fatigue (self-report), resistance (unable to rise from a chair five times), ambulation (slow walking speed), illnesses (greater than or equal to five illnesses on CCI), and loss of weight of 5% or more in the past year.
4. The CHS Index defines frailty as three or more of shrinking (unintentional weight loss of greater than or equal to 4.5 kg in the last year), weakness (low grip strength), exhaustion (self-report), slowness, and low physical activity (low walking speed, defined as unable to walk 6 m in 30 seconds).

C. Multidimensional indices
1. A frailty index can be constructed using different numbers and types of health deficits.
2. The DI based on a set of 48 deficits, including multiple chronic medical conditions, health attitudes, symptoms, functional impairments, ADL, depression and other mental health problems, eyesight/hearing difficulties, and social support
3. The FI-CGA comprises 52 items covering the following: cognition, mood, motivation, health attitude, communication, strength, mobility, continence, nutrition, instrumental and basic ADL, sleep, medical problems, and medications.
4. The FI-CD includes 50 multidimensional health-related deficits largely obtained from patients' CGAs.
5. SHERPA dimensions include age, falls in the previous year before hospitalization, Mini-Mental State Exam (first 21 questions), perception of health, and IADL.
6. The MPI components include ADL, IADL, mental status, nutrition, pressure ulcer risk assessment, number of medications, and living status.
7. The 9-point Clinical Frailty Scale is easy to use and classifies frailty status on a range from very fit to terminally ill. The scale has shown to be valid and reliable, highly correlated (r = .80) with the Frailty Index.
8. The five-item FRAIL scale is another tool used to screen for frailty and the risk for disability.

V. CARE OF THE HOSPITALIZED FRAIL OLDER ADULT

A. Multifaceted plans of care: require multidisciplinary collaboration
1. Evaluate need for nutritional supplements, including fortified food and supplements of essential vitamins and minerals mass.
2. Oral assessment and adequate oral hygiene
3. Promote self-care, continence, mobility, cognitive stimulation. Avoid restraints.
4. Avoid indwelling urinary catheters.
5. Implement strategies to decrease fall risk.

B. Involvement of patient and family in decision making
1. Establish clear goals of care based on patient preferences and needs.
2. For patients with advanced frailty, offer palliative care focused on relief of discomfort and enhancement of quality of life.
3. Whenever possible, combine discharge planning and discharge support (postacute follow-up).
4. Plan to prevent future disability: (i) exercise, including resistance, strength, physical movement (gait and balance) training, and lingual exercise; (ii) nutritional maintenance and/or supplement; (iii) maintenance of oral health; (iv) environmental modifications; and (v) family and professional caregiver education.

C. Referral to postacute services is warranted to address rehabilitative needs, dental care, assistive serves, social engagement, and environmental home safety.

D. Communication to the postacute provider details the treatment of acute problems as well as supportive measures to promote functional recovery.

E. Family and caregiver education is needed to address the need for use of medications, nutritional approaches, oral health, promotion of socialization, and engagement in physical activity.

(continued)

Protocol 27.1: Frailty in the Hospitalized Older Adult *(continued)*

VI. EVALUATION/EXPECTED OUTCOMES

A. Patient outcomes
   1. Improved functional and nutritional outcomes
   2. Delirium detection, avoidance, and abatement
   3. Prevention of complications: falls, pressure ulcers, adverse drug events
   4. Less hospital readmissions and decreased length of stay

B. Clinician outcomes
   1. Assessment, identification, and management of older adults susceptible to or experiencing frailty
   2. Documentation and communication of the patient's functional and cognitive capacity, interventions used, and outcomes
   3. Competence in preventive and restorative strategies for preserving independence and function
   4. Educate older adult and family caregiver(s) on intervention strategies to preserve function and reduce task demand in the preferred home or care setting.

C. Organizational outcomes
   1. Assessment of frailty as indicated
   2. Prompt and accurate referral for evaluation of frailty
   3. Increase in prevalence of patients who leave hospital care facility or professional homecare with baseline or improved functional status
   4. Support of institutional policies programs that promote function, for example, caregiver educational efforts and walking programs
   5. Evidence of continued interdisciplinary assessments and evaluation of care
   6. Environmental approaches that support function and comfort

ABBREVIATIONS

ADL	Activities of daily living
CCI	Charlson's comorbidity index
CHS	Cardiovascular Health Study
DI	Cumulative Deficit Index
FI-CD	Frailty Index of Cumulative Deficits
FI-CGA	Frailty Index based on a comprehensive geriatric assessment
FRAIL scale	Fatigue, Resistance, Ambulation, Illnesses, & Loss of Weight scale
IADL	Instrumental activities of daily living
MACCE	Major adverse cardiac and cerebrovascular events
MPI	Multidimensional Prognostic Index
SHERPA	Score Hospitalier d'Evaluation du Risque de Perte d'Autonomie
SOF	Study of Osteoporotic Fractures

RESOURCES

FRAILTY.NET
www.frailty.net

Frailty Project
www.frailtyproject.com

International Conference on Frailty and Sarcopenia Research
frailty-sarcopenia.com

REFERENCES

Abellan van Kan, G., Rolland, Y., Bergman, H., Morley, J. E., Kritchevsky, S. B., & Vellas, B. (2008). The I.A.N.A Task Force on frailty assessment of older people in clinical practice. *Journal of Nutrition Health and Aging,* 12(1), 29–37. *Evidence Level V.*

Adler, P. A., & Roberts, B. L. (2006). The use of tai chi to improve health in older adults. *Orthopaedic Nursing, 25*(2), 122–126. *Evidence Level V.*

Afilalo, J., Eisenberg, M. J., Morin, J. F., Bergman, H., Monette, J., Noiseux, N., . . . Boivin, J. F. (2010). Gait speed as an incremental predictor of mortality and major morbidity in elderly patients undergoing cardiac surgery. *Journal of the American College of Cardiology, 56*(20), 1668–1676. *Evidence Level IV.*

Bandeen-Roche, K., Xue, Q. L., Ferrucci, L., Walston, J., Guralnik, J. M., Chaves, P., . . . Fried, L. P. (2006). Phenotype of frailty: Characterization in the women's health and aging studies. *Journals of Gerontology. Series A, Biological Sciences and Medical Sciences, 61*(3), 262–266. *Evidence Level IV.*

Barzilay, J. I., Blaum, C., Moore, T., Xue, Q. L., Hirsch, C. H., Walston, J. D., & Fried, L. P. (2007). Insulin resistance and inflammation as precursors of frailty: The Cardiovascular Health Study. *Archives of Internal Medicine, 167*(7), 635–641. *Evidence Level IV.*

Bauer, M., Fitzgerald, L., Haesler, E., & Manfrin, M. (2009). Hospital discharge planning for frail older people and their family. Are we delivering best practice? A review of the evidence. *Journal of Clinical Nursing, 18*(18), 2539–2546. *Evidence Level V.*

Bell, J. (2010). Redefining disease. *Clinical Medicine, 10*(6), 584–594. *Evidence Level V.*

Benefield, L. E., & Higbee, R. L. (n.d.). *Frailty and its implications for care.* Retrieved from http://consultgerirn.org/topics/frailty_and_its_implications_for_care_new/want_to_know_more. *Evidence Level V.*

Bergstrom, N. (2007). Oral nutritional supplements during acute illness and recovery reduced non-elective hospital readmissions in older patients. *Evidence-Based Nursing, 10*(3), 81. *Evidence Level II.*

Blaum, C. S., Xue, Q. L., Michelon, E., Semba, R. D., & Fried, L. P. (2005). The association between obesity and the frailty syndrome in older women: The Women's Health and Aging Studies. *Journal of the American Geriatrics Society, 53*(6), 927–934. *Evidence Level IV.*

Boockvar, K. S., & Meier, D. E. (2006). Palliative care for frail older adults: "There are things I can't do anymore that I wish I could." *Journal of the American Medical Association, 296*(18), 2245–2253. *Evidence Level V.*

Cappola, A. R., Xue, Q. L., & Fried, L. P. (2009). Multiple hormonal deficiencies in anabolic hormones are found in frail older women: The Women's Health and Aging studies. *Journal of Gerontology. Series A, Biological Sciences and Medical Sciences, 64*(2), 243–248. *Evidence Level IV.*

Carr, D. B., Flood, K., Steger-May, K., Schechtman, K. B., & Binder, E. F. (2006). Characteristics of frail older adult drivers. *Journal of the American Geriatrics Society, 54*(7), 1125–1129. *Evidence Level IV.*

Chaves, P. H., Semba, R. D., Leng, S. X., Woodman, R. C., Ferrucci, L., Guralnik, J. M., & Fried, L. P. (2005). Impact of anemia and cardiovascular disease on frailty status of community-dwelling older women: The Women's Health and Aging Studies I and II. *Journals of Gerontology. Series A, Biological Sciences and Medical Sciences, 60*(6), 729–735. *Evidence Level IV.*

Chaves, P. H., Varadhan, R., Lipsitz, L. A., Stein, P. K., Windham, B. G., Tian, J., . . . Fried, L. P. (2008). Physiological complexity underlying heart rate dynamics and frailty status in community-dwelling older women. *Journal of the American Geriatrics Society, 56*(9), 1698–703. *Evidence Level IV.*

Clegg, A., Young, J., Iliffe, S., Rikkert, M. O., & Rockwood, K. (2013). Frailty in elderly people. *Lancet, 381,* 752–762. *Evidence Level V.*

Cornette, P., Swine, C., Malhomme, B., Gillet, J. B., Meert, P., & D'Hoore, W. (2006). Early evaluation of the risk of functional decline following hospitalization of older patients: Development of a predictive tool. *European Journal of Public Health, 16,* 203–208. *Evidence Level IV.*

Crews, D. E., & Zavotka, S. (2006). Aging, disability, and frailty: Implications for universal design. *Journal of Physiological Anthropology, 25*(1), 113–118. *Evidence Level V.*

Dalhouse University Faculty of Medicine Geriatric Medicine Research. (n.d.). *Clinical Frailty Scale.* Retrieved from http://geriatricresearch.medicine.dal.ca/clinical_frailty_scale.htm. *Evidence Level V.*

de Morton, N. A., Keating, J. L., & Jeffs, K. (2007). Exercise for acutely hospitalized older medical patients. *Cochrane Database of Systematic Reviews, 2007*(1), CD005955. *Evidence Level I.*

Dent, E., Chapman, I., Howell, S., Piantadosi, C., & Visvanathan, R. (2014). Frailty and functional decline indices predict poor outcomes in hospitalized older people. *Age and Ageing, 43,* 477–484. *Evidence Level IV.*

Ensrud, K. E., Ewing, S. E., Taylor, B. C., Fink, H. A., Cawthon, P. M., Stone, K. L., . . . Cummings, S. R. (2008). Comparison of 2 frailty indexes for prediction of falls, disability, fractures, and death in older women. *Archives of Internal Medicine, 168*(4), 382–389. *Evidence Level IV.*

Fairhall, N., Aggar, C., Kurrle, S. E., Sherrington, C., Lord, S., Lockwood, K., . . . Cameron, I. D. (2008). Frailty Intervention Trial (FIT). *BMC Geriatrics, 8.* Retrieved from http://bmcgeriatr.biomedcentral.com/articles/10.1186/1471-2318-8-27. *Evidence Level II.*

Fedarko, N. S. (2011). The biology of aging and frailty. *Clinical Geriatric Medicine, 7*(1), 27–37. *Evidence Level V.*

Ferrucci, L., Penninx, B. W., & Volpato, S. (2002). Change in muscle strength explains accelerated decline of physical function in older women with high interleukin-6 serum levels. *Journal of the American Geriatrics Society, 50,* 1947–1955. *Evidence Level IV.*

Fiatarone, M. A., O'Neill, E. F., Ryan, N. D., Clements, K. M., Solares, G. R., Nelson, M. E., . . . Evans, W. J. (1994). Exercise training and nutritional supplementation for physical frailty in very elderly people. *New England Journal of Medicine, 330*(25), 1769–1775. *Evidence Level II.*

Fried, L. P., Ferrucci, L., Darer, J., Williamson, J. D., & Anderson, G. (2004). Untangling the concepts of disability, frailty, and comorbidity: Implications for improved targeting and care. *Journals of Gerontology. Series A, Biological Sciences and Medical Sciences 59,* 255–263. *Evidence Level IV.*

Fried, L. P., Tangen, C. M., Walston, J., Newman, A. B., Hirsch, C., Gottdiener, J., . . . McBurnie, M. A. (2001). Frailty in older adults: Evidence for a phenotype. *Journals of Gerontology. Series A, Biological Sciences and Medical Sciences, 56*(3), M146–M156. *Evidence Level IV.*

Fried, L. P., Xue, Q. L., Cappola, A. R., Ferrucci, L., Chaves, P., Varadhan, R., . . . Bandeen-Roche, K. (2009). Nonlinear multisystem physiological dysregulation associated with frailty in older women: Implications for etiology and treatment. *Journals of Gerontology. Series A, Biological Sciences and Medical Sciences, 64*(10), 1049–1057. *Evidence Level IV.*

Gill, T. M., Gahbauer, E. A., Han, L., & Allore, H. G. (2015). The role of intervening hospital admissions on trajectories of disability in the last year of life: Prospective cohort study of older people. *British Medical Journal, 350,* h2361. *Evidence Level IV.*

Hubbard, R. E., Eeles, E. M. P., Rockwood, M. R. H., Fallah, N., Ross, E., Mitnitski, A., & Rockwood, K. (2011). Assessing balance and mobility to track illness and recovery in older inpatients. *Journal of General Internal Medicine, 26*(12), 1471–1478. *Evidence Level IV.*

Kulminski, A. M., Ukraintseva, S. V., Kulminskaya, I. V., Arbeev, K. G., Land, K., & Yashin, A. I. (2008). Cumulative deficits better characterize susceptibility to death in elderly people than phenotypic frailty: Lessons from the Cardiovascular Health Study. *Journal of the American Geriatrics Society, 56,* 898–903. *Evidence Level IV.*

Lahousse, L., Maes, B., Ziere, G., Loth, D. W., Verlinden, V. J., Zillikens, M. C., . . . Stricker, B. H. (2014). Adverse outcomes of frailty in the elderly: The Rotterdam Study. *European Journal of Epidemiology, 29,* 419–427. *Evidence Level IV.*

Lee, D. H., Buth, K. J., Martin, B. J., Yip, A. M., & Hirsch, G. M. (2010). Frail patients are at increased risk for mortality and prolonged institutional care after cardiac surgery. *Circulation, 121,* 973–978. *Evidence Level IV.*

Lee, S. J., Lindquist, K., Segal, M. R., & Covinsky, K. E. (2006). Development and validation of a prognostic index for 4-year mortality in older adults. *Journal of the American Medical Association, 295,* 801–808. *Evidence Level IV.*

Makary, M. A., Segev, D. L., Pronovost, P. J., Syin, D., Bandeen-Roche, K., Patel, P., . . . Fried, L. P. (2010). Frailty as a predictor of surgical outcomes in older patients. *Journal of the American College of Surgeons, 210,* 901–908. *Evidence Level IV.*

Mistiaen, P., Francke, A., & Poot, E. (2007). Interventions aimed at reducing problems in adult patients discharged from hospital to home: A systematic meta-review. *BMC Health Services Research, 7*(1), 47. *Evidence Level I.*

Morley, J. E., Vellas, B., van Kan, G. A., Anker, S. D., Bauer, J. M., Roberto Bernabei, R., . . . Walston, J. (2013). Frailty consensus: A call to action. *Journal of the American Medical Directors Association, 14*(6), 392–397. *Evidence Level VI.*

Myint, M. W., Wu, J., Wong, E., Chan, S. P., To, T. S., Chau, M. W., & Au, K. S. (2013). Clinical benefits of oral nutritional supplementation for elderly hip fracture patients: A single blind randomized controlled trial. *Age and Ageing, 42,* 39–45. *Evidence Level II.*

Nishiguchi, S., Yamada, M., Fukutani, N., Adachi, D., Tashiro, Y., Hotta, T., . . . Aoyama, T. (2014). Differential association of phenotypic frailty with two key outcomes: Cognitive decline and sarcopenia. *Journal of the American Medical Directors Association, 16*(2), 1–5. *Evidence Level IV.*

O'Caoimh, R., Gao, Y., Svendrovski, A., Healy, E., O'Connell, E., O'Keeffe, G., . . . Molloy, W. D. (2014). Screening for markers of frailty and perceived risk of adverse outcomes using the Risk Instrument for Screening in the Community (RISC). *BMC Geriatrics, 14,* 104. *Evidence Level IV.*

Parker, S. G., Fadayevatan, R., & Lee, S. D. (2006). Acute hospital care for frail older people. *Age & Ageing, 35,* 551–552. *Evidence Level V.*

Pilotto, A., Ferrucci, L., Franceschi, M., Sancarlo, D., Bazzano, S., Copetti, M., . . . Ferrucci, L. (2008). Development and validation of a multidimensional prognostic index for one-year mortality from comprehensive geriatric assessment in hospitalized older patients. *Rejuvenation Research, 11,* 151–161. *Evidence Level IV.*

Robbins, J., Gangnon, R. E., Theis, S. M., Kays, S. A., Hewitt, A. L., & Hind, J. A. (2005). The effects of lingual exercise on swallowing in older adults. *Journal of the American Geriatrics Society, 53*(9), 1483–1489. *Evidence Level III.*

Rockwood, K., & Mitnitski A. (2008). Frailty in relation to the accumulation of deficits. *Journals of Gerontology. Series A, Biological Sciences and Medical Sciences, 62,* 722–727. *Evidence Level IV.*

Rockwood, K., & Mitnitski, A. (2011). Frailty defined by deficit accumulation and geriatric medicine defined by frailty. *Clinical Geriatric Medicine, 27*(1), 17–26. *Evidence Level V.*

Rockwood, K., Song, X., MacKnight, C., Bergman, H., Hogan, D. B., McDowell, I., & Mitnitski, A. (2005). A global clinical measure of fitness and frailty in elderly people. *Canadian Medical Association Journal, 173,* 489–549. *Evidence Level IV.*

Rockwood, K., Stadnyk, K., MacKnight, C., McDowell, I., Hebert, R., & Hogan, D. B. (1999). A brief clinical instrument to classify frailty in elderly people. *Lancet, 353,* 205–206. *Evidence Level IV.*

Rothman, M. D., Leo-Summers, L., & Gill, T. M. (2008). Prognostic significance of potential frailty criteria. *Journal of the American Geriatrics Society, 56,* 2211–2216. *Evidence Level IV.*

Roy, C. N. (2011). Anemia in frailty. *Clinical Geriatric Medicine, 27*(1), 67–78. *Evidence Level V.*

Searle, S. D., Mitnitski, A., Gahbauer, E. A., Gill, T. M., & Rockwood, K. (2008). A standard procedure for creating a frailty index. *BMC Geriatrics, 8,* 24. *Evidence Level IV.*

Semba, R. D., Ferrucci, L., Sun, K., Walston, J., Varadhan, R., Guralnik, J. M., & Fried, L. P. (2007). Oxidative stress and severe walking disability among older women. *American Journal of Medicine, 120*(12), 1084–1089. *Evidence Level IV.*

Sepehri, A., Beggs, T., Hassan, A., Rigatto, C., Shaw-Daigle, C., Tangri, N., & Arora, R. C. (2014). Systematic review: The impact of frailty on outcomes after cardiac surgery. *Journal of Thoracic and Cardiovascular Surgery, 148*(6), 3110–3117. *Evidence Level I.*

Shardell, M., Hicks, G. E., Miller, R. R., Kritchevsky, S., Andersen, D., Bandinelli, S., . . . Ferrucci, L. (2009). Association of low vitamin D levels with the frailty syndrome in men and women. *Journals of Gerontology. Series A, Biological Sciences and Medical Sciences, 64*(1), 69–75. *Evidence Level IV.*

Singer, P. A., Martin, D. K., & Kelner, M. (1999). Quality end-of-life care: Patients' perspectives. *Journal of the American Medical Association, 281,* 163–168. *Evidence Level IV.*

Smith, R. (1994). Validation and reliability of the Elderly Mobility Scale. *Physiotherapy, 80*(11), 744–747. *Evidence Level IV.*

Song, X., Mitnitski, A., & Rockwood, K. (2010). Prevalence and 10-year outcomes of frailty in older adults in relation to deficit accumulation. *Journal of the American Geriatrics Society, 58*(4), 681–687. *Evidence Level IV.*

Steinhauser, K. E., Christakis, N. A., Clipp, E. C., McNeilly, M., McIntyre, L., & Tulsky, J. A. (2000). Factors considered important at the end of life by patients, family, physicians, and other care providers. *Journal of the American Medical Association, 284*, 2476–2482. *Evidence Level IV.*

Sundermann, S., Dademasch, A., Praetorius, J., Kempfert, J., Dewey, T., Falk, V., . . . Walther, T. (2011). Comprehensive assessment of frailty for elderly high-risk patients undergoing cardiac surgery. *European Journal of Cardiothoracic Surgery, 39*, 33–37. *Evidence Level IV.*

Torpy, J. M., Lynm, C., & Glass, R. M. (2006). Frailty in older adults. *Journal of the American Medical Association, 296*(18), 2280. *Evidence Level V.*

Varadhan, R., Chaves, P. H., Lipsitz, L. A., Stein, P. K., Tian, J., Windham, B. G., . . . Fried, L. P. (2009). Frailty and impaired cardiac autonomic control: New insights from principal components aggregation of traditional heart rate variability indices. *Journals of Gerontology. Series A, Biological Sciences and Medical Sciences, 64*(6), 682–687. *Evidence Level IV.*

Varadhan, R., Walston, J., Cappola, A. R., Carlson, M. C., Wand, G. S., & Fried, L. P. (2008). Higher levels and blunted diurnal variation of cortisol in frail older women. *Journals of Gerontology, Series A, Biological Sciences and Medical Sciences, 63*, 190–195. *Evidence Level IV.*

Walston, J., McBurnie, M. A., Newman, A., Tracy, R. P., Kop, W. J., Hirsch, C. H., . . . Fried, L. P. (2002). Frailty and activation of the inflammation and coagulation systems with and without clinical comorbidities: Results from the Cardiovascular Health Study. *Archives of Internal Medicine, 162*(20), 2333–2341. *Evidence Level IV.*

Wang, G. C., Talor, M. V., Rose, N. R., Cappola, A. R., Chiou, R. B., & Weiss, C. (2010). Thyroid autoantibodies are associated with a reduced prevalence of frailty in community-dwelling older women. *Journal of Clinical Endocrinology and Metabolism, 95*, 1161–1168. *Evidence Level IV.*

Xue, Q. L., Fried, L. P., Glass, T. A., Laffan, A., & Chaves, P. H. (2008). Life-space constriction, development of frailty, and the competing risk of mortality: The Women's Health and Aging Study I. *American Journal of Epidemiology, 167*(2), 240–248. *Evidence Level IV.*

Yao, X., Li, H., & Leng, S. X. (2011). Inflammation and immune system alterations in frailty. *Clinical Geriatric Medicine, 27*(1), 79–87. *Evidence Level V.*

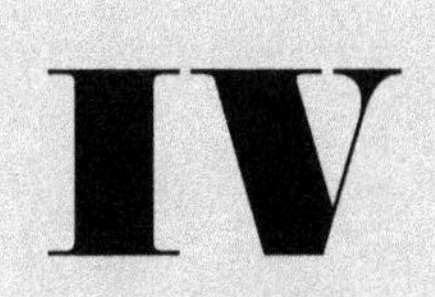

Interventions in Specialty Practice

Substance Misuse and Alcohol Use Disorders

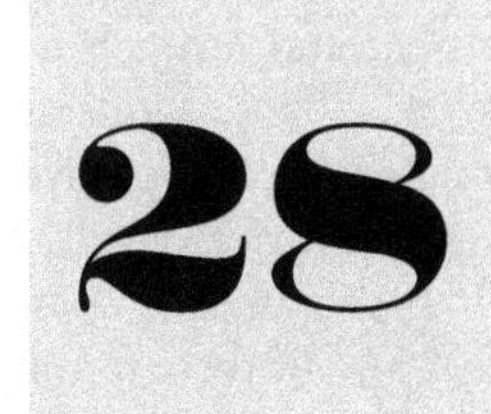

Madeline A. Naegle and Donna McCabe

EDUCATIONAL OBJECTIVES

On completion of this chapter, the reader should be able to:

1. Describe common patterns of substance use in older adults
2. Recognize common substance use disorders diagnosed in older adults
3. Outline steps for screening for substance use disorders in older adults
4. Discuss the stepwise assessment and rationale for identifying a substance use disorder
5. Analyze intervention strategies for substance use disorders in older adults
6. List potential resources on substance-related disorders for older adults and their families

OVERVIEW

Evidence of alcohol and drug use by persons aged 50 years and older is increasing as more people live longer, continue community living, and continue substance use habits established in youth and middle adulthood. Approximately, 57 million persons aged 50 to 64 years now live in the United States, and there are another 37.8 million persons aged 65 years and older. The projected increase in persons aged 65 years and older is expected to double from 40.3 million in 2010 reaching 83.7 million by 2050 (U.S. Census Bureau, 2014). Population growth predicts greater numbers of older adults with substance-related problems, perhaps as many as 5.7 million by 2020, and nurses should be prepared to identify and intervene with these health problems (Han, Gfroerer, Colliver, & Penne, 2009). The estimated one third of the older population who are minority group members will also grow. Drug and alcohol use in minorities are grossly understudied and nursing interventions with these groups of older adults should be culturally competent and tailored to substance use patterns (Andrews, 2008; Grant et al., 2004).

BACKGROUND AND STATEMENT OF PROBLEM

Health care problems linked to substance use and excess alcohol consumption are costly to society with direct and indirect economic costs, including costs of illness ($24.6 billion) and crime ($21 billion) estimated in 2006 (Bouchery, Harwood, Sacks, Simon, & Brewer, 2011). Illicit use of opioids costs another $50 billion (Hansen, Oster, Woody, & Sullivan, 2011). Nearly 22% of community-dwelling older adults use potentially addictive prescription medication (Simoni-Wastila & Yang, 2006), and risks for psychological and/or physical dependence associated with this phenomenon are considerable (Simoni-Wastila, Zuckerman, Singhal, Briesacher, & Hsu, 2005). These costs are anticipated to rise as the middle-aged population, high users of analgesics, grows (Wu & Blazer, 2011).

The drug most commonly misused by older adults is alcohol, followed by nicotine and psychoactive prescription drugs. More and more older people report using marijuana (Moore et al., 2009). Although moderate alcohol use by adults has been inversely associated with the risk

For a description of evidence levels cited in this chapter, see Chapter 1, "Developing and Evaluating Clinical Practice Guidelines: A Systematic Approach."

for cardiovascular heart disease, findings have been inconsistent and research on older adults is limited (Mukamal et al., 2006). Moderate alcohol use has also been linked to improved cognitive function in both older men and women (McDougall, Becker, Delville,Vaughn, & Acee, 2010; Stampfer, Kang, Chen, Cherry, & Grodstein, 2005), but these findings should not be the basis for nonalcohol consumers to begin drinking in late life. Similarly, older adults treated for alcohol use disorders earlier in life are at risk if they return to drinking. Excess alcohol use can result in high personal and medical costs at all ages but especially so for older adults. Alcohol-attributable conditions are often not recognized and reported as such, resulting in underestimation, although almost 12% of nursing home admissions are attributable to excessive drinking (Substance Abuse and Mental Health Services Administration [SAMHSA], 2010). Of persons seen in primary care who are older than 60 years, 15% of men and 12% of women regularly drank in excess of the National Institute Alcohol Abuse and Alcoholism (NIAAA) recommended levels (i.e., one drink per day and no more than three drinks on any one occasion; Fink, Elliott, Tsia, & Beck, 2005). Heavy consumption has been shown to decrease the likelihood that older people will use preventive medical services, such as glaucoma screening, vaccinations, and mammograms (Fink et al., 2005). This population is at risk for falls, motor vehicle accidents, and other unintentional injuries (NIAAA, 2015). Looking to the future, of the estimated 57 million late middle-aged persons (50–64 years old), 14% are drinking heavily, with 9% of them "at-risk" drinkers, and 23% reporting binge drinking (consumption of four to five drinks on an occasion; Blazer & Wu, 2009; Merrick et al., 2008).

The burden of disease linked to tobacco use is the heaviest among older individuals and the leading cause of premature death for those (Sachs-Ericsson, Collins, Schmidt, & Zvolensky, 2011) who have smoked the longest and have the most health problems. In 2004, 18.5 million Americans older than 45 years smoked, (about 42% of all adult smokers) and in 2001/2002, 14% of adults older than 65 years reported tobacco use in the prior month (Moore et al., 2009). Smoking-related deaths number 300,000 annually in this age group (Centers for Disease Control and Prevention [CDC], 2009).

As baby boomers age, their lifetime illicit drug use is anticipated to continue at levels similar to their use in younger years, increasing the number of persons 55 years and older using illicit drugs like marijuana and cocaine; (National Institute on Drug Abuse [NIDA], 2010). The number of persons aged 50 years and older who use marijuana is projected to increase from 4.2%. Use of illicit drugs will increase from 4.7% (4.3 million), and nonmedical use of psychotherapeutic drugs is projected to increase from 4.2% (SAMHSA, 2010). There have been dramatic increases in prescribing and use of opioid analgesics and synthetic opioids over the past decade. There is evidence of accidental overdose in adolescent, adult, and older adults. Although the rates of prescription drug misuse and abuse is lower among older adults, associated mortality rates for drugs like oxycodone, fentanyl, oxymorphone, tramadol, and related drugs has been higher among persons of older age. The drugs most commonly used in this age group are tranquilizers, sedatives, and opioids obtained by prescription. This pattern is more common for those in palliative care, and persons with noncommunicable diseases accompanied by chronic pain, placing them at high risk for negative outcomes (Moore et al., 2009; West, Severtson, Green, & Dart, 2015).

Patterns of substance use vary in subpopulations and some differences among groups are noteworthy. The success of antiretroviral therapies has extended life, and more than half of HIV cases in the United States will soon be persons 50 years and older (Justice, 2010). Older individuals who are HIV positive report higher rates of both alcohol and illicit drug use. One American sample recorded rates of substance use at 22%, alcohol use at 14% and tobacco use at 39.5% in HIV-positive persons aged 50 to 59 years (Vance, Mugavero, Willig, & Raper, 2011).

Differences in alcohol use by race, for example, are more evident with age. Although Caucasian adults outnumber African American drinkers, low-income, older African American males have the highest risk for alcoholism and related problems as well as more legal problems than Whites (Zapolski, Pedersen, McCarthy, & Smith, 2014) this is evident in men older than 50 years.

Given the need for treatment, coupled with older adults' reluctance to seek help for mental health problems (less than 3% of older people visit a mental health professional) nurses and health professionals caring for older adults in all settings need to know how to screen for a substance use disorder (Bartels et al., 2004). Psychiatric disorders often co-occur with alcohol use and misuse in older adults, with prevalence rates ranging from 12% to 30% (Oslin, 2005); depression occurrs both independently and as a consequence of excess drinking, and is frequent in male smokers (Kinnunen et al., 2006).

The metabolic changes of aging are key to health problems related to drug or alcohol use, resulting in increased morbidity in advancing age. Older persons respond differently to alcohol because of decreased total body water and rates of alcohol metabolism in the gastrointestinal tract; increased sensitivity to alcohol combined with decreased tolerance (U.S. Department of Health and Human Services [USDHHS], 2004a). Most alcohol consumers drink less as they age, and only 4.1% of those 65% to 75% and 1.6% of those older than 75 years report a lifetime alcohol use disorder (Wu & Blazer, 2014). More dramatic behavioral changes are evident at lower doses of all drugs and adverse physical responses result in morbidity or mortality, curtailing intake. Social and legal problems occur more frequently and are more pronounced than in younger people, especially for older women (Blow & Barry, 2003). Because the *Diagnostic and Statistical Manual of Mental Disorders* (*DSM-5*; American Psychiatric Association, 2013) criteria may be less applicable to older adults, these criteria must be interpreted and applied in age-appropriate ways. Even when a person does not meet the *DSM-5* criteria for a moderate or severe use disorder, alcohol consumption at levels of more than seven drinks weekly and more than three drinks at a time for persons older than 65 years can result in health consequences. Excess alcohol use compromises health by interfering with the absorption and utilization of prescribed drugs and nutrients. Excessive alcohol consumption may place the older individual at risk for falls, self-neglect, and diminished cognitive capacity. Long-term excess alcohol use is related to the development of common medical problems such as sleep disorders, restlessness and agitation, liver function abnormalities, pneumonia, pancreatitis, gastrointestinal bleeding, and trauma as well as chronic diseases, particularly neuropsychiatric and digestive disorders, diabetes, cardiovascular disease, and pancreatic or head and neck cancer (Rehm et al., 2009).

ASSESSMENT OF SUBSTANCE USE DISORDERS

Substance use and related disorders involve 10 classes of drugs and are categorized as mild, moderate, or severe according to the number of symptoms described in 11 diagnostic criteria (see as follows). Older people may treat negative and physical and psychological symptoms by "self-medicating" with alcohol and other drugs. A significant number of older adults continue heavy alcohol consumption at 60 years and older (Merrick et al., 2008).Whether a disorder is diagnosed and categorized as mild, moderate, or severe depends on the nature and number of symptoms demonstrated. Pathological patterns of use, including social and health problems, can be linked to frequency of the substance used; the length of time of use (a 12-month period or more), and the specific substance. Most individuals who have severe substance use disorders have developed patterns of alcohol/and or drug use before age 60 years, with one half to two thirds of older adult alcoholics having developed moderate to severe problems early in life. "Late-onset alcoholism" and patterns of prescription drug abuse, marked by increased use and/or overreliance on either, can emerge secondary to losses, chronic illness, and psychological traumas. Social use of alcohol, for example, may change to "at risk" drinking or prescription use to drug misuse when someone has lost a spouse, partner, or job; is estranged from family or is facing serious illness. Risks are higher for those with any combination of circumstances listed.

Alcohol Use Disorders

The most common substance use disorders in older adults are those of alcohol use, including interactions of alcohol with prescription and over-the-counter (OTC) drugs (Wu & Blazer, 2014).

A substance use disorder is diagnosed when a maladaptive pattern of use is evidenced by 11 criteria occurring over a 12-month period (modified from American Psychiatric Association [APA], 2013). Behaviors indicate impaired control over use of a substance (Criteria 1–4), with an inability to cut down on use, and persistent failures at control (Criterion 2), the use and recovery from use may occupy significant periods of time (Criterion 3) with the result that other role obligations are neglected (Criterion 5). Craving or an intense desire to use a drug may occur (Criterion 4) and use persists despite social and interpersonal problems worsened by use (Criterion 6); there is a growing tendency to withdraw from work or recreational activities (Criterion 7).

"At-risk" drinking is a pattern that may not appear to cause alcohol-related problems at first but, with this continued pattern, can result in harmful consequences to the user or others. Regular alcohol and tobacco use, for example, is linked to insomnia (Tibbitts, 2008), a common complaint of older persons. Negative consequences of use include accidents, physical and/or mental health problems, and/or social and legal problems. For people older than 60 years, continuing to drink the same amounts of alcohol that did not appear to cause problems earlier in life can result in adverse consequences. Such outcomes are determined by the individual's response to alcohol, the use of prescription drugs (alcohol interacts with at least 50% of prescription drugs), and co-occurrence of other chronic medical or psychiatric disorders. Similarly, a decline in visual, auditory, or other perceptual capacities make alcohol consumption hazardous. Heavy drinking has been correlated with ulcers, respiratory disease, stroke, and myocardial infarction.

Severe substance use disorders are chronic, recurring illnesses. One may achieve sobriety and recovery, using medication, self-help, and psychotherapy. Sobriety may be interrupted by brief "slips" and "relapses," after which the individual returns to efforts toward recovery. Severe substance use disorders have two components. First, physiological dependence, induced by certain drugs, such as alcohol, tobacco, benzodiazepines, barbiturates, amphetamines, and opioids, which is evidenced in "tolerance," the need for increasing amounts of a substance to achieve the desired effect, and "withdrawal," a characteristic pattern of symptoms after use of a substance is suddenly stopped. Second, craving accompanies withdrawal, so there is also psychological dependence, the perceived need to use the drug. Psychological dependence is evidenced in moderate and severe substance disorder and is more difficult to resolve than physiologic dependence.

Illicit Drug Use

Illicit drug use is less prevalent than excess alcohol use or prescription drug misuse in late adulthood. Recent trends seen in the baby boomer generation, however, suggest that this may be changing. Marijuana use, for example, is now more prevalent among persons aged 55 years and older than among adolescents with 3 million adults older than 50 years reporting marijuana use and 2.1 million or 2.3% reporting nonmedical use of prescription drugs (West et al., 2015; SAMHSA, 2010). Of drug users 50 years and older, approximately 10% to 12% have a drug use disorder (Wu & Blazer, 2014). Recent data from emergency room admissions indicate growing numbers of older adults (largely male) using heroin and cocaine as well as marijuana (SAMHSA, 2008). Clinical observation suggests that older people are rarely asked about illicit drugs, that is, cocaine, despite strong evidence of its associated cardiovascular risks. The result is an absence of accurate information on prevalence of illicit drug use among older adults, estimated to be in excess of 5.2% among persons 50 years and older (Chait, Fahmy, & Caceres, 2010; SAMHSA, 2012).

Recovery From Severe Substance Use Disorders

Many older persons are "in recovery" or have established long sobriety from the use of alcohol, cocaine, heroin, or other drugs. The components of recovery have been described by the Betty Ford Institute Consensus Panel (2007). *Recovery* is defined as a lifestyle voluntarily maintained by an individual that includes sobriety, varying levels of personal health, and citizenship. Adverse circumstances and life stressors may contribute to an individual's relapse to alcohol or drug use. Transitions that come with aging, the numbers of losses with increased age, and the onset of chronic illness may all be "triggers," to return to drug use posing threats to recovery and risks for a return to regular, maladaptive patterns of use (relapse). On a positive note, good treatment outcomes and rates of recovery for older persons are higher than in any age group. Nurses can contribute positively by supporting the patient's attendance at self-help group meetings, continued involvement in treatment such as methadone or buprenorphine maintenance, active community and family involvement, and/or group or individual psychotherapy.

In this chapter, the term *drug* applies to OTC medications, prescription medications, nicotine, alcohol, and illicit drugs. Herbs and food supplements are also used frequently by older adults. Although knowing the chemical composition of drugs of abuse is essential to understanding their effects on mind and body, this chapter focuses primarily on substance use disorders, and the effects and consequences for health of excessive use and using drugs in combination, as well as nursing assessment and intervention strategies. Please refer to www.drugabuse.gov for a full listing of drugs of abuse and their chemical properties.

Psychoactive Drug Misuse and Abuse

Drug misuse, defined as use of a drug for reasons other than for which it was intended, occurs with increasing frequency with advancing age because (a) prescriptions for multiple medications and cognitive changes, ranging from early signs of dementia, can lead to medication misuse; (b) failure to discard expired medications; (c) trading medications with friends and companions; and (d) combining both nonprescription and prescription medications and alcohol. The most common resulting problems are related to (a) overdose, (b) additive effects, (c) adverse reactions to drugs used, or (d) drug interactions, especially with alcohol. Older adults account for 30% of national expenditures on all prescription drugs, and nonmedical use of prescription drugs increases in persons older than 60 years (NIDA, 2015). A recent rise in trends of opioid misuse has resulted in higher rates of mortality for older adults than for younger users. Opioid and synthetic opioids as factors in suicide among older adults is an increasing trend (West et al., 2015).

The regular use of numerous drugs for multiple medical conditions (i.e., polypharmacy) is complicated by the older adult's use of alcohol or illicit drugs (Letizia & Reinbolz, 2005). In persons aged 18 to 70 years treated for falls, 40% of men and 8% of women tested positive for alcohol and/or benzodiazepines (9% and 3%, respectively), or both (Boyle & Davis, 2006).

Prescription drug use or misuse contributes to falls and cognitive impairment. Abuse of psychoactive drugs is a growing health problem for older adults and the few research findings listed factors correlating with drug abuse are isolation, history of substance-related or mental health disorder, bereavement, chronic medical disorders, female gender, and exposure to prescription drugs with abuse potential. Few older adults are lifetime illicit drug users (Wu & Blazer, 2014), other than marijuana users, who are growing in number. However, substance abuse by older adults, one in four of whom receives prescriptions for drugs with abuse potential, is becoming more common. Drugs—other than nicotine or tobacco—most commonly misused are benzodiazepines, sedative hypnotics, and opioid analgesics (Wu & Blazer, 2014).

Smoking and Nicotine Dependence

Today's older Americans have smoked at rates among the highest of any U.S. generation (American Lung Association [ALA], 2010), resulting in many health problems and contributing to the estimated 438,000 American deaths annually caused by smoking. Nearly 20 of every 100 American adults aged 45 to 64 years (19.9%) and nearly 9 of every 100 adults aged 65+ years (8.8%) are current smokers (CDC, 2015).

Although these rates in older adults have decreased in recent years, vulnerability to the effects of smoking is evident. Men have been found to be more than twice as likely as women to die of stroke secondary to smoking (ALA, 2006). The risk of dying of a heart attack for men aged 65 years and older is twice that for women smokers and 60% higher than for nonsmoking men of the same age. Smokers also have significantly higher risks than nonsmokers for Alzheimer's disease and other types of dementia, and smoking plays a role in heart and lung disease, cancer, osteoporosis, diabetes, erectile dysfunction, and visual disorders like macular degeneration and nuclear cataracts (ALA, 2010; Whitmer, Sidney, Selby, Johnston, & Yaffe, 2005).

Polysubstance Abuse

Polysubstance abuse, the misuse, abuse, or regular use of three or more drugs, is common in older adults. Prescription analgesics are frequently prescribed for chronic pain, a common complaint in older persons, and depending on the class of drug, can induce dependence. Older problem drinkers, as well, report more severe pain, greater disruption of activities caused by pain, and frequent use of alcohol to manage pain (Brennan, Schutte, & Moos, 2005). These findings underscore the importance of monitoring drinking and medication use in patients who present with complaints of pain, especially those with histories of any heavy drug use or substance use disorders, including alcohol and nicotine.

ASSESSMENT OF SUBSTANCE USE

The nurse should review data collected on the most recent nursing and medical histories and the most recent physical examination. When patients are using alcohol, there may be deviations in standard liver function tests (LFTs) and elevations in gamma-glutamyl transferase (GGT) and carbohydrate-deficient transferrin (CDT) levels; 50% to 70% of heavy drinkers will have percentage of CDT greater than 2.6 (Miller, Cluver, & Anton, 2009). Physical signs, such as ecchymosis, spider angiomas, flushing, palmar erythema, or sarcopenia may be evidence of heavy use. The patient may have an altered level of consciousness, changes in mental status or mood, poor coordination, tremor, increased deep tendon reflexes, or a positive Romberg sign. Increased lacrimal secretions, nystagmus, and sluggish pupil reactivity may also be noted on examination (Letizia & Reinbolz, 2005). Patients who report use of marijuana and/or other drugs should have toxicology tests to establish baseline use level. Findings can be effectively used in a motivational interview and brief interventions and/or counseling.

Nurses need to assess and document frequent changes in drug-using habits and record these in substance use histories, dating from first use to the current situation. Ask whether the individual ever experienced problems related to drug or alcohol use, spontaneously stopped using a drug or alcohol, or is in recovery and participating in self-help programs such as Alcoholics Anonymous or Narcotics Anonymous.

In taking the patient history, ask about a history of smoking, alcohol use in the form of number of standard drinks, OTC medications, prescription and recreational drugs, herbal, and food and drink supplements. Record this information using the Quantity Frequency (QF) Index (Khavari & Farber, 1978). Another helpful technique in assessing drug use is the "brown bag" technique. Ask the client to bring in a brown bag containing all the prescribed OTC, food supplements, and other legal or illicit drugs that he or she consumes weekly. Use these to develop the history and to open a discussion about the implications of drug use with the patient. Be sure to talk with the client about how using the drug is meaningful or helpful (i.e., relieves pain, relieves feelings of loneliness, anxiety, or comfort).

Screening, brief intervention, and referral to treatment (SBIRT) has been found to be effective with adults and older adults for smoking, illicit drug and prescription drug abuse, and alcohol use, and should be part of the nursing evaluation (Schonfeld et al., 2010). Despite federal agency guidelines supporting its use, it is rarely used with older adults. SBIRT has demonstrated efficacy and feasibility in reducing patients' alcohol consumption, decreasing dependence symptoms (Babor et al., 2007; SAMHSA, 2008), and improving general and mental health (Madras et al., 2009) following its use by nurses and nurse practitioners.

How to Use SBIRT

SBIRT begins with screening an individual using a valid and age-appropriate screening tool. The goal of the *screening* is to identify alcohol use behaviors that place the individual at risk for health problems. Short, well-tested questionnaires that identify risk include the Alcohol, Smoking, and Substance Involvement Screening Test (ASSIST), the Short Michigan Alcohol Screening Test-Geriatric version (SMAST-G), the Alcohol Use Disorder Identification Test (AUDIT), the Drug Abuse Screening Test (DAST), and so forth.

Although screens can often be done by paper and pencil, older adults may respond to administration by the nurse or trained personnel. A positive score on the screening tool for excess alcohol use or for smoking, can be determined by a brief 3- to 5-minute session, including advice to cut down. SBIRT is not effective with individuals with severe substance use disorders and physiological dependence on alcohol.

Blow et al. (2005) recommend modifying the *brief intervention* for older adults to include the following points:

1. Help the individual identify future goals for health, activities, and relationships.
2. Give feedback that is customized to the individual's patterns of substance use, health habits, emotional and cognitive function.
3. Discuss norms of drinking habits. Define drinking patterns (light, moderate, and heavy).
4. Help the client weigh the pros and cons of drinking.
5. Explore the consequences of heavy drinking.
6. Explore the reasons to cut down on or quit drinking.
7. Help the client to set a sensible drinking standard using strategies to cut down or quit.
8. Help the client anticipate and plan for coping in risky situations (Blow et al., 2005).

If the patient declines change at this time, the discussion is dropped. The topic of possible change, however, should be raised at the next visit. When the screening instrument (AUDIT, SMAST-G) score indicates dependence on alcohol or nicotine, referrals to specialty treatment and information needed to access a provider or a specialty health care agency are in order.

Referral: For in-depth assessment and/or diagnosis and/or treatment,

Treatment: Depending on the health care setting, between 1% and 10% of patients may need some level of treatment—to ensure safe withdrawal and reinforce decreased intake of cessation.

Although the U.S. Preventive Services Task Force recommends screening older adults for excess alcohol use, screening is not frequently done. Health providers, family members, and friends may overlook excess use because no one identifies how drug use is disrupting their lives. They may feel, based on advanced age, the patient should be free to engage in whatever behavior he or she wishes. Health professionals may be pessimistic that older persons can change long-standing behaviors, so they may not ask about drug and alcohol use. Evidence suggests that many health professionals doubt the effectiveness of alcohol or drug treatment (Vastag, 2003). In addition, health care providers may not recognize the association of drug use, smoking, or excessive alcohol use and health problems like chronic obstructive pulmonary disease (COPD), stroke, or depression.

Recurrent and prolonged substance use disorders are now recognized as chronic conditions, characterized by slips and relapses, and conditions that respond to treatment (McLellan, Lewis, O'Brien, & Kleber, 2000). Interventions and treatment can be matched to stages of the disease (acute phases, exacerbations, and stages of recovery) for improved outcomes.

Screening Tools for Alcohol and Drug Use

Screening for alcohol and other drug use is equally important in the community and hospital setting. A QF Index, such as the Khavari Alcohol Test (KAT), asks respondents to report their (a) usual frequency of drinking, (b) usual amount consumed per occasion, (c) maximum amount consumed on any one occasion, and (d) frequency of consumption of the maximum amount (Allen & Wilson, 2003). The KAT consists of the four questions noted previously that are asked for each type of beverage (beer, wine, spirits, and liqueurs) and can be administered in 6 to 8 minutes (Khavari & Farber, 1978). The amounts are then compared with NIAAA norms for persons older than 65 years, which are one drink per day for men and women and no more than three drinks per occasion. Additional questions, such as (a) "Did you ever feel you had a problem related to alcohol or other drug use?" and (b) "Have you ever been treated for an alcohol or drug problem?" will yield important additional information.

Short Michigan Alcohol Screening Test-Geriatric Version

The SMAST-G is an effective tool for screening older adults in all settings. The complete drug use history can be obtained in the comprehensive assessment. The original instrument from which this version was derived has a sensitivity of 93.9% and a specificity of 78.1% (Blow et al., 1992). The SMAST-G is composed of 10 questions and is quickly administered. It has outcomes equal to the parent instrument. Each positive response counts as 1 point.

Alcohol Use Disorders Indentification Test (AUDIT)

This 10-item questionnaire has good validity in ethnically mixed groups and scores classify alcohol use as hazardous, harmful, or dependent; administration: 2 minutes (Saunders, Ashland, Babur, de la Fuente, & Grant, 1993). The AUDIT has been found to have high specificity in adults older than 65 years (Babur, Higgins-Biddle, Saunders, & Monteiro, 2001).

Fagerström Test for Nicotine Dependence-Revised

This six-question scale provides an indicator of the severity of nicotine dependence: scores less than 4 (*low to moderate dependence*), 4 to 6 (*moderate dependence*), and 7 to 10 (*highly dependent on nicotine*). The questions inquire about first use early in the day, amount and frequency, inability to refrain, and smoking despite illness. This instrument has good internal consistency and reliability in culturally diverse, mixed-gender samples (Pomerleau, Carton, Lutzke, Flessland, & Pomerleau, 1994).

INTERVENTIONS AND CARE STRATEGIES

Interdisciplinary collaboration is essential to providing a range of treatment modalities for substance use disorders and related problems because drug and alcohol use affects physical, mental, spiritual, and emotional health. Primary care providers, psychologists, dentists, nurses, and social workers should all be equipped to detect and refer a problem, and all dimensions of health should be addressed in treatment and aftercare. The least intensive approaches to treatment for older adults should be implemented first and should be flexible, individualized, and implemented over time. Older persons are disinclined to seek or continue care with mental health or addictions specialists. Brief interventions and motivational interviewing have been found effective in producing short-term reduction in alcohol consumption for older persons, both for men and women. There are some findings that motivational interviewing is more effective with smoking than brief advice (Ballesteros, González-Pinto, Querejeta, & Ariño, 2004; Wutzke, Conigrave, Saunders, & Hall, 2002). Research findings also suggest that once enrolled in treatment for a substance use disorder, older people treated for alcohol or opioid dependence with medications, such as naltrexone, methadone, or buprenorphine; as well as individualized, supportive, and medically based psychosocial interventions have better outcomes than younger people (Satre, Mertens, Arean, & Weisner, 2004).

Inpatient Hospitalization

Older adults who report using alcohol should be screened for alcohol use (Nicholas & Hall, 2011) on admission to any care facility. A small but important percentage will be at risk for the development of acute alcohol withdrawal syndrome (AWS) on sudden cessation of drinking. Patients at highest risk have (a) a history of consuming large amounts of alcohol, (b) coexisting acute illness, (c) previous episodes of AWS or seizure activity, (d) a history of detoxification, and (e) intense cravings for alcohol (Letizia & Reinbolz, 2005). Symptoms of withdrawal are intense and of greater duration than in younger persons with onset of withdrawal as early as 4 to 8 hours after the last drink and persisting up to 72 hours. The clinical symptoms determine the need for detoxification and determine medical and nursing decisions. Clinical judgments follow a history, including history of drug and alcohol use, and physical and mental status assessments.

A 10- to 28-day period of acute care hospitalization in a mental health unit or alcohol and drug treatment center is indicated for the older person addicted to alcohol, benzodiazepines, heroin, amphetamines, or cocaine when (a) living situations and access to the drug makes abstinence unlikely; (b) there is a likelihood of severe withdrawal symptoms; (c) comorbid physical or psychiatric diagnoses, such as depression and accompanying suicidal ideation or a chronic physical illness, are present; (d) daily ingestion of alcohol or a sedative hypnotic has been higher than recommended doses for 4 weeks or more; and (e) mixed addiction, as in alcohol and benzodiazepines or cocaine and alcohol, is present. It is helpful if programs specifically designed to meet the needs of older persons are available (USDHHS, 2004a).

Ambulatory Care

Persons dependent on alcohol, tobacco, and heroin can be successfully withdrawn in community-based care through the collaboration of a medical doctor or nurse practitioner and family members and friends. Specialists in addiction should be sought as supervisors or collaborators in the process. Older persons drinking at risky levels or abusing alcohol or other drugs are generally treated in the community. Tobacco-cessation protocols are now available directly to consumers as well as to primary care providers and mental health professionals.

Residential Treatment

Residential treatment is available in specialty care centers, therapeutic communities, and some long-term care facilities. Programs designed specifically for the older person are beneficial in their focus on the specific health care needs and challenges to abstinence faced by older people. These long-standing habits of use, a diminished social network, and the risks of social isolation, and health implications of heavy alcohol and prescription drug use make behavioral change particularly challenging.

Therapeutic Communities

Therapeutic communities provide long-term (up to 18 months) treatment and are abstinence-oriented programs. They use the 12-step Alcoholics Anonymous model of individual and group counseling, as well as participation in a social community, to address drug-related problems. For the isolated, older drug user with a history of frequent relapse, these are good treatment options.

Pharmacological Treatment

Agents for pharmacological treatment of substance abuse and dependence are more available but not all are appropriate for use with older adults, because of metabolic changes with aging. The best outcomes of pharmacological interventions are achieved by the combination of medication with individual and/or group counseling. Attendance at 12-step programs also supports adherence to treatment regimens.

Severe Alcohol Use Disorder and Medication-Assisted Treatment

There is strong evidence that naltrexone can decrease cravings and consumption in heavy drinkers. It is available in liquid form for oral use and is now available in injectable, long-acting form. It is marketed as Vivitrol or Vivitrex. These extended-release formulations of naltrexone act up to 28 days to decrease the euphoric effects of, and craving for alcohol (Bartus et al., 2003). Evidence suggests that this treatment is well tolerated by older people (Oslin, Pettinati, & Volpicelli, 2002). Contraindications for its use include renal problems, acute hepatitis, or liver failure. Study findings stress the importance of psychosocial interventions to improve adherence to pharmacological interventions for alcohol dependence, a finding similar to those regarding smoking cessation (Mayet, Farrell, Ferri, Amato, & Davoli, 2005). Acamprosate calcium (Campral), a recent addition to prescription drug choices, has variable outcomes in reducing the craving for and consumption of alcohol. Disulfiram (Antabuse), used to deter alcohol consumption, produces an elevation in vital signs and severe gastrointestinal symptoms if alcohol is ingested and is poorly tolerated by alcoholics older than 55 years. In addition, it must be taken every day to achieve aversive effects on consumption. The best outcomes with this medication occur when working with the patient's family members and support persons.

Opioid Dependence

The use of methadone, an opioid agonist, assists the opioid-dependent person to focus on psychological and life problems. The drug buprenorphine—both an opioid antagonist and agonist—is longer acting and now available. Both are dispensed in institution-based clinic settings or by physicians specifically credentialed to prescribe and monitor buprenorphine. Evidence supports added benefit of psychosocial treatment for patient adherence to pharmacological treatment (Amato et al., 2008).

Smoking

Bupropion in doses of 75 mg with administration begun 2 weeks before the smoker intends to quit has proved a helpful adjunct to smoking cessation. Nicorette transdermal patches and nicotine gum are now available OTC and there is research support for their pharmacological contribution to smoking cessation. The dosage of transdermal patches is determined by the number of cigarettes smoked (level of substance use disorder). The best outcomes with smoking cessation result from a combination of individual or group psychosocial support and medication (CDC, 2014).

Models of Care

Individualized care plans should be developed for older adults at risk for substance use disorders in accordance with the classes of drugs used and the mild, moderate, or severe nature of the disorder. Individualizing care allows flexibility for patient and nurse. Evidence is emerging, however, on models of care for older adults with complex health problems. For example, in one study, the integration of mental health into primary care increased access to mental health and substance abuse treatment for both Black and White older adult patients who are offered both enhanced specialist services and mental health services at the primary care site (Ayalon, Areán, Linkins, Lynch, & Estes, 2007). Case management has also demonstrated effective outcomes with older adults with multiple social, mental health, and physical needs with problems accessing community services, including substance abuse (Hesse, Vanderplasschen, Rapp, Broekaert, & Fridell, 2007). Guidelines for all interventions should include the following:

- A nonjudgmental, health-oriented approach to substance-related problems is needed. Drug and alcohol use and abuse are highly stigmatized in American society, particularly in minority communities, leading to denial and/or rejection by family members. Understanding addiction as a disease helps nurses and other providers adopt attitudes and approaches similar to care required for other chronic illness.
- A supportive, encouraging approach to changing use habits must be fostered. The patient or client is taught that change occurs in stages and that support and assistance are available at each stage.
- Patient and family need education on the risks associated with drug misuse. Because older persons use so many medications, the potential health consequences of medication misuse and drug abuse may be minimized in the eyes of family members and caretakers.
- Assessment of substance use in relation to lifestyle, existing chronic illnesses, nutritional patterns, sleep, exercise, sexual patterns, and recreation is needed. Counsel the patient and/or family about the effects of substances used on these areas of the patient's life.
- Set the goal of "harm reduction" in the form of decreased use and supervised use if abstinence is not imperative or achievable.
- Monitor substance use patterns at each encounter or visit, documenting changes and providing reinforcement of positive changes and/or movement toward treatment.
- Enhance the involvement of members of the patient's support system, including family and friends identified by the patient, community-based groups, support groups, appropriate clergy, or organizational groups such as senior centers.
- Support the development of coping mechanisms, including modifications in social, housing, and recreational environments, to minimize associations with settings and groups in which substance use and abuse are common (USDHHS, 2004a).

Counseling and Psychotherapy

Older persons tend to seek care from their primary care, medical specialist, or nurse/nurse practitioner provider for mental health and substance-related problems. This practice derives from long-held beliefs that mental health problems like depression or anxiety indicate weakness or lack of character.

Older persons, more than others, stigmatize the excess use of alcohol or use of an illicit drug and problems with prescription drugs. Counseling done by the nurse using SBIRT is likely to be more readily accepted by older patients than referral to mental health or substance abuse clinics.

Optimal treatment involves short-term psychotherapy by a practitioner with education about abuse and addiction. Following the model of cognitive behavioral therapy, in particular, has demonstrated good outcomes with excessive drinking and marijuana use (Cooney, Babor, & Litt, 2001). These approaches help the older adult to modify behavior and to deal with negative feelings and/or chronic pain that often motivate use.

Treatment Outcomes

Health care providers and older persons may feel pessimistic about the possibilities of changing their substance use behavior. Health providers often do not intervene because they believe that older people do not change. Treatment outcomes for older persons with substance use problems, however, have been shown to be as good as or better than those for younger people (USDHHS, 2004b). Good treatment outcomes, however, can be compromised by inconsistency of follow-up and limited access to aftercare for community-dwelling older adults.

CASE STUDY

Joseph and Mary P, both 71 years old, reside in a small, rural community where Mr. P owned the only pharmacy. Retired for 5 years, Mr. P is in good health except for osteoarthritis and Mrs. P has heart failure, which is usually well managed when she adheres to her diet and medication regimen. She is also being treated for depression and generalized anxiety disorder for which she has been prescribed paroxetine (Paxil). The couple enjoys a nightly cocktail hour at which Mr. P consumes two scotch whiskies and Mrs. P has "wine." Recently, the visiting nurse who has been monitoring Mrs. P's recovery from an episode of congestive heart failure received a phone call from the couple's daughter who stated that on her last three evening phone calls to her parents, Mrs. P sounded somewhat confused and her speech was slurred. She also reports that her father had a fall in the evening last week. When the daughter questioned her parents about their drinking, Mr. P became irritable and defensive.

The nurse was concerned that the Ps were at risk related to their alcohol use. She made it a point to visit

(continued)

CASE STUDY *(continued)*

the P's in the early evening on her way home She found them enjoying their cocktails and took the opportunity to conduct a drug and alcohol use screen using the SMAST-G. This indicated a problem with alcohol use and potential for associated negative health outcomes. She conducted a brief intervention, giving them information about their respective chronic diseases, including the benefits of reducing their drinking. The nurse discussed how decreasing alcohol intake can reduce the gastric distress Mr. P experiences and the benefits of improving depression symptoms and effectiveness of paroxetine hydrochloride (Paxil). The nurse taught them (building on autonomy and responsibility) about the relationship between physical changes and the effects of alcohol on their sleep patterns, mood, balance, and fall risk. She also pointed out that both were consuming alcohol more than one daily drink and recommended that they cut down to one standard drink (Figure 28.1) a day (1.5 oz. spirits, 4–5 oz. wine, or 12 oz. of beer). At first, they seemed unhappy about the recommendation but both committed to attempting to reduce their intake for the sake of their overall health. When the nurse visited 2 weeks later, they had begun to journal their drinking and both were recording consistent declines in the amount of alcohol consumed. Thus, this is a successful example of the SBIRT intervention.

SUMMARY

Two current trends are predicted to result in an increase in the already significant number of men and women older than 55 years who experience various substance use disorders: the growing numbers of older persons in America and the continuation of tobacco, drug, and alcohol use patterns established earlier in life. Although most people decrease the amount of alcohol and kinds of drugs they use with age, anywhere from 10% to 24% of older persons do not (USDHHS, 2004a). The most common of substance use disorders is heavy drinking, especially by Caucasian men older than 65 years and living alone (USDHHS, 2004a). The frequency of heavy drinking is closely followed by smoking, which causes the highest number of premature deaths among older people. The high numbers of prescription drugs used by older adults pose serious problems related to misuse and drug interactions. Health professionals are disinclined to query older adults about substance use, but the substance use problems emerge with the diagnosis and treatment of other medical disorders. Nurses in daily contact with institutionalized and community-dwelling older adults must be skilled in screening and counseling on the use of nicotine, alcohol, prescription, illicit, and OTC drugs. Educating patient and family about health risks and referring patients to specialists and community resources are essential "best practices."

FIGURE 28.1

Standard drink.

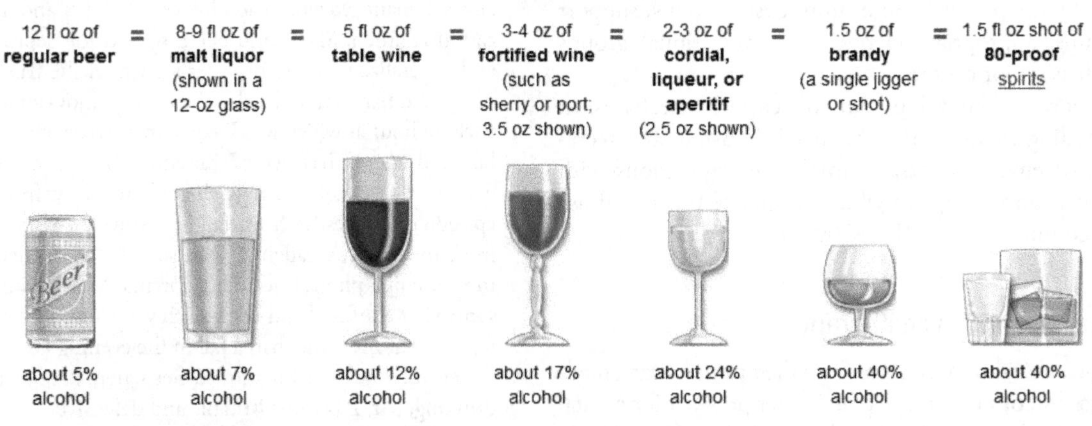

The percentage of "pure" alcohol, expressed here as alcohol by volume (alc/vol), varies by beverage.

Source: Maki and Tambyah (2001).

NURSING STANDARD OF PRACTICE

Protocol 28.1: Substance Misuse and Alcohol Use Disorders

I. GOAL

To implement best nursing practices in older persons with drug, alcohol, tobacco, or other drug use disorders

II. OVERVIEW

A. Several factors increase the risks associated with alcohol and drug use for the older individual; continuing drug use patterns that earlier in life were commonplace can be potentially harmful. Constitutional risk factors include changes in body composition such as decreased muscle mass, decreased organ efficiency (especially kidney and liver), and increased vulnerability of the CNS.
B. Alcohol use in combination with other drugs or used excessively may result in falls, impaired cognition, malnourishment, and decreased resistance to disease, as well as interpersonal and legal problems.
C. At-risk drinking (more than one drink per day or more than three drinks on one occasion) by older adults increases the likelihood of negative health consequences.
D. Any smoking is considered drug abuse and places the person at risk for negative health consequences; advancing age increases the likelihood of respiratory and cardiovascular illnesses.

III. BACKGROUND AND STATEMENT OF THE PROBLEM

A. The use of alcohol, tobacco, illicit drugs, and the misuse of prescription drugs, can result in substance use disorders. These are classified on a continuum of mild, moderate, and severe based on the number of symptoms associated with drug use.
   1. Symptoms include mental or physical health problems; impairment in the performance of social, family, work, and civil role relationships because of excessive and frequent use of a substance or multiple substances. For 25% of the U.S. population *at-risk drinking*—defined as more than one drink per day, 7 days a week or more than three drinks on any one occasion for persons 65 years and older—is an example of drug use that results in short- and long-term health problems. For older adults, at-risk drinking increases the likelihood of negative health consequences including depression, falls, impaired motor function, and interactions with prescription drugs.
   2. The frequency and quantity of the drug used generally determines the extent of a substance use disorder. For example, heavy drinking—5 or more drinks (4 for women) every day for more than 5 days in the past 30 days—can result in health, safety, and social problems. In addition, some drugs, including alcohol opioids, nicotine, benzodiazepines, and barbiturates, induce *tolerance*; defined as
      a. A need for markedly increased amounts of alcohol to achieve intoxication or desired effect
      b. A markedly diminished effect with continued use of the same amount of the drug
   3. Tolerance drives the need to increase amounts of a drug in an effort to achieve the "high" experienced on early use and is indicative of physiologic dependence.
   4. When physiologic dependence has developed, sudden cessation of use of the drug precipitates *withdrawal*, characteristic signs and symptoms derived from the chemical properties of the drug. The continuous use of alcohol, opioids, and sedating drugs results in central nervous system depression and withdrawal symptoms can be nausea, agitation (mild) to seizure, and fluid and electrolyte disorder (severe).
   5. Untreated withdrawal from depressant drugs can be life threatening. Older adults, especially those with comorbid conditions, must be monitored closely and appropriately medicated.
   6. Decreased metabolic capacity for any drug places older adults at risk for *intoxication* and interaction or potentiation of other prescription or illicit drugs. Intoxication is evidenced in signs such as drowsiness, slurred speech, and uneven gait following consumption of sedative drugs such as opioids, alcohol, or barbiturates or agitation, anxiety, and mania associated with the use of cocaine or other stimulants. The symptoms derive from the effects of the drug properties. Of note, women develop more pathology from lower levels of alcohol consumption than

(continued)

Protocol 28.1: Substance Misuse and Alcohol Use Disorders *(continued)*

men of the same age as a function of their physiologic vulnerability. Intoxication will have an earlier onset even with tolerance and withdrawal can be more severe. An aging metabolism complicates these constitutional traits.

7. *Drug misuse* is a common practice among older adults, but is not limited to this population. Drug misuse is defined as taking a drug for purposes other than which the drug was prescribed or intended to achieve a desired effect. Because older adults are often prescribed five or more drugs as common practice in the treatment of chronic illness and common health problems, reliance on pharmacotherapy to address pain, sleep disorders, depression, and general malaise is not uncommon. A comprehensive drug use (including tobacco and alcohol) history is important in identifying this problem as well as *polysubstance-related disorder*, defined as misuse, abuse, or dependence on three or more drugs that have psychotropic effects. For older adults this is often a combination of illicit and prescription drugs and often includes nicotine and/or alcohol.
8. Older adults, once engaged in treatment for a substance use disorder, have good rates of recovery. Recovery means learning and maintaining a lifestyle of sobriety at various levels of personal health, and the capacity to engage productively with society. Early recovery spans a first year and, beyond 1 year, recovery is referred to as "sustained." *Relapse*, or returning to regular use of a substance in a maladaptive pattern, is a lifetime concern, which is why persons often self-refer as "recovering." Substance use disorders are chronic illnesses that require ongoing monitoring and self-care and may include medication.

B. Etiology and/or epidemiology: Of persons older than 50 years, 16.7% reported drinking two or more drinks per day (risky drinking) and 19.6% reported binge drinking on occasion. Among primary care patients older than 60 years, 15% of men and 12% of women regularly drank in excess of the NIAAA recommended levels (one drink per day and no more than three drinks on any one occasion).
   1. The drugs used and misused most frequently by older adults are nicotine, alcohol, and prescription drugs, particularly analgesics and benzodiazepines.
   2. Excessive drinking by individuals of all ethnic groups ages 65 years and older is approximately 7%, down from 12% in persons aged 55 to 64 years.
   3. Five hundred thousand persons aged 55 years and older reported monthly use of illicit drugs in the National Household Survey on Drug Use, NIDA.
   4. Approximately 11% of women older than 59 years misuse psychoactive drugs.

C. Risk factors (USDHHS, 2004a)
   1. Family history of dependence on alcohol, tobacco, prescription, or illicit drugs
   2. Co-occurring moderate to severe substance use disorder dependency or abuse of another substance (i.e., alcohol and tobacco)
   3. Lifelong pattern of substance use, including heavy drinking
   4. Male gender
   5. Social isolation
   6. Recent and multiple losses
   7. Chronic pain
   8. Co-occurrence with depression
   9. Unpartnered and/or living alone

IV. PARAMETERS OF ASSESSMENT

A. Screening for alcohol, tobacco, and other drug use is recommended for all community-dwelling and hospitalized older adults. It is essential that the nurse:
   1. State the purpose of questions about substances used and link them to health and safety
   2. Be empathic and nonjudgmental; avoid stigmatic terms such as *alcoholic*
   3. Ask the questions when the patient is alcohol and drug free
   4. Inquire about the patient's understanding of the question (Aalto, Pekuri, & Seppä, 2003).

B. Assessment and screening tools
   1. The QF Index (Khavari & Farber, 1978): *Review all classes* of drugs; alcohol, nicotine, illicit drugs, prescription drugs, OTC drugs, and vitamin supplements, for each drug used. *Record the types* of drugs, including the kinds of beverages.

(continued)

Protocol 28.1: Substance Misuse and Alcohol Use Disorders *(continued)*

Frequency: The number of occasions on which the drug is consumed (daily, weekly, and monthly). *Amount of drug consumed* on each occasion over the past 30 days. The psychological function, what the drugs does for the individual, is also important to identify. The QF Index tool should be part of the intake nursing history. The brown bag approach is also useful. Ask the patient to bring all drugs and supplements he or she uses in a brown bag to the interview.

2. SMAST-G: Highly valid and reliable, this is a 10-item tool that can be used in all settings. Two to 3 minutes needed for administration. This instrument is derived from the SMAST-G with a sensitivity of 93.6% and a positive predictive value of 87.2% (Blow et al., 1992).
3. The AUDIT: This 10-item questionnaire has good validity in ethnically mixed groups, and scores classify alcohol use as hazardous, harmful, or dependent; administration: 2 minutes. Sensitivity scores range from 0.74% to 0.84% and specificity around 0.90% in groups of mixed age and ethnicity (Allen, Litten, Fertig, & Babor, 1997). This instrument is highly effective for use with older adults (Roberts, Marshall, & MacDonald, 2005). Its derivative, the AUDIT-C, is composed of three questions that have proved equally valid in detecting an alcohol-related problem.
4. Fagerström Test for Nicotine Dependence (Pomerleau et al., 1994): This six-question scale provides an indicator of the severity of nicotine dependence: scores of less than 4 (*very low*); 4 to 6 (*moderate*), and 7 to 10 (*very high*). The questions inquire about first use early in the day, amount and frequency, inability to refrain, and smoking despite illness. This instrument has good internal consistency and reliability in culturally diverse, mixed-gender samples (Pomerleau et al., 1994).

C. Atypical presentation
   1. Men and women older than 65 years may have substance-related disorder problems even though the signs and symptoms may be less numerous than those listed in the *DSM-5* (APA, 2013).

D. Signs of CNS intoxication (i.e., slurred speech, drowsiness, unsteady gait, decreased reaction time, impaired judgment, disinhibition, ataxia)
   1. Assess by individual or collateral (speaking with family members) data collection, detail the consumption of amount and type of depressant medications, including alcohol, sedatives, hypnotics, and opioid or synthetic opioid analgesics.
   2. Obtain a blood alcohol level. Marked intoxication at 0.3% to 0.4%, toxic effects occur at 0.4% to 0.5%, and coma and death at 0.5% or higher.
   3. Assess vital signs and determine respiratory, cardiac, or neurological depression.
   4. Assess for existing medical conditions, including depression.
   5. Arrange for emergency room or hospitalization treatment as necessary.
   6. Obtain urine for toxicology, if possible.
   7. Assess for delirium, which can be confused with intoxication and withdrawal in the older adult.

E. At-risk drinking is regular consumption of alcohol in excess of one drink per day for 7 days a week or more than three drinks on any one occasion.
   1. Assess for readiness to change behavior using SBIRT.
   2. Is the drinker concerned about amount or consequences of the drinking? Has he or she contemplated cutting down?
   3. Does he or she have a plan for cutting down or stopping consumption?
   4. Has he or she previously stopped but then resumed risky drinking?
   5. Personalized feedback and education on "at-risk drinking" results in a reduction in at-risk drinking among older primary care patients.

F. Treatment of acute AWS (guidelines are modified for other CNS-depressant drugs such as barbiturates, heroin, sedative hypnotics)
   1. Assess for risk factors: (a) previous episodes of detoxification; (b) recent heavy drinking; (c) medical comorbidities, including liver disease, pneumonia, and anemia; and (d) previous history of seizures or delirium (Wetterling, Weber, Depfenhart, Schneider, & Junghanns, 2006).
   2. Assess for extreme CNS stimulation and a minor withdrawal syndrome evidenced in tremors, disorientation, tachycardia, irritability, anxiety, insomnia, and moderate diaphoresis. When these signs are not detected, life-threatening situations for older adults often result. Withdrawal, occurring 24 to 72 hours after the last drink, can progress to seizures, hallucinosis, withdrawal delirium, extreme hypertension, and profuse diarrhea from 4 to 8 hours and for up to 72 hours following cessation of alcohol intake (DTs).

(continued)

Protocol 28.1: Substance Misuse and Alcohol Use Disorders *(continued)*

3. Assess neurological signs, using the CIWA-Ar. The CIWA-Ar is a 10-item rating scale that delineates symptoms of gastric distress, perceptual distortions, cognitive impairment, anxiety, agitation, and headache (Sullivan, Sykora, Schneiderman, Naranjo, & Sellers, 1989).
4. Medicate with a short-acting benzodiazepine (lorazepam or oxazepam) in doses titrated to patient's score on the CIWA-Ar, patient's age and weight; use one third to one half recommended dose (Amato, Minozzi, Vecchi, & Davoli, 2010). Continue CIWA-Ar to monitor treatment response.
5. Provide emotional support and frequent reorientation in a cool, low-stimulation setting; monitor hydration and nutritional intake. Give therapeutic dose of thiamine and multivitamins.

G. Report sleep disturbance, anxiety, depression, and problems with attention and concentration (acute care)
1. Assess for neuropsychiatric conditions using the mental status exam, Geriatric Depression Scale, or Hamilton Anxiety Scale.
2. Obtain sleep history because drugs disrupt sleep patterns in older persons.
3. Assess intake of all drugs, including alcohol, OTC, prescription, herbal and food supplements, and nicotine. Use the "brown bag" strategy.
4. If positive for alcohol use, assess for last time of use and amount used.
5. Assess for alcohol or sedative drug withdrawal as indicated.

H. Smoking cigarettes, e-cigarettes, hookah, or using smokeless tobacco
1. Assess for level of dependence using the Fagerström Test (see Screening Tools for Alcohol and Drug Use section).

V. NURSING CARE STRATEGIES

A. At-risk drinking (consumption of alcohol in excess of one drink per day for 7 days a week or more than three drinks on any one occasion) or excess alcohol consumption (more than three to four drinks on frequent occasions):
1. Conduct screening, brief intervention, and, as indicated, referral to treatment: (SAMHSA, 2008)
   a. Screen using the AUDIT-C, AUDIT, or SMAST-G
   b. Feedback information to the client about current health problems or potential problems associated with the level of alcohol or other drug consumption
   c. Stress client's responsible choice about actions in response to the information provided
   d. Advice must be clear about reducing his or her amount of drinking or total consumption
   e. Recommend drinking according to NIAAA levels for older adults.
   f. Provide a menu of choices to the patient or client regarding future drinking behaviors.
   g. Offer information based on scientific evidence, acknowledge the difficulty of change, and avoid confrontation. Empathy is essential to the exchange.

B. Support self-efficacy. Help client explore options for change.
1. Assist client in identifying options to solve the identified problem.
2. Review the pros and cons of behavior change options presented.
3. Help client weigh potential decisions by considering outcomes.

C. Smoking cigars, cigarettes, e-cigarettes, or using smokeless tobacco
1. Apply the five A's Intervention (Agency for Healthcare Research and Quality [formerly the Agency for Healthcare Policy and Research] Guidelines)
   a. Ask: Identify and document all tobacco use.
   b. Advise: Urge the user to quit in a strong personalized manner.
   c. Assess: Is the tobacco user willing to make a quit attempt at this time?
   d. Assist: If user is willing to attempt, refer for individual or group counseling and pharmacotherapy. Refer to telephone "quit lines" in region or state.
   e. Arrange referrals to providers, agencies, and self-help groups. Monitor pharmacotherapy once quit date is established. The U.S. FDA-approved pharmacotherapies for smoking cessation are the following:
      i. Bupropion SR (Zyban) and nicotine replacement products, such as nicotine gum, nicotine inhalers, nicotine nasal spray, and nicotine patch. Nurse-initiated education about these medications is essential.

(continued)

Protocol 28.1: Substance Misuse and Alcohol Use Disorders *(continued)*

ii. Zyban, for example, should not be combined with alcohol. Nurses working with inpatients in a case management model were found to produce outcomes in smoking cessation (Smith, Reilly, Houston Miller, DeBusk, & Taylor, 2002).

iii. Show caring, concern, and provide ongoing support.

2. Communicate care and concern
   a. Encourage moderate-intensity exercise to reduce cravings for nicotine because 5 minutes of such exercise is associated with short-term reduction in the desire to smoke and in tobacco withdrawal symptoms (Daniel, Cropley, Ussher, & West, 2004).
   b. Schedule follow-up contact in person or by telephone within 1 week after planned quit date. Continue telephone counseling, especially with those using medications and nicotine patches (Boyle et al., 2005; Cooper et al., 2004).

D. Alcohol dependence
1. Assess the patient for psychological dependence.
2. Assess the patient for (a) physiological dependence and (b) “tolerance.” Psychological dependence occurs with both abuse and dependence and is more difficult to resolve.
3. Assess need for medical detoxification (see alcohol withdrawal in Inpatient Hospitalization section).
4. Refer patient and family to addictions or mental health nurse practitioner or physician.
5. Evaluate patient and family capacity to implement referral.
6. On successful detoxification, monitor use of medications, interpersonal therapies, and participation in self-help groups.

E. Marijuana dependence: Little research on effective intervention for psychological dependence on marijuana is available. Some guidance can be found for smoking cessation and self-help approaches.
1. Refer to steps for smoking cessation (see section C of Nursing Care Strategies).
2. Refer patient to addiction specialist for counseling for psychological dependence and/or treatment with cognitive behavioral therapy.
3. Refer to community-based self-help groups such as Narcotics Anonymous, Alcoholics Anonymous, or Al-Anon.
4. Encourage development or expansion of patient’s social support system.

F. Heroin or opioid dependence
1. Older long-term opioid users may continue use, relapse, and seek treatment. Methadone or buprenorphine are current pharmacological treatment options that are effective in conjunction with self-help programs and/or psychosocial interventions.
2. Treatment with methadone, a synthetic narcotic agonist, suppresses withdrawal symptoms and drug cravings associated with opioid dependence but requires daily dosing of 60 mg, minimum. It is dispensed only in state-licensed clinics.
3. Treatment with buprenorphine (Subutex or Suboxone): Treatment occurs in office practice by trained physicians, with this opioid partial agonist–antagonist. Alone and in combination with naloxone (Suboxone), it can prevent withdrawal when someone ceases use of an opioid drug and then be used for long-term treatment. Naloxone is an opioid antagonist used to reverse depressant symptoms in opiate overdose and at different dosages to treat dependence (CSAT, 2010).
   a. Close collaboration with the prescriber is required because these drugs should not be abruptly terminated, used with antidepressants, and interact negatively with many prescription medications.
4. Naltrexone, a long-acting opioid antagonist, blocks opioid effects and is most effective with those who are no longer opioid dependent but are at high risk for relapse (Srisurapanont & Jarusuraisin, 2005).
5. Treatment of the older patient who has become addicted to Oxycontin or other opioids should be done in consultation with an addictions specialist nurse or physician.
   a. It is recommended that prescribers avoid opioids and synthetic opioids (Demerol, Dilaudid, and Oxycontin). Opioids have high potential for addiction and Demerol has been associated with delirium in older adults (CSAT, 2010).
   b. Barbiturates should be avoided as hypnotics and the use of benzodiazepines for anxiety should be limited to 4 months (USDHHS, 2004a).

(continued)

Protocol 28.1: Substance Misuse and Alcohol Use Disorders *(continued)*

G. Treatment and relapse prevention
   1. Monitor pharmacological treatment. The benefits of this treatment are dependent on adherence and psychosocial treatment should accompany its use (World Health Organization, 2000). Methadone or buprenorphine should be used for long-term treatment of opioid dependence.
   2. In limited studies using a cognitive behavioral approach, group psychotherapy has produced good outcomes with older adults (Payne & Marcus, 2008).
   3. Refer to community-based groups, such as Alcoholics Anonymous, Narcotics Anonymous, Al-Anon groups, and encourage attendance.
   4. Educate family and patient regarding signs of risky use or relapse to heavy drinking or alcohol-dependent behavior.
   5. Counsel patient to reduce drug use (harm reduction) and engage in relationship healing or building, to engage in community or intellectually rewarding activities, spiritual growth, and so on that increase valued nondrinking rewards.
   6. Counsel in the development of coping skills
      a. Anticipate and avoid temptation.
      b. Learn cognitive strategies to avoid negative moods.
      c. Make lifestyle changes to reduce stress, improve the quality of life, and increase pleasure.
      d. Learn cognitive and behavioral activities to cope with cravings and urges to use.
      e. Encourage development or expansion of patient's social support system.

VI. EVALUATION AND EXPECTED OUTCOMES

A. Patient will have:
   1. Improved physical health and function
   2. Improved quality of life, sense of well-being, and mental health
   3. More satisfying interpersonal relationships
   4. Enhanced productivity and mental alertness
   5. Decreased likelihood of falls and other accidents
B. Nurses will demonstrate:
   1. Increased accuracy in detecting patient problems related to use or misuse of substances.
   2. More evidence-based interventions resulting in better outcomes.
C. Institution will have:
   1. Increased number of referrals to ambulatory substance abuse and mental health treatment programs.
   2. Improved links with community-based organizations engaged in prevention, education, and treatment of older adults with substance-related disorders.

VII. FOLLOW-UP MONITORING OF CONDITION

A. Evaluate for increase in substance use or misuse associated with growing numbers of aging adults.
B. Increase outreach to targeted vulnerable populations.
C. Document chronic care needs of older adults diagnosed with substance-related disorders.
D. Monitor alcohol use among older adults with chronic pain.
E. Communicate findings to all members of the caregiver team.

VIII. GUIDELINES

The National Quality Forum has published *Evidence-Based Practices to Treat Substance Use Disorders.* These guidelines are inclusive of primary care, the settings in which older adults seek treatment (National Quality Forum [NQF], 2007).

ABBREVIATIONS

APA	American Psychiatric Association
AUDIT	Alcohol Use Disorders Identification Test

Protocol 28.1: Substance Misuse and Alcohol Use Disorders *(continued)*

AUDIT-C	Alcohol Use Disorders Identification Test-Condensed
AWS	Alcohol withdrawal syndrome
CIWA-Ar	Clinical Institute Withdrawal Assessment for Alcohol, Revised
CNS	Central nervous system
CSAT	Center for Substance Abuse Treatment
DSM-5	*Diagnostic and Statistical Manual of Mental Disorders, 5th Edition*
DTs	delirium tremens
FDA	Food and Drug Administration
NIAAA	National Institute Alcohol Abuse and Alcoholism
NIDA	National Institute on Drug Abuse
NQF	National Quality Forum
OTC	Over the counter
QF	Quantity frequency
SAMHSA	Substance Abuse and Mental Health Services Administration
SBIRT	Screening, brief intervention, and referral to treatment
SMAST-G	Short Michigan Alcohol Screening Test-Geriatric version
USDHHS	U.S. Department of Health and Human Services

RESOURCES

Important Websites

Agency for Healthcare Research and Quality (AHRQ) Guidelines
AHRQ clinical practice guidelines are available to download.
www.ahrq.gov

American Lung Association
www.ffsonline.org

American Nurses Association
www.ana.org

American Psychiatric Association
www.apa.org

American Psychiatric Nursing Association
www.apna.org

Centers for Disease Control and Prevention
www.cdc.gov/tobacco/how2quit.htm

International Nurses Society on Addictions
www.intnsa.org

National Institute of Mental Health
Patient teaching materials for panic disorders, obsessive compulsive disorder, posttraumatic stress, acute stress, and general anxiety disorders.
www.niaaa.nih.gov

National Institute on Aging
Age page: Medications: Use them safely
www.nia.nih.gov/healthinformation/publications/medicine.htm

National Institute on Alcohol Abuse and Alcoholism (NIAAA)
www.drugabuse.gov

National Institute on Drug Abuse (NIDA)
www.nida.nih.gov

New York City Department of Health and Mental Hygiene
www.nyc.gov/html/doh/html/home/home/shtml

Assessment Tools

Alcohol Use Disorders Identification Test (AUDIT) Tool. Saunders, J. B., Ashland, O. G., Babur, T. F., de la Fuente, J. R., & Grant, M. (1993).

American Psychiatric Association. (2002). *Fagerström test for nicotine dependence (FTND).*

American Psychiatric Association's PsychNET 2002
www.apa.org/videos/fagerstrom.html

Comorbidity Alcohol Risk Evaluation Tool CARET

Dyehouse, J., Howe, S., & Ball, S. (1996). *FRAMES model in the training manual for nursing using brief intervention for alcohol problems.* Rockville, MD: U.S. Department of Health and Human Services.

Fagerström Test for Nicotine Dependence (FTND)

Hartford Institute for Geriatric Nursing
Substance abuse
consultgerirn.org/resources

Naegle, M. A. (2003). *Try this: Best practices in nursing care of older adults: Alcohol use screening and assessment*, Issue # 17. A series provided by The Hartford Institute for Geriatric Nursing.

Retrieved from http://consultgerirn.org/uploads/File/trythis/try_this_17.pdf

Quantity-Frequency Index. Khavari, K. A., & Farber, P. D. (1978).

SBIRT (Screening, Brief Intervention and Referral to Treatment)

SBIRT Toolkit: A Step-by-Step Guide. Massachusetts Bureau of Substance Abuse Services

www.masbirt.org/sites/www.masbirt.org/files/documents/toolkit.pdf

SMAST-G (Short Michigan Alcoholism Screening Test-Geriatric Version)

https://www.nccdp.org/resources/_PDF_.pdf

Guidelines

Agency for Healthcare Research and Quality. (2011). *Treating tobacco use and dependence: 2008 update.* Retrieved from http://www.ahrq.gov/path/tobbaco.htm

Blow, F. C., Bartels, S. J., Brockmann, L. M., & Van Citters, A. S. (2005). *Evidence-based practices for preventing substance abuse and mental health problems in older adults.* Older Americans Substance Abuse and Mental Health Technical Assistance Center. Retrieved from http://store.samhsa.gov/product/KAPT26

Michigan Quality Improvement Consortium (2015). *MQIC Guidelines for Substance Use: SAMHSA-HRSA Center for Integrated Health Care Solutions/Screening Tools; Tobacco Cessation Provider Resources.* Retrieved from http://www.mqic.org/

National Quality Forum is completing a review for "Evidence-Based Treatment Practices for Substance Use Disorders." These guidelines are inclusive of primary care, the settings in which most older adults seek treatment.

http://www.qualityforum.org/projects/substance_use_2009.aspx

REFERENCES

Aalto, M., Pekuri, P., & Seppä, K. (2003). Primary health care professionals' activity in intervening in patients' alcohol drinking during a 3-year brief intervention implementation project. *Drug and Alcohol Dependence, 69*(1), 9–14. *Evidence Level III.*

Allen, J. P., Litten, R. Z., Fertig, J. B., & Babor, T. (1997). A review of research on the Alcohol Use Disorders Identification Test (AUDIT). *Alcoholism, Clinical and Experimental Research, 21*(4), 613–619. *Evidence Level III.*

Allen, J. P., & Wilson, V. (Eds.). (2003). *Assessing alcohol problems: A guide for clinicians and researchers* (2nd ed., pp. 667–671). Bethesda, MD: U.S. Department of Health and Human Services. *Evidence Level VI.*

Amato, L., Minozzi, S., Davoli, M., Vecchi, S., Ferri, M. M., & Mayet, S. (2008). Psychosocial and pharmacological treatments versus pharmacological treatments for opioid detoxification. *Cochrane Database of Systematic Reviews, 2008*(3), CD005031. *Evidence Level I.*

Amato, L., Minozzi, S., Vecchi, S., & Davoli, M. (2010). Benzodiazepines for alcohol withdrawal. *Cochrane Database of Systematic Reviews, 2010*(3), CD005063. *Evidence Level I.*

American Lung Association. (2010). *Smoking among older adults.* Retrieved from http://www.lungusa.org/site/apps/s. *Evidence Level IV.*

American Psychiatric Association. (2013). *Diagnostic and statistical manual of mental disorders* (5th ed). Arlington, VA: American Psychiatric Press. *Evidence Level VI.*

Andrews, C. (2008). An exploratory study of substance abuse among Latino older adults. *Journal of Gerontological Social Work, 51*(1–2), 87–108. *Evidence Level IV.*

Ayalon, L., Areán, P. A., Linkins, K., Lynch, M., & Estes, C. L. (2007). Integration of mental health services into primary care overcomes ethnic disparities in access to mental health services between Black and White elderly. *American Journal of Geriatric Psychiatry, 15*(10), 906–912. *Evidence Level IV.*

Babor, T. F., Higgins-Biddle, J. C., Saunders, J. B., & Monteiro, M. G. (2001). *AUDIT: The alcohol use disorders identification test. Guidelines for use in primary care* (2nd ed.). Geneva, Switzerland: World Health Organization. *Evidence Level IV.*

Babor, T. F., McRee, B. G., Kassebaum, P. A., Grimaldi, P. L., Ahmed, K., & Bray, J. (2007). Screening, brief intervention, and referral to treatment (SBIRT): Toward a public health approach to the management of substance abuse. *Substance Abuse, 28*(3), 7–30. *Evidence Level III.*

Ballesteros, J., González-Pinto, A., Querejeta, I., & Ariño, J. (2004). Brief interventions for hazardous drinkers delivered in primary care are equally effective in men and women. *Addictions, 99*(1), 103–108. *Evidence Level III.*

Bartels, S. J., Coakley, E. H., Zubritsky, C., Ware, J. H., Miles, K. M., Areán, P. A., & PRISM-E Investigators. (2004). Improving access to geriatric mental health services: A randomized trial comparing treatment engagement with integrated versus enhanced referral care for depression, anxiety, and at-risk alcohol use. *American Journal of Psychiatry, 161*(8), 1455–1462. *Evidence Level III.*

Bartus, R. T., Emerich, D. F., Hotz, J., Blaustein, M., Dean, R. L., Perdomo, B., & Basile, A. S. (2003). Vivitrex, an injectable, extended-release formulation of naltrexone, provides pharmokinetic and pharmacodynamic evidence of efficacy for 1 month in rats. *Neuropsychopharmacology, 28*(11), 1973–1982. *Evidence Level II.*

Betty Ford Institute Consensus Panel. (2007). What is recovery? A working definition from the Betty Ford Institute. *Journal of Substance Abuse Treatment, 33*(3), 221–228. *Evidence Level VI.*

Blazer, D. G., & Wu, L. T. (2009). The epidemiology of at-risk and binge drinking among middle-aged and elderly community adults: National Survey on Drug Use and Health. *American Journal of Psychiatry, 166*(10), 1162–1169. *Evidence Level IV.*

Blow, F. C., & Barry, K. L. (2003). Use and misuse of alcohol among older women. National Institutes of Alcohol and Alcohol Abuse. Retrieved from http://pubs.niaaa.nih.gov/publications/arh26–4/308–315.htm. *Evidence Level V.*

Blow, F. C., Bartels, S. J., Brockmann, L. M., & Van Citters, A. S. (2005). *Evidence-based practices for preventing substance abuse and mental health problems in older adults.* Older Americans

Substance Abuse and Mental Health Technical Assistance Center. Retrieved from http://store.samhsa.gov/product/KAPT26. *Evidence Level IV.*

Blow, F. C., Brower, K. J., Schulenberg, J. E., Demo-Dananberg, L. M., Young, J. P., & Beresford, T. P. (1992). The Michigan Alcoholism Screening Test–Geriatric Version (MAST-G): A new elderly-specific screening instrument. *Alcoholism: Clinical and Experimental Research, 16*(2), 372. *Evidence Level III.*

Boyle, A. R., & Davis, H. (2006). Early screening and assessment of alcohol and substance abuse in the elderly: Clinical implications. *Journal of Addictions Nursing, 17*(2), 95–103. *Evidence Level VI.*

Boyle, R. G., Solberg, L. I., Asche, S. E., Boucher, J. L., Pronk, N. P., & Jensen, C. J. (2005). Offering telephone counseling to smokers using pharmacotherapy. *Nicotine & Tobacco Research, 7*(Suppl. 1), S19–S27. *Evidence Level III.*

Bouchery, E. E., Harwood, H., Sacks, J. J. Simon, C. J., & Brewer, R. D. (2011). Economic costs of excessive alcohol consumption in the U.S., 2006. *American Journal of Preventive Medicine* (5), 516–524. doi:10,1016/j.ampre.2011.06.045. *Evidence Level IV.*

Brennan, P. L., Schutte, K. K., & Moos, R. H. (2005). Pain and use of alcohol to manage pain: Prevalence and 3-year outcomes among older problem and non-problem drinkers. *Addiction, 100*(6), 777–786. *Evidence Level III.*

Census Bureau Reports. (2014). *Fueled by aging baby boomers, nation's older population to nearly double in the next 20 Years.* Release Number CB 14-84. Retrieved from http://www.census.gov/news- room/releases/2014/cb14-84.html. *Evidence Level IV.*

Center for Substance Abuse Treatment. (2010). *Clinical guidelines for the use of buprenorphine in the treatment of opioid addiction: A treatment improvement protocol, series 40* (DHHS Publication [SMA] 04–3939). Rockville, MD: Substance Abuse and Mental Health Services Administration. Retrieved from http://www.samhsa.gov. *Evidence Level VI.*

Centers for Disease Control and Prevention. (2009). Annual smoking-attributable mortality, years of potential life lost, and productivity losses—United States, 1997–2001. *Morbidity and Mortality Weekly Report, 54*(25), 625–628. *Evidence Level V.*

Centers for Disease Control and Prevention. (2014). *Best practices for comprehensive tobacco control programs–2014.* Retrieved from http:www.cedc.gov/tobacco/state and community/interventions. *Evidence Level VI.*

Centers for Disease Control and Prevention. (2015). Current cigarette smoking among adults—United States, 2005–2013. *Morbidity and Mortality Weekly Report, 2014,* 63(47), 1108–1112. Retrieved from http://www.cdc.gov/mmwr/preview/mmwrhtml/mm6347a4.htm. *Evidence Level IV.*

Chait, R., Fahmy, S., & Caceres, J. (2010). Cocaine abuse in older adults: An underscreened cohort. *Journal of the American Geriatrics Society, 58*(2), 391–392. *Evidence Level IV.*

Cooney, N. L., Babor, T. F., & Litt, M. D. (2001). Matching clients to alcoholism treatment based on severity of alcohol dependence. In R. H. Longabaugh & P. W. Wirtz (Eds.), *Project MATCH hypotheses. Results and causal chain analyses.* (*NIAAA Project MATCH monograph series, 8,* pp. 134–148). Rockville, MD: NIAAA. *Evidence Level III.*

Cooper, T. V., DeBon, M. W., Stockton, M., Klesges, R. C., Steenbergh, T. A., Sherrill-Mittleman, D., & Johnson, K. C. (2004). Correlates of adherence with transdermal nicotine. *Addictive Behaviors, 29*(8), 1565–1578. *Evidence Level III.*

Daniel, J., Cropley, M., Ussher, M., & West, R. (2004). Acute effects of a short bout of moderate versus light intensity exercise versus inactivity on tobacco withdrawal symptoms in sedentary smokers. *Psychopharmacology, 174*(3), 320–326. *Evidence Level II.*

Fink, A., Elliott, M. N., Tsia, M., & Beck, J. C. (2005). An evaluation of an intervention to assist primary care physicians in screening and educating older patients who use alcohol. *Journal of the American Geriatrics Society, 53*(11), 1937–1943. *Evidence Level III.*

Grant, B. F., Dawson, D. A., Stinson, F. S., Chou, S. P., Dufour, M. C., & Pickering, R. P. (2004). The 12-month prevalence and trends in *DSM-IV* alcohol abuse and dependence: United States, 1991–1992 and 2001–2002. *Drug and Alcohol Dependence, 74*(3), 223–234. *Evidence Level IV.*

Han, B., Gfroerer, J. C., Colliver, J. D., & Penne, M. A. (2009). Substance use disorder among older adults in the United States in 2020. *Addiction, 104*(1), 88–96. *Evidence Level VI.*

Hansen, R. N., Edelsberg, O. G., Woody, G. E., & Sullivan, S. D (2011). Economic costs of onmedical use of prescription opioids. *Clinical Journal of Pain, 3,* 194–201. doi:10.1097/AJP.Ob013e3181ffD4ca. *Evidence Level IV.*

Hesse, M., Vanderplasschen, W., Rapp, R. C., Broekaert, E., & Fridell, M. (2007). Case management for persons with substance use disorders. *Cochrane Database of Systematic Reviews, 2007*(4), CD006265. *Evidence Level I.*

Justice, A. (2010). HIV and aging: Time for a new paradigm. *Current HIV/AIDS Reports, 7,* 69–76. *Evidence Level IV.*

Khavari, K. A., & Farber, P. D. (1978). A profile instrument for the quantification and assessment of alcohol consumption. The Khavari Alcohol Test. *Journal of Studies on Alcohol, 39*(9), 1525–1539. *Evidence Level VI.*

Kinnunen, T., Haukkala, A., Korhonen, T., Quiles, Z. N., Spiro, A., III, & Garvey, A. J. (2006). Depression and smoking across 25 years of the Normative Aging Study. *International Journal of Psychiatry in Medicine, 36*(4), 413–426. *Evidence Level III.*

Letizia, M., & Reinbolz, M. (2005). Identifying and managing acute alcohol withdrawal in the elderly. *Geriatric Nursing, 26*(3), 176–183. *Evidence Level VI.*

Madras, B. K., Compton, W. M., Avula, D., Stegbauer, T., Stein, J. B., & Clark, H. W. (2009). Screening, brief interventions, referral to treatment (SBIRT) for illicit drug and alcohol use at multiple healthcare sites: Comparison at intake and 6 months later. *Drug and Alcohol Dependence, 99*(1–3), 280–295. *Evidence Level III.*

Mayet, S., Farrell, M., Ferri, M., Amato, L., & Davoli, M. (2005). *Psychosocial treatment for opiate abuse and dependence.* The Cochrane Collaboration. Retrieved from http://www.thecochranelibrary.com. *Evidence Level I.*

McDougall, G. J., Becker, H., Delville, C. L.,Vaughn, P. W., & Acee, T. W. (2010). Alcohol use and older adults: A little goes a long way. *International Journal of Disabilities in Human Development, 6*(4), 431. doi:10,1901/jaba.2007 6–431. *Evidence Level II.*

McLellan, A. T., Lewis, D. C., O'Brien, C. P., & Kleber, H. D. (2000). Drug dependence, a chronic medical illness: Implications for treatment, insurance, and outcomes evaluation. *Journal of the American Medical Association, 284*(13), 1689–1695. *Evidence Level VI.*

Merrick, E. L., Horgan, C. M., Hodgkin, D., Garnick, D. W., Houghton, S. F., Panas, L., & Blow, F. C. (2008). Unhealthy drinking patterns in older adults: Prevalence and associated characteristics. *Journal of the American Geriatrics Society, 56*(2), 214–223. *Evidence Level III.*

Miller, P. M., Cluver, J., & Anton, R. F. (2009). A useful test for monitoring alcohol use. *Behavioral healthcare.* Retrieved from http://behavioral.net/article/useful-test-monitoring-alcohol-use. *Evidence Level VI.*

Moore, A. A., Karno, M. P., Grella, C. E., Lin, J. C., Warda, U., Liao, D. H., & Hu, P. (2009). Alcohol, tobacco, and nonmedical drug use in older U.S. adults: Data from the 2001/02 National Epidemiologic Survey on Alcohol and Related Conditions. *Journal of the American Geriatrics Society, 57*(12), 2275–2281. *Evidence Level IV.*

Mukamal, K. J., Chung, H., Jenny, N. S., Kuller, L. H., Longstreth, W. T., Mittleman, . . . Siscovick, D. S. (2006). Alcohol consumption and risk of coronary heart disease in older adults: The cardiovascular health study. *Journal of the American Geriatrics Society, 54*(1), 30–37. doi:10.1111/j.1532-5415.2005.00561. *Evidence Level III.*

National Institute on Alcohol Abuse and Alcoholism. (2015). *Older adults.* Retrieved from http://www.niaaa.nih.gov/alcohol-helath/special-populations-co-occurring-disorders. *Evidence Level IV.*

National Institute on Drug Abuse. (2010). *Drug abuse in the 21st century: What problems lie ahead for the baby boomers?* Retrieved from http://archives/drugabuse.gov/meetings.bbsr/prevalence.html. *Evidence Level V.*

National Institute on Drug Abuse. (2015). Prescription drug abuse: Older adults. Retrieved from http://www.drugabuse.gov/publications/research=-reports/prescription. *Evidence Level IV.*

National Quality Forum. (2007). *Evidence-based Treatment Practices for Substance Use Disorders: A Workshop.* Washington, DC: National Quality Forum. Retrieved from http://www.qualityforum.org. *Evidence Level VI.*

Nicholas, J. A., & Hall, W. J. (2011) Screening and preventive services for older adults. *Mt. Sinai Journal of Medicine, 78* (4), 198–508.

Oslin, D. W. (2005). Treatment of late-life depression complicated by alcohol dependence. *American Journal of Geriatric Psychiatry, 13*(6), 491–500. *Evidence Level III.*

Oslin, D. W., Pettinati, H., & Volpicelli, J. R. (2002). Alcoholism treatment adherence: Older age predicts better adherence and drinking outcomes. *American Journal of Geriatric Psychiatry, 10*(6), 740–747. *Evidence Level III.*

Payne, K. T., & Marcus, D. K. (2008). The efficacy of group psychotherapy for older adult clients: A meta-analysis. *Group Dynamics: Theory, Research, and Practice, 12*(4), 268–278. *Evidence Level III.*

Pomerleau, C. S., Carton, S. M., Lutzke, M. L., Flessland, K. A., & Pomerleau, O. F. (1994). Reliability of the Fagerstrom Tolerance Questionnaire and the Fagerstrom Test for Nicotine Dependence. *Addictive Behaviors, 19*(1), 33–39. *Evidence Level V.*

Rehm, J., Mathers, C., Popova, S., Thavorncharoensap, M., Teerawattananon, Y., & Petra, J. (2009). Global burden of disease and injury and economic cost attributable to alcohol use and alcohol use disordrs. *Lancet, 373*(9682), 2223–2233. *Evidence Level VI.*

Roberts, A. M., Marshall, E. J., & MacDonald, A. J. (2005). Which screening test for alcohol consumption is best associated with "at risk" drinking in older primary care attenders? *Primary Care Mental Health, 3*(2), 131–138. *Evidence Level III.*

Sachs-Ericsson, N., Collins, N., Schmidt, B., & Zvolensky, M. (2011). Older adults and smoking: Characteristics, nicotine dependence and prevalence of *DSM-IV* 12-month disorders. *Aging & Mental Health, 15*(1), 132–141. Retrieved from http://www.informaworld.com/smpp/content. *Evidence Level III.*

Satre, D. D., Mertens, J. R., Areán, P. A., & Weisner, C. (2004). Five-year alcohol and drug treatment outcomes of older adults versus middle-aged and younger adults in a managed care program. *Addiction, 99*(10), 1286–1297. *Evidence Level III.*

Saunders, J. B., Aasland, O. G., Babor, T. F., de la Fuente, J. R., & Grant, M. (1993). Development of the Alcohol Use Disorders Identification Test (AUDIT): WHO Collaborative Project on Early Detection of Persons with Harmful Alcohol Consumption—II. *Addiction, 88*(6), 791–804. *Evidence Level III.*

Schonfeld, L., King-Kallimanis, B. L., Duchene, D. M., Etheridge, R. L., Herrera, J. R., Barry, K. L., & Lynn, N. (2010). Screening and brief intervention for substance misuse among older adults: The Florida BRITE project. *American Journal of Public Health, 100*(1), 108–114. *Evidence Level IV.*

Simoni-Wastila, L., & Yang, H. K. (2006). Psychoactive drug abuse in older adults. *American Journal of Geriatric Pharmacotherapy, 4*(4), 380–392. *Evidence Level IV.*

Simoni-Wastila, L., Zuckerman, I. H., Singhal, P. K., Briesacher, B., & Hsu, V. D. (2005). National estimates of exposure to prescription drugs with addiction potential in community-dwelling elders. *Substance Abuse, 26*(1), 33–42. *Evidence Level III.*

Smith, P. M., Reilly, K. R., Houston Miller, N., DeBusk, R. F., & Taylor, C. B. (2002). Application of a nurse-managed inpatient smoking cessation program. *Nicotine & Tobbacco Research, 4*(2), 211–222. *Evidence Level III.*

Srisurapanont, M., & Jarusuraisin, N. (2005). Naltrexone for the treatment of alcoholism: A meta-analysis of randomized controlled trials. *International Journal of Neuropsychopharmacology, 8*(2), 267–280. *Evidence Level III.*

Stampfer, M. J., Kang, J. H., Chen, J., Cherry, R., & Grodstein, F. (2005). Effects of moderate alcohol consumption on cognitive function in women. *New England Journal of Medicine, 352*, 245–253. doi:10.1056/NEJMoa041152. *Evidence Level III.*

SAMHSA. (2010). *Treatment episode data: 2000-2010 (2012).* Retrieved from http://www.samhsa.gov/data/sites/default/files/2010_Treatment_Episode_Data. *Evidence Level III.*

Substance Abuse and Mental Health Services Administration. (2012). *Results from the 2011 National Survey on Drug Use and*

Health. NSDUH Series H-44. HHS Publication No. (SMA) 12–4713. Rockville, MD: Author. *Evidence Level III.*

Sullivan, J. T., Sykora, K., Schneiderman, J., Naranjo, C. A., & Sellers, E. M. (1989). Assessment of alcohol withdrawal: The revised Clinical Institute Withdrawal Assessment for Alcohol scale (CIWA-Ar). *British Journal of Addiction, 84*(11), 1353–1357. *Evidence Level III.*

Tibbitts, G. M. (2008). Sleep disorders: Causes, effects, and solutions. *Primary Care, 35*(4), 817–837. *Evidence Level VI.*

U.S. Department of Health and Human Services. (2004a). *Substance abuse among older adults: A guide for physicians.* (DHHS Publication No. SMA 00–3394). Rockville, MD: Author, Substance Abuse and Mental Health Services Administration, Center for Substance Abuse Treatment. *Evidence Level VI.*

U.S. Department of Health and Human Services. (2004b). *Substance abuse among older adults: A guide for social service providers* (DHHS Publication No. SMA 00–3393). Rockville, MD: Author, Substance Abuse and Mental Health Services Administration, Center for Substance Abuse Treatment. *Evidence Level VI.*

U.S. Preventative Services Task Force. (2015). *Alcohol misuse: Screening and brief intervention in primary care.* Retrieved from http://www.uspreventiveservicestaskforce.org

Vance, D. E, Mugavero, M., Willig, J., & Raper, J. L. (2011). A cross-sectional study of comorbidity prevalence and clinical characteristics across decades of life. *Journal of Nurses in AIDS Care, 22*(1), 17–26. doi:10.1016/j.jana2010.04.002. *Evidence Level III.*

Vastag, B. (2003). Addiction poorly understood by clinicians: Experts say attitudes, lack of knowledge hinder treatment. *Journal of the American Medical Association, 290*(10), 1299–1303. *Evidence Level III.*

West, N. A., Severtson, S. G., Green, J. L., & Dart, R. C. (2015). Trends in abuse and misuse of prescription opioids among older adults. *Drug and Alcohol Dependence, 149,* 117–121. *Evidence Level III.*

Wetterling, T., Weber, B., Depfenhart, M., Schneider, B., & Junghanns, K. (2006). Development of a rating scale to predict the severity of alcohol withdrawal syndrome. *Alcohol and Alcoholism, 41*(6), 611–615. *Evidence Level III.*

Whitmer, R. A., Sidney, S., Selby, J., Johnston, S. C., & Yaffe, K. (2005). Midlife cardiovascular risk factors and risk of dementia in late life. *Neurology, 64*(2), 277–281. *Evidence Level IV.*

World Health Organization. (2000). *A systematic review of opioid antagonists for alcohol dependence. Management of substance dependence: Review series.* Retrieved from http://www.who.int/entity/substance_abuse/publications/en/opioid.pdf. *Evidence Level I.*

Wu, L. T., & Blazer, D. G. (2011). Illicit and nonmedical drug use among older adults: A review. *Journal of Aging and Health, 23*(3), 481–504. *Evidence Level IV.*

Wu, L. T., & Blazer, D. G. (2014). Substance use disorders and psychiatric comorbidity in mid and later life: A review. *International Journal of Epidemiology, 43,* 304–317. *Evidence Level IV.*

Wutzke, S. E., Conigrave, K. M., Saunders, J. B., & Hall, W. D. (2002). The long-term effectiveness of brief interventions for unsafe alcohol consumption: A 10-year follow-up. *Addiction, 97*(6), 665–675. *Evidence Level I.*

Zapolski, T. C. B., Pedersen, S. L., McCarthy, D. M., & Smith, G. T. (2014). Less drinking, yet more problems: Understanding African American drinking and related problems. *Psychological Bulletin, 140*(1), 188–223. doi:10.1037/a0032113. *Evidence Level III.*

29

Comprehensive Assessment and Management of the Critically Ill

Michele C. Balas, Colleen M. Casey, Lauren Crozier, and Mary Beth Happ

EDUCATIONAL OBJECTIVES

On completion of this chapter, the reader will be able to:

1. Identify factors that influence an older adult's ability to survive and rehabilitate from a catastrophic illness
2. List examples of atypical presentation of illness in critically ill older adults
3. Describe geriatric-specific assessment and physical examination of critically ill older adults
4. Identify nursing interventions that decrease critically ill older adults' risk for adverse outcomes

OVERVIEW

More than half (55.8%) of all intensive care unit (ICU) days are incurred by patients older than 65 years of age (Angus et al., 2006) and this number is expected to increase to unprecedented levels over the next few years as our population ages. For example, it is projected that by the year 2020, more than 350,000 older adults will annually require acute mechanical ventilation for more than 4 days (Zilberberg & Shorr, 2008). Evidence suggests that the characteristics and intensity of treatment for older adults admitted to the ICU have changed significantly over the past decade. The intensity of treatments has increased (e.g., greater use of renal replacement therapy and vasopressors) and ICU survival has vastly improved. There remains, however, a large population of older adults who survive their initial ICU stay and hospitalization but who have high morbidity and mortality over the subsequent years in excess of that seen in comparable controls (Wunsch et al., 2010).

Although critically ill older adults are an extremely heterogeneous group, they do share some age-related characteristics and are susceptible to a variety of geriatric syndromes and complications that may influence ICU treatments and outcomes (Milbrandt, Eldadah, Nayfield, Hadley, & Angus, 2010; Pisani, 2009). In addition to high ICU, hospital, and long-term mortality rates, critically ill older adults are at increased risk for substantial physical, functional, and neurocognitive impairment, psychological distress (e.g., posttraumatic stress disorder, depression, and anxiety), sleep disturbances, and postdischarge institutional care (Balas, Happ, Yang, Chelluri, & Richmond, 2009; Balas et al., 2011; Barr et al., 2013; Brummel et al., 2014; de Rooij et al., 2008; Esteban et al., 2004; Ford, Thomas, Cook, Whitley, & Peden, 2007; Hennessy, Juzwishin, Yergens, Noseworthy, & Doig, 2005; Hopkins & Jackson, 2006; Kaarlola, Tallgren, & Pettile, 2006; Pandharipande et al., 2013; Wunsch et al., 2010). Older age is also one of the factors that may lead to physician

For a description of evidence levels cited in this chapter, see Chapter 1, "Developing and Evaluating Clinical Practice Guidelines: A Systematic Approach."

bias in refusing ICU admission (Joynt et al., 2001; Mick & Ackerman, 2004), the decision to withhold mechanical ventilation, surgery, or dialysis (Hamel et al., 1999), and an increased frequency of do-not-resuscitate orders (Hakim et al., 1996). Despite these findings, most critically ill older adults demonstrate resiliency, report being satisfied with their quality of life (QOL) after discharge, and, if needed, would reaccept ICU care and mechanical ventilation (Guentner et al., 2006; Hennessy et al., 2005; Kleinpell & Ferrans, 2002). Given their knowledge and expertise, nurses play a key role in facilitating older adult's ability to survive and successfully rehabilitate from a catastrophic illness.

BACKGROUND AND STATEMENT OF PROBLEM

Chronological age *alone* is not an acceptable or accurate predictor of poor outcomes after critical illness (Milbrandt et al., 2010). Factors influencing an older adult's ability to survive a critical illness are multifactorial and include severity of illness, nature and extent of comorbidities, medical diagnosis, mechanical ventilation use, complications, preexisting frailty, malnutrition, and patient preference (de Rooij, Abu-Hanna, Levi, & de Jonge, 2005; Marik, 2006; Baldwin et al., 2014; Wunsch et al., 2010). Other, less well investigated variables include senescence, vasoactive drug use, ageism, decreased social support, and the critical care environment (Ford et al., 2007; Mick & Ackerman, 2004; Tullmann & Dracup, 2000). The onset of new geriatric syndromes for an older hospitalized adult, such as delirium, urinary incontinence, infection, or falls, is also a harbinger of decline that can often be prevented with appropriate and timely ICU nursing interventions (for more information visit www.GeroNurseOnline.org). This chapter presents strategies and rationale for comprehensive assessment of critically ill older adults to guide optimal care management.

ASSESSMENT OF PROBLEM AND NURSING CARE STRATEGIES

Assessment of Baseline Health Status

The performance of a comprehensive assessment of a critically ill older adult's preadmission health status, functional and cognitive ability, and social support systems helps nurses identify the multiple risk factors that make older adults susceptible to a variety of life-threatening conditions, complications, and frequently encountered geriatric syndromes. Nurses can use these initial assessments to develop an evidence-based, holistic, and individualized plan of care that meets both the elder's and her or his family's needs and the goals of care throughout hospitalization. This baseline assessment is also useful to other members of the interdisciplinary ICU team as they develop their own profession-specific plans of care.

Preexisting Cognitive Impairment

Several anatomic and physiological changes occur in the aged central nervous system (Table 29.1; Miller, 2009). When these age-related changes are combined with the stress of acute pathology, multiple comorbidities, and polypharmacy, critically ill older adults are particularly vulnerable to a number of commonly encountered ICU syndromes such as pain, oversedation, and delirium (Balas et al., 2007; Barr et al., 2013; McNicoll et al., 2003; Pisani, Murphy, Van Ness, Araujo, & Inouye, 2007). High rates of preexisting cognitive impairment (31%–42%) are also reported in older adults admitted to both medical and surgical ICUs (Balas et al., 2007; Pisani, Redlich, McNicoll, Ely, & Inouye, 2003). It is unfortunate that this cognitive impairment is often unrecognized by both the older adults' family and health care providers (Balas et al., 2007; Pisani et al., 2003). Dementia, a progressive terminal illness, is commonly seen in the ICU setting with one recent study finding that nearly one in 10 nursing home residents with advanced cognitive impairment and severe functional impairment had an ICU stay before death (Fulton, Gozalo, Mitchell, Mor, & Teno, 2014). Given these collective findings, relatives or other caregivers should be asked for baseline information about memory, executive function (problem solving, planning, organization of information), and overall functional ability in daily living before the critical care admission (Kane, Ouslander, & Abrass, 2004). (See Chapter 6, "Assessing Cognitive Function.") Because knowledge of an older adult's preadmission cognitive status may also assist in treatment decisions, ICU clinicians should consider familiarizing themselves with dementia screening tools, such as the Informant Questionnaire of Cognitive Decline in the Elderly (IQCODE), which were specifically designed for proxy administration (Jorm, 1994).

Psychosocial Factors

Critical illness often renders older adults physically unable to effectively communicate with the health care team. The inability to communicate may stem from multiple factors, including physiological instability, tracheal intubation, and/or sedative and narcotic use (Happ, 2000, 2001). Family members or significant others are therefore a crucial source for obtaining important preadmission information such as the older adult's past medical and surgical history,

TABLE 29.1

Age-Associated Changes by Body System in the Older ICU Patient

System	Age-Associated Changes
Respiratory	**Decrease in:** chest wall compliance, rib mobility, lung size/elasticity, ventilatory response to hypoxia and hypercapnia, strength of respiratory muscles, PaO_2 level, mucociliary clearance, total lung capacity (minimal), forced vital capacity, forced inspiratroy and expiratory volume, peak and maximal expiratory flow rate, tidal volume (slight), diffusing capacity, maximal inspiratory and expiratory pressure **Increase in:** residual volume, closing volume, ventilation/perfusion (VQ) imbalance, chest wall stiffness **Physical assessment findings:** Possible kyphosis and an increased anteroposterior diameter of the chest; on auscultation, a few bibasilar crackles that clear with deep breathing and coughing
Gastrointestinal	**Decrease in:** number of mucus-secreting cells, mucosal prostaglandin concentrations, bicarbonate secretion, transit time of feces, pepsin and acid secretion, gastric emptying and thinning of smooth muscle in gastric mucosa, decrease in the number and velocity of peristaltic contractions in esophagus, enteric nervous system neurons, capacity to repair gastric mucosa, calcium absorption, lean muscle mass and strength, daily energy expenditure, intracellular water, number of hepatocytes and overall weight and size of liver (compensatory increase in cell size and proliferation of bile ducts), hepatic blood flow, metabolism of and sensitivity to drugs **Increase in:** body fat, changes to interstitial tissue (predisposing to soft tissue injury and increasing the time and course for mobilization of extra cellular water)
Genitourinary	**Increase in:** proportion of sclerotic nephrons/glomeruli, functional unit hypertrophy, afferent and efferent arteriole atrophy, collagen in the bladder, benign prostatic hypertrophy (men), hypertrophy of bladder muscle, thickening of the bladder **Decline in:** number of functioning nephrons; glomerular filtration rate; renal tubular cell function and number; renal blood flow and creatinine clearance; ability to conserve sodium and excrete hydrogen ions; ability to excrete salt and water loads, ammonia, and certain drugs in the activity of the renin-angiotensin system and end-organ responsiveness to antidiuretic hormone; tone of sphincters; alterations in estrogen cause further changes in urethral sphincter of women
Skin	**Decrease in:** surface area between dermis and epidermis, subcutaneous and connective tissue; number of eccrine and sebaceous glands; sebum amount; vascular supply to dermis; epidermal turnover; skin turgor; moisture content, dermal thickness **Physical assessment findings:** thin, fragile, wrinkled, loose or transparent dry, flaky, rough, and often itchy skin
Neurologic	**Decrease in:** size of brain/brain weight; number of neurons and dendrites; length of dendrite spines; cerebral blood flow; neurotransmitters or their binding sites in dopaminergic function, visual acuity and depth perception (secondary to anatomic and functional changes to the auditory and vestibular apparatus) and proprioception; balance and postural control and tactile and vibratory sensation **Increase in:** liposuscins, neuritic plaques, neurofibrillary bodies, ventricle size, sulci widening **Physical assessment findings:** decreased papillary response to penlight, decrease in near and peripheral vision, loss of visual acuity to dim light, evidence of muscle wasting and atrophy, presentation of a benign essential tumor, slower and less agile movement as compared to younger adults, diminished peripheral reflexes, a decreased vibratory sense in the feet and ankles
Cardiovascular	**Decrease in:** number of myocytes/pacemaker cells, ventricular compliance, rate of relaxation, baroreceptor sensitivity, vein elasticity, compliance of arteries, response of myocardium to catecholamine stimulation, resting heart rate, heart rate with stress, cardiac reserve **Increase in:** myocardial collagen content, amyloid deposits, myocardial irritability, stiffening of the outflow tract and great vessels (causing resistance to vascular emptying), ventricular hypertrophy (slight), pulse wave velocity, time required to complete the cycle of diastolic filling and systolic emptying, vein dilation, valvular stiffening **Physical assessment findings:** On auscultation many healthy older adults display a fourth heart sound (S_4), an aortic systolic murmur, higher systolic blood pressure with a widening pulse pressure, and a slower resting heart rate.
Immune/hematopoietic	Change in T-cell populations, products, and response to stimuli; defects in B-cell function; mix of immunoglobulins change (i.e., IgM decreases, IGG and IGA increase), and decline in neutrophil function

ICU, intensive care unit; IGA, immunoglobulin A; IGG, immunoglobulin G; IGM, immunoglobulin M.

Sources: Bickley (2008); Marik (2006); Menaker and Scalea (2010); Miller (2009); Pisani (2009); Rosenthal and Kavic (2004); Urden et al. (2002).

drug and alcohol use, nutritional status, home environment, infectious disease exposure, medication use, religious preference, and social support systems. Further, the lack of presence of family or a significant other threatens the nurse's ability to obtain accurate data about the person, which is often needed to make important care management decisions and end-of-life discussions (see Chapter 4, "Health Care Decision Making").

Functional Ability and Frailty

Assessing preadmission frailty and functional status is essential when caring for critically ill older adults because many studies have found them to be important prognostic indicators in this population (Baldwin et al., 2014; Daubin et al., 2011; Magnette et al., 2015). The Katz Index of Activities of Daily Living (KATZ ADL; Katz, Ford, Moskowitz, Jackson, & Jaffe, 1963), the Functional Independence Measure (FIM; Kidd et al., 1995), and Fried's Frailty Index (Fried et al., 2001) have been recommended for use with an older critically ill population (see Chapter 7, "Assessment of Physical Function"). On admission to the ICU, nurses should also investigate whether the older adult uses glasses, hearing aids, or other devices to perform activities of daily living. Having these assistive devices available to the older adult while he or she is in the ICU is important to enhance both communication, cognition, and rehabilitation.

Assessment and Interventions During the ICU Stay

Although a full discussion of the physiological changes that accompany normal aging is beyond the scope of this chapter, in the following sections we aim to provide readers with (a) an overview of the major age-related changes to organ systems and description of how these changes often manifest on physical examination (see Table 29.1), (b) a discussion of atypical presentations of some common ICU diagnoses, and (c) a description of interventions that may decrease risk for untoward medical events for critically ill older adults (also see Protocol 29.1). Common nursing interventions that benefit multiple organ systems will only be discussed in the first section in which the intervention is introduced. These interventions include encouraging early, frequent mobilization/ambulation; obtaining timely and appropriate consults (e.g., physical, occupational, speech, respiratory, and nutritional therapy); providing proper oral hygiene and adequate pain control; securing and ensuring the proper functioning of tubes/catheters; maintaining normothermia, deep vein thrombosis (DVT) prophylaxis, and reviewing/assessing medication appropriateness. The importance of these interventions and vigilance to these elements of nursing care cannot be overstated.

Respiratory System

Because respiratory reserve decreases with aging (see Table 29.1; Pisani, 2009), respiratory status can become the most tenuous component of an older adult ICU patient's recovery. Common pulmonary changes in aging elevate an older adult's risk for aspiration, atelectasis, pneumonia, and acute lung injury (Pisani, 2009; Rosenthal, 2004; Rosenthal & Kavic, 2004; Urden, Stacy, & Lough, 2002). These risks are further heightened in older adults who undergo thoracic or abdominal surgery; sustain rib fractures or chest injury; receive narcotics or sedatives; have tubes that bypass the oropharyngeal airway; or who are weak, deconditioned, dehydrated, and have poor oral hygiene (Menaker & Scalea, 2010; Nagappan & Parkin, 2003; Rosenthal, 2004; Rosenthal & Kavic, 2004; Urden et al., 2002).

Caring for the older adult who requires mechanical ventilation is particularly challenging. Although debate exists as to whether age influences outcomes in this population, evidence suggests that chronic ventilator dependency disproportionately affects older patients, whether as a complication of a critical illness or as a result of a chronic respiratory system limitation (Esteban et al., 2004; Zilberberg, de Wit, & Shorr, 2012). Patients who require 4 or more days of mechanical ventilation are more likely to die in the hospital, or, if they survive, to spend a considerable amount of time in an extended care facility on discharge, experience an increased risk for hospital readmission, suffer from continued morbidity, and experience a decreased QOL (Carson, Bach, Brzozowski, & Leff, 1999; Chelluri et al., 2004; Douglas, Daly, Brennan, Gordon, & Uthis, 2001; Douglas, Daly, Gordon, & Brennan, 2002; Kahn et al., 2013). These patients, and their family members, frequently experience symptoms of depression and posttraumatic stress disorder (PTSD) following discharge from the ICU (Douglas, Daly, O lylas, & Hickman, 2010; Griffiths, Fortune, Barber, & Young, 2007; Jubran et al., 2010). Of the few studies that specifically examined the effect of age on outcomes in *prolonged* mechanical ventilation, researchers recently found that 87% of individuals aged 65 years and older requiring prolonged mechanical ventilation in the long-term acute care hospital (LTACH) setting either died in the LTACH or were transferred back to an acute care hospital (Dermot Frengley, Sansone, Shakya, & Kaner, 2014). Only 22% of the older adults in this study were "successfully weaned" (i.e., removed from mechanical ventilation), and of those "weaned," 38% had to be placed back on the ventilator and only 41% were able to have their tracheostomies removed. Equally discouraging is the fact that only 4% of the entire cohort was ever discharged home, an exceedingly important patient- and family-centered outcome. These potential consequences should be included as part of a discussion of treatment options and postdischarge follow-up with older adults and their families.

The aforementioned findings also highlight the need for the ICU team to aggressively pursue means of early ventilator liberation. Fortunately, the evidence base supporting effective ventilator discontinuation strategies has strengthened substantially over the past decade. For example, we now know that daily interruption of sedative and analgesic infusions until a patient is awake and able to follow simple instruction (now referred to as spontaneous awakening trials [SATs]), leads to significant reductions in the duration of mechanical ventilation and ICU length of stay (LOS; Kress, Pohlman, O hlmang, & Hall, 2000), less use of diagnostic tests for unexplained mental status changes (Kress et al., 2000), and fewer complications (Schweickert, Gehlbach, Pohlman, Hall, & Kress, 2004). Further benefit is found when SATs are coordinated with spontaneous breathing trials (SBTs), and daily checks to determine a patient's ability to breathe spontaneously without ventilator assistance (Ely et al., 1996, 1999). Patients receiving both SATs and SBTs, in a well-designed, multisite randomized controlled trial (RCT), spent significantly more days breathing without ventilator assistance, were discharged from the ICU and hospital earlier, had shorter duration of coma, and were less likely to die compared to patients treated with SBTs alone (Girard et al., 2008). It is important to note that SATs and SBTs are associated with few adverse events and no known long-term cognitive or psychological harm (Jackson et al., 2010; Kress et al., 2003). An even more recent study from the Centers for Disease Control's Wake Up and Breathe Collaborative found enhanced performance of paired, daily SATs and SBTs was associated with a 2.4-day decrease in mean duration of mechanical ventilation, a 3.0-day decrease in ICU LOS, a 6.3-day decrease in hospital LOS, and a 37% decrease in the odds of ventilator-associated events (VAEs; Klompas et al., 2015).

Older patients with preexisting obstructive or restrictive lung disease who are mechanically ventilated either in the ICU or in long-term care facilities are also at increased risk for ventilator-assisted pneumonia (VAP) and VAEs (Buczko, 2010). To minimize these complications, nurses should aggressively exercise standard VAP precautions, including elevating the head of the bed to at least 30°, providing frequent oral care, maintaining adequate cuff pressures, using continuous subglottic suctioning, avoiding the routine changing of ventilator circuit tubing, assessing the need for stress ulcer and DVT prophylaxis, turning the patient as tolerated, providing optimal hygiene, and advocating for weaning trials as early as possible (American Association of Critical Care, 2004; Munro & Ruggiero, 2014; Sinuff et al., 2013; Torres, Ferrer, & Badia, 2010). One recent pilot RCT also found that a new standardized oral care program for poststroke survivors led to reductions in methicillin-resistant *Staphylococcus aureus* and methicillin-sensitive *Staphylococcus aureus* colonization (from 20.8% to 16.7%; Chipps et al., 2014). Finally, recent advances in techniques and applications of noninvasive ventilation provide an exceedingly useful means of managing respiratory compromise, thus potentially avoiding mechanical ventilation, in the older adult population (Muir, Lamia, Molano, & Cuvelier, 2010).

Nurses should consider that older adults with common respiratory pathology often do not present with symptoms traditionally considered "hallmarks of infection"—fever, chills, and other constitutional symptoms. In fact, the typical signs of pneumonia—fever, cough, and sputum production—can be absent in older adults, with only 33% to 60% of older patients presenting with a fever (Bellmann-Weiler & Weiss, 2009). Instead, older patients with either sepsis or pneumonia can often present with acute confusion, tachypnea, and tachycardia (Girard & Ely, 2007). This vague symptomatology can delay diagnosis, and important antibiotic administration, leading to poorer outcomes (Iregui, Ward, Sherman, Fraser, & Kollef, 2002).

Cardiovascular System

Because so many older adults live with hypertension, peripheral vascular disease, or coronary artery disease (CAD), individual responses to treatment can dramatically differ depending on the severity of the illness and any preexisting comorbidities. Even the "disease free" older adult may experience a decrease in the ability to respond to stressful situations as a result of the many changes that accompany cardiovascular aging (see Table 29.1; Pisani, 2009).

Cardiovascular-associated aging changes ultimately render the myocardium less compliant and responsive to catecholamine stimulation, can cause ventricular hypertrophy, and predispose the older adult to the development of a number of different types of arrhythmias (Nagappan & Parkin, 2003; Rosenthal & Kavic, 2004; Urden et al., 2002). During times of stress, an older adult achieves an increase in cardiac output by increasing diastolic filling rather than increasing heart rate (Nagappan & Parkin, 2003; Rosenthal

& Kavic, 2004; Urden et al., 2002). The practical implication of this finding is that older adults often require higher filling pressures (i.e., central venous pressures in the 8–10 range, pulmonary artery occlusion pressures in the 14–18 range) to maintain adequate stroke volume and may be especially sensitive to hypovolemia (Rosenthal & Kavic, 2004). However, over hydration of the older adult should also be avoided as it can lead to systolic failure, poor organ perfusion, and hypoxemia with subsequent diastolic dysfunction (Rosenthal & Kavic, 2004). Careful monitoring of hemodynamic and fluid status is therefore essential to optimize the older patient's cardiac status (see Chapter 30, "Fluid Overload: Identifying and Managing Heart Failure Patients at Risk of Hospital Readmission").

Cardiac complications are among the highest causes of mortality in the older surgical patient, not only because of the increased likelihood of coronary disease but also because of the effects of aging on the myocardium (Fleisher et al., 2009). The 2009 the American College of Cardiology Foundation/American Heart Association (ACCF/AHA) Focused Update on Perioperative Beta Blockade incorporates important new information regarding the risks and benefits of perioperative beta blockade (Fleisher et al., 2009). In this update, a Class I indication for perioperative beta-blocker use exists, for continuation of a beta blocker in patients already taking the drug. In addition, several Class IIa recommendations exist for patients with inducible ischemia, CAD, or multiple clinical risk factors who are undergoing vascular (i.e., high risk) surgery and for patients with CAD or multiple clinical risk factors who are undergoing intermediate-risk surgery. It is important to note that initiation of beta-blocker therapy in lower risk groups requires careful consideration. Initiation well before a planned procedure with careful titration perioperatively to achieve adequate heart rate control, while avoiding frank bradycardia or hypotension, is suggested. Finally, routine administration of perioperative beta- blockers, particularly in higher fixed-dose regimens begun on the day of surgery, is no longer advocated.

Symptoms of a myocardial infarction and congestive heart failure may be blunted in critically ill older adults (Menaker & Scalea, 2010; Pisani, 2009), requiring the need to monitor for nonspecific and atypical presentations in this patient population, including shortness of breath, acute confusion, or syncope. Worsening clinical status or difficulty weaning from mechanical ventilation should prompt the ICU team to investigate the possibility of myocardial ischemia in this population (Pisani, 2009).

Neurological System

The central and peripheral nervous system changes that accompany aging may partially explain why older adults often present to emergency departments or the ICU with acute mental status changes. These acute mental status changes often represent an atypical presentation of an acute illness, including alterations caused by infection, an imbalance of electrolytes, or drug toxicity. A thorough physical examination, with follow-up testing, must be conducted in order to accurately diagnose the etiology of an older adult's new-onset neurological/mental status changes as well as a thorough review of medication use.

Age-related changes to the neurological system, when coupled with acute pathology and the ICU environment, increase a critically ill older adult's risk for cognitive dysfunction, falls, restraint use, oversedation, alterations in body temperature, and anorexia. Most important, these changes also elevate the risk for delirium, which occurs in up to 70% of older adults admitted to an ICU (Balas et al., 2007; McNicoll et al., 2003; Peterson et al., 2006) and is associated with increased morbidity, mortality, length of hospital stay, and poor functional outcomes (Balas et al., 2009; Ely, Inouye, et al., 2001; Morandi, Jackson, & Ely, 2009). Pain, sleep deprivation, visual impairment, illness severity, prior cognitive impairment, dehydration, comorbidities, laboratory abnormalities, multiple medications, chemical withdrawal syndromes, infections, fever, windowless units, and ICU length of stay place the critically ill older adult at risk for delirium (Morandi et al., 2009). Although management of delirium in hospitalized patients is discussed more fully in Chapter 17, "Delirium: Prevention, Early Recognition, and Treatment, clinicians must be particularly aware of the interconnectedness of delirium, mechanical ventilation, and immobility in the critical care environment. Nurse-led, interdisciplinary, multicomponent strategies, such as the Awakening/Breathing Coordination, Delirium Monitoring/Management, and Early Mobility (ABCDE) bundle have been shown to improve outcomes in the critically ill population. One recent study found patients treated with the ABCDE bundle, spent 3 more days breathing without mechanical ventilator assistance, experienced a near halving of the odds of delirium, lower mortality, and increased odds of mobilizing out of bed at least once during their ICU stay (Balas et al., 2014).

In addition to the physical barriers to speech imposed by mechanical ventilation, older adult patients are at greater risk for impaired communication than their younger counterparts because of preexisting vision and hearing impairments and cognitive or language impairments (Bartlett, Blais, Tamblyn, Clermont, & MacGibbon, 2008; Happ et al., 2015; Happ, Tate, & Garrett, 2006; Patak et al., 2009). Accurate interpretation of patient messages, including pain and symptom descriptions, may be difficult and frustrating for patients and care providers. Partnering with speech–language pathologists on tools and techniques to facilitate patient comprehension and communication can improve this process (Happ et al., 2006).

A multilevel communication intervention, composed of nurse training, algorithm-guided assessment and communication tool selection, and the provision of communication tools to the ICU, demonstrated improved frequency of communication, successfulness of communication about pain and other symptoms, and less patient-reported difficulty with communication (Happ et al., 2014). Age and delirium status effected communication performance and content. When patients tested positive for delirium, communication exchanges with their nurses were less successful. Delirium was also associated with the identification of fewer patient symptoms and more complaints of dry mouth (*OR*: 3.60, 95% CI [1.1, 11.83]; $p = .03$). Older age was associated with more symptom complaints of pain (*OR*: 2.12, 95% CI [1.12, 4.00]; $p = .02$), drowsiness (*OR*: 0.41, 95% CI [0.17, 0.98]; $p = .04$), and feeling cold (*OR*: 0.31, 95% CI [0.11, 0.88]; $p = .03$; Tate et al., 2013).

Achieving adequate pain control for critically ill older adults is of utmost importance, both related to and independent of its relationship to delirium; however, the nurse also needs to avoid over sedation and undertreatment of pain in this population as both are associated with multiple negative outcomes, including distress, delirium, sleep disturbances, and impaired mobility (Barr et al., 2013; see Chapter 18 "Pain Management"). A number of tools exist to assess a critically ill patient's level of sedation and delirium status. The Richmond Agitation and Sedation Scale (RASS; Sessler et al., 2002) and the Confusion Assessment Method-ICU (CAM-ICU; Ely, Margolin, et al., 2001) are two of the most common in the critical care setting. (See Resources for additional information on these tools and Protocol 29.1 for interventions to reduce delirium.)

Gastrointestinal System

Common age-related changes to the gastrointestinal (GI) system can predispose older ICU patients to complications during their ICU stay, ranging from altered presentation of illness to issues of medication effectiveness (see Table 29.1). Older adults also experience changes in their body composition (i.e., decrease in lean body mass) and energy use that can potentiate the effect of medications on these GI-system changes.

It is ironic that although many conditions affecting the GI system are more common in older adults (e.g., constipation, under- and malnutrition, gastritis) their presence is not fully explained by the aging processes (Urden et al., 2002). When assessing the GI function of a critically ill older adult, it is important for the nurse to realize that age may blunt the manifestations of acute abdominal disease. For example, pain may be less severe, fever less pronounced or absent, and signs of peritoneal inflammation, such as muscle guarding and rebound tenderness, may be diminished or even absent (Bickley, 2008). Because of changes in the secretion of gastric enzymes, the stomach wall of older adults can be more susceptible to acid injury, especially in the face of critical illness. The practice of routine stress ulcer prophylaxis in the critically ill patient, part of the VAP bundle and common in many ICUs, however, has more recently been challenged as a potential contributor to pneumonia with more narrow indications that have been assumed, even in mechanically ventilated patients (Herzig, Howell, Ngo, & Marcantonio, 2009; Logan, Sumukadas, & Witham, 2010; Marik, Vasu, Hirani, & Pachinburavan, 2010).

Delayed gastric emptying may predispose older adults to abdominal distension, nausea, vomiting, aspiration, and constipation. This delayed motility is especially true in the postoperative period, when many older adults are immobile and receiving narcotics. Many older adults take multiple medications, which along with age-related changes such as altered thresholds for taste and smell, a hypersensitive hypothalamic satiety center, and oropharyngeal atrophy, can inhibit their intake of solids and liquids (Menaker & Scalea, 2010). This baseline GI functionality, in combination with their critical illness, must be proactively addressed. The nurse needs to be alert for ill-fitting dentures, swallowing difficulties, silent aspiration, and the possibility of decreased saliva production (either resulting from salivary dysfunction or the use of drugs, such as sympathomimetics). These alterations can lead to insufficient mastication and can combine with other risk factors that put the older ICU patient at risk for aspiration. Aspiration should be considered a life-threatening situation, requiring immediate nursing intervention. Consultation with a speech–language pathologist may also be warranted.

Older adults facing stress from illness, injury, or infection are also at high risk for protein-calorie malnutrition, as evidenced by low serum albumin and prealbumin levels, a decline in hepatic function, decreased muscle mass and strength, and dysfunction in those tissues with high cell turnover (Nagappan & Parkin, 2003; Rosenthal & Kavic, 2004). These changes lead to a breakdown in barrier function, increased susceptibility to infection, delayed wound healing, fluid shifts, deconditioning, and further impairment in absorption of essential nutrients (Rosenthal, 2004). Thus, early enteral or parental nutritional support is crucial (see Chapter 10, "Nutrition").

Reductions with age in the activity of the drug-metabolizing enzyme system and blood flow through the liver influences the liver's capacity to metabolize various drugs (Kane et al., 2004; Menaker & Scalea, 2010). Splanchnic blood flow is further compromised in states of shock or even mild hypotension. These changes may predispose older adults to adverse drug reactions (Urden et al., 2002). For example, drugs, like warfarin, that work directly on hepatocytes may reach their therapeutic effect at lower doses (Rosenthal & Kavic, 2004). Common pharmacological agents used in the critical care setting and their common side effects often experienced by the gerontological patient are given in Table 29.2 (see Chapter 20, "Reducing Adverse Drug Events").

Last, many older adults have diabetes and even those older adults without preexisting diabetes may experience elevated blood glucose levels as a result of medications and a stress response to critical illness. Therefore, glycemic control in the older ICU patient may be more difficult because of a declining glucose tolerance associated with aging. Although initial studies indicated tight control of blood sugar, with blood glucose levels of 80 to 110, optimized recovery and outcomes (Humbert, Gallagher, Gabbay, & Dellasega, 2008; van den Berghe et al., 2001), a more recent study has revealed that this tight control actually increases mortality (Bouillon et al., 2009).

Genitourinary System

Preservation of the older adult's preadmission renal status is one of the goals of ICU care. Common age-related changes in the genitourinary (GU) system decrease the older adult's ability to excrete ammonia and drugs, diminish his or her capacity to regulate fluid and acid–base balance, and often impair their ability to properly empty the

TABLE 29.2

High-Risk Medications Commonly Used in Older ICU Patients[a]

Drug	Severity Rating[b]	Potential Adverse Effects
Amiodarone (Cordarone)[c]	High	May provoke torsades de pointes and QT interval problems; lack of efficacy in older adults
[c]Clonidine (Catapres)	Low	Orthostatic hypotension, CNS adverse effects
[c]Diazepam (Valium)	High	Increased sensitivity to benzodiazepines; long half-life in older patients (can be several days); prolonged sedation; increasing risk of falls/fractures; short- and intermediate-acting benzodiazepines preferred
Digoxin (Lanoxin)	Low	Decreased renal clearance may lead to increased risk of toxic effects; dose should not exceed > .125 mg/d except when treating atrial arrhythmias
Diphenhydramine (Benadryl)	High	Strong anticholinergic effects, confusion, oversedation; also can cause dry mouth, urinary retention; aggravates benign prostatic hypertrophy and glaucoma; use smallest possible dose
[c]Ketorolac (Toradol)	High	Peptic ulceration, GI bleeding, perforation; GI effects can be asymptomatic
[c]Meperidine (Demerol)	High	Active metabolite accumulation may cause CNS toxicity, tremor, confusion, irritability; other narcotics preferred
[c]Promethazine (Phenergan)	High	Highly anticholinergic; confusion, oversedation; also can cause dry mouth, urinary retention; aggravates benign prostatic hypertrophy and glaucoma
Propofol (Diprivan)	Unrated	Lipophilic drug; decreased clearance in older adults related to increased total body fat
Cimetidine (Tagamet) and Ranitidine (Zantac)	Low	CNS effects, confusion

CNS, central nervous system; GI, gastrointestinal.

[a]Adapted from Beers (1997); Bonk, Krown, Matuszewski, and Oinonen (2006); Fick et al. (2003).

[b]Severity rating—Adverse effects of medications rated as high or low severity based on the probability of event occurring and significance of the outcome (Logan et al., 2010; van den Berghe et al., 2001).

[c]Identified in Logan et al. (2010) as seven most commonly prescribed Beers medications used in older hospitalized patients.

bladder (Nagappan & Parkin, 2003; Rosenthal & Kavic, 2004; Urden et al., 2002). The coupling of these common age-related changes with conditions commonly seen in the ICU environment, such as hypovolemia, shock, sepsis, and polypharmacy, render the older adult at increased risk for acute renal failure, metabolic acidosis, and adverse drug events (Yilmaz & Erdem, 2010). The increased prevalence in the older population of asymptomatic bacteriuria also exacerbates an older ICU patient's infection risk related to Foley catheter use (Richards, 2004; see Chapter 22, "Prevention of Catheter-Associated Urinary Tract Infection").

The nurse must take into consideration an older patient's baseline cardiovascular status relative to his or her renal function. If an older patient was typically hypertensive before hospitalization, for example, this patient's renal vasculature may be accustomed to a pressure to perfuse the kidneys that is higher than normal. Furthermore, common indicators of dehydration, such as skin turgor, should be considered an unreliable sign in an older adult, related to loss of subcutaneous tissue (Sheehy, Perry, & Cromwell, 1999). Although the Cockroft and Gault formula (see Chapter 20) has been derived to estimate creatinine clearance in the healthy aged, care must be taken when applying this formula to critically ill older patients or to those patients on medications that directly affect renal function (Rosenthal & Kavic, 2004). Finally, the nurse should be especially cognizant of medications known to contribute to renal failure, including aminoglycosides, certain antibiotics, and contrast dyes, and closely monitor laboratory results as warranted (Urden et al., 2002).

Immune/Hematopoietic System

The changes that occur in the aged immune and hematological system mainly involve altered T and B cell functioning and a decrease in hematopoietic reserve (Nagappan & Parkin, 2003; Rosenthal & Kavic, 2004; Urden et al., 2002; see Table 29.1). The consequences of these changes include an increased susceptibility to infection, increases in autoantibodies and monoclonal immunoglobulins, and tumorigenesis (Rosenthal & Kavic, 2004). These common aging changes, coupled with the stress, malnutrition, and number of invasive procedures seen in the critical care environment, may heighten the older adult's risk for a nosocomial infection. Furthermore, because an older adult's ability to mount a febrile response to infection diminishes with age (related to a decline in hypothalamic function), the older patient may even be septic without the warning of a fever (Urden et al., 2002) and instead may exhibit only a decline in mental status. Close assessment of other nonfebrile signs of infection (restlessness, agitation, delirium, hypotension, and tachycardia) is essential and warranted.

Although recent research suggests that giving blood more liberally to patients may be associated with worse patient outcomes, these findings may not necessarily apply to the older adult population for several reasons: (a) the chronic anemia often seen in aging; (b) the exclusion of many older adults from previous clinical trials; (c) research findings that suggest higher transfusion triggers in older patients with acute myocardial infarction actually decreases mortality; and (d) the association of low hemoglobin levels with increased incidence of delirium, functional decline, and decreased mobility (Rosenthal & Kavic, 2004).

Skin and Wounds

Older adults are at high risk for skin breakdown in the ICU setting resulting from of elastic, subcutaneous, and connective tissues; a decrease in sweat gland activity; and a decrease in capillary arterioles supplying the skin with age (Bickley, 2008; Urden et al., 2002; see Table 29.1). Because the skin changes that occur in older adults can cause difficulty with thermoregulation, can heighten the risk for skin breakdown and intravenous (IV) infiltrations, may delay wound healing, and can make hydration assessment difficult, the nurse should make every effort to prevent heat loss, carefully monitor hydration status, and conduct thorough skin assessments (Bickley, 2008; Urden et al., 2002; see Chapter 24 "Preventing Pressure Ulcers and Skin Tears").

Another important intervention related to the prevention of skin and muscle breakdown in critically ill older adults is early, frequent mobilization. A strategy for whole-body rehabilitation, achieved by the use of SATs, SBTs, and physical therapy-driven early exercise and mobilization, has proven to be safe and well tolerated by mechanically ventilated patients (Schweickert et al., 2009). Patients treated with this intervention experienced significantly shorter duration of delirium and coma, had more ventilator-free days, and were more likely to return to independent functional status at hospital discharge than were controls. Numerous studies have shown active mobilization can be initiated safely in ICU settings (Li, Peng, Zhu, Zhang, & Xi, 2013), resulting in improved physical function (Li et al., 2013), reduced duration of mechanical ventilation (Chen et al., 2012; Malkor, Karadibak, & Yildirim, 2009), shorter LOS (Malkor et al., 2009; Morris et al., 2008), and lower 1-year mortality (Chen et al., 2012) (see Chapter 14, "Preventing Functional Decline in the Acute Care Setting").

Family Engagement

Interactions with family members can be therapeutic for critically ill patients (Black, Boore, & Parahoo, 2011), and help them to make sense of the experience (Davidson, Daly, Agan, Brady, & Higgins, 2010); they may also ameliorate the stress and trauma experienced by patients and family during and after ICU hospitalization (Bergbom & Askwall, 2000; Jones et al., 2010). Family members support patients' psychological well-being by providing reassurance, hope, information, a sense of normality, and distraction from the ICU environment and illness experience (Black et al., 2011; Happ, Swigart, Tate, Hoffman, & Arnold, 2007; Karlsson, Forsberg, & Bergbom, 2010; Morse & Pooler, 2002; Riggio, Singer, Hartman, & Sneider, 1982; Williams, 2005). They also provide reorientation, detect signs of delirium, and serve as proxy or shared decision makers (Black et al., 2011; Happ, 2000; Happ, Swigart, Tate, Arnold, et al., 2007; Happ, Swigart, Tate, Hoffman, et al., 2007; White, Braddock, Bereknyei, & Curtis, 2007; White et al., 2007; Williams, 2005). Family presence has been associated with significantly longer duration of ventilator weaning trials among adult patients weaning from prolonged mechanical ventilation in the ICU (Miller, 2009). Family interventions in the ICU have focused on providing basic information about the environment, patient condition and treatment (Azoulay et al., 2002; Black et al., 2011; Medland & Ferrans, 1998), advice and coaching on family presence or caregiving (Black et al., 2011; Daly et al., 2010; Davidson et al., 2010), and decision-making support (Curtis et al., 2011; Daly et al., 2010; Lautrette, Ciroldi, Ksibi, & Azoulay, 2006; White et al., 2007) with mixed results on patient–family anxiety, depression, and PTSD. For example, an information leaflet improved family members' comprehension of the ICU patient's diagnosis and prognosis but did not affect anxiety or depression (Azoulay et al., 2002).

Black et al. (2011) tested the effect of a family psychological support intervention facilitated by nurses on patient delirium and psychological recovery. Intervention group patients showed less delirium than usual care (29%–77%), and had significantly lower Sickness Impact Profile scores at 4, 8, and 12 weeks after the intervention ($p < .001$). The use of diaries written by health providers and family visitors to help patients to make sense of the memories and ICU experience following discharge were associated with a decrease in patients' PTSD (Jones et al., 2010); however, the impact on family caregivers' anxiety has been equivocal (Kloos & Daly, 2008). Davidson tested the feasibility and acceptability of a family visiting kit and supportive coaching intervention with family members of mechanically ventilated patients in an ICU (Davidson et al., 2010). Families found the kit materials (workbook, cognitive recovery tools, personal care items and information on available services) helpful. The toolkit did not, however, meet their communication needs; the effect on patient or family outcomes was not tested.

Family members are commonly required to act as decisional surrogates for older adult patients in the ICU. This role is known to confer emotional stress, burden, and psychological sequelae (depression, anxiety, PTSD) for some family caregivers, particularly for those family members involved in decisions to limit or withdraw life-sustaining treatments (Gries et al., 2010; McAdam, Fontaine, White, Dracup, & Puntillo, 2012). Nurses play a crucial role in integrating palliative care in the ICU and improving end-of-life care and support for critically ill older adults and their family members (Krimshtein et al., 2011; Nelson et al., 2010; White et al., 2012). Skills-training programs and resources for nurses include the End-of-Life Nursing Education Consortium (ELNEC-Critical Care and ELNEC Geriatric), Improving Palliative Care in the ICU (IPAL-ICU), and the American Association of Critical-Care Nurses E-learning program on Palliative and End-of-Life Care.

CASE STUDY

Ned Saunders is a 71-year-old man who fell off of a ladder while stringing holiday lights and suffered serious complications, including ventilator-associated pneumonia and adult respiratory distress syndrome (ARDS), after laminectomy. He required a second back surgery (revision of the laminectomy) during the same hospital stay, and developed a *Clostridium difficile* infection and nutritional problems secondary to the severe diarrhea. Infection with antibiotic-resistant organisms necessitated the use of isolation protocol. Tracheostomy placement occurred on the 17th ICU day.

Preadmission

Mr. Saunders was a former smoker and his past medical history included mild chronic obstructive pulmonary disease (COPD) and hypertension. His medications before admission were albuterol inhaler two puffs every 6 hours and hydrochlorothiazide 50 mg for blood pressure. He smoked ½ pack per day for 30 years. A retired

(continued)

CASE STUDY *(continued)*

school teacher, Mr. Saunders was slightly overweight but active around the house and enjoyed an active social life, especially dancing with his wife at local dance halls. He was a "social drinker," as reported by his wife, having three to four glasses of wine per week. Mr. Saunders was completely independent in all ADL before this hospitalization. The Mini-Mental State Examination (MMSE) score on admission before surgery was 29. CAM-ICU (for delirium) on admission to the ICU was positive for delirium.

Cognitive/Psychosocial

Mr. Saunders was unable to focus attention for more than 5 seconds at a time and was intermittently agitated during the early stages of his ICU stay. He was diagnosed as delirious via CAM-ICU administration. Delirium was treated with nonpharmacological interventions and discontinuity of any potentially deliriogenic medications. Benzodiazepines, in particular, were avoided in an attempt to clear the delirium. He received a fentanyl patch for pain and intravenous fentanyl as needed for breakthrough pain.

Anxiety and communication difficulties were problems possibly influencing his "mental state" during ventilator weaning. Communication was inhibited by respiratory tract intubation, cognition problems, and lack of dentures and eyeglasses. Because his thinking was unclear, nurses used visual cues in the form of written words, gestures, and pictures to augment their messages to Mr. Saunders. They cued him to use a simple communication board and asked yes/no questions by categories (e.g., family, your body, comfort needs) whenever possible. When the delirium cleared, Mrs. Saunders brought in his iPad, which was placed in a clear protective plastic sheath. With assistance from the speech–language pathologist, he was able to access a voice output communication application and communicate reliably with his wife and caregivers using the iPad mounted on a movable bedside stand. After the tracheostomy procedure was completed, his wife was advised to bring in his dentures to improve lip reading. Mr. Saunders began using a tracheostomy speaking valve after 5 ½ weeks of hospitalization.

The patient's wife was his sole support. They had no children or close relatives. A reserved woman, she remained positive when at the patient's bedside. Nurses coached her to use touch and encouragement at the bedside. Mrs. Saunders asked the therapists to teach her range-of-motion exercises and she performed these during afternoon visits. She provided calm and distracting talk during weaning trials, reading get-well cards from friends.

Cardiac

Mr. Saunders remained in a sinus tachycardia through most of the hospitalization with occasional premature venticular contractions. His hemoglobin and hematocrit dropped to 10/36 during the hospitalization with no identified source of bleeding. He received one unit of packed RBCs and diuretics before SBTs were resumed.

Respiratory

Mr. Saunders progressed from dependence on mechanical ventilation in assist-control mode (FiO_2 = 40%, continuous positive airway pressure = 5, pressure support = 10) to tracheostomy mask oxygen at 50% FiO_2 over a 10-day period.

GI

Nutritional balance was particularly challenging with Mr. Saunders as a result of impaired absorption of nutrients during *C. difficile* infection. The infection was treated with intravenous vancomycin. A jejunostomy tube was placed for continuous tube feeding and caloric requirements adjusted frequently, with careful attention to albumin levels. Vancomycin drug levels must also be monitored.

Skin

Meticulous attention to wound healing at the back surgery site and the fit of a "turtle shell" to prevent friction or skin tears was provided.

Rehabilitation

Mr. Saunders received early physical therapy, beginning in the passive range during the most critical phase of his illness and progressing to active range of motion and chair sitting. His mobility was limited by the protective turtle shell appliance required for healing of his spine during any out-of-bed activity. A daily chair-sitting period was arranged, requiring coordination between physical therapy and nursing. Once medically cleared, he began progressive physical therapy-guided mobilization. The team initiated speech and swallowing rehabilitation (speech and swallowing evaluation), beginning with lollipops to reestablish swallowing.

(continued)

CASE STUDY *(continued)*

Discharge Planning

Mr. Saunders's progress was slow and respiratory status still tenuous at the end of his ICU stay. He required significant physical rehabilitation following his critical illness. An LTACH was the best choice for continued care and rehabilitation. As Mr. Saunders's respiratory status and speaking ability improved, his anxiety diminished. Because Mr. Saunders had multiple risk factors for delirium, the exact cause of the delirium was unknown at discharge. Attention to normalizing the fluid and electrolyte balance, reestablishing and maintaining normal sleep–wake cycles, and avoiding the use of benzodiazepines continued as care was transferred to the LTACH. His mental status improved as evidenced by less frequent periods of inattention and confusion. Short-term memory problems persisted and required frequent cueing and reminders from staff and his wife.

SUMMARY

Nurses in the acute care setting must recognize and respond to the many factors that influence a critically ill older adult's ability to survive and rehabilitate from a catastrophic illness. In order to identify some of these risk factors, it is essential that the nurse perform a comprehensive assessment of each older adult's preadmission health status, functional and cognitive ability, and social support systems. It is equally important that the nurse understand the implications of common aging changes, comorbidities, and acute pathology that interacts with and heightens the risk for adverse and often preventable medical outcomes. The application of evidence-based interventions aimed at restoring physiological stability, preventing complications, maintaining comfort and safety, and preserving preillness functional ability and QOL are crucial components of caring for this extremely vulnerable population.

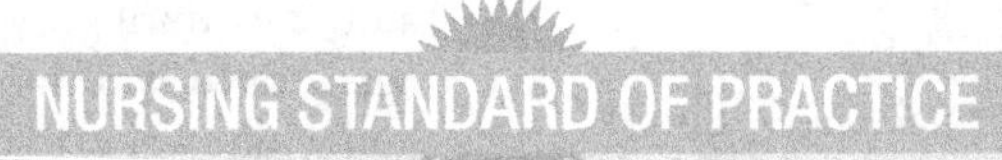

Protocol 29.1: Comprehensive Assessment and Management of the Critically Ill

I. GOAL

To restore physiological stability, prevent complications, maintain comfort and safety, and preserve preillness functional ability and QOL in older adults admitted to critical care units

II. OVERVIEW

Caring for an older adult who is experiencing a serious or life-threatening illness often poses significant challenges for critical care nurses. Although older adults are an extremely heterogeneous group, they share some age-related characteristics that leave them susceptible to a variety of geriatric syndromes and diseases. This vulnerability may influence both their ICU utilization rates and outcomes. Critical care nurses caring for this population must not only recognize the importance of performing ongoing, comprehensive physical, functional, and psychosocial assessments tailored to the older ICU patient, but also must be able to identify and implement evidence-based interventions designed to improve the care of this extremely vulnerable population.

III BACKGROUND

A. Definition
   A critically ill older adult is a person, aged 65 years or older, who is currently experiencing, or at risk for, some form of physiological instability or alteration warranting urgent or emergent, advanced, nursing/medical interventions and monitoring.

(continued)

Protocol 29.1: Comprehensive Assessment and Management of the Critically Ill *(continued)*

B. Etiology/epidemiology
   1. More than one half (55.8%) of all ICU days are incurred by patients older than 65 years of age (Angus et al., 2006).
   2. Older adults are living longer, are more racially and ethnically diverse, often have multiple chronic conditions, and more than one quarter report difficulty performing one or more ADL. These factors may affect both the course and outcome of critical illness.
   3. Once hospitalized for a life-threatening illness, older adults often:
      a. Experience high ICU, hospital, and long-term crude mortality rates and are at risk for deterioration in functional ability and postdischarge institutional care (de Rooij et al., 2005; Esteban et al., 2004; Ford et al., 2007; Hennessy et al., 2005; Hopkins & Jackson, 2006; Kaarlola et al., 2006; Marik, 2006).
      b. Older age is also a factor that may lead to:
         i. Physician bias in refusing ICU admission (Joynt et al., 2001; Mick & Ackerman, 2004)
         ii. The decision to withhold mechanical ventilation, surgery, or dialysis (Hamel et al., 1999)
         iii. An increased likelihood of an established resuscitation directive (Hakim et al., 1996)
      c. Most critically ill older adults:
         i. Demonstrate resiliency
         ii. Report being satisfied with their postdischarge QOL
         iii. Would reaccept ICU care and mechanical ventilation if needed (Guentner et al., 2006; Hennessy et al., 2005; Kleinpell & Ferrans, 2002)
      d. Chronological age *alone* is not an acceptable, or accurate, predictor of poor outcomes after critical illness (Milbrandt et al., 2010; Nagappan & Parkin, 2003).
      e. Factors that may influence an older adult's ability to survive a catastrophic illness include (Ford et al., 2007; de Rooij et al., 2005; Marik, 2006; Mick & Ackerman, 2004):
         i. Severity of illness
         ii. Nature and extent of comorbidities
         iii. Diagnosis, reason for/duration of mechanical ventilation
         iv. Complications
         v. Others
            a) Prehospitalization functional ability
            b) Vasoactive drug use
            c) Preexisting cognitive impairment
            d) Senescence
            e) Ageism
            f) Decreased social support
            g) The critical care environment

IV. PARAMETERS OF ASSESSMENT

A. Preadmission—Comprehensive assessment of a critically ill older adult's preadmission health status, cognitive and functional ability, and social support systems helps identify risk factors for cascade iatrogenesis, the development of life-threatening conditions, and frequently encountered geriatric syndromes. Factors the nurse needs to consider when performing the admission assessment include:
   1. Preexisting cognitive impairment—Many older adults admitted to ICUs suffer from high rates of unrecognized, preexisting cognitive impairment (Balas et al., 2007; Pisani et al., 2003).
      a. Knowledge of preadmission cognitive ability could aid practitioners in:
         i. Assessing decision-making capacity, informed-consent issues, and evaluation of mental status changes throughout hospitalization
         ii. Making anesthetic and analgesic choices
         iii. Considering one-to-one care options
         iv. Weaning from mechanical ventilation

(continued)

Protocol 29.1: Comprehensive Assessment and Management of the Critically Ill *(continued)*

v. Assessing fall risk
vi. Planning for discharge from the ICU

b. On admission to the ICU the nurse should ask relatives or other caregivers for baseline information about the older adult's:
   i. Memory, executive function (e.g., fine motor coordination, planning, organization of information, etc.), and overall cognitive ability (Kane et al., 2004)
   ii. Behavior on a typical day, how the patient interacts with others; his or her responsiveness to stimuli, how able he or she is to communicate (reading level, writing, and speech) and his or her memory, orientation, and perceptual patterns before the illness (Milisen & DeGeest, 2001)
   iii. Medication history to assess for potential withdrawal syndromes (Broyles, Colbert, Tate, Swigart, & Happ, 2008)
c. Psychosocial factors—Critical illness can render older adults unable to effectively communicate with the health care team, often related to physiological instability, technology that leaves them voiceless, and sedative and narcotic use (Happ, 2000, 2001). Family members are therefore often a crucial source for obtaining important preadmission information. On ICU admission the nurse needs to determine:
   i. What is the elder's past medical, surgical, and psychiatric history? What medication was the older adult taking before coming to the ICU? Does the elder regularly use illicit drugs, tobacco, or alcohol? Does he or she have a history of falls, physical abuse, or confusion?
   ii. What is the older adult's marital status? Who is the patient's significant other? Will this person be the one responsible to make decisions for the elder if he or she is unable to do so? Does the elder have an advance directive for health care? Is the elder a primary caregiver to an aging spouse, child, grandchild, or other person?
   iii. How would the elder describe his or her ethnicity? Does he or she they practice a particular religion or have spiritual needs that should be addressed? What was his or her QOL like before becoming ill?
d. Preadmission functional ability/nutritional status—Limited preadmission functional ability and poor nutritional status are associated with many negative outcomes for critically ill older adults. Therefore, the nurse should assess the following:
   i. Did the elder suffer any limitations in the ability to perform their ADL preadmission? If so, what were these limitations?
   ii. Does the elder use any assistive devices to perform ADL? If so, what type?
   iii. Where did the patient live before admission? Did he or she live alone or with others? What was the elder's physical environment like (i.e., house, apartment, stairs, multiple levels, etc.)?
   iv. What was the older adult's nutritional status like preadmission? Does he or she have enough money to buy food? Does he or she need assistance with making meals/obtaining food? Does he or she have any particular food restrictions/preferences? Was he or she using supplements/vitamins on a regular basis? Does he or she have any signs of malnutrition, including recent weight loss/gain, muscle wasting, hair loss, skin breakdown?

B. During ICU stay—There are many anatomic/physiological changes that occur with aging (see Table 29.1). The interaction of these changes with the acute pathology of a critical illness, comorbidities, and the ICU environment leads not only to atypical presentation of some of the most commonly encountered ICU diagnoses; but may also elevate the older adults' risk for complications. The older adult must be systematically assessed for the following:
   1. Comorbidities/common ICU diagnoses
      a. Respiratory: COPD, pneumonia, acute respiratory failure, adult respiratory distress syndrome, rib fractures/flail chest
      b. Cardiovascular: Acute myocardial infarction, coronary artery disease, peripheral vascular disease, hypertension, coronary artery bypass grafting, valve replacements, abdominal aortic aneurysm, dysrhythmias
      c. Neurologic: Cerebral vascular accident, dementia, aneurysms, Alzheimer's disease, Parkinson's disease, closed head injury, transient ischemic attacks

(continued)

Protocol 29.1: Comprehensive Assessment and Management of the Critically Ill *(continued)*

   d. Gastrointestinal: Biliary tract disease, peptic ulcer disease, gastrointestinal cancers, liver failure, inflammatory bowel disease, pancreatitis, diarrhea, constipation, and aspiration
   e. GU: Renal cell cancer, chronic renal failure, acute renal failure, urosepsis, and incontinence
   f. Immune/Hematopoietic: Sepsis, anemia, neutropenia, and thrombocytopenia
   g. Skin: Necrotizing fasciitis, pressure ulcers
2. Acute pathology—Thoracic or abdominal surgery, hypovolemia, hypervolemia, hypo/hyperthermia, electrolyte abnormalities, hypoxia, arrhythmias, infection, hypo/hypertension, delirium, ischemia, bowel obstruction, ileus, blood loss, sepsis, disrupted skin integrity, multisystem organ failure
3. ICU/environmental factors—Deconditioning, poor oral hygiene, sleep deprivation, pain, immobility, nutritional status, mechanical ventilation, hemodynamic monitoring devices, polypharmacy, high-risk medications (e.g., narcotics, sedatives, hypnotics, nephrotoxins, vasopressors), lack of assistive devices (e.g., glasses, hearing aids, dentures), noise, tubes that bypass the oropharyngeal airway, poorly regulated glucose control, Foley catheter use, stress, invasive procedures, shear/friction, intravenous catheters
4. Atypical presentation—Commonly seen in older adults experiencing the following: myocardial infarction, acute abdomen, infection, and hypoxia

V. NURSING CARE STRATEGIES

A. Preadmission: Based on their preadmission assessment findings, the nurse should consider:
   1. Obtaining appropriate consults (i.e., dietitian, physical/occupational/speech therapist)
   2. Implementing safety precautions
   3. Using pressure-relieving devices
   4. Organizing family meetings
   5. Providing the older adult with a consistent primary nurse
B. During ICU: Nursing interventions that may benefit
   1. Multiple organ systems
      a. Encouraging early, frequent mobilization/ambulation
      b. Providing proper oral hygiene
      c. Ensuring adequate pain control
      d. Reviewing/assessing medication appropriateness
      e. Avoiding polypharmacy/high-risk medications (see Table 29.2)
      f. Securing and ensuring the proper functioning of tubes/catheters
      g. Actively taking measures to maintain normothermia
      h. Closely monitoring fluid volume status
   2. Respiratory
      a. Encourage and assist with coughing, deep breathing, incentive spirometer use
      b. Assess for signs of swallowing dysfunction and aspiration
      c. Closely monitor pulse oximetry and arterial blood gas results
      d. Consider the use of specialty beds
      e. Advocate for daily SBTs and extubation as soon as possible
      f. Exercise standard VAP precautions (American Association of Critical Care, 2004; Institute for Healthcare Improvement, 2012)
         i. Keep the head of the bed elevated to greater than 30°
         ii. Provide frequent oral care
         iii. Maintain adequate cuff pressures
         iv. Use continuous subglottic suctioning devices
         v. Do not routinely change ventilator circuit tubing
         vi. Assess the need for stress ulcer and DVT prophylaxis

(continued)

Protocol 29.1: Comprehensive Assessment and Management of the Critically Ill *(continued)*

- vii. Turn the patient as tolerated
- viii. Maintain general hygiene practices

3. Cardiovascular
   - a. Carefully monitor the older adult's hemodynamic and electrolyte status.
   - b. Closely monitor the older adult's EKG with an awareness of many conduction abnormalities seen in aging. Consult with physician regarding prophylaxis when appropriate.
   - c. Advocate for the removal of invasive devices as soon as the patient's condition warrants. The least restrictive device may include long-term access.
   - d. Recognize that both preexisting pulmonary disease and manipulations of the abdominal and thoracic cavities may lead to unreliability of traditional values associated with central venous and pulmonary artery occlusion pressures (Rosenthal & Kavic, 2004).
   - e. Because of age-related changes to the CV system, the nurse should acknowledge (Rosenthal & Kavic, 2004)
     - i. Older adults often require higher filling pressures (i.e., CVPs in the 8–10 range; PAOPs in the 14–18 range) to maintain adequate stroke volume and may be especially sensitive to hypovolemia.
     - ii. Over-hydration of the older adult should also be avoided as it can lead to systolic failure, poor organ perfusion, and hypoxemia with subsequent diastolic dysfunction.
     - iii. Certain drugs commonly used in the ICU setting may prove to be either not as effective (e.g., isoproterenol and dobutamine) or more effective (e.g., afterload reducers).
4. Neurological/pain
   - a. Closely monitor the older adult's neurological/mental status.
   - b. Screen for delirium and sedation level at least once per shift.
   - c. Implement interventions to reduce delirium
     - i. Promote sleep, mobilize as early as possible, review medications that can lead to delirium, treat dehydration, reduce noise or provide "white noise," close doors/drapes to allow privacy, provide comfortable room temperature, encourage family and friends to visit, allow the older adult to assume his or her preferred sleeping positions, discontinue any unnecessary lines or tubes, and avoid the use of physical restraints using least restraint for minimum time only when absolutely necessary.
     - ii. Maximize the older adult's ability to effectively manage and interpret his or her environment.
       - a) Promote the older adult wearing glasses, hearing aids, and other appropriate assistive devices
       - b) Face the patient when speaking, get his or her attention before talking, speak clearly and loud enough for him or her to understand, allow enough time (pause time) for the patient to respond to questions, use a consistent provider (i.e., a primary nurse), use visual clues to remind him or her of the date and time, and provide written or visual input for a message (Garett et al., 2007).
       - c) Provide the older adult with alternate means of communication (e.g., providing them with a pen/paper, using nonverbal gestures, and/or using specially designed boards with alphabet letters, words, or pictures; Happ et al., 2010; Garett et al., 2007).
       - d) Provide translators/interpreters as needed.
   - d. Provide adequate pain control while avoiding over-or undersedation. For full discussion, see Chapter 18.
5. Gastrointestinal
   - a. Monitor for signs of GI bleeding and delayed gastric emptying/motility.
     - i. Encourage adequate hydration, assess for signs of fecal impaction, and implement a bowel regimen.
     - ii. Avoid use of rectal tubes.
   - b. Advocate for stress ulcer prophylaxis
   - c. Provide dentures as soon as possible
   - d. Implement aspiration precautions
     - i. Keep the head of the bed elevated to a high Fowler's position, frequently suction copious oral secretions, assess bedside swallowing ability by a speech therapist, assess phonation and gag reflex, monitor for tachypnea

(continued)

Protocol 29.1: Comprehensive Assessment and Management of the Critically Ill *(continued)*

   e. Advocate for early enteral/parental nutrition
   f. Ensure tight glucose control
6. GU
   a. Assess any GU tubes to ensure patency and adequate urinary output. If the older adult should experience an acute decrease in urinary output, consider using bladder scanner (if available), rather than automatic straight catheterization, to check for distension.
   b. Advocate for early removal of Foley catheters. Use other less invasive devices/methods to facilitate urine collection (i.e., external or condom catheters, offering the bedpan on a scheduled basis.
   c. Monitor blood levels of nephrotoxic medications as ordered.
7. Immune/Hematopoietic
   a. Ensure the older adult is ordered appropriate DVT prophylaxis (i.e., heparin, sequential compression devices).
   b. Monitor laboratory results and assess for signs of anemia relative to patient baseline.
   c. Recognize early signs of infection—restlessness, agitation, delirium, hypotension, tachycardia—as older adults are less likely to develop fever as a first response to infection.
   d. Meticulously maintain infection control/prevention protocols.
8. Skin
   a. Conduct thorough skin assessment.
   b. Vigilantly monitor room temperature, make every effort to prevent heat loss, and carefully use and monitor rewarming devices.
   c. Use methods known to reduce the friction and shear that often occur with repositioning in bed.
   d. In severely compromised patients, the use of specialty beds may be appropriate.
   e. Techniques, such as frequent turning, pressure-relieving devices, early nutritional support, as well as frequent ambulation, may not only protect an older adult's skin but promote the health of cardiovascular, respiratory, and gastrointestinal systems.
   f. Closely monitor IV sites, frequently check for infiltrations and use of nonrestrictive dressings and paper tape.

VI. EVALUATION/EXPECTED OUTCOMES

A. Patient
   1. Hemodynamic stability will be restored.
   2. Complications will be avoided/minimized.
   3. Preadmission functional ability will be maintained/optimized.
   4. Pain/anxiety will be minimized.
   5. Communication with the health care team will be improved.
B. Provider
   1. Employ consistent and accurate documentation of assessment relevant to the older ICU patient.
   2. Provide consistent, accurate, and timely care in response to deviations identified through ongoing monitoring and assessment of the older ICU patient.
   3. Provide patient/caregiver with information and teaching related to his or her illness as well as news of transfer of care and/or discharge.
C. Institution—include QA/QI
   1. Evaluate staff competence in the assessment of older critically ill patients.
   2. Use unit-specific, hospital-specific, and national standards of care to evaluate existing practice.
   3. Identify areas for improvement and work collaboratively across disciplines to develop strategies for improving critical care to older adults.

VII. RELEVANT PRACTICE GUIDELINES

Barr, J., Fraser, G. L., Puntillo, K., Ely, E. W., G. W.ll, C., Dasta, J. F., . . . Jaeschke, R. (2013). Clinical practice guidelines for the management of pain, agitation, and delirium in adult patients in the intensive care unit. *Critical Care Medicine, 41*(1), 263–306.

(continued)

Protocol 29.1: Comprehensive Assessment and Management of the Critically Ill *(continued)*

Fleisher, L. A., Beckman, J. A., Brown, K. A., Calkins, H., Chaikof, E. L., Fleischmann, K. E.,... Robb, J. F. (2009). 2009 ACCF/AHA focused update on perioperative beta blockade incorporated into the ACC/AHA 2007 guidelines on perioperative cardiovascular evaluation and care for noncardiac surgery: A report of the American college of cardiology foundation/American heart association task force on practice guidelines. *Circulation, 120*(21), e169–e276.

ABBREVIATIONS

ACCF/AHA	American College of Cardiology/American Heart Association
ADL	Activities of daily living
COPD	Chronic obstructive pulmonary disease
CV	Cardiovascular
CVP	Central venous pressure
DVT	Deep vein thrombosis
EKG	Electrocardiogram
GI	Gastrointestinal
GU	Genitourinary
ICU	Intensive care unit
PAOP	Pulmonary artery occlusion pressure
QA	Quality assurance
QI	Quality improvement
QOL	Quality of life
SBT	Spontaneous breathing trial
VAP	Ventilator-assisted pneumonia

NOTE

1. This chapter was adapted from the American Association of Colleges of Nursing "Preparing Nursing Students to Care for Older Adults: Enhancing Gerontology in Senior-level Undergraduate Courses" curriculum module, Assessment and Management of Older Adults with Complex Illness in the Critical Care Unit, prepared by Michele C. Balas, Colleen M. Casey, Mary Beth Happ.

ACKNOWLEDGMENTS

The authors would like to acknowledge the continual support and commitment to improving nursing care of older adults provided by the John A. Hartford Foundation. Case study provided by the Study of Ventilator Weaning: Care and Communication Processes database using composite patient information and pseudonyms (R01-NR007973, M. Happ).

RESOURCES

American Association of Critical Care Nurses E-learning program on Palliative and End of Life Care.

http://www.aacn.org/wd/elearning/content/palliative/palliative.pcms?menu=elearning&lastmenu=divheader_courses_for_individuals

End of Life Nursing Education Consortium (ELNEC- Critical Care and ELNEC Geriatric).

http://www.aacn.nche.edu/elnec/about/critical-care and
http://www.aacn.nche.edu/elnec/about/geriatric

GeroNurseOnline.org
http://www.geronurseonline.org

Hartford Institute for Geriatric Nursing
http://www.consultgerirn.org/resources

Improving Palliative Care in the ICU (IPAL-ICU).
https://www.capc.org/ipal/ipal-icu

The Richmond Agitation and Sedation Scale (RASS) and The Confusion Assessment Method-ICU (CAM-ICU). Training manual includes information for administering both the RASS and the CAM-ICU.

http://www.icudelirium.org/docs/CAM_ICU_training.pdf

Topics relevant to this chapter include:

- Falls
- Urinary Incontinence
- Abrupt Change in Mental Status
- Atypical Presentation
- Delirium
- Pain
- Medications

Other topics relevant to the care of the older adult also available through this website.

Topics relevant to this chapter include:
Brief Evaluation of Executive Dysfunction: An Essential Refinement in the Assessment of Cognitive Impairment
Decision Making and Dementia
Recognition of Dementia in the Hospitalized Older Adult
Beers' Criteria for Potentially Inappropriate Medication Use in the Elderly Assessing Pain in Older Adults
Katz Index of Independence in Activities of Daily Living

REFERENCES

American Association of Critical-Care Nurses (2004). *Ventilator-associated pneumonia, AACN practice alert.* Retrieved from http://www.aacn.org/wd/practice/docs/practicealerts/vap.pdf. *Evidence Level I.*

Angus, D. C., Shorr, A. F., White, A., Dremsizov, T. T., Schmitz, R. J., & Kelley, M. A.; Committee on Manpower for Pulmonary and Critical Care Societies (COMPACCS). (2006). Critical care delivery in the United States: Distribution of services and compliance with Leapfrog recommendations. *Critical Care Medicine, 34*(4), 1016–1024. *Evidence Level II.*

Azoulay, E., Pochard, F., Chevret, S., Jourdain, M., Bornstain, C., Wernet, A.,... Lemaire, F. (2002). Impact of a family information leaflet on effectiveness of information provided to family members of intensive care unit patients: A multicenter, prospective, randomized, controlled trial. *American Journal of Respiratory and Critical Care Medicine, 165*(4), 438–442. *Evidence Level II.*

Balas, M. C., Chaperon, C., Sisson, J. H., Bonasera, S., Hertzog, M., Potter, J.,... Burke, W. J. (2011). Transitions experienced by older survivors of critical care. *Journal of Gerontological Nursing, 37*(12), 14–25; quiz 26. *Evidence Level IV.*

Balas, M. C., Deutschman, C. S., Sullivan-Marx, E. M., Strumpf, N. E., Alston, R. P., & Richmond, T. S. (2007). Delirium in older patients in surgical intensive care units. *Journal of Nursing Scholarship: An Official Publication of Sigma Theta Tau International Honor Society of Nursing/Sigma Theta Tau, 39*(2), 147–154. *Evidence Level IV.*

Balas, M. C., Happ, M. B., Yang, W., Chelluri, L., & Richmond, T. (2009). Outcomes associated with delirium in older patients in surgical ICUs. *Chest, 135*(1), 18–25. *Evidence Level III.*

Balas, M. C., Vasilevskis, E. E., Olsen, K. M., Schmid, K. K., Shostrom, V., Cohen, M. Z.,... Burke, W. J. (2014). Effectiveness and safety of the awakening and breathing coordination, delirium monitoring/management, and early exercise/mobility bundle. *Critical Care Medicine, 42*(5), 1024–1036. *Evidence Level VI.*

Baldwin, M. R., Reid, M. C., Westlake, A. A., Rowe, J. W., Granieri, E. C., Wunsch, H.,... Lederer, D. J. (2014). The feasibility of measuring frailty to predict disability and mortality in older medical intensive care unit survivors. *Journal of Critical Care, 29*(3), 401–408. *Evidence Level II.*

Barr, J., Fraser, G. L., Puntillo, K., Ely, E. W., G. W.ll, C., Dasta, J. F.,... Jaeschke, R.; American College of Critical Care Medicine. (2013). Clinical practice guidelines for the management of pain, agitation, and delirium in adult patients in the intensive care unit. *Critical Care Medicine, 41*(1), 263–306. *Evidence Level VI.*

Bartlett, G., Blais, R., Tamblyn, R., Clermont, R. J., & MacGibbon, B. (2008). Impact of patient communication problems on the risk of preventable adverse events in acute care settings. *Canadian Medical Association Journal = Journal de l'Association Medicale Canadienne, 178*(12), 1555–1562. *Evidence Level IV.*

Beers, M. H. (1997). Explicit criteria for determining potentially inappropriate medication use by the elderly. An update. *Archives of Internal Medicine, 157*(14), 1531–1536. *Evidence Level IV.*

Bellmann-Weiler, R., & Weiss, G. (2009). Pitfalls in the diagnosis and therapy of infections in elderly patients—A mini-review. *Gerontology, 55*(3), 241–249. *Evidence Level VI.*

Bergbom, I., & Askwall, A. (2000). The nearest and dearest: A lifeline for ICU patients. *Intensive & Critical Care Nursing: The Official Journal of the British Association of Critical Care Nurses, 16*(6), 384–395. *Evidence Level IV.*

Bickley, L. S. (2008). *Bates guide to physical examination and history taking* (10th vol.). Philadelphia, PA: Wolters Kluwer Health Lippincott Willlams & Wilkins. *Evidence Level VI.*

Black, P., Boore, J. R., & Parahoo, K. (2011). The effect of nurse-facilitated family participation in the psychological care of the critically ill patient. *Journal of Advanced Nursing, 67*(5), 1091–1101. *Evidence Level III.*

Bonk, M. E., Krown, H., Matuszewski, K., & Oinonen, M. (2006). Potentially inappropriate medications in hospitalized senior patients. *American Journal of Health-System Pharmacy: Official Journal of the American Society of Health-System Pharmacists, 63*(12), 1161–1165. *Evidence Level IV.*

Bouillon, R., et al. (2009). Glucose control in critically ill patients... The NICE-SUGAR Study Investigators. Intensive versus conventional glucose control in critically ill patients. *New England Journal of Medicine, 361*(1), 89–92. *Evidence Level II.*

Broyles, L. M., Colbert, A. M., Tate, J. A., Swigart, V. A., & Happ, M. B. (2008). Clinicians' evaluation and management of mental health, substance abuse, and chronic pain conditions in the intensive care unit. *Critical Care Medicine, 36*(1), 87–93. *Evidence Level IV.*

Brummel, N. E., Jackson, J. C., Pandharipande, P. P., Thompson, J. L., Shintani, A. K., Dittus, R. S.,... Girard, T. D. (2014). Delirium in the ICU and subsequent long-term disability among survivors of mechanical ventilation. *Critical Care Medicine, 42*(2), 369–377. *Evidence Level II.*

Buczko, W. (2010). Ventilator-associated pneumonia among elderly Medicare beneficiaries in long-term care hospitals. *Health Care Financing Review, 31*(1), 1–10. *Evidence Level IV.*

Carson, S. S., Bach, P. B., Brzozowski, L., & Leff, A. (1999). Outcomes after long-term acute care. An analysis of 133 mechanically ventilated patients. *American Journal of Respiratory and Critical Care Medicine, 159*(5 Pt 1), 1568–1573. *Evidence Level III.*

Chelluri, L., Im, K. A., Belle, S. H., Schulz, R., Rotondi, A. J., Donahoe, M. P.,... Pinsky, M. R. (2004). Long-term mortality and quality of life after prolonged mechanical ventilation. *Critical Care Medicine, 32*(1), 61–69. *Evidence Level IV.*

Chen, Y. H., Lin, H. L., Hsiao, H. F., Chou, L. T., Kao, K. C., Huang, C. C., & Tsai, Y. H. (2012). Effects of exercise training on pulmonary mechanics and functional status in patients with prolonged mechanical ventilation. *Respiratory Care, 57*(5), 727–734. *Evidence Level II.*

Chipps, E., Gatens, C., Genter, L., Musto, M., Dubis-Bohn, A., Gliemmo, M., . . . Landers, T. (2014). Pilot study of an oral care protocol on poststroke survivors. *Rehabilitation Nursing: The Official Journal of the Association of Rehabilitation Nurses, 39*(6), 294–304. *Evidence Level II.*

Curtis, J. R., Nielsen, E. L., Treece, P. D., Downey, L., Dotolo, D., Shannon, S. E., . . . Engelberg, R. A. (2011). Effect of a quality-improvement intervention on end-of-life care in the intensive care unit: A randomized trial. *American Journal of Respiratory and Critical Care Medicine, 183*(3), 348–355. *Evidence Level II.*

Daly, B. J., Douglas, S. L., O'Toole, E., Gordon, N. H., Hejal, R., Peerless, J., . . . Hickman, R. (2010). Effectiveness trial of an intensive communication structure for families of long-stay ICU patients. *Chest, 138*(6), 1340–1348. *Evidence Level II.*

Daubin, C., Chevalier, S., S.eval, A., Gaillard, C., Valette, X., Prlette, F., . . . Charbonneau, P. (2011). Predictors of mortality and short-term physical and cognitive dependence in critically ill persons 75 years and older: A prospective cohort study. *Health and Quality of Life Outcomes, 9*, 35. *Evidence Level III.*

Davidson, J. E., Daly, B. J., Agan, D., Brady, N. R., & Higgins, P. A. (2010). Facilitated sensemaking: A feasibility study for the provision of a family support program in the intensive care unit. *Critical Care Nursing Quarterly, 33*(2), 177–189. *Evidence Level V.*

Dermot Frengley, J., Sansone, G. R., Shakya, K., & Kaner, R. J. (2014). Prolonged mechanical ventilation in 540 seriously ill older adults: Effects of increasing age on clinical outcomes and survival. *Journal of the American Geriatrics Society, 62*(1), 1–9. *Evidence Level III.*

de Rooij, S. E., Abu-Hanna, A., Levi, M., & de Jonge, E. (2005). Factors that predict outcome of intensive care treatment in very elderly patients: A review. *Critical Care, 9*(4), R307–R314. *Evidence Level V.*

de Rooij, S. E., Govers, A. C., Korevaar, J. C., Giesbers, A. W., Levi, M., & de Jonge, E. (2008). Cognitive, functional, and quality-of-life outcomes of patients aged 80 and older who survived at least 1 year after planned or unplanned surgery or medical intensive care treatment. *Journal of the American Geriatrics Society, 56*(5), 816–822. *Evidence Level V.*

Douglas, S. L., Daly, B. J., Brennan, P. F., Gordon, N. H., & Uthis, P. (2001). Hospital readmission among long-term ventilator patients. *Chest, 120*(4), 1278–1286. *Evidence Level IV.*

Douglas, S. L., Daly, B. J., Gordon, N., & Brennan, P. F. (2002). Survival and quality of life: Short-term versus long-term ventilator patients. *Critical Care Medicine, 30*(12), 2655–2662. *Evidence Level IV.*

Douglas, S. L., Daly, B. J., O'Toole, E., & Hickman, R. L. (2010). Depression among white and nonwhite caregivers of the chronically critically ill. *Journal of Critical Care, 25*(2), 364.e11–364.e19. *Evidence Level IV.*

Ely, E. W., Baker, A. M., Dunagan, D. P., Burke, H. L., Smith, A. C., Kelly, P. T., . . . Haponik, E. F. (1996). Effect on the duration of mechanical ventilation of identifying patients capable of breathing spontaneously. *New England Journal of Medicine, 335*(25), 1864–1869. *Evidence Level V.*

Ely, E. W., Bennett, P. A., Bowton, D. L., Murphy, S. M., Florance, A. M., & Haponik, E. F. (1999). Large scale implementation of a respiratory therapist-driven protocol for ventilator weaning. *American Journal of Respiratory and Critical Care Medicine, 159*(2), 439–446. *Evidence Level II.*

Ely, E. W., Inouye, S. K., Bernard, G. R., Gordon, S., Francis, J., May, L., . . . Dittus, R. (2001). Delirium in mechanically ventilated patients: Validity and reliability of the confusion assessment method for the intensive care unit (CAM-ICU). *Journal of the American Medical Association, 286*(21), 2703–2710. *Evidence Level IV.*

Ely, E. W., Margolin, R., Francis, J., May, L., Truman, B., Dittus, R., . . . Inouye, S. K. (2001). Evaluation of delirium in critically ill patients: Validation of the Confusion Assessment Method for the Intensive Care Unit (CAM-ICU). *Critical Care Medicine, 29*(7), 1370–1379. *Evidence Level I.*

Esteban, A., Anzueto, A., Frutos-Vivar, F., Alut, I., Ely, E. W., Brochard, L., . . . Abroug, F.; Mechanical Ventilation International Study Group. (2004). Outcome of older patients receiving mechanical ventilation. *Intensive Care Medicine, 30*(4), 639–646. *Evidence Level IV.*

Fick, D. M., Cooper, J. W., Wade, W. E., Waller, J. L., Maclean, J. R., & Beers, M. H. (2003). Updating the Beers criteria for potentially inappropriate medication use in older adults: Results of a US consensus panel of experts. *Archives of Internal Medicine, 163*(22), 2716–2724. *Evidence Level I.*

Fleisher, L. A., Beckman, J. A., Brown, K. A., Calkins, H., Chaikof, E. L., Fleischmann, K. E., . . . Robb, J. F. (2009). 2009 ACCF/AHA focused update on perioperative beta blockade incorporated into the ACC/AHA 2007 guidelines on perioperative cardiovascular evaluation and care for noncardiac surgery: A report of the American College of Cardiology Foundation/American Heart Association Task Force on Practice Guidelines. *Circulation, 120*(21), e169–e276. *Evidence Level I.*

Ford, P. N., Thomas, I., Cook, T. M., Whitley, E., & Peden, C. J. (2007). Determinants of outcome in critically ill octogenarians after surgery: An observational study. *British Journal of Anaesthesia, 99*(6), 824–829. *Evidence Level IV.*

Fried, L. P., Tangen, C. M., Walston, J., Newman, A. B., Hirsch, C., Gottdiener, J., . . . McBurnie, M. A.; Cardiovascular Health Study Collaborative Research Group. (2001). Frailty in older adults: Evidence for a phenotype. *Journals of Gerontology. Series A, Biological Sciences and Medical Sciences, 56*(3), M146–M156. *Evidence Level IV.*

Fulton, A. T., Gozalo, P., Mitchell, S. L., Mor, V., & Teno, J. M. (2014). Intensive care utilization among nursing home residents with advanced cognitive and severe functional impairment. *Journal of Palliative Medicine, 17*(3), 313–317. *Evidence Level IV.*

Garett, K. L., Beukelman, D. R., Garrett, K. L. & Yorkston, K. N. (2007). AAC in intensive care units. In D. R. Beukelman, K. L. Garrett, & K. M. Yorkston (Eds.), *Augmentative communication strategies for adults with acute or chronic medical conditions.* Baltimore, MD: Brookes Publishing. *Evidence Level VI.*

Girard, T. D., & Ely, E. W. (2007). Bacteremia and sepsis in older adults. *Clinics in Geriatric Medicine, 23*(3), 633–47, viii. *Evidence Level VI.*

Girard, T. D., Kress, J. P., Fuchs, B. D., Thomason, J. W., Schweickert, W. D., Pun, B. T.,... Ely, E. W. (2008). Efficacy and safety of a paired sedation and ventilator weaning protocol for mechanically ventilated patients in intensive care (Awakening and Breathing Controlled trial): A randomised controlled trial. *Lancet, 371*(9607), 126–134. *Evidence Level II.*

Gries, C. J., Engelberg, R. A., Kross, E. K., Zatzick, D., Nielsen, E. L., Downey, L., & Curtis, J. R. (2010). Predictors of symptoms of posttraumatic stress and depression in family members after patient death in the ICU. *Chest, 137*(2), 280–287. *Evidence Level IV.*

Griffiths, J., Fortune, G., Barber, V., & Young, J. D. (2007). The prevalence of post traumatic stress disorder in survivors of ICU treatment: A systematic review. *Intensive Care Medicine, 33*(9), 1506–1518. *Evidence Level V.*

Guentner, K., Hoffman, L. A., Happ, M. B., Kim, Y., Dabbs, A. D., Mendelsohn, A. B., & Chelluri, L. (2006). Preferences for mechanical ventilation among survivors of prolonged mechanical ventilation and tracheostomy. *American Journal of Critical Care: An Official Publication, American Association of Critical-Care Nurses, 15*(1), 65–77. *Evidence Level IV.*

Hakim, R. B., Teno, J. M., Harrell, F. E., Knaus, W. A., Wenger, N., Phillips, R. S.,... Lynn, J. (1996). Factors associated with do-not-resuscitate orders: Patients' preferences, prognoses, and physicians' judgments. SUPPORT Investigators. Study to understand prognoses and preferences for outcomes and risks of treatment. *Annals of Internal Medicine, 125*(4), 284–293. *Evidence Level III.*

Hamel, M. B., Teno, J. M., Goldman, L., Lynn, J., Davis, R. B., Galanos, A. N.,... Phillips, R. S. (1999). Patient age and decisions to withhold life-sustaining treatments from seriously ill, hospitalized adults. SUPPORT Investigators. Study to understand prognoses and preferences for outcomes and risks of treatment. *Annals of Internal Medicine, 130*(2), 116–125. *Evidence Level II.*

Happ, M. B. (2000). Interpretation of nonvocal behavior and the meaning of voicelessness in critical care. *Social Science & Medicine (1982), 50*(9), 1247–1255. *Evidence Level IV.*

Happ, M. B. (2001). Communicating with mechanically ventilated patients: State of the science. *AACN Clinical Issues, 12*(2), 247–258. *Evidence Level IV.*

Happ, M. B., Baumann, B. M., Sawicki, J., Tate, J. A., George, E. L., & Barnato, A. E. (2010). SPEACS-2: Intensive care unit "communication rounds" with speech language pathology. *Geriatric Nursing, 31*(3), 170–177. *Evidence Level V.*

Happ, M. B., Garrett, K. L., Tate, J. A., DiVirgilio, D., Houze, M. P., Demirci, J. R.,... Sereika, S. M. (2014). Effect of a multi-level intervention on nurse-patient communication in the intensive care unit: Results of the SPEACS trial. *Heart & Lung: Journal of Critical Care, 43*(2), 89–98. *Evidence Level IV.*

Happ, M. B., Seaman, J. B., Nilsen, M. L., Sciulli, A., Tate, J. A., Saul, M., & Barnato, A. E. (2015). The number of mechanically ventilated ICU patients meeting communication criteria. *Heart & Lung: Journal of Critical Care, 44*(1), 45–49. *Evidence Level III.*

Happ, M. B., Swigart, V. A., Tate, J. A., Hoffman, L. A., & Arnold, R. M. (2007). Patient involvement in health-related decisions during prolonged critical illness. *Research in Nursing & Health, 30*(4), 361–372. *Evidence Level IV.*

Happ, M. B., Swigart, V. A., Tate, J. A., Arnold, R. M., Sereika, S. M., & Hoffman, L. A. (2007). Family presence and surveillance during weaning from prolonged mechanical ventilation. *Heart & Lung: Journal of Critical Care, 36*(1), 47–57. *Evidence Level III.*

Happ, M. B., Tate, J., & Garrett, K. (2006). Nursing counts. Focus on: Nonspeaking older adults in the ICU: Communication will require special strategies. *American Journal of Nursing, 106*(5), 37. *Evidence Level IV.*

Hennessy, D., Juzwishin, K., Yergens, D., Noseworthy, T., & Doig, C. (2005). Outcomes of elderly survivors of intensive care: A review of the literature. *Chest, 127*(5), 1764–1774. *Evidence Level V.*

Herzig, S. J., Howell, M. D., Ngo, L. H., & Marcantonio, E. R. (2009). Acid-suppressive medication use and the risk for hospital-acquired pneumonia. *Journal of the American Medical Association, 301*(20), 2120–2128. *Evidence Level VI.*

Hopkins, R. O., & Jackson, J. C. (2006). Long-term neurocognitive function after critical illness. *Chest, 130*(3), 869–878. *Evidence Level VI.*

Humbert, J., Gallagher, K., Gabbay, R., & Dellasega, C. (2008). Intensive insulin therapy in the critically ill geriatric patient. *Critical Care Nursing Quarterly, 31*(1), 14–18. *Evidence Level VI.*

Institute for Healthcare Improvement. (2012). *How-to guide: Prevent ventilator-associated pneumonia.* Cambridge, MA: Institute for Healthcare Improvement. Retrieved from http://www.ihi.org. *Evidence Level III.*

Iregui, M., Ward, S., Sherman, G., Fraser, V. J., & Kollef, M. H. (2002). Clinical importance of delays in the initiation of appropriate antibiotic treatment for ventilator-associated pneumonia. *Chest, 122*(1), 262–268. *Evidence Level IV.*

Jackson, J. C., Girard, T. D., Gordon, S. M., Thompson, J. L., Shintani, A. K., Thomason, J. W.,... Ely, E. W. (2010). Long-term cognitive and psychological outcomes in the awakening and breathing controlled trial. *American Journal of Respiratory and Critical Care Medicine, 182*(2), 183–191. *Evidence Level II.*

Jones, C., B.nessi, C., Capuzzo, M., Egerod, I., Flaatten, H., Granja, C.,... Griffiths, R. D.; RACHEL group. (2010). Intensive care, diaries reduce new onset post traumatic stress disorder following critical illness: A randomised, controlled trial. *Critical Care, 14*(5), R168. *Evidence Level II.*

Jorm, A. F. (1994). A short form of the Informant Questionnaire on Cognitive Decline in the Elderly (IQCODE): Development and cross-validation. *Psychological Medicine, 24*(1), 145–153. *Evidence Level IV.*

Joynt, G. M., Gomersall, C. D., Tan, P., Lee, A., Cheng, C. A., & Wong, E. L. (2001). Prospective evaluation of patients refused admission to an intensive care unit: Triage, futility and outcome. *Intensive Care Medicine, 27*(9), 1459–1465. *Evidence Level IV.*

Jubran, A., Lawm, G., Duffner, L. A., Collins, E. G., Lanuza, D. M., Hoffman, L. A., & Tobin, M. J. (2010). Post-traumatic stress disorder after weaning from prolonged mechanical ventilation. *Intensive Care Medicine, 36*(12), 2030–2037. *Evidence Level IV.*

Kaarlola, A., Tallgren, M., & Pettile, V. (2006). Long-term survival, quality of life, and quality-adjusted life-years among critically ill elderly patients. *Critical Care Medicine, 34*(8), 2120–2126. *Evidence Level IV.*

Kahn, J. M., Werner, R. M., David, G., Ten Have, T. R., Benson, N. M., & Asch, D. A. (2013). Effectiveness of long-term acute care hospitalization in elderly patients with chronic critical illness. *Medical Care, 51*(1), 4–10. *Evidence Level III.*

Kane, R. L., Ouslander, J. G., & Abrass, I. B. (2004). *Essentials of clinical geriatrics* (5th vol.). New York, NY: McGraw-Hill. *Evidence Level VI.*

Karlsson, V., Forsberg, A., & Bergbom, I. (2010). Relatives' experiences of visiting a conscious, mechanically ventilated patient—A hermeneutic study. *Intensive & Critical Care Nursing: The Official Journal of the British Association of Critical Care Nurses, 26*(2), 91–100. *Evidence Level III.*

Katz, S., Ford, A. B., Moskowitz, R. W., Jackson, B. A., & Jaffe, M. W. (1963). Studies of illness in the aged. The Index of ADL: A standardized measure of biological and psychosocial function. *Journal of the American Medical Association, 185,* 914–919. *Evidence Level IV.*

Kidd, D., Stewart, G., Baldry, J., Johnson, J., Rossiter, D., Petruckevitch, A., & Thompson, A. J. (1995). The Functional Independence Measure: A comparative validity and reliability study. *Disability and Rehabilitation, 17*(1), 10–14. *Evidence Level III.*

Kleinpell, R. M., & Ferrans, C. E. (2002). Quality of life of elderly patients after treatment in the ICU. *Research in Nursing & Health, 25*(3), 212–221. *Evidence Level IV.*

Klompas, M., Anderson, D., Trick, W., Babcock, H., Kerlin, M. P., Li, L., . . . Platt, R.; CDC Prevention Epicenters. (2015). The preventability of ventilator-associated events. The CDC Prevention Epicenters Wake Up and Breathe Collaborative. *American Journal of Respiratory and Critical Care Medicine, 191*(3), 292–301. *Evidence Level III.*

Kloos, J. A., & Daly, B. J. (2008). Effect of a family-maintained progress. Journal on anxiety of families of critically ill patients. *Critical Care Nursing Quarterly, 31*(2), 96–107; quiz 108. *Evidence Level II.*

Kress, J. P., Gehlbach, B., Lacy, M., Pliskin, N., Pohlman, A. S., & Hall, J. B. (2003). The long-term psychological effects of daily sedative interruption on critically ill patients. *American Journal of Respiratory and Critical Care Medicine, 168*(12), 1457–1461. *Evidence Level II.*

Kress, J. P., Pohlman, A. S., O'Connor, M. F., & Hall, J. B. (2000). Daily interruption of sedative infusions in critically ill patients undergoing mechanical ventilation. *New England Journal of Medicine, 342*(20), 1471–1477. *Evidence Level II.*

Krimshtein, N. S., Luhrs, C. A., Puntillo, K. A., Cortez, T. B., Livote, E. E., Penrod, J. D., & Nelson, J. E. (2011). Training nurses for interdisciplinary communication with families in the intensive care unit: An intervention. *Journal of Palliative Medicine, 14*(12), 1325–1332. *Evidence Level V.*

Lautrette, A., Ciroldi, M., Ksibi, H., & Azoulay, E. (2006). End-of-life family conferences: Rooted in the evidence. *Critical Care Medicine, 34*(Suppl. 11), S364–S372. *Evidence Level IV.*

Li, Z., Peng, X., Zhu, B., Zhang, Y., & Xi, X. (2013). Active mobilization for mechanically ventilated patients: Atilated, criticall. *Archives of Physical Medicine and Rehabilitation, 94*(3), 551–561. *Evidence Level I.*

Logan, I. C., Sumukadas, D., & Witham, M. D. (2010). Gastric acid suppressants—Too much of a good thing? *Age and Ageing, 39*(4), 410–411. *Evidence Level VI.*

Magnette, C., De Saint Hubert, M., Swine, C., Bouhon, S., Jamart, J., Dive, A., & Michaux, I. (2015). Functional status and medium-term prognosis of very elderly patients after an ICU stay: A prospective observational study. *Minerva Anestesiologica, 81*(7), 743–751. *Evidence Level III.*

Malkor, M., Karadibak, D., & Yildirim, Y. (2009). The effect of physiotherapy on ventilatory dependency and the length of stay in an intensive care unit. *International Journal of Rehabilitation Research. Internationale Zeitschrift fuut Rehabilitationsforschung. Revue internationale de recherches de ree rechesnal, 32*(1), 85–88. *Evidence Level III.*

Marik, P. E. (2006). Management of the critically ill geriatric patient. *Critical Care Medicine, 34*(Suppl. 9), S176–S182. *Evidence Level VI.*

Marik, P. E., Vasu, T., Hirani, A., & Pachinburavan, M. (2010). Stress ulcer prophylaxis in the new millennium: A systematic review and meta-analysis. *Critical Care Medicine, 38*(11), 2222–2228. *Evidence Level I.*

McAdam, J. L., Fontaine, D. K., White, D. B., Dracup, K. A., & Puntillo, K. A. (2012). Psychological symptoms of family members of high-risk intensive care unit patients. *American Journal of Critical Care: An Official Publication, American Association of Critical-Care Nurses, 21*(6), 386–393; quiz 394. *Evidence Level IV.*

McNicoll, L., Pisani, M. A., Zhang, Y., Ely, E. W., Siegel, M. D., & Inouye, S. K. (2003). Delirium in the intensive care unit: Occurrence and clinical course in older patients. *Journal of the American Geriatrics Society, 51*(5), 591–598. *Evidence Level IV.*

Medland, J. J., & Ferrans, C. E. (1998). Effectiveness of a structured communication program for family members of patients in an ICU. *American Journal of Critical Care: An Official Publication, American Association of Critical-Care Nurses, 7*(1), 24–29. *Evidence Level III.*

Menaker, J., & Scalea, T. M. (2010). Geriatric care in the surgical intensive care unit. *Critical Care Medicine, 38*(Suppl. 9), S452–S459. *Evidence Level V.*

Mick, D. J., & Ackerman, M. H. (2004). Critical care nursing for older adults: Pathophysiological and functional considerations. *Nursing Clinics of North America, 39*(3), 473–493. *Evidence Level VI.*

Milbrandt, E. B., Eldadah, B., Nayfield, S., Hadley, E., & Angus, D. C. (2010). Toward an integrated research agenda for critical illness in aging. *American Journal of Respiratory and Critical Care Medicine, 182*(8), 995–1003. *Evidence Level VI.*

Milisen, K., & DeGeest, S. A. I. L. D. H. H. (2001). Delirium. *Critical care nursing of the elderly.* New York, NY: Springer Publishing Company. *Evidence Level VI.*

Milisen, K., Foreman, M. D., Abraham, I. L., De Geest, S., Godderis, J., Vandermeulen, E., . . . Broos, P. L. (2001). A nurse-led interdisciplinary intervention program for delirium in elderly hip-fracture patients. *Journal of the American Geriatrics Society, 49*(5), 523–532. *Evidence Level III.*

Miller, C. A. (2009). *Nursing for wellness in older adults* (5th vol.). Philadelphia, PA: Wolters Kluwer Health/Lippincott, Willams, & Wilkins. *Evidence Level VI.*

Morandi, A., Jackson, J. C., & Ely, E. W. (2009). Delirium in the intensive care unit. *International Review of Psychiatry, 21*(1), 43–58. *Evidence Level VI.*

Morris, P. E., Goad, A., Thompson, C., Taylor, K., Harry, B., Passmore, L., . . . Haponik, E. (2008). Early intensive care unit mobility therapy in the treatment of acute respiratory failure. *Critical Care Medicine, 36*(8), 2238–2243. *Evidence Level III.*

Morse, J. M., & Pooler, C. (2002). Patient-family-nurse interactions in the trauma-resuscitation room. *American Journal of Critical Care: An Official Publication, American Association of Critical-Care Nurses, 11*(3), 240–249. *Evidence Level IV.*

Muir, J. F., Lamia, B., Molano, C., & Cuvelier, A. (2010). Respiratory failure in the elderly patient. *Seminars in Respiratory and Critical Care Medicine, 31*(5), 634–646. *Evidence Level VI.*

Nagappan, R., & Parkin, G. (2003). Geriatric critical care. *Critical Care Clinics, 19*(2), 253–270. *Evidence Level III.*

Nelson, J. E., Bassett, R., Boss, R. D., Brasel, K. J., Campbell, M. L., Cortez, T. B., . . . Weissman, D. E.; Improve Palliative Care in the Intensive Care Unit Project. (2010). Models for structuring a clinical initiative to enhance palliative care in the intensive care unit: A report from the IPAL-ICU Project (Improving Palliative Care in the ICU). *Critical Care Medicine, 38*(9), 1765–1772. *Evidence Level VI.*

Pandharipande, P. P., Girard, T. D., Jackson, J. C., Morandi, A., Thompson, J. L., Pun, B. T., . . . Ely, E. W.; BRAIN-ICU Study Investigators. (2013). Long-term cognitive impairment after critical illness. *New England Journal of Medicine, 369*(14), 1306–1316. *Evidence Level II.*

Patak, L., Wilson-Stronks, A., Costello, J., Kleinpell, R. M., Henneman, E. A., Person, C., & Happ, M. B. (2009). Improving patient-provider communication: A call to action. *Journal of Nursing Administration, 39*(9), 372–376. *Evidence Level IV.*

Peterson, J. F., Pun, B. T., Dittus, R. S., Thomason, J. W., Jackson, J. C., Shintani, A. K., & Ely, E. W. (2006). Delirium and its motoric subtypes: A study of 614 critically ill patients. *Journal of the American Geriatrics Society, 54*(3), 479–484. *Evidence Level IV.*

Pisani, M. A. (2009). Considerations in caring for the critically ill older patient. *Journal of Intensive Care Medicine, 24*(2), 83–95. *Evidence Level VI.*

Pisani, M. A., Murphy, T. E., Van Ness, P. H., Araujo, K. L., & Inouye, S. K. (2007). Characteristics associated with delirium in older patients in a medical intensive care unit. *Archives of Internal Medicine, 167*(15), 1629–1634. *Evidence Level VI.*

Pisani, M. A., Redlich, C., McNicoll, L., Ely, E. W., & Inouye, S. K. (2003). Underrecognition of preexisting cognitive impairment by physicians in older ICU patients. *Chest, 124*(6), 2267–2274. *Evidence Level IV.*

Richards, C. L. (2004). Urinary tract infections in the frail elderly: Issues for diagnosis, treatment and prevention. *International Urology and Nephrology, 36*(3), 457–463. *Evidence Level VI.*

Riggio, R. E., Singer, R. D., Hartman, K., & Sneider, R. (1982). Psychological issues in the care of critically ill respirator patients: Differential perceptions of patients, relatives, and staff. *Psychological Reports, 51*(2), 363–369. *Evidence Level IV.*

Rosenthal, R. A. (2004). Nutritional concerns in the older surgical patient. *Journal of the American College of Surgeons, 199*(5), 785–791. *Evidence Level VI.*

Rosenthal, R. A., & Kavic, S. M. (2004). Assessment and management of the geriatric patient. *Critical Care Medicine, 32*(Suppl. 4), S92–S105. *Evidence Level VI.*

Schweickert, W. D., Gehlbach, B. K., Pohlman, A. S., Hall, J. B., & Kress, J. P. (2004). Daily interruption of sedative infusions and complications of critical illness in mechanically ventilated patients. *Critical Care Medicine, 32*(6), 1272–1276. *Evidence Level III.*

Schweickert, W. D., Pohlman, M. C., Pohlman, A. S., Nigos, C., Pawlik, A. J., Esbrook, C. L., . . . Kress, J. P. (2009). Early physical and occupational therapy in mechanically ventilated, critically ill patients: A randomised controlled trial. *Lancet, 373*(9678), 1874–1882. *Evidence Level II.*

Sessler, C. N., Gosnell, M. S., Grap, M. J., Brophy, G. M., O'Neal, P. V., Keane, K. A., . . . Elswick, R. K. (2002). The Richmond Agitation-Sedation Scale: Validity and reliability in adult intensive care unit patients. *American Journal of Respiratory and Critical Care Medicine, 166*(10), 1338–1344. *Evidence Level I.*

Sheehy, C. M., Perry, P. A., & Cromwell, S. L. (1999). Dehydration: Biological considerations, age-related changes, and risk factors in older adults. *Biological Research for Nursing, 1*(1), 30–37. *Evidence Level V.*

Sinuff, T., Muscedere, J., Cook, D. J., Dodek, P. M., Anderson, W., Keenan, S. P., . . . Heyland, D. K.; Canadian Critical Care Trials Group. (2013). Implementation of clinical practice guidelines for ventilator-associated pneumonia: A multicenter prospective study. *Critical Care Medicine, 41*(1), 15–23. *Evidence Level III.*

Tate, J. A., Sereika, S., Divirgilio, D., Nilsen, M., Demerci, J., Campbell, G., & Happ, M. B. (2013). Symptom communication during critical illness: The impact of age, delirium, and delirium presentation. *Journal of Gerontological Nursing, 39*(8), 28–38. *Evidence Level II.*

Torres, A., Ferrer, M., & Badia, J. R. (2010). Treatment guidelines and outcomes of hospital-acquired and ventilator-associated pneumonia. *Clinical Infectious Diseases: An Official Publication of the Infectious Diseases Society of America, 51*(Suppl. 1), S48–S53. *Evidence Level VI.*

Tullmann, D. F., & Dracup, K. (2000). Creating a healing environment for elders. *AACN Clinical Issues, 11*(1), 34–50; quiz 153. *Evidence Level VI.*

Urden, L. D., Stacy, K. M., & Lough, M. E. (2010). The older adult population. *Critical care nursing: Diagnosis and management (Thelans Critical Care Nursing Diagnosis)* (7th ed.). *Evidence Level VI.*

van den Berghe, G., Wouters, P., Weekers, F., Verwaest, C., Bruyninckx, F., Schetz, M., . . . Bouillon, R. (2001). Intensive insulin therapy in critically ill patients. *New England Journal of Medicine, 345*(19), 1359–1367. *Evidence Level II.*

White, D. B., Braddock, C. H., Bereknyei, S., & Curtis, J. R. (2007). Toward shared decision making at the end of life in intensive care units: Opportunities for improvement. *Archives of Internal Medicine, 167*(5), 461–467. *Evidence Level III.*

White, D. B., Cua, S. M., Walk, R., Pollice, L., Weissfeld, L., Hong, S.,...Arnold, R. M. (2012). Nurse-led intervention to improve surrogate decision making for patients with advanced critical illness. *American Journal of Critical Care: An Official Publication, American Association of Critical-Care Nurses, 21*(6), 396–409. *Evidence Level IV.*

Williams, C. M. A. (2005). The identification of family members' contribution to patients' care in the intensive care unit: A naturalistic inquiry. *Nursing in Critical Care,* 10(1), 6–14. *Evidence Level IV.*

Wunsch, H., Guerra, C., Barnato, A. E., Angus, D. C., Li, G., & Linde-Zwirble, W. T. (2010). Three-year outcomes for Medicare beneficiaries who survive intensive care. *Journal of the American Medical Association, 303*(9), 849–856. *Evidence Level I.*

Yilmaz, R., & Erdem, Y. (2010). Acute kidney injury in the elderly population. *International Urology and Nephrology, 42*(1), 259–271. *Evidence Level VI.*

Zilberberg, M. D., de Wit, M., & Shorr, A. F. (2012). Accuracy of previous estimates for adult prolonged acute mechanical ventilation volume in 2020: Update using 2000–2008 data. *Critical Care Medicine, 40*(1), 18–20. *Evidence Level IV.*

Zilberberg, M. D., & Shorr, A. F. (2008). Prolonged acute mechanical ventilation and hospital bed utilization in 2020 in the United States: Implications for budgets, plant and personnel planning. *BMC Health Services Research, 8,* 242. *Evidence Level IV.*

Fluid Overload: Identifying and Managing Heart Failure Patients at Risk of Hospital Readmission

30

Judith E. Schipper

EDUCATIONAL OBJECTIVES

On completion of this chapter, the reader should be able to:

1. Describe the older adult with heart failure (HF) who is at risk of hospital readmission
2. Conduct a comprehensive cardiac history
3. Identify three physical findings that may be associated with fluid overload in the older adult patient with HF
4. Name three key symptoms associated with fluid overload in the older adult patient with HF
5. Define cardiovascular stability in relation to the five key indicators
6. Plan monitoring strategies to reduce fluid overload in the older adult with HF

OVERVIEW

HF is the most common cause of hospital admission in the older adult (Funk & Krumholz, 1996; Krumholz, Wang, et al., 1997; Roger et al., 2012). Hospitalizations for HF account for approximately 50% of all cardiovascular hospital admissions (Krumholz, Wang, et al., 1997; Lloyd-Jones et al., 2010). The evidence-based literature demonstrates that as many as half of these admissions are readmissions and are preventable (Lloyd-Jones et al., 2004; Rich et al., 1995; Ross et al., 2008). The epidemic in HF prevalence is commensurate with an aging population and has stimulated a focus of research to identify those patients at high risk of hospitalization and readmission. Early identification of patients at risk of rehospitalization during the hospital stay provides opportunity for interventions to impact the readmission rate. Symptoms of HF compel patients to seek medical aid; however, evidence to date has shown that HF patients postpone seeking medical assistance 12 hours to 14 days before recognition of these changes as harmful to bodily functioning (Koenig, 1998; Rich & Kitman, 2005). The delay causes further deterioration in cardiac status requiring acute hospitalization. This chapter presents the complex nature and pathophysiology of HF symptoms, with nursing management strategies to reduce hospital readmission rates. A detailed protocol for nursing practice of the aging population is presented highlighting the nursing assessment and management of HF.

For a description of evidence Levels cited in this chapter, see Chapter 1, "Developing and Evaluating Clinical Practice Guidelines: A Systematic Approach."

BACKGROUND AND STATEMENT OF PROBLEM

HF is a public health problem affecting an estimated 5.8 million Americans yearly (Lloyd-Jones et al., 2010; Thom et al., 2006). Cardiovascular disease (CVD), which includes hypertension (HTN) and HF, valvular heart disease and arrhythmias, along with the atherosclerotic disease that causes coronary heart disease (Hay et al., 1993), stroke, and peripheral vascular disease (PVD), is the major contributor to mortality and comorbidity in older adults. CVD accounts for 40% of all deaths in those aged 75 to 85 years, and 48% of all deaths in those 85 years and older (Lloyd-Jones et al., 2010; Thom et al., 2006). Acute or chronic HF is the leading cause of hospital admission in patients older than 65 years, with readmission rates to acute care facilities averaging 17.2% nationally in 1996, which increased to 23.6% in 2010 (Funk & Krumholz, 1996; Lloyd-Jones et al., 2010). Risk of readmission has been shown to be four times higher in older adults aged 80 years and older, higher in ethnicities other than Whites, and higher with lower economic status (Giamouzis et al., 2011).

The prevalence of HF increases with age, and more than 75% of those affected are older than 65 years of age. Development of HF is higher with male sex, lower level of education, low levels of physical activity, cigarette smoking, overweight, diabetes mellitus (DM), HTN, valvular heart disease, left ventricular hypertrophy (LVH), and atherosclerosis of the coronary arteries (coronary heart disease [CHD]). HTN is a precursor in 75% of individuals diagnosed with HF (Thom et al., 2006). Both the incidence and prevalence of HF continue to increase as the population ages.

Risk Factors for Developing HF in Older Adults

The primary clinical risk factors for developing HF are advancing age, male sex, HTN, myocardial infarction (MI), DM, valvular heart disease, and obesity. HTN is the most common cause of HF in patients without CHD, accounting for 24% of the cases of HF (Ho, Pinsky, Kannel, & Levy, 1993). HTN is also extremely common in type 2 DM, as it occurs in 40% to 60% of older adults with type 2 DM (Hypertension in Diabetes Study Group, 1993). Women with DM are at extremely high risk for developing HF (Levy, Larson, Vasan, Kannel, & Ho, 1996). Individuals with HTN and DM often develop HF with preserved left ventricular (LV) systolic function (heart failure with a preserved ejection fraction [HFpEF]) or so-called diastolic HF, rather than LV systolic dysfunction (heart failure with reduced ejection fraction [HFrEF]; Piccini, Klein, Gheorghiade, & Bonow, 2004). HFpEF is a clinical syndrome in which LV filling pressures are elevated, the LV ejection fraction (LVEF) is normal, and yet the heart is unable to satisfy the systemic oxygen needs of an individual.

Other related clinical risk factors of HF include smoking, dyslipidemia of genetic and dietary etiology, sleep-disordered breathing or obstructive sleep apnea (OSA), chronic kidney disease, albuminuria, sedentary lifestyle, low socioeconomic status, and psychological stress. Toxic substances, such as chemotherapeutic agents (anthracyclines, cyclophosphamide, 5-FU, trastuzumab), illicit drugs (amphetamines, cocaine), and medications (nonsteroidal anti-inflammatory drugs [NSAIDs], thiazolidinediones [TZDs], alcohol), can precipitate HF (Schocken et al., 2008).

DM is a CVD equivalent and, as such, is an important contributor to HF. Women and those individuals treated with insulin are at the greatest risk for ischemic etiology of both HFrEf and HFpEF. In a sample of older Medicare patients with type 2 DM, 22% had a diagnosis of HF, and this prevalence increased with advancing age (Bertoni et al., 2004). In addition, the presence of type 2 DM is associated with higher HF-related morbidity and mortality. After MI or coronary revascularization procedures, individuals with type 2 DM also have a high morbidity and mortality, which is largely caused by the development of HF. An earlier analysis of outcomes in Medicare patients 1 year after an MI revealed that 11% of patients without DM had HF, whereas 17% of patients with DM on oral agents and 25% of those treated with insulin were admitted for HF exacerbation (Chyun, Vaccarino, Murillo, Young, & Krumholz, 2002).

The initial diagnosis of HF is most often an acute index event requiring hospitalization. Patients at risk of readmission after initial diagnosis of HF include the following (Bertoni et al., 2004; Chyun et al., 2002; Lewis et al., 2003):

- Age 65 years and older, and even more so for age 80 years and older
- Newly diagnosed HF with hospitalization (Krumholz, Parent, et al., 1997)
- Low systolic blood pressure (SBP; Pocock et al., 2006)
- OSA and/or chronic obstructive pulmonary disease (COPD)
- Renal dysfunction
- Rheumatoid arthritis
- Increased heart rate (HR; Stefenelli, Bergler-Klein, Globits, Pacher, & Glogar, 1992; Triposkiadis et al., 2009) or arrhythmia atrial fibrillation (Koitabashi et al., 2005)
- Hospitalizations for any reason in the past 5 years (Kossovsky et al., 2000)
- Social isolation (Faris, Purcell, Henein, & Coats, 2002)

- HF related to acute MI or uncontrolled HTN
- History of alcohol abuse (Evangelista, Doering, & Dracup, 2000)
- HF with acute infection
- HF with an exacerbation of a comorbidity; anemia with hemoglobin of less than 12 (Young et al., 2008), kidney disease (Metra et al., 2008), COPD (Braunstein et al., 2003; Mascarenhas, Lourenço, Lopes, Azevedo, & Bettencourt, 2008), and sleep apnea (Kasai et al., 2008)
- History of depression or anxiety (Faris et al., 2002; Rumsfeld et al., 2003)
- Nonadherence to diet, fluid intake, respiratory treatments or medications

Pathophysiology of HF

Understanding the pathophysiology of HF provides insight into the rationale for treatment. HF is defined as the inability of the heart to pump blood sufficient to metabolic needs of the body or the inability to do so without significantly elevated filling pressures (Miller & Piña, 2009). The inability of the left ventricle to eject blood sufficiently represents LV systolic HF or HFrEF and is diagnosed with a measurement of EF less than 50%. Diastolic dysfunction and failure result in high LV filling pressures, yet inadequate ability of LV to deliver oxygenated blood to fulfill the body's needs. Diastolic HF is also more descriptively named HF with preserved systolic function or HFpEF because the EF is essentially normal: approximately 60%. The symptoms of HF are directly related to impairment in the filling and ejecting of the blood in the left ventricle (Owan et al., 2006).

All of the risk factors and disease entities listed previously can cause direct damage to the myocardium, as in MI and toxic exposure, or subject it to an increased level of wall stress, as in HTN or valvular lesions. Such an insult initiates compensatory actions by the heart that are mediated by the neurohormones of the sympathetic nervous system (SNS) and the renin–angiotension–aldosterone system (RAAS), which are active, both systemically and directly, in the myocardium. Rather than offering benefit, the SNS (epinephrine and norepinephrine) and RAAS (angiotensin II, vasopressin, aldosterone) hormones promote cardiac remodeling and hypertrophy, causing dilatation of the ventricle and buildup of fibrous tissue that weakens the cardiomyocytes. These changes occur during compensated (asymptomatic) as well as decompensated (symptomatic) failure. The overexpression of neurohormones causes salt and water retention and vasoconstriction, which in turn produces increased hemodynamic stress on the left ventricle. These factors are cyclical unless treated. Untreated, there is further disruption of left ventricle architecture and performance (Miller & Piña, 2009).

Because this process begins without symptoms, for patients at risk, it is essential to identify factors that are a hazard to cardiovascular health and initiate treatment before significant damage to the myocardium occurs. The American College of Cardiology/American Heart Association Task Force (ACC/AHA) developed guidelines to classify HF in four stages (Hunt et al., 2005) based on the structural changes and damage to the heart:

Stage A is considered a pre-HF stage or an "at-risk" stage. It includes patients with HTN, atherosclerotic disease, DM, obesity, metabolic syndrome, those using cardiotoxic substances, or those with a family history of cardiomyopathy.

Stage B includes asymptomatic individuals with previous MI, LVH, decreased EF, and asymptomatic valvular disease.

Stage C includes individuals with known heart disease and symptoms—shortness of breath, fatigue, and reduced exercise tolerance—or those who, after treatment, are now asymptomatic for their heart disease.

Stage D includes individuals with refractory HF requiring the use of specialized interventions and includes patients with marked symptoms at rest despite maximal medical therapy.

Atherosclerosis and ischemia in CHD are the most common etiology of HF in the United States, followed closely by HTN alone and valvular disease. Thyroid dysfunction and excessive alcohol intake may also lead to HF. In the absence of known CVD, systolic function of the heart remains relatively unchanged in older adults, as does exercise tolerance. Diastolic dysfunction, however, is predominately a disease of older adults and may be present even in the absence of HTN or cardiomyopathy, which are also known to contribute to diastolic failure (Bhatia et al., 2006; Olsson et al., 2006; Yancy, Lopatin, Stevenson, De Marco, & Fonarow, 2006). The prevalence of HFpEF is increasing as the population of those older than 65 years grows along with the burden of lifestyle risk factors of diabetes and obesity (Anderson & Vasan, 2014; Butler et al., 2014). The archetypical patient presenting with diastolic HF is 70 to 80 years of age, female, obese, diabetic, and often has atrial fibrillation (Coats, 2001). Diastolic dysfunction is characterized by an exaggerated HR with activity, which is often one of the first clinical findings. The severity of symptoms varies among patients and may not correlate with LVEF as exercise capacity and quality of life are similarly reduced in HFrEF and HFpEF (Brucks et al., 2005; Farr et al., 2008; Lewis et al., 2007).

HTN, CHD, and hypertrophic cardiomyopathy are all abnormalities that are exacerbated by tachycardia, underscoring the importance of avoiding a high HR in all older individuals. Diastolic abnormalities caused by HTN, aortic stenosis, hypertrophic cardiomyopathy, or CHD may precipitate HF. Patients with either systolic or diastolic HF are at risk of fluid overload. Although discussed as two separate entities, many older adults have components of both systolic and diastolic dysfunction (Gheorghiade et al., 2010).

ASSESSMENT OF THE PROBLEM

For older adults diagnosed with HF, the health history and physical assessment are directed at monitoring symptoms and assessing cardiovascular function. For the nurse assessing and managing the patient with HF, it is important to note that the recognition of fluid overload is not always straightforward. Unlike the classic picture of HF observed in younger adults, the symptoms of fluid overload can be subtle and elusive in older adults (Coviello, 2004). Once symptoms become pronounced in the older adult, the nurse has a challenging task to resolve the HF, especially if it is of a long-standing duration (Giamouzis et al., 2011). Monitoring parameters must be established in which the patient and nurse actively identify subtle changes and seek intervention as early as possible (Grady et al., 2000).

The Health History

HF has both symptomatic and nonsymptomatic phases. When symptoms occur, they are related to intravascular and interstitial fluid overload and inadequate tissue perfusion. Symptoms become evident with exertion and in severe HF, even at rest. The New York Heart Association (NYHA) functional capacity is an important standardized classification of the HF patient according to how much activity patients are able to accomplish without symptoms (Table 30.1). Classifying patients according to their physical symptoms offers evidence of the extent of volume overload and limitation caused by symptoms, which then leads the nurse to recognize the severity of the disease. Patients, with proper treatment, can improve their functional status and classification as their symptoms improve from a NYHA class III to class II or even class I; however, once identified at an advanced stage, C or D, earlier stages are not reclaimed. For example, a stage C patient does not return to stage B. Although current therapies are shown in studies to improve mortality, success in returning diseased myocardium to health has not yet been achieved.

Both patients and providers frequently attribute symptoms of fluid overload to aging. When symptoms occur during exertion, senior patients may simply decrease their activities to prevent symptoms, yet when asked, they report activity from a memory of months earlier. Because of inaccurate reporting of activity, HF in older adults is often difficult to recognize and, therefore, goes untreated. Thus, the nurse should routinely ask questions related to activity-limiting dyspnea. A key indicator in establishing a baseline for functional capacity is to ask the patient what his or her maximal asymptomatic activity is now, what it was 6 months ago, and what it was 1 year ago. Other important questions include "How far can you walk without getting short of breath?" The answer to a question, such as "How far is the bathroom from your bed?" can elicit information about symptoms in walking, sleep habits, and nocturia. "What is the activity that commonly produces shortness of breath?" Try to avoid questions that can be answered "yes" or "no" (e.g., "Do you experience shortness of breath when simply sitting?" "Do you wake at night feeling short of breath?"). Rather, say, "tell me about what you do during a typical day." Repeating these questions in subsequent interviews will help monitor changes in activity associated with treatment or with suspected fluid gain. The goal is to identify whether the patient is physically capable of performing activities of daily living (ADL).

TABLE 30.1

New York Heart Association Functional Capacity Classification

Class I	No limitation of physical activity. Ordinary physical activity does not cause undue fatigue, palpitation, dyspnea, or angina.
Class II	Slight limitation of physical activity. Ordinary physical activity results in fatigue, palpitation, dyspnea, or angina.
Class III	Marked limitation of physical activity. Comfortable at rest, but less than ordinary physical activity results in fatigue, palpitation, dyspnea, or angina.
Class IV	Unable to carry on any physical activity without discomfort. Symptoms present at rest. With any physical activity, symptoms increase.

Adapted from American Heart Association (1994).

HFrEF is a pathophysiological process in which LV dysfunction occurs independent of symptom development (Brucks et al., 2005). Symptom expression is dependent on compensatory mechanisms and the length of time HF has been present. Patients with acute HF, as seen with MI, may be more symptomatic because their compensatory mechanisms have not fully developed. In comparison, the patient with long-standing HF may have severe dysfunction but may not become symptomatic until consuming a high-sodium meal or experiencing physical stress. Fluid overload can then occur rapidly, oftentimes overnight. In this case, compensatory mechanisms are now exhausted and, as a result, fail. The window of opportunity to successfully intervene is narrow, as is the margin of error. Treatment for fluid overload in this case must be swift and brisk but gentle enough to maintain BP (Grady et al., 2000). Nurses need to be aware of the importance of both early recognition and early intervention in the patient with fluid overload. A few hours delay in providing treatment can mean the difference between successful management at home or need for hospital admission with variable outcomes.

Knowledge of past medical history will help to anticipate problems related to other conditions because their presence may complicate assessment and management of HF. Cardiac risk factors; levels of physical activity; and control of lipids, HTN, obesity, DM, and smoking need to be determined. Additionally, it is important to consider that older adult responses to HF medications and treatment are variable. Other drugs commonly used in this age group, such as over-the-counter NSAIDs, can actually exacerbate fluid overload by increasing sodium retention. Previous questions related to cardiovascular functional capacity may have already provided some information, but additional information on musculoskeletal and neurological function can add needed insight.

Assessment for additional symptoms will assist in identifying the patient with HF. *Orthopnea* is the most sensitive and specific symptom of elevated filling pressures, and it tends to reliably parallel filling pressures in patients with this symptom (Anker et al., 2003; Stevenson & Perloff, 1989). Nocturnal or exertional cough is often a dyspnea equivalent and should not be confused with the cough from an angiotensin-converting enzyme (ACE) inhibitor, which is not associated with activity or position. Individual patients generally exhibit patterns of fluid overload that reoccur in subsequent exacerbations. These should be documented, be made available to all on the care team, and be used in patient education for self-monitoring and for early recognition by the health care team. Questions related to symptoms and function should be part not only of the initial assessment, but also of subsequent visits as a means of surveillance (Stevenson & Perloff, 1989).

The clinical presentation of HF may include a variety of symptoms reflective of pulmonary congestion and decreased cardiac output. The questions related to health history are important to include and/or observe during the health encounter. Although the presence of any one major symptom is sufficient to warrant consideration of HF, symptoms occurring with other physical findings of orthopnea, paroxysmal nocturnal dyspnea, and progressive dyspnea on exertion are virtually diagnostic of fluid overload. The Framingham criteria (Margolis et al., 1974) are validated and are most often used to identify congestive HF or HF exacerbation. If two major criteria or one major with two minor criteria are present, the professional can have reasonable certainty that the patient has HF. These criteria are listed as follows.

Major:

- Paroxysmal nocturnal dyspnea
- Neck vein distension
- Rales
- Enlarged heart on chest x-ray
- Acute pulmonary edema
- S3 gallop
- Increased central venous pressure
- Hepatojugular reflux
- Weight loss greater than or equal to 4.5 kg (10 pounds) in response to treatment

Minor:

- Bilateral ankle edema
- Nocturnal cough
- Dyspnea on ordinary exertion
- Hepatomegaly
- Pleural effusion
- Tachycardia greater than or equal to 120 beats per minute

The presence of other comorbidities, such as DM, renal dysfunction, and liver disease, along with systemic physiological changes associated with aging, further complicates the assessment and management of HF in the older adult. Comorbidities should also be carefully assessed by reviewing laboratory data. DM may necessitate monitoring of blood glucose because wide variations in glucose can affect the ischemic threshold. Renal dysfunction and liver disease may affect pharmacodynamics of drugs used to treat HF. Inclusion of the pharmacist on the health care team or at least a consultation with the pharmacist will assist in ensuring the efficacy and safety of medications in the aging population. Anemia, a common medical condition in older adults, affects oxygenation, activity tolerance, and subsequent fluid balance (Young et al., 2008). The presence of COPD, as well as other comorbidities, may necessitate special precautions when assessing and managing oxygen therapy and beta blockers.

As overuse of salt in the diet may precipitate fluid overload, a comprehensive dietary history is absolutely essential.

The nurse should include specific questions about what the patient eats for meals and who prepares those meals realizing that it may be more important to discuss food preparation and sodium restriction with the patient's primary caregiver. Additionally, does the patient use the saltshaker or salt substitutes at the table or in cooking? How often does the patient eat out at a restaurant or order in food? A review of foods high in sodium on a printed list often reveals foods the patient is eating but previously did not admit to. For instance, important dietary questions related to use of canned products or deli meats, which contain higher amounts of sodium, should be included. A list of the sodium and the potassium content of a variety of foods, including fruits and vegetables, can be helpful in providing the information necessary for the patient to make appropriate daily choices. Because assessment of nutritional status is critical to elicit accurate fluid and sodium intake, it is prudent in the acute care setting for the older adult to have a dietician consultation. Additionally, as cachexia is a harbinger of a downward spiral in patients with HF, questions need to be included on the health history related to appetite and weight loss (Evangelista et al., 2000; Lavie, Osman, Milani, & Mehra, 2003).

Current prescription and over-the-counter medication use should be assessed, along with any alternative or herbal therapies. Many older adults who are eligible for aspirin, beta blockers, and ACE inhibitors (ACEIs) do not receive these medications despite the important role that these agents have in reducing CHD-related morbidity and mortality (Anker et al., 2003; Colucci et al., 1996, 2007; Packer, 1998; Packer, Bristow, et al., 1996; Schocken et al., 2008).

Included in the health history should be questions related to medication adherence and the patient's decision to either take or not to take medications (Grady et al., 2000; Riegel et al., 2009). Understanding a patient's rationale to selectively not take certain medications at certain times will help reveal ways for the nurse to intervene. Patients may wish to adjust their diuretic dose so that they can function socially during the day. This is not an adherence issue but a sound decision based on the patient's rationale as to how to fit the medication regimen into his or her lifestyle. The interview can reveal whether "nonadherence" has such a rationale. If a cause is not found, other issues need to be explored, such as cost, number of medications, and/or the frequency of the doses. Ways to simplify the drug regimen should be explored as the older adult can become overwhelmed because of cognitive impairment, lack of health literacy with poor understanding of medication importance, and when symptomatic, for example, simply unable to do more than breathe.

Psychosocial factors, personal beliefs and behaviors, along with cultural and environmental influences, all contribute to management of chronic disease. The importance of depression and social support has been well documented in the older adult; therefore, all of these factors need to be assessed (Davos et al., 2003; Faris et al., 2002). The nursing assessment in individuals with HF should identify the individual's response to treatment, which can then be used to assist the individual in subsequent management of symptoms and the underlying condition, health-promotion and disease prevention activities, and chronic disease management. Awareness of the patient's own perception of why he or she sought medical care and a detailed analysis of the symptoms will assist in assessing the individual's or caregiver's ability to identify symptoms, his or her knowledge regarding the condition, its prognosis, and general health beliefs, along with the prior ability to manage this or other medical conditions.

The Physical Assessment of the Older Adult With Fluid Overload

Physical assessment of the patient with suspected fluid overload includes inspection; palpation; and auscultation of the peripheral vasculature, heart, lungs, abdomen, and extremities. Orientation, functional limitations, and mental clarity are observed during examination of vital signs, which include height and weight and waist circumference.

A patient's height and baseline weight are important indicators of both nutritional and fluid status. Patients may know their ideal weight or "dry weight." Ascertain this when obtaining the health history to establish initial goals in diuretic treatment. Hospitalized patients with HF should have a weight measurement each day. The importance of daily weights should be emphasized with each weight in the hospital setting to reinforce the need to continue this practice at home. At home, weights should be taken daily, typically the first thing in the morning on arising, before breakfast, and with no clothes or wearing light clothing to avoid false fluctuations (Grady et al., 2000; Riegel et al., 2009; Riegel, Naylor, Stewart, McMurray, & Rich, 2004). This provides the best baseline for consistency. A 2-lb weight gain overnight or a 3-lb weight gain in a week is an indication that medical management must change. Measurement of a senior's waist circumference is also important to determine at baseline, because many times, this is the location for fluid accumulation (Grady et al., 2000). Once height and weight are measured, a body mass index (BMI) should be calculated. Research has shown that higher BMIs (25–30 kg/m^2) are associated with longer survival (Horwich et al., 2001; Lavie et al., 2003; Pickering et al., 2005, 2008).

A thorough evaluation of the BP should be performed. A variety of environmental factors can influence BP determination; therefore, the room should be a comfortable temperature, the patient as relaxed as possible, and a 5-minute rest allowed before taking the first reading. Clothing that covers the area where the cuff will be placed should be removed, and the individual should be seated comfortably, with legs uncrossed, with the back and arm supported; the middle of the cuff on the upper arm should be at a level of the right atrium (Sansevero, 1997). The initial BP reading should be taken in both arms. Proper cuff size is critical to obtaining an accurate measurement. Obese individuals with large arm circumference need to have the appropriate cuff size for accuracy. Conversely, thin, cachectic patients will also have inaccurate readings with a standard cuff. The bladder length should be 80% of the arm circumference and width at least 40%. The midline of the bladder should be placed above the brachial artery, 2 to 3 cm above the antecubital fossa, where the artery should have first been palpated. When using the auscultatory method, which remains the "gold standard" for BP measurement, palpating the radial pulse first while inflating the cuff will identify the point at which the pulse disappears. For the subsequent auscultatory measurement, the cuff should then be inflated to at least 30 mmHg above this point. The rate of deflation is also extremely important with a rate of 2 to 3 mmHg/sec recommended. The first and last audible sounds are the SBP and diastolic BP (DBP), respectively. Two readings, taken 5 minutes apart should be averaged and if there is greater than 5 mmHg difference, additional readings should be obtained (Pickering et al., 2005, 2008; Sansevero, 1997).

Pseudohypertension is a rare phenomenon resulting from noncompressibility of thickened arteries and will result in the recording of falsely high BP when indirect methods are used. A high BP over time without any indication of end-organ damage and treatment of the BP creating symptoms of hypotension, such as dizziness, confusion, and decreased urine output, point to a diagnosis of pseudohypertension. This tendency for peripheral arteries to become rigid with aging may result in a need to increase cuff pressure in order to compress the artery. If suspected, an intra-arterial reading has been suggested to avoid overmedication with antihypertensives; however, this is an extreme measure and is rarely done. Most providers, who treat HTN in older adults, consider 160/90 mmHg as a hypertensive BP and will treat gently with appropriate antihypertensives and pull back on treatment if symptoms of hypotension or orthostasis occur. Isolated systolic HTN is also common in the older adult and is defined by an SBP greater than 140 mmHg and a DBP less than 90 mmHg. Care must be taken not to overtreat in this population, especially if aortic stenosis or other valvular disease is present. Older adults are also more likely to exhibit white-coat HTN, in which the BP may be elevated more than 140/90 mmHg in the presence of a health care worker and an actual reading at home is usually 135/85 mmHg or less. Therefore, assessment of the BP not only requires careful attention to technique but also consideration of the physiological abnormalities associated with aging. Home BP monitoring has been suggested as a means for patients to partner with their providers to provide care. For those patients who are unable for whatever reason, 24-hour ambulatory BP monitoring is available to more accurately assess BP fluctuations during the day (Arzt et al., 2006).

In addition, the standing BP should be assessed because older adults have a tendency for postural hypotension. Orthostatic hypotension is diagnosed when the SBP falls by at least 20 mmHg or the DBP by 10 mmHg within 3 minutes. The presence of orthostatic hypotension may also reveal early dehydration in a patient who is usually otherwise stable (Arzt & Bradley, 2006). Because dehydration is the second most common admission for the older adult with HF, with falls following closely behind, standing BPs should be part of the routine assessment. In addition, patients should be assessed for dehydration during diuresis and whenever a condition exists in which fluid loss could occur. This includes not only with vomiting or diarrhea but also with diaphoresis caused by extremes in temperature and humidity.

Inspection is the first step of the physical assessment. General inspection of the periphery includes the following:

- Observing color of the skin and mucous membranes
- Inspecting the patient's nails, including nail beds, and the angle between the base of the nail and the skin of the cuticle (normally less than 160°). An angle of 180° is called *clubbing*; the distal phalanx appears rounded. Clubbing is associated with chronic hemoglobin desaturation.
- If cachexic, check dependent areas for decubiti.
- Evaluate hair on distal extremities (indication of adequate arterial perfusion)

Palpation of the extremities occurs following inspection of the skin color for temperature and turgor as well as the color of the nail beds. Capillary refill of the nail should be assessed by compressing the nail for 2 to 3 seconds and then releasing. Note the time elapsed until the original color returns. Normally, the nail bed is pink; capillary refill occurs within 2 to 3 seconds. A pale or cyanotic nail with delayed capillary refill may indicate decreased peripheral perfusion. The peripheral pulses should be palpated bilaterally, including radial, femoral, pedal, and posterior tibial pulse. Note pulse rate, rhythm, and symmetry.

Respiratory rate and effort should be assessed before auscultation of the lungs. If possible, oxygen saturation during rest and activity should be recorded. Patients whose oxygen level desaturates during activity to 86% or lower may require oxygen support at home. In addition, surveillance of oxygen saturation during sleep may be required if the patient or family reports difficulty with sleep at night. Sleep apnea can be the etiology of HF in patients with HF and, if untreated or treated ineffectively, can be the cause of exacerbation and decompensation in HF (Bennett & Sauvé, 2003; Cormican & Williams, 2004; Kaneko, Hajek, Zivanovic, Raboud, & Bradley, 2003; Lanfranchi & Somers, 2003; Maisel, 2001a; Mansfield et al., 2003). Use the diaphragm of the stethoscope to assess the lungs. Listen in all the lobes for diminished sounds, crackles, wheezes, or rhonchi. Lung sounds are an important part of the assessment, particularly in patients with a history of HF.

The cardiovascular assessment begins by locating the apex and apical pulse by feeling for the point of maximal impulse (PMI). In systolic HF, the PMI is displaced laterally and indicates the heart is dilated. Assessment of apical pulse rate and regularity, with attention to fullness and amplitude, also are important. Heart sounds should be ascertained with both the diaphragm and the bell of the stethoscope. Note the presence of S1 and S2 and of extra sounds, S3 gallop, S4 murmurs, clicks, or rubs. If extra heart sounds are present, also examine the carotid arteries by listening on both sides of the neck with the bell. Bruits sound like murmurs, so it is important to differentiate between the two. Some aortic murmurs will radiate into the neck and may even be audible when auscultating the lungs posteriorly. Always listen to the heart before listening for extra sounds in the neck. Carotids should be palpated unilaterally, never simultaneous bilaterally, to avoid occlusion of blood flow to the brain.

Jugular veins are assessed best with the patient in semi-Fowler's position but, if the patient is severely dyspneic, Fowler's position may be necessary. With the patient's head in straight alignment, observe the jugular neck veins for the presence of jugular venous distention (JVD). Turning the head slightly to the left and shining a penlight angularly on the vein allows for easier visualization of JVD and "a" and "v" waves, particularly in obese patients with thick necks. The jugular venous pulse waves will vary with respiration and decrease during inspiration. The jugular vein is compressible and varies with the angle of the neck. In the absence of pathology, venous distention is not present. JVD is the most sensitive sign of elevated filling pressures and is present with fluid overload, cor pulmonale, or high venous pressure (Stevenson et al., 1989).

The abdomen should then be examined. First, auscultate for bowel sounds in a distended abdomen to assess for other pathology-causing distention. Next, palpate to determine whether the abdomen is soft and nontender. A protuberant abdomen with bulging flanks suggests the possibility of ascites. Because ascitic fluid characteristically sinks with gravity, whereas gas-filled loops of bowel float to the top, percussion gives a dull note in dependent areas of the abdomen. Look for such a pattern by percussing outward in several directions from the central area of tympany. Map the area between tympany and dullness. To palpate the liver, place your hand behind the patient, parallel to and supporting the right 11th and 12th ribs and adjacent soft tissues below. Remind the patient to relax. By pressing your left hand forward, the patient's liver may be felt more easily by the other hand. Patients who are sensitive to palpation can rest their hand on your palpating hand. Note any tenderness. If at all palpable, the edge of the liver is soft, sharp, and regular. The liver can be enlarged in HF because of congestion. To further assess for volume excess, place the patient in semi-Fowler's position at the highest level at which the jugular neck pulsations remain visible. Firmly apply pressure with the palmar surface of the hand over the right upper quadrant of the patient's abdomen for 1 minute. A 1-cm rise in the jugular distention called *hepatojugular reflux* confirms the presence of fluid overload. Hepatojugular reflux may be associated with or without tenderness. Patients may also complain of a feeling of fullness.

The presence of *peripheral edema*, a symptom that can be related to fluid overload from cardiac renal disease or PVD, should be evaluated. Edema can also occur in response to medications such as calcium channel blockers. Dependent parts of the body, such as the feet, the ankles, and the sacrum, are the most likely locations to find edema. The presence and location of edema, and whether it is pitting or nonpitting, should be assessed. Depress an edematous area over a bony prominence for 5 to 15 seconds, then release. Grading scale for edema is as follows:

0 = *no pitting*
1+ = *trace*
2+ = *moderate*, disappears in 10 to 45 seconds
3+ = *deep*, disappears in 1 to 2 minutes
4+ = *very deep*, disappears in 3 to 5 minutes

The neurological assessment cannot be overlooked because changes in HR and rhythm, a decrease in cardiac output, and side effects of cardiac medications may cause significant changes in mental status. The nurse can observe and assess the patient's mood, thought processes, thought content, abnormal perceptions, insight, judgment, memory, and retention throughout the examination from intake of history and throughout treatment. Because depression is common among both the older adult and the chronically ill, signs of depression should be assessed (Koenig, 1998; Maisel, 2001b). Examples of signs of depression include feelings of hopelessness and sadness (also see Chapter 15, "Late-Life Depression"). The time, the day, and the year, as well as orientation to place, should be included. Memory of hospitalization, teaching that occurred while hospitalized, and subsequent events postdischarge can be addressed depending on whether the patient is hospitalized or being seen as an outpatient (Grady et al., 2000; Wang, FitzGerald, Schulzer, Mak, & Ayas, 2005).

To summarize, the physical examination findings consistent with HF include the following:

- JVD
- Basilar crackles, bronchospasm, and wheezing
- Displaced apical impulse
- Presence of S3 or S4; heart murmur
- Elevated HR and BP
- Hepatomegaly/splenomegaly
- Hepatojugular reflux
- Elevated HR and BP
- Temperature of extremities, warm versus cool

Laboratory and Diagnostic Studies

The initial laboratory evaluation of patients presenting with symptoms of HF should include complete blood count, serum electrolytes, including calcium and magnesium; blood urea nitrogen (BUN); serum creatinine; fasting blood glucose; glycosylated hemoglobin A1c (HbA_{1c}); lipid profile; liver function tests; thyroid-stimulating hormone; and urinalysis.

B-type natriuretic peptide (BNP) is useful in the evaluation of symptomatic patients presenting in the urgent care setting in whom the clinical diagnosis of HF is uncertain (Cygankiewicz et al., 2009; Huang et al., 2007; Hunt et al., 2005). A baseline BNP in the patient with a confirmed diagnosis of HF in the compensated state can provide a comparison measurement when the presence of fluid overload is suspected. A BNP level below 100 indicates a very low probability of HFrEF; however, a symptomatic patient may have diastolic HF or HFpEF. A level between 100 and 400 pg/mL should begin to raise suspicion of either HFrEf or HFpEF or right ventricular systolic dysfunction. Levels greater than 400 pg/mL have a 95% probability of HF and congestion caused by volume overload (Cygankiewicz et al., 2009; Hunt et al., 2005).

Electrolyte abnormalities are common in the older adult, particularly in individuals on chronic diuretic therapy. The serum potassium level should be monitored and supplemented so that it does not drop below 3.8 mmol/L. Renal function, as well as electrolyte levels, should remain current and test repeated whenever a patient has to increase diuretic therapy for longer than 3 days because of fluid overload. Anemia is frequently observed especially in renal insufficiency and poor nutritional status and may contribute to hypoxia, myocardial ischemia, and fluid overload.

The index episode or first acute HF is most often ischemic in etiology. Cardiac enzymes assist in determining the presence of acute MI when an acute fluid overload event occurs (Bertoni et al., 2004; Chyun et al., 2002; Lewis et al., 2003). Older adults may have an MI in the total absence of symptoms or with atypical symptoms. It is important to know also that patients who are congested may leak troponin at low levels and not be acutely ischemic. All of these factors make a review of diagnostic test results very important.

A 12-lead electrocardiogram (EKG) and chest x-ray (posterioranterior [PA] and lateral) should be performed initially in all patients presenting with symptoms of HF. A baseline EKG is vital so that ST and T waves; axis changes; prolongation in PR, QRS, and QT intervals can be assessed for indication of ongoing ischemia and response to medications. A new-onset arrhythmia heralded by an episode of fluid overload is not uncommon. The excess volume in HF can cause a stretch of the atrium, which, in turn, can precipitate atrial fibrillation, a common arrhythmia in patients with chronic HF. Two-dimensional echocardiography with Doppler should be performed during the initial evaluation to assess LVEF, LV size, wall thickness, and valve function. Radionucleotide ventriculography (multigated acquisition [MUGA] scan) can be performed to assess ventricular volumes, LVEF, and myocardial perfusion abnormalities although the current advanced technology of echocardiography makes the radionucleotide method of MUGA unnecessary. Cardiac catheterization should be performed on patients presenting with symptoms of HF who have angina or significant ischemia or who have known, suspected, or are at high risk of CHD, unless the patient is not eligible for revascularization of any kind.

Holter monitoring may be considered in patients presenting with HF who have a history of MI and/or syncope and are being considered for an electrophysiology study to document an inducible ventricular tachycardia. In addition, other candidates for electrophysiology referral include those with an LVEF of 30% or less with a QRS complex duration that exceeds 130 msec. Patients who meet this criteria should receive a biventricular pacemaker in combination with an automatic implantable defibrillator in order to prevent sudden death from ventricular arrhythmia (Prystowsky & Nisam, 2000), as well as improve cardiac output (Bonds et al., 2010; Chobanian et al., 2003; Glandt & Raz, 2010).

INTERVENTIONS AND CARE STRATEGIES

Initial goals in the acute management of HF are to alleviate symptoms and improve oxygenation, improve circulation, and correct the underlying causes of the HF. Longer term goals are to improve exercise tolerance and functional capacity, and through treatment improve ventricular function. Guideline-directed medical therapies (GDMT) are evidence-based therapies (EBT) that demonstrate reductions in the morbidity and mortality in HF and as such are recommended in the guidelines for managing HF. Effective treatment with EBT can also assist in reducing admission and readmission rates. The management of HF follows standard ACC/AHA Task Force expert consensus recommendations, including intensive treatment of coexistent HTN, CHD, and renal disease (Chobanian et al., 2003). It is important to note that optimal treatment of HTN is critical to both the prevention and treatment of HF. Although the level at which medication should be started is often still debated (Lee, Lindquist, Segal, & Covinsky, 2006), the treatment goal in HTN for those older than 60 years, according to Eighth Joint National Committee (JNC-8), is 150/90 mmHg (Baruch et al., 2004; James et al., 2014). There is compelling evidence for patients with coronary disease to continue to treat to the lower targets recommended in the previous commission, JNC-7 (Bangalore, Gong, Cooper-DeHoff, Pepine, & Messerli, 2014; Dinicolantonio et al., 2013).

Key prognostic indicators of 4-year mortality for older adults diagnosed with HF include renal dysfunction, pulmonary disease, a BMI of less than 25 kg/m^2, diabetes, HTN, and cancer. Patients who continue to smoke have a greater risk of mortality. Those individuals with a functional deficit in ADL, such as difficulty bathing, managing finances, walking several blocks, or pushing or pulling heavy objects, combined with one or more of the earlier mentioned factors are at greater risk not only for mortality but additionally the need for hospitalization. A chart review and history during hospitalization should include the standard accepted cardiac risk factors and the key indicators as listed previously. Detecting these additional prognostic indicators can aid in developing interventions that can affect quality of life and survival (Carson, Tognoni, & Cohn, 2003). Goals for therapy should include reaching goals for fasting blood sugar and HbA$_{1c}$, BP, cholesterol, and HF therapy through the use of evidence-based standards of care.

In *stage A*, HF, HTN, and lipid disorders are treated with lifestyle modification and medication as indicated to achieve guideline-recommended goals for BP and cholesterol. Smoking-cessation assistance, in the form of counseling and medication, is offered at every interaction with a patient who smokes. A goal of increasing activity or exercise should be mutually established with patients. For some, this may be as little as standing and sitting during television commercials, whereas for others, it may mean a walk before or after dinner or more for others. The control of metabolic syndrome is achieved through lifestyle modification. Alcohol is a simple sugar, and in excess contributes to the development of insulin resistance and diabetes, increasing cardiovascular risk. Illicit drug use must be identified, treatment offered, and encouraged. Both ACEIs and angiotensin-receptor blockers (ARBs; Maggioni et al., 2005) treat HTN and HFrEF but, it is important to note that they, have been shown to prevent cardiovascular events, cerebrovascular events, and progression of renal disease in stage A. Their use is especially important in patients with vascular disease or in those with DM.

In *stage B*, these same cited measures are used with ACEIs, ARBs, and beta-blockers in certain patients. All ACEIs are indicated in HFrEF; however, there are only two ARBs with evidence strong enough to be GDMT in HFrEF. Valsartan and candesartan, both ARBs, obtained recognition for benefit in HFrEF in their respective studies (Cohn, 1999; Cohn & Tognoni, 2001; Ostergren, 2006; Packer, 1998; Packer, Bristow, et al., 1996; Packer, Colucci, et al., 1996; Shah, Desai, & Givertz, 2010).

In *stage C*, dietary sodium restriction is added to this regimen, and as a symptomatic stage, diuretics are needed to be added to treat the fluid retention that causes symptoms, along with ACEIs or ARBs and beta blockers. Carvedilol and metoprolol, in the extended-release form of metoprolol succinate, are the two drugs in the beta-blocker category that are evidence based and guideline recommended in the treatment of HFrEF. (Barrella & Della Monica, 1998; Carmody & Anderson, 2007; Colucci et al., 1996, 2007; Goldstein & Hjalmarson, 1999; Hjalmarson et al., 2000; Hjalmarson & Fagerberg, 2000; M. Naylor et al., 1994). Aldosterone antagonists are also GDMT in HFrEF with some evidence of benefit in HFpEF as well. In certain patients, digitalis can also be effective (Baruch et al., 2004; Carson et al., 2003; Cohn & Tognoni, 2001; Maggioni et al., 2005). Hydralazine in combination with isordil or other nitrates is beneficial and GDMT in the African American population (Rich & Nease, 1999). Many of the *stage C* patients qualify for a biventricular pacemaker and/or implantable defibrillators to treat life-threatening arrhythmias.

In *stage D*, patients younger than 70 years without significant comorbidities may be offered advanced therapy options, such as cardiac transplant or LV assist device (LVAD; ventricular assist device [VAD]). A trial of inotropic therapy, such as milrinone or dobutamine, may serve as a temporary boost to end-stage patients but also may be treatment as palliative therapy, offering patients at end of life an improved quality and ability to be with their family. Palliative care offers the end-stage patient comfort that affords the patient a quality of life in an environment where the patient can be at ease rather than enduring the frequent and recurrent hospital visits on an emergent basis. Although the LVAD first was designed as a bridge to transplant, VADs are now offered as a bridge to decision about transplant. Additionally, the LVAD as destination therapy is a palliative measure, again offering the patients a quality of life their heart is unable to give. Hospice care is also offered to the end-stage HF patient who is not a candidate for any further therapy. The nurse has an important role in assisting the individual and his or her caregivers in understanding the disease process and treatment options, including end-of-life care (Coviello, Hricz-Borges, & Masulli, 2002).

Open and honest discussion regarding the chronic, progressive nature of HF must begin early in the disease process as the natural history of HF involves declining physical as well as psychological functioning. Although depression is commonly seen in the older adult, as well as individuals with CVD, there are few studies that have addressed this important problem in older adults with HF (Faris et al., 2002). In a study of patients older than 60 years at Duke University, Koenig found that 107 patients of 342 depressed patients had HF, with 36.5% having a major depression and 25.5% having a minor depression (Koenig, 1998). Because pharmacotherapy and behavioral interventions have demonstrated effectiveness, all older individuals should be screened for depression and treated appropriately. Early discussions related to the goals of care and advance directives with frequent revisiting of patient understanding of the disease course and patient preferences as the illness progresses ensure patient and care partner participation in decision making. A multidisciplinary team, including a spiritual and/or a psychological representative, should be developed to offer support for all involved: the patient, family, and all caregivers.

The benefits of the multidisciplinary team providing care to HF patients have been discussed for the past several years. In most cases, this has been related to the use of the team approach to help keep patients stable in order to prevent hospital readmissions (Naylor, 2006; Naylor, Griffiths, & Fernandez, 2004; Naylor & Keating, 2008). Comprehensive transitional care interventions have been shown not only to reduce costs and cardiac outcomes, but also have a beneficial effect on hospitalization for comorbid conditions (Chriss, Sheposh, Carlson, & Riegel, 2004; Coviello et al., 2002; Dickson, Deatrick, & Riegel, 2008; Naylor et al., 2009; Riegel et al., 2004). In the case of the patient in end-stage HF, a multidisciplinary team—either for inpatient or outpatient management—can provide cost-effective service for patients with the care in the environment of choice (Grady et al., 2000; Riegel et al., 2006).

Once the initial history and physical assessment have been completed, an individualized care plan to monitor and treat fluid overload should be implemented. The care plan should include teaching that begins early in the hospital stay while the patient's memory of a decompensated state is fresh. The teaching of principles of HF self-care relies on the patient's ability to learn to recognize the beginnings of decompensation. Techniques to prevent a congested state and manage self-care to maintain euvolemia are crucial to begin as early as possible (Cavallari et al., 2004; Lancaster, Smiciklas-Wright, Heller, Ahern, & Jensen, 2003; Riegel et al., 2009; Taylor et al., 2004). A 3-lb weight gain in 1 to 2 days or a 5-lb weight gain in the course of the week is a reason to alter diuretic dosage for up to 3 days. If the patient returns to baseline weight before the 3-day period, he or she may reduce the dose back to the standard daily dose (Grady et al., 2000). Patients can be taught how to regulate their diuretic doses based on their symptoms and weight. The nurse and patient can construct a self-care algorithm that gives them a sound "recipe" to follow if fluid overload occurs. The important factor here is early recognition and swift, brief action. Clear guidelines as to when to contact caregivers, if they are not living with the patient, should also be provided. Consideration should be given to the patient's baseline functional capacity, as well as renal function. Diuretics are used in both systolic and diastolic HF to relieve congestive symptoms by promoting the excretion of sodium and water and by decreasing cardiac filling pressures, thereby decreasing preload. They should be used effectively but cautiously in the older adult with diastolic dysfunction, when maintaining an adequate cardiac output is required in order to avoid syncope, falls, or confusion.

A doubled dose of oral diuretics for up to 3 days is usually well tolerated in congested patients with systolic or diastolic HF. When diuretics are used, serum potassium levels should be monitored because of an increased risk of hypokalemia with loop diuretics and of hyperkalemia with potassium-sparing agents, especially if renal impairment exists. Patients should be forewarned about signs of hypokalemia such as profound weakness. Loop diuretics may be useful for patients who are volume sensitive or who have a tendency to retain fluid because of renal impairment. Aldosterone antagonists are potassium-sparing diuretics, which abate some degree of hypokalemia seen with loop diuretics; however, serum potassium levels should be monitored. In some patients, ACEIs can cause hyperkalemia and, in combination with aldosterone inhibitors, this may be exacerbated. Recent evidence suggests that many individuals, particularly African Americans, may still require potassium supplementation (Gonseth, Guallar-Castillón, Banegas, & Rodríguez-Artalejo, 2004). In addition, dehydration is an important problem in older adults taking diuretics and appears to be an even greater concern in African Americans (McKelvie et al., 2002), making assessment of hydration status an important nursing concern (Arzt & Bradley, 2006).

Use of diuretic agents increases the risk of sudden loss of urinary control (urinary incontinence) in older adults. This is a very common, potentially reversible geriatric syndrome (see Chapter 21 "Urinary Incontinence"). The older adult population requires frequent monitoring and detection of symptoms related to the onset of urinary incontinence, which is often signaled by symptoms of urinary frequency, urgency, or nocturia. These symptoms may actually be present in the older adult from other coexisting comorbidities. Nocturia is particularly evident in patients with heart disease because the supine position increases vascular return and precipitates frequent rising at night to urinate. Nighttime falls in the older adult often occur when the patient wakes to advance to the bathroom. Preexisting comorbidities, such as visual impairment or osteoarthritis of the hip and/or knees, as well as prostate hypertrophy in men, make safety strategies a priority in urgent bathroom requirements. Overall, management considerations for the older adult with heart disease and a new development of urinary incontinence or falls include reevaluation of medication regimen, activity considerations, and the use of additional adaptive aides to assist in avoidance of preventable events. Use of a nighttime bedpan, urinal, or commode with frequent toileting rounds and reduction of nighttime fluids, are all possible and worthwhile solutions. Furosemide, as the most commonly used diuretic, has a half-life of 6 hours. In patients who are at a falling risk, timing the completion of diuresis before bedtime can decrease nocturia.

Beta blockers are useful in the management of diastolic HF because of their inhibition of the SNS and resultant negative chronotropic effect, which decreases HR and increases time for diastolic filling. Beta blockers are beneficial in the treatment of systolic HFrEF and are initiated in a euvolemic state after symptoms have resolved (Cohn, 1999; Colucci et al., 1996, 2007; Goldstein & Hjalmarson, 1999; Hjalmarson & Fagerberg, 2000; Ostergren, 2006; Packer, 1998; Packer, Bristow, et al., 1996; Packer, Colucci, et al., 1996; Shah et al., 2010). These agents should be initiated at low doses and titrated up to an optimal tolerated dose. Use of beta blockers in combination with ACEIs has demonstrated both an improvement in LVEF and functional capacity once optimized. Although beta blockers may potentially worsen insulin resistance, mask hypoglycemia, or aggravate orthostatic hypotension in older individuals with DM, these agents have been shown to contribute to improved outcomes. Therefore, careful monitoring for adverse effects is required with beta-blocker treatment to realize the beneficial effects of this important medication.

Digoxin increases contractility and decreases HR. It is not routinely indicated; however, it may be useful in those patients with persistent symptoms despite diuretic and ACEI therapy and in those patients who also have atrial fibrillation. Blood levels of digoxin should be monitored for toxicity and interactions with other medications such as amiodarone, verapamil, and vasodilators. Quinidine is no longer indicated or used therapeutically. The narrow therapeutic range for potassium is extremely important to monitor to prevent hypokalemia, which can precipitate arrhythmias in older adult patients with HF who are predisposed to both atrial and ventricular arrhythmias. Other medications that have a positive inotropic effect are dopamine and dobutamine. Both of these drugs can improve contractility and subsequent cardiac output; however, they also increase myocardial oxygen demand. *Milrinone* is a phosphodiesterase inhibitor that has been shown to be beneficial in the management of the hospitalized patient with HF, providing a positive inotropic effect, as well as a vasodilation (see Chapter 20, "Reducing Adverse Drug Events," for potential sequelae to several CV medications).

Vasodilators are also useful in the treatment of systolic and diastolic failure through reduction in preload. As with diuretics, they should be used cautiously in those with diastolic HF. Hydralazine and isosorbide reduce both preload and afterload, relieving symptoms and improving exercise tolerance. This combination is commonly used when patients do not tolerate ACE therapy. African Americans, in particular, had reduction in morbidity and mortality with hydralazine/nitrate combination (Piepoli, Davos,

Francis, & Coats, 2004). Morphine sulfate, often used in an emergent situation, also has a peripheral vasodilating effect and is useful with pulmonary edema or in patients with breathlessness at end of life.

With appropriate titration of these medications, an improvement in both LV function and functional capacity can be achieved. Medications to treat HTN and lipid abnormalities may not be well tolerated, and the potential for side effects and drug interactions is increased in the setting of polypharmacy. An antihypertensive agent should be used in the lowest dose to bring about the desired goal for BP treatment. Lipid-lowering agents should be offered as they were found to be effective in studies; however, patients may not be able to tolerate high doses. Use the highest dose that the patient can tolerate to achieve cholesterol lowering.

Patients and caregivers need to understand the warning signs of HF decompensation and recurrent MI such as chest pain, pressure, shortness of breath, indigestion, nausea, dizziness, palpitations, confusion, weakness, and weight gain. A clear plan for obtaining immediate medical attention should be developed. This is especially important if the older person lives alone; some type of "medical alert" system may be needed. Telemonitoring may be an option for some patients to consider. Understanding and ability to follow the medication regimen is paramount. A thorough assessment of the patient and his or her caregivers is therefore vital. The older individual may be on multiple medications and the schedule may be confusing. The need to maintain cardiac medications must be stressed and the risk of the patient abruptly discontinuing beta blocker, nitrates, and antiarrhythmics must be assessed. All medications should be reviewed with the patient and caregivers, stressing desired effects, common side effects, and possible interactions with over-the-counter medications (see Chapter 20). The nurse should also review what to do if medications are accidentally omitted or become too costly to maintain.

Long-term management of HF requires a multidisciplinary team approach (Lloyd-Jones et al., 2004) and disease management programs have been effective in reducing readmission rates (Taylor et al., 2006). Furthermore, even though many of these individuals are debilitated, exercise training has been shown to improve functional ability (Masoudi et al., 2005; Nesto et al., 2004). Referral to inpatient cardiac rehabilitation is an important stepping stone to reconditioning patients so they can better function at home when discharged.

Optimization of the medication for HF, coupled with activity progression, can enhance the patient's capacity for ADL and quality of life. An active patient may notice early signs of fluid overload when unable to accomplish standard activities done the previous week. Therefore, questions related to activity tolerance can provide insight for the nurse who monitors the patient. The patient with gradual fluid gain will first notice a change in his or her level of fatigue, which will translate into a change in daily routine. Previous experience with fluid overload will also reveal to the nurse the patient's own unique signs and symptoms because not every patient has the same indicators. It is not only important to assess these factors directly with the patient during the interview but also to reinforce that these symptoms are important for the patient to monitor as well (Grady et al., 2000). In addition to changes in weight, deviation from the baseline functional ability is an early clue, even before peripheral edema or lung congestion is present.

The prevention and treatment of HF in patients with DM requires optimal management of coexistent HTN, CHD, and LV dysfunction. Additionally, control of hyperglycemia is an important issue because the presence of HF affects the choice of medications used to treat type 2 DM. Although insulin and insulin secretagogues are considered safe for use in individuals with HF, TZDs are contraindicated, and metformin should be used only cautiously with careful monitoring of renal function (Hope-Ross, Buchanan, Archer, & Allen, 1990). Decreased clearance of metformin in individuals with HF caused by hypoperfusion or renal insufficiency can lead to potentially dangerous lactic acidosis. TZDs are associated with fluid retention, pedal edema, and weight gain, particularly when used in conjunction with insulin, and contribute to HF (Yusuf et al., 2000). Careful clinical assessment and ongoing monitoring should be implemented in the presence of known structural heart disease or a prior history of HF.

Adequate control of BP is also essential in the management of HF. Treatment of older persons with HTN has been shown to reduce CVD morbidity and mortality (Bari et al., 2004). An important nursing consideration is to monitor for adverse effects of medications used to manage HF, as well as HTN, along with patient and caregiver education. ACEIs are important in the management of systolic HF and may also be helpful in diastolic failure. In the Heart Outcomes Prevention Evaluation Study (Wing et al., 2003), ACEIs prevented cardiac events in high-risk patients without HF or known low EFs (Brenner et al., 2001). In addition, ACEIs have a renal protective benefit that is extremely important in preventing the development or worsening of HF, especially in patients with DM. Recent evidence suggests that use of ACEIs is associated with a larger lower extremity muscle mass, which may have benefit in wasting syndromes and prevention of disability

(Riegel, Lee, Dickson, & Carlson, 2009) and that they are particularly efficacious in older adults (Bonow et al., 2006). ARBs are also used widely for the prevention and treatment of HFrEF, particularly when patients are unable to use ACEIs because of the development of cough (Bonow et al., 2006). Renal function and hyperkalemia should be assessed when using both classes of agents, especially in the presence of underlying renal dysfunction.

CASE STUDY

CTG is a 72-year-old woman with a history of diet-controlled glucose intolerance and HFrEF of 38% with normal renal function. She is seen in the geriatric clinic with a 3-day history of poor appetite, nausea, and occasional vomiting. She complains of a constant feeling of fullness. She was last hospitalized 3 months ago because of fluid overload related to newly diagnosed HF. Her diuretic was increased 6 weeks ago for mild ankle swelling. She denies recent lower extremity swelling, orthopnea, or paroxysmal nocturnal dyspnea. Her blood sugars have been well controlled in the 90 to 130 range without hypoglycemic episodes. She denies fever, chills, cough, or urinary symptoms. She says she never misses her medications. Until 5 days ago, she was able to walk 30 minutes a day without difficulty. She had noticed a gradual increase in fatigue over the last 10 days and found herself too tired to attend several social and church events in the evening. When asked what her daily weights have been, she confessed that since she had been feeling so good she had abandoned this as a daily practice. Concerned, however, about her recent symptoms, she weighed herself this morning and found that she had gained 6 pounds since she last weighed herself 2 weeks ago despite being compliant to her medications for HF, which include the following:

Coreg 6.25 mg twice a day
Altace 5 mg daily
Aldactone 12.5 mg daily
Lasix 20 mg daily
Imdur 15 mg daily

She has not taken a double dose of Lasix with the additional weight gain as shown in her self-care action plan. She had been unaware of that weight gain because she had not been weighing herself. In addition, she had attended two social events 2 weekends ago that included eating out. Her self-care action plan had shown that she should increase her diuretic for 1 day following eating out the day before.

On physical examination, her BP is 132/86 mmHg with a HR of 88 beats per minute. She is afebrile. She has fine crackles in the lower bases bilaterally. There is 1+ lower extremity edema. Heart sounds demonstrate S1, S2, and S3. Her apical impulse is displaced to the left. There is jugular neck vein distention. Her abdominal girth has increased 2 inches since her last visit.

Lasix was increased to 40 mg for a maximum of 3 days. If at any point during the 3 days her weight returned to baseline, she was instructed to return to her usual dose of Lasix. She was advised of the importance of daily weights in order to maintain her baseline weight. She was referred back to her self-care action plan for changes in diuretic depending on her daily weight and the maintenance of her low-sodium diet in light of her social schedule. She will return to the clinic in 1 week.

Discussion

This patient exemplifies the need for educational reinforcement in a newly diagnosed patient with HF, who is just learning how to incorporate a self-care action plan. Like many patients who have had to take antibiotics in the past, compliance can wane when the patient feels well. Assessment of self-care knowledge and ability should be ongoing throughout the hospital stay, but is critical at the time of discharge in order to provide appropriate focus in outpatient care and support. The use of a tool to quantify knowledge and ability of self-care, such as the Self-Care in Heart Failure Index, is useful to identify patients who have continued needs for assistance after discharge (Riegel, Lee, et al., 2009). It is important to make contact with a newly diagnosed patient with HF fairly frequently in order to address questions that might influence the self-care decision making of the patient.

SUMMARY

Hospital admissions can be reduced in older adults with HF:

1. When care is taken in identifying the patients' own unique signs and symptoms of fluid overload
2. By creating monitoring parameters for the nurse in the form of history and physical assessment
3. By creating monitoring parameters for the patient in the form of a self-care algorithm with clear guidelines for self-care action
4. By achieving goals for clinical stability

NURSING STANDARD OF PRACTICE

Protocol 30.1: Heart Failure: Early Recognition and Treatment of the Patient at Risk of Hospital Readmission

I. GOAL

To reduce the incidence of hospital readmission of older adult patients with HF

II. OVERVIEW

A. HF is the most common cause of hospitalization of adults older than 65 years (Funk & Krumholz, 1996; Krumholz, Parent, et al., 1997) and is the cause of functional impairment and ultimate morbidity and mortality as well as significant hospital costs (Lloyd-Jones et al., 2010; Thom et al., 2006).

B. Hospitalization can be prevented by identifying the high-risk HF patient, early recognition of sign and symptoms of decompensation, and timely initiation or regulation of medical therapy (Lloyd-Jones et al., 2004; Rich et al., 1995; Ross et al., 2008).

C. Recognition of risk factors and routine monitoring for potential HF decompensation should be part of comprehensive nursing care of older adults (Lloyd-Jones et al., 2004; Rich et al., 1995; Ross et al., 2008).

III. BACKGROUND AND STATEMENT OF PROBLEM

A. Definition
   HF is the inability of the heart to pump blood sufficient to metabolic needs of the body or it cannot do so without significantly elevated filling pressures (Miller & Pina, 2009). Acute HF can develop swiftly or over the preceding weeks as the primary initial event. Acute decompensated HF is the result of chronic HF (Brucks et al., 2005).

B. Etiology and epidemiology
   1. *Prevalence and incidence:* There are more than 5.8 million individuals with HF in the United States and approximately half a million new cases develop every year (Lloyd-Jones et al., 2010; Thom et al., 2006).
   2. *Etiology:* Deficiency in myocardial pump function as a result of nonischemic progressive cardiomyopathy or more prevalent ischemic causes, such as coronary heart disease and MI with a resulting development of signs and symptoms, such as edema, dyspnea, and orthopnea (Bertoni et al., 2004; Chyun et al., 2002; Lewis et al., 2003).
   3. *Risk factors*
      a. *Predisposing* age (65 years and older); severity of illness; comorbidities, such as HTN, coronary artery disease, diabetes, valvular heart disease, and obesity. Additionally, cognitive impairment, depression, sensory impairment, fluid and electrolyte disturbances, and polypharmacy also impose an increased risk (Ho et al., 1993; Hypertension in Diabetes Study Group, 1993; Levy et al., 1996; Piccini et al., 2004).
      b. *Precipitating*: High-sodium diet; excess fluid intake; sleep-disordered breathing; chronic kidney disease; anemia; cardiotoxins, such as chemotherapeutic agents, NSAIDs, illicit drugs, or alcohol (Schocken et al., 2008).
      c. *Environmental factors*: Low socioeconomic status, psychological stress, and inadequate social support (Schocken et al., 2008).
   4. *Outcomes:* HF has a downward trajectory that through preventative measures can be delayed; however, not without considerable impact on quality of life (Grady et al., 2000).

IV. PARAMETERS OF ASSESSMENT

A. Assess at initial encounter and every shift
   1. *Baseline:* Health history NYHA classification of functional status and stage of HF, cognitive and psychosocial support systems (Brucks et al., 2005)
   2. *Symptoms:* Dyspnea, orthopnea, cough, edema; vital signs: BP, HR, and RR (Pickering et al., 2005, 2008; Sansevero, 1997); physical assessment with signs: rales or "crackles"; peripheral edema, ascites, or pulmonary vascular congestion of chest x-ray (Stevenson & Perloff, 1989)
   3. *Medications review*: Optimal medical regimen according to ACC/AHA/HFSA guideline unless contraindicated (Brenner et al., 2001; Riegel et al., 2009; Wing et al., 2003)

(continued)

Protocol 30.1: Heart Failure: Early Recognition and Treatment of the Patient at Risk of Hospital Readmission *(continued)*

4. *Electrocardiogram/telemetry review*: HR, rhythm, QRS duration, QT interval (Bertoni et al., 2004; Chyun et al., 2002)
5. Review echocardiography, cardiac angiogram, MUGA scan, cardiac CT or MRI for left ventricle and valve function: LVEF (Bertoni et al., 2004; Chyun et al., 2002; Lewis et al., 2003)
6. Laboratory value review (Cygankiewicz et al., 2009; Huang et al., 2007; Hunt et al., 2005)
   Metabolic evaluation: Electrolytes (hyponatremia, hypokalemia), thyroid function, liver function, kidney function
   Hematology: Evaluation for anemia: hemoglobin, hematocrit, iron, iron-binding capacity, and B12 folic acid
   Evaluation for infection (fever, WBCs with differential, cultures)
7. *Impaired mobility/deconditioned status*: Physical therapy or structured cardiac rehabilitation inpatient or outpatient

B. Sensory impairment—vision, hearing—limitations in ability for self-care (Davos et al., 2003; Faris et al., 2002)
C. Signs and symptoms—assess for changes in mental status every shift (Davos et al., 2003; Faris et al., 2002)

V. NURSING CARE STRATEGIES

A. Obtain HF/cardiology and geriatric consultation (Naylor, 2006; Naylor & Keating, 2008; Naylor et al., 2004; Rich et al., 1995).
B. Eliminate or minimize risk factors
   1. Administer medications according to guidelines and patient assessment (Brenner et al., 2001; Riegel et al., 2009; Wing et al., 2003).
   2. Avoid continuous intravenous infusion especially of saline (Cavallari et al., 2004; Lancaster et al., 2003; Riegel et al., 2009; Taylor et al., 2004).
   3. Maintain euvolemia once fluid overload is treated. Prevent/promptly treat fluid overload, dehydration, and electrolyte disturbances. Maximize oxygen delivery (supplemental oxygen, blood, and BP support as needed [Cavallari et al., 2004; Lancaster et al., 2003; Riegel et al., 2009; Taylor et al., 2004]).
   4. Ensure daily weights accurately charted (Grady et al., 2000; Riegel et al., 2004, 2009).
   5. Provide adequate nutrition with a 2-g per day sodium diet (see Chapter 10, "Nutrition").
   6. Provide adequate pain control (see Chapter 18, "Pain Management").
   7. Use sensory aids as appropriate.
   8. Regulate bowel/bladder function.

D. Provide self-care education with maintenance and management strategies (Masoudi et al., 2005; Nesto et al., 2004; Piotrowicz, Kucharska, Skalska, Kwater, Bhagavatula, & Gasowski, 2014).
   1. Encourage activity recommendation as appropriate to functional status. Assess for safety in ambulation hourly rounds with encouragement to toilet.
   2. Facilitate rest with schedule of diuretic medications for limited nocturia.
   3. Maximize mobility: involve occupational therapy and physical therapy and limit use of urinary catheters.
   4. Communicate clearly; provide explanations.
   5. Emphasize purpose and importance of daily weights.
   6. Arrange dietician referral for educational needs regarding sodium.

E. Identify primary care partner. Reassure and educate.
   1. Foster care support of family/friends.
   2. Assess willingness and ability of care partner to assist with self-care: dietary needs of sodium restriction, daily weight logging, symptom recognition, and medical follow-up.

VI. EVALUATION/EXPECTED OUTCOMES

A. Patient
   1. Absence of symptoms of congestion
   2. Hemodynamic status remains stable
   3. Functional status returned to baseline (before acute decompensation)
   4. Improved adherence to medical and self-care regimen
   5. Discharged to same destination as prehospitalization

(continued)

Protocol 30.1: Heart Failure: Early Recognition and Treatment of the Patient at Risk of Hospital Readmission *(continued)*

B. Health care provider
   1. Regular use of self-care HF index screening tool
   2. Increased detection of symptoms of acute decompensation
   3. Implementation of appropriate interventions to prevent/treat volume overload
   4. Improved nurse awareness of patient/caregiver self-care confidence and ability
   5. Increased management using guideline-directed therapy
C. Institution
   1. Staff education and interprofessional care planning
   2. Implementation of HF specific treatments
   3. Decreased overall cost
   4. Decreased preventable readmission and length of hospital stay
   5. Decreased morbidity and mortality
   6. Increased referrals and consultation to previously-specified specialists
   7. Improved satisfaction of patients, families, and nursing staff

VII. FOLLOW-UP MONITORING OF CONDITION

A. Decreased frequency of readmission as a measure of quality care
B. Incidence of decompensated HF to decrease
C. Patient days with symptoms of congestion to decrease
D. Staff competence in prevention, recognition, and treatment of HF
E. Documentation of a variety of interventions for HF

ABBREVIATIONS

ACC/AHA/HFSA	American College of Cardiology/American Heart Association Task Force/Heart Failure Society of America
BP	Blood pressure
BUN/Cr	Blood urea nitrogen/creatinine ratio
Hgb/Hct	Hemoglobin and hematocrit
HF	Heart failure
HR	Heart rate
HTN	Hypertension
LVEF	Left ventricular ejection fraction
Na^+	Sodium
NSAIDs	Nonsteroidal anti-inflammatory drugs
NYHA	New York Heart Association
ROM	Range of motion
RR	Respiratory rate
SpO_2	Pulse oxygen saturation
URI	Upper respiratory infection
UTI	Urinary tract infection
WBCs	White blood cells

NOTE

1. This chapter was adapted from the American Association of Colleges of Nursing, Preparing Nursing Students to Care for Older Adults: Enhancing Gerontology in Senior-Level Undergraduate Courses curriculum module, *Assessment and Management of Hypertension and Heart Failure,* prepared by Deborah A. Chyun and Jessica Coviello.

RESOURCES

American Association of Heart Failure Nurses
http://aahfn.org

Heart Failure Society of America
http://www.hfsa.org

REFERENCES

American Heart Association. (1994). Revisions to classification of functional capacity and objective assessment of patients with disease of the heart. *Circulation, 90*, 644–645. *Evidence Level VI.*

Anderson, C., & Vasan, R. S. (2014). Epidemiology of heart failure with preserved ejection fraction. *Heart Failure Clinics, 10*, 377–388. *Evidence Level V.*

Anker, S. D., Negassa, A., Coats, A. J., Afzal, R., Poole-Wilson, P. A., Cohn, J. N., & Yusuf, S. (2003). Prognostic importance of weight loss in chronic heart failure and the effect of treatment with angiotension-converting-enzyme inhibitors: An observational study. *Lancet, 361*(9363), 1077–1083. *Evidence Level III.*

Arzt, M., & Bradley, T. D. (2006). Treatment of sleep apnea in heart failure. *American Journal of Respiratory and Critical Care Medicine, 173*(12), 1300–1308. *Evidence Level V.*

Arzt, M., Young, T., Finn, L., Skatrud, J. B., Ryan, C. M., Newton, G. E., . . . Bradley, T. D. (2006). Sleepiness and sleep in patients with both systolic heart failure and obstructive sleep apnea. *Archives of Internal Medicine, 166*(16), 1716–1722. *Evidence Level III.*

Bangalore, S., Gong, Y., Cooper-DeHoff, R. M., Pepine, C. J., & Messerli, F. H. (2014). 2014 Eighth Joint National Committee panel recommendation for blood pressure targets revisited: Results from the INVEST study. *Journal of the American College of Cardiology, 64*(8), 784–793. *Evidence Level VI.*

Bari, M. D., Pozzi, C., Cavallini, M. C., Innocenti, F., Baldereschi, G., Alfieri, W. D., . . . Marchionni, N. (2004) The diagnosis of heart failure in the community. *Journal of the American College of Cardiology, 44*(8), 1601–1608. *Evidence Level VI.*

Barrella, P., & Della Monica, E. (1998). Managing congestive heart failure at home. *AACN Clinical Issues, 9*(3), 377–388. *Evidence Level VI.*

Baruch, L., Glazer, R. D., Aknay, N., Vanhaecke, J., Heywood, J. T., Anand, I., . . . Cohn, J. N. (2004). Morbidity, mortality, physiologic and functional parameters in elderly and non-elderly patients in the Valsartan Heart Failure Trial (Val-HeFT). *American Heart Journal, 148*(6), 951–957. *Evidence Level I.*

Bennett, S. J., & Sauvé, M. J. (2003). Cognitive deficits in patients with heart failure: A review of the literature. *Journal of Cardiovascular Nursing, 18*(3), 219–242. *Evidence Level VI.*

Bertoni, A. G., Hundley, W. G., Massing, M. W., Bonds, D. E., Burke, G. L., & Goff, D. C., Jr. (2004). Heart failure prevalence, incidence, and mortality in the elderly with diabetes. *Diabetes Care, 27*, 699–703. *Evidence Level IV.*

Bhatia, R. S., Tu, J. V., Lee, D. S., Austin, P. C., Fang, J., Haouzi, A., . . . Liu, P. P. (2006). Outcome of heart failure with preserved ejection fraction in a population-based study. *New England Journal of Medicine, 355*(3), 260–269. *Evidence Level III.*

Bonds, D. E., Miller, M. E., Bergenstal, R. M., Buse, J. B., Byington, R. P., Cutler J. A., . . . Sweeney, M. E. (2010). The association between symptomatic, severe hypoglycaemia and mortality in type 2 diabetes: Retrospective epidemiological analysis of the ACCORD study. *British Medical Journal, 340*, b4909. doi:10.1136/bmj.b4909. *Evidence Level II.*

Bonow, R. O., Carabello, B. A., Chatterjee, K., de Leon, A. C., Jr., Faxon, D. P., Freed, M. D., . . . Riegel, B. (2006). ACC/AHA 2006 guidelines for the management of patients with valvular heart disease. *Circulation, 114*(5), e84–e131. *Evidence Level I.*

Braunstein, J. B., Anderson, G. F., Gerstenblith, G., Weller, W., Niefeld, M., Herbert, R., & Wu, A. W. (2003). Noncardiac comorbidity increases preventable hospitalizations and mortality among Medicare beneficiaries with chronic heart failure. *Journal of the American College of Cardiology, 42*(7), 1226–1233. *Evidence Level IV.*

Brenner, B. M., Cooper, M. E., de Zeeuw, D., Keane, W. F., Mitch, W. E., Parving, H. H., & Shahinfar, S. (2001). Effects of losartan on renal and cardiovascular outcomes in patients with type 2 diabetes and nephropathy. *New England Journal of Medicine, 345*(12), 861–869. *Evidence Level I.*

Brucks, S., Little, W. C., Chao, T., Kitzman, D. W., Wesley-Farrington, D., Gandhi, S., & Shihazabi, Z. K. (2005). Contribution of left ventricular diastolic dysfunction to heart failure regardless of ejection fraction. *American Journal of Cardiology, 95*(5), 603–606. *Evidence Level II.*

Butler, J., Fonarow, G., Zile, M. R., Lam, C. S., Roessig, L., Schelbert, E. B., . . . Gleorghiade, M. (2014). Developing therapies for heart failure with preserved ejection fraction. *Journal of the American College of Cardiology, 2*(2), 95–112. *Evidence Level V.*

Carmody, M. S., & Anderson, J. R. (2007). BiDil (isosorbide dinitrate and hydralazine): A new fixed-dose combination of two older medications for the treatment of heart failure in black patients. *Cardiology Review, 15*(1), 46–53. *Evidence Level I.*

Carson, P., Tognoni, G., & Cohn, J. N. (2003). Effect of Valsartan on hospitalization: Results from Val-HeFT. *Journal of Cardiac Failure, 9*(3), 164–171. *Evidence Level II.*

Cavallari, L. H., Fashingbauer, L. A., Beitelshees, A. L., Groo, V. L., Southworth, M. R., Viana, M. A., . . . Dunlap, S. H. (2004). Racial differences in patients' potassium concentrations during spironolactone therapy for heart failure. *Pharmacotherapy, 24*(6), 750–756. *Evidence Level III.*

Chobanian, A. V., Bakris, G. L., Black, H. R., Cushman, W. C., Green, L. A., Izzo, J. L., Jr., . . . Rocella, E. J. (2003). The seventh report of the Joint National Committee on Prevention, Detection, Evaluation, and Treatment of High Blood Pressure. *Journal of the American Medical Association, 289*, 1560–1572. *Evidence Level VI.*

Chriss, P. M., Sheposh, J., Carlson, B., & Riegel, B. (2004). Predictors of successful heart failure self-care maintenance in the first three months after hospitalization. *Heart Lung, 33*(6), 345–353. *Evidence Level III.*

Chyun, D., Vaccarino, V., Murillo, J., Young, L. H., & Krumholz, H. M. (2002). Mortality, heart failure and recurrent myocardial infarction in the elderly with diabetes. *American Journal of Critical Care, 11*, 504–519. *Evidence Level II.*

Coats, A. J. (2001). Heart failure: What causes the symptoms of heart failure? *Heart, 86*(5), 574–578. *Evidence Level V.*

Cohn, J. N. (1999). Improving outcomes in congestive heart failure: Val-HeFT. Valsartan in Heart Failure Trial. *Cardiology, 91*(Suppl. 1), 19–22. *Evidence Level II.*

Cohn, J. N., & Tognoni, G. (2001). A randomized trial of the angiotensin-receptor blocker valsartan in chronic heart failure.

New England Journal of Medicine, 345(23), 1667–1675. *Evidence Level I.*

Colucci, W. S., Kolias, T. J., Adams, K. F., Armstrong, W. F., Ghali, J. K., Gottlieb, S. S., . . . Sugg, J. E. (2007). Metoprolol reverses left ventricular remodeling in patients with asymptomatic systolic dysfunction: The REversal of VEntricular Remodeling with Toprol-XL (REVERT) trial. *Circulation, 116*(1), 49–56. *Evidence Level II.*

Colucci, W. S., Packer, M., Bristow, M. R., Gilbert, E. M., Cohn, J. N., Fowler, M. B., . . . Lukas, M. A. (1996). Carvedilol inhibits clinical progression in patients with mild symptoms of heart failure. US Carvedilol Heart Failure Study Group. *Circulation, 94*(11), 2800–2806. *Evidence Level II.*

Cormican, L. J., & Williams, A. (2005). Sleep disordered breathing and its treatment in congestive heart failure. *Heart, 91*(10), 1265–1270. *Evidence Level V.*

Coviello, J. S. (2004). Cardiac assessment 101: A new look at the guidelines for cardiac homecare patients. *Home Healthcare Nurse, 22*(2), 116–123. *Evidence Level VI.*

Coviello, J. S., Hricz-Borges, L., & Masulli, P. S. (2002). Accomplishing quality of life in end-stage heart failure: A hospice multidisciplinary approach. *Home Healthcare Nurse, 20*(3), 195–198. *Evidence Level VI.*

Cygankiewicz, I., Gillespie, J., Zareba, W., Brown, M. W., Goldenberg, I., Klein, H., . . . Moss, A. J. (2009). Predictors of long-term mortality in Multicenter Automatic Defibrillator Implantation Trial II (MADIT II) patients with implantable cardioverter-defibrillators. *Heart Rhythm, 6*(4), 468–473. *Evidence Level II.*

Davos, C. H., Doehner, W., Rauchhaus, M., Cicoira, M., Francis, D. P., Coats, A. J., . . . Anker, S. D. (2003). Body mass and survival in patients with chronic heart failure without cachexia: The importance of obesity. *Journal of Cardiac Failure, 9*(1), 29–35. *Evidence Level IV.*

Dickson, V. V., Deatrick, J. A., & Riegel, B. (2008). A typology of heart failure self-care management in non-elders. *European Journal of Cardiovascular Nursing, 7*(3), 171–181. *Evidence Level IV.*

Dinicolantonio, J. J., Lavie, C. J., Fares, H., Menezes, A. R., O'Keefe, J. H., Bangalore, S., & Messerli, F. H. (2013). Meta-analysis of cilostazol versus aspirin for the secondary prevention of stroke. *American Journal of Cardiology, 112*(8), 1230–1234. *Evidence Level IV.*

Evangelista, L. S., Doering, L. V., & Dracup, K. (2000). Usefulness of a history of tobacco and alcohol use in predicting multiple heart failure readmissions among veterans. *American Journal of Cardiology, 86*(12), 1339–1342. *Evidence Level III.*

Faris, R., Purcell, H., Henein, M. Y., & Coats, A. J. (2002). Clinical depression is common and significantly associated with reduced survival in patients with non-ischaemic heart failure. *European Journal of Heart Failure, 4*(4), 541–551. *Evidence Level III.*

Farr, M. J., Lang, C. C., Lamanca, J. J., Zile, M. R., Francis, G., Tavazzi, L., . . . Mancini, D; MCC-135 GO1 Investigators. (2008). Cardiopulmonary exercise variables in diastolic versus systolic heart failure. *American Journal of Cardiology, 102*(2), 203–206. *Evidence Level II.*

Funk, M., & Krumholz, H. M. (1996). Epidemiologic and economic impact of advanced heart failure. *Journal of Cardiovascular Nursing, 10*(2), 1–10. *Evidence Level V.*

Gheorghiade, M., Follath, F., Ponikowski, P., Barsuk, J. H., Blair, J. E., Cleland, J. G., . . . Filippatos, G. (2010). Assessing and grading congestion in acute heart failure: A scientific statement from the acute heart failure committee of the heart failure association of the European Society of Cardiology and endorsed by the European Society of Intensive Care Medicine. *European Journal of Heart Failure, 12*(5), 423–433. *Evidence Level VI.*

Giamouzis, G., Kalogeropoulos, A., Georgiopoulou, V., Laskar, S., Smith, A. L., Dunbar, S., . . . Butler, J. (2011). Hospitalization epidemic in patients with heart failure: Risk factors, risk prediction, knowledge gaps, and future directions. *Journal of Cardiac Failure, 17*(1), 54–75. *Evidence Level V.*

Glandt, M., & Raz, I. (2010). Pharmacotherapy: ACCORD blood pressure and ACCORD lipid: How low can we go? *Natural Reviews, Endocrinology, 6*(9), 483–484. *Evidence Level II.*

Goldstein, S., & Hjalmarson, A. (1999). The mortality effect of metoprolol CR/XL in patients with heart failure: Results of the MERIT-HF trial. *Clinical Cardiology, 22*(Suppl. 5), 30–35. *Evidence Level V.*

Gonseth, J., Guallar-Castillón, P., Banegas, J. R., & Rodríguez-Artalejo, F. (2004). The effectiveness of disease management programs in reducing hospital re-admission in older persons with heart failure: A systematic review and meta-analysis of published reports. *European Heart Journal, 25*(18), 1570–1595. *Evidence Level I.*

Grady, K. L., Dracup, K., Kennedy, G., Moser, D. K., Piano, M., Stevenson, L. W., & Young, J. B. (2000). Team management of patients with heart failure: A statement for healthcare professionals from The Cardiovascular Nursing Council of the American Heart Association. *Circulation, 102*(19), 2443–2456. *Evidence Level VI.*

Hay, P., Sachdev, P., Cumming, S., Smith, J. S., Lee, T., Kitchener, P., & Matheson, J. (1993). Treatment of obsessive-compulsive disorder by psychosurgery. *Acta Psychiatrica Scandinavica, 87*(3), 197–207. *Evidence Level III.*

Hjalmarson, A., & Fagerberg, B. (2000). MERIT-HF mortality and morbidity data. *Basic Research in Cardiology, 95*(Suppl. 1), 198–103. *Evidence Level V.*

Hjalmarson, A., Goldstein, S., Fagerberg, B., Wedel, H., Waagstein, F., Kjekshus, J., . . . Deedwania, P. (2000). Effects of controlled-release metoprolol on total mortality, hospitalizations, and well-being in patients with heart failure: The Metoprolol CR/XL Randomized Intervention Trial in congestive heart failure (MERIT-HF). MERIT-HF study group. *Journal of the American Medical Association, 283*(10), 1295–1302. *Evidence Level I.*

Ho, K. K., Pinsky, J. L., Kannel, W. B., & Levy, D. (1993). The epidemiology of heart failure: The Framingham study. *Journal of the American College of Cardiology, 22*(4 Suppl. A), 6A–13A. *Evidence Level V.*

Hope-Ross, M., Buchanan, T. A., Archer, D. B., & Allen, J. A. (1990). Autonomic function in Holmes Adie syndrome. *Eye, 4*(Pt. 4), 607–612. *Evidence Level V.*

Horwich, T. B., Fonarow, G. C., Hamilton, M. A., MacLellan, W. R., Woo, M. A., & Tillisch, J. H. (2001). The relationship between obesity and mortality in patients with heart failure. *Journal of the American College of Cardiology, 38*(3), 789–795. *Evidence Level IV.*

Huang, D. T., Sesselberg, H. W., McNitt, S., Noyes, K., Andrews, M. L., Hall, W. J., . . . Moss, A. J. (2007). Improved survival associated with prophylactic implantable defibrillators in elderly patients with prior myocardial infarction and depressed ventricular function: A MADIT-II substudy. *Journal of Cardiovascular Electrophysiology, 18*(8), 833–888. *Evidence Level II.*

Hunt, S. A., Abraham, W. T., Chin, M. H., Feldman, A. M., Francis, G. S., Ganiats, T. G., . . . Riegel, B. (2005). ACC/AHA 2005 Guideline update for the diagnosis and management of chronic heart failure in the adult. *Circulation, 112*(12), e154–e235. *Evidence Level I.*

Hypertension in Diabetes Study Group. (1993). HDS: 1: Prevalence of hypertension in newly presenting type 2 diabetic patients and the association with risk factors for cardiovascular disease and diabetic complications. *Journal of Hypertension, 11*, 309–317. *Evidence Level III.*

James, P. A., Oparil, S., Carter, B. L., Cushman, W. C., Dennison-Himmelfarb, C., Handler, J., . . . Ortiz, E. (2014). Evidence-based guideline for the management of high blood pressure in adults: Report from the panel members appointed to the Eighth Joint National Committee. *Journal of American Medical Association, 311*(5), 507–520. *Evidence Level VI.*

Kaneko, Y., Hajek, V. E., Zivanovic, V., Raboud, J., & Bradley, T. D. (2003). Relationship of sleep apnea to functional capacity and length of hospitalization following stroke. *Sleep, 26*(3), 293–297. *Evidence Level II.*

Kasai, T., Narui, K., Dohi, T., Yanagisawa, N., Ishiwata, S., Ohno, M., . . . Momomura, S. (2008). Prognosis of patients with heart failure and obstructive sleep apnea treated with continuous positive airway pressure. *Chest, 133*(3), 690–696. *Evidence Level II.*

Koenig, H. G. (1998). Depression in hospitalized older patients with congestive heart failure. *General Hospital Psychiatry, 20*(1), 29–43. *Evidence Level III.*

Koitabashi, T., Inomata, T., Niwano, S., Nishii, M., Takeuchi, I., Nakano, H., . . . Izumi, T. (2005). Paroxysmal atrial fibrillation coincident with cardiac decompensation is a predictor of poor prognosis in chronic heart failure. *Circulation Journal, 69*(7), 823–830. *Evidence Level III.*

Kossovsky, M. P., Sarasin, F. P., Perneger, T. V., Chopard, P., Sigaud, P., & Gaspoz, J. (2000). Unplanned readmissions of patients with congestive heart failure: Do they reflect in-hospital quality of care or patient characteristics? *American Journal of Medicine, 109*(5), 386–390. *Evidence Level III.*

Krumholz, H. M., Parent, E. M., Tu, N., Vaccarino, V., Wang, Y., Radford, M. J., & Hennen, J. (1997). Readmission after hospitalization for congestive heart failure among Medicare beneficiaries. *Archives of Internal Medicine, 157*(1), 99–104. *Evidence Level IV.*

Krumholz, H. M., Wang, Y., Parent, E. M., Mockalis, J., Petrillo, M., & Radford, M. J. (1997). Quality of care for elderly patients hospitalized with heart failure. *Archives of Internal Medicine, 157*(19), 2242–2247. *Evidence Level II.*

Lancaster, K. J., Smiciklas-Wright, H., Heller, D. A., Ahern, F. M., & Jensen, G. (2003). Dehydration in Black and White older adults using diuretics. *Annals of Epidemiology, 13*(7), 525–529. *Evidence Level IV.*

Lanfranchi, P. A., & Somers, V. K. (2003). Sleep-disordered breathing in heart failure: Characteristics and implications. *Respiratory Physiology & Neurobiology, 136*(2–3), 153–165. *Evidence Level VI.*

Lavie, C. J., Osman, A. F., Milani, R. V., & Mehra, M. R. (2003). Body composition and prognosis in chronic systolic heart failure: The obesity paradox. *American Journal of Cardiology, 91*(7), 891–894. *Evidence Level IV.*

Lee, S. J., Lindquist, K., Segal, M. R., & Covinsky, K. E. (2006). Development and validation of a prognostic index for 4-year mortality in older adults. *Journal of the American Medical Association, 295*(7), 801–808. *Evidence Level III.*

Levy, D., Larson, M. G., Vasan, R. S., Kannel, W. B., & Ho, K. K. (1996). The progression from hypertension to congestive heart failure. *Journal of the American Medical Association, 275*(20), 1557–1562. *Evidence Level II.*

Lewis, E. F., Lamas, G. A., O'Meara, E., Granger, C. B., Dunlap, M. E., McKelvie, R. S., . . . Pfeffer, M. A.; CHARM Investigators. (2007). Characterization of health-related quality of life in heart failure patients with preserved versus low ejection fraction in CHARM. *European Journal of Heart Failure, 9*(1), 83–91. *Evidence Level III.*

Lewis, E. F., Moye, L. A., Rouleau, J. L., Sacks, F. M., Arnold, J. M., Warnica, J. W., . . . Pfeffer, M. A. (2003). Predictors of late development of heart failure in stable survivors of myocardial infarction: The CARE study. *Journal of the American College of Cardiology, 42*(8), 1446–1453. *Evidence Level II.*

Lloyd-Jones, D., Adams, R. J., Brown, T. M., Carnethon, M., Dai, S., De Simone G., . . . American Heart Association Statistics Committee and Stroke Statistics Subcommittee. (2004). Comprehensive discharge planning with post discharge support for older persons with congestive heart failure. *Journal of the American Medical Association, 291*(11), 1358–1367. *Evidence Level I.*

Lloyd-Jones, D., Adams, R. J., Brown, T. M., Carnethon, M., Dai, S., De Simone G., . . . Wylie-Rosett, J. (2010). Heart disease and stroke statistics—2010 update: A report from the American Heart Association. *Circulation, 121*(7), e46–e215. *Evidence Level IV.*

Maggioni, A. P., Latini, R., Carson, P. E., Singh, S. N., Barlera, S., Glazer, R., . . . Cohn, J. N. (2005). Valsartan reduces the incidence of atrial fibrillation in patients with heart failure: Results from the Valsartan Heart Failure Trial (Val-HeFT). *American Heart Journal, 149*(3), 548–557. *Evidence Level II.*

Maisel, A. S. (2001a). B-type natriuretic peptide (BNP) levels: Diagnostic and therapeutic potential. *Reviews in Cardiovascular Medicine, 2*(Suppl. 2), S13–S18. *Evidence Level VI.*

Maisel, A. S. (2001b). B-type natriuretic peptide in the diagnosis and management of congestive heart failure. *Cardiology Clinics, 19*(4), 557–571. *Evidence Level VI.*

Mansfield, D. R., Solin, P., Roebuck, T., Bergin, P., Kaye, D. M., & Naughton, M. T. (2003). The effect of successful heart transplant treatment of heart failure on central sleep apnea. *Chest, 124*(5), 1675–1681. *Evidence Level III.*

Margolis, J. R., Gillum, R. F., Feinleib, M., Brasch, R. C., & Fabsitz, R. R. (1974). Community surveillance for coronary heart disease: The Framingham cardiovascular disease survey. *American Journal of Epidemiology, 100*(6), 425–436. *Evidence Level IV.*

Mascarenhas, J., Lourenço, P., Lopes, R., Azevedo, A., & Bettencourt, P. (2008). Chronic obstructive pulmonary disease in heart failure. Prevalence, therapeutic and prognostic implications. *American Heart Journal, 155*(3), 521–525. *Evidence Level IV.*

Masoudi, F. A., Inzucchi, S. E., Wang, Y., Havranek, E. P., Foody, J. M., & Krumholz, H. M. (2005). Thiazolidinediones, metformin, and outcomes in older patients with diabetes and heart failure: An observational study. *Circulation, 111*, 583–590. *Evidence Level II.*

McKelvie, R. S., Teo, K. K., Roberts, R., McCartney, N., Humen, D., Montague, T., . . . Yusuf, S. (2002). Effects of exercise training in patients with heart failure: The exercise rehabilitation trial (EXERT). *American Heart Journal, 144*(1), 23–30. *Evidence Level II.*

Metra, M., Nodari, S., Parrinello, G., Bordonali, T., Bugatti, S., Danesi, R., . . . Dei Cas, L. (2008). Worsening renal function in patients hospitalized for acute heart failure: Clinical implications and prognostic significance. *European Journal of Heart Failure, 10*(2), 188–195. *Evidence Level III.*

Miller, A. B., & Piña, I. L. (2009). Understanding heart failure with preserved ejection fraction: Clinical importance and future outlook. *Congestive Heart Failure, 15*(4), 186–192. *Evidence Level V.*

Naylor, C. J., Griffiths, R. D., & Fernandez, R. S. (2004). Does a multidisciplinary total parenteral nutrition team improve patient outcomes? A systematic review. *Journal of Parenteral and Enteral Nutrition, 28*(4), 251–258. *Evidence Level I.*

Naylor, M., & Keating, S. A. (2008). Transitional care. *American Journal of Nursing, 108*(9 Suppl.), 58–63.

Naylor, M., Brooten, D., Jones, R., Lavizzo-Mourey, R., Mezey, M., & Pauly, M. (1994). Comprehensive discharge planning for the hospitalized elderly. A randomized clinical trial. *Annals of Internal Medicine, 120*(12), 999–1006. *Evidence Level II.*

Naylor, M. D. (2006). Transitional care: A critical dimension of the home healthcare quality agenda. *Journal for Healthcare Quality, 28*(1), 48–54. *Evidence Level VI.*

Naylor, M. D., Feldman, P. H., Keating, S., Koren, M. J., Kurtzman, E. T., Maccoy, M. C., . . . Krakauer, R. (2009). Translating research into practice: Transitional care for older adults. *Journal of Evaluation in Clinical Practice, 15*(6), 1164–1170. *Evidence Level VI.*

Nesto, R. W., Bell, D., Bonow, R. O., Fonseca, V., Grundy, S. M., Horton, E. S., . . . Kahn, R. (2004). Thiazolidinedione use, fluid retention, and congestive heart failure: A consensus statement from the American Heart Association and American Diabetes Association. *Diabetes Care, 27*, 256–263. *Evidence Level V.*

Olsson, L. G., Swedberg, K., Ducharme, A., Granger, C. B., Michelson, E. L., McMurray, J. J., . . . Pfeffer, M. A. (2006). Atrial fibrillation and risk of clinical events in chronic heart failure with and without left ventricular systolic dysfunction: Results from the candesartan in heart failure—Assessment of Reduction in Mortality and Morbidity (CHARM) program. *Journal of the American College of Cardiology, 47*(10), 1997–2004. *Evidence Level I.*

Ostergren, J. B. (2006). Angiotensin receptor blockade with candesartan in heart failure: Findings from the Candesartan in Heart failure—Assessment of reduction in mortality and morbidity (CHARM) programme. *Journal of Hypertension, 24*(1), S3–S7. *Evidence Level II.*

Owan, T. E., Hodge, D. O., Herges, R. M., Jacobsen, S. J., Roger, V. L., & Redfield, M. M. (2006). Trends in prevalence and outcome of heart failure with preserved ejection fraction. *The New England Journal of Medicine, 355*(3), 251–259. *Evidence Level II.*

Packer, M. (1998). Beta-blockade in heart failure. Basic concepts and clinical results. *American Journal of Hypertension, 11*(1 Pt. 2), 23S–37S. *Evidence Level V.*

Packer, M., Bristow, M. R., Cohn, J. N., Colucci, W. S., Fowler, M. B., Gilbert, E. M., & Shusterman, N. H. (1996). The effect of carvedilol on morbidity and mortality in patients with chronic heart failure. U.S. Carvedilol Heart Failure Study Group. *New England Journal of Medicine, 334*(21), 1349–1355. *Evidence Level I.*

Packer, M., Colucci, W. S., Sackner-Bernstein, J. D., Liang, C. S., Goldscher, D. A., Freeman, I., . . . Shusterman, N. H. (1996). Double-blind, placebo-controlled study of the effects of carvedilol in patients with moderate to severe heart failure. The PRECISE trial. Prospective randomized evaluation of carvedilol on symptoms and exercise. *Circulation, 94*(11), 2793–2799. *Evidence Level I.*

Piccini, J. P., Klein, L., Gheorghiade, M., & Bonow, R. O. (2004). New insights into diastolic heart failure: Role of diabetes mellitus. *American Journal of Medicine, 116*(Suppl. 5A), 64S–75S. *Evidence Level V.*

Pickering, T. G., Hall, J. E., Appel, L. J., Falkner, B. E., Graves, J., Hill, M. N., . . . Roccella, E. J. (2005). Recommendations for blood pressure measurements in humans and experimental animals: Part 1: Blood pressure measurement in humans: A statement for professionals from the Subcommittee of Professional and Public Education of the American Heart Association Council on High Blood Pressure Research. *Circulation, 111*, 697–716. *Evidence Level VI.*

Pickering, T. G., Miller, N. H., Ogedegbe, G., Krakoff, L. R., Artinian, N. T., & Goff, D. (2008). Call to action on use and reimbursement for home blood pressure monitoring: Executive summary: A joint scientific statement from the American Heart Association, American Society of Hypertension, and Preventive Cardiovascular Nurses Association. *Hypertension, 52*(1), 1–9. *Evidence Level VI.*

Piepoli, M. F., Davos, C., Francis, D. P., & Coats, A. J. (2004). Exercise training meta-analysis of trials in patients with chronic heart failure (ExTraMATCH). *British Medical Journal, 328*(7433), 189. *Evidence Level II.*

Piotrowicz, K., Kucharska, E., Skalska, A., Kwater, A., Bhagavatula, S, & Gasowski, J. (2014). Pharmacological management of hypertension in the elderly–Certitudes and controversies. *Current Pharm Des, 20*(38), 5963–5967. *Evidence Level V.*

Pocock, S. J., Wang, D., Pfeffer, M. A., Yusuf, S., McMurray, J. J., . . . Granger, C. B. (2006). Predictors of mortality and morbidity in patients with chronic heart failure. *European Heart Journal, 27*(1), 65–75. *Evidence Level IV.*

Prystowsky, E. N., & Nisam, S. (2000). Prophylactic implantable cardioverter defibrillator trials: MUSTT, MADIT, and beyond. Multicenter Unsustained Tachycardia Trial. Multicenter Automatic Defibrillator Implantation Trial. *American Journal of Cardiology, 86*(11), 1214–1215. *Evidence Level I.*

Rich, M. W., & Kitman, D. W. (2005). Third pivotal research in cardiology in the elderly (PRICE-III) symposium: Heart failure in the elderly: Mechanisms and management. *American Journal of Geriatric Cardiology, 14*(5), 250–261. *Evidence Level V.*

Rich, M. W., & Nease, R. F. (1999). Cost-effectiveness analysis in clinical practice: The case of heart failure. *Archives of Internal Medicine, 159*(15), 1690–1700. *Evidence Level IV.*

Rich, M. W., Beckham, V., Wittenberg, C., Leven, C. L., Freedland, K. E., & Carney, R. M. (1995). A multidisciplinary intervention to prevent the readmission of elderly patients with congestive heart failure. *New England Journal of Medicine, 333*(18), 1190–1195. *Evidence Level II.*

Riegel, B., Dickson, V. V., Hoke, L., McMahon, J. P., Reis, B. F., & Sayers, S. (2006). A motivational counseling approach to improving heart failure self-care: Mechanisms of effectiveness. *Journal of Cardiovascular Nursing, 21*(3), 232–241. *Evidence Level II.*

Riegel, B., Lee, C. S., Dickson, V. V., & Carlson, B. (2009). An update on the self-care of heart failure index. *Journal of Cardiovascular Nursing, 24*(6), 485–497. *Evidence Level II.*

Riegel, B., Moser, D. K., Anker, S. D., Appel, L. J., Dunbar, S. B., Grady, K. L., . . . Whellan, D. J. (2009). State of the science: Promoting self-care in persons with heart failure: A scientific statement from the American Heart Association. *Circulation, 120*(12), 1141–1163. *Evidence Level VI.*

Riegel, B., Naylor, M., Stewart, S., McMurray, J. J., & Rich, M. W. (2004). Interventions to prevent readmission for congestive heart failure. *Journal of the American Medical Association, 291*(23), 2816. *Evidence Level II.*

Roger, V. L., Go, A. S., Lloyd-Jones, D. M., Benjamin, E. J., Berry, J. D., Borden, W. B., . . . Turner, M. B.; American Heart Association Statistics Committee and Stroke Statistics Subcommittee.(2012). Executive summary: Heart disease and stroke statistics--2012 update: A report from the American Heart Association. *Circulation, 125*(1), 188–197. *Evidence Level I.*

Ross, J. S., Mulvey, G. K., Stauffer, B., Patlolla, V., Bernheim, S. M., Keenan, P. S., & Krumholz, H. M. (2008). Statistical models and patient predictors of readmission for heart failure: A systematic review. *Archives of Internal Medicine, 168*(13), 1371–1386. *Evidence Level I.*

Rumsfeld, J. S., Havranek, E., Masoudi, F. A., Peterson, E. D., Jones, P., Tooley, J. F., . . . Spertus, J. A. (2003). Depressive symptoms are the strongest predictors of short-term declines in health status in patients with heart failure. *Journal of the American College of Cardiology, 42*(10), 1811–1817. *Evidence Level III.*

Sansevero, A. C. (1997). Dehydration in the elderly: Strategies for prevention and management. *Nurse Practitioner, 22*(4), 41–42, 51–67, 63–66. *Evidence Level VI.*

Schocken, D. D., Benjamin, E. J., Fonarow, G. C., Krumholz, H. M., Levy, D., Mensah, G. A., . . . Hong, Y. (2008). Prevention of heart failure: A scientific statement from the American Heart Association Councils on Epidemiology and Prevention, Clinical Cardiology, Cardiovascular Nursing, and High Blood Pressure Research; Quality of Care and Outcomes Research Interdisciplinary Working Group; and Functional Genomics and Translational Biology Interdisciplinary Working Group. Circulation, *117*(19), 2544–2565. *Evidence Level VI.*

Shah, R. V., Desai, A. S., & Givertz, M. M. (2010). The effect of renin-angiotensin system inhibitors on mortality and heart failure hospitalization in patients with heart failure and preserved ejection fraction: A systematic review and meta-analysis. *Journal of Cardiac Failure, 16*(3), 260–267. *Evidence Level I.*

Stefenelli, T., Bergler-Klein, J., Globits, S., Pacher, R., & Glogar, D. (1992). Heart rate behavior at different stages of congestive heart failure. *European Heart Journal, 13*(7), 902–907. *Evidence Level III.*

Stevenson, L. W., & Perloff, J. K. (1989). The limited reliability of physical signs for estimating hemodynamics in chronic heart failure. *Journal of the American Medical Association, 261*(6), 884–888. *Evidence Level II.*

Taylor, A. L., Ziesche, S., Yancy, C., Carson, P., D'Agostino, R., Jr., Ferdinand, K., . . . Cohn, J. N. (2004). Combination of isosorbide dinitrate and hydralazine in Blacks with heart failure. *New England Journal of Medicine, 351*, 2049–2057. *Evidence Level II.*

Taylor, R. S., Unal, B., Critchley, J. A., & Capewell, S. (2006). Mortality reductions in patients receiving exercise-based cardiac rehabilitation: How much can be attributed to cardiovascular risk factor improvements? *European Journal of Cardiovascular Prevention & Rehabilitation, 13*(3), 369–374. *Evidence Level I.*

Thom, T., Haase, N., Rosamond, W., Howard, V. J., Rumsfeld, J., Manolio, T., . . . Wolf, P. (2006). Heart disease and stroke statistics—2006 update: A report from the American Heart Association Statistics Committee and Stroke Statistics Subcommittee. *Circulation, 113*(6), e85–e151. Retrieved from http://circ.ahajournals.org. *Evidence Level IV.*

Triposkiadis, F., Karayannis, G., Giamouzis, G., Skoularigis, J., Louridas, G., & Butler, J. (2009). The sympathetic nervous system in the heart failure physiology, pathophysiology, and clinical implications. *Journal of the American College of Cardiology, 54*(19), 1747–1762. *Evidence Level I.*

Wang, C. S., FitzGerald, J. M., Schulzer, M., Mak, E., & Ayas, N. T. (2005). Does this dyspneic patient in the emergency department have congestive heart failure? *Journal of the American Medical Association, 294*(15), 1944–1956. *Evidence Level V.*

Wing, L. M., Reid, C. M., Ryan, P., Beilin, L. J., Brown, M. A., Jennings, G. L., . . . West, M. J. (2003). A comparison of outcomes with angiotensin-converting enzyme inhibitors and diuretics for hypertension in the elderly. *New England Journal of Medicine, 348*(7), 583–592. *Evidence Level II.*

Yancy, C. W., Lopatin, M., Stevenson, L. W., De Marco, T., & Fonarow, G. C. (2006). Clinical presentation, management, and in-hospital outcomes of patients admitted with acute decompensated heart failure with preserved systolic function: A report from the Acute Decompensated Heart Failure National Registry (ADHERE) database. *Journal of the American College of Cardiology, 47*(1), 76–84. *Evidence Level I.*

Young, J. B., Abraham, W. T., Albert, N. M., Gattis Stough, W., Gheorghiade, M., Greenberg, B. H., . . . Fonarow, G. C. (2008). Relation of low hemoglobin and anemia to morbidity and mortality in patients hospitalized with heart failure (insight from the OPTIMIZE-HF registry). *American Journal of Cardiology, 101*(2), 223–230. *Evidence Level II.*

Yusuf, S., Sleight P., Pogue, J., Bosch, J., Davies, R., & Dagenais, G. (2000). Effects of an angiotensin-converting enzyme inhibitor, ramipril, on cardiovascular events in high-risk patients. The Heart Outcomes Prevention Evaluation Study Investigators. *New England Journal of Medicine, 342*, 145–153. *Evidence Level I.*

31

Cancer Assessment and Intervention Strategies

Janine Overcash

EDUCATIONAL OBJECTIVES

On completion of this chapter, the reader should be able to:

1. Recognize the incidence and prevalence of U.S. statistics of malignancy in the older adult
2. Identify three common malignancies in the older adult
3. Recognize three common comorbidities in the older adult with cancer
4. Identify three common cancer-related emergencies in the older adult
5. Identify three assessment instruments useful in the assessment of the older person
6. Identify three important elements of a health history specific to the older cancer patient
7. Identify three important elements of a physical examination specific to the older cancer patient
8. Define clinical parameters of frailty of an older adult with cancer

OVERVIEW

The probability of developing a malignancy increases with age. In the years between 2007 and 2011, the National Cancer Institute Surveillance, Epidemiology, and End Results Program (SEER) found that the mean age of a cancer diagnosis is 66 years (Surveillance, Epidemiology, and End Results Program [SEER], 2014). Cancer of any site is most often diagnosed among people aged 65 to 74 years (SEER, 2014). According to the Centers for Disease Control and Prevention, the age-adjusted risk of dying dropped 60% from the years between 1935 and 2010; however, heart disease and cancer are the leading causes of death in the United States and have been for 75 years (Hoyert, 2012).

Older people diagnosed with cancer are often resilient; however, problems associated with comorbid conditions and poor general health status can result in less aggressive cancer treatment options (Williams et al., 2015). Treatment decisions of older cancer patients depend on life expectancy, comorbidity, and health status and not on chronological age (Hurria, 2013). Many older people tolerate chemotherapy as compared with younger people depending on their level of fitness and general health status (Sastre, Puente, García-Saenz, & Díaz-Rubio, 2008). The same is true for surgery (Wildiers et al., 2007) and radiation therapy (Gomez-Millan, 2009).

Acute care nurses must appreciate that cancer is common in older adult patients and be aware of management strategies and potential emergencies associated with the diagnosis and treatment of a malignancy. This chapter presents aspects of health that should be considered when caring for a hospitalized older cancer patient. Geriatric assessment instruments that can be used in an acute care

For a description of evidence Levels cited in this chapter, see Chapter 1, "Developing and Evaluating Clinical Practice Guidelines: A Systematic Approach."

setting and potential medical emergencies associated with the cancer disease process are addressed.

ASSESSMENT OF THE OLDER HOSPITALIZED PATIENT

Comorbid Conditions

A diagnosis of cancer may be one of several diagnoses and it is important to understand how the malignant and nonmalignant conditions affect the health of the older person. Often, nonmalignant conditions can present more risk of mortality as compared with a cancer diagnosis. Breast cancer patients undergoing treatment with chemotherapy or radiation are likely to die of nonmalignant diagnoses (Ording et al., 2015). In early-stage breast cancer, rates of noncancer-related disease death in patients aged 80 years and above are higher compared with people aged 65 to 69 years (Sakurai et al., 2015). In patients with lung cancer, cardiovascular comorbidities have a considerable impact on survival (Kravchenko et al., 2015).

The timing of a nonmalignant diagnosis between 18 and 6 months before a diagnosis of colorectal cancer has been associated with lower 1-year survival (Shack, Rachet, Williams, Northover, & Coleman, 2010). The more severe the degree of comorbidity, the less probability of survival at 1 year and 5 years after a diagnosis of cancer (Iversen, Nørgaard, Jacobsen, Laurberg, & Sørensen, 2009). For patients who are diagnosed with diabetes, there is a twofold risk of recurrence or development of a new breast cancer as compared with people who do not have diabetes (Patterson et al., 2010). Recognition, management, and severity of comorbid conditions are the principal aspects of the acute nursing assessment. Unmanaged or uncontrolled comorbid conditions have the potential to modify cancer treatment and outcomes.

Comprehensive Geriatric Assessment

The comprehensive geriatric assessment (CGA) has been used to predict various risk factors (Klepin et al., 2011), postoperative complications (Fukuse, Satoda, Hijiya, & Fujinaga, 2005), toxicity to cancer chemotherapy treatment (Aaldriks et al., 2011; Freyer et al., 2005; Hurria & Lichtman, 2007), and frailty (Kristjansson et al., 2010), and to identify people who are at risk of falls (Overcash & Beckstead, 2008). The CGA is also helpful in identifying older cancer patients who are most likely to benefit from more aggressive chemotherapy (Tucci et al., 2009) and from various surgical oncology procedures. Postsurgical cognitive changes can be predicted using CGA (Liang et al., 2015). CGA used in oncology has been found to influence cancer treatment decisions in terms of dosing, delaying treatment, and other management considerations (Chaïbi et al., 2011; Wildiers et al., 2014).

The CGA can be a predictor of 2-year mortality (Pilotto et al., 2007) and a 3-year predictor of survival (Stotter, Reed, Gray, Moore, & Robinson, 2015) in older patients. Impairment on various components of the CGA, such as nutrition, functional status, and cognition, is predictive of in-hospital mortality (Avelino-Silva et al., 2014). The American Geriatrics Society recommendations suggest that CGA is an important component of care for older persons who have or are at risk for functional limitations (American Geriatrics Society, 2008). Older patients receiving acute care can benefit from the CGA by revealing health concerns and potential readmissions to an acute care setting (Lee, Chou, et al., 2014).

No one definition of a CGA exists. A CGA can be developed to include screening instruments necessary to meet the needs of a particular older patient population (American Geriatrics Society and the British Geriatrics Society, 2010). The instruments that commonly make up the CGA and that guide screening practices in many health care domains are all found on www.consultgerirn.org and chapters in this text. Although a CGA may be relevant to primary care settings, understanding such issues as medication history and polypharmacy, caregiver situation, and emotional condition is also important to an acute assessment.

A CGA can include various laboratory tests in addition to self-report and performance evaluations. Laboratory data, such as C-reactive protein, are able to predict morbidity or mortality and help identify individual risk factors (Chundadze et al., 2010; Pal, Katheria, & Hurria, 2010). Serum 25-hydroxyvitamin D (25OHD) will assess vitamin D levels to determine whether falls or muscle weakness can be a risk factor. People with lower concentrations of 25OHD have a high probably of falling (Annweiler & Beauchet, 2015). In patients with colorectal cancer, higher levels of 25OHD are related to better survival (Wesa et al., 2015). Serum albumin levels at 3.3 mg/dL on admission, serum creatinine levels at 1.3 mg/dL or higher, history of heart failure, immobility, and advanced age are all predictors of inpatient mortality (Silva, Jerussalmy, Farfel, Curiati, & Jacob-Filho, 2009). Other mortality risk factors in older hospitalized patients are red blood cell and platelet transfusions, which increase the opportunity for venous and arterial thrombotic events (Khorana et al., 2008).

Determining caregiver availability in the home following hospital discharge is another important element of the CGA. For many older cancer patients, lack of a caregiver can be a problem and can impact health and medical treatment. Breast cancer patients who live alone or are unmarried have an increased risk of mortality (Osborne, Ostir, Du, Peek, & Goodwin, 2005). Conversely, older cancer patients who are married tend to live longer than those who are not married (Patel et al., 2010). In general, people who are married report higher perceived health status (Joutsenniemi et al., 2006). It is important for the nurse to determine whether the patient lives with someone and the extent to which that person is able to assist. Of note, often the patient is the caregiver to the spouse or others (Overcash, 2004) and it is important to discuss the caregiver situation before discharge.

Assessment of the older patient should occur on admission to the hospital and before discharge to understand trends in health, as well as in functional and behavioral ability. Discharge planning should include interventions based on the CGA findings and communication is vital with outpatient providers to continue to address the limitations that may affect the health, quality of life, and independence of the older person with cancer.

DEVELOPING A COMPREHENSIVE GERIATRIC ASSESSMENT FOR HOSPITALIZED PATIENTS

The following are instruments that can identify functional, physical, emotional, and medication history and cognitive impairment in the acute care patient and are generally included in a CGA (see Chapters 6, 14, 15, 16, and 19):

A. Assess for depression and/or emotional distress
   1. The Geriatric Depression Scale (Yesavage et al., 1982)
   2. The SF-12 Tool (Ware, Kosinski, & Keller, 1996): The SF-12 is a general health-related quality-of-life instrument that is widely used in research and clinical assessment. Two summary scores are the culmination of the measures from the mental health aspect and the physical health domain. The SF-12 is simple to administer and provides the clinician with a measure of emotional health and physical health.
B. Assessment for cognitive limitations
   1. The Mini-Cog is used in the assessment of cognition (Borson, Scanlan, Brush, Vitaliano, & Dokmak, 2000; Borson, Scanlan, Chen, & Ganguli, 2003). The instrument comprises the Clock Draw test and recall.
   2. Assess the number and indications of medications. Look for medications with the same indications, potential harmful interactions and consider any difficulty with cancer treatment, agents. (For more information on polypharmacy screening, visit www.consultgeriRN.org and select "Try This: The Beers Medication Screen, Criteria for Potentially Inappropriate Medication Use in the Elderly.")
C. Assess for geriatric syndromes (such as urinary incontinence, falls, or depression; for more information, visit www.consultgerirn.org/resources and select "Try This: Urinary Incontinence Assessment, Fall Risk Assessment or the Geriatric Depression Scale")
D. Assess functional status and potential for falls
   1. Ask the patient whether a fall had been experienced within the past year.
   2. The Physical Performance Test battery (Simmonds, 2002) has age-related norms and is a valid and reliable tool used with cancer patients.
   3. The 6-minute walk that assesses the speed and ability to ambulate for the entire time (Enright et al., 2003)
      a. The Timed Get Up & Go Test considers rising from a chair, walking 3 m and returning to the chair in a sitting position (Podsiadlo & Richardson, 1991).
      b. Assessment of physical status can take place on observation of gait using the Gait Assessment Scale (Tinetti, 1986; Tinetti, Mendes de Leon, Doucette, & Baker, 1994).
      c. Berg Balance Scale (BBS) is a 14-item scale developed for use in a clinical setting (Berg, Wood-Dauphinee, Williams, & Maki, 1992). The BBS can be helpful in predicting falls and functional-status problems.
F. Assess the ability to perform self-care activities
   1. Activities of Daily Living Scale (Katz, Downs, Cash, & Grotz, 1970)
   2. Instrumental Activities of Daily Living Scale (Lawton & Brody, 1969)

Health History

The subjective information obtained from the older adult is a critical factor in the development of the plan of care. Respect and confidence are not only prudent, but standard practice for the acute care nurse, and can set the stage for a productive health-centered dialogue. The nurse should assess the reason(s) for seeking care (chief complaint) and include the family and support person(s). The following are issues that should be considered when conducting a health history of the older adult with cancer:

A. Assess history of present illness in regard to cancer diagnosis, cancer stage at diagnosis, current cancer stage, and cancer treatment (surgical, chemotherapy, radiation therapy, and hormonal therapy).

B. Assess past medical history as related to a diagnosis of cancer (include dates of diagnosis and treatments and regular oncological assessment continue).
C. Assess family medical history of malignancy and ages on diagnosis (some families have strong familial histories of malignancy and perhaps younger generations should consider genetic counseling).
D. Assess regular cancer screening examinations.
E. Assess for common geriatric syndromes (issues, such as incontinence or falls, that have many motivating factors).

Physical Examination

Conducting a physical examination of an older adult must orchestrate an understanding of normative aging changes and knowledge of pathology. The physical examination is also an opportunity to teach about the importance of self-examination (breast and skin exams) and provide relevant health information. The physical exam is not only an empirical evaluation, but an opportunity to determine current health status and trends over time.

Evaluation of functional status should be performed with the physical examination of the older patient. Understanding level of fitness (healthy, vulnerable, frail, or terminally ill) can help identify appropriate cancer treatment options (Droz et al., 2014). Physical examination and functional status assessment can help reveal a clinical presentation of frailty. According to a classic study by Fried et al. (2001), frailty can, in part, be defined as:

1. Older than 85 years
2. Dependent in one or more activities of daily living (ADL)
3. The presence of one or more geriatric syndromes (Fried et al., 2001)

Determining whether a person is "frail" in the primary care setting can help make important decisions before a patient is admitted to an acute care unit (Lee, Heckman, & Molnar, 2015). When frailty is considered in the physical examination, discussions concerning advance directives, palliative versus curative treatment, and many other critical conversations can occur before an acute situation is realized (Sanchis et al., 2014).

MEDICAL EMERGENCIES ASSOCIATED WITH CANCER AND CANCER TREATMENT

A diagnosis of cancer can lead to medical emergencies, such as electrolyte imbalances, unstable fractures, and neutropenia leading to infection. It is important to obtain cancer-related history and physical information concerning the type of treatment and the exact diagnosis with metastasis (spread of the malignancy from the original site). It is also important for the acute care nurse to know the chemotherapy administration schedule, the dosage, and when it was last administered. Often chemotherapy, such as doxorubicin and cyclophosphamide, is administered four times, 3 weeks apart. As the chemotherapy proceeds, various issues, such as nausea and vomiting, low white cell counts (neutropenia), and mouth sores, may occur and be present on acute evaluation. The following are considered oncological emergencies and require acute care.

Hypercalcemia

Hypercalcemia is a reasonably common complication associated with multiple myeloma, breast, and lung cancers. A common cause of hypercalcemia is malignancy (Reagan, Pani, & Rosner, 2014) and is generally found in 3% to 5% of emergency admission patients (Lee et al., 2006). In primary hypercalcemia, hyperparathyroidism is the most common cause (Ahmad, Kuraganti, & Steenkamp, 2015). Survival can be markedly improved with early recognition in the emergency department (Royer, Maclellan, Stanley, Willingham, & Giles, 2014).

Hypercalcemia is defined as calcium concentration greater than 10.2 mg/dL (Lee et al., 2006). Signs and symptoms of hypercalcemia are often not evident in patients with mild or moderate hypercalcemia (calcium levels of 10.3–14.0 mg/dL). Gastrointestinal discomfort, changes in level of consciousness, and general nonspecific discomfort can be experienced in cases of moderate hypercalcemia (Reagan et al., 2014). Other signs and symptoms are lethargy, confusion, anorexia, nausea, constipation, polyuria, and polydipsia (Halfdanarson, Hogan, & Moynihan, 2006).

Treatment of hypercalcemia depends on the severity. Thiazide diuretics should be discontinued. Hydration must be maintained to diminish the risk of exacerbation of hypercalcemia. Severe hypercalcemia should be considered a medical emergency. Intravenous normal saline and loop diuretics should be implemented but will only last as long as the treatments are infusing. Bisphosphonates can help reduce bone reabsorption resulting in low serum calcium levels (Fallah-Rad & Morton, 2013). Calcitonin can also be administered subcutaneously or intramuscularly and can also reduce calcium levels (Halfdanarson et al., 2006). 25OHD levels and vitamin D supplementation may also reduce the risk of hypercalcemia (Fallah-Rad & Morton, 2013).

Tumor Lysis Syndrome

Tumor lysis syndrome (TLS) is caused when a tumor breaks down rapidly as a result of treatment or decompensation leading to massive cell death (Wagner & Arora, 2014). TLS is often detected in hematological malignancies (Rasool et al., 2014) and can be associated with high proliferation rate, bulky tumor (Mughal, Ejaz, Foringer, & Coiffier, 2010), high tumor burden, and sensitivity to chemotherapy (Rasool et al., 2014). TLS causes hyperkalemia, hyperuricemia, and hyperphosphatemia, which can enhance the risk of renal failure, reduced cardiac function, and mortality (Cantril & Haylock, 2004; Mughal et al., 2010; Shah, 2014). As chemotherapy agents become more effective, the risks increase for TLS.

Hyperphosphatemia and hypocalcemia can occur about 24 to 48 hours following the first chemotherapy administration. Signs and symptoms, such as muscle cramps, anxiety, depression, confusion, hallucinations, cardiac arrhythmia, and seizures, can result (Cantril & Haylock, 2004). The use of biomarkers (superoxide dismutase, malondialdehyde, glutathione, and catalase) may help one to recognize TLS so that treatment can be started (Rasool et al., 2014).

Other issues associated with TLS are hyperkalaemia, which is created by a release of potassium from the debilitation of the tumor cells. High serum potassium levels can cause severe arrhythmias and sudden death (Cairo & Bishop, 2004). Hyperuricemia (uric acid > 10 mg/dL) can result in acute obstruction uropathy and cause hematuria, flank pain, hypertension, edema, lethargy, and restlessness (Cairo & Bishop, 2004; Cantril & Haylock, 2004) and is caused by underexcretion (Oka et al., 2014). Hydration, administration of allopurinol, and diuresis are generally the first-line treatment (Ahmad et al., 2015; Cantril & Haylock, 2004). Treatment with rasburicase has been found to be effective in the treatment by lowering plasma uric acid levels (Dinnel, Moore, Skiver, & Bose, 2015).

The signs and symptoms associated with TLS include decreased urine output, seizures, and arrhythmias. Electrolytes must be assessed to determine the presence of hyperkalemia, hyperuricemia, and hyperphosphatemia. Electrocardiograms should be obtained to assess arrhythmia.

Spinal Cord Compression

Spinal cord compression (SCC) is not uncommon and can occur when metastasis spreads to the vertebral bodies and invades the spinal cord. The spinal column in the thoracic area is the most common location for this and must be recognized immediately to prevent critical, irreversible damage (Halfdanarson et al., 2006). SCC can lead to long-term neurological deficits and is often detected in solid tumors such as prostate, lung, breast, and kidney cancers (Savage et al., 2014).

Signs and symptoms are numbness, tingling and weakness in the extremities, sensory changes, and upper thorax and back pain (Lowey, 2006; Tsukada et al., 2015). Pain can radiate or localize and may seem chronic, which may disguise the emergent SCC and delay critical treatment. Bowel and bladder dysfunction can also occur. For patients who are experiencing SCC, the inability to walk into the clinic or emergency department often results in a delay of care (Tsukada et al., 2015) and it is important to recognize that the ability to ambulate does not exclude the existence of SCC.

Diagnosis is often made with MRI and CT and sometimes plain radiographic films of the affected area. Treatment is often initiated with glucocorticoids followed by either radiation therapy and/or surgery. For people who are ambulatory, radiation therapy can be considered. Patients with paraplegia, nonradiosensitive tumors, and a predicted survival of more than 3 months may benefit from surgery to decompress the spine (George et al., 2008). In some cases, combination therapy of surgery and radiation therapy can be beneficial to preserving ambulatory status and survival (Lee, Kwon, et al., 2014).

Neutropenic Fever

Neutropenic fever is an oncological medical emergency, which is caused by the diminishment of neutrophils by chemotherapeutic agents. Neutropenia is defined by an oral temperature of 101°F, an absolute neutrophil count (ANC) of less than 1,500 cells/µL. An ANC of less than 500 cells/µL is considered severe (Freifeld et al., 2011). Neutropenia can be the motivator for a severe infection and timely treatment is essential (Villafuerte-Gutierrez, Villalon, Losa, & Henriquez-Camacho, 2014). Generally, fever is the presenting sign; however, skin rashes and mucositis may also be present. For some patients, neutropenic fever can occur after the first cycle of chemotherapy and patients who have undergone aggressive surgery with bowel resections are at enhanced risk (Sharma, Rezai, Driscoll, Odunsi, & Lele, 2006).

Myelosuppression is associated with many chemotherapies, and growth factors, such as granulocyte-colony stimulating factor (G-CSF), work to elevate white blood cell counts necessary in fighting infection (Miller & Steinbach, 2014). A great amount of nursing literature exists on the definition, prevention, and management of neutropenic fever. Prevention of neutropenia and neutropenic fever should be proactive in the administration of G-CSFs in patients who are considered at high risk (Aapro et al., 2011). An older cancer patient receiving myelotoxic chemotherapy (cyclophosphamide, doxorubicin, vincristine, and prednisolone) is considered high risk and should receive prophylactic G-CSF administration (Aapro et al., 2011; Repetto et al., 2003), yet many patients are not treated with growth factors despite the potential positive outcomes (Lugtenburg et al., 2012).

CASE STUDY

A 76-year-old woman presents to the emergency department with delirium and trauma to her left hip. The patient's daughter reports that the patient fell in the bathroom several hours earlier. She has a diagnosis of breast cancer and is currently undergoing chemotherapy and has received four cycles of adriamycin and cyclophosphamide. She also has a history of osteoarthritis, hypertension, and gastric reflux disease. Presenting signs and symptoms are delirium, cracked mucous membranes, low blood pressure at 88/42 mmHg, and tachycardia.

Situations, such as dehydration, are not uncommon in an older person undergoing chemotherapy. Patients may have vomiting or diarrhea and become dehydrated as a result. Seniors have less functional reserve and are therefore more likely to suffer from complications of cancer treatment (Balducci, 2006). Older adults require careful examination and intervention in order to maintain and enhance health and independence.

1. In this clinical scenario, which geriatric syndromes are present?
   Answer: Falls, delirium, pain associated with trauma, functional status limitations, and ambulatory difficulty.
   Rationale: This patient has multiple geriatric syndromes and is at risk of further deconditioning. It is important to recognize the geriatric syndromes present and anticipate any additional injuries. Ensure caregiver support and help facilitate a plan for care while at home.
2. In this clinical scenario, which oncological emergency is this patient at greatest risk to develop?
   Answer: This clinical scenario is not written for an oncological emergency. Let us give the patient bone metastasis in her thoracic spine. Then she can be at risk for SCC.
   Rationale: Based on the signs and symptoms of dehydration, hypercalcemia is of concern. Hydrate to prevent hypercalcemia and to reduce signs and symptoms of dementia. Falls are also of concern because the risk of future falls is associated with prior falls. Dehydration in an older adult cancer patient can be associated with many problematic health and functional limitations.

SUMMARY

Acute care of the older patient requires nurses' health assessment skills be proactive in detecting and addressing limitations that can result from a cancer diagnosis and treatment. Nonmalignant comorbidities and geriatric syndromes play a role in the diagnosis and treatment of cancer and should be assimilated into the critical thinking involved in developing the nursing plan of care. Careful health assessment and evaluation are critical to the acute care nurse in understanding the disease progress, treatment tolerance, and the presence of oncological emergencies. Nurses working in acute settings must be acquainted with principles of geriatric care, which should be applied to patients with any type of diagnosis and not limited to malignancy. Understanding normative aging changes versus pathology can help facilitate a specialized plan of care with enhanced health and independence as the intended patient outcomes.

NURSING STANDARD OF PRACTICE

Protocol 31.1: Cancer Assessment and Interventions

I. GOAL

Improve the care of the older person diagnosed with cancer

II. OVERVIEW

Older adults have an increased risk of malignancy (SEER, 2014). Seniors often tolerate cancer treatment as well as younger people depending on functional and general health status (Sastre et al. 2008, Wildiers et al., 2007; Gomez-Millan, 2009).

(continued)

Protocol 31.1: Cancer Assessment and Interventions *(continued)*

III. BACKGROUND

Cancer is most often diagnosed in people aged 65 years and over (SEER, 2014). Nurses must be aware of management options and some potential emergencies associated with the diagnosis and treatment of a malignancy.

IV. PRINCIPLES OF CANCER CARE IN THE OLDER PERSON

A. Assessment of comorbid conditions
   1. Cancer may be one of several chronic conditions.
   2. The more severe the comorbidity, the less probability of survival after a diagnosis of cancer (Iversen et al. 2009).

B. Assess the patient using a comprehensive geriatric assessment
   1. The CGA is a battery of clinical measures used to assess functional, emotional, cognitive, falls, medications and general health status (AGS, 2010).
   2. Functional status can be measured using an Activity of Daily Living Scale (Katz et al., 1970), Instrumental Activities of Daily Living Scale (Lawton & Brody, 1969), Gait Assessment Scale (Tinetti, 1986), Berg Balance Scale (Berg et al., 1992).
   3. Risk of falls can be assessed using the Timed Up and Go Test (Podsiadlo & Richardson, 1991).
   4. Emotional status is often assessed using the Geriatric Depression Scale (Yesavage et al., 1982).
   5. Cognitive status is assessed using a mini-cog (Borson et al., 2000).
   6. General health status is assessed with a complete history and physical exam.
   7. Medication evaluation using the Beers Medication Screen (American Geriarics Society, 2012).

C. Assessment of medical emergencies associated with cancer
   1. Hypercalcemia
      a. Defined as calcium concentrations greater than 10.2 mg/mL (Lee et al., 2006)
      b. Signs and symptoms are not often noticeable.
      c. Gastrointestinal discomfort, lethargy, confusion, anorexia, nausea, constipation, polyuria, polydipsia (Halfdanarson et al., 2006)
      d. Treatment depends on severity.
      e. Thiazide diuretics should be discontinued.
      f. Hydration with intravenous normal saline
      g. Bisphosphonates (Fallah-Rad & Morton, 2013).
   2. Tumor lysis syndrome
      a. Caused when a tumor breaks down rapidly (Wagner & Arora, 2014).
      b. Causes hyperkalemia, hyperuricemia, hyperphosphatemia which can cause renal failure and reduced cardiac function
      c. Signs and symptoms are muscle cramps, anxiety, depression, confusion, hallucinations, cardiac arrhythmia and seizures (Cantril & Haylock, 2004).
      d. Treatment with hydration, administration of allupurinol and diuresis are generally the first line treatment (Cantril & Haylock, 2004).
      e. Treatment with rasburicase has been found to be effective in the treatment and prevention of hyperuricemia and tumor lysis syndrome (Dinnel et al., 2015).
   3. Spinal cord compression
      a. Occurs when metastasis spreads to the vertebral bodies and invades the spinal cord (Halfdanarson et al., 2006).
      b. Signs and symptoms are numbness, tingling and weakness in the extremities, sensory changes, upper thorax and back pain (Lowey, 2006; Tsukada et al., 2015).
      c. Pain can radiate or localize and may seem chronic which may disguise the emergent spinal cord compression and delay critical treatment.
      d. Bowel and bladder dysfunction can also occur (Tsukada et al., 2015).
      e. Treatment is often initiated with glucocorticoids followed by either radiation therapy and/or surgery (George et al., 2008).

(continued)

Protocol 31.1: Cancer Assessment and Interventions *(continued)*

4. Neutropenia fever
   a. Caused by the diminishment of neutrophils by chemotherapeutic agents
   b. Neutropenia is defined by an oral temperature of 101°F, an absolute neutrophil count (ANC) of < 1500 cells/microL. An ANC of < 500 cells/microL is considered severe (Freifeld et al., 2011).
   c. Generally fever is the presenting sign; however skin rashes and mucositis may also be present.
   d. Prevention of neutropenia and neutropenic fever should be proactive in the administration of G-CSFs in patients who are considered at high risk (Aapro et al., 2011).
   e. Treatment of neutropenia is to stop chemotherapy until white counts elevate

V. PARAMETERS OF ASSESSMENT

A. Older patients with cancer require comprehensive geriatric assessment and monitoring during diagnosis and treatment of malignancy.

RESOURCES

American Geriatric Society offers clinical guidelines in using the CGA in older persons.
http://www.americangeriatrics.org

National Comprehensive Cancer Network offers Clinical Practice Guidelines, including Senior Adult Oncology:
http://www.nccn.org/professionals/physician_gls/default.asp

Oncology Nursing Society offers recommendations for practice of the oncology patient.
www.ons.org

REFERENCES

Aaldriks, A. A., Maartense, E., le Cessie, S., Giltay, E. J., Verlaan, H. A., van der Geest, L. G., . . . Nortier, J. W. (2011). Predictive value of geriatric assessment for patients older than 70 years, treated with chemotherapy. *Critical Reviews in Oncology/Hematology, 79*(2), 205–212. *Evidence Level IV.*

Aapro, M. S., Bohlius, J., Cameron, D. A., Dal Lago, L., Donnelly, J. P., Kearney, N., . . . Zielinski, C.; European Organisation for Research and Treatment of Cancer. (2011). 2010 update of EORTC guidelines for the use of granulocyte-colony stimulating factor to reduce the incidence of chemotherapy-induced febrile neutropenia in adult patients with lymphoproliferative disorders and solid tumours. *European Journal of Cancer, 47*(1), 8–32. *Evidence Level V.*

Ahmad, S., Kuraganti, G., & Steenkamp, D. (2015). Hypercalcemic crisis: A clinical review. *American Journal of Medicine, 128*(3), 239–245. *Evidence Level V.*

American Geriatrics Society. (2006). Comprehensive geriatric assessment position statement. *Annals of Long-Term Care, 14*(3), 54–57. *Evidence Level VI.*

American Geriatrics Society and the British Geriatrics Society. (2010). *Summary of the updated American Geriatrics Society/British Geriatrics Society practice guideline for prevention of falls in older persons.* Retrieved from http://geriatricscareonline.org/ProductAbstract/updated-american-geriatrics-societybritish-geriatrics-society-clinical-practice-guideline-for-prevention-of-falls-in-older-persons-and-recommendations/CL014. *Evidence Level V.*

Annweiler, C., & Beauchet, O. (2015). Questioning vitamin D status of elderly fallers and nonfallers: A meta-analysis to address a "forgotten step." *Journal of Internal Medicine, 277*(1), 16–44. *Evidence Level I.*

Avelino-Silva, T. J., Farfel, J. M., Curiati, J. A., Amaral, J. R., Campora, F., & Jacob-Filho, W. (2014). Comprehensive geriatric assessment predicts mortality and adverse outcomes in hospitalized older adults. *BMC Geriatrics, 14*, 129. *Evidence Level IV.*

Balducci, L. (2006). Management of cancer in the elderly. *Oncology, 20*(2), 135–143; discussion 144, 146, 151–152. *Evidence Level V.*

Berg, K. O., Wood-Dauphinee, S. L., Williams, J. I., & Maki, B. (1992). Measuring balance in the elderly: Validation of an instrument. Canadian *Journal of Public Health, 83*(Suppl. 2), S7–S11. *Evidence Level IV.*

Borson, S., Scanlan, J., Brush, M., Vitaliano, P., & Dokmak, A. (2000). The Mini-Cog: A cognitive "vital signs" measure for dementia screening in multi-lingual elderly. *International Journal of Geriatric Psychiatry, 15*(11), 1021–1027. *Evidence Level IV.*

Borson, S., Scanlan, J. M., Chen, P., & Ganguli, M. (2003). The Mini-Cog as a screen for dementia: Validation in a population-based sample. *Journal of the American Geriatrics Society, 51*(10), 1451–1454. *Evidence Level IV.*

Cairo, M. S., & Bishop, M. (2004). Tumour lysis syndrome: New therapeutic strategies and classification. *British Journal of Haematology, 127*(1), 3–11. *Evidence Level V.*

Cantril, C. A., & Haylock, P. J. (2004). Emergency. Tumor lysis syndrome. *American Journal of Nursing, 104*(4), 49–52; quiz 52. *Evidence Level V.*

Chaïbi, P., Magné, N., Breton, S., Chebib, A., Watson, S., Duron, J. J., . . . Spano, J. P. (2011). Influence of geriatric consultation with comprehensive geriatric assessment on final therapeutic decision in elderly cancer patients. *Critical Reviews in Oncology/Hematology, 79*(3), 302–307. *Evidence Level V.*

Chundadze, T., Steinvil, A., Finn, T., Saranga, H., Guzner-Gur, H., Berliner, S.,... Paran, Y. (2010). Significantly elevated C-reactive protein serum levels are associated with very high 30-day mortality rates in hospitalized medical patients. *Clinical Biochemistry, 43*(13–14), 1060–1063. *Evidence Level V.*

Dinnel, J., Moore, B. L., Skiver, B. M., & Bose, P. (2015). Rasburicase in the management of tumor lysis: An evidence-based review of its place in therapy. *Core Evidence, 10*, 23–38. *Evidence Level V.*

Droz, J. P., Aapro, M., Balducci, L., Boyle, H., Van den Broeck, T., Cathcart, P.,... Sugihara, T. (2014). Management of prostate cancer in older patients: Updated recommendations of a working group of the International Society of Geriatric Oncology. *Lancet. Oncology, 15*(9), e404–e414. *Evidence Level V.*

Enright, P. L., McBurnie, M. A., Bittner, V., Tracy, R. P., McNamara, R., Arnold, A., & Newman, A. B.; Cardiovascular Health Study. (2003). The 6-min walk test: A quick measure of functional status in elderly adults. *Chest, 123*(2), 387–398. *Evidence Level IV.*

Fallah-Rad, N., & Morton, A. R. (2013). Managing hypercalcaemia and hypocalcaemia in cancer patients. *Current Opinion in Supportive and Palliative Care, 7*(3), 265–271. *Evidence Level V.*

Freifeld, A. G., Bow, E. J., Sepkowitz, K. A., Boeckh, M. J., Ito, J. I., Mullen, C. A.,... Wingard, J. R.; Infectious Diseases Society of America. (2011). Clinical practice guideline for the use of antimicrobial agents in neutropenic patients with cancer: 2010 update by the infectious diseases society of America. *Clinical Infectious Diseases, 52*(4), e56–e93. *Evidence Level IV.*

Freyer, G., Geay, J. F., Touzet, S., Provencal, J., Weber, B., Jacquin, J. P.,... Pujade-Lauraine, E. (2005). Comprehensive geriatric assessment predicts tolerance to chemotherapy and survival in elderly patients with advanced ovarian carcinoma: A GINECO study. *Annals of Oncology, 16*(11), 1795–1800. *Evidence Level IV.*

Fried, L. P., Tangen, C. M., Walston, J., Newman, A. B., Hirsch, C., Gottdiener, J.,... McBurnie, M. A.; Cardiovascular Health Study Collaborative Research Group. (2001). Frailty in older adults: Evidence for a phenotype. *Journals of Gerontology, 56*(3), M146–M156. *Evidence Level IV.*

Fukuse, T., Satoda, N., Hijiya, K., & Fujinaga, T. (2005). Importance of a comprehensive geriatric assessment in prediction of complications following thoracic surgery in elderly patients. *Chest, 127*(3), 886–891. *Evidence Level V.*

George, R., Jeba, J., Ramkumar, G., Chacko, A. G., Leng, M., & Tharyan, P. (2008). Interventions for the treatment of metastatic extradural spinal cord compression in adults. *Cochrane Database of Systematic Reviews, 2008*(4), CD006716. *Evidence Level I.*

Gomez-Millan, J. (2009). Radiation therapy in the elderly: More side effects and complications? *Critical Reviews in Oncology/Hematology, 71*(1), 70–78. *Evidence Level V.*

Halfdanarson, T. R., Hogan, W. J., & Moynihan, T. J. (2006). Oncologic emergencies: Diagnosis and treatment. *Mayo Clinic Proceedings, 81*(6), 835–848. *Evidence Level V.*

Hoyert, D. L. (2012). 75 years of mortality in the United States, 1935–2010. *NCHS Data Brief*, (88), 1–8. *Evidence Level IV.*

Hurria, A. (2013). Management of elderly patients with cancer. *Journal of the National Comprehensive Cancer Network, 11* (Suppl. 5), 698–701. *Evidence Level V.*

Hurria, A., & Lichtman, S. M. (2007). Pharmacokinetics of chemotherapy in the older patient. *Cancer Control, 14*(1), 32–43. *Evidence Level V.*

Iversen, L. H., Nørgaard, M., Jacobsen, J., Laurberg, S., & Sørensen, H. T. (2009). The impact of comorbidity on survival of Danish colorectal cancer patients from 1995 to 2006—A population-based cohort study. *Diseases of the Colon and Rectum, 52*(1), 71–78. *Evidence Level IV.*

Joutsenniemi, K. E., Martelin, T. P., Koskinen, S. V., Martikainen, P. T., Härkänen, T. T., Luoto, R. M., & Aromaa, A. J. (2006). Official marital status, cohabiting, and self-rated health-time trends in Finland, 1978–2001. *European Journal of Public Health, 16*(5), 476–483. *Evidence Level IV.*

Katz, S., Downs, T. D., Cash, H. R., & Grotz, R. C. (1970). Progress in development of the index of ADL. *The Gerontologist, 10*(1), 20–30. *Evidence Level IV.*

Khorana, A. A., Francis, C. W., Blumberg, N., Culakova, E., Refaai, M. A., & Lyman, G. H. (2008). Blood transfusions, thrombosis, and mortality in hospitalized patients with cancer. *Archives of Internal Medicine, 168*(21), 2377–2381. *Evidence Level IV.*

Klepin, H. D., Geiger, A. M., Tooze, J. A., Kritchevsky, S. B., Williamson, J. D., Ellis, L. R.,... Powell, B. L. (2011). The feasibility of inpatient geriatric assessment for older adults receiving induction chemotherapy for acute myelogenous leukemia. *Journal of the American Geriatrics Society, 59*(10), 1837–1846. *Evidence Level IV.*

Kravchenko, J., Berry, M., Arbeev, K., Kim Lyerly, H., Yashin, A., & Akushevich, I. (2015). Cardiovascular comorbidities and survival of lung cancer patients: Medicare data based analysis. *Lung Cancer, 88*(1), 85–93. *Evidence Level IV.*

Kristjansson, S. R., Nesbakken, A., Jordhøy, M. S., Skovlund, E., Audisio, R. A., Johannessen, H. O.,... Wyller, T. B. (2010). Comprehensive geriatric assessment can predict complications in elderly patients after elective surgery for colorectal cancer: A prospective observational cohort study. *Critical Reviews in Oncology/Hematology, 76*(3), 208–217. *Evidence Level IV.*

Lawton, M. P., & Brody, E. M. (1969). Assessment of older people: Self-maintaining and instrumental activities of daily living. *The Gerontologist, 9*(3), 179–186. *Evidence Level IV.*

Lee, C. H., Kwon, J. W., Lee, J., Hyun, S. J., Kim, K. J., Jahng, T. A., & Kim, H. J. (2014). Direct decompressive surgery followed by radiotherapy versus radiotherapy alone for metastatic epidural spinal cord compression: A meta-analysis. *Spine, 39*(9), E587–E592. *Evidence Level I.*

Lee, C. T., Yang, C. C., Lam, K. K., Kung, C. T., Tsai, C. J., & Chen, H. C. (2006). Hypercalcemia in the emergency department. *American Journal of the Medical Sciences, 331*(3), 119–123. *Evidence Level V.*

Lee, L., Heckman, G., & Molnar, F. J. (2015). Frailty: Identifying elderly patients at high risk of poor outcomes. *Canadian Family Physician, 61*(3), 227–231. *Evidence Level IV.*

Lee, W. J., Chou, M. Y., Peng, L. N., Liang, C. K., Liu, L. K., Liu, C. L., . . . Wu, Y. H.; VAIC Study Group. (2014). Predicting clinical instability of older patients in post-acute care units: A nationwide cohort study. *Geriatrics & Gerontology International, 14*(2), 267–272. *Evidence Level IV.*

Liang, C. K., Chu, C. L., Chou, M. Y., Lin, Y. T., Lu, T., Hsu, C. J., . . . Chen, L. K. (2015). Developing a prediction model for post-operative delirium and long-term outcomes among older patients receiving elective orthopedic surgery: A prospective cohort study in Taiwan. *Rejuvenation Research, 18*(4), 347–355. *Evidence Level IV.*

Lowey, S. E. (2006). Spinal cord compression: An oncologic emergency associated with metastatic cancer: Evaluation and management for the home health clinician. *Home Healthcare Nurse, 24*(7), 439–46; quiz 447. *Evidence Level V.*

Lugtenburg, P., Silvestre, A. S., Rossi, F. G., Noens, L., Krall, W., Bendall, K., . . . Jaeger, U. (2012). Impact of age group on febrile neutropenia risk assessment and management in patients with diffuse large B-cell lymphoma treated with R-CHOP regimens. *Clinical Lymphoma, Myeloma & Leukemia, 12*(5), 297–305. *Evidence Level IV.*

Miller, R. C., & Steinbach, A. (2014). Growth factor use in medication-induced hematologic toxicity. *Journal of Pharmacy Practice, 27*(5), 453–460. *Evidence Level V.*

Mughal, T. I., Ejaz, A. A., Foringer, J. R., & Coiffier, B. (2010). An integrated clinical approach for the identification, prevention, and treatment of tumor lysis syndrome. *Cancer Treatment Reviews, 36*(2), 164–176. *Evidence Level V.*

Oka, Y., Tashiro, H., Sirasaki, R., Yamamoto, T., Akiyama, N., Kawasugi, K., . . . Fujimori, S. (2014). Hyperuricemia in hematologic malignancies is caused by an insufficient urinary excretion. *Nucleosides Nucleotides Nucleic Acids, 33*(4–6), 434–438. *Evidence Level V.*

Ording, A. G., Boffetta, P., Garne, J. P., Nystrom, P. M., Cronin-Fenton, D., Froslev, T., . . . Lash, T. L. (2015). Relative mortality rates from incident chronic diseases among breast cancer survivors—A 14 year follow-up of five-year survivors diagnosed in Denmark between 1994 and 2007. *European Journal of Cancer,* 51(6), 767–775. *Evidence Level IV.*

Osborne, C., Ostir, G. V., Du, X., Peek, M. K., & Goodwin, J. S. (2005). The influence of marital status on the stage at diagnosis, treatment, and survival of older women with breast cancer. *Breast Cancer Research and Treatment, 93*(1), 41–47. *Evidence Level IV.*

Overcash, J. A. (2004). Using narrative research to understand the quality of life of older women with breast cancer. *Oncology Nursing Forum, 31*(6), 1153–1159. *Evidence Level V.*

Overcash, J. A., & Beckstead, J. (2008). Predicting falls in older patients using components of a comprehensive geriatric assessment. *Clinical Journal of Oncology Nursing, 12*(6), 941–949. *Evidence Level IV.*

Pal, S. K., Katheria, V., & Hurria, A. (2010). Evaluating the older patient with cancer: Understanding frailty and the geriatric assessment. *CA: A Cancer Journal for Clinicians, 60*(2), 120–132. *Evidence Level IV.*

Patel, M. K., Patel, D. A., Lu, M., Elshaikh, M. A., Munkarah, A., & Movsas, B. (2010). Impact of marital status on survival among women with invasive cervical cancer: Analysis of population-based surveillance, epidemiology, and end results data. *Journal of Lower Genital Tract Disease, 14*(4), 329–338. *Evidence Level IV.*

Patterson, R. E., Flatt, S. W., Saquib, N., Rock, C. L., Caan, B. J., Parker, B. A., . . . Pierce, J. P. (2010). Medical comorbidities predict mortality in women with a history of early stage breast cancer. *Breast Cancer Research and Treatment, 122*(3), 859–865. *Evidence Level II.*

Pilotto, A., Ferrucci, L., Scarcelli, C., Niro, V., Di Mario, F., Seripa, D., . . . Franceschi, M. (2007). Usefulness of the comprehensive geriatric assessment in older patients with upper gastrointestinal bleeding: A two-year follow-up study. *Digestive Diseases, 25*(2), 124–128. *Evidence Level IV.*

Podsiadlo, D., & Richardson, S. (1991). The timed "Up & Go": A test of basic functional mobility for frail elderly persons. *Journal of the American Geriatrics Society, 39*(2), 142–148. *Evidence Level IV.*

Rasool, M., Malik, A., Qureshi, M. S., Ahmad, R., Manan, A., Asif, M., . . . Pushparaj, P. N. (2014). Development of tumor lysis syndrome (TLS): A potential risk factor in cancer patients receiving anticancer therapy. *Bioinformation, 10*(11), 703–707. *Evidence Level V.*

Reagan, P., Pani, A., & Rosner, M. H. (2014). Approach to diagnosis and treatment of hypercalcemia in a patient with malignancy. *American Journal of Kidney Diseases, 63*(1), 141–147. *Evidence Level V.*

Repetto, L., Biganzoli, L., Koehne, C. H., Luebbe, A. S., Soubeyran, P., Tjan-Heijnen, V. C., & Aapro, M. S. (2003). EORTC Cancer in the Elderly Task Force guidelines for the use of colony-stimulating factors in elderly patients with cancer. *European Journal of Cancer, 39*(16), 2264–2272. *Evidence Level V.*

Royer, A. M., Maclellan, R. A., Stanley, J. D., Willingham, T. B., & Giles, W. H. (2014). Hypercalcemia in the emergency department: A missed opportunity. *American Surgeon, 80*(8), 732–735. *Evidence Level V.*

Sakurai, K., Muguruma, K., Nagahara, H., Kimura, K., Toyokawa, T., Amano, R., . . . Hirakawa, K. (2015). The outcome of surgical treatment for elderly patients with gastric carcinoma. *Journal of Surgical Oncology, 111*(7), 848–854. *Evidence Level IV.*

Sanchis, J., Bonanad, C., Ruiz, V., Fernández, J., García-Blas, S., Mainar, L., . . . Núñez, J. (2014). Frailty and other geriatric conditions for risk stratification of older patients with acute coronary syndrome. *American Heart Journal, 168*(5), 784–791. *Evidence Level IV.*

Sastre, J., Puente, J., García-Saenz, J. A., & Díaz-Rubio, E. (2008). Irinotecan in the treatment of elderly patients with advanced colorectal cancer. *Critical Reviews in Oncology/Hematology, 68*(3), 250–255. *Evidence Level IV.*

Savage, P., Sharkey, R., Kua, T., Schofield, L., Richardson, D., Panchmatia, N., . . . Ulbricht, C. (2014). Malignant spinal cord compression: NICE guidance, improvements and challenges. *QJM, 107*(4), 277–282. *Evidence Level V.*

Shack, L. G., Rachet, B., Williams, E. M., Northover, J. M., & Coleman, M. P. (2010). Does the timing of comorbidity affect colorectal cancer survival? A population based study. *Postgraduate Medical Journal, 86*(1012), 73–78. *Evidence Level IV.*

Shah, B. K. (2014). Hypercalcemia in tumor lysis syndrome. *Indian Journal of Hematology & Blood Transfusion, 30*(Suppl. 1), 88–89. *Evidence Level V.*

Sharma, S., Rezai, K., Driscoll, D., Odunsi, K., & Lele, S. (2006). Characterization of neutropenic fever in patients receiving first-line adjuvant chemotherapy for epithelial ovarian cancer. *Gynecologic Oncology, 103*(1), 181–185. *Evidence Level IV.*

Silva, T. J., Jerussalmy, C. S., Farfel, J. M., Curiati, J. A., & Jacob-Filho, W. (2009). Predictors of in-hospital mortality among older patients. *Clinics, 64*(7), 613–618. *Evidence Level IV.*

Simmonds, M. J. (2002). Physical function in patients with cancer: Psychometric characteristics and clinical usefulness of a physical performance test battery. *Journal of Pain and Symptom Management, 24*(4), 404–414. *Evidence Level IV.*

Stotter, A., Reed, M. W., Gray, L. J., Moore, N., & Robinson, T. G. (2015). Comprehensive Geriatric Assessment and predicted 3-year survival in treatment planning for frail patients with early breast cancer. *British Journal of Surgery, 102*(5), 525–533; discussion 533. *Evidence Level IV.*

Surveillance, Epidemiology, and End Results Program (SEER). (2014). *Cancer fact sheets.* Retrieved from http://seer.cancer.gov. *Evidence Level IV.*

Tinetti, M. E. (1986). Performance-oriented assessment of mobility problems in elderly patients. *Journal of the American Geriatrics Society, 34*(2), 119–126. *Evidence Level IV.*

Tinetti, M. E., Mendes de Leon, C. F., Doucette, J. T., & Baker, D. I. (1994). Fear of falling and fall-related efficacy in relationship to functioning among community-living elders. *Journal of Gerontology, 49*(3), M140–M147. *Evidence Level IV.*

Tsukada, Y., Nakamura, N., Ohde, S., Akahane, K., Sekiguchi, K., & Terahara, A. (2015). Factors that delay treatment of symptomatic metastatic extradural spinal cord compression. *Journal of Palliative Medicine, 18*(2), 107–113. *Evidence Level IV.*

Tucci, A., Ferrari, S., Bottelli, C., Borlenghi, E., Drera, M., & Rossi, G. (2009). A comprehensive geriatric assessment is more effective than clinical judgment to identify elderly diffuse large cell lymphoma patients who benefit from aggressive therapy. *Cancer, 115*(19), 4547–4553. *Evidence Level IV.*

Villafuerte-Gutierrez, P., Villalon, L., Losa, J. E., & Henriquez-Camacho, C. (2014). Treatment of febrile neutropenia and prophylaxis in hematologic malignancies: A critical review and update. *Advances in Hematology, 2014*, 986938. *Evidence Level IV.*

Wagner, J., & Arora, S. (2014). Oncologic metabolic emergencies. *Emergency Medicine Clinics of North America, 32*(3), 509–525. *Evidence Level V.*

Ware, J., Kosinski, M., & Keller, S. D. (1996). A 12-item Short-Form Health Survey: Construction of scales and preliminary tests of reliability and validity. *Medical Care, 34*(3), 220–233. *Evidence Level IV.*

Wesa, K. M., Segal, N. H., Cronin, A. M., Sjoberg, D. D., Jacobs, G. N., Coleton, M. I., . . . Cassileth, B. R. (2015). Serum 25-hydroxy vitamin D and survival in advanced colorectal cancer: A retrospective analysis. *Nutrition and Cancer, 67*(3), 424–430. *Evidence Level IV.*

Wildiers, H., Heeren, P., Puts, M., Topinkova, E., Janssen-Heijnen, M. L., Extermann, M., . . . Hurria, A. (2014). International Society of Geriatric Oncology consensus on geriatric assessment in older patients with cancer. *Journal of Clinical Oncology, 32*(24), 2595–2603. *Evidence Level V.*

Wildiers, H., Kunkler, I., Biganzoli, L., Fracheboud, J., Vlastos, G., Bernard-Marty, C., . . . Aapro, M.; International Society of Geriatric Oncology. (2007). Management of breast cancer in elderly individuals: Recommendations of the International Society of Geriatric Oncology. *Lancet. Oncology, 8*(12), 1101–1115. *Evidence Level V.*

Williams, T. A., McConigley, R., Leslie, G. D., Dobbs, G. J., Phillips, M., Davies, H., & Aoun, S. (2015). A comparison of outcomes among hospital survivors with and without severe comorbidity admitted to the intensive care unit. *Anaesthesia and Intensive Care, 43*(2), 230–237. *Evidence Level IV.*

Yesavage, J. A., Brink, T. L., Rose, T. L., Lum, O., Huang, V., Adey, M., & Leirer, V. O. (1982). Development and validation of a geriatric depression screening scale: A preliminary report. *Journal of Psychiatric Research, 17*(1), 37–49. *Evidence Level IV.*

32

Perioperative Care of the Older Adult

Fidelindo Lim and Larry Z. Slater

EDUCATIONAL OBJECTIVES

On completion of this chapter, the reader should be able to:

1. Identify unique multifactorial challenges affecting the older adult perioperative patient
2. Synthesize current best practices from related geriatric themes in the assessment and management of the older adult perioperative patient
3. Describe geriatric-specific, evidence-based, and collaborative interventions to improve outcomes among older adult perioperative patients

OVERVIEW

The confluence of advancing age, geriatric syndromes, regulatory changes, and advances in medical technology has made perioperative care scenarios of older adults more complex. Surgical procedures performed on older adults are expected to rise. About one third of all procedures and one half of surgical procedures on the cardiovascular and digestive systems in nonfederal short-term hospitals are performed on inpatients aged 65 years and older (Hall, DeFrances, Williams, Golosinskiy, & Schwartzman, 2010). Factors, such as polypharmacy, diabetes, presurgical cognitive status, use of general anesthesia, and increasing number of procedures done in ambulatory care settings, will continue to impact postsurgical outcomes, particularly the development of postoperative delirium, a significant determinant of poor outcomes (Brooks, 2012).

Perioperative nursing is defined as the "delivery of comprehensive care within preoperative, intraoperative and postoperative periods of the patient's experience during operative and other invasive procedures" (Steelman, 2015, p. 1). The high stake demands of perioperative patient care, the increasing number of older adults undergoing surgery, and the unique vulnerabilities of this population require the translation of science-based interprofessional collaboration. The use of the nursing process, critical thinking, and evidence-based practice models will ensure patient safety and quality for older adult patients and their families.

The discussion about perioperative care of older adults comes at an opportune time, when there is growing recognition that the educational background of nursing staff directly impacts mortality of surgical patients. Aiken et al. (2014) found that a 10% increase in the proportion of staff nurses holding a bachelor's degree is associated with a 7% decrease in the risk of death among patients following common surgeries in an acute care setting. This finding supports earlier evidence of lower mortality among surgical patients when there is a higher proportion of bachelor's-prepared nurses on staff (Aiken, Clarke, Cheung, Sloane, & Silber, 2003). Lower rates of postoperative deep vein thrombosis (DVT) or pulmonary

For a description of evidence levels cited in this chapter, see Chapter 1, "Developing and Evaluating Clinical Practice Guidelines: A Systematic Approach."

embolism (PE) and shorter length of stay have also been found in hospitals with a higher percentage of registered nurses (RNs) with baccalaureate or higher degrees (Blegen, Goode, Park, Vaughn, & Spetz, 2013).

As fall rate remains high in medical–surgical units and a predictor of poorer outcomes, it is important to note that there is an inverse relationship between nurse certification and fall rate (Boltz, Capezuti, Wagner, Rosenberg, & Secic, 2013).

The improvement of care outcomes in older adult surgical patients will draw from an array of evidence not only from clinical studies but also from research in nursing policy, management, and health professions education. Specific safety and quality benchmarks for the general surgical care of older adults are described in Chapter 33, "General Surgical Care of the Older Adult." The inevitable aging of the population will result in greater demand for surgical care. Comprehensive geriatric assessment that takes into account patient's participation is an established clinical approach in optimizing positive outcomes for the perioperative older adult patient (Partridge, Harari, Martin, & Dhesi, 2014).

BACKGROUND AND STATEMENT OF PROBLEM

The number and type of surgical procedures performed in the past decade vary according to the body systems involved. A total of 51.4 million all-listed procedures for discharges from short-stay hospitals were performed in 2010 (Centers for Disease Control and Prevention [CDC], 2010). Of these, 19.2 million were performed among patients 65 years and older (CDC, 2010). In 2011, more than 15 million operating room (OR) procedures were performed in U.S. hospitals (Weiss & Elixhauser, 2014). Earlier estimates reported that patients aged 65 years and older were two to three times more likely to experience OR procedures (Elixhauser & Andrews, 2010). The authors reported that more than 4 million major operations are performed annually in the United States in patients 65 years and older. However, those who are 85 years and older are noted to be less likely to undergo an OR procedure compared with younger older adults (Weiss & Elixhauser, 2014). The following are the highlights of the characteristics of OR procedures in U.S. hospitals in 2011(Weiss & Elixhauser, 2014):

- Hospitalizations that involved OR procedures constituted 29% of the total 38.6 million hospital stays and 48% of the total $387 billion in hospital costs.
- Hospital stays that involved an OR procedure were about twice as costly as stays that did not involve an OR procedure.
- Compared with hospital admissions that did not include an OR procedure, admissions involving an OR procedure resulted in a longer length of stay, and were more likely to be elective admissions.
- Hospital stays involving OR procedures were about half as likely to result in patient death compared with stays without an OR procedure.
- The 20 most common procedures accounted for more than half of all OR procedures with a substantial majority being musculoskeletal and cardiac procedures.
- Twenty procedures accounted for more than half of all costs for stays involving OR procedures. Spinal fusion, knee arthroplasty, and percutaneous coronary angioplasty (PTCA) were the procedures with the highest hospital costs.

Although trends in operative procedures vary over time, trends in U.S. hospitals operative procedures between 2001 and 2011 show that the current mix may disproportionately affect older adults (except caesarian section and circumcision).

Going for surgery, whether an outpatient or inpatient procedure, emergent or elective, marks an important health care transition, particularly among vulnerable older adults, because of the increased morbidity and mortality risks. A study involving 24,216 patients reported that failures-to-rescue were more than two times higher in patients older than 75 years compared with those younger than 75 years (26.0% vs. 10.3% at high-mortality hospitals, $p < .001$; Sheetz et al., 2014). It is interesting to note that higher nurse–patient ratio (odds ratio [*OR*]: 0.99, 95% confidence interval [CI] [0.98–1.00]) did not influence failure-to-rescue (Sheetz et al., 2014).

Overall mortality among older adults presenting with trauma is higher among those older than 74 years than in younger geriatric cohorts (Hashmi et al., 2014). Furthermore, severe and extremely severe injuries and systolic hypotension at presentation are associated with significant mortality risks (Hashmi et al., 2014). Higher mortality trends have also been noted among older adults who had cardiac surgery (Sepehri et al., 2014), kidney transplant (Knoll, 2013), hip-fracture surgery (Carpintero et al., 2014), and colectomy (Visser, Keegan, Martin, & Wren, 2009), and among surgical oncology patients (Korc-Grodzicki et al., 2014). Among cardiac surgical patients, age more than 75 years is an independent risk factor for intensive care unit (ICU) mortality, and these patients have a higher risk of multiorgan dysfunction syndrome (MODS; Curiel-Balsera et al., 2013).

In general, high surgical mortality among older adults is closely linked with increased risk of falls, prolonged hospitalization, and frailty (Green et al., 2012; Sepehri et al., 2014). However, advanced age alone does not correlate or predict higher mortality postsurgery (Green et al., 2012). Similar findings have been noted among patients in critical care settings (Balas et al., 2012). This is important for nurses to consider in their assessment and they should be aware of personal or professional biases (e.g., ageism) that might impact the overall quality of care provided among older adult perioperative patients. Consideration of the overall health scenario, including the typical age-related physiologic changes, baseline health status, severity of present illness, and potential risks of perioperative complications, rather than age alone, should guide the realistic care decisions for perioperative older adult patients (Oresanya, Lyons, & Finlayson, 2014).

Failure-to-rescue, resulting in death among surgical inpatients with treatable serious complications, and the percentage of major surgical inpatients who experience hospital-acquired complications (e.g., sepsis, pneumonia, gastrointestinal bleeding, shock/cardiac arrest, DVT/PE) are nursing-sensitive measures and publicly reportable events (National Quality Forum [NQF], 2004). As a result, there have been numerous collaborative safety initiatives, both from governmental and nonregulatory agencies, in the past decade.

ASSESSMENT OF PROBLEM AND NURSING CARE STRATEGIES

Preoperative Considerations

Successful perioperative care of the older adult begins at the time surgery has been determined to be a safe option. What distinguishes older adults from their younger counterparts is the former's loss of functional reserve and a general decline in organ function (White, Khan, & Smitham, 2011). Older patients may present with a host of comorbidities involving any organ system and these must be evaluated and optimized before surgery to improve the postoperative outcome. This highlights the crucial roles played by anesthetists, geriatricians, and nurses in the preoperative management of this challenging patient population. Functional and cognitive impairment, malnutrition, facility residence, and frailty have been associated with adverse surgical outcomes (Oresanya et al., 2014).

As part of the comprehensive preoperative assessment of older patients, "it is useful to determine whether a patient is physiologically 'young' (i.e., exhibiting only changes associated with normal aging) or 'old' (i.e., exhibiting aging effects due to comorbidities in addition to normal aging)" (White et al., 2012, p. 1191).

Consent for Surgery

Determining the patient's capacity to consent for surgery is another challenge for the provider. Age alone does not predict incapacity to consent for surgery (Oresanya et al., 2014). It is important to view capacity within a continuum. It can be evanescent, and can be optimized with careful consideration of situational, psychosocial, medical, psychiatric, and neurological factors (Sessums, Zembrzuska, & Jackson, 2011). Reliable capacity assessment can also be influenced by problematic relationships between patients and providers, as well as cultural, linguistic, and educational barriers (Ivashkov & Van Norman, 2009). It is best to assume that patients have the capacity to make medical decisions unless proven otherwise (Barton, Mallik, Orr, & Janofsky, 1996). From a legal and medical standpoint, competence to consent to treatment may require the following criteria (Appelbaum & Grisso, 1995; Welie & Welie, 2001):

- Ability to appreciate the nature of one's situation and the consequences of one's choices
- Ability to understand the relevant information
- Ability to reason about the risks and benefits of potential options
- Ability to communicate a choice

The use of validated tools, such as the Standardized Mini-Mental State Examination (SMMSE) or the Mini-Cog must be used to evaluate the medical decision-making capacity of the patient (see Chapter 4, "Health Care Decision Making," and Chapter 6, "Assessing Cognitive Function"). A review of 43 prospective studies to determine the prevalence of incapacity and assessment accuracy in adult medical patients without severe mental illnesses found that only 2.8% of healthy older adult control subjects lacked decision-making capacity, compared with 20% in those with mild cognitive impairment and 54% among persons with Alzheimer's disease (Sessums et al., 2011). The authors also noted that SMMSE scores of less than 20 are associated with increased likelihood of incapacity (Likelihood ratio [LR]: 6.3; 95% CI [3.7–11]). Other validated tools that can be used to assess capacity are the Aid to Capacity Evaluation (ACE) tool, the Hopkins Competency Assessment Test, and the Understanding Treatment Disclosure (Sessums et al., 2011). Competency to use any assessment tools is paramount. Therefore, clinicians must have sufficient training and ongoing validation on how to use these tools.

Preoperative Optimization

It is ideal if the process of obtaining an informed consent includes a discussion of treatment goals, risks, and benefits, with full participation of the patient, family, and other caregivers. If surgery is unlikely to satisfy the patient's goals and preferences, nonoperative treatments may be pursued (Oresanya et al., 2014). A comprehensive geriatric assessment is called for not only for its benefits in reducing adverse postoperative outcomes, but to aid clinicians in optimizing function before surgery (Oresanya et al., 2014; Partridge et al., 2014). Experts recommend the following four domains as the focus of preoperative optimization: cognition, functional status, nutrition, and frailty (Oresanya et al., 2014). Evidence suggests that poor functional status (e.g., inability to climb two flights of stairs or walk four blocks) is associated with an increased risk of postoperative cardiopulmonary complications after major noncardiac surgery (Girish, Trayner, Dammann, Pinto-Plata, & Celli, 2001).

For older adults with hip fractures, optimization requires estimating perioperative risks and performing the surgery early, as well as focusing on intravascular volume restoration, pain management, and prevention of perioperative hypotension (Nicholas, 2014a). Advanced preoperative cardiac testing (e.g., echocardiography and stress testing) does not seem to improve outcomes and may inappropriately delay surgical repair (Nicholas, 2014b). Regardless of the surgery needed, older adults with active cardiac conditions, such as unstable coronary syndromes, decompensated heart failure, significant arrhythmia, and severe valvular disease, require evaluation and treatment before nonurgent or noncardiac surgery (Fleisher et al., 2014).

Admission

Unless the patient is coming in for an elective or ambulatory surgery, inpatient surgeries usually necessitate a visit to the emergency department (ED), partly because of the nature of clinical scenarios requiring surgical interventions (e.g., hip fracture, gastrointestinal bleeding, subdural hematoma, etc.). The time spent in the ED, particularly among vulnerable older adults, is an important consideration because of its positive correlation with negative patient-oriented outcomes, from worse patient satisfaction to higher inpatient mortality rates (Singer, Thode, Viccellio, & Pines, 2011).

A retrospective cohort study (N = 41,256 with 37% of subjects older than 65 years) reported higher mortality correlates with increased ED boarding time (2.5% inpatients boarded less than 2 hours; 4.5% inpatients boarded 12 hours or more ($p < .001$; Singer et al., 2011). The authors also noted longer hospital stay correlates with longer boarding time in the ED. On average, those who stayed in the ED for less than 2 hours had 5.6 days of hospitalization (SD ± 11.4) compared with 8.7 days (SD ± 16.3 days) for those who boarded for more than 24 hours (Singer, Thode, Viccellio, & Pines, 2011). Similar negative findings have been reported in ED nursing case studies of older adult patients (Donatelli, Gregorowicz, & Somes, 2013). Among orthopedic patients, surgical delay is associated with a significant increase in the risk of death and pressure sores (Moja et al., 2012)—both are nursing-sensitive indicators. Clinical and administrative nursing personnel play a pivotal role in expediting patient transfer from the ED to the surgical unit or the OR and in facilitating timely performance of diagnostic procedures and other inpatient preoperative screening to minimize unwanted delays.

Assessment of Surgical Risk

Comprehensive preoperative assessment of older adults needs to consider calculating surgical risks in order for the patient and his or her family and the provider to come up with an informed decision to operate. Although there are currently no validated tools specific to the older adult population, various available surgical-risk calculators may be applied, particularly in evaluating cardiac risk before noncardiac surgery (Bilimoria et al., 2013). The *Assessment of an Older Patient With a Condition Potentially Amenable to Surgery* is an algorithm intended to guide the surgeon and the patient in determining the appropriateness of surgery (Oresanya et al., 2014). Table 32.1 shows examples of surgical-risk assessment tools and their descriptions.

Based on the synthesis of existing evidence, the following clinical factors have been associated with increased perioperative risk of a cardiovascular event (Fleisher et al., 2014): history of ischemic heart disease, heart failure, cerebrovascular disease, insulin-dependent diabetes mellitus, preoperative serum creatinine greater than 1.5 mg/dL, increasing age, American Society of Anesthesiologists (ASA) class, and preoperative functional status. Emergency surgery is associated with higher risk, as cardiac complications are two to five times more likely than with elective procedures (Fleisher et al., 2014). Frailty and resiliency are two vital concepts to consider in the comprehensive assessment of older surgical patients. Use of a validated frailty scoring tool can be used in preoperative assessment where applicable (Chow, Rosenthal, Merkow, Ko, & Esnaola, 2012).

Intraoperative Considerations

Anesthesia

The physiological changes that accompany aging may put the older adult surgical patient at risk of adverse effects of anesthetics. Loss of skeletal muscle mass, decrease in total body water and increased adipose tissue, especially in women, can lead to an expansion of the lipid reservoir

TABLE 32.1
Examples of Surgical Risk Assessment Tools

Surgical Risk Assessment Tool	Description
Revised Goldman Cardiac Risk Index (RCRI; Devereaux et al., 2005; Lee et al., 1999)	Referred to as the Lee Index, the tool offers significant predictive value for cardiac complications and mortality after major noncardiac surgery in various populations and settings, except for abdominal aortic aneurysm surgery.
Vascular Study Group of New England (VSGNE; Bertges et al., 2010)	The risk index predicts in-hospital cardiac events after vascular surgeries such as nonemergent carotid endarterectomy, lower extremity bypass, endovascular abdominal aortic aneurysm repair, and open infrarenal abdominal aortic aneurysm repair.
American College of Surgeons—National Surgery Quality Improvement Program (ACS-NSQIP) Universal Surgical Risk Calculator (Bilimoria et al., 2013)	A universal decision-support tool based on 21 preoperative factors. It is used as a morbidity and mortality risk calculator for patients undergoing surgery and includes several geriatric variables, such as age, functional health status, albumin level, type of procedure, demographics, and comorbidities. The tool can be used to estimate risks for postoperative complications.
Gupta MICA (myocardial infarction or cardiac arrest) NSQIP Database Risk Model (Gupta et al., 2011)	This cardiac risk calculator provides a risk estimate of intraoperative or postoperative myocardial infarction or cardiac arrest. Five factors identified as predictors of MICA include type of surgery, dependent functional status, abnormal creatinine, American Society of Anesthesiologists class, and increased age.

for centrally active anesthetic drugs (e.g., benzodiazepines, volatile agents, opioid analgesics, and sedative hypnotics) contributing to delayed elimination and increased duration of action of these drugs (White et al., 2012). Among malnourished older adults with hypoalbuminemia there is a higher risk of toxicity for albumin-bound anesthetic agents, such as propofol and diazepam, because of increased free-drug concentrations, contributing to increased sensitivity to these drugs (Aymanns, Keller, Maus, Hartmann, & Czock, 2010). Anesthetic agents are also known to decrease cardiac output, arterial pressure, and microvascular perfusion (Bentov & Reed, 2014), which can further strain the patient's limited physiologic reserve.

To assess postoperative risks, the ASA Classification of Physical Health remains the most common tool used in appraising preoperative health of surgical patients. The patient's preoperative health is categorized into five classes (I–V). An "E" for emergency surgery is placed after the Roman numeral (Dripps, 1963):

I. Patient is a completely healthy, fit patient.
II. Patient has mild systemic disease.
III. Patient has severe systemic disease that is not incapacitating.
IV. Patient has incapacitating disease that is a constant threat to life.
V. A moribund patient who is not expected to live 24 hours with or without surgery.

An ASA score of VI is designated for patients who are declared brain dead and coming to the OR for organ procurement. An ASA score of III or higher is a predictor of greater blood loss and need for transfusion in total hip replacement patients (Grosflam, Wright, Cleary, & Katz, 1995). The ASA score has been shown to have a predictive value in long-term mortality after a hip fracture (Bjorgul, Novicoff, & Saleh, 2010). In a prospective study of 1,635 patients with hip fracture, survival for those rated with ASA I was 8.5 years versus only 1.6 years for those rated as ASA IV (Bjorgul et al., 2010). A prospective study of 168 hip-fracture patients (age range: 50–98 years) reported that an ASA score of III or higher is a predictive factor of postoperative delirium (Zakriya et al., 2002).

Although this grading system is widely used, there has been notable criticism of its value. Variations of the classification systems are available. Perioperative nurses need to inform themselves of what system is used in their facility. Use of the ASA classification to predict postoperative mortality risk can be further enhanced by complementing it with the Short Potable Mental Status Questionnaire (SPMSQ) for assessing cognitive function. Söderqvist et al. (2009), in a prospective cohort study of 1,944 patients aged 66 years or older, reported that the combination of ASA score and SPMSQ provides greater information about survival times compared with the ASA score alone. Nurses are encouraged to be an active participant in evaluating the patient's surgical risk and in communicating with the provider any changes in patient's condition that may impact the use of anesthetics. In order to safely monitor patients, nurses need to have a stable knowledge of pharmacokinetics and pharmacodynamics of the common anesthetic agents used and the unique precautions related to older adults.

Intraoperative Medication Safety

Although the exact number of medication errors taking place throughout the perioperative continuum cannot be fully known, medication safety continues to be a challenge (Treiber & Jones, 2012). Based on voluntary sentinel event reporting, 428 medication errors resulting in death or permanent loss of function were reported between 2004 and 2014 (The Joint Commission [TJC], 2014a). Potential factors in medication errors include medications in unlabeled containers or removed from their original containers and placed into unlabeled containers. This unsafe practice neglects basic principles of safe medication management, yet it is routine in many organizations (TJC, 2015). In one qualitative study, preoperative medication errors were the most frequently reported perioperative medication error (Treiber & Jones, 2012). To maintain medication safety within the perioperative settings see Protocol 32.1 for details of TJC's guidelines.

Antibiotic Prophylaxis

The high prevalence of surgical site infection (SSI) is an ongoing challenge. Among the many strategies to prevent SSI is the use of antibiotic prophylaxis. The current guidelines are an interprofessional collaboration espoused by the American Society of Health-System Pharmacists (ASHP), the Infectious Diseases Society of America (IDSA), the Surgical Infection Society (SIS), and the Society for Healthcare Epidemiology of America (SHEA). The guidelines include specific recommendations for various surgeries (e.g., neurosurgery, cardiac, thoracic, gastroduodenal, bowel, and biliary) that disproportionately affect older adults. The key recommendation is to administer intraoperative antibiotic within 60 minutes before surgical incision. Antibiotics requiring longer infusion times, such as fluoroquinolones and vancomycin, should begin within 120 minutes before surgical incision (Bratzler et al., 2013).

Time Out/Universal Protocol

In a 10-year period between 2004 and 2014, the TJC reported 1,071 sentinel events related to wrong-patient, wrong-site, wrong-procedure events (TJC, 2014a). Seen within the overall number of surgeries done annually (51.4 million procedures performed in the United States in 2010 [CDC, 2010]), these incidences are considered rare, though they have very serious consequences. Older adults can be seen as having high vulnerability for such events because of higher prevalence of cognitive or memory impairment, which might affect their full participation in the Time Out procedure.

A Cochrane Review that evaluated the effectiveness of organizational and professional interventions for reducing wrong-site surgery reported that preoperative verification using Universal Protocol, site marking, Time Out, and targeted educational interventions has been demonstrated to reduce the incidence of wrong-site surgery events (Algie et al., 2015). Recognizing the complexities of the work processes involved in Universal Protocol, TJC offers some guidelines for its implementation (see Protocol 32.1 for details).

POSTANESTHESIA CARE UNIT CONSIDERATIONS

Perioperative Delirium

Delirium is a high-impact, high-volume complication of surgery among older adults that is associated with a host of negative outcomes (Brooks, Spillane, Dick, & Stuart-Shor, 2014). Underlying cognitive impairment predisposes the patient to postoperative delirium, which cascades to a host of adverse care trajectories such as longer hospitalization and ICU stay, higher costs, increased mortality, greater use of continuous sedation and physical restraints, increased unintended removal of catheters and self-extubation, functional decline, new institutionalization, and new onset of cognitive impairment (Balas et al., 2012; Brooks, 2012). A narrative review of 54 studies of surgical patients older than 60 years reported an adjusted *OR* of 17 (CI [1.2–239.8]; $p < .05$), associating preoperative cognitive impairment with postoperative delirium (Oresanya et al., 2014).

Current best practice guidelines recommend the use of validated clinical protocols to assist in preventing episodes of delirium. Specialized delirium units that concentrate on assessment of delirium risk factors and targeted risk-factor modification represent a best practice model and should be a mainstay of clinical care (Sieber & Barnett, 2011). Because of its significant impact, preoperative discussions among patients, their families, and providers may include the use of preoperative delirium prophylaxis. Findings from a meta-analysis suggest that perioperative use of prophylactic antipsychotics may effectively reduce the overall risk of postoperative delirium in the elderly (Teslyar et al., 2013). In all decisions, patients' preference must be taken into account. See Chapter 17, "Delirium: Prevention, Early Recognition, and Treatment," for more detailed discussion and current guidelines.

Pain Management

There is evidence that pain management of older adults is inadequate, particularly among the cognitively impaired and those with altered mental states, in spite of the availability of validated tools for pain assessment and management (Schofield, 2014). High compliance with implementation of assessment tools will result in increased identification of postoperative pain as well as delirium (Brooks et al., 2014). The American Society of PeriAnesthesia Nurses (ASPAN) has issued guidelines on how to manage pain and promote comfort (ASPAN, 2003). Please refer to Chapter 18, "Pain Management," for a detailed discussion of pain in older adults.

Medication Reconciliation and Perioperative Beta Blocker

Medication reconciliation of perioperative older adults should pay close attention to making sure that beta blockers are part of the patient's ongoing medications. The Beers Criteria for Potentially Inappropriate Medication Use in Older Adults (American Geriatrics Society [AGS], 2012) should be used as a guide in reviewing medications during medication reconciliation and bedside rounds. The continuation of beta blocker therapy perioperatively decreases the risk of in-hospital death among high-risk, but not low-risk, patients undergoing major noncardiac surgery. Patient safety may be enhanced by increasing the use of beta blockers in high-risk patients (Lindenauer et al., 2005). For patients who cannot take oral beta blockers, the intravenous equivalent needs to be given.

Postoperative and Postdischarge Nausea and Vomiting

The ASPAN has published practice guidelines on how to manage the common perioperative complication of nausea and vomiting. Potential trajectories of postoperative nausea and vomiting (PONV) and postdischarge nausea and vomiting (PDNV) include aspiration, wound dehiscence, prolonged postoperative hospital stays, unanticipated hospital admission after outpatient surgery, delayed return of a patient's functional ability in the 24-hour period after surgery, and lost time from work for patients and care providers at home (ASPAN, 2006). A weblink to the ASPAN guidelines is provided in Protocol 32.1 practice guidelines section.

GENERAL PERIOPERATIVE CONSIDERATIONS

A Culture of Safety

Maintaining safety and quality patient care in a high-stress environment, such as the perioperative unit, enables the unit to flourish in a culture of safety based on nonpunitive principles. The use of an evidence-based teamwork system to improve communication and collaborative skills (e.g., TeamSTEPPS) will empower staff to self-advocate for safety (Agency for Healthcare Research and Quality [AHRQ], n.d.). Nurse-led initiatives, such as unit practice councils and appointing "champions" for specific perioperative core measures, are essential in this process (Institute for Healthcare Improvement [IHI], n.d.). Hardwiring a culture of safety would require a concerted systematic approach across all levels of care.

Handoff Communication

The transition between preoperative (preop) to postoperative (postop) is a high-stake event that might require multiple location changes (from the admitting area to the holding area, from the OR to the postanesthesia care unit [PACU], from the PACU to the surgical ward or specialty care units, from the surgical inpatient unit to a rehabilitation unit and other transitions). Essential to safe transition is high-quality handoff. This is defined as "the process of transferring primary authority and responsibility for providing clinical care to a patient from one departing caregiver to one oncoming caregiver" (Patterson & Wears, 2010, p. 53). Handoff communication has now become a proxy measure of the overall communication quality among providers (Riesenberg, Leisch, & Cunningham, 2010).

The Joint Commission accreditation evaluates the effectiveness of communication among caregivers as part of its National Patient Safety Goals (TJC, 2015). Perioperative sentinel event (e.g., resulting in death or permanent loss of function) data root-cause analysis from 2004 to 2014 reveals communication failure and human factors as leading causes of errors (greater than 60%) in anesthesia-related events, wrong-site/procedures; operative and postoperative complications, transfer-related events, transfusion-related events, and unintended retention of foreign object events (TJC, 2014a). Communication skills have been measured as the worst aspect of teamwork behavior in the OR (Wahr et al., 2013).

Although handoff varies according to unique institution process (e.g., use of electronic health record), it is imperative to use a standardized form or checklist coupled with preoperative and postoperative debriefings (Wahr et al., 2013). The Association of periOperative Registered Nurses (AORN) website has extensive resources and tools to guide design and implementation of quality handoff (AORN, 2012). For guidance on how to implement quality-improvement projects in handoff, the Handoff Communications Targeted Solutions Tool by TJC is an excellent starting point (see the Resources section for the website).

SSI Prevention

SSIs are reported to be the most prevalent health care–associated infections (HAIs), accounting for 31% of all HAIs among hospitalized patients (Magill et al., 2012). HAI is estimated to affect 2% to 5% of inpatient surgery, with 3% mortality, while increasing the risk of death two to 11 times compared to those who did not acquire an SSI (Anderson et al., 2014). *Staphylococcus aureus* is the most common pathogen causing SSIs, accounting for 30% of SSIs in the United States (Bratzler et al., 2013). Standards and guidelines to prevent SSI have been espoused by the Surgical Care Improvement Project (SCIP) supported by key stakeholders. Comprehensive SSI prevention strategies include well-established measures, such as surgical hand asepsis and other collaborative measures, such as antibiotic prophylaxis, glycemic control, maintaining normothermia, and skin and bowel prep (Fry, 2008). A comprehensive policy on SSI prevention includes environmental and engineering policies such as keeping the OR doors closed during surgery except as needed for passage of equipment, personnel, and the patient (Berríos-Torres, 2009). The CDC standard and transmission-based precautions should be followed where applicable. See Protocol 32.1 for SSI practice guidelines.

Deep Vein Thrombosis Prophylaxis

Venous thromboembolism (VTE) is defined as having either a DVT and/or a PE (He et al., 2014). The rate of postoperative VTE after hip-fracture surgery is low, estimated at 1.34%, 95% (CI [1.04–1.64]) with PE actuarial rate of 0.25% at 3 months; however, the overall mortality is 14.7% (Rosencher et al., 2005). Indeed, hip fracture patients belong to a vulnerable group of old people with comorbid diseases that put them at a high risk of postoperative VTE morbidity and mortality. Residents in long-term care (LTC) facilities and hospitals account for about 60% of diagnosed VTE events (Heit et al., 2002).

Well-known risk factors for VTE include advanced age; obesity; trauma; hypertension; those with a diagnosis of cancer, congestive heart failure, chronic obstructive pulmonary disease, or chronic kidney disease, especially nephrotic syndrome; trauma; and those undergoing major surgery, including laparoscopic surgery (Buesing, Mullapudi, & Flowers, 2015). Appropriate screening using evidence-based clinical decision rules (CDRs) is warranted among perioperative older adults (Siccama et al., 2011) in the light of the 2008 Surgeon General's office call to action to prevent the estimated 350,000 to 600,000 annual VTE cases in the United States (Leavitt, 2008). To maintain the safety and reduce harm, nurses need to observe TJC's guidelines related to the use of anticoagulants (TJC, 2015). VTE prophylaxis should be initiated 24 hours before surgery and continued thereafter as clinically indicated (Cataife, Weinberg, Wong, & Kahn, 2014; TJC, 2014b).

Special Population: Bariatric Surgery

Current U.S. estimates indicate approximately one third of persons older than 65 years are obese (CDC, 2012). As result, there is a consequent rise of bariatric surgery among this age group (Dorman et al., 2012). Although there has been some debate on the safety of bariatric surgery among older adults, a systematic review and meta-analysis declared the procedure to be safe for those 55 years and older (Lynch & Belgaumkar, 2012). VTE prophylaxis is essential in the perioperative management of bariatric surgery patients (Buesing et al., 2015).

Preoperative Fasting Guidelines

Traditional practice of not letting patients eat or drink after midnight ("NPO after midnight") before general anesthesia aims to reduce the volume and acidity of stomach contents during surgery, thus reducing the risk of regurgitation or aspiration. Prolonged fasting has been associated with adverse physical and psychological perioperative complications such as irritability, headache, dehydration, emesis, hypotension, hypovolemia, and hypoglycemia (Brady, Kinn, & Stuart, 2003).

Current guidelines recommend fasting of 2 hours for clear liquid and 6 hours for a light meal (ASA, 2011). Nurses need to get familiarized with institutional fasting procedures and be proactive in evaluating outdated policies that might impact the well-being of older adult patients. Another important consideration is determining which medications (e.g., beta blockers) the patient should continue taking in spite of fasting requirements.

Surgery and Do-Not-Resuscitate Orders

Although information on advance directives, such as health care proxies, is now routinely collected during patient interviews, the discussion on do not resuscitate (DNR) orders remains a sensitive topic. This highlights the importance of clear communication among the patient or designated surrogate and the provider. According to a position statement by the American College of Surgeons (ACS):

> Once a decision is reached on the patient's DNR status . . . the surgeon must continue his or her leadership role in the following areas: (1) documenting

and conveying the patient's advance directive and DNR status to the members of the operating room team; (2) helping the operating room team members understand and interpret the patient's advance directive; and (3) if necessary, finding an alternate team member to replace an individual who has an ethical or professional conflict with the patient's advance directive instructions. (ACS, 2014)

The nursing staff provides high-quality care regardless of the patient's DNR status. Nurses need to communicate advance directive information during handoff and care transitions. In patient teaching, nurses may interpret for the patient and designated surrogate unfamiliar language of advance directives and related institutional policies.

CASE STUDY

Mr. P is an 85-year-old male patient who was brought in by ambulance after falling in his apartment, where he lives alone. He reported to have slipped while getting out of bed. He remained conscious but felt pain on his right hip. He denied headache, loss of consciousness, chest pain, palpitation, and dizziness. After he managed to get up from the floor, he called his son on the phone who, in turn, called the emergency medical service (EMS). Mr. P's past medical history includes coronary artery disease (CAD), coronary artery bypass graft in 2005, atrial fibrillation (on Coumadin), permanent pacemaker, peripheral vascular disease, end-stage renal disease (ESRD; on hemodialysis on Mondays, Wednesdays, and Fridays), and anemia of chronic disease. He has an allergy to sulfa drugs (rash). Mr. P is a resident of an assisted living facility.

On arrival to the ED, he was awake, alert, and oriented to self and place, but not to time. His right arm and forehead have multiple bruises and abrasions. Up until very recently, he has been mostly independent in performing his activities of daily living (ADL) and can ambulate using a walker. He gets physical therapy at home five times a week and his last hospitalization was 6 months ago for pneumonia.

In the ED, his vital signs were as follows: blood pressure (BP): 124/76 mmHg, heart rate (HR): 60 per minute (paced rhythm), respiratory rate (RR): 17 regular, temperature: 36.9°C, and his oxygen saturation was 97% on room air. His current body mass index (BMI) is 25. His physical examination was unremarkable other than an external rotation and abduction of his right leg and exertional pain on the right hip area (6/10) as well as bruising on the hip area. An x-ray of the right hip revealed a comminuted intertrochanteric fracture with mild displacement of bone fragments. The head CT scan showed no evidence of acute intracranial trauma. Mr. P has a right brachial arteriovenous fistula for dialysis. His baseline lab values are shown in Table 32.2.

TABLE 32.2
Mr. P's Current Lab Results

Na: 139 mEq/L	WBC: 6.9 × 10^3/μL	Albumin: 3.6 g/dL
K: 4.6 mEq/L	Hemoglobin: 11.1 g/dL	Calcium: 10 mg/dL
Cl: 98 mEq/L	Hematocrit: 34.1%	Magnesium: 2.0 mEq/L
CO_2: 25 mEq/L	Platelets: 140 × 10^9/L	Phosphorus: 4.0 mg/dL
BUN: 40 mg/dL	Prothrombin time: 25.4 seconds	Troponin: 0.2 μg/L
Creatinine: 4.0 mg/dL	INR: 2.2	

BUN, blood urea nitrogen; Cl, chlorine; CO_2, carbon dioxide; INR, international normalized ratio; K, potassium; Na, sodium; WBC, white blood cells.

Mr. P's current home medications include Coumadin, sevelamer carbonate, Zyrtec, baby aspirin, docusate sodium, Senna, and multivitamins. He denied alcohol or other chemical dependency issues. His son, who is named in the patient's health care proxy, lives nearby and is actively involved in his care.

Discussion

1. What are the priority assessments and interventions for Mr. P in the ED?

   Given that Mr. P was not in acute distress and his vital signs were stable when he arrived in the ED, the care team would conduct a comprehensive geriatric assessment and request consult with an orthopedic surgeon as soon as possible. If available within the facility, a call for a geriatric consult (MD or APRN [advanced practice registered nurse]) should also be arranged. Assessment and evaluation of his right hip pain should be performed. The choice for pain medication needs to take into consideration his ESRD. For mild to moderate pain, acetaminophen may be prescribed. Drugs, such as meperidine and ketorolac, are best avoided in treating pain in older adult patients. Nonpharmacologic

(continued)

CASE STUDY *(continued)*

interventions for pain should also be explored. Because of Mr. P's elevated international normalized ratio (INR), his Coumadin should be stopped and he should be monitored for bleeding, including changes in neurological status. In anticipation for surgery, his aspirin should also be held.

Preoperative Optimization

2. Describe the best practices for preoperative optimization for Mr. P.

Maintaining patient safety is a priority for Mr. P. Once a hospital bed has been assigned, he should be transferred as soon as possible. Stabilizing his fracture might require the use of an abduction pillow. A bedside discussion with his son and the orthopedic surgeon determined that a closed reduction and intramedullary nailing will be performed once the INR is less than 1.5 and a cardiology clearance is obtained. Mr. P expressed optimism and understanding of the operative procedure and he signed the consent himself.

A comprehensive preoperative workup should include assessment of Mr. P's cognitive status (using the Mini-Cog tool), depression screening, and identifying risk factors for developing postoperative delirium. The cardiology consult would entail obtaining a 12-lead EKG, serial Troponin, an echocardiogram, and a chest x-ray. Mr. P's telemetry reading shows a paced rhythm. Routine blood tests would include a complete blood count, renal profile, and coagulation profile. In anticipation of possible fresh frozen plasma (FFP) transfusion, a blood type and screen would be needed. A urinalysis is not recommended because Mr. P is anuric and has no risk of urinary tract infection. Mr. P's current lab values are consistent with his ESRD diagnosis with no critical levels requiring immediate intervention.

Initial medication reconciliation revealed Mr. P takes metoprolol 25 mg twice a day, though this was not reflected in his original list of medications. Metoprolol is added to his current medication orders. A physical therapy consult determined a plan for postop bedside therapy. As a result of increased risk of VTE, pneumatic sequential compression sleeves were applied. Because of his ESRD, heparin 5,000 units every 12 hours, instead of low-molecular-weight heparin, was ordered for VTE prophylaxis.

Bedside hemodialysis was scheduled and a renal/cardiac diet was ordered. To optimize and to prevent further reduction of physiologic reserve, it is essential that Mr. P consumes enough calories and adequate hydration within the context of his ESRD. A nutrition consultation recommended two cans per day of high-calorie supplemental drink for renal patients and multivitamins. It is important that the nursing staff assist and encourage Mr. P to eat. Nursing handoff should include findings on how well Mr. P is meeting caloric requirements as well as intake and output balance. Taking all the relevant clinical data, a frailty score can be calculated for Mr. P and this information should be shared during interprofessional rounds.

Intraoperative Considerations

Five days after admission, Mr. P was scheduled for a 9 a.m. closed reduction and intramedullary nailing under general anesthesia. Hemodialysis was done in the late afternoon before surgery. His latest INR was 1.4. He did not require any FFP transfusion and his vital signs reflected baseline patterns. He remained alert and oriented to self, place, and time. Morphine 2 mg intravenous (IV) push every 4 hours as needed was ordered for pain, although Mr. P hardly requested medication for pain. The nursing staff continued to perform turning every 2 hours to prevent pressure ulcers.

3. Describe safety and quality benchmarks for the care of older adults within the intraoperative continuum.

A standardized electronic preoperative checklist was used to ensure that key assessment parameters were met. A copy of the consent was kept in the chart. The nursing staff verified that Mr. P had correct name and allergy bands. On the evening before the surgery, patient education using teach-back was reinforced to verify Mr. P's comprehension of the procedure. This is also an opportunity to reinforce postoperative teaching topics, such as using the incentive spirometer, and to provide reassurance to the patient and family. Mr. P was informed that he could continue to drink and eat a light meal after midnight if desired. He was notified that in the morning he could take his metoprolol with a sip of water. Parameters for withholding the metoprolol dose have been included in the medication order.

The nursing care focus was to allow Mr. P a restful night, continue VTE prophylaxis using the pneumatic sleeves, discontinue heparin the day before surgery, and continue delirium surveillance. The nurse anesthetist and orthopedic surgeon examined

(continued)

CASE STUDY *(continued)*

Mr. P and reviewed his latest lab values. Based on the nature of the procedure, hair removal was not indicated. A gauge-22 IV needle was placed on his left arm for intermittent or emergency use. The patient care technician assisted Mr. P with his bedbath.

An RN-to-RN handoff report using a standardized form took place before Mr. P was picked up for the OR. His son and grandson accompanied him to the OR entrance and were notified where to wait until Mr. P's return from the PACU. During the bedside handoff, the plan of care was communicated using the electronic health record.

Within 60 minutes before the surgical incision, Mr. P received an IV infusion of cefazolin (adjusted renal dose based on his latest glomerular filtration rate [GFR]) with no untoward reactions. Throughout his stay in the OR, his temperature was kept within normal limits through the use of warm blankets and a head covering. The circulating nurse made sure that the SCIP Core Measures were followed at all times.

Immediate Postoperative Considerations

4. Discuss key parameters of assessment and intervention of older adults in PACU.

When the surgery was completed, an RN-to-RN handoff report took place using a standardized form. On arrival to the PACU, the priority focus was to maintain a patent airway and adequate oxygenation because Mr. P was just extubated. Mr. P's vital signs, telemetry rhythm, and pain were assessed, followed by a comprehensive head-to-toe examination, focusing on the surgical site and signs of delirium. A warming blanket was used to maintain Mr. P's temperature at greater than or equal to 96.8°F. Pneumatic sequential compression devices for both legs were continued. The RN reviewed Mr. P's current medication orders particularly focusing on starting the patient-controlled analgesia (PCA) morphine and continuation of beta blockers. Cefazolin 1 g IV piggyback once daily was to be continued for another 24 hours. During his stay in the PACU, Mr. P was monitored for signs of pain, agitation, and delirium using validated tools such as the confusion assessment method for the ICU (CAM-ICU). The PACU nurse notified Mr. P's family of his current status and his expected return to his surgical room.

SUMMARY

The perioperative period is a highly vulnerable time for older adults. Safe, quality patient care requires meaningful implementation of various evidence-based guidelines discussed in this chapter. The benefits of high-quality interprofessional team collaboration cannot be overemphasized. Regardless of the type of surgery, a comprehensive plan of care that takes into account the patient's values and preferences is desirable. Meeting the various perioperative core measures unique to the older adult population will rely on a seamless, albeit challenging, synthesis of various specialty practice recommendations, models of care, and understanding of geriatric syndromes; as well as clinical judgment and provider expertise.

NURSING STANDARD OF PRACTICE

Protocol 32.1: Perioperative Care of the Older Adult

I. GOAL

To restore physiological stability, prevent complications, maintain comfort and safety, and preserve pre-illness functional ability and QOL in older adults throughout the perioperative continuum

II. OVERVIEW

A. About one third of all procedures and one half of surgical procedures on the cardiovascular and digestive systems in nonfederal short-term hospitals were performed on inpatients aged 65 years and above (Hall et al., 2010).
B. A 10% increase in the proportion of staff nurses holding a bachelor's degree is associated with a 7% decrease in the risk of death among patients following common surgeries in an acute care setting (Aiken et al., 2014).

(continued)

Protocol 32.1: Perioperative Care of the Older Adult *(continued)*

C. Lower rates of postoperative VTE and shorter length of stay have also been found in hospitals with a higher percentage of RNs with baccalaureate or higher degrees (Blegen et al., 2013).
D. Comprehensive preoperative geriatric assessment correlates with positive postoperative outcomes in older patients (Partridge et al., 2014).

III. BACKGROUND

A. Definition
   1. *Perioperative nursing* is defined as the "delivery of comprehensive care within preoperative, intraoperative and postoperative periods of the patient's experience during operative and other invasive procedure" (Steelman, 2015, p. 1). The high-stake demands of perioperative patient care, the increasing number of older adults undergoing surgery, and the unique vulnerabilities of this population require the translation of science-based interprofessional collaboration. The use of the nursing process, critical thinking, and evidence-based practice models will ensure patient safety and quality for older adult patients and their families.
B. Etiology/epidemiology
   1. The demand for surgical procedures is expected to rise with the aging population.
   2. In 2010, 19.2 million surgeries were performed among patients 65 years and older (CDC, 2010).
   3. Procedures that place the patient at the most risk include those that involve general anesthesia or deep sedation (TJC, 2015).
   4. Failure-to-rescue was more than two times higher in patients older than 75 years compared with those younger than 75 years (26.0% vs. 10.3% at high-mortality hospitals, $p < .001$; Sheetz et al., 2014).
   5. Death (failure-to-rescue) among surgical inpatients with treatable serious complications and the percentage of major surgical inpatients who experience hospital-acquired complications (e.g., sepsis, pneumonia, gastrointestinal bleeding, shock/cardiac arrest, VTE) are nursing-sensitive measures and publicly reportable events (NQF, 2004).
   6. A 10% increase in the proportion of staff nurses with bachelor's degree is associated with a 7% decrease in the risk of death among patients following common surgeries in an acute care setting (Aiken et al., 2014).
   7. Lower postoperative VTE and shorter length of stay are associated with higher percentage of RNs with baccalaureate or higher degrees (Blegen et al., 2013).
   8. Perioperative beta blocker therapy is associated with a reduced risk of in-hospital death among high-risk, but not low-risk, patients undergoing major noncardiac surgery. Patient safety may be enhanced by increasing the use of beta blockers in high-risk patients (Lindenauer et al., 2005)

IV. PARAMETERS OF ASSESSMENT

A. The ACS-NSQIP and the AGS's *Best Practices Guidelines for Optimal Preoperative Assessment of the Geriatric Surgical Patient* recommend the following preoperative assessment parameters (Chow et al., 2012):
   1. Assess the patient's cognitive ability and capacity to understand the anticipated surgery.
   2. Screen the patient for depression.
   3. Identify the patient's risk factors for developing postoperative delirium.
   4. Screen for alcohol and other substance abuse/dependence.
   5. Perform a preoperative cardiac evaluation according to the ACC/AHA algorithm for patients undergoing noncardiac surgery.
   6. Identify the patient's risk factors for postoperative pulmonary complications and implement appropriate strategies for prevention.
   7. Document functional status and history of falls.
   8. Determine baseline frailty score.
   9. Assess patient's nutritional status and consider preoperative interventions if the patient is at severe nutritional risk.
   10. Take an accurate and detailed medication history and consider appropriate perioperative adjustments. Monitor for polypharmacy.

(continued)

Protocol 32.1: Perioperative Care of the Older Adult *(continued)*

11. Determine the patient's treatment goals and expectations in the context of the possible treatment outcomes.
12. Determine patient's family and social support system.
13. Order appropriate preoperative diagnostic tests based on unique clinical scenarios of elderly patients.

B. For comprehensive preoperative evaluation, the provider should inquire about symptoms, such as angina, dyspnea, syncope, and palpitations, as well as history of heart disease, including ischemic, valvular, or myopathic disease; and history of hypertension, diabetes, chronic kidney disease, and cerebrovascular or peripheral artery disease (Bilimoria et al., 2013).

C. For geriatric fracture patients, recommended preoperative optimization focus includes (Nicholas, 2014a):
  1. Assurance of adequate intravascular volume
  2. Medication adjustment in anticipation of intraoperative hypotension
  3. Judicious continuation of beta blockers and other antiarrhythmic chronotropic drugs for selected patients
  4. Pain management
  5. Prevention of polypharmacy and excessive laboratory testing

D. Orthopedic surgery services should ensure that patients are operated within 1 or 2 days of admission when cleared for surgery (Moja et al., 2012).

E. In patients assessed to be at intermediate or high cardiovascular risk, a referral to a cardiologist for further evaluation is recommended (Fleisher et al., 2014).

F. Adjust dose of medications according to renal function using GFR parameters.

G. Implement the 2014 SCIP Core Measure Set (TJC, 2014b)
  1. Prophylactic antibiotic received within 1 hour before surgical incision
  2. Prophylactic antibiotics discontinued within 24 hours after surgery end time
  3. Cardiac surgery patients with controlled postoperative blood glucose
  4. Surgery patients with appropriate hair removal
  5. Urinary catheter removed on POD 1 or 2 with day of surgery being day 0
  6. Perioperative temperature management
  7. Those who were under beta blocker therapy before arrival received a beta blocker during the perioperative period.
  8. Received appropriate VTE prophylaxis within 24 hours before surgery to 24 hours after surgery

H. Improve medication safety within the perioperative settings by (TJC, 2015)
  1. Label all medications, medication containers, and other solutions on and off the sterile field in perioperative and other procedural settings.
  2. Label medications and solutions that are not immediately administered. This applies even if there is only one medication being used.
  3. Label any medication or solution transferred from the original packaging to another container.
  4. Verify all medication or solution labels both verbally and visually.
  5. Label each medication or solution as soon as it is prepared, unless it is immediately administered.
  6. Discard immediately any medication found unlabeled.
  7. Remove all labeled containers on the sterile field and discard their contents at the conclusion of the procedure.
  8. Review all medications and solutions both on and off the sterile field.

I. Implement SSI prevention guidelines (TJC, 2015)
  1. Educate staff and licensed independent practitioners involved in surgical procedures about SSIs and the importance of prevention.
  2. Educate patients who are undergoing a surgical procedure and their families about SSI prevention as needed.
  3. Implement policies and practices aimed at reducing the risk of SSI.
  4. Conduct periodic risk assessments for SSI.
  5. Select SSI measures using best practices or evidence-based guidelines.
  6. Monitor compliance with best practices or evidence-based guidelines.
  7. Evaluate the effectiveness of prevention efforts.

(continued)

Protocol 32.1: Perioperative Care of the Older Adult *(continued)*

J. Consistently implement TJC's Time Out and Universal Protocol guidelines that include the following (TJC, 2015):
   1. Implement a preprocedure process to verify the correct procedure, for the correct patient, at the correct site. Involve the patient in the verification process when possible.
   2. Identify the items that must be available for the procedure and use a standardized list to verify their availability.
   3. Match the items that are to be available in the procedure area to the patient.
   4. Identify those procedures that require marking of the incision or insertion site. At a minimum, sites are marked when there is more than one possible location for the procedure and when performing the procedure in a different location would negatively affect quality or safety.
   5. Mark the procedure site before the procedure is performed and, if possible, with the patient involved.

V. NURSING CARE STRATEGIES

Synthesis of perioperative best practices guidelines (AORN, 2006; Bratzler, et al., 2013; Chow et al., 2012; Fleisher et al., 2014; TJC, 2014b, 2015) provides collaborative nursing opportunities across the perioperative continuum.

A. Preoperative
   1. Perform a comprehensive assessment: history and physical examination, cognitive and functional assessment, medication reconciliation, nutrition, advance directives, and so on, using validated tools and checklists (Chow et al., 2012).
   2. Collect nursing-sensitive data during interview with patient and family.
   3. Review, document, and interpret pertinent laboratory and diagnostic findings, specific to patient's clinical scenario.
   4. Assess, review, and document vital signs, including glucose finger stick (e.g., blood sugar goal) and other disease-specific lab values as appropriate.
   5. Educate patient and family using teach-back method on routine (e.g., consent, fasting requirement [2 hours for clear liquid and 6 hours for light meal], patient escort) and special topics (e.g., bowel preparation or withholding specific drugs, such as Metformin, after an angiogram).
   6. Conduct medication reconciliation (TJC, 2015), focusing on Beers Criteria for Potentially Inappropriate Medication Use in Older Adults (AGS, 2012).
   7. Evaluate use of cardiac drugs throughout perioperative continuum. In particular, the guidelines for perioperative use of beta blockers recommend to (Fleisher et al, 2014):
      a. Continue beta blockers, particularly those with independent cardiac indications such as arrhythmia or history of myocardial infarction.
      b. Continue beta blockers in patients undergoing intermediate risk or vascular surgery with known coronary artery disease or with multiple clinical risk factors for ischemic heart disease.
      c. Titrate to a heart rate of 60 to 80 beats per minute in the absence of hypotension.
      d. Titrated rate control with beta blockers should continue during the intraoperative and postoperative periods.
      e. Beta blockers should be tapered off slowly to minimize risk of withdrawal.
   8. Inform patient or caregiver to bring all home medications on the day of procedure, especially for outpatient same-day surgery.
   9. Reinforce appropriate VTE prophylaxis within 24 hours before surgery (Cataife et al., 2014; TJC, 2014b).
   10. Facilitate appropriate hair removal before surgery (TJC, 2014b).

B. Intraoperative
   1. Participate in interprofessional Time Out and handoff procedure.
   2. Safely administer antibiotics within 60 minutes before surgical incision. For some agents that require longer administration time, such as fluoroquinolones and vancomycin, infusion can begin 120 minutes before incision. Redosing of antibiotic is recommended if the procedure exceeds two half-lives of the drug or if there is excessive blood loss during surgery (Bratzler et al., 2013).
   2. Safely administer beta blocker during the perioperative period if applicable.
   3. Assess and manage patient temperature intraoperatively (e.g., active warming to maintain greater than or equal to 96.8°F 30 minutes before anesthesia or 15 minutes postanesthesia end time).
   4. Maintain asepsis and sterility of the operative field.

(continued)

Protocol 32.1: Perioperative Care of the Older Adult *(continued)*

5. Keep OR doors closed during surgery except as needed for passage of equipment, personnel, and the patient (Berríos-Torres, 2009).
6. Monitor intraoperative systems processes throughout the procedure.
7. Follow procedure and policy related to prevention on unintended retention of foreign objects intraoperatively.
8. Follow CDC infection control guidelines in handling infectious materials (e.g., specimen, equipment).

C. Immediate postoperative period (PACU)
   1. Perform high-quality handoff during care transitions (e.g., between the OR and PACU using standardized forms or checklists (TJC, 2015).
   2. Maintain patient safety during transfer.
   3. Monitor vital signs per institution protocol, including hemodynamic profile and glucose finger stick, if applicable.
   4. Assess and document pain, including pharmacologic and nonpharmacologic interventions.
   5. Maintain patient temperature at greater than or equal to 96.8°F.
   6. Monitor blood sugar as clinically applicable (e.g., SCIP measure for cardiac surgery patients is to keep serum glucose greater than or equal to 200 mg/dL 18 to 24 hours postoperation [Fry, 2008]).
   7. Monitor patient's GFR, assess patient's urine output and weight; and follow standard protocol/procedures in administering nephrotoxic medications.
   8. Coordinate medication reconciliation, with special attention to beta blockers (TJC, 2015) and antidiabetic medications.
   9. Implement safe VTE prophylaxis within 24 hours before surgery or 24 hours postoperation (e.g., compression stockings or pneumatic compression devices, heparin, low-dose heparin; Buesing et al., 2015; TJC, 2014b).
   10. Protect primary closure incisions with sterile dressing for 24 to 48 hours postoperation (Fry, 2008).
   11. Discontinue antibiotics within 24 hours after surgery end time (48 hours for cardiac surgery; Fry, 2008).
   12. Provide timely and accurate information to patient and family members.
   13. Resume diet as clinically appropriate.

VI. EVALUATION/EXPECTED OUTCOMES

A. Patient outcomes
   1. Maintain patient safety across the perioperative continuum.
   2. Assess patient decision-making capacity and honor patient and family care decision choices.
   3. Receive a comprehensive preoperative screening, including, but not limited to, the following domains: cognitive and behavioral, cardiopulmonary, functional status, nutrition, medication, and frailty.
   4. Undergo clinically relevant preoperative testing (e.g., blood, urine, radiologic, EKG, etc.) based on best practice evidence (see ACS-NSQIP/AGS Best Practice Guidelines Optimal Preoperative Assessment of the Geriatric Surgical Patient).
   5. Optimize function across the perioperative continuum.
   6. Receive timely and accurate information related to plan of care, including transitional care and long-term follow-up.
   7. Patient will not develop postoperative complications such as SSI, DVT, cardiopulmonary adverse events, falls, and pressure ulcers.
   8. Patient will be free from adverse events such as medication errors, wrong site-procedure events, anesthesia-related events, and issues.

B. Provider outcomes
   1. Receive education and ongoing training on best practices in the care of the geriatric surgical patient.
   2. Assess patient's decision-making capacity and obtain informed consent.
   3. Implement latest guidelines for antimicrobial prophylaxis in surgery (e.g., receive antibiotics within 60 minutes before surgical incision).
   4. Participate in high-quality interprofessional collaboration across the perioperative continuum including rounding, handoff, Time Out/Universal Protocol, pain management, SSI prevention, early mobility, nutrition, medication reconciliation, and transitional care.

(continued)

Protocol 32.1: Perioperative Care of the Older Adult *(continued)*

5. Use an evidence-based teamwork system to improve communication and teamwork skills (e.g., TeamSTEPPS) for patient safety (AHRQ, n.d.).
6. Apply teach-back method in all patient education encounters that are culturally competent and patient centered.
7. Employ consistent and accurate documentation of care throughout the perioperative continuum.
8. Provide patient and caregivers timely and accurate information of patient's condition and plan of care, including care transitions.
9. Perioperative nurses achieve a minimum of bachelor's degree and obtain practice-specific certification (e.g., gerontological nursing, CNOR).
10. Organize and participate in unit-based practice and quality-improvement councils.

C. Systems outcomes
1. Uphold patient safety and quality in the care of older adults through policy and social statements (e.g., safety language in hospital's mission).
2. Review and align existing institutional policies and procedures with latest national standards (see Practice Guidelines section).
3. Facilitate and sustain interprofessional geriatrics care teams.
4. Monitor, evaluate, and disseminate hospital performance in perioperative benchmarks such as Time Out/Universal Protocol, antibiotic prophylaxis, DVT prophylaxis, and other site-specific parameters.
5. Establish a system of reporting patient safety issues (e.g., falls, medication errors, unintended retention of foreign object, wrong patient, wrong site, wrong procedure, etc.) across the perioperative continuum to identify opportunities for improvement.
6. Adopt specific patient safety initiatives for older adults that include use of informatics, algorithms, checklists, and personnel oversight.
7. Develop ongoing quality-improvement initiatives consistent with SCIP core measures and other practice guidelines.
8. Facilitate clinical rotation for nursing students across the perioperative units to promote experiential learning for prelicensure students.
9. Enforce SSI prevention policies and conduct SSI surveillance based on CDC and TJC guidelines.
10. Organize and support interprofessional unit-based practice and quality-improvement councils (IHI, n.d.).
11. Demonstrate a commitment to culture of safety based on openness and mutual trust (e.g., patient safety leadership walk rounds; IHI, n.d.).

VII. RELEVANT PRACTICE GUIDELINES

A. AORN Guidance Statement. (2006). Safe Medication Practices in Perioperative Settings Across the Life Span: www.aornjournal.org/article/S0001–2092(08)00719–9/pdf

B. ACC/AHA. (2014). Guideline on Perioperative Cardiovascular Evaluation and Management of Patients Undergoing Noncardiac Surgery. A Report of the American College of Cardiology/American Heart Association Task Force on Practice Guidelines:
content.onlinejacc.org/article.aspx?articleid=1893784

C. ACS-NSQIP and the AGS (2012). Best Practices Guidelines for Optimal Preoperative Assessment of the Geriatric Surgical Patient:
https://www.facs.org//media/files/quality%20programs/nsqip/acsnsqipagsgeriatric2012guidelines.ashx

D. ASHP (2013). Antimicrobial Prophylaxis in Surgery:
www.idsociety.org/uploadedFiles/IDSA/Guidelines-Patient_Care/PDF_Library/2013%20Surgical%20Prophylaxis%20ASHP,%20IDSA,%20SHEA,%20SIS(1).pdf

E. The Joint Commission. (2015). National Patient Safety Goals:
www.jointcommission.org/assets/1/6/2015_NPSG_HAP.pdf

F. PeriAnesthesia Pain and Comfort Clinical Guidelines (ASPAN):
www.aspan.org/Clinical-Practice/Clinical-Guidelines/Pain-and-Comfort

(continued)

Protocol 32.1: Perioperative Care of the Older Adult *(continued)*

G. PONV/PDNV Guidelines: www.aspan.org/Portals/6/docs/ClinicalPractice/Guidelines/PONV-PDNV_Clinical_Guideline_Aug_2006_JoPAN.pdf
H. 2014 SCIP Core Measure Set: www.jointcommission.org/assets/1/6/SCIP-Measures-012014.pdf
I. AORN. (2015). Guidelines for Perioperative Practice: www.aorn.org/guidelines/#NewIn2015
J. ASA. (2011). Practice Guidelines for Preoperative Fasting and the Use of Pharmacologic Agents to Reduce the Risk of Pulmonary Aspiration: Application to Healthy Patients Undergoing Elective Procedures.
K. VTE Prophylaxis Guidelines for Surgical Patients: www.clinicalkey.com/#!/content/playContent/1-s2.0-S0039610914002126

ABBREVIATIONS

ACC/AHA	American College of Cardiology/American Heart Association
ACS-NSQIP	American College of Surgeons—National Surgical Quality Improvement Program
AGS	American Geriatrics Society
AORN	Association of periOperative Registered Nurses
ASA	American Society of Anesthesiologists
ASHP	American Society of Health-System Pharmacists
ASPAN	American Society of PeriAnesthesia Nurses
CDC	Centers for Disease Control and Prevention
CNOR	Operative Nursing Certification
DVT	Deep vein thrombosis
GFR	Glomerular filtration rate
OR	Odds ratio
PACU	Postanesthesia care unit
POD	Postoperative day
PONV/PDNV	Postoperative and postdischarge nausea and vomiting
QOL	Quality of life
SCIP	Surgical Care Improvement Project
SSI	Surgical site infection
TJC	The Joint Commission
VTE	Venous thromboembolism

RESOURCES

ACS NSQIP Surgical Risk Calculator
http://riskcalculator.facs.org

Advancing Effective Communication, Cultural Competence, and Patient- and Family-Centered Care (Joint Commission)
http://www.jointcommission.org/assets/1/6/ARoadmapforHospitalsfinalversion727.pdf

American Geriatrics Society (AGS) Updated Beers Criteria for Potentially Inappropriate Medication Use in Older Adults
http://onlinelibrary.wiley.com/doi/10.1111/j.1532-5415.2012.03923.x/pdf

American Society of PeriAnesthesia Nurses (ASPAN)
http://www.aspan.org

Association of periOperative Registered Nurses (AORN)
https://www.aorn.org

Institute for Healthcare Improvement (IHI)—Develop a Culture of Safety
http://www.ihi.org/resources/Pages/Changes/DevelopaCultureofSafety.aspx

Online Vascular Surgery Clinical Calculators
http://www.qxmd.com/calculate-online/vascular-surgery

Perioperative Assessment of the Older Adult
http://consultgerirn.org/uploads/File/trythis/try_this_sp6.pdf

Perioperative Cardiac Risk Calculator
http://www.surgicalriskcalculator.com/miorcardiacarrest

Surgical Site Infection (SSI) Toolkit (CDC)
http://www.cdc.gov/HAI/pdfs/toolkits/SSI_toolkit021710SIBT_revised.pdf

Targeted Solutions Tool for Hand Hygiene, Hand-off Communications and Safe Surgery by The Joint Commission
http://www.centerfortransforminghealthcare.org/tst.aspx

REFERENCES

Agency for Healthcare Research and Quality (AHRQ). (n.d.). *TeamSTEPPS: National implementation.* Retrieved from http://teamstepps.ahrq.gov. *Evidence Level VI.*

Aiken, L. H., Clarke, S. P., Cheung, R. B., Sloane, D. M., & Silber, J. H. (2003). Educational levels of hospital nurses and surgical patient mortality. *Journal of the American Medical Association, 290*(12), 1617–1623. *Evidence Level IV.*

Aiken, L. H., Sloane, D. M., Bruyneel, L., Van den Heede, K., Griffiths, P., Busse, R.,... Sermeus, W. (2014). Nurse staffing and education and hospital mortality in nine European countries: A retrospective observational study. *Lancet, 383*(9931), 1824–1830. doi:10.1016/S0140–6736(13)62631–8. *Evidence Level IV.*

Algie, C. M., Mahar, R. K., Wasiak, J., Batty, L., Gruen, R. L., & Mahar, P. D. (2015). Interventions for reducing wrong-site surgery and invasive clinical procedures. *Cochrane Database of Systematic Reviews, 2015*(3), CD009404. doi:10.1002/14651858.CD009404.pub3. *Evidence Level I.*

American College of Surgeons (ACS). (2014). *Statement on advance directives by patients: "Do not resuscitate" in the operating room.* Retrieved from http://www.facs.org/aboutacs/statements/19-advance-directives. *Evidence Level VI.*

American Geriatrics Society (AGS). (2012). Updated Beers Criteria for potentially inappropriate medication use in older adults. *Journal of the American Geriatrics Society, 60*(4), 616–631. doi:10.1111/j.1532–5415.2012.03923.x. *Evidence Level VI.*

American Society of Anesthesiologists (ASA). (2011). Practice guidelines for preoperative fasting and the use of pharmacologic agents to reduce the risk of pulmonary aspiration: Application to healthy patients undergoing elective procedures: an updated report by the American Society of Anesthesiologists Committee on Standards and Practice Parameters. *Anesthesiology, 114*(3), 495–511. doi:10.1097/ALN.0b013e3181fcbfd9. *Evidence Level V.*

American Society of Health-System Pharmacists (ASHP). (2013). *Antimicrobial prophylaxis in surgery.* Retrieved from http://www.idsociety.org/uploadedFiles/IDSA/GuidelinesPatient_Care/PDF_Library/2013%20Surgical%20Prophylaxis%20ASHP,%20IDSA,%20SHEA,%20SIS(1).pdf. *Evidence Level V.*

American Society of PeriAnesthesia Nurses (ASPAN). (2003). *Pain and comfort clinical guidelines.* Retrieved from http://www.aspan.org/Portals/6/docs/ClinicalPractice/Guidelines/ASPAN_ClinicalGuideline_PainComfort.pdf. *Evidence Level V.*

American Society of PeriAnesthesia Nurses (ASPAN). (2006). ASPAN'S evidence-based clinical practice guideline for the prevention and/or management of PONV/PDNV. *Journal of PeriAnesthesia Nursing, 4*(21), 230–250. *Evidence Level V.*

Anderson, D. J., Kaye, K. S., Classen, D., Arias, K. M., Podgorny, K., Burstin, H.,... Yokoe, D. S. (2014). Strategies to prevent surgical site infections in acute care hospitals. *Infection Control and Hospital and Epidemiology, 35*(6), 605–627. doi:10.1086/676022. *Evidence Level V.*

Appelbaum, P. S., & Grisso, T. (1995). The MacArthur treatment competence study I: Mental illness and competence to consent to treatment. *Law and Human Behavior, 19*(2), 105. *Evidence Level IV.*

Association of periOperative Registered Nurses. (2006). AORN guidance statement: Safe medication practices in perioperative settings across the life span. *AORN Journal, 84*(2), 276–283. doi:http://dx.doi.org/10.1016/S0001-2092(06)60495-X. *Evidence Level VI.*

Association of periOperative Registered Nurses (AORN). (2012). *Patient hand-off tool kit.* Retrieved from http://www.aorn.org/toolkits/patienthandoff/. *Evidence Level VI.*

Association of periOperative Registered Nurses (AORN). (2015). *Comprehensive surgical checklist.* Retrieved from https://www.aorn.org/Clinical_Practice/ToolKits/Correct_Site_Surgery_Tool_Kit/Comprehensive_checklist.aspx. *Evidence Level VI.*

Aymanns, C., Keller, F., Maus, S., Hartmann, B., & Czock D. (2010). Review on pharmacokinetics and pharmacodynamics and the aging kidney. *Clinical Journal of the American Society of Nephrology, 5*(2), 314 –27. doi:10.2215/CJN.03960609. *Evidence Level IV.*

Balas, M. C., Rice, M., Chaperon, C., Smith, H., Disbot, M., & Fuchs, B. (2012). Management of delirium in critically ill older adults. *Critical Care Nurse, 32*(4), 15–26. doi:10.4037/ccn2012480. *Evidence Level V.*

Barton, C. D., Jr., Mallik, H. S., Orr, W. B., & Janofsky, J. S. (1996). Clinicians' judgment of capacity of nursing home patients to give informed consent. *Psychiatric Services, 47*(9), 956–960. *Evidence Level II.*

Bentov, I., & Reed, M. J. (2014). Anesthesia, microcirculation, and wound repair in aging. *Anesthesiology, 120*(3), 760–772. doi:10.1097/ALN.0000000000000036. *Evidence Level V.*

Berríos-Torres, S. I. (2009). *CDC surgical site infection (SSI) toolkit.* Retrieved from http://www.cdc.gov/HAI/pdfs/toolkits/SSI_toolkit021710SIBT_revised.pdf. *Evidence Level VI.*

Bertges, D. J., Goodney, P. P., Zhao, Y., Schanzer, A., Nolan, B. W., Likosky, D. S.,... Cronenwett, J. L.; Vascular Study Group of New England. (2010). The Vascular Study Group of New England Cardiac Risk Index (VSG-CRI) predicts cardiac complications more accurately than the Revised Cardiac Risk Index in vascular surgery patients. *Journal of Vascular Surgery, 52*(3), 674–683. doi:10.1016/j.jvs.2010.03.03. *Evidence Level IV.*

Bilimoria, K. Y., Liu, Y., Paruch, J. L., Zhou, L., Kmiecik, T. E., Ko, C. Y., & Cohen M. E. (2013). Development and evaluation of the universal ACS NSQIP surgical risk calculator: A decision aid and informed consent tool for patients and surgeons. *Journal of the American College of Surgeons, 217*(5), 833–842. doi:10.1016/j.jamcollsurg.2013.07.385. *Evidence Level IV.*

Bjorgul, K., Novicoff, W. M., & Saleh, K. J. (2010). American Society of Anesthesiologist Physical Status score may be used as a comorbidity index in hip fracture surgery. *Journal of Arthroplasty, 25*(6), 134–137. doi:10.1016/j.arth.2010.04.010. *Evidence Level IV.*

Blegen, M. A., Goode, C. J., Park, S. H., Vaughn, T., & Spetz, J. (2013). Baccalaureate education in nursing and patient outcomes. *Journal of Nursing Administration, 43*(2), 89–94. doi:10.1097/NNA.0b013e31827f2028. *Evidence Level IV.*

Boltz, M., Capezuti, E., Wagner, L., Rosenberg, M. C., & Secic, M. (2013). Patient safety in medical-surgical units: Can nurse certification make a difference. *Medsurg Nursing, 22*(1), 26–37. *Evidence Level IV.*

Brady, M., Kinn, S., & Stuart, P. (2003). Preoperative fasting for adults to prevent perioperative complications. *Cochrane Database of Systematic Reviews, 2003*(4), CD004423. *Evidence Level I.*

Bratzler, D. W., Dellinger, E. P., Olsen, K. M., Perl, T. M., Auwaerter, P. G., Bolon, M. K., . . . Weinstein, R. A. (2013). American Society of Health-System Pharmacists; Infectious Disease Society of America; Surgical Infection Society; Society for Healthcare Epidemiology of America. Clinical practice guidelines for antimicrobial prophylaxis in surgery. *American Journal of Health-System Pharmacy, 70*(3):195–283. doi:10.2146/ajhp120568. *Evidence Level VI.*

Brooks, P., Spillane, J. J., Dick, K., & Stuart-Shor, E. (2014). Developing a strategy to identify and treat older patients with postoperative delirium. *AORN Journal, 99*(2), 256–726. doi:10.1016/j.aorn.2013.12.009. *Evidence Level V.*

Brooks, P. B. (2012). Postoperative delirium in elderly patients. *American Journal of Nursing, 112*(9), 38–49. doi:10.1097/01.NAJ.0000418922.53224.36. *Evidence Level V.*

Buesing, K. L., Mullapudi, B., & Flowers, K. A. (2015). Deep venous thrombosis and venous thromboembolism prophylaxis. *Surgical Clinics of North America, 95*(2), 285–300. doi:10.1016/j.suc.2014.11.005. *Evidence Level V.*

Carpintero, P., Caeiro, J. R., Carpintero, R., Morales, A., Silva, S., & Mesa, M. (2014). Complications of hip fractures: A review. *World Journal of Orthopedics, 5*(4), 402. doi:10.5312/wjo.v5.i4.402. *Evidence Level V.*

Cataife, G., Weinberg, D. A., Wong, H. H., & Kahn, K. L. (2014). The effect of surgical care improvement project (SCIP) compliance on surgical site infections (SSI). *Medical Care, 52*(2 Suppl. 1), S66–S73. doi:10.1097/MLR.0000000000000028. *Evidence Level IV.*

Centers for Disease Control and Prevention (CDC). (2010). *National Center for Health Statistics national hospital discharge survey 2010.* Retrieved from http://www.cdc.gov/nchs/data/nhds/4procedures/2010pro4_numberprocedureage.pdf. *Evidence Level VI.*

Centers for Disease Control and Prevention (CDC). (2012). *Prevalence of obesity among older adults in the United States, 2007–2010.* Retrieved from http://www.cdc.gov/nchs/data/databriefs/db106.htm. *Evidence Level V.*

Chow, W. B., Rosenthal, R. A., Merkow, R. P., Ko, C. Y., & Esnaola, N. F. (2012) Optimal preoperative assessment of the geriatric surgical patient: A best practices guideline from the American College of Surgeons National Surgical Quality Improvement Program and the American Geriatrics Society. *Journal of the American College Surgeons, 215*(4), 453–466. doi:10.1016/j.jamcollsurg.2012.06.017. *Evidence Level VI.*

Curiel-Balsera, E., Mora-Ordoñez, J. M., Castillo-Lorente, E., Benitez-Parejo, J., Herruzo-Avilés, A., Ravina-Sanz, J. J., . . . Rivera-Fernandez, R. (2013). Mortality and complications in elderly patients undergoing cardiac surgery. *Critical Care, 28*(4), 397–404. doi:10.1016/j.jcrc.2012.12.011. *Evidence Level III.*

Devereaux, P. J., Goldman, L., Cook, D. J., Gilbert, K., Leslie, K., & Guyatt, G. H. (2005). Perioperative cardiac events in patients undergoing noncardiac surgery: A review of the magnitude of the problem, the pathophysiology of the events and methods to estimate and communicate risk. *Canadian Medical Association Journal, 173*(6), 627–634. *Evidence Level V.*

Donatelli, N. S., Gregorowicz, J., & Somes, J. (2013). Extended ED stay of the older adult results in poor patient outcome. *Journal of Emergency Nursing, 39*(3), 268–272. doi:10.1016/j.jen.2013.02.005. *Evidence Level V.*

Dorman, R. B., Abraham, A. A., Al-Refaie, W. B., Parsons, H. M., Ikramuddin, S., & Habermann, E. B. (2012). Bariatric surgery outcomes in the elderly: An ACS NSQIP study. *Journal of Gastrointestinal Surgery, 16*(1), 35–44. doi:10.1007/s11605-011-1749-6. *Evidence Level IV.*

Dripps, R. D. (1963). New classification of physical status. *Anesthesiology, 24*(1), 111. *Evidence Level VI.*

Elixhauser, A., & Andrews, R. M. (2010). Profile of inpatient operating room procedures in US hospitals in 2007. *Archives of Surgery, 145*(12), 1201–1208. doi:10.1001/archsurg.2010.269. *Evidence Level IV.*

Fleisher, L. A., Fleischmann, K. E., Auerbach, A. D., Barnason, S. A., Beckman, J. A., Bozkurt, B., . . . Wijeysundera, D. N. (2014). ACC/AHA guideline on perioperative cardiovascular evaluation and management of patients undergoing noncardiac surgery: A report of the American College of Cardiology/American Heart Association Task Force on Practice Guidelines. *Journal of the American College of Cardiologists, 64*(22), e77–e173. doi:10.1016/j.jacc.2014.07.944. *Evidence Level VI.*

Fry, D. E. (2008). Surgical site infections and the surgical care improvement project (SCIP): Evolution of national quality measures. *Surgical Infections, 9*(6), 579–584. doi:10.1089/sur.2008.9951. *Evidence Level V.*

Girish, M., Trayner, E., Jr., Dammann, O., Pinto-Plata, V., & Celli, B. (2001). Symptom-limited stair climbing as a predictor of postoperative cardiopulmonary complications after high-risk surgery. *Chest, 120*(4), 1147–1151. *Evidence Level III.*

Green, P., Woglom, A. E., Genereux, P., Daneault, B., Paradis, J. M., Schnell, S., . . . Williams, M. (2012). The impact of frailty status on survival after transcatheter aortic valve replacement in older adults with severe aortic stenosis: A single-center experience. *JACC Cardiovascular Interventions, 5*(9), 974–981. doi:10.1016/j.jcin.2012.06.011. *Evidence Level IV.*

Grosflam, J. M., Wright, E. A., Cleary, P. D., & Katz, J. N. (1995). Predictors of blood loss during total hip replacement surgery. *Arthritis Care Research, 8*(3), 167–173. *Evidence Level IV.*

Gupta, P. K., Gupta, H., Sundaram, A., Kaushik, M., Fang, X., Miller, W. J., . . . Mooss A. N. (2011). Development and validation of a risk calculator for prediction of cardiac risk after surgery. *Circulation, 124*(4), 381–387. doi:10.1161/CIRCULATIONAHA.110.015701. *Evidence Level IV.*

Hall, M. J., DeFrances, C. J., Williams, S. N., Golosinskiy, A., & Schwartzman, A. (2010). National hospital discharge survey: 2007 summary. *National Health Statistics Report,* (29), 1–20, 24. *Evidence Level IV.*

Hashmi, A., Ibrahim-Zada, I., Rhee, P., Aziz, H., Fain, M. J., Friese, R. S., & Joseph, B. (2014). Predictors of mortality in geriatric trauma patients: A systematic review and meta-analysis.

Journal of Trauma and Acute Care Surgery, 76(3), 894–901. doi:10.1097/TA.0b013e3182ab0763. *Evidence Level I.*

He, M. L., Xiao, Z. M., Lei, M., Li, T. S., Wu, H., & Liao, J. (2014). Continuous passive motion for preventing venous thromboembolism after total knee arthroplasty. *Cochrane Database Systematic Reviews, 2014*(7). doi:10.1002/14651858.CD008207.pub3. *Evidence Level I.*

Heit, J., O'Fallon, W., Petterson, T., Lohse, C., Silverstein, M., Mohr, D., & Melton, L. (2002). Relative impact of risk factors for deep vein thrombosis and pulmonary embolism: A population-based study. *Archives of Internal Medicine, 162*, 1245–1248. *Evidence Level IV.*

Institute for Healthcare Improvement (IHI). (n.d.). *Changes for improvement.* Retrieved from http://www.ihi.org/resources/Pages/Changes/default.aspx. *Evidence Level VI.*

Ivashkov, Y., & Van Norman, G. A. (2009). Informed consent and the ethical management of the older patient. *Anesthesiology Clinics, 27*(3), 569–580. doi:10.1016/j.anclin.2009.07.016. *Evidence Level V.*

Knoll, G. A. (2013). Kidney transplantation in the older adult. *American Journal of Kidney Diseases, 61*(5), 790–797. doi:10.1053/j.ajkd.2012.08.049. *Evidence Level V.*

Korc-Grodzicki, B., Downey, R. J., Shahrokni, A., Kingham, T. P., Patel, S. G., & Audisio, R. A. (2014). Surgical considerations in older adults with cancer. *Journal of Clinical Oncology, 32*(24), 2647–2653. doi:10.1200/JCO.2014.55.0962. *Evidence Level V.*

Leavitt, M. O. (2008). Message from the Secretary, US Department of Health and Human Services. In *Office of the Surgeon General, the surgeon general's call to action to prevent deep vein thrombosis and pulmonary embolism.* Rockville, MD: Office of the Surgeon General. *Evidence Level VI.*

Lee, T. H., Marcantonio, E. R., Mangione, C. M., Thomas, E. J., Polanczyk, C. A., Cook, E. F., . . . Goldman, L. (1999). Derivation and prospective validation of a simple index for prediction of cardiac risk of major noncardiac surgery. *Circulation, 100*(10), 1043–1049. *Evidence Level IV.*

Lindenauer, P. K., Pekow, P., Wang, K., Mamidi, D. K., Gutierrez, B., & Benjamin, E. M. (2005). Perioperative beta-blocker therapy and mortality after major noncardiac surgery. *New England Journal of Medicine, 353*(4), 349–361. *Evidence Level IV.*

Lynch, J., & Belgaumkar, A. (2012). Bariatric surgery is effective and safe in patients over 55: A systematic review and meta-analysis. *Obesity Surgery, 22*(9), 1507–1516. doi:10.1007/s11695–012-0693–1. *Evidence Level I.*

Magill, S. S., Hellinger, W., Cohen, J., Kay, R., Bailey, C., Boland, B., . . . Fridkin, S. (2012). Prevalence of healthcare-associated infections in acute care hospitals in Jacksonville, Florida. *Infection Control and Hospital Epidemiology, 33*(3), 283–391. doi:10.1086/664048. *Evidence Level IV.*

Moja, L., Piatti, A., Pecoraro, V., Ricci, C., Virgili, G., Salanti, G., . . . Banfi, G. (2012). Timing matters in hip fracture surgery, patients operated within 48 hours have better outcomes: A meta-analysis and meta-regression of over 190,000 patients. *PloS One, 7*(10), e46175. doi:10.1371/journal.pone.0046175. *Evidence Level I.*

National Quality Forum (NHQ). (2004). *National voluntary consensus standards for nursing-sensitive care: An initial performance measure set.* Retrieved from http://www.qualityforum.org/Publications/2004/10/National_Voluntary_Consensus_Standards_for_Nursing-Sensitive_Care__An_Initial_Performance_Measure_Set.aspx. *Evidence Level VI.*

Nicholas, J. A. (2014a). Preoperative optimization and risk assessment. *Clinics in Geriatric Medicine, 30*(2), 207–218. doi:10.1016/j.cger.2014.01.003. *Evidence Level V.*

Nicholas, J. A. (2014b). Management of postoperative complications: Cardiovascular disease and volume management. *Clinics in Geriatric Medicine, 30*(2), 293–301. doi:10.1016/j.cger.2014.01.008. *Evidence Level V.*

Oresanya, L. B., Lyons, W. L., & Finlayson, E. (2014). Preoperative assessment of the older patient: A narrative review. *Journal of the American Medical Association, 311*(20), 2110–2120. doi:10.1001/jama.2014.4573. *Evidence Level V.*

Partridge, J. S. L., Harari, D., Martin, F. C., & Dhesi, J. K. (2014). The impact of pre-operative comprehensive geriatric assessment on postoperative outcomes in older patients undergoing scheduled surgery: A systematic review. *Anaesthesia, 69*(Suppl. 1), 8–16. doi:10.1111/anae.12494. *Evidence Level I.*

Patterson, E. S., & Wears, R. L. (2010). Patient handoffs: Standardized and reliable measurement tools remain elusive. *Joint Commission Journal on Quality and Patient Safety, 36*(2), 52–61. *Evidence Level V.*

Riesenberg, L. A., Leisch, J., & Cunningham, J. M. (2010). Nursing handoffs: A systematic review of the literature. *American Journal of Nursing, 110*(4), 24–34. doi:10.1097/01.NAJ.0000370154.79857.09. *Evidence Level I.*

Rosencher, N., Vielpeau, C., Emmerich, J., Fagnani, F., & Samama, C. M.; ESCORTE Group. (2005). Venous thromboembolism and mortality after hip fracture surgery: The ESCORTE study. *Journal of Thrombosis and Haemostasis, 3*(9), 2006–2014. *Evidence Level III.*

Schofield, P. A. (2014). The assessment and management of perioperative pain in older adults. *Anaesthesia, 69*(Suppl. 1), 54–60. doi:10.1111/anae.12520. *Evidence Level V.*

Sepehri, A., Beggs, T., Hassan, A., Rigatto, C., Shaw-Daigle, C., Tangri, N., & Arora, R. C. (2014). The impact of frailty on outcomes after cardiac surgery: A systematic review. *Journal of Thoracic and Cardiovascular Surgery, 148*(6), 3110–3117. doi:10.1016/j.jtcvs.2014.07.087. *Evidence Level I.*

Sessums, L. L., Zembrzuska, H., & Jackson, J. L. (2011). Does this patient have medical decision-making capacity? *Journal of the American Medical Association, 306*(4), 420–427. doi:10.1001/jama.2011.1023. *Evidence Level V.*

Sheetz, K. H., Guy, K., Allison, J. H., Barnhart, K. A., Hawken, S. R., Hayden, E. L., . . . Englesbe, M. J. (2014). Improving the care of elderly adults undergoing surgery in Michigan. *Journal of the American Geriatrics Society, 62*(2), 352–357. doi:10.1111/jgs.12643. *Evidence Level IV.*

Siccama, R. N., Janssen, K. J., Verheijden, N. A., Oudega, R., Bax, L., van Delden, J. J., & Moons, K. G. (2011). Systematic review: Diagnostic accuracy of clinical decision rules for venous thromboembolism in elderly. *Ageing Research Review, 10*(2), 304–313. doi:10.1016/j.arr.2010.10.005. *Evidence Level I.*

Sieber, F. E., & Barnett, S. R. (2011). Preventing postoperative complications in the elderly. *Anesthesiology Clinics, 29*(1), 83–97. doi:10.1016/j.anclin.2010.11.011. *Evidence Level V.*

Singer, A. J., Thode, H. C., Jr., Viccellio, P., & Pines, J. M. (2011). The association between length of emergency department boarding and mortality. *Academic Emergency Medicine, 18*(12), 1324–1329. doi:10.1111/j.1553–2712.2011.01236.x. *Evidence Level IV.*

Söderqvist, A., Ekström, W., Ponzer, S., Pettersson, H., Cederholm, T., Dalén, N.,... Tidermark, J. (2009). Prediction of mortality in elderly patients with hip fractures: A two-year prospective study of 1,944 patients. *Gerontology, 55*(5), 496–504. doi:10.1159/000230587. *Evidence Level IV.*

Steelman, V. M. (2015). Concepts basic to perioperative nursing. In J. C. Rothrock (Ed.), *Alexander's care of the patient in surgery* (15th ed., pp. 1–15). St. Louis, MO: Elsevier Mosby. *Evidence Level VI.*

Teslyar, P., Stock, V. M., Wilk, C. M., Camsari, U., Ehrenreich, M. J., & Himelhoch, S. (2013). Prophylaxis with antipsychotic medication reduces the risk of post-operative delirium in elderly patients: A meta-analysis. *Focus, 11*(4), 544–551. doi:10.1016/j.psym.2012.12.004. *Evidence Level I.*

The Joint Commission (TJC). (2014a). *Sentinel event data root causes by event type 2004–2Q 2014*. Retrieved from http://www.jointcommission.org/assets/1/18/Root_Causes_by_Event_Type_2004-2Q_2014.pdf. *Evidence Level VI.*

The Joint Commission (TJC). (2014b). *Surgical care improvement project core measure set 2014*. Retrieved from http://www.jointcommission.org/assets/1/6/SCIP-Measures-012014.pdf. *Evidence Level VI.*

The Joint Commission (TJC). (2015). *Hospital national patient safety goals*. Retrieved from http://www.jointcommission.org/assets/1/6/2015_NPSG_HAP.pdf. *Evidence Level VI.*

Treiber, L. A., & Jones, J. H. (2012). Medication errors, routines, and differences between perioperative and non-perioperative nurses. *AORN Journal, 96*(3), 285–94. doi:10.1016/j.aorn.2012.06.013. *Evidence Level V.*

Visser, B. C., Keegan, H., Martin, M., & Wren, S. M. (2009). Death after colectomy: It's later than we think. *Archives of Surgery, 144*(11), 1021–1027. doi:10.1001/archsurg.2009.197. *Evidence Level IV.*

Wahr, J. A., Prager, R. L., Abernathy, J. H., III, Martinez, E. A., Salas, E., Seifert, P. C.,... Nussmeier, N. A. (2013). American Heart Association Council on Cardiovascular Surgery and Anesthesia, Council on Cardiovascular and Stroke Nursing, and Council on Quality of Care and Outcomes Research. Patient safety in the cardiac operating room: Human factors and teamwork: A scientific statement from the American Heart Association. *Circulation, 128*(10), 1139–1169. doi:10.1161/CIR.0b013e3182a38efa. *Evidence Level VI.*

Weiss, A. J., & Elixhauser, A. (2014). *Trends in operating room procedures in U.S. hospitals, 2011–2011* (HCUP Statistical Brief No. 171). Retrieved from http://www.hcup-us.ahrq.gov/reports/statbriefs/sb171-Operating-RoomProcedure-Trends.pdf. *Evidence Level VI.*

Welie, J. V., & Welie, S. P. (2001). Patient decision making competence: Outlines of a conceptual analysis. *Medicine, Health Care and Philosophy, 4*(2), 127–138. *Evidence Level V.*

White, J. J., Khan, W. S., & Smitham, P. J. (2011). Perioperative implications of surgery in elderly patients with hip fractures: An evidence-based review. *Journal of Perioperative Practice, 21*(6), 192–197. *Evidence Level V.*

White, P. F., White, L. M., Monk, T., Jakobsson, J., Raeder, J., Mulroy, M. F.,... Bettelli G. (2012). Perioperative care for the older outpatient undergoing ambulatory surgery. *Anesthesia & Analgesia, 114*(6), 1190–1215. doi:10.1213/ANE.0b013e31824f19b8. *Evidence Level V.*

Zakriya, K. J., Christmas, C., Wenz, J. F., Sr., Franckowiak, S., Anderson, R., & Sieber, F. E. (2002). Preoperative factors associated with postoperative change in confusion assessment method score in hip fracture patients. *Anesthesia & Analgesia, 94*(6), 1628–1632. *Evidence Level IV.*

33

General Surgical Care of the Older Adult

Larry Z. Slater and Fidelindo Lim

EDUCATIONAL OBJECTIVES

On completion of this chapter, the reader will be able to:

1. Identify the unique challenges associated with the care of older adults following surgery
2. Integrate preoperative and perioperative assessment and plans into the postoperative care plan for older adults following surgery
3. Synthesize current best practices in the assessment and interdisciplinary management of the older adult surgical patient
4. Describe evidence-based nursing and collaborative interventions to improve outcomes among older adult surgical patients

OVERVIEW

Older adult surgical patients offer unique challenges for the multidisciplinary team from the postoperative period to discharge. Physiological changes of aging (e.g., decreased cardiac and respiratory reserve, impaired kidney and liver function, and loss of muscle mass) can significantly affect the recovery time of older adult surgical patients and put them at greater risk of postoperative complications (Leung & Dzankic, 2001; Makary et al., 2010). In addition, older adults often present for elective and nonelective or emergent surgeries with a number of medical comorbidities that place them at further risk of postoperative morbidity and mortality (Dasgupta, Rolfson, Stolee, Borrie, & Speechley, 2009). The risk of complications and mortality continues to increase with advancing age, with those aged 90 years and older experiencing twice the rate of mortality at less than 48 hours postsurgery as compared to those younger than 65 years (Deiner, Westlake, & Dutton, 2014).

As the number of surgeries for older adults continues to rise, with adults aged 65 years and older currently accounting for 34% of all surgeries (Deiner et al., 2014), it is imperative that nurses in intensive care, step-down, and medical–surgical units develop competencies in working with a multidisciplinary team to provide patient-centered care for older adult surgical patients. Such care can help maximize recovery, facilitate a return to baseline functioning, and decrease the time to discharge. Longer lengths of stay have been consistently linked to increased postoperative adverse outcomes (Leung & Dzankic, 2001; Makary et al., 2010). Blegen, Goode, Park, Vaughn, and Spetz (2013) found that surgical patients at hospitals with a higher percentage of nurses with a baccalaureate or higher degree experienced shorter lengths of stay and less postoperative complications. Similarly, Aiken et al. (2014) demonstrated that a higher education level for nursing staff decreased mortality risk among surgical patients. These studies underscore the importance of nurses receiving

For a description of evidence levels cited in this chapter, see Chapter 1, "Developing and Evaluating Clinical Practice Guidelines: A Systematic Approach."

initial and ongoing education and training in providing evidence-based care to older adult surgical patients.

BACKGROUND AND STATEMENT OF PROBLEM

In 2010, older adults (aged 65 years and older) had a total of 19.2 million operative procedures performed in acute care settings (Centers for Disease Control and Prevention [CDC], 2010). In addition, they accounted for more than 37% of all procedures and 45% of total hospital days of care (CDC, 2010). As the population continues to age, comprising an estimated 16.8% of the total population by 2020 and 20.3% by 2030 (Ortman, Velkoff, & Hogan, 2014), the number of operative procedures and hospital stays for older adults will only increase. Hospital stays that involve surgical procedures have been shown to be more costly, require longer lengths of stay, and result in higher morbidity and mortality (Weiss & Elixhauser, 2014), so it is imperative that nurses address the specific needs of older adult surgical patients.

The American Geriatrics Society (AGS, 2007) developed quality indicators related to care of vulnerable elders (Assessing Care of Vulnerable Elders [ACOVE]), which include sections on hospital care, surgery, and perioperative care. The indicators address several key areas that fall under the purview of nurses providing general surgical care of the older adult: venous thromboembolism (VTE) prophylaxis, infection prevention, delirium screening and prevention, mobilization, fall prevention, and discharge assessment (AGS, 2007). An expert panel, with funding from the National Institute of Aging (NIA), also developed a list of process-based quality indicators for older adult surgical patients, applicable across disciplines, to improve surgical care and outcomes (McGory et al., 2009). The panel rated 91 indicators as valid for surgical management of the older adult, which direct the assessment and management of critical areas in order to prevent postoperative complications, decrease lengths of stay, and facilitate discharge transitions (McGory et al., 2009). The report highlighted the need for comprehensive baseline status assessment and the use of an interdisciplinary team with surgical and geriatric expertise to follow the patient from preop to discharge, facilitating as quick a return as possible to presurgery functioning (McGory et al., 2009). The indicators were similar to the ACOVE indicators: nutrition, hydration, pain management, delirium, respiratory function, infection prevention, mobility/ambulation, functional status, fall prevention, skin integrity, and restraint use (McGory et al., 2009).

This chapter provides the latest evidence and guidelines for the management of the stable older surgical patient in each of these key areas outlined by the ACOVE (AGS, 2007) and NIA Expert Panel (McGory et al., 2009) quality indicators. In addition, the nurse's responsibilities related to discharge planning will be highlighted. The discussion also provides, where applicable, the identification of applicable Joint Commission (TJC) National Patient Safety Goals (TJC, 2015) and National Quality Forum (NQF) National Database of Nursing Quality Indicators (NDNQI; Montalvo, 2007). For a discussion on the comprehensive management of critically ill, older patients, please refer to Chapter 29, "Comprehensive Assessment and Management of the Critically Ill."

ASSESSMENT OF THE PROBLEM AND NURSING CARE STRATEGIES

The Patient Safety Indicators (PSIs) espoused by the Agency for Healthcare Research and Quality (AHRQ) guide assessment and screening for adverse events that patients experience as a result of exposure to the health care system (AHRQ, 2014). PSIs that are directly related to postsurgical care include:

- Death among surgical inpatients
- Central venous catheter (CVC)-related bloodstream infection
- Postoperative hemorrhage or hematoma rate, physiological and metabolic derangements, respiratory failure, pulmonary embolism or deep vein thrombosis (DVT), sepsis, and wound dehiscence
- Transfusion reaction

These high-risk and high-impact events are deemed amenable to prevention by changes at the system or provider level (AHRQ, 2014). Nurses play a pivotal role in the prevention and management of these events. In the next section, specific care topics directly or indirectly related to the PSIs are explored.

Postoperative Delirium and Cognitive and Sensory Function

Postoperative delirium can occur in up to 50% of high-risk older adult surgical patients, leading to prolonged and more costly hospitalizations, functional decline, and death (AGS, 2014). Older adult surgical patients are at a high risk of delirium for a number of causes, including medication side effects; immobility; infection; inadequate pain management; and cardiac, renal, and respiratory complications (Hughes, Leary, Zweizig, & Cain, 2013). In addition, routine hospital care may contribute to delirium resulting from effects on the patient's sleep–wake cycle and sleep deprivation, often related to routine procedures and hospital noise, and inattention to visual and hearing deficits, including lack of appropriate corrective lenses and hearing aids (Hughes et al., 2013).

The management of postoperative delirium begins presurgery. The ACOVE and NIA Expert Panel recommend that this assessment be performed 8 weeks before surgery (AGS, 2007; McGory et al., 2009). The AGS Expert Panel on Postoperative Delirium in Older Adults (2014) emphasizes the assessment of risk factors for postoperative delirium, with the presence of two or more factors placing the patient at a greater risk of delirium after surgery. Moreover, patients should receive a comprehensive evaluation of cognitive and sensory (vision/hearing) function 8 weeks before surgery (McGory et al., 2009). Chapter 6, "Assessing Cognitive Function," discusses the assessment of cognitive function and Chapter 5, "Sensory Changes," outlines sensory changes in older adults. For more on preoperative (as well as intraoperative) management of delirium in surgical patients, see Chapter 32, "Perioperative Care of the Older Adult."

Postoperatively, health care professionals with adequate training in the assessment and diagnosis of delirium should screen patients using validated screening instruments, at least daily or as clinically indicated, to diagnose postoperative delirium and institute early interventions (AGS, 2014). ACOVE recommends screening to occur for at least the first 3 days after surgery (AGS, 2007). Table 33.1 provides more specific medical evaluations, which include both nursing and collaborative assessments, as listed by the AGS Expert Panel on Postoperative Delirium. These evaluations are also highlighted in the British Geriatric Society (BGS, 2006) guidelines for management of delirium and the NIA Expert Panel quality indicators (McGory et al., 2009) for older surgical patients. Lagoo-Deenadayalan, Newell, and Pofahl (2011) also provide a useful mnemonic, *I'm Confused*, to summarize etiologies of delirium in surgical older adult patients. This mnemonic is provided in Table 33.2.

Chapter 17, "Delirium: Prevention, Early Recognition, and Treatment," outlines in greater detail the prevention, recognition, and treatment of delirium in the older adult population. For the older surgical patient, however, there are some specific management dos and don'ts that need to be highlighted here. Given the breadth of factors that may lead to postoperative delirium, adequate nursing care, as emphasized in the rest of this chapter, that addresses the general surgical care of the older adult may help prevent delirium; it will also be essential in the management of delirium, should it occur. Although evidence has not demonstrated that specific units designed for older adult surgical patients or those with delirium improve patient outcomes, environmental adjustments remain an important component of care (AGS, 2014). These may include continuity of care (familiar residents, nurses, and care technicians), continuous environmental and personal orientation, availability of working hearing and vision aids, minimization of noise and interruptions to promote adequate sleep, and involvement of family and caregivers (BGS, 2006). In addition, the AGS (2014) and BGS (2006) emphasize the following pharmacologic and nonpharmacological interventions.

TABLE 33.1

Evaluation of Precipitating Factors for Postoperative Delirium

Precipitating Factors	Evaluation
Environmental factors	
■ Inadequate pain control	Physical examination
■ Sleep deprivation	Pain assessment
■ Use of restraints	Review of records, nursing notes
■ Urinary catheterization	
■ Poor vision/hearing	
Infection	
■ Urinary tract infection	Physical examination
■ Pneumonia	Urinalysis with white blood cell count
■ Central-line and bloodstream infections	Chest x-ray
■ Surgical site infection	Blood, sputum, and urine cultures
	Surgical site imaging, as needed
	Medication reconciliation
Delirium-inducing medications	Medication reconciliation
Metabolic derangement	
■ Hypoxia and acidosis	Vital signs and pulse oximetry
■ Electrolyte imbalances	Laboratory evaluation, including electrolytes, creatinine, blood urea nitrogen, glucose, hematocrit, and blood gas analysis
■ Hypoglycemia	
■ Dehydration	
■ Anemia	
■ Hypotension and shock	
Substance withdrawal	
■ Alcohol	Physical examination
■ Benzodiazepines	Social history
■ Illicit drugs	Preadmission medication reconciliation

Adapted from the American Geriatrics Society Expert Panel on Postoperative Delirium in Older Adults Best Practices Statement (2014).

TABLE 33.2
Mnemonic for Etiology of Postoperative Delirium in Older Adult Surgical Patients

I	Infection
M	Metabolism
C	Cognitive, sensory
O	Oxygenation
N	Nutrition, swallowing
F	Function, pharmacy, Foley catheter
U	Unfamiliar environment
S	Stress, pain
E	Electrolytes, fluids
D	Dysfunction—lung, liver, kidney, brain

Adapted from Lagoo-Deenadayalan, Newell, and Pofahl, (2011).

Pharmacologic

- Adequate pain management, preferably with nonopioid pain medications
- Avoidance of delirium-inducing medications such as benzodiazepines, anticholinergics, diphenhydramine, histamine$_2$-receptor antagonists, sedative-hypnotics, and meperidine (see also the AGS Beers Criteria [AGS, 2012])
- Avoidance of routine sedation or prophylactic antipsychotics

Nonpharmacologic

- Use of nonpharmacologic pain management strategies
- Adequate fluid and nutrition intake
- Promotion of early ambulation/mobility, physical and occupational therapy
- Initiation of plans to prevent pressure ulcers, falls, and infection
- Prevention of complications (respiratory, cardiac, gastrointestinal, and renal)
- Avoidance of unnecessary catheterization and restraint use

Pain Management

A large majority of hospitalized older adults experience pain or discomfort, but they are consistently less likely to receive adequate pain management than their younger counterparts (Schofield, 2014). Pain may be postoperative, but could also include the patient's chronic pain issues, which may be exacerbated as a result of the stress of surgery and/or hospitalization. A study in the United Kingdom found that although 81% of older adults were being treated in a hospital that had an acute pain service, only a small minority of them actually had a pain assessment chart (National Confidential Enquiry into Perioperative Deaths [NCEPOD], 1999). One reason may be the misconception that older adults have a higher pain threshold (Doerflinger, 2009). This may be compounded by the fact that older adults may be more hesitant to report pain, feeling that it is just a fact of life or possibly not wanting to be a bother to the nursing staff (Panprese & Johnson, 2014), or they may be concerned about becoming dependent on pain medications (Hughes et al., 2013). Pain management is further complicated if the older adult has cognitive or communication issues.

Adequate assessment and management of pain are the nurse's imperative for the older surgical patient, as a lack of pain control can lead to a host of complications, including delirium, depression, fluid imbalances, atelectasis, and fatigue (AGS, 2014; Bashaw & Scott, 2012). Pain assessments should be performed with each set of vital signs, at a minimum (McGory et al., 2009; Schofield, 2014), but are most effective when performed as part of hourly rounding. Assessments should include a rating of intensity (using numeric, verbal, or visual scales), a pain description (to address sensory and affective dimensions as well as the impact of pain on function), and observations of signs of pain, which are especially important for patients with cognitive or communication issues (Royal College of Physicians, British Geriatrics Society, & British Pain Society, 2007). For patients with dementia, a rating scale, such as Patient Assessment in Advanced Dementia (PAINAD), may be used to systematically gather pain data (Warden, Hurley, & Volicer, 2003). In addition, a family member or caregiver may be able to assist in identifying signs of pain in the person with dementia as they are often more experienced in recognizing subtle clues (Hughes et al., 2013).

Although pain assessment is a critical component of TJC Hospital Accreditation Standards (2014b), and pain has been assessed as the fifth vital sign since the Veterans Health Administration launched its initiative in 1999, there has been little improvement in the overall quality of pain management (Mularski et al., 2006). The NIA Expert Panel recommends that a comprehensive pain management plan should be offered to any patient with a pain score greater than 5 (McGory et al., 2009). However, it is best to set pain management plans and goals according to the individualized needs of the patient and the plans must take into account any chronic pain-related conditions that already exist. ACOVE states that for complaints of moderate to severe pain, an intervention should be performed, reassessment of pain should occur within 4 hours, and documentation of the intervention and reassessment should be placed in the medical chart (AGS, 2007). In practice, pain reassessment often occurs within 15 minutes for intravenous (IV) medications and 1 hour for oral (PO) medications.

Chapter 18, "Pain Management," provides specific protocols for management of pain in older adult populations. When applying these protocols to the surgical patient, the nurse must also take into account medication side effects that can contribute to postoperative complications (e.g., morphine and constipation). ACOVE specifically recommends interventions to address constipation when the older adult surgical patient is on opioid therapy (AGS, 2007). These are described in greater detail in the following section on Nutrition and Gastrointestinal Complications. TJC (2014a) provided a clarification to their pain management standard to express the many nonpharmacologic strategies, such as massage, acupuncture, and cognitive behavioral therapy, which may be used as part of the pain management arsenal. These methods may be preferred over the use of nonsteroidal anti-inflammatory drugs (NSAIDs) because of the potential gastrointestinal (GI) and renal complications associated with these medications (Griffiths et al., 2014).

Nutrition and Gastrointestinal Complications

Poor preoperative nutritional status can put the older adult surgical client at risk of serious postoperative complications, including impaired skin integrity, delayed wound healing, wound or other infections, sepsis, and death (Lagoo-Deenadayalan et al., 2011; Scandrett, Zuckerbraun, & Peitzman, 2015). As older adults may have several factors that put them at risk of malnutrition, such as financial constraints, social isolation, poor oral health, depression, alcohol use, or difficulties with meal preparation (Volkert, 2002), nutritional screening before surgery is of vital importance. In the American College of Surgeons National Surgical Quality Improvement Program (ACS NSQIP) and AGS *Best Practice Guidelines* on preoperative assessment, Chow, Rosenthal, Merkow, Ko, and Esnaola (2012) list a body mass index (BMI) less than 18.5 kg/m^2, a serum albumin less than 3.0 g/dL, and unintentional weight loss greater than 10% to 15% within 6 months as placing the surgical patient at severe nutritional risk; they advise that a comprehensive nutritional plan be developed to address deficits through the postoperative period. As approximately 86% of older hospitalized adults are malnourished or are at risk of malnutrition (Kaiser et al., 2010), early nutritional intervention is imperative in preventing complications, decreasing length of stay, and promoting a quick return to baseline functioning.

Chapter 10, "Nutrition," provides a detailed discussion of nutrition assessment and nursing care strategies for older adults and Chapter 25, "Mealtime Difficulties in Dementia," discusses mealtime difficulties. Nutritional care requires collaboration with the multidisciplinary health care team, including the nurse, surgical resident, and dietitian, as well as the speech therapist and occupational therapist. The goal is to provide early and adequate nutritional intake, preferably by mouth, which may be enhanced through the use of nutritional supplements (e.g., Ensure®). If oral intake is not possible, the team may consider the use of other forms of enteral nutrition (e.g., percutaneous endoscopic gastrostomy [PEG] tube and Dobhoff tube) or parenteral nutrition. Although parenteral nutrition may temporarily be the only option for some postsurgical older adults, especially those with a prolonged postoperative ileus (POI), it is important to note that enteral nutrition offers better outcomes than parenteral, as the former is associated with shorter hospital stays, lower incidence of infection, and lower severity of complications (Wheble, Knight, & Khan, 2012).

Several issues could possibly prevent early postsurgical nutrition intake, including postoperative nausea and vomiting (PONV) and dysphagia. PONV affects about one third of surgical patients (Apfel, Kranke, & Eberhart, 2004). Not only does PONV affect nutritional status, but it can also lead to further complications for the older surgical patient, including aspiration, wound dehiscence, and prolonged length of stay (American Society of PeriAnesthesia Nurses [ASPAN], 2006). The risk of PONV increases with age and duration of surgery (ASPAN, 2006). PONV should be continually monitored, especially within the first 24 hours of arrival to the unit. If PONV is present, it should be quantified using a descriptive or visual scale and then rescue interventions should be implemented, including the administration of antiemetic agents, verification of adequate hydration, and use of aromatherapy (ASPAN, 2006). For older adults, however, it is important to steer clear of metoclopramide, which can lead to extrapyramidal effects (AGS, 2012).

Older adults may experience age-related decreases in swallowing function (Scandrett et al., 2015). Additionally, swallowing difficulties take longer to resolve following extubation for older adults, particularly after long surgeries (El Solh, Okada, Bhat, & Peitrantoni, 2003), predisposing the older adult patient to postoperative dysphagia. As such, swallowing ability should be assessed early to address the need for fluid and caloric intake and to lower the risk of aspiration and debilitating aspiration pneumonia (Lagoo-Deenadayalan et al., 2011). If the swallowing assessment shows signs of aspiration, modification of the diet, including alterations in food consistency, upright positioning during and up to 1 hour after feeding, speech therapy, and aggressive oral care should be implemented to improve intake (Marik & Kaplan, 2003; McGory et al., 2009). For patients who may need to receive tube feedings because of swallowing difficulties or other postoperative complications, a documented plan to reduce the risk of aspiration should be incorporated into the medical record (AGS, 2007).

Constipation or diarrhea can also complicate postsurgical nutritional interventions and may signify more serious complications. Constipation can occur postoperatively as a result of immobility, altered (or lack of) diet, and excessive use of opioid pain medications (Doerflinger, 2009). In addition, the use of anticholinergics, particularly first-generation antihistamines (e.g., diphenhydramine), may initiate or exacerbate constipation and should be avoided in the older postsurgical patient (AGS, 2012). Preventive methods for constipation should be instituted for older adult surgical patients on opioid pain management regimens. This typically includes the use of bowel stimulants (senna and bisacodyl) and osmotic agents (polyethylene glycol); however, bulk-forming agents (psyllium) should be avoided as they are ineffective and may worsen symptoms, especially in a patient without adequate fluid intake (AGS, 2007; Malec & Shega, 2015). Quick transitioning from opioid medications to acetaminophen for mild to moderate pain may help reduce the risk of constipation.

The presence of diarrhea might trigger assessment for fecal impaction (following unaddressed constipation) or a more serious complication, such as *Clostridium dificile* infection (Doerflinger, 2009). A study by Zerey et al. (2008) showed that *C. dificile* infection occurs in about 1% of older adults undergoing a general surgical procedure. The occurrence of *C. dificile* infection can increase length of stay by 16 days and triple the mortality risk (Zerey et al., 2008). Universal precautions and proper handwashing are essential in reducing the risk of *C. difficile* infection. If *C. difficile* infection is suspected, then stool samples should be taken and prompt treatment initiated if samples test positive (Doerflinger, 2009).

Special Consideration: POI Following Gastrointestinal Surgery

Older adult surgical patients have a higher incidence of POI following surgeries involving manipulation of the bowel (Hamel, Henderson, Khuri, & Daley, 2005). Prolonged POI (lasting more than 5 days) occurs in 40% of patients and leads to prolonged hospital stays and increased medical costs (Delaney, 2004; Schuster et al., 2006). Management for POI has routinely included bowel rest and bowel decompression (through placement of a nasogastric [NG] tube (Lagoo-Deenadayalan et al., 2011). However, evidence has shown that early enteral feeding is often well tolerated and may decrease POI, whereas NG decompression has not been shown to reduce incidence of POI and may actually place the patient at risk of aspiration and other postoperative pulmonary complications (Lubawski & Saclarides, 2008). In addition to early return to feeding, early mobilization and avoiding unnecessary use of opioids can reduce incidence of prolonged POI (Lagoo-Deenadayalan et al., 2011, Lubawski & Saclarides, 2008).

Hydration and Renal Complications

Older adults are at greater risk of fluid and electrolyte imbalances caused by physiological changes that lead to decreased total body water and poorer kidney function (lower glomerular filtration rate [GFR] and decreased ability to concentrate urine; Luckey & Parsa, 2003). Older adults are more susceptible to experiencing dehydration resulting from changes in thirst response, functional disability leading to decreased intake, and polypharmacy, including the overuse of diuretics (El-Sharkaway, Sahota, Maughan, & Lobo, 2014). However, surgical stress and excessive fluid resuscitation during the perioperative period could have the opposite effect, leading to water, sodium, and chloride excess, all of which have been shown to be independent risk factors for mortality, postoperative renal injury, and increased lengths of stay (El-Sharkaway et al., 2014).

Given this dichotomy, fluid management during the perioperative period is of vital importance. However, fluid orders are often delegated to the most junior member of the medical team who may lack an understanding of the importance of maintaining fluid balance for the older adult surgical patient (El-Sharkaway et al., 2014). In a report by the NCEPOD in the United Kingdom (1999), the authors noted that fluid management in older adult surgical patients was poor and contributed to serious postoperative morbidity and mortality. After conducting chart reviews, the report cited both doctors and nurses as being remiss in providing accurate documentation in fluid balance charts and recommended that working practices be developed, including elevating fluid management to the same importance as drug prescribing, to address the problem (NCEPOD, 1999).

During the postoperative period, the older adult is most at risk of dehydration and acute renal failure. Gajdos et al. (2013) reported that approximately 1.5% of adults older than 60 years undergoing nonemergent surgery developed postoperative renal insufficiency and, of those, the mortality rate was more than 31%. The nurse plays a vital role in the assessment of fluid status, monitoring for signs and symptoms of fluid volume deficit and providing accurate documentation of fluid balance. The NIA Expert Panel recommends that fluid status be monitored for at least the first 5 days after surgery using daily weights and/or daily intake and output (McGory et al., 2009). However, Sullivan (2011) notes that because fluid volume shifts may take up to twice as long to resolve in the older surgical patient, urine output alone may not be enough to determine whether the patient has low blood volume leading to poor perfusion. The nurse should also be on the lookout for drops in blood pressure, changes in mental status, and new-onset atrial fibrillation, all of which could signify poor perfusion (Sullivan, 2011). Hughes et al. (2013) stress the importance of routine screening of serum electrolytes, urea nitrogen, and creatinine, although in older adults creatinine levels may not change even with significant drops in GFR.

As with nutrition, oral hydration should begin as soon as feasibly possible. Similarly, PONV and dysphagia must be addressed in order for the postoperative older adult to maintain adequate fluid balance. Chapter 9, "Managing Oral Hydration," addresses the management of oral hydration in the older adult, much of which is applicable to the older postsurgical patient. However, if the patient is unable to maintain adequate oral intake, IV fluids or adequate hydration through tube feeding may be required (with appropriate aspiration precautions instituted).

Respiratory Complications

Age-related changes in respiratory function include weakened swallowing and cough responses, chest wall stiffness, a weakened diaphragm, and decreased vital capacity and forced expiratory volume in 1 second (Bashaw & Scott, 2012; Hughes et al., 2013). These changes predispose the older adult surgical patient to respiratory complications. For patients with preexisting respiratory conditions, such as chronic obstructive pulmonary disease or asthma or for those who are smokers, the risk of complications is even greater (Lagoo-Deenadayalan et al., 2011). Preoperative assessment of pulmonary function is vital to delineating postoperative risk and the promotion of preoperative smoking cessation, even just 24 to 48 hours before surgery, may help lessen postoperative sequelae (AGS, 2007; Hughes et al., 2013).

Pulmonary complications occur in approximately 10% of older adult surgical patients and account for up to 40% of postoperative complications and nearly 20% of preventable deaths (Lagoo-Deenadayalan et al., 2011). Magill et al. (2014) estimated that there were approximately 157,500 cases of hospital-acquired pneumonia (HAP) in the United States in 2011, of which 39% were ventilator-associated pneumonia (VAP). Gajdos et al. (2013) found that pulmonary complications, including pneumonia, failure to wean from a ventilator, and unplanned intubation, occurred in 7% of patients aged 60 years and older undergoing nonemergent surgery, with a mortality rate of 23% among those that had such complications.

Nursing interventions are essential in the prevention of respiratory complications through implementation of an aggressive pulmonary toilet regimen (Lagoo-Deenadayalan et al., 2011). In order to promote lung expansion and prevent postoperative atelectasis, the nurse should promote the use of an incentive spirometer (with adequate education and reinforcement on use) at least 10 times per hour; turning, coughing, and deep breathing every 2 hours; and chest percussion or other chest physiotherapy as needed (Doerflinger, 2009; McGory et al., 2009). Early ambulation should also be encouraged, as should proper positioning when in bed with the head of the bed elevated (Bashaw & Scott, 2012; Doerflinger, 2009). Adequate pain control is imperative as pain may reduce respiratory effort and may limit coughing to clear secretions (Lagoo-Deenadayalan et al., 2011). The health care team should also avoid the excessive use of narcotics and sedatives that could lead to respiratory depression (Lagoo-Deenadayalan et al., 2011).

VAP is a key nursing-sensitive indicator listed by the NDQNI and also endorsed by the NQF as the nurse plays a pivotal role in its prevention (Montalvo, 2007). For patients who are mechanically ventilated, the Institute of Healthcare Improvement (IHI; 2012c) lists five components of care (a ventilator bundle) to be instituted in order to prevent VAP. These components include (a) elevation of the head of the bed between 30° and 45°, (b) daily sedative interruptions and assessment of readiness to extubate, (c) peptic ulcer disease prophylaxis, (d) deep vein thrombosis (DVT) prophylaxis, and (e) daily oral care with chlorhexidine (IHI, 2012c). Despite the evidence, Munaco, Dumas, and Edlund (2014) noted that lack of staff education and limitations of the electronic medical record (EMR) affected overall compliance with a VAP bundle. AGS (2007) emphasizes the need of a documented care plan to reduce VAP. Therefore, facilities must address EMR limitations and provide ongoing education and training of nurses and nursing assistants to adequately implement VAP prevention.

Infection Prevention

Older adults are at increased infection risk postsurgery because of immune system changes and delayed wound healing (Panprese & Johnson, 2014). In 2011, it was estimated that approximately 4% of hospitalized patients had at least one hospital-acquired infection (HAI; Magill et al., 2014). In addition to pneumonia (22% of HAI) and GI infection (17%), the remaining common HAI included surgical site infection (SSI; 22%), urinary tract infection (UTI; 13%), and primary blood stream infection (10%; Magill et al., 2014). Older age and increased length of stay were related to increased risk of HAI (Magill et al., 2014). One of the most consistently cited ways to reduce HAI is through improving hand hygiene in the hospital setting. TJC (2015) specifies that current CDC or World Health Organization (WHO) guidelines should be used as a basis for hand-hygiene programs.

A localized infection could potentially become systemic, putting the patient at risk of increased morbidity/mortality resulting from sepsis, which can occur in up to 2% of postoperative older adults (Lagoo-Deenadayalan et al., 2011). The NIA Expert Panel on quality indicators for older adult surgical patients recommends the following for any patient who has a fever greater than 38.0°C after postoperative (postop) day 2: urinalysis and urine culture, examination of wound, blood culture from central venous line (if one is in place), peripheral vein blood culture, and chest radiograph (McGory et al., 2009). Older adults, however, may not necessarily mount a febrile response to systemic infection (Norman, 2000). Therefore, it is also important to monitor for other manifestations of sepsis, including altered mental status, agitation, respiratory distress, tachycardia, and hypotension (Lee, Chen, Chang, Chen, & Wu, 2007). If the older adult does have a significant febrile response, it often indicates severe infection with increased morbidity and mortality (Norman, 2000).

The Centers for Medicare & Medicaid Services (CMS) list several HAI as hospital-acquired conditions for which hospitals will receive no reimbursement (CMS, 2014). The HAI include SSIs following coronary artery bypass graft, bariatric surgery, and orthopedic procedures; catheter-associated urinary tract infections (CAUTI); and vascular catheter-associated infections (CMS, 2014). As reimbursement will not be provided for HAI, it is imperative that the multidisciplinary health care team works to prevent HAI from occurring in the hospital.

Zingg et al. (2015) performed a comprehensive systematic literature review and identified 10 key components that can impact HAI prevention. Some of the components addressed system issues, such as availability and ease of access to equipment (poorer access is related to higher risk); bed occupancy, staffing, and workload (high occupancy, low staffing levels, and high workload correlated with increased risk); and modeling a culture of infection control at the organizational level (Zingg et al., 2015). The study group also noted that adequate education and training on the appropriate use of guidelines, as well as proper auditing, surveillance, and feedback, reduced HAI risk (Zingg et al., 2015). In reviewing HAI programs from a national collaborative, Welsh, Flanagan, Hoke, Doebbeling, and Herwaldt (2012) had similar findings. They highlighted the importance of engaging front-line staff by involving them in projects and enlisting champions to further complement the education, surveillance, and feedback required to succeed in reduction of HAI (Welsh et al., 2012). In sum, a system-wide, multidisciplinary, collaborative effort is required to reduce HAI and thus reduce morbidity and mortality in older adult surgical patients.

Surgical Site Infection

Approximately 2% to 5% of surgical patients develop an SSI (Anderson et al., 2014). Among older surgical patients (aged 60 years and older), SSI occurred in 8%, with a 7% mortality rate for those developing an SSI (Gajdos et al., 2013). The occurrence of an SSI, of which approximately 60% are preventable, can lead to an additional 11 days of postoperative hospital days and two to 11 times the mortality rate of those who do not acquire an SSI (Anderson et al., 2014). SSI, which are typically defined as those that occur within 30 days of surgery but may occur up to 90 days after, are classified into three categories: superficial incisional SSI, which affects only the skin or subcutaneous tissue; deep incisional SSI, which involves deep soft tissues such as fascia or muscle; and organ/space SSI, which involves any other part of the body that was manipulated during surgery (Anderson et al., 2014).

The Surgical Care Improvement Project (SCIP) was developed to decrease SSI and develop performance measures to improve outcomes (Fry, 2008). SCIP built on previous work by the Surgical Infection Prevention Project (SIP) that identified three quality-performance measures, which related to use of prophylactic antibiotics (Fry, 2008). SCIP added three additional measures: glucose control in cardiac patients, proper hair removal before incision, and maintenance of normothermia in colorectal surgery patients (Fry, 2008). The ACOVE quality indicators also identified prophylactic antibiotics for the prevention of SSI (AGS, 2007).

These measures relate more specifically to the perioperative phase, which is discussed in Chapter 32, with the exception of glucose monitoring, which should occur for each of the first two postoperative days, with an attempt to maintain serum glucose levels below 200 mg/dL (IHI, 2012b). Compliance to appropriate antibiotic selection and administration within 60 minutes of time of incision has been associated with lower SSI rate (Cataife, Weinberg, Wong, & Kahn, 2014).

A majority of TJC (2015) National Patient Safety Goals for SSI, as well as the TJC (2013) Implementation Guide for SSI, relate to implementation of education and training of health care providers and patients/families on SSI and how to prevent them, as well as ongoing monitoring and reporting of SSI occurrences. However, other than hand hygiene, TJC provides no clear postoperative procedures for prevention of SSI. For hand hygiene, the WHO identified five key moments that require adequate hand hygiene: (a) before touching a patient, (b) before clean and aseptic procedures (which would include clean and sterile dressing changes), (c) after contact with bodily fluids, (d) after touching a patient, and (e) after touching a patient's surroundings (Tsai & Caterson, 2014). Hand hygiene should include hand rubbing with alcohol-based products or, if hands are visibly soiled, then scrubbing with soap and water (Tsai & Caterson, 2014).

For incisional care, the CDC recommends that closed incisions, those with approximated edges after surgery, be covered with a sterile dressing for 24 to 48 hours and that dressing changes be done using a sterile technique (Mangram, Horan, Pearson, Silver, & Jarvis, 1999). Beyond 48 hours, the CDC did not provide any guidance on continued use of sterile dressings or the effects of bathing/showering (Mangram et al., 1999). For open surgical incisions, the CDC recommended that the wound should be packed with sterile moist gauze and covered with a sterile dressing (Mangram et al., 1999). Some conventional wound care regimens have specified dressing changes up to 7 days postoperatively, which could also require patient education if the patient was discharged before that time (Akagi et al., 2012). In a study by Akagi et al. (2012), the authors found that the CDC recommendation of dressing changes up to 48 hours showed no increased risk of SSI compared with a standard 7-day regimen. A Cochrane Review also found no difference in SSI risk for early dressing removal (48 hours) when compared with delayed removal (after 48 hours; Toon, Ramamoorthy, Davidson, & Gurusamy, 2013). Furthermore, early removal could result in shorter hospital stays and decreased costs (Akagi et al., 2012; Toon et al., 2013).

In addition to wound care and dressing changes, the nurse must be vigilant in assessing for signs of infection, including redness around the wound edges, warmth, tenderness to palpation, and purulent drainage from the site (Lagoo-Deenadayalan et al., 2011). If an SSI occurs, treatment may include reopening of the incision to allow for drainage and frequent monitoring for signs of systemic infection; antibiotic use is typically discouraged unless the infection becomes systemic (Lagoo-Deenadayalan et al., 2011). A wound culture will identify any infection with multi-drug-resistant organisms (MDRO). If an MDRO is the infectious agent, contact isolation precautions will be instituted along with adequate cleaning and disinfecting of equipment and the patient's environment (TJC, 2015).

Catheter-Associated Urinary Tract Infections

Up to 25% of all hospitalized patients receive urinary catheterization (IHI, 2011a). However, studies have shown that approximately 21% of patients with urinary catheters lacked a proper indication for insertion and up to 58% of catheters that were in place were subsequently found to be unnecessary (IHI, 2011a). The risk of developing a CAUTI increases as the length of catheterization increases, with a daily UTI risk of 5% (Bhardwaj, Pickard, Carrick-Sen, & Brittain, 2012; IHI, 2011a). Magill et al. (2014) noted that 68% of all UTIs in 2011 were CAUTI. In a survey of postoperative complications following nonemergent surgery, Gajdos et al. (2013) found that UTI occurred in 4% of adults aged 60 years and older, with a 5% mortality rate for those experiencing a UTI. The occurrence of a postoperative CAUTI can result in longer lengths of stay, increased hospital costs, and increased morbidity/mortality for the older adult surgical patient (Gajdos et al., 2013; Lagoo-Deenadayalan et al., 2011). CAUTI is listed as a nursing-sensitive indicator by NDNQI (Montalvo, 2007) and is a target for TJC National Patient Safety Goals (2015).

The IHI (2011a) provides four components of care to prevent or reduce the risk of CAUTI. They include (a) avoidance of unnecessary catheterizations, (b) insertion of catheters using an aseptic technique, (c) maintenance of catheters based on recommended guidelines, and (d) daily review of catheter necessity and prompt removal. TJC's National Patient Safety Goals (2015) address these same components. Hospitals should have specific protocols outlining the criteria for appropriate catheter insertion. For the older adult surgical client, catheterization will most likely occur in the perioperative period. However, catheters should be removed as soon as possible postsurgery to prevent infection risk. IHI (2011a) recommends developing protocols that allow nurses to remove catheters if criteria for necessity are no longer met and if there are no contraindications to removal. Additionally, automatic stop orders can be used in the EMR to promote removal within 48 to 72 hours after surgery (IHI, 2011a). The NIA Expert Panel also specified that the catheter should be removed by postop day 3 (McGory et al., 2009). If the catheter remains in place, documentation should be provided to indicate the need for continued catheterization (IHI, 2011a). ACOVE quality indicators recommend documentation at least every 3 days indicating the continued need for use until the catheter is removed (AGS, 2007).

Involving the patient in catheter-related decision making could also lead to decreased length of catheterization. Bhardwaj et al. (2012) found that patients who underwent short-term catheterization for surgery lacked knowledge about the reason for catheterization, often did not provide consent, and were not included in the decision to remove the catheter. Patients also felt that their catheter remained in longer than was necessary because of a lack of easily accessible toileting options, even though they would have preferred to use a bedpan or bedside commode over continued catheterization (Bhardwaj et al., 2012). Therefore, the nurse should advocate for patient participation in the decision-making process for catheter removal as part of CAUTI-prevention practices.

Chapter 22, "Prevention of Catheter-Associated Urinary Tract Infection," provides further protocols on the prevention of CAUTI in older adults. The chapter discusses proper insertion using an aseptic technique as well as evidence-based maintenance of catheters that are in place. Guidelines for proper insertion include adequate hand hygiene, use of sterile equipment and an aseptic technique, and use of as small a catheter as possible that still allows for proper drainage (IHI, 2011a). Routine maintenance should include, at a minimum, maintaining a closed, sterile drainage system; properly securing the catheter and collection bag, which should be below the level of the bladder at all times; maintaining unobstructed urine flow; and emptying the collection bag regularly, using a separate container for each patient and not allowing the nozzle to touch the collection device (IHI, 2011a).

Central Line–Associated Bloodstream Infections

Approximately 84% of the estimated 72,000 primary bloodstream infections in the United States in 2011 were central line–associated bloodstream infections (CLABSI; Magill et al., 2014). For older adults, CLABSI is associated with more than twice the mortality risk, longer lengths of stay (up to 10 additional hospital days), and increased health care costs (Kaye et al., 2014). Most CVC days, approximately 15 million in the United States, occur in the intensive care setting (CDC, 2011). However, some older adult surgical patients on step-down or medical–surgical floors may have peripherally inserted central catheters (PICC) or other tunneled lines that can also place them at risk of CLABSI. As with other HAI, nurses play an integral role in the prevention of CLABSI, which is listed as an NDNQI nursing-sensitive indicator (Montalvo, 2007) and specified as a National Patient Safety Goal by TJC (2015).

The IHI (2012a) describes five key components of its central line bundle aimed at preventing CLABSI. The components include: (a) hand hygiene; (b) maximal barrier precautions, which includes sterile operator procedures and equipment and sterile patient draping from head to toe; (c) chlorhexidine skin antisepsis before insertion; (d) optimal catheter site selection, avoiding the use of the femoral vein; and (e) daily review of line necessity and prompt removal when indicated. The CDC, in its 2011 guidelines, also recommended implementing bundle strategies, which incorporate hand hygiene and aseptic, appropriate catheter and site selection, and maximum barrier precautions. The guidelines also highlight the need for adequate education, training, and staffing in the prevention of CLABSI. The ACOVE quality indicators for vulnerable elders include documentation in the EMR of the use of maximal barrier protection.

For nursing care, the CDC (2011) specifies dressing-change regimens, which include the following:

- Use sterile gauze (if patient is diaphoretic or the site is bleeding or oozing) and a transparent, semipermeable dressing to cover the site.
- Replace dressing if it becomes damp, loosened, or visibly soiled.
- Replace gauze dressings every 2 days and transparent dressings every 7 days for short-term sites.
- Use chlorhexidine-impregnated sponge dressing for temporary catheters if basic prevention measures are not working.

The nurse should also replace IV administration sets at the appropriate intervals: no less than 96-hour intervals but at least every 7 days for continuous or secondary infusion tubing; within 24 hours for tubing involving blood, blood products, or fat emulsions; or every 6 to 12 hours for propofol infusion tubing (CDC, 2011). When accessing catheter hubs, needleless injectors, and injection ports, the nurse should disinfect (scrub) using an appropriate antiseptic and access the site using only sterile devices/equipment (CDC, 2011).

Other important nursing functions are to ensure that the patient is not showering or submerging the CVC site in water (adequate patient education and monitoring) and to palpate the site through an intact dressing regularly to assess for tenderness (CDC, 2011). If tenderness is noted, the dressing should be removed for full visual inspection and, if indicated, provider notification made to address possible CLABSI (CDC, 2011). ACOVE indicators specify daily documentation of examination of the site for signs of infection as well as documentation of the continued need for use (AGS, 2007). The NIA Expert Panel offers the same quality indicators as ACOVE, but also adds daily examination for swelling in the extremity on the side of line placement (McGory et al., 2009).

Mobility, Function, and Frailty

Older adults experience loss of muscle mass, muscle strength, and bone mass as they age (Bashaw & Scott, 2012). Further deconditioning can occur following periods of inactivity, such as prolonged immobility during surgical procedures and bed rest during the immediate postoperative period (Lagoo-Deenadayalan et al., 2011). Postsurgical deconditioning can slow recovery in older adults, including restoration of activities of daily living (ADL), and put the patient at increased risk of DVT, delirium, incontinence, constipation, pressure ulcers, and falls (Lagoo-Deenadayalan et al., 2011). Early mobilization has been shown to combat deconditioning, decrease length of stay, and increase discharges to home (Engel, Tatebe, Alonzo, Mustille, & Rivera, 2013).

Frailty is defined as having decreased physiological and functional reserve (Scandrett et al., 2015). Frailty has been shown to be an independent risk factor for postoperative complications, increased length of hospital stay, and discharge to a skilled or assisted-living facility after previously living at home (Dasgupta et al., 2009; Makary et al., 2010). Chapter 27, "The Frail Hospitalized Older Adult," provides a more thorough discussion of frailty in older adult populations.

To address postoperative risks for issues with mobility and functional decline, it is imperative to develop a preoperative baseline assessment. The ACS NSQIP/AGS *Best Practice Guidelines* specifically address assessment of functional/performance status and frailty risk (Chow et al., 2012). If the patient is unable to perform any ADL, a full screening of ADL and instrumental ADL (IADL) should be performed (Chow et al., 2012). Performance is assessed using the Timed Up and Go Test (TUGT) and also includes inquiring about a history of falls (see the following section on Fall Prevention; Chow et al., 2012). The TUGT is performed by the patient using normal walking aids and without any assistance in the following manner (Chow et al., 2012). The patient:

1. Rises from a chair, if possible without using armrests
2. Walks 10 feet down a line on the floor
3. Turns
4. Returns to the chair and
5. Sits down again

If the patient takes longer than 15 seconds to complete the exercise, the patient is considered to have a high risk of falls and a more detailed gait assessment should be completed (Chow et al., 2012).

Frailty can be measured using a number of validated tools. ACS NSQIP/AGS (Chow et al., 2012) recommend the use of the Frailty Phenotype, which assesses five domains: weight loss, weakness, exhaustion, low physical activity, and slowness (Makaray et al., 2010). Each domain is scored 0 to 1 and then scores are totaled; scores of 2 to 3 indicate prefrailty and 4 to 5 indicate frailty (Chow et al., 2012). Panprese and Johnson (2014) recommend using the Braden Scale because, although it is typically used for pressure ulcer risk, its six domains of sensory perception, moisture, mobility, nutrition, activity, and skin friction and shearing characterize frailty vulnerabilities. Another reason for its use is that nurses are familiar with the tool and it is already incorporated into many EMR systems (Panprese & Johnson, 2014).

The NAI Expert Panel recommends that function and mobility screening be performed 8 weeks before surgery (McGory et al., 2009). The assessment should include the TUGT with a comprehensive assessment of mobility if it is abnormal, and assessment of hearing/visual impairment, ADL, and IADL (McGory et al., 2009). For any abnormalities, including with the TUGT, the panel recommends that a written plan be developed for postoperative care before surgery (McGory et al., 2009). Chapter 7, "Assessment of Physical Function," provides further discussion about the assessment of physical function in older adults.

Re-enablement after surgery describes the process of returning the patient to presurgery functioning (Griffiths et al., 2014). During the postoperative period, the nurse participates with a multidisciplinary team to prevent functional decline and the development of frailty and allow for re-enablement before discharge. The team includes the nurse, nursing assistant, physician resident, physical therapist, and occupational therapist. It is imperative that each member of the team understands his or her role in patient re-enablement, as confusion has been shown to be a significant barrier to mobility and activity program implementation (Markey & Brown, 2002). Other potential caregiver and patient barriers must also be addressed. Some patient barriers include dependent behavior and daytime sleepiness; the nurse and nursing assistant as well as family members should encourage independence and discourage daytime sleeping (Markey & Brown, 2002). For further information on excessive sleepiness in older adults, refer to Chapter 26, "Excessive Sleepiness." Caregiver barriers include scheduling conflicts and the use of equipment (i.e., IV poles and tubing, urinary catheters, and sequential compression devices [SCDs]) that make ambulation and mobility activities more complex (Markey & Brown, 2002).

A physical therapy consult should provide an early assessment of the patient to develop a mobility and strengthening plan, including the potential need for assistive devices (Hughes et al., 2013). ACOVE and the NIA Expert Panel stress that ambulation should occur by postop day 2 and, if not, documentation should be provided in the EMR about why ambulation could not occur (AGS, 2007; McGory et al., 2009). The NIA Expert Panel further specifies that if the patient cannot ambulate, mobilization (e.g., range-of-motion [ROM] exercises) should be performed by postop day 2 and, if not, documentation should be provided about why it could not be done (McGory et al., 2009).

The nurse, nursing assistant, and occupational therapist will address the patient's ADL and IADL. Independent performance of ADL should be encouraged, but if the patient needs assistance, the level of assistance should be documented, relayed to the occupational therapist, and communicated during handoff (Markey & Brown, 2002). If the level of assistance indicates a change from baseline functioning, a plan should be developed and documented in the EMR to facilitate re-enablement (McGory et al., 2009). A final assessment of ambulation, mobility, ADL, and IADL should also be completed and documented at discharge, with appropriate documentation provided to the skilled or assisted-living facility, home health agency, or family/caregivers, depending on the discharge destination (McGory et al., 2009). Chapter 14, "Preventing Functional Decline in the Acute Care Setting," provides further information on preventing functional decline in the acute care setting.

Fall Prevention

In the acute care setting, up to 20% of patients fall at least once over the course of their hospitalization (IHI, 2012d). Falls are the most frequently reported adverse event in hospitals, reaching approximately 1 million per year, with 90,000 serious injuries and 11,000 deaths occurring as a result (Currie, 2008). Falls can lead to head injuries, hip fracture, reduced mobility (caused by pain or added fear of falling), longer length of stay, unplanned discharge to assisted-living facilities, and increased medical costs (IHI, 2012d). Studies have consistently identified unsteady gait, confusion, increased need for toileting, use of sedative-hypnotics, and history of falling as key risk factors for falling in an acute care setting (Currie, 2008). Although it is inconclusive whether older age is a risk factor for falls, it does place the surgical patient at greater risk of injury from a fall (Currie, 2008). NQF (2011) placed falls resulting in serious injury on its list of serious reportable events (SRE). NDNQI lists falls and falls with injury as key nursing-sensitive indicators (Montalvo, 2007). CMS (2014) lists trauma related to falls as a nonreimbursable hospital-acquired condition.

Similar to mobility and function, preoperative fall-risk assessment is critical to identifying those who may be at risk for falls and developing a multidisciplinary plan to prevent falls postoperatively. The NIA Expert Panel specifies that an assessment should be performed 8 weeks before surgery on an older adult and, if the patient has reported two or more falls in the past year or one fall with injury, referral should be made for a comprehensive preoperative fall evaluation as well as inpatient physical therapy (McGory et al., 2009). There are a number of tools that have been developed to assess fall risk, including the Morse Falls Risk Assessment Tool, the Hendrich Falls Risk Model II, or the STRATIFY instrument (Currie, 2008). Although research has demonstrated that the Hendrich Falls Risk Model II may be more robust, it is more important that assessment remains consistent from preoperative screening through discharge (Currie, 2008).

Chapter 19, "Preventing Falls in Acute Care," provides a comprehensive discussion on preventing falls in acute care settings. A number of intervention strategies have been examined, including staff education, armband identification, bed alarms, exercise and toileting regimens, and vitamin D supplementation (Cameron et al., 2012). Although some have shown to be effective, multifaceted prevention strategies have been shown to be more effective (Cameron et al., 2012). IHI (2012d) highlights six key areas to address in its guide on preventing falls: fall risk screening on admission, injury and injury risk factors screening on admission, in-depth admission screening for any positive findings, communication and education about the patient's fall risk, standardized interventions for those at risk for falls, and customized interventions for those at highest risk. The final three areas address postoperative care and may incorporate such interventions as signage to identify those at risk; teach-back education to patients and family members about fall risk; and rounding every hour or 2 to address the patient's need for pain relief, toileting, and positioning (IHI, 2012d). TJC and the AHRQ have similar guidelines and also provide educational and training materials for preventing falls on their websites. If a fall does occur, ACOVE recommends that an inpatient fall evaluation should occur within 24 hours to include the presence or absence of any signs/symptoms of injury and a review of medications that could potentially contribute to a fall.

Skin Integrity

With advancing age, older adults experience thinning of the dermis, loss of collagen and adipose tissue, and decreased skin elasticity (Bashaw & Scott, 2012). As the skin becomes more friable, older adults are at increased risk for bruising, tearing, shearing, and infection, especially over bony prominences (Panprese & Johnson, 2014). If the older adult is malnourished or dehydrated, the risk of skin breakdown and pressure ulcer development increases (Bashaw & Scott, 2012). Approximately 2.5 million patients are treated for pressure ulcers each year, and about 15% of patients in hospitals at any given time have a pressure ulcer (IHI, 2011b). Pressure ulcers lead to increased morbidity (pain, delayed functional recovery, infection, and sepsis), increased length of stay, and increased hospital costs (IHI, 2011b). It is estimated that 60,000 patients die in hospitals each year as a result of complications from pressure ulcers (IHI, 2011b). Because of the nurse's specific role in assessing and maintaining skin integrity, pressure ulcers are listed by NDQNI as a nursing-sensitive quality indicator (Montalvo, 2007). Additionally, CMS (2014) lists stage 3 and 4 pressure ulcers as nonreimbursable hospital-acquired conditions.

The IHI (2011b) identifies six essential elements for pressure ulcer prevention: (a) pressure ulcer admission assessment, (b) daily reassessment of pressure ulcer risk, (c) daily skin inspection, (d) moisture management, (e) adequate nutrition and hydration, and (f) minimization of pressure. The NIA Expert Panel dictates admission screening for pressure ulcer risk using the Braden or Norton Scales (McGory et al., 2009).This is in line with admission assessments as recommended by TJC and NQF (IHI, 2011b). The remaining five elements fall under the nurse's purview during postoperative care. Chapter 24, "Preventing Pressure Ulcers and Skin Tears, outlines nursing protocols for preventing pressure ulcers and skin tears in older adults. Daily risk assessment should be completed using the same tool as was used on admission and should be documented in the EMR along with the visual skin inspection (IHI, 2011b). Some other key interventions include the following (IHI, 2011b):

- *Management of moisture*: (a) skin cleaning routinely and at times of soiling with mild cleansing agents; (b) use of skin moisturizes for dry skin; (c) use of absorbent underpads for excessive incontinence, perspiration, or wound drainage
- *Pressure relief*: (a) turn/reposition the patient every 2 hours; (b) use mattresses and cushions to redistribute pressure

Additional care should be focused on pressure caused by medical devices as well as caution when removing dressings, pads, tape, or leads in order to prevent skin tears (Bashaw & Scott, 2012).

The NIA Expert Panel recommends daily screening and repositioning/pressure reduction at least until the patient is ambulatory (McGory et al., 2009). Additionally, if the surgical patient has an existing stage 2, stage 3, or stage 4 pressure ulcer, a treatment plan should be outlined and documented before surgery (McGory et al., 2009). For patients undergoing cardiac surgery, it is recommended to continue skin assessment and interventions up until the postop day 5 (Pokorny, Koldjeski, & Swanson, 2003).

Prevention of VTE

Older adult surgical patients may have many factors, including age, that place them at risk of VTE, including obesity, prolonged immobility, lengthy surgery (longer than 2 hours), presence of varicose veins, and smoking history (Bashaw & Scott, 2012). VTE occurs in approximately 1 million patients each year (Dobesh, 2009). In a study of nonemergent surgeries, Gajdos et al. (2013) found that 2% of adults aged 60 years and older experienced VTE, and 10% of those with VTE died. The occurrence of VTE leads to increased length and cost of stay, and also puts the patient at risk of other potentially life-threatening complications (Dobesh, 2009). In addition, there may be significant long-term complications and related costs, often caused by recurrent VTE, postthrombotic syndrome, or pulmonary hypertension (Dobesh, 2009). According to the CMS (2014), the occurrence of VTE following certain orthopedic surgeries (e.g., total knee replacement and hip replacement) is a nonreimbursable hospital-acquired condition.

The AHRQ (2012) guidelines for VTE prophylaxis list four interventions and practices to consider: (a) assessment of VTE risk factors, (b) patient education and early ambulation, (c) mechanical prophylaxis, and (d) pharmacologic prophylaxis (AHRQ, 2012). The guidelines also address special situations, such as prophylaxis for patients with hip/knee arthroplasty and hip fracture (see Chapter 34, "Care of the Older Adult With Fragility Hip Fracture"). For VTE screening of surgical patients, AHRQ (2012) recommends the use of the Caprini Risk Assessment Model. The Caprini Model uses a checklist of factors scored as 1 point (e.g., swollen legs and acute myocardial infarction), 2 points (e.g., age 61–74 years and central venous access), 3 points (e.g., age 75 years or more and history of DVT), or 5 points (e.g., stroke within the past month); the scores for the checked boxes are then summed for an overall Caprini score (Caprini, 2009).

Mechanical prophylaxis measures include early ambulation and the use of SCDs (AHRQ, 2012). Compression stockings have been shown to reduce VTE risk when used effectively, but are not necessarily recommended because tight fit can impair circulation and lead to additional complications (Bashaw & Scott, 2012). The BGS cautions against the use of compression stockings in older adults but

TABLE 33.3
VTE Prophylaxis

VTE Risk Category	Low Bleeding Risk	High Risk for Major Bleeding
Very low risk		
(Caprini score 0)	Early ambulation	Early ambulation
Low risk		
(Caprini score 1–2)	SCDs	SCDs
Moderate risk		
(Caprini score 3–4)	LMWH/LUDH *or* SCDs	SCDs
High risk		
(Caprini score greater than or equal to 5)	LMWH/LUDH *and* SCDs	SCDs until bleeding risk diminishes then addition of LMWH/ LUDH

LMWH, low-molecular-weight heparin; LUDH, low-dose unfractionated heparin SCD, sequential compression device; VTE, venous thromboembolism.

Adapted from the Agency for Healthcare Research and Quality (2012).

if they are used, skin integrity needs to be regularly and carefully monitored (Donald, 2010). ROM exercises can also be effective if the patient is unable to ambulate (Bashaw & Scott, 2012). Inferior vena cava (IVC) filters may be placed in critically ill adults to prevent pulmonary embolism related to DVT; however, AHRQ (2012) does not recommend their use. Pharmacologic prophylaxis measures include the use of low-molecular-weight heparin (LMWH) or low-dose unfractionated heparin (LDUH). However, the BGS purports that major bleeding risk may outweigh VTE risk in older adults, thus use of LMWH or LDUH may not be the best choice for prophylaxis (Donald, 2010).

The AHRQ (2012) stratifies mechanical and pharmacologic prophylaxis based on the Caprini Risk score and a comprehensive assessment of bleeding risk. Table 33.3 provides the measures based on score and bleeding risk for patients undergoing nonorthopedic surgery. The ACOVE quality indicators also emphasize the use of SCDs and pharmacologic prophylaxis in vulnerable elders at high risk of VTE (AGS, 2007).

Restraint Use

Restraints are often used in an acute care setting to prevent falls and patient interference with therapy (Minnick, Mion, Johnson, Catrambone, & Leipzig, 2007). Restraints may also be used on patients who are confused or agitated, wander, or are perceived to have behavioral problems (Evans & Fitzgerald, 2002). Use may also be a result of inadequate staffing (Evans & Fitzgerald, 2002). Although rates of restraint use among older and younger adults in intensive care settings are similar, older adults represent much higher rates on medical units than their younger counterparts (Minnick et al., 2007). The use of restraints has been shown to increase the risk of falls, pressure ulcers, and delirium in older adult surgical patients, which could lead to increased morbidity, mortality, and length of stay (Baumgarten et al., 2008; Inouye et al., 2007; Shorr et al., 2002). Restraint use is a key NDNQI nursing-sensitive indicator endorsed by the NQF (Montalvo, 2007).

If restraints are used, the NIA Expert Panel quality indicators specify that the target behavioral or safety issue must be addressed with the patient or legal guardian and documented in the chart, along with methods other than restraints implemented as part of the plan of care (McGory et al., 2009). In order to prevent or lessen restraint use, the health care provider should certify the continued need for invasive lines as removal of unnecessary lines may eliminate the need for restraints. In addition, the NIA Expert Panel advises implementation of the following care measures (McGory et al., 2009):

- Release from restraints and repositioning at least every 2 hours
- Face-to-face reassessment by the nurse at least every 4 hours and by the physician before renewal of the restraint order
- 15-minute observations; more if the patient's condition warrants more frequent assessment
- Nurse-related interventions every 2 hours to address nutrition, hydration, toileting, personal hygiene, and ROM

Additional information on the use of restraints in the acute care setting is provided in Chapter 23, "Physical Restraints and Side Rails in Acute and Critical Care Settings."

Discharge Planning

Adequate discharge planning begins before surgery, including assessment of the need for social support or home health expected after discharge (McGory et al., 2009). Comprehensive discharge planning involves the multidisciplinary team to address patient status before discharge as well as follow-up care after discharge (Palmer, 2009). ACOVE quality indicators specify that an assessment of cognition and function should be performed and compared with preoperative levels and that the level of independence, along with the need for home health services, be documented in the EMR (AGS, 2007). The NIA Expert Panel includes assessment of nutrition, cognition, ambulation, and ADL in its discharge planning criteria (McGory et al., 2009).

A comprehensive medication reconciliation addressing chronic medications as well as new prescriptions will help facilitate discharge and, along with adequate care transition planning and communication with outpatient providers, can help reduce rehospitalizations and emergency room visits (Legrain et al., 2011). For new medications, the nurse will facilitate patient education with regard to the purpose of the drug, how to take it, expected side effects, as well as possible adverse effects (McGory et al., 2009). Medication education is just one of many patient and family education tasks of the nurse. Others include a detailed explanation of the plan of care, which may include home health visits, physical or occupational therapy appointments, follow-up appointments; education on the use of new equipment or devices; or demonstration on the performance of activities such as dressing changes and wound care. Effective nursing education using teach-back and return demonstration has been shown to increase patient and family confidence and decrease nonscheduled health care visits postdischarge (Henderson & Zernike, 2001; Williams, 2008). For further information on discharge planning, refer to Chapter 36 "Transitional Care."

CASE STUDY

Admission and Preoperative Course

KL is a 72-year-old Asian female admitted from home because of intermittent vomiting and poor oral intake. No other associated symptoms were reported. The history was obtained from the patient's daughter via an interpreter. KL has no known drug allergies and is full-code status. The remainder of her admission history includes:

- *Home medications*: Aspirin, ascorbic acid, docusate sodium, folic acid, multivitamins, ferrous sulfate, pantoprazole, senna, metoprolol, and lisinopril
- *Past medical history*: Anemia, constipation, hypertension, chronic kidney disease, non-ST-segment elevation myocardial infarction (NSTEMI)
- *Past surgical history*: "Bowel surgery many years ago" (unknown date)
- *Psychosocial history*: KL is widowed. She lives with her daughter in a single-family house. She has no history of tobacco or alcohol use and was independent with ADL until this admission.

General overview revealed a frail-looking, non-English speaking female who looks her stated age. Her general physical examination is mostly unremarkable except for a distended and tympanic abdomen with hypoactive bowel sounds. An episode of vomiting of bilious liquid was noted in the emergency department (ED) for which she was given metoclopramide 10-mg IV push. A Salem sump tube attached to low continuous intermittent suction (LCS) was draining yellow-greenish liquid. Normal saline at 100 mL/hr was started via a left peripheral IV line and an indwelling urinary catheter was inserted.

KL was oriented to self and place but not to time. She denied any abdominal pain but referred to feeling bloated and nauseated. Her vital signs were blood pressure = 141/71 mmHg, heart rate = 7,090/min, respiratory rate = 18–20/min, temperature = 98.2°F, and a 96% oxygen saturation on room air. Her latest lab results were:

Na = 145 mEq/L	WBC = 16,100 × 10^3/μL	Albumin = 3.9 g/dL
K = 4.4 mEq/L	Hemoglobin = 9.6 g/dL	Calcium = 9.0 mg/dL
Cl = 103 mEq/L	Hematocrit = 31.3%	Magnesium = 2.5 mEq/L
CO_2 = 24 mEq/L	Platelets = 360 × 10^9/L	Phosphorus = 4.2 mg/dL
BUN = 33 mg/dL	Prothrombin time = 16.1 seconds	Troponin = 0.0 μg/L
Creatinine = 2.0 mg/dL	International normalized ratio (INR) = 1.2	Creatinine clearance (CrCl) = 23.2

BUN, blood urea nitrogen; Cl, chlorine; CO_2, carbon dioxide; K, potassium; Na, sodium; WBC, white blood cells.

A 12-lead electrocardiogram (EKG) revealed sinus rhythm. KL's chest x-ray showed an enlarged cardiac silhouette but no signs of consolidation or infiltrates. The abdominal CT scan findings reported marked gaseous distention of stomach; small and large bowels without definite transition point identified; and mild colonic stool retention within the rectosigmoid up to 4.2 cm in transverse diameter. After a 6-hour stay in the ED, KL was moved to the surgical ward. She was kept at nothing-by-mouth status, continued on normal saline at 100 mL/hr, and the Salem sump to LCS. VTE prophylaxis with pneumatic compressions was initiated. Routine lab work, including urinalysis, blood type, and screening, were ordered for the

(continued)

CASE STUDY *(continued)*

following morning. Once cleared by cardiology, KL was scheduled for exploratory laparotomy.

Intraoperative Course

After routine universal protocol procedure, KL had an uneventful induction and administration of general anesthesia. No adverse events were noted intraoperatively. The surgery performed was small bowel resection with anastomosis and lysis of adhesion. After extubation, she was transported to the postanesthesia care unit (PACU) for 4 hours and subsequently transferred to the surgical step-down unit.

Postoperative Course

KL's postop orders include oxygen 4 L via nasal cannula; Lactated Ringers at 100 mL/hr for 24 hours; Salem sump to LCS; SCD to both legs; bedside telemetry; Foley to side drainage; patient-controlled analgesia (PCA) morphine 1-mg continuous dose, 1-mg demand dose, 6-minute lock out, and 20 mg 4-hour limit; metoprolol 5 mg IV piggy back (IVPB) every 6 hours; famotidine 20 mg IVPB once daily; metoclopramide 10 mg IVPB every 6 hours as needed for nausea and vomiting; Benadryl 25 mg IVPB every 12 hours as needed for itchiness; out-of-bed to chair in a.m.; and physical therapy and nutrition consults.

1. Describe the application of best practice guidelines for KL's transition from PACU to the surgical unit. Patient safety is an utmost consideration.
   Transitions between the various operative units should be marked by high-quality handoff between providers using standardized forms, both in paper and electronically. Bedside safety checks are best done with both the giving and receiving providers present using a checklist. Specific institutional procedures and protocols should be followed (e.g., who should accompany the patient during transport).
2. Describe key assessment parameters for KL's post-surgical care.
   When KL arrives on the surgical unit, a priority is to ensure she has a patent airway and is hemodynamically stable. A thorough head-to-toe assessment is essential, giving special attention to abdominal and operative wound assessment and ensuring that KL's vital signs are within baseline. It is important to ensure that the Salem sump tube is attached to suction and VTE prophylaxis is maintained (SCD). As KL has baseline chronic kidney disease (CKD), a close monitoring or her urine output and implementing the CAUTI bundle are important considerations.
3. Describe the importance of medication reconciliation in postop older adult patients.
   Medication reconciliation should be performed during every transition in order to prevent inadvertent omission of essential medications (e.g., beta blockers) and use of inappropriate medications. In KL's case, it is important to raise clinical concern regarding the order of metoclopramide for postop nausea and vomiting. It is best avoided among older adults as it can cause extrapyramidal effects, including tardive dyskinesia (AGS, 2012). The use of diphenhydramine, chlorpromazine, and H_2-receptor antagonist is also considered inappropriate in older adults because of increased risk of confusion/delirium (AGS, 2012). In KL's case, famotidine can be replaced with pantoprazole and metoclopramide with ondansetron. If KL develops itchiness as a result of the morphine, nonpharmacological interventions should be tried first (e.g., applying lotion to her skin). For mild to moderate pain, acetaminophen can be ordered for KL.
4. Describe ongoing best practices for postop older adult patients.
   The postop period is a vulnerable time that can set back the older patient from major gains such as overcoming general anesthesia. Essential to achieving positive outcomes is hardwired interprofessional collaboration across all disciplines. In addition to focused assessments, purposeful hourly rounding (e.g., addressing pain, positioning, elimination, and comfort needs) will enable the staff to address the patient's routine needs and avert potentially high-risk events such as a fall. Fall risk assessment and interventions need to be reviewed as per hospital protocol. The removal of catheters or other nonessential invasive devices will reduce the overall risk for infection. Key postop complications that require special attention are listed in the following.
   A. *Postop ileus*—Preventing postop ileus can be a challenge for KL because of the use of morphine. Using the lowest dose and transitioning from PCA to "as needed" status might be considered. Early mobilization and active range-of-motion exercises will be beneficial in promoting peristalsis, preventing VTE, and improving general well-being. The nurse needs to continue focused GI surveillance for signs of ileus. When listening for bowel sounds, KL's Salem sump

(continued)

CASE STUDY (continued)

tube should be disconnected from the LCS in order not to confuse the negative pressure from the suction as bowel sounds.

B. *Postop atelectasis*—The nature of abdominal surgeries puts the patient at a greater risk for atelectasis. Although KL has no pulmonary comorbidities, she should be encouraged and coached to use the incentive spirometer (e.g., 10 times every hour while awake). Nursing measures to improve compliance with breathing and coughing exercises include splinting wound with a binder, premedicating with pain relievers, and empowering the patient.
C. *Postop VTE*—KL's abdominal surgery and her comorbidities make her vulnerable to VTE. Early mobilization, adequate hydration, the use of SCD and pharmacologic prophylaxis (e.g., heparin) will help reduce the risk.
D. *Surgical site infection*—The implementation of evidence-based practices listed in this chapter will eliminate the risk of SSI. The operative wound should have a sterile dressing for 24 to 48 hours postop. Monitoring and reporting changes in KL's mental status that might signal an infection are essential. Trend of KL's white blood cell count and wound appearance should be monitored. Hand hygiene remains the most cost-effective and most effective way to prevent the transmission of infection.

5. Describe best practices in patient/family education for postop patients.

Patients' active participation in their care is now recognized as an essential element for positive health outcomes. For surgical patients, physical (e.g., wound) and psychological healing continues on discharge. This endeavor requires high-quality patient education using proven methods such as the teach-back approach. KL and her daughter should be provided easy-to-understand handouts on wound care, nutrition, and exercise at home. Providing KL and her daughter a script from the National Patient Safety Foundation (e.g., What is my main problem? What do I need to do? Why is it important for me to do this?) for use when they visit the surgical provider will help them feel empowered and improve follow-up care. For best practices in transitional care, please refer to Chapter 36.

SUMMARY

Older adult surgical patients are at higher risk of morbidity and mortality following surgery due to age-related changes that lead to limited physiological reserve as well as a potential number of medical comorbidities that may further complicate recovery. As such, the nurse must work diligently with the interprofessional team to develop a comprehensive plan of care postsurgery. Frequent assessment and early intervention are necessary to prevent debilitating complications, including postoperative delirium, functional decline, HAIs, pressure ulcers, and falls. Pain management, early ambulation, and adequate nutrition and hydration can help prevent complications or lessen the intensity or duration of their effects. With an appropriate plan of care, the older adult surgical patient will experience shorter lengths of stay, be discharged with baseline cognitive and physical functioning, and transition to the location from which they were admitted.

NURSING STANDARD OF PRACTICE

Protocol 33.1: General Surgical Care of the Older Adult

I. GOAL

To restore physiological stability, prevent complications, maintain safety and comfort, and preserve presurgical functional ability and QOL in older adult surgical patients

II. OVERVIEW

A. Physiological changes of aging can significantly affect the recovery time of older adult surgical patients and put them at greater risk for postoperative complications (Leung & Dzankic, 2001; Makary et al., 2010).

(continued)

Protocol 33.1: General Surgical Care of the Older Adult *(continued)*

B. Older adults often present for elective and nonelective or emergent surgeries with a number of medical comorbidities that place them at further risk of postoperative morbidity and mortality (Dasgupta et al., 2009).
C. The risk of complications and mortality increase with advancing age, with those aged 90 years and older experiencing twice the rate of mortality at less than 48 hours postsurgery as compared with those younger than 65 years (Deiner et al., 2014).
D. Longer lengths of stay have been consistently linked to increased postoperative adverse outcomes (Leung & Dzankic, 2001; Makary et al., 2010).
E. Surgical patients at hospitals with a higher percentage of nurses with a baccalaureate or higher degree experienced shorter lengths of stay and fewer postoperative complications (Blegen et al., 2013).
F. A proportionate increase of staff nurses with bachelor's degrees decreases the risk of death among patients following common surgeries in acute care settings (Aiken et al., 2014).

III. BACKGROUND

A. Definition
   1. The patient is discharged from the PACU following an established protocol, such as the Aldrete Score, a post-anesthesia recovery score. Patients with scores of 9 or 10 may be discharged to the surgical or equivalent units, those with 8 require further observation, those with 7 or less require admission to the ICU (Aldrete & Kroulik, 1970). Another tool in use is the PADSS (Chung, Chan, & Ong, 1995). No matter which tool is used, collaborative ongoing assessment and clinical judgment are required.
   2. Nursing priorities when the patient arrives from the PACU to the surgical unit include high-quality handoff; focus on airway, breathing and circulation; assessment of vital signs based on specific protocol; monitoring of complications; and discharge readiness (Odom-Forren, 2015).

B. Etiology/epidemiology
   1. In 2010, 19.2 million operative procedures were performed among older adults in acute care settings. These accounted for more than 37% of all procedures and 45% of total hospital days of care (CDC, 2010).
   2. Hospital stays that involve surgical procedures have been shown to be more costly, required longer lengths of stay, and resulted in higher morbidity and mortality (Weiss & Elixhauser, 2014).
   3. The need for comprehensive baseline status assessment and the use of an interdisciplinary team with surgical and geriatric expertise to follow the patient from preop to discharge are essential for achieving positive outcomes (McGory et al., 2009).
   4. Postoperative delirium can occur in up to 50% of high-risk older adult surgical patients, leading to prolonged and more costly hospitalizations, functional decline, and death (AGS, 2014).
   5. Older adult surgical patients are at a higher risk of delirium resulting from medication side effects; immobility; infection; inadequate pain management; and cardiac, renal, and respiratory complications (Hughes et al., 2013).
   6. Hospitalized older adults are consistently less likely to receive adequate pain control compared with younger adult patients (Schofield, 2014).
   7. A lack of pain control for the older surgical patient can lead to delirium, depression, fluid imbalances, atelectasis, and fatigue (AGS, 2014; Bashaw & Scott, 2012).
   8. A large majority of hospitalized older adults are malnourished or at risk of malnutrition, placing them at risk of impaired skin integrity, wound or other infections, sepsis, and death (Kaiser et al., 2010; Lagoo-Deenadayalan et al., 2011; Scandrett et al., 2015).
   9. Approximately 1.5% of older surgical patients develop postoperative renal insufficiency, with a mortality rate of greater than 31% (Gajdos et al., 2013).
   10. Postoperative pulmonary complications occur in about 10% of older adult surgical patients, accounting for 40% of postoperative complications and 20% of preventable deaths (Lagoo-Deenadayalan et al., 2011).
   11. Among older surgical patients, SSI occurred in 8%, with a 7% mortality rate for those developing an SSI (Gajdos et al., 2013).
   12. Approximately 60% of SSIs are preventable. Developing an SSI can lead to an additional 11 postoperative hospital days and a two- to 11-fold increase in mortality risks (Anderson et al., 2014).

(continued)

Protocol 33.1: General Surgical Care of the Older Adult *(continued)*

13. The risk for developing CAUTI increases 5% per day of catheterization (Bhardwaj et al., 2012; IHI, 2011a).
14. CLABSI has been shown to double mortality risk, add up to 10 additional hospital days, and increase health care costs (Kaye et al., 2014).
15. Postsurgical deconditioning can slow recovery, delay in restoring independence with ADL, and increase risk for VTE, delirium, incontinence, constipation, pressure ulcers, and falls (Lagoo-Deenadayalan et al., 2011).
16. The postsurgical period is a vulnerable time for increased risk of falls (Currie, 2008).
17. Approximately 15% of hospitalized patients in hospitals at any given time have pressure ulcers, with 60,000 dying per year (IHI, 2011b).
18. The postsurgical older adult is at increased risk of VTE, which occurs in about 1 million patients each year (Bashaw & Scott, 2012; Dobesh, 2009).
19. Restraint use increases the risk of falls, pressure ulcers, and delirium, leading to increased morbidity, mortality, and length of stay (Baumgarten et al., 2008; Inouye et al., 2007; Shorr et al., 2002).

IV. PARAMETERS OF ASSESSMENT

A. The PSIs are the key drivers of assessment and screening of surgical older adult patients. PSIs that are relevant to surgical patients include (AHRQ, 2014):
   1. Death among surgical inpatients
   2. CVC-related bloodstream infection
   3. Postoperative hemorrhage or hematoma, physiological and metabolic derangements, respiratory failure, pulmonary embolism or DVT, sepsis, and wound dehiscence
   4. Transfusion reaction

B. A seamless synthesis of various practice guidelines, such as those recommended in the Assessing Care of Vulnerable Elders-3 (ACOVE) Quality Indicators (AGS, 2007), Beers Criteria for Potentially Inappropriate Medication Use in Older Adults (AGS, 2014), and Clinical Practice Guideline for Postoperative Delirium in Older Adults (AGS, 2014), will be essential in achieving positive outcomes. All older adult postsurgical patients must be assessed and screened for:
   1. Falls (AGS, 2007)
   2. Frailty (AGS, 2007)
   3. Inappropriate medication use (AGS, 2012)
   4. Postoperative atelectasis (AGS, 2007)
   5. Postoperative delirium (AGS, 2007, 2014)
   6. Postoperative ileus (AGS, 2007)
   7. PONV (ASPAN, 2006)
   8. Postoperative pain (AGS, 2007, 2014)
   9. Pressure ulcers (AGS, 2007)
   10. SSI (TJC, 2013)
   11. VTE (AHRQ, 2012; AGS, 2007)
   12. Restraint use (McGory et al., 2009)

C. Other epidemiologically significant assessment parameters, depending on the specific patient scenario, would include screening patients for CAUTI, CLABSI, and VAP. The nurse is encouraged to be familiar with the current best practices related to these HAIs.

V. NURSING CARE STRATEGIES

A. Unit admission
   1. Provide for high-quality handoff to include the following information:
      a. Preoperative assessment of cognitive and functional status
      b. List of comorbidities and preoperative home medications
      c. Preoperative assessment for falls and pressure ulcers

(continued)

Protocol 33.1: General Surgical Care of the Older Adult *(continued)*

- d. Course of surgery, including any surgical complications and interventions for such, blood loss, blood transfusions, and intraoperative fluid use
- e. Description of surgical sites, including dressings and instructions for care
- f. Identification of invasive lines, including arterial and/or venous catheters, urinary catheters, GI tubes, chest tubes, and any other drainage devices (e.g., Jackson–Pratt, t-tube)
- g. Patient's respiratory, cardiovascular, and cognitive status before transfer
- h. Patient's current pain level and description of pharmacologic and nonpharmacologic interventions (used since surgery) before transfer

2. Perform comprehensive admission assessment to include:
   - a. Airway, breathing, circulation, and cognitive status
   - b. Pain and/or PONV, with immediate intervention if necessary
   - c. Surgical site or surgical dressing if in place and intact
   - d. Invasive lines, including line patency and visual inspection of site and dressing
   - e. Thorough skin examination, particularly on bony prominences that may have been damaged during surgery
   - f. ROM, mobility, and functional status
3. Discuss plan of care with patient and caregivers, addressing pain management, mobility, nutrition, hydration, and functional status.

B. Duration of stay—comprehensive management to prevent postoperative complications and sentinel events

1. Postoperative delirium/cognitive and sensory function
   - a. Use a validated tool to assess for delirium at least once per shift for up to 3 days postop
   - b. Provide for continuity of care (familiar residents, nurses, and care technicians)
   - c. Provide continuous environmental and personal orientation
   - d. Adequately manage pain (see Pain Management in subsequent discussion)
   - e. Avoid delirium-inducing medications such as benzodiazepines and anticholinergics (see also the AGS Beers Criteria [AGS, 2012])
   - f. Avoid use of routine sedation
   - g. Provide for adequate fluid and nutrition intake (see Nutrition and Hydration in the following)
   - h. Avoid use of restraints (see Restraints)
   - i. Avoid urinary catheterization or ensure prompt removal if in place (see HAIs in the following discussion)
   - j. Promote adequate sleep, including involving family and caregivers in managing daytime sleepiness
   - k. Promote appropriate use of glasses, hearing aids, and other assistive devices
   - l. Provide for adequate communication as necessary, including the use of pen/paper, nonverbal communication, or translators
   - m. Minimize noise and patient care activities, as much as possible, during nighttime hours
2. Pain management
   - a. Perform comprehensive pain assessment during hourly rounding or, at a minimum, with each set of vital signs
     - i. Rating of intensity (numeric, verbal, or visual scales)
     - ii. Pain description to include location, characteristics, and impact of pain on function
     - iii. Observation of signs of pain
     - iv. Use appropriate scales (e.g., PAINAD) for patients with dementia
   - b. For pain scores greater than 5, initiate comprehensive pain management plan
     - i. Pharmacologic strategies
       - a) Preferable use of nonopioid pain medications
       - b) Address medication side effects, as necessary (e.g., morphine and constipation)
       - c) Avoid NSAIDs, if possible
     - ii. Nonpharmacologic strategies (e.g., massage, acupuncture, cognitive behavioral therapy, and distraction)
     - iii. See Chapter 18 for specific protocols on the management of pain in older adults

(continued)

Protocol 33.1: General Surgical Care of the Older Adult *(continued)*

- c. Reassess pain post-intervention
  - i. At 15 minutes, for IV medication interventions
  - ii. At 1 hour for by-mouth medication interventions
  - iii. Within 4 hours, at a minimum, for other interventions

3. Nutrition and gastrointestinal complications
   - a. Assess for postoperative dysphagia
     - i. Assessment by speech therapist if patient is at high risk of aspiration
     - ii. Modification of diet as necessary (e.g., alteration in food consistency)
   - b. Assess for and aggressively manage PONV
   - c. Implement a comprehensive nutrition plan
     - i. Assessment by a registered dietitian specializing in geriatric care
     - ii. Include adequate nutritional intake with supplementation as necessary
   - d. Implement a collaborative feeding plan, involving care technicians, family, and caregivers
     - i. Maintain upright position while feeding and for at least 1 hour after
     - ii. Provide comprehensive oral care
     - iii. See Chapters 10 and 25 for further discussion on nutrition and mealtime difficulties in older adults, respectively
   - e. Assess for and manage constipation
     - i. Avoid excessive use of anticholinergics and opioid medications, with quick transition to acetaminophen for mild to moderate pain
     - ii. Administer bowel stimulants (e.g., senna and bisacodyl) and osmotic agents (e.g., polyethylene glycol) as needed
     - iii. Provide adequate hydration (see Hydration)
     - iv. Promote early ambulation and mobilization (see Mobility)
   - f. Assess for and manage diarrhea
     - i. Maintain adequate hydration (see Hydration) and nutritional intake
     - ii. Collect stool samples, as ordered, to assess for *C. difficile* infection
     - iii. Provide prompt treatment if positive for *C. difficile,* including implementation of contact precautions and maintenance of adequate hand-hygiene regimens
   - g. Manage postoperative ileus for GI surgery patients
     - i. Promote early feeding and mobilization
     - ii. If NG decompression is used, continuously monitor for aspiration and postoperative pulmonary complications
4. Hydration and renal complications
   - a. Initiate oral hydration as soon as feasibly possible
     - i. Promptly manage PONV
     - ii. Provide adequate hydration through IV fluids or tube feedings if oral hydration is not possible
     - iii. Provide comprehensive oral care
   - b. Monitor fluid status at least once per shift for the first 5 days postop
     - i. Weigh patient daily
     - ii. Accurately assess and document intake and output
     - iii. Assess for changes in blood pressure, mental status, and new-onset atrial fibrillation that could indicate dehydration
   - c. Perform routine screening of serum electrolytes, urea nitrogen, and creatinine
5. Respiratory complications
   - a. Implement an aggressive pulmonary toilet regimen
     - i. Promote use of incentive spirometer 10 times per hour
     - ii. Perform turn, cough, and deep-breathing exercises every 2 hours

(continued)

Protocol 33.1: General Surgical Care of the Older Adult *(continued)*

iii. Provide chest percussion or chest physiotherapy as needed
iv. Promote early mobilization and ambulation (see Mobility)
v. Maintain head of bed in an elevated position
vi. Adequately manage pain (see earlier section on Pain Management)
vii. Avoid excessive use of narcotics and sedatives

b. Prevent VAP for intubated patients
  i. Implement a VAP bundle, including:
    a) Elevation of the head of the bed between 30° and 45°
    b) Daily sedative interruptions and assessment of readiness to extubate
    c) Peptic ulcer disease prophylaxis
    d) DVT prophylaxis
    e) Daily oral care with chlorhexidine

6. Infection prevention
  a. Implement unit-wide HAI prevention programs
    i. Continuing education on the appropriate use of guidelines for HAI prevention
    ii. Enforce universal precaution and contact precaution protocols
    iii. Hand-hygiene protocols, including hand rubbing with alcohol-based products or scrubbing with soap and water if hands are visibly soiled:
      a) Before touching the patient
      b) Before clean and aseptic procedures
      c) After contact with body fluids
      d) After touching a patient
      e) After touching a patient's surroundings
  b. Assess for signs/symptoms of infection
    i. Local signs/symptoms, including redness, tenderness, swelling, and warmth
    ii. Systemic signs/symptoms, including:
      a) Fever greater than 38.0°C after postop day 2
      b) Altered mental status, agitation, respiratory distress, tachycardia, and hypotension
      c) Elevated white blood cell count
  c. SSI
    i. Perioperative prevention protocols, including prophylactic antibiotics and proper hair removal before incision (see Chapter 32 on the perioperative care of older adult surgical patients)
    ii. For closed surgical incisions
      a) Maintain sterile dressing for closed surgical incisions up to 48 hours
      b) Perform dressing changes using sterile technique
      c) Remove dressing after 48 hours, unless instructed otherwise
    iii. For open surgical incisions
      a) Pack wound with sterile gauze and cover with sterile dressing
      b) Consult with wound ostomy continence nurse for dressing change regimen, which may continue postdischarge.
    iv. Continue to assess for local and systemic signs/symptoms of infection
    v. Aggressively treat SSI
      a) Reopening and drainage of incision
      b) Wound culture
      c) Antibiotic treatment of infection if it becomes systemic
      d) Contact precautions and adequate cleaning and disinfecting of equipment/environment if infectious agent is an MDRO

(continued)

Protocol 33.1: General Surgical Care of the Older Adult *(continued)*

d. CAUTI
   i. Implement CAUTI bundle
      a) Avoid unnecessary catheterizations
      b) Insert catheters using an aseptic technique, using the smallest possible catheter
      c) Review catheter necessity daily and remove promptly if use is no longer indicated
   ii. Remove catheters placed during surgery by postop day 3. If not removed, provide documentation of the need for continued use
   iii. Provide bedpan, urinal, bedside commode, and/or ambulation to the bathroom as an alternative to catheterization
   iv. Involve the patient, family, and caregivers in catheter plan of care
   v. Continue to assess for local and systemic signs/symptoms of infection
   vi. See Chapter 22 for further information on the prevention of CAUTI
e. CLABSI
   i. Implement a CLABSI bundle
      a) Maintain adequate hand hygiene regimens
      b) Provide maximal barrier precautions when inserting lines
      c) Use chlorhexidine skin antiseptic before insertion
      d) Optimize site selection, avoiding the use of the femoral vein
      e) Review necessity of line daily and provide for prompt removal if no longer indicated
   ii. Institute appropriate dressing change regimens
      a) Use sterile gauze and a transparent, semipermeable dressing to cover the site
      b) Replace dressing if it becomes damp, loosened, or visibly soiled
      c) Replace gauze dressings every 2 days and transparent dressings every 7 days for short-term sites
      d) Use chlorhexidine-impregnated sponge dressing for temporary catheters if other measures are not working
   iii. Replace administration sets at appropriate intervals
      a) At least every 7 days (but not less than 96 hours) for continuous or secondary infusion tubing
      b) Within 24 hours for tubing involving blood, blood products, or fat emulsions
      c) Every 6 to 12 hours for propofol infusion tubing
   iv. Disinfect (scrub) using an appropriate antiseptic when accessing catheter hubs, needleless injectors, and injection ports, using only sterile devices/equipment
   v. Educate the patient and monitor to prevent submersion of CVC sites in water during showering or bathing
   vi. Continue to assess for local and systemic signs/symptoms of infection

7. Mobility, function, and frailty
   a. Work with interprofessional team to develop a plan for re-enablement after surgery
   b. Incorporate the patient, family, and caregivers in the development of the plan of care for re-enablement
   c. Address barriers to plan, including lack of understanding of roles among health care team members, patient dependence and daytime sleepiness, scheduling conflicts, and patient care equipment (e.g., IV tubing, catheters, and SCDs)
   d. Ensure physical therapy provides early assessment of the patient postsurgery and develops a mobility and strengthening plan, including the need for assistive devices
   e. Provide ambulation by postop day 2
      i. If ambulation is not possible, then documentation should be provided as to why ambulation did not occur
      ii. Provide ROM exercises for patients unable to ambulate
      iii. If ROM exercises cannot be performed, then documentation should be provided as to why they did not occur
   f. Assist patient with ADL and IADL, while allowing for as much independence as possible

(continued)

Protocol 33.1: General Surgical Care of the Older Adult *(continued)*

8. Fall prevention
   a. Routine screening of fall risk, at least once per shift, using validated assessment tools
   b. Use a multipronged approach to address falls, including:
      i. Fall risk screening on admission
      ii. Injury and injury risk-factors screening on admission
      iii. In-depth admission screening for any positive findings
      iv. Communication and education about the patient's fall risk
      v. Standardized interventions (e.g., armband identification, bed alarms, exercise and toileting regimens, pain relief) for any positive findings
      vi. Customized interventions for those at highest risk
   c. If a fall occurs, perform a comprehensive fall evaluation within 24 hours to include the presence or absence of any signs/symptoms of injury and a review of medications that may have contributed to the fall
   d. See Chapter 19 for a more detailed discussion on fall prevention in the older adult
9. Skin integrity
   a. Address pressure ulcer prevention from admission to discharge, including:
      i. Perform a comprehensive skin assessment and adequately document findings on admission to the unit
      ii. Complete a pressure ulcer risk assessment at least daily using a validated assessment tool (e.g., Braden Scale)
      iii. Daily comprehensive assessment of skin integrity
      iv. Moisture management
         a) Skin cleaning routinely and at times of soiling with mild cleansing agents
         b) Use of skin moisturizers for dry skin
         c) Use of absorbent underpads for excessive incontinence, perspiration, or wound drainage
      v. Maintenance of adequate nutrition and hydration (see earlier sections Nutrition and Hydration)
      vi. Minimize pressure on skin and bony prominences
         a) Turn and reposition the patient every 2 hours
         b) Use mattresses and cushions to redistribute pressure
         c) Address pressure from medical devices
      vii. Use care when removing dressings, pads, tape, or leads in order to prevent skin tears
   b. See Chapter 24 for further information on the prevention of pressure ulcers in older adults
10. VTE prevention
   a. Institute VTE prophylaxis, including:
      i. Assessment of VTE risk factors using validated measures (e.g., Caprini Risk Score)
      ii. Patient education about VTE risk
      iii. Early ambulation (see earlier section, Mobility)
      iv. Mechanical prophylaxis
         a) Use of SCDs
         b) Caution when using compression stockings as tight fit may impair circulation and lead to complications
         c) ROM exercises for patients unable to ambulate
      v. Pharmacologic prophylaxis
         a) Use of LMWH or LDUH, as indicated
         b) Monitor for signs/symptoms of bleeding
11. Restraint use
   a. Restraint use should be avoided if at all possible
   b. If restraints must be used, address the target behavioral or safety issue with the patient and caregivers and document in the chart
   c. Use and document methods other than restraints that can be used as part of the plan of care

(continued)

Protocol 33.1: General Surgical Care of the Older Adult *(continued)*

d. Seek early removal of devices or lines that will allow for the discontinuation of restraint use
e. Implement a care plan for the management of the patient in restraints
    i. Release from restraints and reposition every 2 hours
    ii. Perform face-to-face assessment at least every 4 hours (with physician assessment before renewal of restraint order)
    iii. Provide 15-minute observations, more frequently if warranted by the patient's condition
    iv. Perform nurse-related interventions every 2 hours to address nutrition, hydration, toileting, personal hygiene, and ROM
f. See Chapter 23 for further information on the use of restraints in the hospitalized older adult.

C. Discharge
1. Assess the need for social support or home health care expected after discharge
2. Perform comprehensive discharge assessment of cognition and function (mobility, ADL, IADL) and compare with preoperative levels
3. Assess nutritional status before discharge
4. Perform comprehensive medication reconciliation
    a. Address both prior-use and new medications
    b. Facilitate education for new medications, including purpose of the drug, how to take it, expected side effects, and adverse side effects
5. Provide detailed explanation to patient, family, and caregivers about the plan of care, including:
    a. Home health visits
    b. Physical or occupational therapy appointments
    c. Follow-up appointments
    d. Education on the use of new equipment or devices, and activity
    e. Education using teach-back strategies on performance of activities such as dressing changes, wound care, and medication administration

VI. EVALUATION/EXPECTED OUTCOMES

A. Patient outcomes
1. Maintain patient safety across the postoperative continuum
2. Assess patient decision-making capacity and honor patient and family care decision choices
3. Receive a comprehensive unit admission screening and ongoing assessment, including, but not limited to, the following domains: cognitive and behavioral, cardiopulmonary, functional status, nutrition, medication, and frailty
4. Receive adequate pain control through implementation of a patient-centered pain management plan
5. Restore mobility and functioning to preoperative levels before discharge
6. Receive timely and accurate information related to plan of care, including transitional care and long-term follow-up
7. Patient will not develop postop complications such as delirium, HAI, VTE, cardiopulmonary adverse events, GI or renal complications, and pressure ulcers
8. Patient will be free from adverse events such as medication errors and falls
9. Comprehensive discharge planning, including discharge assessment of cognitive, functional, and nutritional status; medication reconciliation; discharge location; and home health or other follow-up care

B. Provider outcomes
1. Receive education and ongoing training on best practices in the care of the geriatric surgical patient
2. Assess patient's and family's decision-making capacity and involve the patient and family in the development of the plan of care
3. Provide patient and caregivers timely and accurate information of patient's condition and plan of care, including transitions

(continued)

Protocol 33.1: General Surgical Care of the Older Adult *(continued)*

4. Participate in high-quality interprofessional collaboration throughout the postoperative stay, including rounding, handoff, pain management, early mobility, nutrition and hydration, medication reconciliation, and transitional care
5. Use an evidence-based teamwork system to improve communication and teamwork skills (e.g., TeamSTEPPS) for patient safety (AHRQ, n.d.)
6. Employ consistent and accurate documentation throughout the postoperative stay
7. Apply teach-back method in all patient and family education encounters that are culturally competent and patient centered
8. Staff nurses achieve a minimum of a bachelor's degree and obtain practice-specific certification (e.g., gerontological nursing)
9. Organize and participate in unit-based practice and quality-improvement councils

C. Systems outcomes
1. Uphold patient safety and quality in the care of older adults through policy and social statements (e.g., safety language in hospital's mission)
2. Review and align existing institutional policies and procedures with latest national standards (see Relevant Practice Guidelines section)
3. Facilitate and sustain interprofessional geriatric care teams
4. Establish a system of reporting patient safety issues (e.g., falls, medication errors, HAI, restraint use, etc.) across the postoperative continuum to identify opportunities for improvement
5. Adopt specific patient safety initiatives for older adults that include use of informatics, algorithms, checklists, and personnel oversight
6. Develop ongoing quality-improvement initiatives consistent with practice guidelines
7. Facilitate clinical rotations for nursing students across postoperative units to promote experiential learning for prelicensure students
8. Enforce SSI, CAUTI, CLABSI, and VAP prevention policies and conduct SSI surveillance based on CDC and TJC guidelines
9. Organize and support interprofessional unit-based practice and quality-improvement councils (IHI, n.d.)
10. Demonstrate a commitment to culture of safety based on openness and mutual trust (e.g., patient safety leadership walk rounds; IHI, n.d.)

VII. RELEVANT PRACTICE GUIDELINES

A. ACS NSQIP and the AGS's Best Practices Guidelines for Optimal Preoperative Assessment of the Geriatric Surgical Patient (2012): http://site.acsnsqip.org/wp-content/uploads/2011/12/ACS-NSQIP-AGS-Geriatric-2012-Guidelines.pdf
B. AGS Clinical Practice Guideline for Postoperative Delirium in Older Adults (2014): http://onlinelibrary.wiley.com/doi/10.1111/jgs.13281/epdf
C. AGS Assessing Care of Vulnerable Elders-3 Quality Indicators (2007)
D. CDC—Guideline for Prevention of Surgical Site Infection: http://www.cdc.gov/hicpac/pdf/SSIguidelines.pdf
E. Evidence-Based Guidelines for Selected, Candidate, and Previously Considered Hospital-Acquired Conditions (2014): http://www.cms.gov/Medicare/Medicare-Fee-for-Service-Payment/HospitalAcqCond/Downloads/Evidence-Based-Guidelines.pdf
F. IHI—How-to Guide: Prevent Surgical Site Infections: http://www.ihi.org/resources/Pages/Tools/HowtoGuidePreventSurgicalSiteInfection.aspx
G. National Patient Safety Goals by TJC (2015): http://www.jointcommission.org/assets/1/6/2015_NPSG_HAP.pdf
H. Surgical Care Improvement Guidelines (2014): http://www.jointcommission.org/assets/1/6/SCIP-FactSheet_010114v4.3.pdf
I. SCIP Core Measure Set (2014): http://www.jointcommission.org/assets/1/6/SCIP-Measures-012014.pdf
J. WHO Guidelines for Safe Surgery (2009): http://whqlibdoc.who.int/publications/2009/9789241598552_eng.pdf

(continued)

Protocol 33.1: General Surgical Care of the Older Adult *(continued)*

K. VTE Prophylaxis Guidelines for Surgical Patients: https://www.clinicalkey.com/#!/content/playContent/1-s2.0-S0039610914002126

ABBREVIATIONS

ACS	American College of Surgeons
ADL	Activities of daily living
AGS	American Geriatrics Society
CAUTI	Catheter-associated urinary tract infections
CDC	Centers for Disease Control and Prevention
CLABSI	Central line–associated bloodstream infections
CVC	Central venous catheter
DVT	Deep vein thrombosis
GI	Gastrointestinal
HAI	Hospital-acquired infection
IADL	Instrumental activities of daily living
ICU	Intensive care unit
IV	Intravenous
LDUH	Low-dose unfractionated heparin
LMWH	Low-molecular-weight heparin
MDRO	Multidrug-resistant organisms
NG	Nasogastric
NSAIDs	Nonsteroidal anti-inflammatory drugs
NSQIP	National Surgical Quality Improvement Program
PACU	Postanesthesia care unit
PADSS	Post-Anesthetic Discharge Scoring System
PAINAD	Patient Assessment in Advanced Dementia
PONV	Postoperative nausea and vomiting
PSI	Patient Safety Indicators
QOL	Quality of life
ROM	Range of motion
SCD	Sequential compression device
SCIP	Surgical Care Improvement Project
SSI	Surgical site infection
TJC	The Joint Commission
VAP	Ventilator-associated pneumonia
VTE	Venous thromboembolism
WHO	World Health Organization

RESOURCES

Advancing Effective Communication, Cultural Competence, and Patient- and Family-Centered Care (Joint Commission)
http://www.jointcommission.org/assets/1/6/ARoadmapforHospitalsfinalversion727.pdf

Always Use Teach-Back
http://www.teachbacktraining.org

American Geriatrics Society (AGS) Updated Beers Criteria for Potentially Inappropriate Medication Use in Older Adults
http://onlinelibrary.wiley.com/doi/10.1111/j.1532–5415.2012.03923.x/pdf

Ask Me Three—National Patient Safety Foundation (NPSF)
http://www.npsf.org/?page=askme3

Frequently Asked Questions About SSI
http://www.cdc.gov/HAI/pdfs/ssi/SSI_tagged.pdf

Institute for Healthcare Improvement (IHI)—Develop a Culture of Safety
http://www.ihi.org/resources/Pages/Changes/DevelopaCultureofSafety.aspx

Surgical Site Infection (SSI) Toolkit (CDC)
http://www.cdc.gov/HAI/pdfs/toolkits/SSI_toolkit021710SIBT_revised.pdf

Targeted Solutions Tool for Hand Hygiene, Hand-off Communications and Safe Surgery by TJC
http://www.centerfortransforminghealthcare.org/tst.aspx

REFERENCES

Agency for Healthcare Research and Quality (AHRQ). (n.d.). TeamSTEPPS: National implementation. Retrieved from http://teamsteppsahrq.gov. *Evidence Level VI.*

Agency for Healthcare Research and Quality (AHRQ). (2012). *Venous thromboembolism prophylaxis* (Guideline NGC-9541). Bloomington, MN: Institute for Clinical Systems Improvement. *Evidence Level I.*

Agency for Healthcare Research and Quality (AHRQ). (2014). *Fact sheet on patient safety indicators.* Retrieved from http://www.ahrq.gov/sites/default/files/wysiwyg/professionals/systems/hospital/qitoolkit/a1b_psifactsheet.pdf. *Evidence Level V.*

Aiken, L. H., Sloane, D. M., Bruyneel, L., Van de Heede, K., Griffiths, P., Busse, R., . . . Sermeus, W. (2014). Nurse staffing and education and hospital mortality in nine European countries: A retrospective observational study. *Lancet, 383*(9931), 1824–1830. doi:10.1016/S0140-6736(13)62631-8. *Evidence Level IV.*

Akagi, I., Furukawa, K., Miyashita, M., Kyama, T., Matsuda, A., Nomura, T., . . . Uchida, E. (2012). Surgical wound management made easier and more cost-effective. *Oncology Letters, 4*(1), 97–100. doi:10.3892/ol.2012.687. *Evidence Level III.*

Aldrete, J., & Kroulik, D. A. (1970). Postanesthetic recovery score. *Anesthesia and Analgesia, 49*(6), 924–934. *Evidence Level II.*

American Geriatrics Society (AGS). (2007). Assessing care of vulnerable elders-3 quality indicators. *Journal of the American Geriatrics Society, 55*(Suppl. 2), S464–S487. *Evidence Level VI.*

American Geriatrics Society (AGS). (2012). American Geriatrics Society updated Beers Criteria for potentially inappropriate medication use in older adults. *Journal of the American Geriatrics Society, 60*(4), 616–631. doi:10.1111/j.1532-5415.2012.03923.x. *Evidence Level I.*

American Geriatrics Society (AGS). (2014). *Clinical practice guideline for postoperative delirium in older adults.* Retrieved from http://geriatricscareonline.org/ProductAbstract/american-geriatrics-society-clinical-practice-guideline-for-postoperative-delirium-in-older-adults/CL018. *Evidence Level I.*

American Society of PeriAnesthesia Nurses (ASPAN). (2006). ASPAN'S evidence-based clinical practice guideline for the prevention and/or management of PONV/PDNV. *Journal of PeriAnesthesia Nursing, 21*(4), 230–250. *Evidence Level I.*

Anderson, D. J., Kaye, K. S., Classen, D., Arias, K. M., Podgorny, K., Burstin, H., . . . Yokoe, D. S. (2014). Strategies to prevent surgical site infections in acute care hospitals. *Infection Control and Hospital and Epidemiology, 35*(6), 605–627. doi:10.1086/676022. *Evidence Level V.*

Apfel, C. C., Kranke, P., & Eberhart, L. H. J. (2004). Comparison of surgical site and patient's history with a simplified risk score for the prediction of postoperative nausea and vomiting. *Anaesthesia, 59*(11), 1078–1082. doi:10.1111/j.1365-2044.2004.03875.x. *Evidence Level IV.*

Bashaw, M., & Scott, D. N. (2012). Surgical risk factors in geriatric perioperative patients. *AORN Journal, 96*(1), 58–73. doi:10.1016/j.aorn.2011.05.025. *Evidence Level V.*

Baumgarten, M., Margolis, D. J., Localio, A. R., Kagan, S. H., Lowe, R. A., Kinosian, B., . . . Mehari, T. (2008). Extrinsic risk factors for pressure ulcers early in the hospital stay: A nested case–control study. *Journal of Gerontology, 63*(4), 408–413. *Evidence Level III.*

Bhardwaj, R., Pickard, R., Carrick-Sen, D., & Brittain, K. (2012). Patients' perspectives on timing of urinary catheter removal after surgery. *British Journal of Nursing, 21*(18), S4–S9. *Evidence Level IV.*

Blegen, M. A., Goode, C. J., Park, S. H., Vaughn, T., & Spetz, J. (2013). Baccalaureate education in nursing and patient outcomes. *Journal of Nursing Administration, 43*(2), 89–94. doi:10.1097/NNA.0b013e31827f2028. *Evidence Level IV.*

British Geriatric Society (BGS). (2006). *Guidelines for the prevention, diagnosis, and management of delirium in older people in the hospital.* Retrieved from http://www.bgs.org.uk/index.php/clinicalguides/170-clinguidedeliriumtreatment. *Evidence Level I.*

Cameron, I. D., Gillespie, L. D., Robertson, M. C., Murray, G. R., Hill, K. D., Cumming, R. G., & Kerse, N. (2012). Interventions for preventing falls in older people in care facilities and hospitals. *Cochrane Database of Systematic Reviews, 12,* CD005465. doi:10.1002/14651858.CD005465.pub3. *Evidence Level I.*

Caprini, J. A. (2010). Risk assessment as a guide for the prevention of the many faces of venous thromboembolism. *American Journal of Surgery, 199*(Suppl. 1), S3–S10. doi:10.1016/j.amjsurg.2009.10.006. *Evidence Level IV.*

Cataife, G., Weinberg, D. A., Wong, H. H., & Kahn, K. L. (2014). The effect of surgical care improvement project (SCIP) compliance on surgical site infections (SSI). *Medical Care, 52*(2 Suppl. 1), S66–S73. doi:10.1097/MLR.0000000000000028. *Evidence Level IV.*

Centers for Disease Control and Prevention (CDC). (2010). *National Center for Health Statistics National Hospital Discharge Survey 2010.* Retrieved from http://www.cdc.gov/nchs/data/nhds/4procedures/2010pro4_numberprocedureage.pdf. *Evidence Level IV.*

Centers for Disease Control and Prevention (CDC). (2011). *Guidelines for the prevention of intravascular catheter-related infections, 2011.* Retrieved from http://www.cdc.gov/hicpac/pdf/guidelines/bsi-guidelines-2011.pdf. *Evidence Level I.*

Centers for Medicare & Medicaid Services (CMS). (2014). *Hospital-acquired conditions.* Retrieved from http://www.cms.gov/Medicare/Medicare-Fee-for-Service-Payment/HospitalAcqCond/Hospital-Acquired_Conditions.html. *Evidence Level VI.*

Chow, W. B., Rosenthal, R. A., Merkow, R. P., Ko, C. Y., & Esnaola, N. F. (2012) Optimal preoperative assessment of the geriatric surgical patient: A best practices guideline from the American College of Surgeons National Surgical Quality Improvement Program and the American Geriatrics Society. *Journal of the American College Surgeons, 215*(4), 453–466. doi:10.1016/j.jamcollsurg.2012.06.017. *Evidence Level I.*

Chung, F., Chan, V., & Ong, D. (1995). A post anaesthetic discharge scoring system for home readiness after ambulatory surgery. *Journal of Clinical Anesthesia, 7*(6), 500–506. doi:10.1016/0952–8180(95)00130-A. *Evidence Level II.*

Currie, L. (2008). Fall and injury prevention. In R. G. Hughes (Ed.), *Patient safety and quality: An evidence-based handbook for nurses* (Chapter 10). Rockville, MD: Agency for Healthcare Research and Quality. *Evidence Level V.*

Dasgupta, M., Rolfson, D. B., Stolee, P., Borrie, M. J., & Speechley, M. (2009). Frailty is associated with postoperative complications in older adults with medical problems. *Archives of Gerontology and Geriatrics, 48*(1), 78–83. doi:10.1016/j.archger.2007.10.007. *Evidence Level IV.*

Deiner, S., Westlake, B., & Dutton, R. P. (2014). Patterns of surgical care and complications in elderly adults. *Journal of the American Geriatrics Society, 62*(5), 829–835. doi:10.1111/jgs.12794. *Evidence Level IV.*

Delaney, C. P. (2004). Clinical perspective on postoperative ileus and the effect of opiates. *Neurogastroenterology and Motility, 16*(Suppl. 2), 61–66. *Evidence Level VI.*

Dobesh, P. P. (2009). Economic burden of venous thromboembolism in hospitalized patients. *Pharmacotherapy, 29*(8), 943–953. doi:10.1592/phco.29.8.943. *Evidence Level V.*

Doerflinger, D. M. (2009). Older adult surgical patients: Presentation and challenges. *AORN Journal, 90*(2), 223–240. *Evidence Level V.*

Donald, I. (2010). *Prophylaxis for venous thromboembolism.* Retrieved from http://www.bgs.org.uk/index.php/topresources/publicationfind/goodpractice/845-prophylaxisvenousthromboembolism. *Evidence Level I.*

El-Sharkaway, A. M., Sahota, O., Maughan, R. J., & Lobo, D. N. (2014). The pathophysiology of fluid and electrolyte balance in the older surgical patient. *Clinical Nutrition, 33*(1), 6–13. doi:10.1016/j.clnu.2013.11.010. *Evidence Level I.*

El Solh, A., Okada, M., Bhat, A., & Peitrantoni, C. (2003). Swallowing disorders post orotracheal intubation in the elderly. *Intensive Care Medicine, 29*(9), 1451–1455. doi:10.1007/s00134–003-1870–4. *Evidence Level III.*

Engel, H. J., Tatebe, S., Alonzo, P. B., Mustille, R. L., & Rivera, M. J. (2013). Physical therapist-established intensive care unit early mobilization program: Quality improvement project for critical care at the University of California San Francisco Medical Center. *Physical Therapy, 93*(7), 975–985. *Evidence Level III.*

Evans, D., & Fitzgerald, M. (2002). Reasons for physically restraining patients and residents: A systematic review and content analysis. *International Journal of Nursing Studies, 39*(7), 735–743. doi:10.1016/S0020–7489(02)00015–9. *Evidence Level V.*

Fry, D. E. (2008). Surgical site infections and the surgical care improvement project (SCIP): Evolution of national quality measures. *Surgical Infections, 9*(6), 579–584. doi:10.1089/sur.2008.9951. *Evidence Level V.*

Gajdos, C., Kile, D., Hawn, M., Finlayson, E., Henderson, W. G., & Robinson, T. N. (2013). Advancing age and 30-day adverse outcomes after nonemergent general surgeries. *Journal of the American Geriatrics Society, 61*(9), 1608–1614. doi:10.1111/jgs.12401. *Evidence Level IV.*

Griffiths, R., Beech, F., Brown, A., Dhesi, J., Foo, I., Goodall, J., . . . White, S. (2014). Peri-operative care of the elderly 2014. *Anaesthesia, 69*(Suppl. 1), 81–98. doi:10.1111/anae.12524. *Evidence Level I.*

Hamel, M. B., Henderson, W. G., Khuri, S. F., & Daley, J. (2005). Surgical outcomes for patients aged 80 and older: Morbidity and mortality from major noncardiac surgery. *Journal of the American Geriatrics Society, 53*(3), 424–429. doi:10.1111/j.1532–5415.2005.53159.x. *Evidence Level IV.*

Henderson, A., & Zernike, W. (2001). A study of the impact of discharge information for surgical patients. *Journal of Advanced Nursing, 35*(3), 435–441. *Evidence Level III.*

Hughes, S., Leary, A., Zweizig, S., & Cain, J. (2013). Surgery in elderly people: Preoperative, operative and postoperative care to assist healing. *Best Practice & Research: Clinical Obstetrics & Gynecology, 27*(5), 753–765. doi:10.1016/j.bpobgyn.2013.02.006. *Evidence Level I.*

Inouye, S. K., Zhang, Y., Jones, R. N., Kiely, D. K., Yang, F., & Marcantonio, E. R. (2007). Risk factors for delirium at discharge: Development and validation of a predictive model. *Archives of Internal Medicine, 167*(13), 1406–1413. doi:10.1001/archinte.167.13.1406. *Evidence Level III.*

Institute for Healthcare Improvement (IHI). (n.d.). *Changes for improvement.* Retrieved from http://www.ihi.org/resources/Pages/Changes/default.aspx. *Evidence Level VI.*

Institute for Healthcare Improvement (IHI). (2011a). *How-to guide: Prevent catheter-associated urinary tract infections.* Cambridge, MA: Author. *Evidence Level I.*

Institute for Healthcare Improvement (IHI). (2011b). *How-to guide: Prevent pressure ulcers.* Cambridge, MA: IHI. *Evidence Level I.*

Institute for Healthcare Improvement (IHI). (2012a). *How-to guide: Prevent central line-associated bloodstream infections (CLABSI).* Cambridge, MA: Author. *Evidence Level I.*

Institute for Healthcare Improvement (IHI). (2012b). *How-to guide: Prevent surgical-site infections.* Cambridge, MA: IHI. *Evidence Level I.*

Institute for Healthcare Improvement (IHI). (2012c). *How-to guide: Prevent ventilator-associated pneumonia.* Cambridge, MA: Author. *Evidence Level I.*

Institute for Healthcare Improvement (IHI). (2012d). *How-to guide: Reducing patient injuries from falls.* Cambridge, MA: Author. *Evidence Level I.*

Kaiser, M. J., Bauer, J. M., Rämsch, C., Uter, W., Guigoz, Y., Cederholm, T., . . . Sieber, C. C. (2010). Frequency of malnutrition in older adults: A multinational perspective using the Mini Nutritional Assessment. *Journal of the American Geriatrics Society, 58*(9), 1734–1783. doi:10.1111/j.1532–5415.2010.03016.x. *Evidence Level IV.*

Kaye, K. S., Marchaim, D., Chen, T., Baures, T., Anderson, D. J., Choi, Y., . . . Schmader, K. E. (2014). Effect of nosocomial bloodstream infections on mortality, length of stay, and hospital costs in older adults. *Journal of the American Geriatrics Society, 62*(2), 306–311. doi:10.1111/jgs.12634. *Evidence Level IV.*

Lagoo-Deenadayalan, S. A., Newell, M. A., & Pofahl, W. E. (2011). Common perioperative complications in older patients. In R. A. Rosenthal, M. E. Zenilman, & M. R. Katlic (Eds.) *Principles and practice of geriatric surgery* (pp. 361–376). New York, NY: Springer Publishing Company. *Evidence Level V.*

Lee, C., Chen, S., Chang, I., Chen, S., & Wu, S. (2007). Comparison of clinical manifestations and outcome of community-acquired bloodstream infections among the oldest old, elderly, and adult patients. *Medicine, 86*(3), 138–144. doi:10.1097/MID.0b013e31806a754c. *Evidence Level IV.*

Legrain, S., Tubach, F., Bonnet-Zamponi, D., Lemaire, A., Aquino, J., Paillaud, E., & Lacaille, S. (2011). A new multimodal geriatric discharge-planning intervention to prevent emergency room visits and rehospitalizations of older adults: The Optimization of Medication in AGEd Multicenter Randomized Control Trial. *Journal of the American Geriatrics Society, 59*(11), 2017–2028. doi:10.1111/j.1532-5415.2011.03628.x. *Evidence Level II.*

Leung, J. M., & Dzankic, S. (2001). Relative importance of preoperative health status versus intraoperative factors in predicting postoperative adverse outcomes in geriatric surgical patients. *Journal of the American Geriatrics Society, 49*(8), 1080–1085. *Evidence Level IV.*

Lubawski, J., & Saclarides, T. (2008). Postoperative ileus: Strategies for reduction. *Therapeutics and Clinical Risk Management, 4*(5), 913–917. *Evidence Level V.*

Luckey, A. E., & Parsa, C. J. (2003). Fluid and electrolytes in the aged. *Archives of Surgery, 138*(1), 1055–1060. *Evidence Level V.*

Magill, S. S., Edwards, J. R., Bamberg, W., Beldavs, Z. G., Dumyati, G., Kainer, M. A.,... Fridkin, S. K. (2014). Multistate point-prevalence survey of health care-associated infections. *New England Journal of Medicine, 370*(13), 1198–208. doi:10.1056/NEJMoa1306801. *Evidence Level IV.*

Makary, M. A., Segev, D. L., Pronovost, P. J., Syin, D. Bandeen-Roche, K. Patel, P.,... Fried, L. P. (2010). Frailty as a predictor of surgical outcomes in older patients. *Journal of the American College of Surgeons, 210*(6), 901–908. doi:10.1016/j.archger.2007.10.007. *Evidence Level IV.*

Malec, M., & Shega, J. W. (2015). Pain management in the elderly. *Medical Clinics of North America, 99*(2), 337–350. *Evidence Level V.*

Mangram, A. J., Horan, T. C., Pearson, M. L., Silver, L. C., & Jarvis, W. R. (1999). Guideline for prevention of surgical site infection, 1999: Centers for Disease Control and Prevention (CDC) Hospital Infection Control Practices Advisory Committee. *American Journal of Infection Control, 27*(2), 97–132. *Evidence Level I.*

Marik, P. E., & Kaplan, D. (2003). Aspiration pneumonia and dysphagia in the elderly. *Chest, 124*(1), 328–336. *Evidence Level V.*

Markey, D. W., & Brown, R. J. (2002). An interdisciplinary approach to addressing patient activity and mobility in the medical-surgical patient. *Journal of Nursing Care Quality, 16*(4), 1–12. *Evidence Level IV.*

McGory, J. L., Kao, K. K., Shekelle, P. G., Rubenstein, L. Z., Leonardi, M. J., Parikh, J. A.,... Ko, C. Y. (2009). Developing quality indicators for elderly surgical patients. *Annals of Surgery, 250*(2), 338–347. doi:10.1097/SLA.0b013e3181ae575a. *Evidence Level I.*

Minnick, A. F., Mion, L. C., Johnson, M. E., Catrambone, C., & Leipzig, R. (2007). Prevalence and variation of physical restraint use in acute care settings in the US. *Journal of Nursing Scholarship, 39*(1), 30–37. *Evidence Level IV.*

Montalvo, I. (2007). The National Database of Nursing Quality Indicators (NDNQI). *Online Journal of Issues in Nursing, 12*(3), Manuscript 2. doi:10.3912/OJIN.Vol12No03Man02. *Evidence Level I.*

Mularski, R. A., White-Chu, F., Overbay, D., Miller, L., Asch, S. M., & Ganzini, L. (2006). Measuring pain as the 5th vital sign does not improve quality of pain management. *Journal of General Internal Medicine, 21*(6), 607–612. doi:10.1111/j.1525-1497.2006.00415.x. *Evidence Level IV.*

Munaco, S. S., Dumas, B., & Edlund, B. J. (2014). Preventing ventilator-associated events: Complying with evidence-based practice. *Critical Care Nurse Quarterly, 37*(4), 384–392. doi:10.1097/CNQ.0000000000000039, *Evidence Level III.*

National Confidential Enquiry into Perioperative Deaths (NCEPOD). (1999). *Extremes of age: The 1999 Report of the National Confidential Enquiry into Perioperative Deaths.* London, UK: NECPOD. *Evidence Level IV.*

National Quality Forum (NQF). (2011). *Serious reportable events in healthcare—2011 update: A consensus report.* Washington, DC: Author. *Evidence Level VI.*

Norman, D. C. (2000). Fever in the elderly. *Clinical Infectious Diseases, 31*(1), 148–151. doi:10.1086/313896. *Evidence Level V.*

Odom-Forren, J. (2015). Concepts basic to perioperative nursing. In J. C. Rothrock (Ed.), *Alexander's care of the patient in surgery* (15th ed., pp. 270–294). St. Louis, MO: Mosby. *Evidence Level VI.*

Ortman, J. M., Velkoff, V. A., & Hogan, H. (2014). *An aging nation: The older population in the United States* (Report No. P25-1140). Retrieved from http://www.census.gov/prod/2014pubs/p25-1140.pdf. *Evidence Level VI.*

Palmer, R. M. (2009). Perioperative care of the elderly patient: An update. *Cleveland Clinic Journal of Medicine, 76*(Suppl. 4), S16–S21. doi:10.3949/ccjm.76.s4.03. *Evidence Level V.*

Panprese, B., & Johnson, C. (2014). Optimizing the perioperative nursing role for the older adult surgical patient. *OR Nurse, 8*(4), 26–33. doi:10.1097/01.orn.0000451047.90117.7a. *Evidence Level V.*

Pokorny, M. W., Koldjeski, D., & Swanson, M. (2003). Skin care intervention for patients having cardiac surgery. *American Journal of Critical Care, 12*(6), 535–544. *Evidence Level IV.*

Royal College of Physicians, British Geriatrics Society, & British Pain Society. (2007). *The assessment of pain in older people: National guidelines* (Concise guidance to good practice series, No. 8). London, UK: Royal College of Physicians. *Evidence Level I.*

Scandrett, K. G., Zuckerbraun, B. S., & Peitzman, A. B. (2015). Operative risk stratification in the older adult. *Surgical Clinics of North America, 95*(1), 149–172. doi:10.1016/j.suc.2014.09.014. *Evidence Level IV.*

Schofield, P. A. (2014). The assessment and management of perioperative pain in older adults. *Anaesthesia, 69*(Suppl. 1), 54–60. doi:10.1111/anae.12520. *Evidence Level V.*

Schuster, R., Grewal, N., Greaney, G. C., & Waxman, K. (2006). Gum chewing reduces ileus after elective open sigmoid colectomy. *Archives of Surgery, 141*(2), 174–176. *Evidence Level II.*

Shorr, R. I., Guillen, M. K., Rosenblatt, L. C., Walker, K., Caudle, C. E., & Kritchevsky, S. B. (2002). Restraint use, restraint orders, and the risk of falls in hospitalized patients. *Journal of the American Geriatrics Society, 50*(3), 526–529. *Evidence Level III.*

Sullivan, J. M. (2011). Caring for older adults after surgery. *Nursing, 41*(4), 48–51. doi:10.1097/01.NURSE.0000394459.56297.85. *Evidence Level VI.*

The Joint Commission (TJC). (2013). *The Joint Commission's implementation guide for NPSG.07.05.01 on surgical site infections: The SSI Change Project.* Retrieved from http://www.jointcommission.org/assets/1/18/Implementation_Guide_for_NPSG_SSI.pdf. *Evidence Level VI.*

The Joint Commission (TJC). (2014a). Clarification of the pain management standard. *Joint Commission Perspectives®, 34*(11), 11. *Evidence Level I.*

The Joint Commission (TJC). (2014b). *2015 Hospital accreditation standards.* Oakbrook Terrace, IL: Joint Commission Resources. *Evidence Level I.*

The Joint Commission (TJC). (2015). *National patient safety goals effective January 1, 2015: Hospital accreditation program.* Retrieved from http://www.jointcommission.org/assets/1/6/2015_NPSG_HAP.pdf. *Evidence Level I.*

Toon, C. D., Ramamoorthy, R., Davidson, B. R., & Gurusamy, K. S. (2013). Early versus delayed dressing removal after primary closure of clean and clean-contaminated surgical wounds. *Cochrane Database Systematic Reviews, 9*, CD010259. doi:10.1002/14651858.CD010259.pub2. *Evidence Level I.*

Tsai, D. M., & Caterson, E. J. (2014). Current preventive measures for health-care associated surgical site infections: A review. *Patient Safety in Surgery, 8*(1), 42. doi:10.1186/s13037-014-0042-5. *Evidence Level V.*

Volkert, D. (2002). Malnutrition in the elderly: Prevalence, causes and corrective strategies. *Clinical Nutrition, 21*(Suppl. 1), 110–112. doi:10.1016/S0261–5614(02)80014–0. *Evidence Level IV.*

Warden, V., Hurley, A. C., & Volicer, L. (2003). Development and psychometric evaluation of the Pain Assessment in Advanced Dementia (PAINAD) scale. *Journal of the American Medical Directors Association, 4*(1), 9–15. doi:10.1097/01.JAM.0000043422.31640.F7. *Evidence Level III.*

Weiss, A. J., & Elixhauser, A. (2014). *Trends in operating room procedures in U.S. hospitals, 2011–2011* (HCUP Statistical Brief No. 171). Retrieved from http://www.hcup-us.ahrq.gov/reports/statbriefs/sb171-Operating-RoomProcedure-Trends.pdf. *Evidence Level VI.*

Welsh, C. A., Flanagan, M. E., Hoke, S. C., Doebbeling, B. N., & Herwaldt, A. (2012). Reducing health care-associated infections (HAIs): Lessons learned from a national collaborative of regional HAI programs. *American Journal of Infection Control, 40*(1), 29–34. doi:10.1016/j.ajic.2011.02.017. *Evidence Level IV.*

Wheble, G. A., Knight, W. R., & Khan O. A. (2012). Enteral vs total parenteral nutrition following major upper gastrointestinal surgery. *International Journal of Surgery, 10*(4), 194–197. doi:10.1016/j.ijsu.2012.02.015. *Evidence Level III.*

Williams, B. (2008). Supporting self-care of patients following general abdominal surgery. *Journal of Clinical Nursing, 17*(5), 584–592. doi:10.1111/j.1365–2702.2006.01857.x. *Evidence Level III.*

Zerey, M., Paton, B. L., Lincourt, A. E., Gersin, K. S., Kercher, K. W., & Heniford, B. T. (2007). The burden of *Clostridium dificile* in surgical patients in the United States. *Surgical Infections, 8*(6), 557–566. doi:10.1089/sur.2006.062. *Evidence Level IV.*

Zingg, W., Holmes, A., Dettenkofer, M., Goetting, T., Secci, F., Clack, L., . . . Pittet, D. (2015). Hospital organization, management, and structure for prevention of health-care-associated infection: A systematic review and expert consensus. *Lancet: Infectious Diseases, 15*(2), 212–224. doi:10.1016/S1473–3099(14)70854–0. *Evidence Level I.*

34

Care of the Older Adult With Fragility Hip Fracture

Anita J. Meehan, Ami Hommel, Karen Hertz, Valerie MacDonald, and Ann Butler Maher

EDUCATIONAL OBJECTIVES

On completion of this chapter, the reader should be able to:

1. Discuss the impact of fragility hip fracture on global health care systems
2. Describe methods to assess bone health and fracture risk
3. Identify common complications associated with care of older adults with fragility hip fracture
4. Articulate specific nursing management strategies to address common complications
5. Discuss fracture liaison service as a process for secondary fracture prevention

OVERVIEW

The global incidence of fragility hip fractures continues to rise on an annual basis making it one of the most common causes of hospital admission following trauma for older adults. In 1990, the global incidence of hip fracture was approximately 1.26 million; conservative estimates indicate that this number will burgeon to between 4.5 and 6.3 million by 2050 (Gullberg, Johnell, & Kanis, 1997). Fragility fracture treatment is expensive. Annual cost to treat fragility fractures in the United States in 2005 was $17 billion, with hip fractures accounting for 72% of these expenses (Burge et al., 2007); these costs will increase with the growing aging population. Rehabilitation is not always successful. A study by Bertram, Norman, Kemp, and Vos (2011) found that 1 year after fragility hip fracture, 29% of patients did not achieve their prefracture level of function for activities of daily living (ADL).

Despite advances in anesthesia, nursing care, and surgical techniques, this injury can be overwhelming for both patient and family, often resulting in permanent disability and increased reliance on others. Evidence-based interventions to reduce common complications and prevent secondary fractures are crucial to maximize recovery for individuals as well as decrease mortality and contain health care costs. Nurses are in an optimal position to make a significant difference for patients who suffer a fragility fracture.

BACKGROUND AND STATEMENT OF PROBLEM

Hip fracture is the most devastating of all fragility fractures with risk of long-lasting disability and significant morbidity and mortality (Bass, French, Bradham, & Rubenstein, 2007). Although the vast majority of people who suffer a hip fracture are older females, the number of men suffering from fragility hip fracture is increasing, with as many as one third of all hip fractures occurring in men (Gullberg et al., 1997).

As the age of patients sustaining hip fracture continues to trend upward and include more of the very old (older than 90 years), the incidence of coexisting medical problems and subsequent complications will increase (Bergström et al., 2009). Studies show that many of those who survive do not regain their prefracture level of independence (Andrew, Freter, & Rockwood, 2005; Bentler et al., 2009;

For a description of evidence levels cited in this chapter, see Chapter 1, "Developing and Evaluating Clinical Practice Guidelines: A Systematic Approach."

Bertram et al., 2011). According to the American Academy of Orthopaedic Surgeons (AAOS) position statement on hip fractures in seniors (AAOS, 1999), 44% of nursing home admissions for fracture are result from a hip fracture; as many as 50% of these individuals lived independently before hip fracture, but were unable to walk unaided after fracture.

Mortality rates after hip fracture are significant as well, with rates reported as 10% within 1 month and from 18% to 33% after 1 year (Bentler et al., 2009). Functional decline and subsequent death are attributable to the complex interplay of surgical stress, comorbidity, prefracture frailty, and level of physical and cognitive functions. Although the fracture itself is responsible for less than half of the deaths (Parker & Johansen, 2006), families often identify the hip fracture as playing a central role in the patient's decline.

Decades of research shows that half of those who sustain a fragility hip fracture have had a previous fragility fracture (Edwards, Bunta, Simonelli, Bolander, & Fitzpatrick, 2007; Gallagher, Melton, Riggs, & Bergstrath, 1980). Despite evidence demonstrating benefits of early detection of osteoporosis and implementation of strategies to reduce fracture risk (Akesson et al., 2013, Greene & Dell, 2010; Newman, Ayoub, Starkey, Diehl, & Wood, 2003), studies reveal that these recommendations are not being applied in practice (Ellanti et al., 2014; Mitchell, 2013; Sobolev, Sheehan, Kuramoto, & Guy, 2015).

Nurses are ideally positioned to play a pivotal role in preventing or ameliorating common complications associated with fragility hip fracture, such as pain, delirium, venous thromboembolism (VTE), malnutrition, pressure ulcers, infections, fluid and electrolyte imbalances, and functional decline, and to manage programs focused on secondary fracture prevention.

DEFINITION OF FRAGILITY HIP FRACTURE

A fragility fracture is defined as a break in the bone resulting from low-impact trauma, such as falling from a standing height or less, or one that occurs in the absence of significant trauma. Hip fracture is a collective term for different types of fractures in the proximal end of the femur. The type and location of the fracture will determine how the fracture is repaired, specific postoperative restrictions, and how quickly healing will progress. Hip fracture location can be broadly categorized into two areas: intracapsular and extracapsular. Intracapsular fractures occur within the capsule that forms the hip joint and involve the head and neck of the femur. Fractures outside the capsule are further described as trochanteric or subtrochanteric fractures.

The most common location for a fragility hip fracture is the femoral neck (45%–53%) followed by intertrochanteric fractures (38%–49%) and, less often, subtrochanteric fractures (5%–15%; Marks, Allegrante, Ronald MacKenzie, & Lane, 2003; Figure 34.1). A large prospective study of more than 220,000 persons found that people who suffered fractures around the trochanters tended to be older

FIGURE 34.1

Common sights of hip fracture.

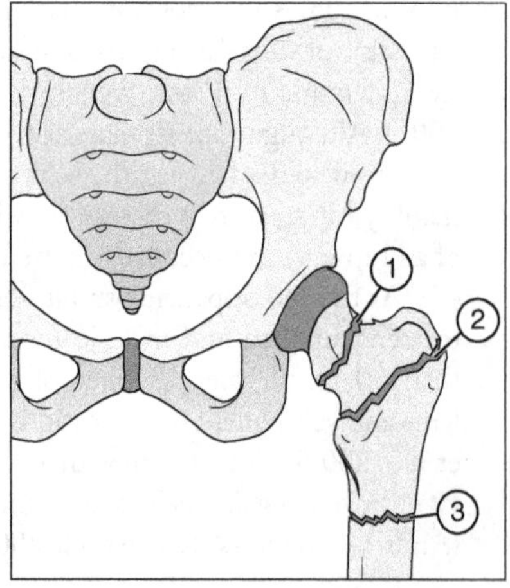

(1) Femoral neck subcapital fracture
(2) Intertrochanteric fracture
(3) Subtrochanteric fracture

Adapted from the Centre for Hip Health and Mobility.

with poorer health status, longer hospital stays, and poorer functional recovery (Fox, Magaziner, Hebel, Kenzora, & Kashner, 1999).

SURGICAL REPAIR OF HIP FRACTURE

When the bone breaks, the broken pieces may remain in their original position and the fracture is said to be nondisplaced. A displaced fracture occurs if the broken pieces move out of alignment. Surgical treatment approaches depend on a variety of factors, including quality of the bone and postsurgical rehabilitation potential. A nondisplaced fracture may be stabilized using percutaneously inserted pins (Figure 34.2). If the fracture is displaced, or out of alignment, the blood supply to the area is often compromised and patients will generally do better if some of the components of the hip are replaced. If both the ball and the socket, or acetabulum, are replaced the procedure is referred to as a total hip replacement (Figure 34.2). If only the head of the femur is replaced, the procedure is referred to as a hemiarthroplasty (Figure 34.3). A nondisplaced fracture around the trochanters may be repaired with a large screw that slides within the barrel of a plate that is screwed to the side of the femur. This type of fixation will stabilize the fracture over time by impacting the broken area on itself, thus stimulating new bone growth, and is called a dynamic or compression hip screw (Figure 34.4). A subtrochanteric fracture, distal to the trochanters is commonly fixed with an intermedullary rod and stabilized with a large screw (Figure 34.5). Regardless of the type of fixation, postoperatively the goal is to advance the patient to maximum weight-bearing status as quickly as possible. The type of surgical fixation and quality of the bone will determine weight-bearing limitations and/or postoperative positioning restrictions.

FIGURE 34.2

Total hip replacement (right hip) and cannulated screws (left hip).

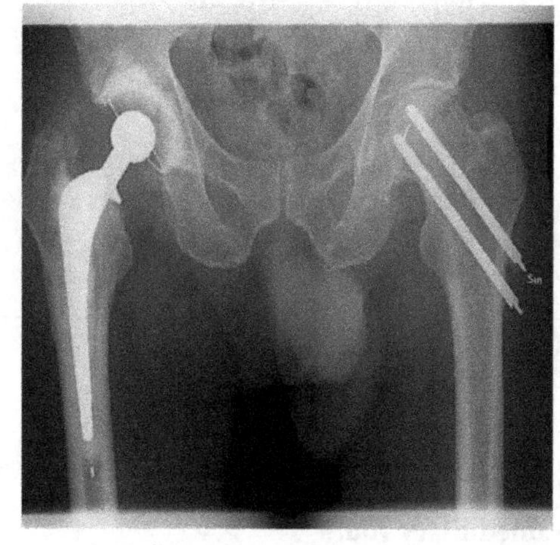

Image courtesy of Dr. K.G. Thorngren, Lund University Hospital.

FIGURE 34.3

Hip procedures.

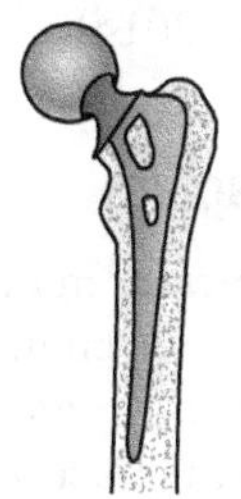

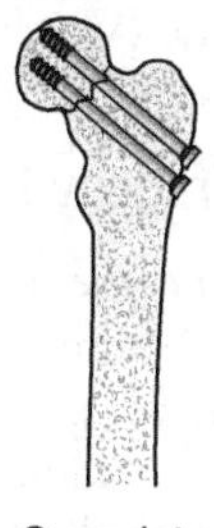

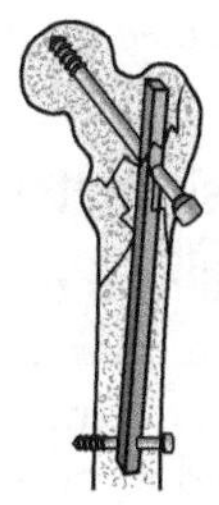

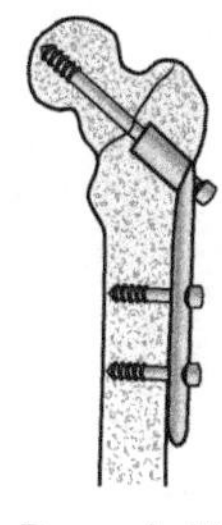

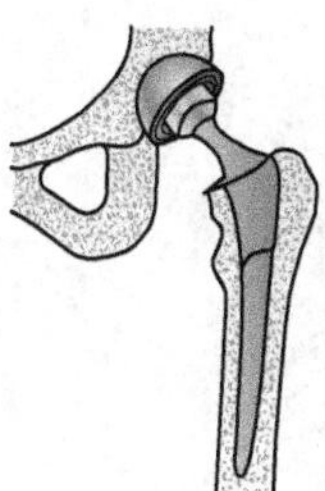

Adapted from the Centre for Hip Health and Mobility.

FIGURE 34.4

Compression or dynamic hip screw.

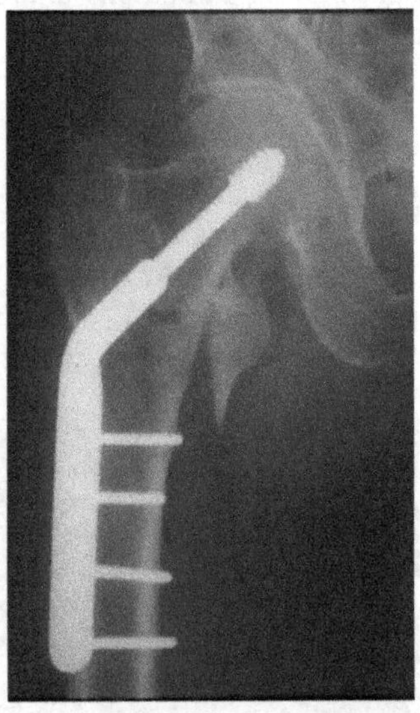

Image courtesy of Mr. Phillip Roberts, University Hospital of North Midlands.

FIGURE 34.5

Intramedullary rod.

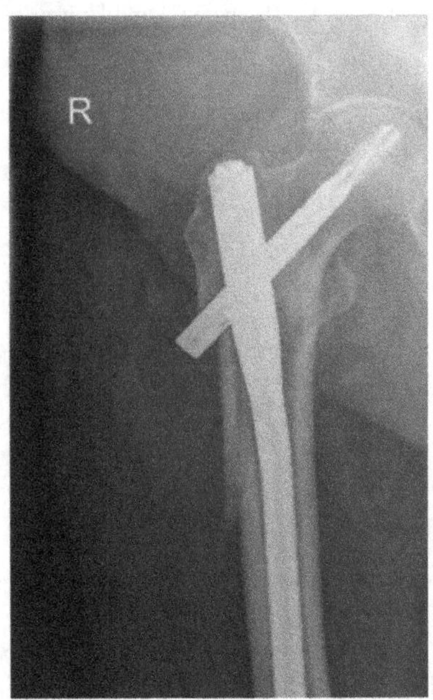

Image courtesy of Mr. Phillip Roberts, University Hospital of North Midlands.

Fracture Repair as a Palliative Measure

The 1-year mortality rate following hip fracture is around 30% (Pugely et al., 2014). Those most likely to die in the first year have advanced age, severe comorbidity, poor ambulation abilities, severe dementia, and reside in a facility (Hu, Jiang, Shen, Tnag, & Wang, 2012; Pugely et al., 2014; Wiles, Moran, Sahota, & Moppett, 2011). The fall and hip fracture may be precipitated by a cardiorespiratory, metastatic, or neurological condition. For patients with advanced age, severe comorbid illness, and high dependency needs, the hip fracture surgery may be viewed as a palliative intervention performed with the goal of reducing pain and improving the quality of life (Ko & Morrison, 2014a, 2014b; Leland, Teno, Gozalo, Bynum, & Mor, 2012). For more detailed information, see Chapter 37, "Palliative Care Models."

PATHOPHYSIOLOGY

Fragility hip fracture is a painful sequela of poor bone quality and a traumatic event, often involving a fall. In adults, small amounts of bone mineral are lost as osteoclast cells clean up old bone, in a process known as resorption. These bone minerals are replaced by bone-building cells called osteoblasts in a process known as remodeling. With aging, the loss of bone occurs progressively and asymptomatically, accelerating in women after menopause. When the balance tips toward excessive resorption, bones weaken (osteopenia) and over time can become brittle and prone to fracture (osteoporosis). Based on a number of factors, men develop greater bone strength as they mature and lose bone strength more slowly, in part because of a more gradual loss in sex hormone levels with aging (Willson, Nelson, Newbold, Nelson, & LaFleur, 2015).

A fracture is often the first indication of diminished bone health. Approximately 10 million people in the United States have osteoporosis and as the population continues to age an increasing number of people will be affected by this disease (Wright et al., 2014).

Risk Factors for Fragility Hip Fracture

Falling is the leading cause of hip fracture in older adults. Determination of the circumstances precipitating a fall and fracture is essential to illuminate underlying issues that need to be addressed in addition to the fracture. Intrinsic factors, such as acute medical conditions, exacerbation of chronic conditions, visual or balance problems as well as extrinsic factors including environmental factors and life style, contribute to increasing the risk of falling.

Intrinsic Fall Risk Factors

Normal age-related changes affecting vision, hearing loss, balance and/or gait disturbances coupled with a slowed reaction time are factors that contribute to increased fall risk in older adults. In addition, many older adults have underlying chronic conditions or an acute event that may result in a fall. A neurologic event, cardiac condition, dehydration, urge incontinence, or underlying infection may contribute to increasing the risk of falling and subsequent fracture. Medications may have anticholinergic side effects that increase fall/fracture risk, for example, dizziness or blurred vision.

Sarcopenia is an age-related decline in muscle bulk and quality that may escalate the risk of fracture, especially if associated with diminished functional mobility, reduced lower quadriceps strength, and poor balance or body sway. Sarcopenia and osteoporosis are linked from a biological and functional perspective and increase fracture risk in the elderly. The elevated fracture risk from sarcopenia and osteoporosis is a result of the decline of muscle mass and strength, the decrease in bone mineral density (BMD), and limited mobility (Tarantino et al., 2015).

Extrinsic Fall Risk Factors

Environmental tripping hazards, for example, small pets, clutter, or poor fitting footwear, may contribute to increasing fall risk. Alcohol or drug use may impair balance and/or cause drowsiness or delirium. Another concern in this population is elder abuse. Inspect the patient as part of the admitting head-to-toe assessment to ensure that the circumstances of the fall are consistent with the pattern of injury. (For more detailed information, see Chapter 13, "Mistreatment Detection"; Chapter 19, "Preventing Falls in Acute Care"; and Chapter 28, "Substance Misuse and Alcohol Use Disorders.")

Diminished Bone Strength

The other risk factor that contributes to increasing the risk of fragility fracture is bone loss associated with aging. There are several factors that increase the risk of bone loss.

- *Age.* Bones weaken as we age. Eighty percent of patients hospitalized for hip fracture are of age 65 years and older (Hall, DeFrances, Williams, Golosinskiy, & Schwartzman, 2010).
- *Gender.* The drop in estrogen levels that occurs with menopause accelerates bone loss in women. The majority of hip fractures occur in women.
- *Nutrition.* Poor nutrition and a diet low in calcium and vitamin D contribute to increasing risk of hip fracture.
- *Heredity.* A family history of osteoporosis or broken bones after age 50 years and people with a low body mass index are at greater risk for fragility fracture.
- *Lifestyle.* Smoking and drinking more than two alcoholic beverages per day can interfere with normal processes of bone remodeling resulting in bone loss. Inactivity can weaken bones.
- *Medications.* Long-term corticosteroid use can weaken bones. Side effects of medications can affect balance and eyesight, which increases fall risk.
- *Medical conditions.* Endocrine disorders, such as hyperparathyroidism, and intestinal disorders, such as Crohn's disease, may reduce absorption of calcium and vitamin D, which negatively impacts bone health.

Assessment of Bone Health and Fracture Risk

There are two widely used measures to determine bone health and fracture risk. The World Health Organization (WHO) developed the Fracture Risk Assessment Tool (FRAX) in 2008 (Kanis, Johnell, Oden, Johansson, & McCloskey, 2008). The FRAX is a major achievement in helping to determine which patients may suffer a fragility fracture (Vernon & King, 2011) as well as those who may be candidates for pharmacological therapy for osteoporosis (Watts, 2011). The FRAX contains 12 variables used to calculate risks such as BMD, including age, low body mass index, previous fragility fracture, parental history of fracture, glucocorticoid treatment, current smoking status, rheumatoid arthritis history, alcohol intake, and other secondary causes of osteoporosis. The FRAX takes approximately 20 minutes to complete, and provides a qualitative estimate of 10-year fracture risk. Its intended use is for those not currently being treated for osteoporosis. The FRAX is commonly administered in conjunction with dual-energy x-ray absorptiometry (DEXA scan; www.shef.ac.uk/FRAX/tool.jsp).

The DEXA scan is the most widely used method to evaluate BMD. The WHO uses BMD measured by the DEXA to define osteoporosis. A DEXA scan measures the density of bone at two areas, the proximal femur and the lumbar spine. The results are reported as a T- and a Z-score. The standard measure T-score is 0.0 representing bone density of a young healthy individual at peak bone health. According to WHO criteria (Kanis et al., 2008) a T-score higher than −0.1 is considered normal bone density, a T-score between −1.0 and −2.5 is considered osteopenia, and a T-score below −2.5 is considered osteoporosis. The Z-score is a comparative measure of persons of the same age and gender as the patient and can be used to evaluate men, children, and premenopausal women. A Z-score measure of −2.0 is considered low bone mass for chronological age and a Z-score of above −2.0 is considered within the expected range for age (National Osteoporosis Foundation [NOF], 2010).

Although BMD using the DEXA is considered the gold standard surrogate marker of bone health, and assessment of fracture risk is completed using the FRAX, there are newer measures being reported in the literature that hold promise as measures of bone health and treatment monitoring (Fitton, Astroth, & Wilson, 2015). Bone turnover markers (BTM) are measures of byproducts of protein secreted by bone-forming osteoblasts, measured in serum, and bone-resorbing osteoclasts, measured in urine. Unlike the DEXA, which evaluates specific skeletal sites, these markers reflect global skeletal activity and have the potential to be used to monitor effectiveness of treatment (Kleerekoper, 2001). Another approach under investigation is the use of MRI to evaluate bone marrow adipose tissue (BMAT). A study conducted by Li et al. (2014) found that women with osteopenia and osteoporosis had a higher marrow fat content compared to those with normal BMD. There is growing attention to the use of bone turnover markers and BMAT as biomarkers for bone quality (Burch et al., 2014; Li et al., 2014; Tang et al., 2010).

COMMON COMPLICATIONS AND EVIDENCE-BASED NURSING CARE STRATEGIES

Although in most cases surgical repair is crucial, optimal outcome depends on an interprofessional approach to care. Advanced age, chronic conditions, and diminished physical and cognitive reserves expose older adults with fragility hip fracture to an increased risk for the development of specific geriatric syndromes. Nursing care that includes evidence-based strategies to engage both patient and family in learning about risk factors, prevention, and management of complications such as delirium, pressure ulcers, VTE, malnutrition, constipation, fluid and electrolyte imbalances, functional decline, infections, and prevention of secondary fractures is crucial (Maher et al., 2012, 2013).

Although many of these complications are experienced by hospitalized older adults and most are discussed elsewhere in this book, they coalesce in the hip fracture patient population to increase morbidity and mortality and significantly reduce the individual's prospects for maximum functional recovery. Nurses play a vital role in ameliorating these risk factors and ensuring optimal outcomes.

PAIN: SIGNIFICANCE IN HIP-FRACTURE PATIENTS

A fall, hip fracture, and surgical repair are painful assaults injuring the skin, muscle, and bone. Older patients with hip fractures are at high risk of unmanaged pain with higher rates of delirium, impaired mobility, and long-term functional impairment as a result (Bjorkelund, Hommel, Thorngren, Lundberg, & Larsson, 2011; Morrison et al., 2003). Unmanaged pain disturbs sleep, diminishes appetite, and may also increase the risk of delirium (American Geriatrics Society Panel on the Pharmacological Management of Persistent Pain in Older Persons, 2009; Vaurio, Sands, Wang, Mullen, & Leung, 2006). Painful conditions, such as osteoarthritis, osteoporotic fractures, degenerative spine disease, cancer, and neuralgias, increase in prevalence with age and may add to the pain experience for patients with hip fracture (American Geriatrics Society Panel on the Pharmacological Management of Persistent Pain in Older Persons, 2009).

Nursing Management Strategies to Address Pain

There is a paucity of evidence on pain management for patients with hip fractures. Studies often exclude those with delirium, dementia, and/or severe comorbid illness because of challenges with communication and obtaining consent. Approximately 40% of the population, the most vulnerable, are often excluded. Expert opinion supplements the evidence for this section.

As functional mobility is the key to recovery, a balanced approach to pain management is required to achieve both mobility and comfort. Frequent evidence-based pain assessment is the foundation for effective pain management. Using an evidence-based pain history tool and screening health records for preexisting painful conditions and prior pain treatments illuminate potential sources of discomfort and considerations for the treatment plan. Assessing and recording pain intensity using a valid scale with vital signs make the pain assessment visible and help ensure that pain is assessed on a regular basis (Purser, Warfield, & Richardson, 2014). The specific pain scale used would be based on the patient's comprehension and preference (Herr & Titler, 2009). For patients with severe cognitive impairment, one should use a validated pain behavior scale (Herr, Coyne, McCaffery, Manworren, & Merkel, 2011). For information on specific pain assessment tools, see Chapter 18, "Pain Management."

A multimodal approach to analgesia helps maximize the synergistic effect of analgesics while decreasing the dose requirement of any one medication, thereby limiting their adverse effects (Kehlet & Dahl, 2003). A combination of a geriatric-appropriate opioid together with acetaminophen and regional analgesia (e.g., nerve block) may manage pain while reducing side-effects such as sedation and delirium (Kang et al., 2013). Nonpharmacological strategies, such as relaxation exercises, physiotherapy, and application of heat or cold, may reduce opioid requirements and improve comfort (Abou-Setta et al., 2011; Pellino et al., 2005). Nonsteroidal anti-inflammatory medications are usually not recommended because of their higher rates of adverse effects, such as bleeding and cardiovascular complications, in older patients (American Geriatrics Society 2012 Beers Criteria Update Expert Panel, 2012).

Minimizing sedation while maximizing pain control is a goal to facilitate mobility. Strategic timing of analgesics can help alleviate the increased pain of mobilization and reduce the need for additional opioid doses. Identify the time of the peak effect of the specific analgesic and route of administration and administer the analgesic when peak effect will coincide with physiotherapy or ambulation.

Nerve block (e.g., femoral and fascial iliacal) is effective in relieving the acute pain of hip fracture compared with standard care (Abou-Setta et al., 2011; AAOS, 2014). The nerve block is typically administered before surgery and provides substantial perioperative pain relief reducing the need for opioid analgesia and the risk of delirium (Beaudoin, Nagdev, Merchant, & Becker, 2010). Nurse-initiated fascial iliacal blocks have improved pain management effectiveness and safety (Dochez et al., 2014).

Managing moderate to severe pain after hip fracture usually involves the administration of opioids. Older adults are more susceptible to the adverse effects of opioids and a "start low/go slow" approach to opioid administration is advised. This approach is not appropriate if the patient was on opioid therapy before admission as a higher dose may be required. An individualized approach considering the patient's opioid use history with careful monitoring and titration of analgesic to achieve an acceptable pain level is essential.

Strategies to Manage Adverse Effects of Analgesics

Oversedation is a serious adverse effect of opioid therapy that could lead to respiratory failure. According to Pasero (2009), the level of sedation increases gradually and is a warning sign requiring a prompt reduction in opioid use with more frequent monitoring. The first 24 hours of opioid therapy are the riskiest time, and sedation assessment using a validated tool every hour is recommended, with reduction to every 4 hours thereafter if the patient is stable (Pasero, 2009). The Pasero Sedation Scale is recommended as a validated tool that defines levels of sedation as well as actions to take for patient comfort and safety.

Constipation is highly likely to occur and increases the risk of abdominal and rectal pain, delirium, agitation, and bowel obstruction (Neighbour, 2014). Although individual bowel habits vary, in general, the goal is that the patient has a moderate to large bowel movement (BM; e.g., at least 8 ounces) every 48 hours (Auron-Gomez & Michota, 2008) and daily monitoring of BMs is required. The pre-emptive use of laxatives, a high-fiber diet, and fluids are recommended (Neighbour, 2014).

Other practice recommendations include:

- Avoid prolonged fasting and delays to surgery.
- Encourage a minimum of 6 cups of oral fluid daily unless otherwise restricted.
- Mobilize frequently, for example, walk to the toilet every 2 hours while awake.
- Avoid the use of bedpans—use a toilet or commode. Ensure privacy for patient dignity.

Nausea and vomiting are potential adverse effects of opioids and are typically managed with antiemetic medication. However, medications with anticholinergic properties should be avoided, as they can cause delirium (American Geriatrics Society 2012 Beers Criteria Update Expert Panel, 2012). Delirium can also be an adverse effect of analgesics; however, delirium is also associated with unmanaged pain. Assessing and adjusting the medication or reducing the dose of analgesics are interventions that may reduce the analgesic contribution to delirium (Maher et al., 2012). For more information on analgesic adverse effects, see Chapter 18.

DELIRIUM: SIGNIFICANCE IN HIP-FRACTURE PATIENTS

Delirium is the most common complication associated with hip fracture. Studies reveal that between 16% and 62% of patients develop delirium following hip fracture (Bitsch, Foss, Kristensen, & Kehlet, 2004; J. J. White, Khan, & Smitham, 2011). One of the strongest predictors of postoperative delirium is preoperative cognitive dysfunction (Oh et al., 2014). Cognitive impairment is common in this population; Griffiths et al. (2012) report that approximately 25% of hip fracture patients have a moderate cognitive impairment. Lundstrom, Stenvall, and Olofsson (2012) studied 129 patients with hip fracture who developed postoperative delirium and found that patients with delirium superimposed on dementia (54%) displayed hyperactive symptoms, while those without base line dementia more commonly displayed symptoms of hypactive delirium.

Multiple studies report that delirium is independently associated with a variety of adverse outcomes including pressure ulcers, functional decline, institutionalization, and death (Andrew et al., 2005; Bellelli et al., 2014; Krogseth, Wyller, Engedal, & Juliebo, 2014; McAvay et al., 2006). Patients with persistent delirium are 2.9 times more likely to die within 1 year than those whose delirium resolves (Kiely et al., 2009). The ability to differentiate between dementia and delirium is important because unlike dementia, the cognitive changes in delirium are potentially preventable, and are likely reversible. Despite its prevalence, significant cost, and negative outcomes, nurses and physicians often fail to recognize delirium, especially when dementia or the hypoactive form of delirium is present (Lemiengre et al., 2006; Steis & Fick, 2008).

Nursing Management Strategies for Delirium

Determination of baseline cognition is an essential first step in the assessment of delirium. In addition, patients who have developed delirium in the past are at increased risk for recurrance so it is important to ask about any prior episodes. It is also important to ask about alcohol or other drug use in order to avoid having the patient experience withdrawal symptoms during hospitalization. Often family is the best source of this information. Although delirium cannot be prevented in every instance, optimal results are achieved by clinicians who are knowledgable of the risk factors and take preventive action. Martinez, Tobar, and Hill (2015), who conducted a systematic review of nonpharmacological, multicomponent interventions for delirium, found that strategies such as ensuring access to sensory aids, providing a restful environment, ensuring adequate hydration and nutiriton, and adequate and appropriate pain control are effective in reducing incident delirium and recommend inclusion as a standard of care for older adult inpatients. Vigilant screening and documenting of cognitive assessment will increase the liklihood that delirium is detected early and underlying causes identified and addressed. Delirium is a frightening experience for the patient and family. Conversations should be initiated with families on admission to educate them on the risks and reinforce the vital role they play in providing a sense of familiarity, comfort, and reassurance (American Geriatrics Society Expert Panel on Postoperative Delirium in Older Adults, 2015).

The management of postoperative pain can be especially challenging in the delirious patient. It is not uncommon for the surgeon to withdraw or reduce analgesia as a way to reduce agitation associated with acute confusion. However, inadequate pain control may also contribute to delirium (Morrison et al., 2003). (For more detailed information, see Chapter 17, "Delirium: Prevention, Early Recognition, and Treatment," and Chapter 18.)

MALNUTRITION: SIGNIFICANCE IN HIP-FRACTURE PATIENTS

It is estimated that as many as 63% of patients with fragility hip fracture are malnourished at the time of admission (Wyers et al., 2010). Circumstances before and surrounding the fall and fracture coupled with processes of care, such as prolonged restriction of solid food while awaiting surgery, combine to increase the risk for malnutrition. The stress of the acute injury and surgical intervention results in postoperative nutritional intake that routinely fails to meet energy and protein requirements, contributing to further deterioration in nutritional status (Bell, Bauer, Capra, & Pulle, 2013). Surveys of dietary intake of patients recovering from hip fracture reveal a less-than-optimal dietary intake (Lumbers, New, Gibson, & Murphy, 2001).

Lack of adequate nutrition leads to lowered cognitive function, lean muscle wasting, weakness, and impaired cardiac function, all of which contribute to impaired mobility and an increased risk of developing postoperative complications (Wyers et al., 2010). Duration of preoperative fasting is also a precipitating and modifiable risk factor for postoperative delirium (Radtke et al., 2010). A descriptive cohort study of 428 older adults with hip fractures revealed that preoperative fasting of 12 hours or longer was a risk factor for development of delirium and an increased risk for mortality at 4 months postoperatively (Bjorkelund et al., 2011). Fry, Pine, Jones, and Meimban (2010) looked at the records of more than 800,000 surgical patients from more than 13,000 hospitals and found that malnutrition was an independent risk factor for developing a number of hospital-acquired infections (Table 34.1).

Although common preoperative fasting time in the United States remains "NPO (nothing by mouth) after midnight," a growing number of organizations have endorsed liberalizing food and fluid restrictions (American Society of Anesthesiologists Committee, 1999; American Society of Anesthesiologists Committee on Preoperative Fasting, 1999; Braga et al., 2009). Evidence supports that patients with no specific risk of aspiration may drink clear fluids up to 2 hours before anesthesia and have solid foods up to 6 hours before surgery. The maximum period of oral fasting should be no greater than 12 hours under any circumstances (Shiga, Wajima, & Ohe, 2008).

TABLE 34.1
Complications Associated With Malnutrition

Complication	Odds Ratio of Developing if Malnourished
Pressure ulcers	3.8
Postoperative pneumonia	2.8
Catheter-associated urinary tract infections	5.1
Surgical site infections	2.5

Adapted from Fry, Pine, Jones, and Meimban (2010).

Emerging evidence suggests that in addition to liberalizing fasting restrictions, in select patients, prescribing a clear carbohydrate-rich beverage, such as apple juice, to be consumed 2 to 3 hours before surgery, can reduce the negative consequences of preoperative fasting, which include postoperative nausea and vomiting, loss of muscle strength, and postoperative insulin resistance (Hausel et al., 2001; Melis et al., 2006; Nygren, Thorell, & Ljungqvist, 2015; Yagci et al., 2008).

The AAOS guidelines for management of hip fractures in the elderly (Roberts & Bronx, 2014), the European Pressure Ulcer Advisory Panel (EPUAP), and National Pressure Ulcer Advisory Panel (NPUAP, 2014) support offering a high-protein oral nutritional supplement in addition to regular diet for patients at nutritional risk caused by chronic or acute illness following surgery. A systematic review of nutritional interventions provided to older adults recovering from hip fracture found only weak evidence to support benefits of protein and energy feedings; however, the authors did note the lack of a consistent definition of malnutrition in the studies reviewed. The reviewers did comment that patients who were malnourished benefitted more from high-protein oral supplements more than those who were not malnourished (Avenell & Handoll, 2010).

Nursing Management Strategies for Malnutrition

Nutritional screening is suggested for all hospitalized patients (Mueller, Compher, Druyan, & American Society for Parenteral and Enteral Nutrition [ASPEN] Board of Directors, 2011). Prompt referral to a registered dietitian for at-risk patients should be a nursing priority and is essential in order to curtail the negative consequences associated with malnutrition (Jefferies, Johnson, & Ravens, 2011). Nurses should be aware of the potential for swallowing problems in this population. A prospective cohort study of 181 patients after hip-fracture surgery found that 34% presented with oropharyngeal dysphasia within 72 hours after surgery. Common factors in those with swelling problems included preexisting dementia, postoperative delirium, and preexisting respiratory problems (Love, Cornwell, & Whitehouse, 2013). Early identification and referral to speech therapy for a more comprehensive swallow evaluation are essential to avoid aspiration pneumonia.

Implementation of protocols that liberalize preoperative fasting in accordance with existing guidelines should be advocated for patients who have no specific risk of aspiration, for example, gastroparesis. Evidence-based protocols should include orders to advance the diet as tolerated after surgery (Association of Anaesthetists of Great Britain & Ireland, 2014). Nursing staff should monitor dietary intake and notify a dietitian if a consistent pattern of consuming less than 50% of meals is observed. For patients who are malnourished, incorporating a high-protein oral nutritional supplement, as part of the daily medication pass, is an effective strategy to enhance the likelihood of consumption and embed a nutritional intervention into the routine process of care (Breedveld-Peters et al., 2012; Dillabough, Mammel & Yee, 2011; Meehan et al., 2016). For more detailed information, see Chapter 10, "Nutrition."

FLUID AND ELECTROLYTE IMBALANCE: SIGNIFICANCE IN HIP-FRACTURE PATIENTS

Patients admitted for hip fracture are at risk of dehydration, electrolyte disturbances, fluid overload, and heart failure because of advanced age and comorbid conditions (Bukata et al., 2011). White, Rashid, and Chakladar (2009) found renal dysfunction in 36% of patients admitted with hip fracture, whereas Carbone et al. (2010) cited the incidence of heart failure as 21% in this patient population.

Dehydration

Older adults admitted with hip fracture often present with dehydration for a variety of reasons. These include preexisting restricted fluid intake, diminished thirst reflex with subsequent diminished fluid intake, and prolonged time from injury to discovery and initiation of care. Many patients who suffer from incontinence or frequency self-regulate fluid intake to reduce the risk of incontinence or they may have difficulty accessing toilet facilities. Diuretic use is high in this patient group and may be partly responsible for altered fluid balance.

Because dehydration diminishes perfusion to both organs and tissues, it is implicated in the development of a range of conditions and complications prevalent in the hip-fracture population, such as delirium, acute kidney injury (AKI), pressure ulcers, falls, VTE, and urinary tract infections.

Fluid Overload/Heart Failure

Preexisting heart failure or renal conditions that increase fluid load will worsen with the stress of the injury and subsequent surgery. This diminished cardiac and renal function renders the frail older adult more susceptible to fluid overload. For a detailed discussion, see Chapter 30, "Fluid Overload: Identifying and Managing Heart Failure Patients at Risk of Hospital Readmission."

Electrolyte Imbalance/Acute Kidney Injury

Electrolyte imbalances, particularly hyponatremia and hypokalemia, are common in the postoperative period, reflecting limited renal reserve (Maher et al., 2013). Diuretics and inappropriate maintenance of intravenous fluids may exacerbate the situation. Limited renal reserve is also reflected in the high risk of AKI in hip-fracture patients, which is estimated to be 16% (Bennet, Berry, Goddard, & Keating, 2010) and is associated with prolonged hospital stay, increased morbidity and mortality, and poor outcome (Ulucay et al., 2012).

Older patients admitted to hospital for emergency surgery are at increased risk of AKI and its associated pre- and postoperative complications. Risk factors include preexisting comorbid conditions, age, complex polypharmacy, and use of diuretics, nephrotoxic medications such as angiotensin-converting enzyme inhibitors (ACE inhibitors) used in the management of hypertension and heart failure, and nonsteroidal anti-inflammatory drugs (NSAIDs) used for pain relief. Time spent down before discovery as well as immobility before surgery also increases the risk of rhabdomyolysis. The most significant complication of rhabdomyolysis is AKI (Torres, Helmstetter, Kaye, & Kaye, 2015).

Nursing Management Strategies: Fluid and Electrolyte Imbalances

Optimized perioperative fluid management helps in controlling the frequent incidence of dehydration in hip-fracture patients while avoiding volume overload, which is crucial as many of these patients have coexisting cardiac disease (Bukata et al., 2011). Strict fluid balance monitoring that begins in the emergency department (ED) and continues throughout the acute hospitalization is essential.

Dehydration

Factors that add to the normal risk of dehydration in this population include preoperative fasting and surgical blood loss. A short period of preoperative fasting supported by intravenous fluids with early resumption of oral intake in the postoperative period is optimal. Environmental factors, such as limited access to fluids, visual impairments, and drinking containers that are difficult to handle, may compound the problem. Hourly rounding that includes proactive offering of fluids as well as mouth care are two important nursing interventions.

Fluid Overload

Ensure that regular diuretics are administered as prescribed, monitor vital signs, maintain accurate documentation of fluid balance, and promptly report alterations in the patient's clinical and cognitive status.

The stress of surgery leads to an increased secretion of the antidiuretic hormone (ADH), which impairs the ability to excrete sodium and water. Symptoms to monitor include urinary output less than 30 mL/hr, increasing blood pressure, shortness of breath, moist breath sounds, and dependent edema.

Electrolyte Imbalance/AKI

AKI, previously referred to as acute renal failure, is an abrupt change in kidney function signaled by a rise in serum creatinine and a reduction in urine output (Pakula & Skinner, 2015). This type of injury usually occurs within 48 hours of one or more precipitating events, such as a hip fracture. Baseline renal function is an independent predictor for AKI (Ulucay et al., 2012), but establishment of this may be difficult in hip-fracture patients, as they may be acutely dehydrated on admission with or without the presence of some chronic renal dysfunction.

Close monitoring of fluid balance, particularly decreasing urine output and rising serum creatinine, is essential to early identification of this significant clinical problem.

AKI is managed with renal replacement therapy, a topic that is beyond the scope of this protocol (Ftouh & Lewington, 2014; Pakula & Skinner, 2015).

PRESSURE ULCER: SIGNIFICANCE IN HIP-FRACTURE PATIENTS

Older adults undergoing surgical repair of a fragility hip fracture constitute a high-risk population for developing pressure ulcer. A major factor that increases risk in this population is the long periods of immobility before, during, and after surgery. A meta-analysis (Simunovic et al., 2010) revealed that earlier surgery was associated with a lower risk of death and lower rates of postoperative complications, such as pneumonia and pressure ulcers, among older patients with hip fracture. Baumgarten et al. (2012)

showed that patients who had surgical repair longer than 24 hours after admission had a higher rate of postsurgical pressure ulcers than those who had surgery within 24 hours of admission, suggesting that reducing delays to surgery may reduce the risk of developing pressure ulcer. Patients with fragility hip fracture are an important group to target for assessment of risk factors and implementation of strategies to prevent these wounds.

Nursing Management Strategies to Avoid Pressure Ulcers

A head-to-toe skin assessment on admission with examination of pressure points every shift is an important strategy to proactively avoid development of pressure ulcers. Before surgery, it is important to ensure that the heels are off loaded and free from pressure. Patients should be cared for on pressure-relieving mattresses throughout the continuum of care, including the ED, the perioperative area, and the nursing unit. Interoperative padding of bony prominences and avoidance of friction and shearing forces are also imperative to avoid skin tears. These patients will require assistance with repositioning, especially before surgery. Adequate pain relief, both before and after surgery, is crucial to reduce fear of repositioning. As patients with hip fracture often have poor nutritional status and are fasting before surgery, the risk of developing pressure ulcer increases. However, it is possible to reduce this risk by introducing an evidence-based pathway that includes early surgery and optimizing fluid and nutritional balance, which is a clinical imperative for these vulnerable patients (Hommel, Bjorkelund, Thorngren, & Ulander, 2007). For a more detailed discussion, see Chapter 24, "Preventing Pressure Ulcers and Skin Tears."

VTE: SIGNIFICANCE IN HIP-FRACTURE PATIENTS

VTE is a serious, potentially fatal, surgical complication in patients operated on for hip fracture and one of the principal causes of perioperative morbidity and mortality (Carpintero et al., 2014). It is, therefore, no surprise that prophylaxis is recommended in evidence-based clinical practice guidelines (AAOS, 2014; Falck-Ytter et al., 2012; National Institute for Health and Clinical Excellence (NICE; 2010) and has long been a part of standard treatment protocols.

Patients sustaining hip fracture are at increased risk of VTE resulting from advanced age, delay to surgery, blood vessel damage secondary to the fracture as well as the operative repair (Prisco, Cenci, Silvestri, Emmi, & Ciucciarelli, 2014), cardiac and respiratory comorbidities (Falck-Ytter et al., 2012), and delay to postoperative mobilization. Patients with orthopedic trauma are also more vulnerable to coagulation activation from tissue and bone injury as well as reduced venous emptying perioperatively (Cionac Florescu, Anastase, Munteanu, Stoica, & Antonescu, 2013).

Nursing Strategies to Avoid VTE

Mobilization

Prevention of VTE is the key. Early mobilization and adequate hydration are *essential* components of VTE prevention. Encourage patients to mobilize as soon as practical after surgery and to undertake leg exercises as instructed in order to get the calf muscles pumping and limit blood stasis. Request that family provide sturdy footwear with a closed heel and toe and ensure that an individually fitted walker is available at the bedside. Offer and encourage fluid intake in accordance with any limitations.

Pharmacologic Prophylaxis

There is no way to predict which patients will develop VTE (Cionac Florescu et al., 2013) and therefore pharmacologic prophylaxis must be administered to all patients with hip fractures unless contraindicated (Marsland, Mears, & Kates, 2010). However, as soon as the hemorrhagic risk is under control, pharmacologic prophylaxis should be started if the thrombotic risk persists (Prisco et al., 2014). Current treatment with aspirin or clopidogrel is not a contraindication for pharmacologic prophylaxis (AAOS, 2014).

Pharmacologic agents recommended for VTE prophylaxis include primarily low-molecular-weight heparin (LMWH) or fondaparinux (Falck-Ytter et al., 2012; NICE, 2010; Prisco et al., 2014). LMWH interrupts the clotting cascade at various levels, whereas fondaparinux is a specific Factor Xa inhibitor. Agents, such as unfractionated heparin and aspirin, among others, may be used depending on individual patient circumstances.

Nursing strategies include administering medications within the prescribed time schedule and monitoring the patient for adverse effects, primarily bleeding. Other complications include liver function abnormalities, skin rashes, and bruising.

Mechanical Prophylaxis

The most important intervention for VTE prevention is the mechanism of walking. Establish mobility goals and stress the importance of mobility in healing and restoring functional recovery as well as VTE prevention.

Until such time as the patient is ambulatory or when resting in bed, mechanical prophylaxis may also include intermittent (or sequential) compression devices and graduated compression stockings. The magnitude of individual benefit from these mechanical treatment methods is unclear as they are usually combined with pharmacologic methods (Cionac Florescu et al., 2013).

Intermittent pneumatic compression devices (IPCD) provide a good alternative to anticoagulation and may be used alone for VTE prophylaxis in patients at high risk of bleeding (Koo, Choi, Ahn, Kwon, & Cho, 2014). They can also be used in conjunction with pharmacologic prophylaxis (Falck-Ytter et al., 2012). However, many IPC units are large and bulky making correct application difficult for patients after discharge and increasing fall risk. Smaller portable, battery-powered units are an alternative. Foot compression requires higher pressures than calf compression so patient cooperation with therapy may be problematic. When part of a patient's treatment plan, ensure correct application and continuous use for the recommended time period daily.

A recent Cochrane Review (Sachdeva, Dalton, Amaragiri, & Lees, 2014) concluded that graduated compression/anti embolic stockings (GCS) diminish the risk of VTE in hospitalized patients with evidence favoring their use in orthopedic surgery. However, in a review of the literature specific to hip-fracture patients, Alsawadi and Loeffler (2012) were unable to find sufficient evidence to support use of GCS in combination with LMWH for VTE prevention. Compression stockings can be difficult and painful for patients and caregivers to apply correctly and thus compliance with their appropriate use is a concern. Most commonly cited adverse effects are skin irritation and skin breakdown. To prevent development of a pressure sore from compression stockings, Bukata et al. (2011) suggest stockings be removed while the patient is in bed. Although rare, pain and numbness could be early warning signs of compartment syndrome or peroneal nerve injury, which have been described in the literature as complications (Güzelküçük, Skempes, & Kumnerddee, 2014; Hinderland, Ng, Paden, & Stone, 2011).

In light of these issues, there is variability in usage. The Institute for Clinical Systems Improvement in the United States (Jobin et al., 2012) notes that GCS are routinely used though there is little evidence supporting their efficacy. They are recommended by the NICE Guidelines in the United Kingdom (NICE, 2011) but national hip fracture care guidance in both Sweden and Canada no longer includes use of compression stockings (A. Hommel, personal communication, March 23, 2015; V. MacDonald, personal communication, March 29, 2015).

It is recommended that stockings are removed at least once daily for hygienic purposes and to inspect skin condition as this is the most notable complication associated with their use. Stockings should be discontinued if there is marking, blistering, or discoloration of skin, particularly over heels and bony prominences, or if the patient has associated pain, numbness, or discomfort. The nurse is advised to use caution and clinical judgment when applying antiembolism stockings over wounds. If edema or postoperative swelling develops, legs are remeasured and stockings refitted.

GCS are contraindicated in patients with diagnoses such as arterial disease, peripheral arterial bypass graft, peripheral neuropathy, leg deformities, and certain skin conditions and cardiac failure (NICE, 2010).

Patient Education

VTE prophylaxis usually continues past the acute care period. In preparation for discharge, patients and/or their families and care providers require both verbal and written information addressing:

- The signs and symptoms of VTE and pulmonary embolism (PE)
- The proper technique for administering injectable medication
- The importance of taking the medication at the appropriate time and for the prescribed duration
- The signs and symptoms of adverse reactions related to VTE prophylaxis and the importance of seeking medical help as well as whom to contact; and for those patients who are discharged with antiembolism stockings or intermittent compression devices, their use and whom to contact for questions

CATHETER-ASSOCIATED URINARY TRACT INFECTION: SIGNIFICANCE IN HIP-FRACTURE PATIENTS

Older adults with fragility hip fracture are at increased risk of developing a urinary tract infection. There is no good-quality evidence to support routine catheterization in this population, although indwelling urinary catheters (IUCs) are commonly inserted on admission to the ED. The clinical indication for the catheter is to avoid movement at the fracture site before surgical repair, which is in compliance with Centers for Disease Control and Prevention (CDC) criteria. The Joint Commission (TJC) and Centers for Medicare & Medicaid Services (CMS) Surgical Care

Improvement Project (SCIP) have developed and implemented standards (core measures) aimed at encouraging early discontinuation of these devices in surgical patients. SCIP core measure related to IUCs states that IUCs are to be removed on postoperative day 1 or 2 with day 0 defined as the day of surgery (TJC, 2015).

Although commonly used, these devices are not innocuous. IUCs are known to be a contributing factor to the development of urinary tract infection, delirium, and they are considered a one-point restraint impacting ease of mobility (Saint, Lipsky, & Goold, 2002). A study by Wald, Epstein, and Kramer (2005) found that patients discharged to a nursing facility after hip-fracture surgery with an IUC in place had greater incidence of readmission with a urinary tract infection and increased rates of mortality at 30 days when compared with those without an IUC.

Nursing Management Strategies to Avoid Catheter-Associated Urinary Tract Infection

The criteria for avoiding the development of a catheter-associated urinary tract infection (CAUTI) include ensuring that insertion is clinically necessary and reflects CDC and Society for Healthcare Epidemiology of America (SHEA)/Infectious Disease Society of America (IDSA) criteria, use of aseptic technique when inserting the device; good/routine perineal hygiene, and removal of the device as soon as no longer needed (Gould et al., 2010; Lo et al., 2014). Nurse-initiated protocols for the management of IUCs have proven beneficial in reducing dwell time and thus reducing the risk of infection (Alexaitis & Broome, 2014; Mori, 2014). For more detailed information see Chapter 22, "Prevention of Catheter-Associated Urinary Tract Infection."

FUNCTIONAL DECLINE: SIGNIFICANCE IN HIP-FRACTURE PATIENTS

Fragility hip fracture in old age is a condition recognized as a major cause of functional decline and disability. The devastating effect on long-term function is described in a review by Bertram et al. (2011), who found that 29% of the patients with hip fracture did not regain their prefracture level of ADL function. Furthermore, at 1 year postoperatively, more than 40% had not regained their prefracture level of function and 47% reported pain. More than one third were unable to walk independently as a result of the fracture. Decreased mobility and pain contribute to functional decline and may lead to frailty. These findings suggest that a significant proportion of the patients will experience disability, a high risk of falls, and are at increased risk of another fracture. Many will become dependent on community care and home care services (Milte & Crotty, 2014).

Nursing Management Strategies to Avoid Functional Decline

The goal of rehabilitation is that the patient will regain as much of his or her prefracture level of function and health-related quality of life as he or she had before the fracture. A nursing strategy to achieve that goal is to adopt a function-focused approach to care, encouraging and supporting hospitalized patients to be active participants in their self-care activities (Boltz, Resnick, Capezuti, Shuluk, & Secic, 2012). Early mobility, transferring in and out of bed, dressing, grooming and walking to the toilet, and being out of bed for meals are essential. Effective interventions also include nutritional therapy and resistance training (Morley et al., 2013). Continued rehabilitation after the patient returns home is also important. In a randomized controlled study, Ziden, Kreuter, and Frandin (2010) focused on early rehabilitation in the home setting. The results showed improved balance confidence, independence, and physical activity in the group participating in the program.

LOSS, GRIEF, AND DEPRESSION: SIGNIFICANCE IN HIP-FRACTURE PATIENTS

Patients vary greatly in the speed and extent of their recovery. For some patients and families, the hip fracture is a catastrophic event that results in diminished function, a loss of independence, and a high risk of death within 1 year. Patients may lose hope for the future and experience loss, grief, and depression. The rate of depression in hip-fracture patients across a review of eight U.S. and U.K. studies ranged from 9% to 47% (Holmes & House, 2000). Hip-fracture patients with depression are less likely to regain function and are prone to longer stays in hospital (Holmes & House, 2000; Lenze et al., 2004).

Nursing Strategies to Address Grief, Loss, and Depression

Nurses play a key role in assessing the patient and family's emotional well-being. Essential functions include screening for depression and ensuring referrals are sent to medical or psychiatric clinicians if warranted.

A positive attitude, social supports, and active participation/movement were findings consistent across two qualitative studies that identified themes reported by patients on what enabled them to recover (Schiller et al., 2015; Young & Resnick, 2009). Nurses can foster a positive attitude and hope by informing patients and families that most patients survive and can regain some or all of their prefracture function through participation in rehabilitation. Facilitating early mobility and encouraging ambulation activity can foster confidence and hope for the future. For more detailed information, see Chapter 15, "Late-Life Depression."

CARE TRANSITIONS: SIGNIFICANCE IN HIP-FRACTURE PATIENTS

Care transition is a term used to describe a patient's movement from one health care setting to the next (Coleman & Berenson, 2004). Leaving the hospital to go home is a perilous time for patients with hip fractures. Without a coordinated plan and clear communication, medication adverse events, complications, emergency room visits, and unnecessary readmissions to hospital can occur (Forster, Murff, Peterson, Gandhi, & Bates, 2003; Glenny, Stolee, Sheiban, & Jaglal, 2013). Although deemed ready for discharge by the health care team, some patients and families feel unprepared to manage independently at home. Interviews of family care provides reveal that they are often confused and distressed about the fracture and surgery, feel uninformed about their medications, and may become overwhelmed with the challenges of coping at home (Sims-Gould, Hicks, Khan, & Stolee, 2012). Older adults report extreme vulnerability following a hip fracture, with the first 12 weeks particularly turbulent (Ziden et al., 2010).

The readmission rate for hip-fracture patients was determined to be 11.9% in a university-affiliated trauma center (Kates, Behrend, Mendelson, Cram, & Friedman, 2015). The 1-year mortality rate for readmitted patients was 56.2% versus 21.8% for those not readmitted. Readmission was attributed to medical causes for 81.4% of patients and surgical causes for 18.6%. It was concluded that 17% of these readmissions were preventable through interventions.

Coleman's Care Transitions Intervention (Coleman & Berenson, 2004; Coleman, Parry Chalmers, & Min, 2006) is a proven model shown to improve the safety and experience for patients and family. In this model, patient and family caregivers engage with the health care team to prevent and address risks by focusing on (a) medication adherence strategies; (b) postdischarge follow-ups, for example, for bone health and medication reviews; (c) detecting and addressing "red flags," indicative of complications or medical deterioration; and (d) keeping a personal health record to aid communication.

Hip fracture represents a major traumatic life change for many patients and families. They may be anxious and distressed and may require emotional support and counseling around loss and grief (Lenze et al., 2007; Ziden et al., 2010).

The following guidelines are derived from the *Fresh Start Toolkit: Hip Fracture Recovery Guide for Patients and Families*, an evidence-based tool developed collaboratively by patients and the interprofessional team (BC Hip Fracture Redesign Committee Centre for Hip Health and Mobility, 2015). Involvement of the interprofessional team is required to address the patient's needs.

1. Apply principles of teaching appropriate to older adults, provide both verbal and written instruction and begin early in the hospital stay; see Chapter 36, "Transitional Care."
2. Include information on the surgical procedure/activity restrictions, the importance of frequent ambulation, healthy diet, sleep strategies, and pain management at home.
3. Educate patients on early warning signs of "red flags" and what to do (e.g., VTE, delirium, infection, dislocation, and constipation).
4. Determine home assistance requirements for ADL, housekeeping, shopping, and banking. Assist patients to arrange the aformentioned.
5. Assess medication management skills and develop a plan for medication review and safety at home.
6. As falls remain a significant risk for these patients, conduct a fall-risk assessment and develop an individualized plan.
7. Evaluate need for home modifications to improve home safety and convenience, for example, a bath or shower bench, grab bars installed for the toilet and bath, setting the bed to knee height, solid handrails on stairs, removing tripping hazards, and good lighting. Specialized equipment, such as a walker, raised toilet seat, and a reacher, may also be required. Assess the individual's needs and facilitate arrangements to procure and install as appropriate.
8. Because so many patients feel overwhelmed at home, a follow-up phone call or home visit from a health care professional is recommended for support, teaching, and problem solving.

SECONDARY PREVENTION: SIGNIFICANCE IN HIP-FRACTURE PATIENTS

It is well known that one of the highest risk factors for sustaining a fragility fracture is the history of a previous fracture (Cooper, Mitchell, & Kanis, 2011). The highest risk period is in the first year following a fracture, but the risk persists for at least 10 years (Sobolev et al., 2015). It has been known for decades that half of all patients who suffer a fragility hip fracture experienced a prior fracture (Edwards et al., 2007; Gallagher et al., 1980; Port et al., 2003). The first fragility fracture should serve as a signal alerting clinicians of the need to evaluate the patient for underlying osteoporosis and, if confirmed, to initiate interventions to prevent the occurrence of future fracture (Port et al., 2003). Although effective treatments and care models have been available for many years, a review of current practice suggests that care gaps continue (Mitchell & Chem, 2013). This gap in secondary care needs to be addressed in order to minimize both the debilitating consequences of subsequent fractures for patients and the associated economic burden to health care systems (Marsh et al., 2011).

Sobolev et al. (2015) reviewed more than 38,000 records of patients aged 60 years or older discharged after hip fracture and found that less than 20% were screened for osteoporosis. An observational cohort study of 51,346 Medicare patients admitted to 318 hospitals in the United States with a diagnosis of osteoporosis found that despite proven therapies for osteoporosis, hip-fracture patients remain grossly undertreated, and only 2% were provided ideal therapy (Jennings et al., 2010).

One of the most commonly used and most effective approaches to fracture management is a fracture liaison service (FLS). This approach has been developed and successfully implemented, both nationally and internationally, with the most mature programs in the United Kingdom. FLS programs center around the use of a dedicated coordinator to identify patients with fragility fracture. Marsh et al. (2011) conducted a systematic review of fracture-management programs and found that 65% included a dedicated coordinator. The role of the coordinator, often an advanced practice nurse, is to identify patients with fragility fracture, and following evidence-based protocols, facilitate BMD testing, provide osteoporosis education, evaluate and address fall risks, initiate osteoporosis treatment, and monitor adherence to therapy. A review of best practices (Mitchell, 2013) and findings of a task force commissioned by the Society of Bone and Mineral Research (Eisman et al., 2012) reports that the most effective tool for change and the optimal approach to fracture management is a program that uses a dedicated fracture liaison coordinator.

Several FLSs have been established in the United States. Kaiser Permanente, a California-based health maintenance organization, established a "Healthy Bones Program" in 2002. Within this fracture-management program, advanced practice nurses identify, stratify risk, treat, and track patients with osteoporosis as well as individuals who have had or are at risk of a fragility fracture. Since its inception, it is estimated that the Healthy Bones Program has reduced incidence of hip fractures by more than 40% (Dell, 2011; Greene & Dell, 2010). The Geisinger Health System, serving a large population in rural central Pennsylvania, developed an osteoporosis disease management program and using a cost–benefit model projected a $7.8 million cost savings over the 5-year period from 1996 to 2000 (Newman et al., 2013). The success of these programs is aided by having integrated electronic medical record systems enhancing the ability to share information and monitor patients.

The International Osteoporosis Foundation (IOF) launched a Capture the Fracture program in 2012 with the goal of promoting coordinator-based FLSs globally (Akesson et al., 2013). In 2012, the National Bone Health Alliance (NBHA) and Kaiser Permanente unveiled their 20/20 vision for reducing hip fractures by 20% by the year 2020. They are lobbying the federal government for reimbursement criteria to be established within the Medicare system that would support the development of secondary fracture-prevention services for Medicare recipients (NBHA, 2012). In addition, the NBHA has developed an online education program for nurses interested in being certified as a fracture liaison nurse. The growing emphasis on quality improvement for reimbursement and accreditation may heighten interest in expanding the number of fragility fracture management services in other institutions (Aizer & Bolster, 2014).

The ultimate goal of a fracture-management program is to capture 100% of fragility-fracture sufferers and prevent a second fragility fracture.

Core objectives include:

1. Inclusive case finding
2. Evidence-based assessment to:
   a. Stratify risk
   b. Identify secondary causes of osteoporosis
   c. Evaluate fall risk
3. Initiate individualized treatment plan in accordance with relevant evidence-based guidelines
4. Improve long-term adherence with treatment plan

These programs ensure that all patients presenting with fragility fractures receive fracture risk assessment, education, and treatment appropriately. The fracture-management program can be based in secondary or primary care health care settings and requires support from a medically qualified practitioner, commonly an advanced practice nurse, with expertise in fragility-fracture prevention or a primary care physician with a specialist interest.

FIGURE 34.6

Hospital-based fracture liaison service algorithm.

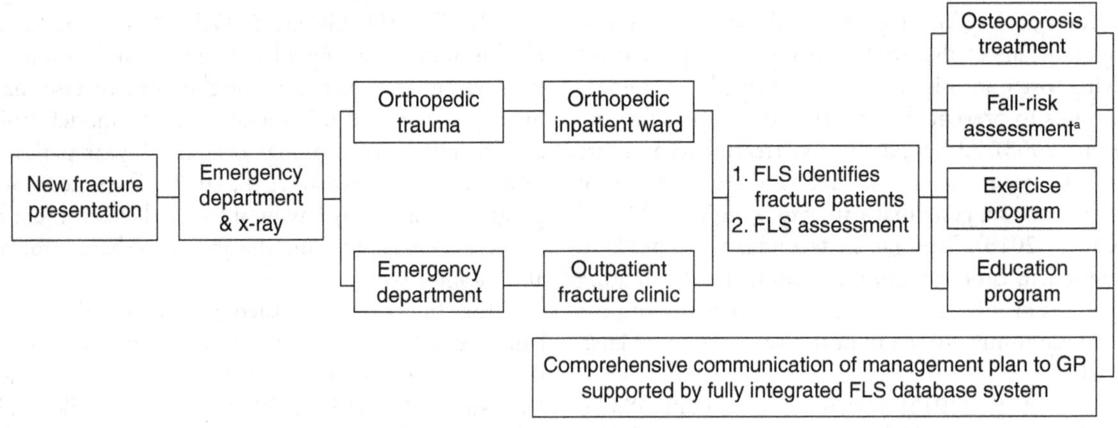

[a]Older patients, where appropriate, are identified and referred for falls assessment.

FLS, fracture liaison service; GP, general practitioner.

Image used with permission from Åkesson et al. (2013). With permission of Springer.

An example of the structure of a hospital-based fracture-management service is illustrated in Figure 34.6.

For more information on secondary prevention and fracture-management programs visit the IOF Capture the Fracture website (http://share.iofbonehealth.org/WOD/2012/report/WOD12-Report.pdf), the National Bone Health Alliance website (http://nbha.org/projects/secondary-fracture-prevention-initiative), and the Fragility Fracture Network website (http://fragilityfracturenetwork.org).

CASE STUDY

Mrs. W is an 84-year-old widow and a retired schoolteacher who lives in a senior apartment complex. Her 80-year-old sister lives in a nearby apartment. Mrs. W is independent in her ADL, she cooks meals and sorts her medications; however, her daughter provides help with bill paying and transportation as Mrs. W voluntarily gave up driving 2 years ago as a result of limited motion in her neck. She wears glasses for reading and distance and she uses a cane for walking outside her apartment. Her medical history includes hypertension, osteoarthritis, and gastroesophageal reflux disease (GERD). She has urge incontinence and chronic pain caused by osteoarthritis, which sometimes interferes with her sleep. Her family will tell you that she has some "occasional forgetfulness." Her medications include a multivitamin, antihypertensive, a proton pump inhibitor, and extra-strength acetaminophen for her arthritic pain, which she takes as needed. Past surgical history includes hysterectomy for fibroids (age 48 years), a non-displaced distal radius fracture that was treated with a cast (age 58 years), and 6 years ago she had a total left hip replacement for degenerative joint disease.

The night of her fall, Mrs. W recalls taking two acetaminophen PM tablets before going to bed. She remembers waking during the night needing to toilet and falling on her way to the bathroom. Unable to get up or summon help she remained on the floor until discovered in the morning by her sister. She presents in the ED complaining of pain in her right hip. Her sister accompanies her in the ambulance to the emergency room and her daughter is on the way. She arrives at your hospital, which has a geriatric section in the ED and protocols based on best practice to care for older adults with hip fracture.

Nursing concerns in the ED will include:

- Medication history

(continued)

CASE STUDY *(continued)*

- Review of circumstances surrounding fall/fracture and pattern of injury
- Assessment and treatment for acute pain and chronic pain
  - Regional pain block would reduce opioid use
- Sensory devices and family at bedside
- Monitoring of fluid balance
- Monitor oxygenation/avoid hypoxia
- Establish baseline cognition
- Awareness of increased risk of delirium
- Skin assessment; pressure ulcer prevention
- Evaluation of need for indwelling catheter before insertion
  - Catheter inserted because of fracture instability and related immobility
- Protocol for fast tracking through ED to the orthopedic unit

An x-ray of Mrs. W's hip confirms a displaced neck of the femur fracture. She is transferred to the orthopedic unit within 4 hours of arrival. Nursing strategies on the *admitting unit* include:

- Monitoring of adequate and appropriate pain relief
- VTE prophylaxis as ordered
- Delirium assessment every 12 hours, more frequent if changes in mentation
- Sensory aids in place
- Invite family involvement/inform of potential risk of delirium
- Pressure-relieving mattress/position changes
- Nutritional assessment, dietary consults
- High-protein oral nutritional supplement with medications
- Protocol in place that liberalizes presurgical fasting restrictions
  - High-carbohydrate drink, such as apple juice, up to 2 hours before surgery
- Avoid overstimulating environment/preserve sleep–wake cycle

Mrs. W is scheduled for surgery within 48 hours of arrival. She is transferred to the *perioperative* area where her fracture is repaired with hemiarthroplasty. She spends a total of 4 hours in the *preoperative, surgery,* and *postoperative* units. Nursing management strategies include:

- Pressure-relieving surfaces in the perioperative area
- Padding of pressure points
- Monitoring of oxygenation
- Administration of ordered antibiotics
- Monitoring of fluid balance/blood loss

Mrs. W returns to the nursing unit after surgery. *Postoperative* nursing management strategies include:

- Continuation of adequate and appropriate pain relief, both acute and chronic
- Sensory aids in place, family involvement
- Nursing begins mobilization day of surgery/physical therapy (PT) occupational therapy (OT) consulted
- VTE prophylaxis continued
- IUCs removed postoperative day 1
- Awareness of increased risk and assessment for delirium and depression
- Pressure-point assessment; pressure-relieving seat cushion when in chair
- Advance diet as tolerated per protocol; continue oral nutritional supplements with medications
- Monitor fluids and electrolytes
- Monitor bowel function

Proactive care strategies designed to avoid risk factors associated with common complications of hip fracture ensured an uneventful course during hospitalization. PT and OT recommend discharge to a rehabilitation facility before returning home with assistance. As part of the care transition process nursing management strategies include:

- With Mrs. W's permission, arrange a meeting with her daughter and her sister to help them prepare for Mrs. W's eventual homecoming.
- Provide both verbal and written instructions on the surgical procedure, activity restrictions, importance of frequent ambulation and early warning signs of "red flags" and what to do if they develop (e.g., VTE, delirium, infection, constipation, and dislocation).
- PT and OT assess Mrs. W's home-equipment needs and provide further information on where to obtain additional items. Review home safety instructions to reduce fall risk.
- Before transfer to rehab unit, a consultation with FLS is initiated for evaluation, and ongoing fracture risk management.
- Follow-up with orthopedic surgeon and family nurse practitioner needed in 6 weeks.

SUMMARY

A hip fracture is a serious injury with a significant impact on the patient, family, and health care system. Health care resources will be strained as the proportion of older adults in the population steadily increases and the incidence of hip fracture reaches unprecedented numbers. Although there is a high rate of mortality and disability postfracture, an interprofessional approach that incorporates best practices can significantly improve the experience and outcomes for these patients.

The risks that lead to death and disability postfracture are foreseeable and, in many cases, preventable. People with fragility hip fractures, with few exceptions, are older than 65 years with comorbid conditions. As such, they are highly susceptible to the stress of the injury, surgery, and immobility. Timely surgery, good pain management, early and frequent mobility, prevention of infection, and fluid balance are associated with improved outcomes. Providing support for loss and grief, goal setting for recovery, and screening and referral for depression when warranted will aid in longer term recovery. Going home is a precarious time and patients are at high risk of readmissions resulting from medical concerns, falls, and subsequent fractures. Patients and families require education and support to prepare their home environments, caregivers, and follow-ups for medical concerns and bone health. Nurses who provide evidence-based care focused on the patient and family ensure the best possible outcomes for patients with fragility hip fractures.

NURSING STANDARD OF PRACTICE

Protocol 34.1: Managing Patients With Hip Fracture

I. GOALS

Patients with hip fracture are susceptible to foreseeable and potentially avoidable complications. An interprofessional team approach to care that uses evidence-based strategies for prevention, early detection, and proactive care to avoid complications is the key to optimal patient outcomes.

II. EMERGENCY ROOM

The majority of these patients will enter the hospital via the emergency room. Considerations must be given to provide an environment that is sensitive to the care needs of this vulnerable population. Increasingly, hospitals are providing spaces in their emergency rooms designed to accommodate the needs of older adults and avoid the negative consequences associated with an overstimulating environment. Early implementation of multifactorial interventions aimed at reducing complications in this vulnerable population, starting in the emergency department, has proven beneficial (Bjorkelund et al., 2011; see Chapter 38, "Care of the Older Adult in the Emergency Department."

III. TIMELY SURGERY

Delays to surgery greater than 24 to 48 hours increase the risk of complications, delirium, and mortality. Hommel et al. (2008) found higher mortality at 4 months among medically fit patients with administrative delay to surgery compared to patients with no delay and longer hospital stays for those with delays greater than 24 hours. In a study of 38,020 patients with hip fractures, Daugaard et al. (2012) concluded that avoiding surgical delay is the most important factor in reducing mortality for hip-fracture patients. Most patients benefit more from early surgery than being delayed for investigations and medical optimization (Holt, Smith, Duncan, & McKeown, 2010). Nurses can play an important role in advocating for timely access to surgery.

IV. DELIRIUM

A. Determine patient's preadmission cognitive status and cognitive presentation on admission using a standardized tool and information from family.
B. Screen for delirium every 12 hours using an evidence-based tool.
C. Educate patient and family on the increased risk of delirium with hip fracture and how they can help prevent and cope with it.

(continued)

Protocol 34.1: Hip Fracture *(continued)*

D. Prevent/address the factors that may contribute to delirium, for example, pain, urine retention, infection, constipation, sensory impairment, sleep, metabolic disturbances, medications, alcohol withdrawal, dehydration, and environmental over/understimulation.
E. Reassess cognitive status before care transition.

V. MALNUTRITION

A. Assess for malnutrition on admission using a standardized screening tool.
B. Consult registered dietitian for comprehensive assessment if malnourished or if the patient is unable to tolerate the diet.
C. Screen for dysphagia and refer to a speech or occupational therapist if dysphagia suspected.
D. Adopt protocols that minimize fasting before surgery. Evidence supports the benefits of:
   1. Solid food up to 8 hours before surgery
   2. Clear fluids up to 2 to 4 hours before surgery
   3. Clear fluid high-carbohydrate drink 2 to 4 hours before surgery, for example, clear juice

E. Postsurgery nutrition
   1. Provide a regular diet as tolerated the day of surgery.
   2. Monitor nutritional intake. Inform dietitian or physician if intake is consistently less than 50% of the diet provided.
   3. Provide scheduled administration of high-protein, high-calorie nutritional supplements in addition to ordered diet.

VI. PAIN

A. Asume your patient has moderate to severe pain. Recognize that unmanaged pain increases complications, impedes recovery, and increases mortality.
B. Assess pain and pain history on admission using a comprehensive validated tool.
C. Consider any painful comorbid conditions and prehospital analgesic use in the pain management plan.
D. Assess valid pain scale with vital signs.
E. Assess using a validated sedation scale every hour for 24 hours and then every 4 hours thereafter. Adjust analgesic dosing according to the scale.
F. Time the administration of analgesics such that their peak effect coincides with physiotherapy and mobility.
G. Use a pharmacological and nonpharmacological multimodal approach to reduce the need for opioids.
H. Advocate for regional blocks (nerve/compartment).
I. Ensure that geriatric-appropriate analgesics/doses are prescribed and administered.
J. Use regularly scheduled doses of analgesics while pain persists.

VII. CONSTIPATION

A. Assess prehospital bowel habits and management.
B. Assess for BM daily, including size, consistency, and color.
C. Assume your patient will be constipated as a result of immobility, analgesics, and pain.
D. Use a standardized geriatric-appropriate bowel protocol.
E. Administer prophylactic laxatives as ordered unless contraindicated, for example, diarrhea, multiple daily moderate to large BMs.
F. Ensure adequate fluid intake and a high-fiber diet where appropriate, for example, bran, prunes, applesauce, and dates.
G. Encourage ambulation to promote bowel function. Avoid bedpans, ambulate to the toilet.

(continued)

Protocol 34.1: Hip Fracture *(continued)*

VIII. CATHETER-ASSOCIATED URINARY TRACT INFECTION

A. Avoid indwelling catheters. Use an indwelling catheter only if evidence-based criteria are met, for example, Centers for Disease Control and Prevention.
B. Reassess the need for the catheter each shift and remove as soon as possible, within 36 hours after surgery.
C. Use an evidence-based nursing protocol to guide insertion, hygiene, and management of the catheter and drainage system.

IX. PRESSURE ULCER PREVENTION

A. Conduct a head-to-toe pressure point assessment on admission and then each shift.
B. Use an evidence-based pressure ulcer risk screening tool (i.e., Braden Scale) to identify areas to be monitored and addressed.
C. Implement a written care plan to address any underlying risk factors as indicated (e.g., immobility, nutrition, moisture, etc.).
D. Consider using pressure reduction mattresses and chair surfaces routinely for hip fracture patients.
E. Ensure that patients are repositioned every 2 hours (some patients may do this independently).
F. Mobilize and assess toileting needs every 2 to 3 hours while awake.
G. Ensure nutrition and hydration are monitored and needs are met.
H. Implement a written care plan to address any skin injury or breakdown as per evidence-based clinical guidelines.

X. VENOUS THROMBOEMBOLISM

A. Recognize that hip fracture patients are at high risk of VTE.
B. Advocate for evidence-based treatment.
C. Ensure that treatment is initiated as prescribed.
D. Monitor for adverse events, for example, bleeding, bruising, or rashes with chemopropylaxis or skin breakdown and circulatory impairment with compression stockings or pneumatic compression sleeves.
E. Encourage leg exercises and early, frequent mobilization.
F. Encourage fluid intake of six cups minimum unless contraindicated.
G. Educate patients and families on detection and prevention of VTE at home and actions to take if VTE suspected.

XI. FLUID AND ELECTROLYE IMBALANCE

A. Monitor fluid balance after surgery.
B. Review lab values and report abnormalities to medical practitioner as indicated.
C. Ensure adequate fluid intake, minimum 6 cups per day or as per fluid restrictions.
D. Assess for clinical signs of dehydration (hypotension, headache, dry mouth, oliguria, and skin turgor) or overload (edema, cough, and coarse breath sounds). Follow-up with medical practitioner as indicated.

XII. MOBILITY

The nurse is responsible to ensure timely and consistent postoperative mobility.

A. Request that family provide sturdy footwear with a closed heel and toe.
B. Ensure that an individually fitted walker is available at the bedside.
C. Teach bed exercises: buttock tightening, foot circles, dorsi and plantar flexion of both feet. Remind patient to do exercises every hour while awake.
D. Teach the importance of mobility in healing and restoring function.
E. Establish mobility goals with patient.
F. Assist patient to:
   1. Sit at the bedside, stand, and/or walk on the day of surgery.
   2. Get up in a chair for at least two meals each day beginning the day after surgery.
   3. Walk every day after surgery at least three times with increasing distances.

(continued)

Protocol 34.1: Hip Fracture *(continued)*

XIII. TRANSITIONS FROM HOSPITAL TO HOME

A. Provide both verbal and written instruction on preparing to go home and begin early in the hospital stay (see Chapter 36).
B. Include information on the surgical procedure/activity restrictions, the importance of frequent ambulation, healthy diet, sleep strategies, bone health, and pain management.
C. Educate patients on early warning signs of "red flags" and what to do (e.g., VTE, delirium, infection, dislocation, and constipation).
D. Determine home-assistance requirements and assist patients to make arrangements.
E. Assess medication management skills and develop a plan for medication review and safety at home.
F. Consult with occupational or physical therapists to assess and address the need for home modifications and equipment.
G. Arrange a home follow-up phone call or home visit from a health care professional for support, teaching, and problem solving.
H. Provide information for follow-up with orthopedic surgeon.

XIV. SECONDARY FRACTURE PREVENTION

A. Ensure consultation with fracture liaison service before discharge.
   1. Evaluation of bone health and fracture risk

ABBREVIATIONS

BM Bowel movement
VTE Venous thromboembolism

ACKNOWLEDGMENT

The authors wish to thank Judy Knight, MLS, AHIP, Health Services Librarian, for her generosity support and expertise. We wish her all the best as she transitions into retirement.

REFERENCES

Abou-Setta, A. M., Beaupre, L. A., Jones, C. A., Rashiq, S., Hamm, M. P., Sadowski, C. A., ... Dryden, D. M. (2011). *AHRQ comparative effectiveness reviews of pain management interventions for hip fracture*. Rockville, MD: Agency for Healthcare Research and Quality. *Evidence Level I.*

Aizer, J., & Bolster, M. B. (2014). Fracture liaison services: Promoting enhanced bone health care. *Current Rheumatology Reports, 16*(11), 455. doi:10.1007/s11926–014-0455–2. *Evidence Level V.*

Akesson, K., Marsh, D., Mitchell, P. J., McLellan, A. R., Stenmark, J., Pierroz, D. D., ... Group, I. F. W. (2013). Capture the fracture: A best practice framework and global campaign to break the fragility fracture cycle. *Osteoporosis International, 24*(8), 2135–2152. doi:10.1007/s00198–013-2348-z. *Evidence Level V.*

Alexaitis, I., & Broome, B. (2014). Implementation of a nurse-driven protocol to prevent catheter-associated urinary tract infections. *Journal of Nursing Care Quality, 29*(3), 245–252. doi:10.1097/ncq.0000000000000041. *Evidence Level V.*

Alsawadi, A., & Loeffler, M. (2012). Graduated compression stockings in hip fractures. *Annals of the Royal College of Surgeons of England, 94*(7), 463–471. doi:10.1308/003588412X13171221592492. *Evidence Level V.*

American Academy of Orthopaedic Surgeons (AAOS). (1999). *Hip fracture in seniors: A call for health system reform*. Retrieved from http://www.aaos.org/about/papers/position/1144.asp. *Evidence Level VI.*

American Academy of Orthopaedic Surgeons (AAOS). (2014). *Management of hip fractures in the elderly: Evidence-based clinical practice guideline*. Retrieved from http://www.aaos.org/Research/guidelines/GuidelineHipFracture.asp. *Evidence Level 1.*

American Geriatrics Society 2012 Beers Criteria Update Expert Panel. (2012). American Geriatrics Society updated Beers Criteria for potentially inappropriate medication use in older adults. *Journal of the American Geriatrics Society, 60*(4), 616–631. doi:10.1111/j.1532–5415.2012.03923.x. *Evidence Level I.*

American Geriatrics Society Expert Panel on Postoperative Delirium in Older Adults. (2015). Postoperative delirium in older adults: Best practice statement from the American Geriatrics Society. *Journal of the American College of Surgeons, 220*(2),

136–148. doi:10.1016/j.jamcollsurg.2014.10.019. *Evidence Level I.*

American Geriatrics Society Panel on the Pharmacological Management of Persistent Pain in Older Persons. (2009). Pharmacological management of persistent pain in older persons. *Journal of the American Geriatrics Society, 57*(8), 1331–1346. doi:10.1111/j.1532–5415.2009.02376.x. *Evidence Level V.*

American Society of Anesthesiologists Committee. (1999). Practice guidelines for preoperative fasting and the use of pharmacologic agents to reduce the risk of pulmonary aspiration: Application to healthy patients undergoing elective procedures: A report by the American Society of Anesthesiologist Task Force on Preoperative Fasting. *Anesthesiology, 90*(3), 896–905. *Evidence Level I.*

Andrew, M. K., Freter, S. H., & Rockwood, K. (2005). Incomplete functional recovery after delirium in elderly people: A prospective cohort study. *BMC Geriatrics, 5*, 5. doi:10.1186/1471–2318-5–5. *Evidence Level III.*

Association of Anaesthetists of Great Britain & Ireland. (2014). *Peri-operative care of the elderly 2014.* Retrieved from http://www.aagbi.org/sites/default/files/perioperative_care_of_the_elderly_2014.pdf. *Evidence Level V.*

Auron-Gomez, M., & Michota, F. (2008). Medical management of hip fracture. *Clinics in Geriatric Medicine, 24*(4), 701–719, ix. doi:10.1016/j.cger.2008.07.002. *Evidence Level III.*

Avenell, A., & Handoll, H. H. (2010). Nutritional supplementation for hip fracture aftercare in older people. *Cochrane Database of Systematic Reviews, 2010*(1), CD001880. doi:10.1002/14651858.CD001880.pub5. *Evidence Level I.*

Bass, E., French, D. D., Bradham, D. D., & Rubenstein, L. Z. (2007). Risk-adjusted mortality rates of elderly veterans with hip fractures. *Annals of Epidemiology, 17*(7), 514–519. doi:10.1016/j.annepidem.2006.12.004. *Evidence Level IV.*

Baumgarten, M., Rich, S. E., Shardell, M. D., Hawkes, W. G., Margolis, D. J., Langenberg, P.,... Magaziner, J. (2012). Care-related risk factors for hospital-acquired pressure ulcers in elderly adults with hip fracture. *Journal of the American Geriatrics Society, 60*(2), 277–283. doi:10.1111/j.1532–5415.2011.03849.x. *Evidence Level III.*

BC Hip Fracture Redesign Committee Centre for Hip Health and Mobility. (2015). *Fresh start toolkit: A hip fracture recovery guide for patients and families.* Retrieved from http://www.hiphealth.ca/blog/FReSHStart. *Evidence Level VI.*

Beaudoin, F. L., Nagdev, A., Merchant, R. C., & Becker, B. M. (2010). Ultrasound-guided femoral nerve blocks in elderly patients with hip fractures. *American Journal of Emergency Medicine, 28*(1), 76–81. doi:10.1016/j.ajem.2008.09.015. *Evidence Level IV.*

Bell, J., Bauer, J., Capra, S., & Pulle, C. R. (2013). Barriers to nutritional intake in patients with acute hip fracture: Time to treat malnutrition as a disease and food as a medicine? *Canadian Journal of Physiology and Pharmacology, 91*(6), 489–495. doi:10.1139/cjpp-2012–0301. *Evidence Level IV.*

Bellelli, G., Mazzola, P., Morandi, A., Bruni, A., Carnevali, L., Corsi, M.,... Annoni, G. (2014). Duration of postoperative delirium is an independent predictor of 6-month mortality in older adults after hip fracture. *Journal of the American Geriatrics Society, 62*(7), 1335–1340. doi:10.1111/jgs.12885. *Evidence Level IV.*

Bennet, S. J., Berry, O. M., Goddard, J., & Keating, J. F. (2010). Acute renal dysfunction following hip fracture. *Injury, 41*(4), 335–338. doi:10.1016/j.injury.2009.07.009. *Evidence Level IV.*

Bentler, S. E., Liu, L., Obrizan, M., Cook, E. A., Wright, K. B., Geweke, J. F.,... Wolinsky, F. D. (2009). The aftermath of hip fracture: Discharge placement, functional status change, and mortality. *American Journal of Epidemiology, 170*(10), 1290–1299. doi:10.1093/aje/kwp266. *Evidence Level IV.*

Bergström, U., Jonsson, H., Gustafson, Y., Pettersson, U., Stenlund, H., & Svensson, O. (2009). The hip fracture incidence curve is shifting to the right. *Acta Orthopaedica, 80*(5), 520–524. doi:10.3109/17453670903278282. *Evidence Level IV.*

Bertram, M., Norman, R., Kemp, L., & Vos, T. (2011). Review of the long-term disability associated with hip fractures. *Injury Prevention, 17*(6), 365–370. doi:10.1136/ip.2010.029579. *Evidence Level I.*

Bitsch, M., Foss, N., Kristensen, B., & Kehlet, H. (2004). Pathogenesis of and management strategies for postoperative delirium after hip fracture: A review. *Acta Orthopaedica Scandinavica, 75*(4), 378–389. doi:10.1080/00016470410001123. *Evidence Level IV.*

Bjorkelund, K. B., Hommel, A., Thorngren, K. G., Lundberg, D., & Larsson, S. (2011). The influence of perioperative care and treatment on the 4-month outcome in elderly patients with hip fracture. *AANA Journal, 79*(1), 51–61. *Evidence Level III.*

Boltz, M., Resnick, B., Capezuti, E., Shuluk, J., & Secic, M. (2012). Functional decline in hospitalized older adults: Can nursing make a difference? *Geriatric Nursing, 33*(4), 272–279. doi:10.1016/j.gerinurse.2012.01.008. *Evidence Level III.*

Braga, M., Ljungqvist, O., Soeters, P., Fearon, K., Weimann, A., Bozzetti, F., & ESPEN. (2009). ESPEN guidelines on parenteral nutrition: Surgery. *Clinical Nutrition, 28*(4), 378–386. doi:10.1016/j.clnu.2009.04.002. *Evidence Level I.*

Breedveld-Peters, J. J., Reijven, P. L., Wyers, C. E., van Helden, S., Arts, J. J., Meesters, B.,... Dagnelie, P. C. (2012). Integrated nutritional intervention in the elderly after hip fracture. A process evaluation. *Clinical Nutrition, 31*(2), 199–205. doi:10.1016/j.clnu.2011.10.004. *Evidence Level II.*

Bukata, S. V., Digiovanni, B. F., Friedman, S. M., Hoyen, H., Kates, A., Kates, S. L.,... Tyler, W. K. (2011). A guide to improving the care of patients with fragility fractures. *Geriatric Orthopaedic Surgery & Rehabilitation, 2*(1), 5–37. doi:10.1177/2151458510397504. *Evidence Level V.*

Burch, J., Rice, S., Yang, H., Neilson, A., Stirk, L., Francis, R., ... Craig, D. (2014). Systematic review of the use of bone turnover markers for monitoring the response to osteoporosis treatment: The secondary prevention of fractures, and primary prevention of fractures in high-risk groups. *Health Technology Assessment, 18*(11), 1–180. doi:10.3310/hta18110. *Evidence Level 1.*

Burge, R. T., Dawson-Hughes, B., Solomon, D., Wong, J. B., King, A. B., & Tosteson, A. N. A. (2007). Incidence and economic burden of osteoporotic fractures in the United States, 2005–2025. *Journal of Bone and Mineral Research, 22*(3), 465–475. *Evidence Level IV.*

Carbone, L., Buzkova, P., Fink, H. A., Lee, J. S., Chen, Z., Ahmed, A.,... Robbins, J. R. (2010). Hip fractures and heart failure: Findings from the Cardiovascular Health Study. *European Heart Journal, 31*(1), 77–84. doi:10.1093/eurheartj/ehp483. *Evidence Level IV.*

Carpintero, P., Caeiro, J. R., Carpintero, R., Morales, A., Silva, S., & Mesa, M. (2014). Complications of hip fractures: A review. *World Journal of Orthodontics, 5*(4), 402–411. doi:10.5312/wjo.v5.i4.402. *Evidence Level V.*

Centre for Hip Health and Mobility and BC Hip Fracture Redesign (2014). *Fresh start toolkit. Fracture recovery for seniors at home: A hip fracture recovery guide for patients and families.* Retrieved from http://www.hiphealth.ca/media/FReSH%20Start%20Manual_Letter_Final_OOP.pdf. *Evidence Level V.*

Cionac Florescu, S., Anastase, D. M., Munteanu, A. M., Stoica, I. C., & Antonescu, D. (2013). Venous thromboembolism following major orthopedic surgery. *Maedica, 8*(2), 189–194. *Evidence Level V.*

Coleman, E. A., & Berenson, R. A. (2004). Lost in transition: Challenges and opportunities for improving the quality of transitional care. *Annals of Internal Medicine, 141*(7), 533–536. *Evidence Level VI.*

Coleman, E. A., Parry, C., Chalmers, S., & Min, S. J. (2006). The care transitions intervention: Results of a randomized controlled trial. *Archives of Internal Medicine, 166*(17), 1822–1828. doi:10.1001/archinte.166.17.1822. *Evidence Level II.*

Cooper, C., Mitchell, P., & Kanis, J. A. (2011). Breaking the fragility fracture cycle. *Osteoporosis International, 22*(7), 2049–2050. doi:10.1007/s00198–011-1643–9. *Evidence Level V.*

Daugaard, C. L., Jørgensen, H. L., Riis, T., Lauritzen, J. B., Duus, B. R., & van der Mark, S. (2012). Is mortality after hip fracture associated with surgical delay or admission during weekends and public holidays? A retrospective study of 38,020 patients. *Acta Orthopaedica, 83*(6), 609–613. doi:10.3109/17453674.2012.747926. *Evidence Level IV.*

Dell, R. (2011). Fracture prevention in Kaiser Permanente Southern California. *Osteoporosis International, 22*(Suppl. 3), 457–460. doi:10.1007/s00198–011-1712–0. *Evidence Level V.*

Dillabough, A., Mammel, J., & Yee, J. (2011). Improving nutritional intake in post-operative hip fracture patients: A quality improvement project. *International Journal of Orthopaedic and Trauma Nursing, 15*(4), 196–201. doi:10.1016/j.ijotn.2011.05.005. *Evidence Level V.*

Dochez, E., van Geffen, G. J., Bruhn, J., Hoogerwerf, N., van de Pas, H., & Scheffer, G. (2014). Prehospital administered fascia iliaca compartment block by emergency medical service nurses, a feasibility study. *Scandinavian Journal of Trauma, Resuscitation and Emergency Medicine, 22*, 38. doi:10.1186/1757–7241-22–38. *Evidence Level III.*

Edwards, B. J., Bunta, A. D., Simonelli, C., Bolander, M., & Fitzpatrick, L. A. (2007). Prior fractures are common in patients with subsequent hip fractures. *Clinical Orthopaedics and Related Research, 461*, 226–230. doi:10.1097/BLO.0b013e3180534269. *Evidence Level IV.*

Eisman, J. A., Bogoch, E. R., Dell, R., Harrington, J. T., McKinney, R. E., Jr., McLellan, A.,... Siris, E. (2012). Making the first fracture the last fracture: ASBMR task force report on secondary fracture prevention. *Journal of Bone and Mineral Research, 27*(10), 2039–2046. doi:10.1002/jbmr.1698. *Evidence Level V.*

Ellanti, P., Cushen, B., Galbraith, A., Brent, L., Hurson, C., & Ahern, E. (2014). Improving hip fracture care in Ireland: A preliminary report of the Irish hip fracture database. *Journal of Osteoporosis*, Article ID 656357. doi:10.1155/2014/656357. *Evidence Level IV.*

Falck-Ytter, Y., Francis, C. W., Johanson, N. A., Curley, C., Dahl, O. E., Schulman, S.,... Colwell, C. W., Jr. (2012). Prevention of VTE in orthopedic surgery patients: Antithrombotic therapy and prevention of thrombosis, 9th ed: American College of Chest Physicians evidence-based clinical practice guidelines. *Chest, 141*(2 Suppl.), e278S–325S. doi:10.1378/chest.11–2404. *Evidence Level I.*

Fitton, L., Astroth, K. S., & Wilson, D. (2015). Changing measures to evaluate changing bone. *Orthopedic Nursing, 34*(1), 12–18; quiz 19–20. doi:10.1097/NOR.0000000000000110. *Evidence Level V.*

Forster, A. J., Murff, H. J., Peterson, J. F., Gandhi, T. K., & Bates, D. W. (2003). The incidence and severity of adverse events affecting patients after discharge from the hospital. *Annals of Internal Medicine, 138*(3), 161–167. *Evidence Level IV.*

Fox, K. M., Magaziner, J., Hebel, J. R., Kenzora, J. E., & Kashner, T. M. (1999). Intertrochanteric versus femoral neck hip fractures: Differential characteristics, treatment, and sequelae. *Journals of Gerontology. Series A, Biological Sciences and Medical Sciences, 54*(12), M635–M640. *Evidence Level III.*

Fry, D. E., Pine, M., Jones, B. L., & Meimban, R. J. (2010). Patient characteristics and the occurrence of never events. *Archives of Surgery, 145*(2), 148–151. doi:10.1001/archsurg.2009.277. *Evidence Level IV.*

Ftouh, S., & Lewington, A. (2014). Prevention, detection and management of acute kidney injury: Concise guideline. *Clinical Medicine, 14*(1), 61–65. doi:10.7861/clinmedicine.14–1-61. *Evidence Level I.*

Gallagher, J. C., Melton, L. J., Riggs, B. L., & Bergstrath, E. (1980). Epidemiology of fractures of the proximal femur in Rochester, Minnesota. *Clinical Orthopaedics and Related Research 150*(July/August), 163–171. *Evidence Level IV.*

Glenny, C., Stolee, P., Sheiban, L., & Jaglal, S. (2013). Communicating during care transitions for older hip fracture patients: Family caregiver and health care provider's perspectives. *International Journal of Integrated Care, 13*, e044. *Evidence Level IV.*

Gould, C. V., Umscheid, C. A., Agarwal, R. K., Kuntz, G., Pegues, D. A., & Healthcare Infection Control Practices Advisory Committee. (2010). Guideline for prevention of catheter-associated urinary tract infections 2009. *Infection Control and Hospital Epidemiology, 31*(4), 319–326. doi:10.1086/651091. *Evidence Level I.*

Greene, D., & Dell, R. M. (2010). Outcomes of an osteoporosis disease-management program managed by nurse practitioners. *Journal of the American Academy of Nurse Practitioners, 22*(6), 326–329. doi:10.1111/j.1745–7599.2010.00515.x. *Evidence Level V.*

Griffiths, R., Alper, J., Beckingsale, A., Goldhill, D., Heyburn, G., Holloway, J., Leaper, E., . . . Wilson, I.; Association of Anaesthetists of Great Britain and Ireland (2012). Management of proximal femoral fractures 2011: Association of Anaesthetists of Great Britain and Ireland. *Anaesthesia, 67*(1), 85–98. doi:10.1111/j.1365–2044.2011.06957.x. *Evidence Level V.*

Gullberg, B., Johnell, O., & Kanis, J. A. (1997). World-wide projections for hip fracture. *Osteoporosis International, 7*(5), 407–413. *Evidence Level IV.*

Güzelküçük, Ü., Skempes, D., & Kumnerddee, W. (2014). Common peroneal nerve palsy caused by compression stockings after surgery. *American Journal of Physical Medicine & Rehabilitation/Association of Academic Physiatrists, 93*(7), 609–611. doi:10.1097/PHM.0000000000000086. *Evidence Level V.*

Hall, M. J., DeFrances, C. J., Williams, S. N., Golosinskiy, A., & Schwartzman, A. (2010). National hospital discharge survey: 2007 summary. *National Health Statistics Reports,* no. 29, 1–20, 24. *Evidence Level IV.*

Hausel, J., Nygren, J., Lagerkranser, M., Hellstrom, P. M., Hammarqvist, F., Almstrom, C., . . . Ljungqvist, O. (2001). A carbohydrate-rich drink reduces preoperative discomfort in elective surgery patients. *Anesthesia and Analgesia, 93*(5), 1344–1350. *Evidence Level II.*

Herr, K., Coyne, P. J., McCaffery, M., Manworren, R., & Merkel, S. (2011). Pain assessment in the patient unable to self-report: Position statement with clinical practice recommendations. *Pain Management Nursing, 12*(4), 230–250. doi:10.1016/j.pmn.2011.10.002. *Evidence Level IV.*

Herr, K., & Titler, M. (2009). Acute pain assessment and pharmacological management practices for the older adult with a hip fracture: Review of ED trends. *Journal of Emergency Nursing, 35*(4), 312–320. doi:10.1016/j.jen.2008.08.006. *Evidence Level V.*

Hinderland, M. D., Ng, A., Paden, M. H., & Stone, P. A. (2011). Lateral leg compartment syndrome caused by ill-fitting compression stocking placed for deep vein thrombosis prophylaxis during surgery: A case report. *Journal of Foot and Ankle Surgery, 50*(5), 616–619. doi:10.1053/j.jfas.2011.04.025. *Evidence Level V.*

Holmes, J. D., & House, A. O. (2000). Psychiatric illness in hip fracture. *Age and Ageing, 29*(6), 537–546. *Evidence Level IV.*

Holt, G., Smith, R., Duncan, K., & McKeown, D. W. (2010). Does delay to theatre for medical reasons affect the perioperative mortality in patients with fracture of the hip? *Journal of Bone and Joint Surgery, 92*(6), 835–841. *Evidence Level III.*

Hommel, A., Bjorkelund, K. B., Thorngren, K. G., & Ulander, K. (2007). Nutritional status among patients with hip fracture in relation to pressure ulcers. *Clinical Nutrition, 26*(5), 589–596. doi:10.1016/j.clnu.2007.06.003. *Evidence Level III.*

Hommel, A., Ulander, K., Bjorkelund, K. B., Norrman, P. O., Wingstrand, H., & Thorngren, K. G. (2008). Influence of optimized treatment of people with hip fracture on time to operation, length of hospital stay, reoperations and mortality within 1 year. *Injury, 39*(10), 1164–1174. doi:10.1016/j.injury.2008.01.048. *Evidence Level III.*

Hu, F., Jiang, C., Shen, J., Tnag, P., & Wang, Y. (2012). Preoperative predictors for mortality following hip fracture surgery: A systematic review and meta-analysis. *Injury, 43*(6), 676–85. *Evidence Level I.*

International Osteoporosis Foundation (IOF). (2012). *Facts and statistics. International Osteoporosis Foundation.* Retrieved from http://www.iofbonehealth.org/facts-statistics. *Evidence Level V.*

Jefferies, D., Johnson, M., & Ravens, J. (2011). Nurturing and nourishing: The nurses' role in nutritional care. *Journal of Clinical Nursing, 20*(3–4), 317–330. doi:10.1111/j.1365–2702.2010.03502.x. *Evidence Level I.*

Jennings, L. A., Auerbach, A. D., Maselli, J., Pekow, P. S., Lindenauer, P. K., & Lee, S. J. (2010). Missed opportunities for osteoporosis treatment in patients hospitalized for hip fracture. *Journal of the American Geriatrics Society, 58*(4), 650–657. doi:10.1111/j.1532–5415.2010.02769.x. *Evidence Level III.*

Jobin, S. K. L., Adebayo, L., Agarwal, Z., Card, R., Christie, B., Haland, T., . . . Morton, C.; Institute for Clinical Systems Improvement. (2012). *Venous thromboembolism prophylaxis.* Retrieved from https://www.icsi.org/_asset/ht2bhd/VTEProphy.pdf. *Evidence Level I.*

Kang, H., Ha, Y. C., Kim, J. Y., Woo, Y. C., Lee, J. S., & Jang, E. C. (2013). Effectiveness of multimodal pain management after bipolar hemiarthroplasty for hip fracture: A randomized, controlled study. *Journal of Bone and Joint Surgery. American Volume, 95*(4), 291–296. doi:10.2106/JBJS.K.01708. *Evidence Level II.*

Kanis, J. A., Johnell, O., Oden, A., Johansson, H., & McCloskey, E. (2008). FRAX and the assessment of fracture probability in men and women from the UK. *Osteoporosis International, 19*(4), 385–397. doi:10.1007/s00198–007-0543–5. *Evidence Level III.*

Kates, S. L., Behrend, C., Mendelson, D. A., Cram, P., & Friedman, S. M. (2015). Hospital readmission after hip fracture. *Archives of Orthopaedic and Traumatic Surgery, 135*(3), 329–337. doi:10.1007/s00402–014-2141–2. *Evidence Level III.*

Kehlet, H., & Dahl, J. B. (2003). Anaesthesia, surgery, and challenges in postoperative recovery. *Lancet, 362*(9399), 1921–1928. doi:10.1016/s0140–6736(03)14966–5. *Evidence Level VI.*

Kiely, D. K., Marcantonio, E. R., Inouye, S. K., Shaffer, M. L., Bergmann, M. A., Yang, F. M., . . . Jones, R. N. (2009). Persistent delirium predicts greater mortality. *Journal of the American Geriatrics Society, 57*(1), 55–61. doi:10.1111/j.1532–5415.2008.02092.x. *Evidence Level IV.*

Kleerekoper, M. (2001). Biochemical markers of bone turnover: Why theory, research, and clinical practice are still in conflict. *Clinical Chemistry, 47*(8), 1347–1349. *Evidence Level V.*

Ko, F. C., & Morrison, R. S. (2014a). Hip fracture: A trigger for palliative care in vulnerable older adults. *JAMA Internal Medicine, 174*(8), 1281–1282. doi:10.1001/jamainternmed.2014.999. *Evidence Level IV.*

Ko, F. C., & Morrison, R. S. (2014b). Hip fracture: A trigger for palliative care in vulnerable older adults. *JAMA Internal Medicine, 174*(8), 1281–1282. doi:10.1001/jamainternmed.2014.999. *Evidence Level IV.*

Koo, K. H., Choi, J. S., Ahn, J. H., Kwon, J. H., & Cho, K. T. (2014). Comparison of clinical and physiological efficacies of different intermittent sequential pneumatic compression devices in preventing deep vein thrombosis: A prospective randomized study. *Clinics in Orthopedic Surgery, 6*(4), 468–475. doi:10.4055/cios.2014.6.4.468. *Evidence Level II.*

Krogseth, M., Wyller, T. B., Engedal, K., & Juliebo, V. (2014). Delirium is a risk factor for institutionalization and functional decline in older hip fracture patients. *Journal of Psychosomatic*

Research, 76(1), 68–74. doi:10.1016/j.jpsychores.2013.10.006. *Evidence Level IV.*

Leland, N. E., Teno, J. M., Gozalo, P., Bynum, J., & Mor, V. (2012). Decision making and outcomes of a hospice patient hospitalized with a hip fracture. *Journal of Pain Symptom Manage, 44*(3), 458–465. doi:10.1016/j.jpainsymman.2011.09.011. *Evidence Level III.*

Lemiengre, J., Nelis, T., Joosten, E., Braes, T., Foreman, M., Gastmans, C., & Milisen, K. (2006). Detection of delirium by bedside nurses using the confusion assessment method. *Journal of the American Geriatrics Society, 54*(4), 685–689. doi:10.1111/j.1532–5415.2006.00667.x. *Evidence Level IV.*

Lenze, E. J., Munin, M. C., Dew, M. A., Rogers, J. C., Seligman, K., Mulsant, B. H., & Reynolds, C. F. (2004). Adverse effects of depression and cognitive impairment on rehabilitation participation and recovery from hip fracture. *International Journal of Geriatric Psychiatry, 19*(5), 472–478. doi:10.1002/gps.1116. *Evidence Level IV.*

Lenze, E. J., Munin, M. C., Skidmore, E. R., Dew, M. A., Rogers, J. C., Whyte, E. M., . . . Reynolds, C. F. (2007). Onset of depression in elderly persons after hip fracture: Implications for prevention and early intervention of late-life depression. *Journal of the American Geriatrics Society, 55*(1), 81–86. doi:10.1111/j.1532–5415.2006.01017.x. *Evidence Level IV.*

Li, G. W., Xu, Z., Chen, Q. W., Tian, Y. N., Wang, X. Y., Zhou, L., & Chang, S. X. (2014). Quantitative evaluation of vertebral marrow adipose tissue in postmenopausal female using MRI chemical shift-based water-fat separation. *Clinical Radiology, 69*(3), 254–262. doi:10.1016/j.crad.2013.10.005. *Evidence Level IV.*

Ljungqvist, O. (2009). Modulating postoperative insulin resistance by preoperative carbohydrate loading. *Best Practice & Research, 23*(4), 401–409. *Evidence Level V.*

Lo, E., Nicolle, L. E., Coffin, S. E., Gould, C., Maragakis, L. L., Meddings, J., . . . Yokoe, D. S. (2014). Strategies to prevent catheter-associated urinary tract infections in acute care hospitals: 2014 update. *Infection Control and Hospital Epidemiology, 35*(5), 464–479. doi:10.1086/675718. *Evidence Level I.*

Love, A. L., Cornwell, P. L., & Whitehouse, S. L. (2013). Oropharyngeal dysphagia in an elderly post-operative hip fracture population: A prospective cohort study. *Age and Ageing, 42*(6), 782–785. doi:10.1093/ageing/aft037. *Evidence Level III.*

Lumbers, M., New, S. A., Gibson, S., & Murphy, M. C. (2001). Nutritional status in elderly female hip fracture patients: Comparison with an age-matched home living group attending day centres. *British Journal of Nutrition, 85*(6), 733–740. *Evidence Level IV.*

Lundstrom, M., Stenvall, M., & Olofsson, B. (2012). Symptom profile of postoperative delirium in patients with and without dementia. *Journal of Geriatric Psychiatry and Neurology, 25*(3), 162–169. *Evidence Level III.*

Maher, A. B., Meehan, A. J., Hertz, K., Hommel, A., MacDonald, V., O'Sullivan, M. P., . . . Taylor, A. (2012). Acute nursing care of the older adult with fragility hip fracture: An international perspective (Part 1). *International Journal of Orthopaedic and Trauma Nursing, 16*(4), 177–194. doi:10.1016/j.ijotn.2012.09.001. *Evidence Level V.*

Maher, A. B., Meehan, A. J., Hertz, K., Hommel, A., MacDonald, V., O'Sullivan, M. P., . . . Taylor, A. (2013). Acute nursing care of the older adult with fragility hip fracture: An international perspective (Part 2). *International Journal of Orthopaedic and Trauma Nursing, 17*(1), 4–18. doi:10.1016/j.ijotn.2012.09.002. *Evidence Level V.*

Marks, R., Allegrante, J. P., Ronald MacKenzie, C., & Lane, J. M. (2003). Hip fractures among the elderly: Causes, consequences and control. *Ageing Research Reviews, 2*(1), 57–93. *Evidence Level V.*

Marsh, D., Akesson, K., Beaton, D. E., Bogoch, E. R., Boonen, S., Brandi, M. L., . . . Group, I. C. F. W. (2011). Coordinator-based systems for secondary prevention in fragility fracture patients. *Osteoporosis International, 22*(7), 2051–2065. doi:10.1007/s00198–011-1642-x. *Evidence Level I.*

Marsland, D., Mears, S. C., & Kates, S. L. (2010). Venous thromboembolic prophylaxis for hip fractures. *Osteoporosis International, 21*(Suppl. 4), S593–S604. doi:10.1007/s00198–010-1403–2. *Evidence Level V.*

Martinez, F., Tobar, C., & Hill, N. (2015). Preventing delirium: Should non-pharmacological, multicomponent interventions be used? A systematic review and meta-analysis of the literature. *Age and Ageing, 44*(2), 196–204. doi:10.1093/ageing/afu173. *Evidence Level I.*

McAvay, G. J., Van Ness, P. H., Bogardus, S. T., Jr., Zhang, Y., Leslie, D. L., Leo-Summers, L. S., & Inouye, S. K. (2006). Older adults discharged from the hospital with delirium: 1-year outcomes. *Journal of the American Geriatrics Society, 54*(8), 1245–1250. doi:10.1111/j.1532–5415.2006.00815. *Evidence Level IV.*

Meehan, A., Loose, C., Bell, J., Partridge, J. Nelson, J., & Goates, S. (2016). Health system quality improvement: Impact of prompt nutritional care on patient outcomes and health care costs. *Journal of Nursing Care Quality* (Epub ahead of print). *Evidence Level III.*

Melis, G. C., van Leeuwen, P. A., von Blomberg-van der Flier, B. M., Goedhart-Hiddinga, A. C., Uitdehaag, B. M., Strack van Schijndel, R. J., . . . van Bokhorst-de van der Schueren, M. A. (2006). A carbohydrate-rich beverage prior to surgery prevents surgery-induced immunodepression: A randomized, controlled, clinical trial. *JPEN. Journal of Parenteral and Enteral Nutrition, 30*(1), 21–26. *Evidence Level I.*

Milte, R., & Crotty, M. (2014). Musculoskeletal health, frailty and functional decline. *Best Practice & Research. Clinical Rheumatology, 28*(3), 395–410. doi:10.1016/j.berh.2014.07.005. *Evidence Level V.*

Mitchell, P. J. (2013). Best practices in secondary fracture prevention: Fracture liaison services. *Current Osteoporosis Reports, 11*(1), 52–60. doi:10.1007/s11914–012-0130–3. *Evidence Level V.*

Mitchell, P. J., & Chem, C. (2013). Secondary prevention and estimation of fracture risk. *Best Practice & Research. Clinical Rheumatology, 27*(6), 789–803. doi:10.1016/j.berh.2013.11.004. *Evidence Level V.*

Mori, C. (2014). Avoiding catastrophe: Implementing a nurse-driven protocol. *Medsurg Nursing: Official Journal of the Academy of Medical-Surgical Nurses, 23*(1), 15–21, 28. *Evidence Level IV.*

Morley, J. E., Vellas, B., van Kan, G. A., Anker, S. D., Bauer, J. M., Bernabei, R.,... Walston, J. (2013). Frailty consensus: A call to action. *Journal of the American Medical Directors Association, 14*(6), 392–397. doi:10.1016/j.jamda.2013.03.022. *Evidence Level V.*

Morrison, R. S., Magaziner, J., Gilbert, M., Koval, K. J., McLaughlin, M. A., Orosz, G.,... Siu, A. L. (2003). Relationship between pain and opioid analgesics on the development of delirium following hip fracture. *Journals of Gerontology. Series A, Biological Sciences and Medical Sciences, 58*(1), 76–81. *Evidence Level III.*

Mueller, C., Compher, C., Druyan, M. E., & American Society for Parenteral and Enteral Nutrition (ASPEN) Board of Directors. (2011). ASPEN clinical guidelines. Nutrition screening, assessment and intervention in adults. *JPEN. Journal of Parenteral and Enteral Nutrition, 35*(1), 16–24. *Evidence Level I.*

National Bone Health Alliance (NBHA). (2012). *Secondary fracture prevention initiative.* Retrieved from http://nbha.org/projects/secondary-fracture-prevention-initiative. *Evidence Level VI.*

National Institute for Health and Clinical Excellence (NICE). (2010). *Venous thromboembolism: Reducing the risk.* Retrieved from http://www.nice.org.uk/guidance/cg92. *Evidence Level I.*

National Institute for Health and Clinical Excellence (NICE). (2011). *The management of hip fracture in adults.* Retrieved from https://www.nice.org.uk/guidance/cg124/evidence/full-guideline-183081997. *Evidence Level I.*

National Osteoporosis Foundation (NOF). (2010). *Clinicians guide to prevention and treatment of osteoporosis.* Washington, DC: National Osteoporosis Foundation. *Evidence Level I.*

National Pressure Ulcer Advisory Panel (NPUAP), European Pressure Ulcer Advisory Panel, Pan Pacific Pressure Injury Alliance. (2014). *Prevention and treatment of pressure ulcers: Quick reference guide.* Retrieved from http://www.npuap.org/resources/educational-and-clinical-resources/prevention-and-treatment-of-pressure-ulcers-clinical-practice-guideline. *Evidence Level I.*

Neighbour, C. (2014). Improving bowel care after surgery for hip fracture. *Nursing Older People, 26*(10), 16–22. doi:10.7748/nop.26.10.16.e649. *Evidence Level III.*

Newman, B., McCarthy, L., Thomas, P. W., May, P., Layzell, M., & Horn, K. (2013). A comparison of pre-operative nerve stimulator-guided femoral nerve block and fascia iliaca compartment block in patients with a femoral neck fracture. *Anaesthesia, 68*(9), 899–903. doi:10.1111/anae.12321. *Evidence Level II.*

Newman, E. D., Ayoub, W. T., Starkey, R. H., Diehl, J. M., & Wood, G. C. (2003). Osteoporosis disease management in a rural health care population: Hip fracture reduction and reduced costs in postmenopausal women after 5 years. *Osteoporosis International, 14*(2), 146–151. doi:10.1007/s00198–002-1336–5. *Evidence Level IV.*

Nygren, J., Thorell, A., & Ljungqvist, O. (2015). Preoperative oral carbohydrate therapy. *Current Opinion in Anaesthesiology, 28*(3), 364–369. doi:10.1097/ACO.0000000000000192. *Evidence Level V.*

Oh, E. S., Li, M., Fafowora, T. M., Inouye, S. K., Chen, C. H., Rosman, L. M.,... Puhan, M. A. (2014). Preoperative risk factors for postoperative delirium following hip fracture repair: A systematic review. *International Journal of Geriatric Psychiatry, 30*(9), 900–910. doi:10.1002/gps.4233. *Evidence Level I.*

Pakula, A. M., & Skinner, R. A. (2015). Acute kidney injury in the critically ill patient: A current review of the literature. *Journal of Intensive Care Medicine.* doi:10.1177/0885066615575699. *Evidence Level V.*

Parker, M., & Johansen, A. (2006). Hip fracture. *BMJ, 333*(7557), 27–30. doi:10.1136/bmj.333.7557.27. *Evidence Level V.*

Pasero, C. (2009). Assessment of sedation during opioid administration for pain management. *Journal of Perianesthesia Nursing, 24*(3), 186–190. doi:10.1016/j.jopan.2009.03.005. *Evidence Level III.*

Pellino, T. A., Gordon, D. B., Engelke, Z. K., Busse, K. L., Collins, M. A., Silver, C. E., & Norcross, N. J. (2005). Use of nonpharmacologic interventions for pain and anxiety after total hip and total knee arthroplasty. *Orthopedic Nursing, 24*(3), 182–190; quiz 191–182. *Evidence Level IV.*

Port, L., Center, J., Briffa, N. K., Nguyen, T., Cumming, R., & Eisman, J. (2003). Osteoporotic fracture: Missed opportunity for intervention. *Osteoporosis International, 14*(9), 780–784. doi:10.1007/s00198–003-1452-x. *Evidence Level IV.*

Prisco, D., Cenci, C., Silvestri, E., Emmi, G., & Ciucciarelli, L. (2014). Pharmacological prevention of venous thromboembolism in orthopaedic surgery. *Clinical Cases in Mineral and Bone Metabolism, 11*(3), 192–195. *Evidence Level I.*

Pugely, A. J., Martin, C. T., Gao, Y., Klocke, N. F., Callaghan, J. J., & Marsh, J. L. (2014). A risk calculator for short-term morbidity and mortality after hip fracture surgery. *Journal of Orthopaedic Trauma, 28*(2), 63–69. doi:10.1097/BOT.0b013e3182a22744. *Evidence Level IV.*

Purser, L., Warfield, K., & Richardson, C. (2014). Making pain visible: An audit and review of documentation to improve the use of pain assessment by implementing pain as the fifth vital sign. *Pain Management Nursing, 15*(1), 137–142. doi:10.1016/j.pmn.2012.07.007. *Evidence Level IV.*

Radtke, F. M., Franck, M., MacGuill, M., Seeling, M., Lutz, A., Westhoff, S.,... Spies, C. D. (2010). Duration of fluid fasting and choice of analgesic are modifiable factors for early postoperative delirium. *European Journal of Anaesthesiology, 27*(5), 411–416. doi:10.1097/EJA.0b013e3283335cee. *Evidence Level III.*

Roberts, K. C., & Brox, W. T. (2015). AAOS clinical practice guideline: Management of hip fractures in the elderly. *Journal of the American Academy of Orthopaedic Surgeons, 23*(2), 138–140. doi:10.5435/jaaos-d-14–00433. *Evidence Level I.*

Sachdeva, A., Dalton, M., Amaragiri, S. V., & Lees, T. (2014). Graduated compression stockings for prevention of deep vein thrombosis. *Cochrane Database of Systematic Reviews (Online), 2014*(12), CD001484. doi:10.1002/14651858.CD001484.pub3. *Evidence Level I.*

Saint, S., Lipsky, B. A., & Goold, S. D. (2002). Indwelling urinary catheters: A one-point restraint? *Annals of Internal Medicine, 137*(2), 125–127. *Evidence Level V.*

Schiller, C., Franke, T., Belle, J., Sims-Gould, J., Sale, J., & Ashe, M. C. (2015). Words of wisdom—Patient perspectives to guide recovery for older adults after hip fracture: A qualitative study. *Patient Prefer Adherence, 9,* 57–64. doi:10.2147/PPA.S75657. *Evidence Level IV.*

Shiga, T., Wajima, Z., & Ohe, Y. (2008). Is operative delay associated with increased mortality of hip fracture patients? Systematic review, meta-analysis, and meta-regression. *Canadian Journal of Anaesthesia, 55*(3), 146–154. doi:10.1007/bf03016088. *Evidence Level I.*

Sims-Gould, J, B. K., Hicks, E., Khan, K., & Stolee P. (2012). Examining "success" in post-hip fracture care transitions: A strengths-based approach. *Journal of Interprofessional Care, 26*(3), 205–211. *Evidence Level V.*

Simunovic, N., Devereaux, P. J., Sprague, S., Guyatt, G. H., Schemitsch, E., Debeer, J., & Bhandari, M. (2010). Effect of early surgery after hip fracture on mortality and complications: Systematic review and meta-analysis. *CMAJ: Canadian Medical Association Journal, 182*(15), 1609–1616. doi:10.1503/cmaj.092220. *Evidence Level I.*

Sobolev, B., Sheehan, K. J., Kuramoto, L., & Guy, P. (2015). Risk of second hip fracture persists for years after initial trauma. *Bone, 75*, 72–76. doi:10.1016/j.bone.2015.02.003. *Evidence Level IV.*

Steis, M. R., & Fick, D. M. (2008). Are nurses recognizing delirium? A systematic review. *Journal of Gerontological Nursing, 34*(9), 40–48. *Evidence Level I.*

Tang, G. Y., Lv, Z. W., Tang, R. B., Liu, Y., Peng, Y. F., Li, W., & Cheng, Y. S. (2010). Evaluation of MR spectroscopy and diffusion-weighted MRI in detecting bone marrow changes in postmenopausal women with osteoporosis. *Clinical Radiology, 65*(5), 377–381. doi:10.1016/j.crad.2009.12.011. *Evidence Level III.*

Tarantino, U., Piccirilli, E., Fantini, M., Baldi, J., Gasbarra, E., & Bei, R. (2015). Sarcopenia and fragility fractures: Molecular and clinical evidence of the bone–muscle interaction. *Journal of Bone and Joint Surgery, 97*(5), 429–437. doi:10.2106/jbjs.n.00648. *Evidence Level V.*

The Joint Commission (TJC). (2014, updated May 2015). *Accountability measure list.* Retrieved from http://www.jointcommission.org/assets/1/18/2014ACCOUNTABILITY_MEASURESfor2015_TPrecognitionMay2015.pdf. *Evidence Level I.*

Torres, P. A., Helmstetter, J. A., Kaye, A. M., & Kaye, A. D. (2015). Rhabdomyolysis: Pathogenesis, diagnosis, and treatment. *Ochsner Journal, 15*(1), 58–69. *Evidence Level V.*

Ulucay, C., Eren, Z., Kaspar, E. C., Ozler, T., Yuksel, K., Kantarci, G., & Altintas, F. (2012). Risk factors for acute kidney injury after hip fracture surgery in the elderly individuals. *Geriatric Orthopaedic Surgery & Rehabilitation, 3*(4), 150–156. doi:10.1177/2151458512473827. *Evidence Level II.*

Vaurio, L. E., Sands, L. P., Wang, Y., Mullen, E. A., & Leung, J. M. (2006). Postoperative delirium: The importance of pain and pain management. *Anesthesia and Analgesia, 102*(4), 1267–1273. doi:10.1213/01.ane.0000199156.59226.af. *Evidence Level III.*

Vernon, S., & King, R. (2011). Using FRAX to assess the risk that an older person will suffer a fragility fracture. *British Journal of Community Nursing, 16*(11), 534, 536, 538–539. doi:10.12968/bjcn.2011.16.11.534. *Evidence Level VI.*

Wald, H., Epstein, A., & Kramer, A. (2005). Extended use of indwelling urinary catheters in postoperative hip fracture patients. *Medical Care, 43*(10), 1009–1017. *Evidence Level III.*

Watts, N. B. (2011). The Fracture Risk Assessment Tool (FRAX): Applications in clinical practice. *Journal of Women's Health/The Official Publication of the Society for the Advancement of Women's Health Research (Larchmt), 20*(4), 525–31. *Evidence Level V.*

White, J. J., Khan, W. S., & Smitham, P. J. (2011). Perioperative implications of surgery in elderly patients with hip fractures: An evidence-based review. *Journal of Perioperative Practice, 21*(6), 192–197. *Evidence Level I.*

White, S. M., Rashid, N., & Chakladar, A. (2009). An analysis of renal dysfunction in 1511 patients with fractured neck of femur: The implications for peri-operative analgesia. *Anaesthesia, 64*(10), 1061–1065. doi:10.1111/j.1365-2044.2009.06012.x. *Evidence Level IV.*

Wiles, M. D., Moran, C. G., Sahota, O., & Moppett, I. K. (2011). Nottingham Hip Fracture Score as a predictor of one year mortality in patients undergoing surgical repair of fractured neck of femur. *British Journal of Anaesthesia, 106*(4), 501–504. doi:10.1093/bja/aeq405. *Evidence Level IV.*

Willson, T., Nelson, S. D., Newbold, J., Nelson, R. E., & LaFleur, J. (2015). The clinical epidemiology of male osteoporosis: A review of the recent literature. *Clinical Epidemiology, 7*, 65–76. doi:10.2147/clep.s40966. *Evidence Level V.*

Wright, N. C., Looker, A. C., Saag, K. G., Curtis, J. R., Delzell, E. S., Randall, S., & Dawson-Hughes, B. (2014). The recent prevalence of osteoporosis and low bone mass in the United States based on bone mineral density at the femoral neck or lumbar spine. *Journal of Bone and Mineral Research, 29*(11), 2520–2526. doi:10.1002/jbmr.226. *Evidence Level IV.*

Wyers, C. E., Breedveld-Peters, J. J., Reijven, P. L., van Helden, S., Guldemond, N. A., Severens, J. L., . . . Dagnelie, P. C. (2010). Efficacy and cost-effectiveness of nutritional intervention in elderly after hip fracture: Design of a randomized controlled trial. *BMC Public Health, 10*, 212. doi:10.1186/1471-2458-10-212. *Evidence Level II.*

Yagci, G., Can, M. F., Ozturk, E., Dag, B., Ozgurtas, T., Cosar, A., & Tufan, T. (2008). Effects of preoperative carbohydrate loading on glucose metabolism and gastric contents in patients undergoing moderate surgery: A randomized, controlled trial. *Nutrition, 24*(3), 212–216. doi:10.1016/j.nut.2007.11.003. *Evidence Level II.*

Young, Y., & Resnick, B. (2009). Don't worry, be positive: Improving functional recovery 1 year after hip fracture. *Rehabilitation Nursing, 34*(3), 110–117. *Evidence Level IV.*

Ziden, L., Kreuter, M., & Frandin, K. (2010). Long-term effects of home rehabilitation after hip fracture—1-year follow-up of functioning, balance confidence, and health-related quality of life in elderly people. *Disability and Rehabilitation, 32*(1), 18–32. doi:10.3109/09638280902980910. *Evidence Level II.*

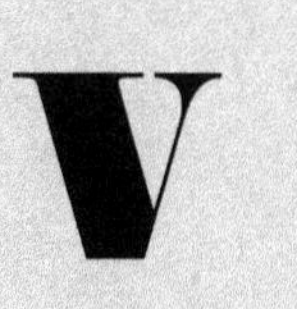

Models of Care

35

Acute Care Models

Elizabeth Capezuti, Ana Julia Parks, Marie Boltz,
Michael L. Malone, and Robert M. Palmer

EDUCATIONAL OBJECTIVES

On completion of this chapter, the reader should be able to:

1. Identify the objectives common to all geriatric acute care models
2. Describe the various types of models employed in North American hospitals
3. Understand the evidence to support implementation of geriatric acute care models

OVERVIEW

Advances in geriatric science, coupled with the increasing older adult patient population, have led to the development of several geriatric models of care across all health care settings. Acute care models addressing the unique needs of older hospitalized patients began with the comprehensive geriatric assessment (CGA) programs first developed in the 1970s (Palmer, 2014).

Geriatric acute care models aim to facilitate improved overall outcomes by promoting a rehabilitative approach while preventing adverse events that occur more commonly in older patients. Also known as geriatric syndromes, these are clinical conditions in older persons that do not fit into discrete disease categories (Palmer, 2014) and include functional decline, pressure ulcers, fall-related injury, undernutrition or malnutrition, urinary tract infection, and delirium (see Part III: Clinical Interventions). These syndromes or complications contribute to prolonged hospital stays as well as increased likelihood for rehospitalization, institutionalization, emergency department (ED) usage, and postacute rehabilitation therapy services. These complications rarely occur alone; the interrelationships among these various syndromes during hospitalization are well documented (Flood, Booth, Danto-Nocton, Kresevic, & Palmer, 2015; Inouye, Studenski, Tinetti, & Kuchel, 2007; Palmer, 2014).

Acute care models attend to the age-specific vulnerabilities (i.e., frailty, comorbidities, and cognitive impairment) of older hospitalized patients. These models also address the role of institutional factors that determine staff practices and the physical environment that can contribute to iatrogenic complications. Thus, the overall goals of acute geriatric models of care are (a) prevention of complications that occur more commonly in older adults and (b) address hospital factors that contribute to complications (Capezuti, Boltz, & Kim, 2011). This chapter provides an overview of care delivery issues that are addressed by acute models of care for older adults and a description of the most commonly employed hospital models.

OBJECTIVES OF GERIATRIC ACUTE CARE MODELS

There are several geriatric acute care models, each with its own approach to prevent complications and address institutional/staff practices that can contribute to complications. All of these models, however, share a common set of general objectives (Hickman, Newton, Halcomb, Chang, & Davidson, 2007; Hickman, Rolley, & Davidson, 2010).

For a description of evidence levels cited in this chapter, see Chapter 1, "Developing and Evaluating Clinical Practice Guidelines: A Systematic Approach."

The six general objectives of geriatric acute care models are discussed herein.

Educate Health Care Providers in Core Geriatric Principles

Many health care providers have not received the core geriatric care principles, such as recognition of age-specific factors that increase the risk of complications, in their basic or continuing education (Berman et al., 2005; Wald, Huddleston, & Kramer, 2006). All acute care models require a coordinator with advanced geriatric education; however, successful implementation depends on direct-care staff with the knowledge and competencies to deliver evidence-based care to older patients. Thus, the coordinator or a clinician with geriatric specialization will facilitate staff learning via individual patient consultation, in-service group education, unit rounds, journal clubs, web-based discussion groups, conferences, and other internal institutional educational venues (Fletcher, Hawkes, Williams-Rosenthal, Mariscal, & Cox, 2007; Smyth, Dubin, Restrepo, Nueva-Espana, & Capezuti, 2001).

Target Risk Factors for Complications

The ideal method to prevent complications is timely screening of potential geriatric syndromes, early identification, and subsequent reduction of risk factors. Some of the models focus on a particular syndrome; however, because of the interrelationship of shared risk factors, reduction of one complication will affect the prevention of other geriatric syndromes. Standardized assessment tools are recommended to properly identify individuals who are at an increased risk of geriatric syndromes. The Portal of Geriatrics Online Education (www.pogoe.org) and the Hartford Institute for Geriatric Nursing websites provide assessment instruments (www.hartfordign.org). At the institutional level, incorporating these risk-assessment tools into the workflow of everyday practice requires hospital policies, procedures, and protocols that will promote usage such as embedding these tools within the electronic health record.

Incorporate Patient or Family Choices and Treatment Goals

Informed patient's choices are essential whether they are decisions about activity level and medication use to more complex issues such as advance directives.

Family members of patients who can no longer participate in decision making must often deal with the complicated balance between quality-of-life considerations and potential length of life. The decision to employ life-sustaining treatments consistent with patients' preferences is often only considered when the patient is hospitalized (Somogyi-Zalud, Zhong, Hamel, & Lynn, 2002). For this reason, many geriatric models work collaboratively or in conjunction with palliative care programs (see Chapter 37, "Palliative Care Models").

Employ Evidence-Based Interventions

The high proportion of complications in older hospitalized patients is partly attributed to the lack of evidence-based geriatric care practices. There is tremendous variability in the adoption of geriatric protocols (Neuman, Speck, Karlawish, Schwartz, & Shea, 2010). Issues with overuse or inappropriate medications (e.g., overuse of psychoactive drugs), unnecessary restraints, inadequate detection of cognitive or affective changes (e.g., delirium and depression), and poor pain control are examples of hospital factors that can lead to adverse outcomes. Thus, geriatric acute care models promote the use of standardized evidence-based protocols described in this book.

Promote Interprofessional Communication

The management of geriatric syndromes is not limited to medical intervention but requires other disciplines, such as nursing, pharmacy, social work, and physical and occupational therapy, to address the complex interaction of medical, functional, psychological, and social issues leading to these complications. Communication of the various disciplines' input, facilitated by geriatric care models, is essential.

Emphasize Proactive Discharge Planning

Older hospitalized patients are more likely to experience delays in discharge, greater emergency service use, hospital readmission, and rehabilitation in an institution or at home (Coleman, Min, Chomiak, & Kramer, 2004). Hospital readmission for older patients is most likely associated with medical errors in medication continuity (Coleman, Smith, Raha, & Min, 2005; Foust, Naylor, Boling, & Cappuzzo, 2005), diagnostic workup, or test follow-up (Forster, Murff, Peterson, Gandhi, & Bates, 2003). Geriatric acute care models address the posthospital care environment and the care transition following hospital discharge by promoting coordination among health care providers, facilitating medication reconciliation, preparing patients and their caregivers to carry out discharge instructions, and making appropriate home care referrals (Bowles, Naylor, & Foust, 2002; Flacker, Park, & Sims, 2007; Moore,

McGinn, & Halm, 2007). Two of the six models consider care transition as the primary focus of their programs.

TYPES OF ACUTE CARE MODELS

Although there are several types of geriatric acute care models that are used in U.S. hospitals, all address both common health problems and care delivery issues. Most consider all geriatric syndromes, whereas others target specific syndromes such as delirium. The models are implemented in various degrees from a hospital-wide to a unit-based approach, whereas others focus on specific processes of hospitalization such as discharge planning.

Geriatric Consultation Service

The consultants in a geriatric service may include a geriatrician, a geropsychiatrist, a geriatric advanced practice nurse (GAPN), or an interprofessional team of geriatric health care providers who conduct a CGA or evaluate a specific condition (older adult mistreatment), symptom (wandering), or situation (adequacy of spouse to care for patient at home). Some hospitals will require that all patients who are screened at high risk for geriatric-related complications or are admitted from a homebound program or a nursing home will receive a geriatric consult, whereas most are requested by another primary service for an individual patient (Hung, Tejada, Soryal, Akbar, & Bowman, 2015). A systematic review/meta-analysis of randomized and nonrandomized studies did not find a statistically significant reduction in functional decline, readmissions, or length of stay but did report fewer consult patients dying at 6 and 8 months following discharge (Deschodt, Flamaing, Haentijens, Boonen, & Millisen, 2013). A geriatric consultation service that proactively provided daily geriatric recommendations for older patients who were receiving care for hip fracture resulted in decreased rate of the development of delirium (Marcantonio, Flacker, Wright, & Resnick, 2001). It is difficult to evaluate any consultation service because their recommendations may not be followed or the hospital may not have the resources or staff to adequately implement the recommendations (Allen et al., 1986).

Acute Care for Elders Units

These discrete geriatric units provide CGA delivered by a multidisciplinary team with a focus on the rehabilitative needs of older patients. Team rounds and patient-centered team conferences are considered essential. The core team includes a geriatrician, GAPN, social worker, as well as specialists from other disciplines providing consultation—occupational and physical therapy, nutrition, pharmacy, audiology, and psychology. Geriatric evaluation and management (GEM) units developed in the U.S. Department of Veterans Affairs (VA) system have documented significant reductions in functional decline and suboptimal medication use as well as return to home post-discharge and, more recent, decreased rate of nursing home placement among hospitalized veterans on GEM units compared with general medical units (Phibbs et al., 2006).

Since the 1990s, acute care for the elderly (ACE) units have been implemented in non-VA hospitals. An interprofessional team consisting of staff with geriatric expertise works collaboratively using strategies such as team rounds and family conferences. Most ACE units have made physical environment adaptations to address age-related changes (e.g., flooring to reduce glare), support orientation (white boards indicating staff names and discharge goals), and promote staff observation (e.g., alarmed exit doors and communal space for meals). Led by geriatricians and/or GAPNs, the interprofessional team facilitates care coordination and identification of modifiable risk factors for geriatric syndromes and prevents avoidable discharge delay (Flood et al., 2015; Fox et al., 2013; Malone, Capezuti, & Palmer, 2014).

Compared with other medical units, patients hospitalized on ACE units have maintained prehospital or demonstrated improved functional status at discharge without increases in hospital or postdischarge costs and are less likely to be discharged to nursing homes (Fox et al., 2012; Landefeld, Palmer, Kresevic, Fortinsky, & Kowal, 1995). Other important positive outcomes associated with ACE units include improved drug prescribing (Spinewine et al., 2007), fewer falls (Fox et al., 2012), less delirium (Bo et al., 2009; Fox et al., 2012), and reduced mortality (Saltvedt, Mo, Fayers, Kaasa, & Sletvold, 2002). In addition, reduced costs have been reported in those on ACE units as a result of shorter hospital stays (Barnes et al., 2012; Fox et al., 2012) and fewer 30-day readmissions (Flood et al., 2013).

These positive outcomes are attributed to processes of care more likely found in ACE units: less restraint use, early mobilization, fewer days to discharge planning, and less use of high-risk medications (Counsell et al., 2000). A 2013 systematic review suggested that the best outcomes from ACE programs were those that included patient-centered care, medical review, and early mobilization (Fox et al., 2012). In a recent shift, more hospitals are using ACE units for those at the highest risk of age-related complications with ACE staff also providing consultation, while exporting ACE principles, throughout the health system to reach a greater number of older hospitalized patients. These "virtual" and/or "ACE without walls" consult teams work similarly to a geriatric consultation service except for the fact that there is also an inpatient ACE unit within the hospital or health system. In another variant, the Mobile Acute Care for Elders (MACE) service, an outpatient geriatric team (attending geriatrician hospitalist, geriatric medicine fellow, social worker, and clinical nurse specialist), also provides primary care to its patients when hospitalized (Hung, Ross, Farber, & Siu, 2013). An evaluation of this model in one hospital reported that MACE service patients experienced fewer adverse events (catheter-associated urinary tract infection, pressure ulcers, restraint use, and falls) and had shorter hospital stays when compared with similar older patients cared for on medical units (Hung et al., 2013).

Nurses Improving Care for Healthsystem Elders

A national program aimed at system improvement to achieve positive outcomes for hospitalized older adults, Nurses Improving Care for Healthsystem Elders (NICHE), seeks to improve the quality of care provided to older patients and improve nurse competence by modifying the nurse practice environment with the infusion of geriatric-specific (a) core values into the mission statement of the institution; (b) special equipment, supplies, and other resources; and (c) protocols and techniques that promote interprofessional collaboration (Boltz et al., 2008b; Bub, Boltz, Malsch, & Fletcher, 2015; Capezuti, Bricoli, & Boltz, 2013; Capezuti et al., 2012). NICHE includes several approaches that promote dissemination of evidence-based geriatric best practices into hospital care. The system-level approach of NICHE provides a structure for nurses to collaborate with other disciplines and to actively participate in or coordinate other geriatric acute care models. A NICHE coordinator acts in a leadership role by facilitating, teaching, and mentoring others and changing systems of care (Fletcher et al., 2007). In some hospitals, a GAPN functions in this role as well as providing direct clinical consultation for evaluating and managing patients. The geriatric resource nurse (GRN) model is foundational to NICHE; it is an educational intervention whereby the NICHE coordinator or the GAPN prepares staff nurses to be the clinical resource person on geriatric issues to other nurses on the unit (Capezuti et al., 2012; Lee, Fletcher, Westley, & Fankhauser, 2004). The GRN model provides staff nurses, via education and role modeling (e.g., nursing bedside rounds) by a GAPN or NICHE coordinator, with content focusing on care management for geriatric syndromes. Application of evidence-based practice at the bedside is facilitated by organizational strategies such as incorporation of institution-wide clinical protocols as provided in this book.

The GRN model fosters professional development and enhanced work satisfaction for nurses who feel that they have institutional support in providing quality care. These supports include geriatric-specific resources (continuing education, equipment, and specialty services); interprofessional collaboration; as well as patient, family, and nurse involvement in treatment-related decision making. Evaluation in NICHE hospitals has reported improved clinical outcomes, rate of compliance with geriatric institutional protocols, cost-related outcomes, and improved nurse knowledge (Boltz et al., 2013; Bub, Boltz, Marlsch, & Fletcher et al., 2015; Capezuti et al., 2013; Hendrix, Matters, West, Stewart, & McConnell, 2011; Pfaff, 2002; Swauger, & Tomlin, 2002; Turner, Lee, Fletcher, Hudson, & Barton, 2001; Wald, Bandle, Richard, Min, & Capezuti, 2014a, 2014b). The GRN model is associated with positive outcomes such as reduced delirium in a NICHE orthopedic unit (Guthrie, Schumacher, & Edinger, 2006) and reduced complications among hospitalized older adults with dementia (Allen & Close, 2010). In studies aggregating results from several NICHE hospitals, NICHE implementation is associated with improved processes of care (Fulmer et al., 2002; Mezey et al., 2004) as well as higher nurse-perceived quality of care (Boltz et al., 2008a).

NICHE also promotes implementation of the ACE model. The ACE model as promoted by NICHE, emphasizes nurse-driven protocols and geriatric continuing education of all nursing staff. Similar to other ACE units, study of a NICHE–ACE unit found lower fall and pressure ulcer rates and lower length of stay when compared with overall hospital rates (LaReau & Raphelson, 2005).

The Hospital Elder Life Program

The Hospital Elder Life Program (HELP) is an intervention program using clinicians (geriatric specialists of various disciplines) working together as an interprofessional team with trained volunteers who target risk factors for delirium (mental orientation, therapeutic activities, early mobilization, vision and hearing adaptations, hydration and feeding assistance, and sleep enhancement). Protocols based on several well-designed clinical trials are employed to reduce incidence of delirium and, among those who did develop delirium, reduce total number of episodes and days with delirium, functional decline, costs of hospital services, and use of long-term nursing home services (Babine, Farrington, & Wierman, 2013; Inouye, Baker, Fugal, Bradley, & for the HELP Dissemination Project, 2006; Inouye, Bogardus, Baker, Leo-Summers, & Cooney, 2000; Inouye et al., 1999; Yue, Kshieh, & Inouye, 2015). The HELP program has also been successfully adapted for the community-hospital setting as well specifically for older surgery patients who have a high occurrence of delirium (Chen et al., 2014; Zaubler et al., 2013). Currently, the HELP protocols have been adapted to incorporate the NICE (National Institute for Health and Clinical Excellence) guidelines (National Clinical Guideline Centre, 2010).

The program depends on hospital volunteers who are well trained and closely supervised to deploy patient care interventions (Bradley, Webster, Schlesinger, Baker, & Inouye, 2006b) that are coordinated by elder life nurse specialists. The elder life nurse specialist typically has advanced geriatric nursing education and will supervise the implementation of nursing-related assessments and tracking of delirium risk-factor-protocol adherence.

Transitional Care Models

Transitional care models address the needs of older adult patients with complex medical and social needs and their caregivers as they move from hospital to postacute care. Two models with demonstrated positive outcomes include the advanced practice nurse (APN) transitional care model (Naylor & Keating, 2008) and the care transitions coaching or care transitions intervention (Coleman, Parry, Chalmers, & Min, 2006; Coleman, Smith, et al., 2004). (These are described in more detail in Chapter 36, "Transitional Care.")

Combination and Specialty Geriatric Acute Care Models

In some hospitals, a combination of geriatric models is implemented such as a geriatric consultation team and transitional care (Arbaje et al., 2010) or inpatient geriatric assessment and intensive home care (Buurman, Parlevliet, van Deelen, de Haan, & de Rooij, 2010). In others, a core geriatric interprofessional team provides direct consultation as well as screens patients for other related services, such as palliative care, rehabilitative services, or pain management programs. Some hospitals have developed dual-function units, such as merging an ACE unit with a palliative care (Gelfman, Meier, & Morrison, 2008; Tomasovic, 2005), stroke (K. R. Allen et al., 2003), or oncology (Flood, Brown, Carroll, & Locher, 2011) unit, as well as incorporating a "delirium room" within an ACE unit (Flaherty et al., 2003), whereas others have developed programs that incorporate geriatric comanagement with other specialties such as rehabilitation, orthopedics, trauma, and oncology (Allen et al., 2003; Gelfman et al., 2008; Kammerlander et al., 2010; Mendelson & Friedman, 2014). These programs have demonstrated increased detection of and reduced incidence of delirium, as well as reduced length of stay, readmission rates, morbidity, and mortality (Flaherty et al., 2003; Flood et al., 2011; Kates, 2014; Milisen et al., 2001; Pareja et al., 2009).

Collaboration With Hospitalists

Considering that hospitalists provide care for an increasing number of older acutely ill Medicare patients, some hospitals have initiated a proactive geriatrics consultation service implemented in collaboration with hospitalists (Sennour, Counsell, Jones, & Weiner, 2009). After 4 years and more than 1,500 consults, this service reported a high level of satisfaction by hospitalists while resulting in a shorter hospital stay and less hospital costs in patients receiving a geriatrics consultation (Sennour et al., 2009). A program in which hospitalists are trained to lead transitional care teams (BOOST—Better Outcomes for Older adults through Safer Transitions) has shown preliminary evidence to suggest prevention of postdischarge complications and readmissions within 30 days and increased confidence in self-management (Dedhia et al., 2009). In an analysis of the initial hospitals participating in the quality-improvement program, BOOST was associated with a modest but significant reduction in 30-day hospital readmissions from 14.7% at baseline to 12.7% after the intervention (Hansen et al., 2013). Administered by the Society of Hospital Medicine, the BOOST program provides technical support to optimize the hospital discharge process and diminish discontinuity and fragmentation of care (Williams & Coleman, 2009).

Models of Senior ED Care

Organizational models have emerged to address the specialized needs of older adults using the ED, and their families. Core components of these models include interprofessional collaboration, the use of evidence-based clinical interventions, and the central role of the nurse in coordinating care. Interprofessional teams (geriatrician, nurse practitioner, rehabilitation therapists, and social worker) evaluate high-risk patients in the ED (and follow them throughout the hospital stay; Gold & Bergman, 1997). A prospective, randomized, controlled trial conducted in a medical school–affiliated urban public hospital in Sydney, Australia, found that older adults sent home from the ED who received a CGA demonstrated positive outcomes. Although there was no difference in admission to nursing homes or mortality, patients randomized to the intervention group maintained a greater degree of physical and mental function (Caplan, Williams, Daly, & Abraham, 2004). In the randomized controlled trial of SIGNET

(Systematic Interventions for a Geriatric Network of Evaluation and Treatment), an intervention (CGA) conducted in the ED by an APN resulted in very modest reductions in the risk of 90-day admission of elderly patients to a nursing home and in the mean number of hospital days among high-risk patients who received the intervention (Mion et al., 2003).

Mobile interprofessional teams in the ED conduct a brief geriatric assessment and develop a comprehensive plan. Two types of recommendations have been made: (a) medical recommendations for diagnosis and treatment of the presenting illnesses, and other geriatrics syndromes; and (b) gerontological recommendations for social and home needs. Outcomes reported include shortened hospital stay and early discharge from the ED (Launay, Decker, Hureaux-Huynh, Annweiler, & Beauchet, 2012).

Geriatric emergency management (GEM) nurses provide targeted geriatric assessment and intervention for older adult patients (aged 65-plus years) in the ED. At-risk patients are identified through the Triage Risk Factor Screening Tool (TRST) and the Identification of Seniors at Risk (ISAR) tool. Interventions include support for staff to implement geriatric care strategies in the ED, linkage to community support services, referral for specialized geriatric services, and collaboration with the family physician. GEM nurses have provided timely development of care plans and initiation of needed referrals (Asomaning, Loftus, & Ramsden, 2012; Rogers, 2009).

The first senior-friendly ED, a self-contained unit within a larger ED, was created by Holy Cross Hospital in Maryland in 2008. The physical environment is adapted to age-related changes (warm colors with select use of color contrast; thick mattresses; indirect light; glare-free floors; large, easy-to-use call light/TV remotes, telephones, and clocks; and documents with larger print). Dedicated, gerontologically prepared nursing staff, nurse practitioners, and social workers staff the unit and volunteers provide comfort measures. Evidence-based clinical protocols are used. A geriatric pharmacist reviews the medications of seniors who receive seven or more medications. The staff provides follow-up calls or home visits after discharge from the ED and care coordination is provided as indicated. The trend of senior-friendly EDs is growing and future research is planned to evaluate clinical and organizational effectiveness (Hwang & Morrison, 2007). The elder-friendly hospital conceptual framework offered by Parke and Brand (2004) provides guidance in efforts to develop a senior-friendly ED. This framework includes four major components to consider when developing a senior-friendly ED, and is described in Table 35.1.

TABLE 35.1
Dimensions of a Senior-Friendly Hospital

Social climate: Evident in the treatment of older people in the hospital and the degree of conflict and stress experienced in the ED environment.
Policies and procedures: Expressed in the conduct of hospital staff, which is influenced by the explicit and implicit bureaucratic rules and regulations.
Care systems and processes: The organization of clinical ED care and how work is completed in the provision of services; access to best practice.
Physical design: The observable built environment and all its architectural features, including equipment, furnishings, and decor, that together enable or disable an older person's independent functioning.

ED, emergency department.
Source: Parke and Brand (2004).

New Model Approaches

The availability of geriatric clinicians is essential to implementing any model; however, there is a significant shortage of fellowship-trained geriatricians, geriatric psychiatrists, master's-prepared geriatric nurse specialists, as well as specialists in other disciplines (Committee on the Future Health Care Workforce for Older Americans, 2008). This is especially true for hospitals located in rural areas as well as small hospitals without the financial capacity to employ geriatric specialists (Jayadevappa, Bloom, Raziano, & Lavizzo-Mourey, 2003). Some hospitals are working with other hospitals in their health system or in their region to create learning collaboratives or "knowledge networks" by using web-based and other long-distance communication strategies. Thus, a geriatrician (Malone et al., 2010) or a GAPN (Capezuti, 2010) can participate in "virtual" rounds with staff in another location (Friedman, Mendelson, Kates, & McCann, 2008; Pallawala & Lun, 2001) to foster communication; that is, the e-geriatrician or e-APN has access to a system-wide electronic health record such as the ACE Tracker and the TeleGeriatric system (Pallawala & Lun, 2001) or similar web-based assessment tool (Gray & Wootton, 2008; Martin-Khan et al., 2012; Meyer, 2011; Vollbrecht et al., 2015). In this way, collaboration and mentoring of professional colleagues are facilitated while enhancing the care provided to older adults.

SUMMARY

Despite differences in approaches or foci, all models share common goals. The model employed in a hospital or health system is based on the unique needs of that hospital's patient population, the resources available (geriatric clinicians, bed size, volunteers, etc.), and especially the senior administrator's commitment to geriatric programming. Because there is currently no direct reimbursement for many components of these models, administrators are motivated by the model's alignment to the institution's strategic plan or mission, consumer or community satisfaction, and costs savings (such as reduced costly and nonreimbursable complications; Adunsky et al., 2005; Boult et al., 2009; Bradley, Webster, Schlesinger, Baker, & Inouye, 2006a; Capezuti et al., 2013; Hart, Frank, Hoffman, Dickey, & Kristjansson, 2006; Kammerlander et al., 2010; Leff et al., 2012; Siu, Spragens, Inouye, Morrison, & Leff, 2009). Although all of the models have demonstrated positive outcomes, only a small number (approximately 750) have been implemented in U.S. acute care facilities. Most are located in academic or teaching hospitals. Implementing and monitoring these acute care models can be seen as a continuous quality-improvement process. Geriatric nurses and geriatricians play a key role in leading these system-based programs to bring best-practice strategies to populations of older individuals. Expansion to more than 3,000 hospitals that serve a high proportion of older adults may depend on advancing the unique contributions of each within an integrated model that will enhance the hospital experience of the older patient (Capezuti & Brush, 2009; Leff et al., 2012; Marcantonio et al., 2001).

REFERENCES

Adunsky, A., Arad, M., Levi, R., Blankstein, A., Zeilig, G., & Mizrachi, E. (2005). Five-year experience with the "Sheba" model of comprehensive orthogeriatric care for elderly hip fracture patients. *Disability and Rehabilitation, 27*(18–19), 1123–1127. *Evidence Level IV.*

Allen, C. M., Becker, P. M., McVey, L. J., Saltz, C., Feussner, J. R., & Cohen, H. J. (1986). A randomized, controlled clinical trial of a geriatric consultation team. Compliance with recommendations. *Journal of the American Medical Association, 255*(19), 2617–2621. *Evidence Level II.*

Allen, J., & Close, J. (2010). The NICHE geriatric resource nurse model: Improving the care of older adults with Alzheimer's disease and other dementias. *Geriatric Nursing, 31*(2), 128–132. *Evidence Level V.*

Allen, K. R., Hazelett, S. E., Palmer, R. R., Jarjoura, D. G., Wickstrom, G. C., Weinhardt, J. A.,... Counsell, S. R. (2003). Developing a stroke unit using the acute care for elders intervention and model of care. *Journal of the American Geriatrics Society, 51*(11), 1660–1667. *Evidence Level V.*

Arbaje, A. I., Maron, D. D., Yu, Q., Wendel, V. I., Tanner, E., Boult, C.,... Durso, S. C. (2010). The geriatric floating interdisciplinary transition team. *Journal of the American Geriatrics Society, 58*(2), 364–370. *Evidence Level III.*

Asomaning, N., Loftus, C., & Ramsden, R. (2012). *Solutions: Supporting hospitalized frail seniors from ED to home.* Retrieved from https://s3.amazonaws.com/Resources2014/NICHESolutions_Loftus_24.pdf. *Evidence Level V.*

Babine, R. L., Farrington, S., & Wierman, H. R. (2013). HELP prevent falls by preventing delirium. *Nursing, 43*(5), 18–21. *Evidence Level V.*

Barnes, D. E., Palmer, R. M., Kresevic, D. M., Fortinsky, R. H., Kowal, J., Chren, M. M., & Landefeld, C. S. (2012). Acute care for elders units produce shorter hospital stays at lower costs while maintaining patient's functional status. *Health Affairs, 31*(6), 1227–1236. *Evidence Level II.*

Berman, A., Mezey, M., Kobayashi, M., Fulmer, T., Stanley, J., Thornlow, D., & Rosenfeld, P. (2005). Gerontological nursing content in baccalaureate nursing programs: Comparison of findings from 1997 and 2003. *Journal of Professional Nursing, 21*(5), 268–275. *Evidence Level V.*

Bo, M., Martini, B., Ruatta, C., Massaia, M., Ricauda, N. A., Varetto, A.,... Torta, R. (2009). Geriatric ward hospitalization reduced incidence delirium among older medical inpatients. *American Journal of Geriatric Psychiatry, 17*(9), 760–768. *Evidence Level IV.*

Boltz, M., Capezuti, E., Bowar-Ferres, S., Norman, R., Secic, M., Kim, H.,... Fulmer, T. (2008a). Changes in the geriatric care environment associated with NICHE (Nurses Improving Care for Healthsystem Elders). *Geriatric Nursing, 29*(3), 176–185. *Evidence Level IV.*

Boltz, M., Capezuti, E., Bowar-Ferres, S., Norman, R., Secic, M., Kim, H.,... Fulmer, T. (2008b). Hospital nurses' perception of the geriatric nurse practice environment. *Journal of Nursing Scholarship, 40*(3), 282–289. *Evidence Level IV.*

Boltz, M., Capezuti, E., Shuluk, J., Brouwer, J., Carolan, D., Conway, S.,... Galvin, J. E. (2013). Implementation of geriatric acute care best practices: Initial results of the NICHE SITE self-evaluation. *Nursing & Health Sciences, 15*(4), 518–524. doi:10.1111/nhs.12067. *Evidence Level IV.*

Boult, C., Green, A. F., Boult, L. B., Pacala, J. T., Snyder, C., & Leff, B. (2009). Successful models of comprehensive care for older adults with chronic conditions: Evidence for the Institute of Medicine's "retooling for an aging America" report. *Journal of the American Geriatrics Society, 57*(12), 2328–2337. *Evidence Level I.*

Bowles, K. H., Naylor, M. D., & Foust, J. B. (2002). Patient characteristics at hospital discharge and a comparison of home care referral decisions. *Journal of the American Geriatrics Society, 50*(2), 336–342. *Evidence Level IV.*

Bradley, E. H., Webster, T. R., Schlesinger, M., Baker, D., & Inouye, S. K. (2006a). Patterns of diffusion of evidence-based clinical programmes: A case study of the Hospital Elder Life Program. *Quality & Safety in Health Care, 15*(5), 334–338. *Evidence Level V.*

Bradley, E. H., Webster, T. R., Schlesinger, M., Baker, D., & Inouye, S. K. (2006b). The roles of senior management in improving hospital experiences for frail older adults. *Journal of Healthcare Management, 51*(5), 323–336. *Evidence Level IV.*

Bub, L., Boltz, M., Malsch, A., & Fletcher, K. (2015). The NICHE program to prepare the workforce to address the needs of older adults. In M. L. Malone, E. Capezuti, & R. M. Palmer (Eds.), *Geriatrics models of care—Bringing "best practice" to an aging America* (1st ed., pp. 57–70). Cham, Switzerland: Springer International Publishing AG. *Evidence Level VI.*

Buurman, B. M., Parlevliet, J. L., van Deelen, B. A., de Haan, R. J., & de Rooij, S. E. (2010). A randomised clinical trial on a comprehensive geriatric assessment and intensive home follow-up after hospital discharge: The transitional care bridge. *BMC Health Services Research, 10,* 296. *Evidence Level II.*

Capezuti, E. (2010). An electronic geriatric specialist workforce: Is it a viable option? *Geriatric Nursing, 31*(3), 220–222. *Evidence Level V.*

Capezuti, E., Boltz, E., Cline, D., Dickson, V., Rosenberg, M., Wagner, L., . . . Nigolian, C. (2012). NICHE—A model for optimizing the geriatric nursing practice environment. *Journal of Clinical Nursing, 21,* 3117–3125. *Evidence Level VI.*

Capezuti, E., Boltz, M., & Kim, H. (2011). Models of care for hospitalized older adults. In R. A. Rosenthal, M. E. Zenilman, & M. R. Katlic (Eds.), *Principles and practice of geriatric surgery* (1st ed., pp. 253–266). New York, NY: Springer-Verlag. *Evidence Level VI.*

Capezuti, E., Boltz, M., Shuluk, J., Denysyk, L., Brouwers, J., Roberts, M. C., . . . Secic, M. (2013). Utilization of a benchmarking database to inform NICHE implementation. *Research in Gerontological Nursing, 6*(3), 198–208. *Evidence Level IV.*

Capezuti, E., Bricoli, B., & Boltz, M. (2013). NICHE: Creating a sustainable business model to improve care of hospitalized older adults. *Journal of the American Geriatrics Society, 61*(8), 1387–1393. *Evidence Level V.*

Capezuti, E., & Brush, B. L. (2009). Implementing geriatric care models: What are we waiting for? *Geriatric Nursing, 30*(3), 204–206. *Evidence Level V.*

Caplan, G. A., Williams, A. J., Daly, B., & Abraham K. (2004). A randomized, controlled trial of comprehensive geriatric assessment and multidisciplinary intervention after discharge of elderly from the emergency department—The DEED II Study. *Journal of the American Geriatrics Society, 52,* 1417–1423. *Evidence Level II.*

Chen, C. C., Chen, C. N., Lai, I. R., Huang, G. H., Saczynski, J. S., & Inouye, S. K. (2014). Effects of a modified Hospital Elder Life Program on frailty in individuals undergoing major elective abdominal surgery. *Journal of the American Geriatrics Society, 62*(2), 261–268. *Evidence Level III.*

Coleman, E. A., Min, S. J., Chomiak, A., & Kramer, A. M. (2004). Posthospital care transitions: Patterns, complications, and risk identification. *Health Services Research, 39*(5), 1449–1465. *Evidence Level IV.*

Coleman, E. A., Parry, C., Chalmers, S., & Min, S. J. (2006). The care transitions intervention: Results of a randomized controlled trial. *Archives of Internal Medicine, 166*(17), 1822–1828. *Evidence Level II.*

Coleman, E. A., Smith, J. D., Frank, J. C., Min, S. J., Parry, C., & Kramer, A. M. (2004). Preparing patients and caregivers to participate in care delivered across settings: The care transitions intervention. *Journal of the American Geriatrics Society, 52*(11), 1817–1825. *Evidence Level III.*

Coleman, E. A., Smith, J. D., Raha, D., & Min, S. J. (2005). Posthospital medication discrepancies: Prevalence and contributing factors. *Archives of Internal Medicine, 165*(16), 1842–1847. *Evidence Level IV.*

Committee on the Future Health Care Workforce for Older Americans. (2008). *Retooling for an aging America: Building the health care workforce.* Washington, DC: National Academies Press. *Evidence Level VI.*

Counsell, S. R., Holder, C. M., Liebenauer, L. L., Palmer, R. M., Fortinsky, R. H., Kresevic, D. M., . . . Landefeld, C. S. (2000). Effects of a multicomponent intervention on functional outcomes and processes of care in hospitalized older patients: A randomized controlled trial of acute care for elders (ACE) in a community hospital. *Journal of the American Geriatrics Society, 48*(12), 1572–1581. *Evidence Level II.*

Dedhia, P., Kravet, S., Bulger, J., Hinson, T., Sridharan, A., Kolodner, K., . . . Howell, E. (2009). A quality improvement intervention to facilitate the transition of older adults from three hospitals back to their homes. *Journal of the American Geriatrics Society, 57*(9), 1540–1546. *Evidence Level V*

Deschodt, M., Flamaing, J., Haentijens, P., Boonen, S., & Millisen, K. (2013). Impact of geriatric consultation teams on clinical outcomes in acute hospitals: a systematic review and meta-analysis. *BMC Medical, 11,* 48. doi:10.1186/1741-7015-11-48. *Evidence Level I.*

Flacker, J., Park, W., & Sims, A. (2007). Hospital discharge information and older patients: Do they get what they need? *Journal of Hospital Medicine, 2*(5), 291–296. *Evidence Level IV.*

Flaherty, J. H., Tariq, S. H., Raghavan, S., Bakshi, S., Moinuddin, A., & Morley, J. E. (2003). A model for managing delirious older inpatients. *Journal of the American Geriatrics Society, 51*(7), 1031–1035. *Evidence Level V.*

Fletcher, K., Hawkes, P., Williams-Rosenthal, S., Mariscal, C. S., & Cox, B. A. (2007). Using nurse practitioners to implement best practice care for the elderly during hospitalization: The NICHE journey at the University of Virginia Medical Center. *Critical Care Nursing Clinics of North America, 19*(3), 321–337. *Evidence Level V.*

Flood, K. L., Booth, E. P., Danto-Nocton, E. S., Kresevic, D. M., & Palmer, R. M. (2015). Acute care for elders. In M. L. Malone, E. Capezuti, & R. M. Palmer (Eds.), *Geriatrics models of care—Bringing "best practice" to an aging America* (1st ed., pp. 3–23). Cham, Switzerland: Springer International Publishing AG. *Evidence Level VI.*

Flood, K. L., Brown, C. J., Carroll, M. B., & Locher, J. L. (2011). Nutritional processes of care for older adults admitted to an oncology-acute care for elders unit. *Critical Reviews in Oncology/Hematology, 78*(1), 73–78. *Evidence Level IV.*

Flood, K. L., MacLennan, P. A., McGrew, D., Green, D., Dodd, C., & Brown, C. J. (2013). An acute care for elders unit reduces costs and 30-day readmissions. *Journal of the American Medical Association Internal Medicine, 173*(11), 981–987. *Evidence Level III.*

Forster, A. J., Murff, H. J., Peterson, J. F., Gandhi, T. K., & Bates, D. W. (2003). The incidence and severity of adverse events affecting patients after discharge from the hospital. *Annals of Internal Medicine, 138*(3), 161–167. *Evidence Level IV.*

Foust, J. B., Naylor, M. D., Boling, P. A., & Cappuzzo, K. A. (2005). Opportunities for improving post-hospital home medication management among older adults. *Home Health Care Services Quarterly, 24*(1–2), 101–122. *Evidence Level V.*

Fox, M. T., Persaud, M., Maimets, I., O'Brien, K., Brooks, D., Tregunno, D., & Schraa, E. (2012). Effectiveness of acute geriatric unit care using acute care for elders components: A systematic review and meta-analysis. *Journal of the American Geriatrics Society, 60*, 2237–2245. *Evidence Level I.*

Fox, M. T., Sidani, S., Persaud, M., Tregunno, D., Maimets, I., Brooks, D., & O'Brien, K. (2013). Acute care for elders components of acute geriatric unit care: Systematic descriptive review. *Journal of the American Geriatrics Society, 61*, 939–946. *Evidence Level I.*

Friedman, S. M., Mendelson, D. A., Kates, S. L., & McCann, R. M. (2008). Geriatric co-management of proximal femur fractures: Total quality management and protocol-driven care result in better outcomes for a frail patient population. *Journal of the American Geriatrics Society, 56*(7), 1349–1356. *Evidence Level V.*

Fulmer, T., Mezey, M., Bottrell, M., Abraham, I., Sazant, J., Grossman, S., & Grisham, E. (2002). Nurses Improving Care for Healthsystem Elders (NICHE): Using outcomes and benchmarks for evidenced-based practice. *Geriatric Nursing, 23*(3), 121–127. *Evidence Level IV.*

Gelfman, L. P., Meier, D. M., & Morrison, R. S. (2008). Does palliative care improve quality? A survey of bereaved family members. *Journal of Pain and Symptom Manage, 36*(1), 22–28. *Evidence Level IV.*

Gold, S., & Bergman, H. (1997). A geriatric consultation team in the emergency department. *Journal of American Geriatrics Society, 45*(6), 764–7. *Evidence Level VI.*

Gray, L., & Wootton, R. (2008). Comprehensive geriatric assessment "online." *Australasian Journal on Ageing, 27*(4), 205–208. *Evidence Level V.*

Guthrie, P. F., Schumacher, S., & Edinger, G. (2006). A NICHE delirium prevention project for hospitalized elders. In N. M. Silverstein & K. Maslow (Eds.), *Improving hospital care for persons with dementia* (pp. 139–157). New York, NY: Springer Publishing Company. *Evidence Level V.*

Hansen L. O., Greenwald, J. L., Budnitz, T., Howell, E., Halasyamani, L., Maynard, G.,... Williams, M. V. (2013). Project BOOST: Effectiveness of a multi-hospital effort to reduce hospitalizations. *Journal of Hospital Medicine, 8*, 421–427. *Evidence Level III.*

Hart, B., Frank, C., Hoffman, J., Dickey, D., & Kristjansson, J. (2006). Senior friendly health services. *Perspectives, 30*(1), 18–21. *Evidence Level V.*

Hendrix, C. C., Matters, L., West, Y., Stewart, B., & McConnell, E. S. (2011). The Duke-NICHE program: An academic practice collaboration to enhance geriatric nursing care. *Nursing Outlook, 59*(3), 149–157. *Evidence Level V.*

Hickman, L., Newton, P., Halcomb, E. J., Chang, E., & Davidson P. (2007). Best practice interventions to improve the management of older people in acute care settings: A literature review. *Journal of Advanced Nursing, 60*(2), 113–126. *Evidence Level V.*

Hickman, L. D., Rolley, J. X., & Davidson, P. M. (2010). Can principles of the Chronic Care Model be used to improve care of the older person in the acute care sector? *Collegian, 17*(2), 63–69. *Evidence Level V.*

Hung, W. W., Tejada, J. A. M., Soryal, S., Akbar, S. T., & Bowman, E. H. (2015). The Acute Care for Elders Consult Program. In M. L. Malone, E. Capezuti, & R. M. Palmer (Eds.). *Geriatrics models of care—Bringing "best practice" to an aging America* (1st ed., pp. 39–49). Cham, Switzerland: Springer International Publishing AG. *Evidence Level VI.*

Hung, W. W., Ross, J. S., Farber, J., & Siu, A. L. (2013). Evaluation of a mobile acute care for the elderly (MACE) service. *JAMA Internal Medicine, 173*(11), 990–996. *Evidence Level III.*

Hwang, U., & Morrison, R. S. (2007). The geriatric emergency department. *Journal of the American Geriatrics Society, 55*(11), 1873–1876. *Evidence Level V.*

Inouye, S. K., Baker, D. I., Fugal, P., Bradley, E. H., & for the HELP Dissemination Project. (2006). Dissemination of the hospital elder life program: Implementation, adaptation, and successes. *Journal of the American Geriatrics Society, 54*(10), 1492–1499. *Evidence Level IV.*

Inouye, S. K., Bogardus, S. T., Jr., Baker, D. I., Leo-Summers, L., & Cooney, L. M., Jr. (2000). The Hospital Elder Life Program: A model of care to prevent cognitive and functional decline in older hospitalized patients. Hospital Elder Life Program. *Journal of the American Geriatrics Society, 48*(12), 1697–1706. *Evidence Level IV.*

Inouye, S. K., Bogardus, S. T., Jr., Charpentier, P. A., Leo-Summers, L., Acampora, D., Holford, T. R., & Cooney, L. M., Jr. (1999). A multicomponent intervention to prevent delirium in hospitalized older patients. *New England Journal of Medicine, 1340*(9), 669–676. *Evidence Level II.*

Inouye, S. K., Studenski, S., Tinetti, M. E., & Kuchel, G. A. (2007). Geriatric syndromes: Clinical, research, and policy implications of a core geriatric concept. *Journal of the American Geriatrics Society, 55*(5), 780–791. *Evidence Level VI.*

Jayadevappa, R., Bloom, B. S., Raziano, D. B., & Lavizzo-Mourey, R. (2003). Dissemination and characteristics of acute care for elders (ACE) units in the United States. *International Journal of Technology Assessment in Health Care, 19*(1), 220–227. *Evidence Level V.*

Kammerlander, C., Roth, T., Friedman, S. M., Suhm, N., Luger, T. J., Kammerlander-Knauer, U.,... Blauth M. (2010). Orthogeriatric service—A literature review comparing different models. *Osteoporosis International, 21*(Suppl. 4), S637–S646. *Evidence Level V.*

Kates, S. L. (2014). Lean business model and implementation of a geriatric fracture center. *Clinics in Geriatric Medicine, 30*(2), 191–205. *Evidence Level V.*

Landefeld, C. S., Palmer, R. M., Kresevic, D. M., Fortinsky, R. H., & Kowal, J. (1995). A randomized trial of care in a hospital medical unit especially designed to improve the functional outcomes of acutely ill older patients. *New England Journal of Medicine, 332*(20), 1338–1344. *Evidence Level II.*

LaReau, R., & Raphelson, M. (2005). The treatment of the hospitalized elderly patient in a specialized acute care of the elderly unit: A southwest Michigan perspective. *Southwest Michigan Medical Journal, 2*(3), 21–27. *Evidence Level V.*

Launay, C., Decker, L., Hureaux-Huynh, R., Annweiler, C., & Beauchet, O. (2012). Mobile geriatric team and length of hospital stay among older inpatients: A case–control pilot study. *Journal of the American Geriatrics Society, 60*(8), 1593–1594. *Evidence Level III.*

Lee, V., Fletcher, K., Westley, C., & Fankhauser, K. A. (2004). Competent to care: Strategies to assist staff in caring for elders. *Medsurg Nursing, 13*(5), 281–288. *Evidence Level V.*

Leff, B., Spragens, L. H., Morano, B., Powell, J., Bickert, T., Bond, C., . . . Siu, A. L. (2012). Rapid reengineering of acute medical care for Medicare beneficiaries: The Medicare innovations collaborative. *Health Affairs, 31*(6), 12014–1215. *Evidence Level V.*

Malone, M. L., Capezuti, E., & Palmer, R. (Eds.). (2014). *Acute care for elders—A model for interdisciplinary care.* Cham, Switzerland: Springer International Publishing AG. *Evidence Level IV.*

Malone, M. L., Vollbrecht, M., Stephenson, J., Burke, L., Pagel, P., & Goodwin, J. S. (2010). Acute Care for Elders (ACE) Tracker and e-Geriatrician: Methods to disseminate ACE concepts to hospitals with no geriatricians on staff. *Journal of the American Geriatrics Society, 58*(1), 161–167. *Evidence Level IV.*

Marcantonio, E. R., Flacker, J. M., Wright, R. J., & Resnick, N. M. (2001). Reducing delirium after hip fracture: A randomized trial. *Journal of the American Geriatrics Society, 49*(5), 516–522. *Evidence Level II.*

Martin-Khan, M., Flicker, L., Wootton, Loh, P., Edwards, H. E., Varghese, P., Byrne, G. J., . . . Gray, L. C. (2012). The diagnostic accuracy of telegeriatrics for the diagnosis of dementia via video conferencing. *Journal of the American Medical Directors Association, 13*(5), 487.e19–487.e24. *Evidence Level III.*

Mendelson, D. A., & Friedman, S. M. (2014). Principles of comanagement and geriatric fracture center. *Clinics in Geriatric Medicine, 30*(2), 183–189. *Evidence Level VI.*

Meyer, H. (2011). Using teams, real-time information, and teleconferencing to improve elders' hospital care. *Health Affairs, 30*(3), 408–411. *Evidence Level V.*

Mezey, M., Kobayashi, M., Grossman, S., Firpo, A., Fulmer, T., & Mitty, E. (2004). Nurses Improving Care to Health System Elders (NICHE): Implementation of best practice models. *Journal of Nursing Administration, 34*(10), 451–457. *Evidence Level V.*

Milisen, K., Foreman, M. D., Abraham, I. L., De Geest, S., Godderis, J., Vandermeulen, E., . . . Broos, P. L. (2001). A nurse-led interdisciplinary intervention program for delirium in elderly hip-fracture patients. *Journal of the American Geriatrics Society, 49*(5), 523–532. *Evidence Level III.*

Mion, L. C., Palmer, R. M., Meldon, S. W., Bass, D. M., Singer, M. E., Payne, S. M. C., . . . Emerman, C. (2003). Case finding and referral model for emergency department elders: A randomized clinical trial. *Annals of Emergency Medicine, 41*, 5–68. *Evidence Level II.*

Moore, C., McGinn, T., & Halm, E. (2007). Tying up loose ends: Discharging patients with unresolved medical issues. *Archives of Internal Medicine, 167*(12), 1305–1311. *Evidence Level IV.*

National Clinical Guideline Centre. (2010). *Delirium: Diagnosis, prevention and management* (full guideline). Retrieved from http://www.nice.org.uk/guidance/CG103. *Evidence Level I.*

Naylor, M., & Keating, S. A. (2008). Transitional care. *American Journal of Nursing, 108*(Suppl. 9), 58–63. *Evidence Level V.*

Neuman, M. D., Speck, R. M., Karlawish, J. H., Schwartz, J. S., & Shea, J. A. (2010). Hospital protocols for the inpatient care of older adults: Results from a statewide survey. *Journal of the American Geriatrics Society, 58*(10), 1959–1964. doi:10.1111/j.1532-5415.2010.03056.x. *Evidence Level IV.*

Pallawala, P. M., & Lun, K. C. (2001). EMR-based TeleGeriatric system. *Studies in Health Technology and Informatics, 84*(Pt. 1), 849–853. *Evidence Level V.*

Palmer, R. (2014). Geriatric evaluation and management units. In E. Capezuti, M. Malone, P. Katz, & M. Mezey (Eds.), *The encyclopedia of elder care* (3rd ed., pp. 337–339). New York, NY: Springer Publishing Company. *Evidence Level VI.*

Pareja, T., Hornillos, M., Rodríguez, M., Martínez, T., Madrigal, M., Mauleón, C., & Alvarez, B. (2009). Unidad de observación de urgencias para pacientes geriátricos: Beneficios clínicos y asistenciales [Medical short stay unit for geriatric patients in the emergency department: Clinical and healthcare benefits]. *Revista Española De Geriatría y Gerontología, 44*(4), 175–179. *Evidence Level IV.*

Parke, B., & Brand, P. (2004). An Elder-friendly hospital: Translating a dream into reality. *Nursing Leadership, 17*, 62–76. *Evidence Level VI.*

Pfaff, J. (2002). The Geriatric Resource Nurse Model: A culture change. *Geriatric Nursing, 23*(3), 140–144. *Evidence Level V.*

Phibbs, C. S., Holty, J. E., Goldstein, M. K., Garber, A. M., Wang, Y., Feussner, J. R., & Cohen, H. J. (2006). The effect of geriatrics evaluation and management on nursing home use and health care costs: Results from a randomized trial. *Medical Care, 44*(1), 91–95. *Evidence Level II.*

Rogers, J. A. (2009). Emergency care: A new model. *Health Progress*, 36–39. *Evidence Level VI.*

Saltvedt, I., Mo, E. S., Fayers, P., Kaasa, S., & Sletvold, O. (2002). Reduced mortality in treating acutely sick, frail older patients in a geriatric evaluation and management unit. A prospective randomized trial. *Journal of the American Geriatrics Society, 50*(5), 792–798. *Evidence Level II.*

Sennour, Y., Counsell, S. R., Jones, J., & Weiner, M. (2009). Development and implementation of a proactive geriatrics consultation model in collaboration with hospitalists. *Journal of the American Geriatrics Society, 57*(11), 2139–2145. *Evidence Level V.*

Siu, A. L., Spragens, L. H., Inouye, S. K., Morrison, R. S., & Leff, B. (2009). The ironic business case for chronic care in the acute care setting. *Health Affairs, 28*(1), 113–125. *Evidence Level V.*

Smyth, C., Dubin, S., Restrepo, A., Nueva-Espana, H., & Capezuti, E. (2001). Creating order out of chaos: Models of GNP practice with hospitalized older adults. *Clinical Excellence for Nurse Practitioners, 5*(2), 88–95. *Evidence Level V.*

Somogyi-Zalud, E., Zhong, Z., Hamel, M. B., & Lynn, J. (2002). The use of life-sustaining treatments in hospitalized persons aged 80 and older. *Journal of the American Geriatrics Society, 50*(5), 930–934. *Evidence Level IV.*

Spinewine, A., Swine, C., Dhillon, S., Lambert, P., Nachega, J. B., Wilmotte, L., & Tulkens, P. M. (2007). Effect of a collaborative approach on the quality of prescribing for geriatric inpatients: A randomized, controlled trial. *Journal of the American Geriatrics Society, 55*(5), 658–665. *Evidence Level II.*

Swauger, K., & Tomlin, C. (2002). Best care for the elderly at Forsyth Medical Center. *Geriatric Nursing, 23*(3), 145–150. *Evidence Level V.*

Tomasovic, N. (2005). Geriatric-palliative care units model for improvement of elderly care. *Collegium Antropologicum, 29*(1), 277–282. *Evidence Level V.*

Turner, J. T., Lee, V., Fletcher, K., Hudson, K., & Barton, D. (2001). Measuring quality of care with an inpatient elderly population: The geriatric resource nurse model. *Journal of Gerontological Nursing, 27*(3), 8–18. *Evidence Level V.*

Vollbrecht, M., Malsch, A., Hook, M. L., Simpson, M. R., Khan, A, & Malone, M. (2015). Acute care for elders tracker, e-geriatrician telemedicine programs. In M. L. Malone, E. Capezuti, & R. M. Palmer (Eds.), *Geriatrics models of care—Bringing "best practice" to an aging America* (1st ed., pp. 51–56). Cham, Switzerland: Springer International Publishing AG. *Evidence Level VI.*

Wald, H., Huddleston, J., & Kramer, A. (2006). Is there a geriatrician in the house? Geriatric care approaches in hospitalist programs. *Journal of Hospital Medicine, 1*(1), 29–35. *Evidence Level IV.*

Wald, H. L., Bandle, B., Richard, A. A., Min, S. J., & Capezuti, E. (2014a). Implementation of electronic surveillance of catheter use and CAUTI at NICHE Hospitals. *American Journal of Infection Control, 42*, S242–S249. *Evidence Level IV.*

Wald, H. L., Bandle, B., Richard, A. A., Min, S. J., & Capezuti, E. (2014b). A trial of electronic surveillance feedback for quality improvement at NICHE hospitals. *American Journal of Infection Control, 42*, S25–S256. *Evidence Level II.*

Walke, L. M., Rosenthal, R. A., Trentalange, M., Perkal, M. F., Maiaroto, M., Jeffery, S. M., & Marottoli, R. A. (2014). Restructuring care for older adults undergoing surgery: Preliminary data from the Co-Management of Older Operative Patients En Route Across Treatment Environments (CO-OPERATE) model of care. *Journal of the American Geriatrics Society, 62* (11), 2185–2190. *Evidence Level V.*

Williams, M. V., & Coleman, E. (2009). BOOSTing the hospital discharge. *Journal of Hospital Medicine, 4*(4), 209–210. *Evidence Level V.*

Yue, J., Kshieh, T. T., & Inouye, S. K. (2015). Hospital Elder Life Program (HELP). In M. L. Malone, E. Capezuti, & R. M. Palmer (Eds.), *Geriatrics models of care—Bringing "best practice" to an aging America* (1st ed., pp. 25–37). Cham, Switzerland: Springer International Publishing AG. *Evidence Level VI.*

Zaubler, T. S., Murphy, K., Rizzuto, L., Santos, R., Skotzko, C., Giordano, J., . . . Inouye, S. K. (2013). Quality improvement and cost savings with multicomponent delirium interventions: Replication of the Hospital Elder Life Program in a community hospital. *Psychosomatics, 54*(3), 219–226. *Evidence Level III.*

36

Transitional Care

Fidelindo Lim, Janice B. Foust, and Janet H. Van Cleave

EDUCATIONAL OBJECTIVES

On completion of this chapter, the reader should be able to:

1. Describe various transitional care models (TCMs) and hospital discharge redesign
2. Identify potential for nurse-led and advanced practice nurse (APN)-led transitional care
3. Identify essential elements of successful transitional care

OVERVIEW

Persons with continuous complex care needs frequently require care in multiple settings. The American Geriatrics Society defines *transitional care* as "a set of actions designed to ensure the coordination and continuity of health care as patients transfer between different locations or different levels of care within the same location" (Coleman, 2003, p. 549). Representative locations include (but are not limited to) hospitals, subacute and postacute nursing facilities, the patient's home, primary and specialty care offices, and long-term care facilities (Coleman, 2003). During transitions between settings, this population is particularly vulnerable to experiencing poor care quality and problems of care fragmentation. For example, among Medicare patients, 20% were hospitalized within 30 days and 34% were rehospitalized within 60 days (Jencks, Williams, & Coleman, 2009) of a care transition. Despite how common these transitions have become, the challenges of improving care transitions have historically received little attention from policy makers, clinicians, and quality improvement entities (Coleman, 2003), until recently.

With hospital readmission now heralded as a quality indicator, there is more incentive to correct transition-related problems. The enactment of the Patient Protection and Affordable Care Act (PPACA) in 2010 has helped formalize and implement transitional care services with federal funding. In addition, the focus on reducing 30-day hospital readmissions is further generating the adoption of TCMs or the redesign of hospital discharge processes (Balaban, Weissman, Samuel, & Woolhandler, 2008).

Many factors contribute to gaps in care during critical transitions. Poor communication, incomplete transfer of information, inadequate education of older adults and their family caregivers, limited access to essential services, and the absence of a single point person to ensure continuity of care all contribute to transition-associated problems (Naylor, 2002; Naylor & Keating, 2008). The practice of nursing is closely tied to health illness transitions in a person's lifetime. The quality of the outcomes during these transitional events is largely determined by the degree of care coordination among health care environments and proactive involvement of the patient and their families in the process, wherein a nurse plays a pivotal role. Success in implementing evidence-based transition-care strategies will help curtail preventable rehospitalizations and save health care dollars.

For a description of evidence levels cited in this chapter, see Chapter 1, "Developing and Evaluating Clinical Practice Guidelines: A Systematic Approach."

This chapter reviews issues and trends associated with transitional care mainly from the acute care setting and presents evidence-based TCMs, redesigned hospital discharge models, as well as strategies to enhance outcome performance.

BACKGROUND AND STATEMENT OF PROBLEM

In 2012, an estimated 43.1 million U.S. residents (13.7% of the U.S. population) were older than 65 years (National Center for Health Statistics, 2013). This population subset remains the core consumer of health care resources. There were 19.6 million emergency department (ED) visits among adults aged 65 years and older reported in 2010 (Albert, McCraig, & Ashman, 2013). Approximately 8.8 million ED visits by patients older than 65 years resulted in hospital admission (Weiss, Wier, Stocks, & Blanchard, 2014). Therefore, the likelihood of older adults being in a state of transition between care environments is very high.

Although current trends indicated a decrease in hospitalization rates from 2008 through 2012 (4% per year) for those aged 65 years and older (Weiss & Elixhauser, 2012), an estimated 13.5 million discharges (38.7% of total discharges) from short-stay hospitals among this age group were reported in 2010 (U.S. Department of Health and Human Services, 2012) and 16% of all hospitalizations in 2012 (National Center for Health Statistics, 2013). This cohort is also reported to have the highest average length of hospital stay of 5.2 days in 2012 (Weiss & Elixhauser, 2012) and the highest mean hospitalization cost ($13,000 per episode in 2012 dollars; Moore, Levit, & Elixhauser, 2014).

The top five most common diagnoses for the hospitalized adult older than 65 years are septicemia, nonhypertensive congestive heart failure (CHF), pneumonia, chronic obstructive pulmonary disease and bronchiectasis, and cardiac dysrhythmias (Weiss et al., 2014). This is notable because evidence-based TCMs have targeted these high-volume, high-risk conditions (Naylor et al., 2013).

Transitions are considered high-stress events for patients, their families, and care providers alike. Evidence suggests that transitions are particularly vulnerable to breakdowns in care and, thus, there is a need for transitional care services (Naylor et al., 2013). Two especially problematic areas are medication discrepancies and poor posthospital follow-up with primary care providers. Forster, Murff, Peterson, Gandhi, and Bates (2003) found that nearly 20% of recently discharged medical patients experienced an adverse event during the first several weeks at home. Of these, 66% involved medications and were the most common type of adverse event (Forster et al., 2003). In a study on home medication discrepancies, Corbett, Setter, Daratha, Neumiller, and Wood (2010) found that the problems were astoundingly widespread, with 94% of the participants having at least one discrepancy. The average number of medication discrepancies identified was 3.3 per patient during hospital-to-home transition (Corbett et al., 2010). Similarly, 71% of the hospital discharge records of older adults with heart failure had at least one type of medication reconciliation problem (i.e., discrepancies, partial discharge instructions, or incomplete discharge summaries; Foust, Naylor, Bixby, & Ratcliffe, 2012). Another major area of breakdown is patient follow-up visits after discharge. For example, one study reported that among Medicare patients rehospitalized within 30 days, up to 50% did not have documentation of physician follow-up visits postdischarge (Jencks et al., 2009). Standardizing handoff processes and developing metrics for transfers of care have been shown to improve transition care to and from the ED (Kessler, Williams, Moustoukas, & Pappas, 2012).

Patients and their caregivers are often unprepared for transitions and are overwhelmed by discharge information. Poor preparation of the patient and his or her informal caregivers for the next level-of-care interface, be it the home or another facility, compromises overall patient safety (Coleman, Parry, Chalmers, & Min, 2006). Follow-up visits after discharges provide opportunities to reinforce discharge education and monitor for changes in conditions.

The 2001 Institute of Medicine (IOM) landmark report, *Crossing the Quality Chasm: A New Health System for the 21st Century*, pointed out that the health care delivery system is poorly organized to meet the challenges at hand. The delivery of care is often overly complex and uncoordinated, requiring steps and patient "handoffs" that slow down care and decrease rather than improve safety (IOM, 2001).

At an increasing rate, patients are being discharged home or to other health care environments with both complex and complicated treatment plans with limited timely follow-through by professionals, causing undue stress to the patient and his or her informal caregivers once they leave the hospital. Levine, Halper, Peist, and Gould (2010) have described informal caregivers' essential role and called for more proactive involvement of caregivers as partners during transitions, especially when they could be the major source of continuity for the patient. The stress of caregiving is likely to be exacerbated during episodes of acute illness (Naylor & Keating, 2008), readmissions, and transfers to various health care environments.

Health care disparity and lack or inadequate access to transition care resources will be more pronounced in the disenfranchised segment of older adults, namely, those who are living alone, have multiple comorbidities, are undomiciled, suffering from mental illness, victims of elder abuse and neglect, the uninsured, and those lacking in legal status.

ASSESSMENT OF THE PROBLEM

Until very recently, sustained transitional care programs outside of funded randomized controlled trials (RCTs) were lacking largely because of limited third-party reimbursement of transitional care services (Naylor & Keating, 2008). Federal funding of transitional care programs was launched in 2012 with the implementation of the Community-Based Care Transitions Program (CCTP), created by Section 3026 of the Affordable Care Act (Centers for Medicare & Medicaid Services [CMS], n.d.). CCTP is currently evaluating various TCMs for high-risk Medicare beneficiaries. The goals of the CCTP are to improve transitions of beneficiaries from the inpatient hospital setting to other care settings, to improve quality of care, to reduce readmissions for high-risk beneficiaries, and to document measurable savings to the Medicare program (CMS, n.d.).

Several studies have delineated the problems that patients encounter during transitions. Coleman, Min, Chomiak, and Kramer (2004) identified four major content areas that patients and caregivers who recently underwent post-hospital care transitions expressed as most essential and most needed: medication self-management, a patient-centered health record, primary care and specialist follow-up, and knowledge of "red-flag" warning symptoms or signs indicative of a worsening condition. Similarly, Miller, Piacentine, and Weiss (2008) identified posthospital difficulties faced by adults during the first 3 weeks at home. Among those patients who had difficulty coping, pain was the most frequent stressor, followed by managing complications and recovery challenges. These recently discharged patients also described relying on family or friends for emotional support, and were concerned about being a burden. A lack of written detail and accessibility of hospital discharge instructions were significant problems described by patients, informal caregivers, and home health care clinicians when patients returned home from the hospital (Foust, Vuckovic, & Henriquez, 2012).

A study that compared the referral decisions of hospital clinicians with those of nurses with expertise in discharge planning and transitional care found that transitional care nurses (TCNs) judged that 96 of 99 of the control-group patients discharged without home care had unmet discharge needs that may have benefited from a postdischarge referral (Bowles, Naylor, & Foust, 2002).

A prospective observational cohort study to evaluate the quality of discharge practices at an academic medical center (N = 395) found that, although the majority of patients (95.6%) reported understanding the reason for their hospitalization, fewer patients (59.6%) were able to accurately describe their diagnosis in postdischarge interviews (Horwitz et al., 2013). Other key findings include deficiencies in follow-up appointments and advance discharge planning, and patient understanding of key aspects of postdischarge care (Horwitz et al., 2013). The impetus to implement high-quality discharge instructions stems from the CMS and The Joint Commission's (TJC) Core Measures to meet accreditation and public reporting requirements.

A retrospective cohort study of age and other risk factors for medication discrepancies reported that 96% of all hospitalized patients have at least one medication or dosage change compared with their home medication regimens (Unroe et al., 2010). Only 44% of them were notified of the changes at hospital discharge. A study of older Chinese Americans, who transitioned from hospital to home care, reported that 24.3% of participants were prescribed at least one potentially inappropriate medication (PIM) at hospital discharge, whereas 67.1% experienced at least one medication discrepancy. A positive correlation was found between the occurrence of PIM and medication discrepancy (Hu, Capezuti, Foust, Boltz, & Kim, 2012). It is imperative that during discharge medication reconciliation and instructions, a standard guideline, such as the Beers Criteria for PIM use in older adults, be hardwired in the transition process (Hu, Foust, Boltz, & Capezuti, 2014).

Another medication-related concern is posthospitalization adverse drug events (Kanaan et al., 2013). Among 1,000 hospital discharges, 19% of them involved an adverse drug event within 45 days among older adults discharged home from the hospital (Kanaan et al., 2013). More than half of these events occurred within 2 weeks of discharge. This highlights the importance of medication reconciliation in care transitions (TJC, 2012).

The current Joint Commission National Patient Safety Goals (NPSG; TJC, 2015a) now focus on the safe use of medicines. The goals include patient education, steps on obtaining an accurate list of medications from patients, and encouraging patients to bring a current medication list to physician or provider visits (TJC, 2015a).

A review of literature noted that direct communication between hospital and community physicians was relatively rare (3%–20%), and available discharge summaries at the first primary care visit were low (12%–34%; Kripalani et al., 2007). Additionally, discharge summaries did not always have essential information (i.e., medications and diagnostic results) when available.

The most common example of communication breakdown is when systems of care fail to ensure that the essential elements of the patient's care plan that were developed in one setting are communicated to the next team of clinicians (i.e., preparation for the goals of care delivered in the next setting, arrangements for follow-up appointments and laboratory testing, and reviewing the current medication regimen; Coleman, 2003). Language and health literacy issues and cultural differences exacerbate the communication breakdowns encountered in health care transition (Hu et al., 2014; Naylor & Keating, 2008). The use of pictographs in discharge instructions for older adults with low-literacy skills has been demonstrated to be effective (Choi, 2011).

INTERVENTIONS AND CARE STRATEGIES

Various TCMs have been described in the literature, and several RCTs have tested interventions. Key outcome variables from these RCTs include rehospitalization rate, cost reduction, patient satisfaction, and quality of care. Specific features of the two well-known evidence-based models are summarized in Table 36.1.

The Two Leading Examples of Transitional Care Interventions

The Advanced Practice Nurses TCM

The TCM developed at the University of Pennsylvania provides a comprehensive in-hospital planning and home follow-up for chronically ill, high-risk older adults hospitalized for common medical and surgical conditions (Naylor & Keating, 2008). The central facilitator of the model is an advanced practice TCN, who follows patients from the hospital into their homes and provides services designed to streamline plans of care, interrupt patterns of frequent acute hospital and ED use, and prevent health status decline. Although the TCM is nurse led, it is a multidisciplinary model that includes physician, other nurses, social workers, discharge planners, pharmacists, and other members of the health care team, all of whom implement tested protocols uniquely focused on increasing the ability of patients and their caregivers to manage their care (Naylor et al., 2009).

This model involves advanced practice nurses who assume a primary role in managing patients and coordinating the transition from hospital to home and vice versa. APNs implement a comprehensive discharge planning and home follow-up protocol. A qualitative analysis highlighted the barriers and facilitators faced by advanced practice TCNs and emphasized how individualized approaches, providing care that exceeds the type of care typically staffed and reimbursed by insurers, and advanced clinical judgment influenced positive outcomes in the implementation of TCM (Bradway et al., 2012). When compared with the control group, members of the intervention group had improved physical function, quality of life, and satisfaction with care. People in the intervention group had fewer rehospitalizations during the year after discharge, resulting in a mean savings in total health care costs of $5,000 per patient (Naylor & Keating, 2008). An RCT using the TCM for older adults hospitalized with heart failure showed an increase in the length of time between hospital discharge and readmission or death, reduced the total number of rehospitalizations, and decreased health care costs (Naylor et al., 2004).

Among cognitively impaired older adults, a comparative effectiveness RCT among three models (Augmented Standard Care [ASC], Resource Nurse Care [RNC], and TCM) has demonstrated a statistically significant decrease in mean 30-day rehospitalization per patient using TCM, with similar effects 90 days after the index hospitalization (Naylor et al., 2014).

There are currently more than 300 health care organizations using the TCM in the United States and ongoing program evaluations are in progress (Lucinda Bertsinger, personal communication, May 4, 2015).

The Care Transitions Intervention Model

Coleman, Parry, Chalmers, and Min (2006) developed the Care Transitions Intervention Model through the Division of Health Care Policy and Research at the University of Colorado Health Sciences Center in Denver. This model involves a nurse (social workers and occupational therapists may also serve as a coach) functioning as a "transition coach," who teaches patients self-management skills and ensures their needs are met during a transition between health care settings. The transition coach helps the patients achieve positive outcomes outlined in the four pillars of care transitions intervention (CTI), which include medication self-management, dynamic patient-centered health record keeping, follow-up care with primary physician, and learning how to recognize and respond to red flags that indicate their condition is worsening.

Providing patients with support and tools to participate in their transitional care using this model has been shown to reduce hospital readmissions and associated

TABLE 36.1

Transition Care—Strategies for Implementation

Model	Transition Interface	Target Population	Implementation	Primary Provider	Duration of Follow-Up
Transitional care model (TCM; Bradway et al., 2012; Naylor, 2002; Naylor & Sochalski, 2010; Naylor et al., 2004, 2009; 2013; 2014)	Hospital to home and home to hospital	Sixty-five years or older, high-risk, adults with a variety of medical and surgical conditions (i.e., CHF and comorbidities)	Initial APN visit within 24 hours of hospital admission. APN visits at least daily at index hospitalization. APN home visits (one within 24 hours of discharge), weekly visits during the first month (with one of these visits coinciding with the initial follow-up visit to the patient's physician). Bimonthly visits during the second and third months. Additional APN visits based on patients' needs and APN telephone availability 7 d/wk. If a patient was rehospitalized for any reason during the intervention period, the APN resumed daily hospital visits to facilitate the transition from hospital to home. Use of care management strategies foundational to the quality-cost model of APN transitional care model, including identification of patients' and caregivers' goals, individualized and collaborative plan of care. Implementation of an evidence-based protocol, guided by national heart failure guidelines.	APN in a "manager coordinator" role	From admission to 3 months postdischarge
Care transitions intervention (CTI; Coleman, Mahoney, & Parry, 2005; Coleman, Parry, Chalmers, & Min, 2006; Gardner et al., 2014; Hung & Leidig, 2015)	Hospital to home and hospital to skilled nursing facility	Sixty-five years or older with at least one of the following diagnoses: stroke, congestive heart failure, coronary artery disease, cardiac arrhythmias, COPD, diabetes mellitus, spinal stenosis, hip fracture, peripheral vascular disease, deep venous thrombosis, and pulmonary embolism.	The transition coach first met with the patient in the hospital before discharge. Arrange a home visit, ideally within 48 to 72 hours after hospital discharge. For those patients transferred to a skilled nursing facility, the transition coach telephoned or visited at least weekly. The home visit involved the transition coach, the patient, and the caregiver. The primary goal of the home visit is to reconcile all of the patient's medication regimens (i.e., prehospitalization and posthospitalization medications).	Nurse "transition coach" in a supportive role (social workers and occupational therapists may also serve as a transition coach)	From admission to 28 days postdischarge

(*continued*)

TABLE 36.1

Transition Care—Strategies for Implementation ***(continued)***

Model	Transition Interface	Target Population	Implementation	Primary Provider	Duration of Follow-Up
			Transition coach imparted skills on how to effectively communicate care needs during subsequent encounters with health care professionals. The patient and transition coach rehearsed or role-played effective communication strategies. The transition coach reviewed with the patient any red flags that indicated a condition was worsening and provided education about the initial steps to take to manage the red flags and when to contact the appropriate health care professional. Following the home visit, the transition coach maintained continuity with the patient and caregiver by telephoning three times during a 28-day posthospitalization discharge period. The first telephone call generally focused on determining whether the patient had received appropriate services (i.e., whether new medications had been obtained or durable medical equipment had been delivered). In the two subsequent telephone calls, the transition coach reviewed the patient's progress toward goals established during the home visit, discussed any encounters that took place with other health care professionals, reinforced the importance of maintaining and sharing the personal health record, and supported the patient's role in chronic illness self-management.		

APN, advanced practice nurses; CHF, congestive heart failure; COPD, chronic obstructive pulmonary disease.

costs (Coleman et al., 2006). An RCT found that patients who received this intervention had lower all-cause rehospitalization rates through 90 and 180 days after discharge compared with control patients. At 6 months, mean hospital costs were approximately $500 less for patients in the intervention group compared with controls (Coleman et al., 2006).

A self-care model of the CTI has been demonstrated to improve outcomes in a Medicare fee-for-service population. There were significantly fewer hospital readmissions at 30, 90, and 180 days in the intervention group as compared with those who did not receive the CTI (Parry, Min, Chugh, Chalmers, & Coleman, 2009). When compared with matched internal controls (N = 321), patients who received the CTI had significantly lower utilization in the 6 months postdischarge and lower mean total health care costs ($14,729 vs. $18,779, p = .03). The cost saving per patient receiving the CTI was $3,752 (Gardner et al., 2014). The CTI has been adopted by more than 900 health care organizations in 44 states (Care Transitions Program, 2014).

A qualitative exploration of the value of CTI has demonstrated that patient-centered coaching interventions improved care transitions in chronically ill older adults, particularly because it fostered the perception of a caring relationship, leading to greater patient investment in the program (Parry, Kramer, & Coleman, 2006). A study aimed at understanding the barriers and facilitators for successful implementation of the CTI has been described in the literature (Hung & Leidig, 2015). Several studies have been conducted to explore quality-improvement processes in CTI implementation, particularly its dissemination and sustainability (Bennett, Coleman, Parry, Bodenheimer, & Chen, 2010; Coleman, Rosenbek, & Roman, 2013; Parrish, O'Malley, Adams, Adams, & Coleman, 2009).

Other Transitional Care Interventions

Naylor et al. (2013) describe the core features of transitional care, which can be used as a guide for program planning and implementation to include the following:

- A comprehensive assessment of an individual's health goals and preferences; physical, emotional, cognitive, and functional capacities and needs; and social and environmental considerations.
- Implementation of an evidence-based plan of transitional care.
- Transition care that is initiated at hospital admission but extends beyond discharge through home visit and telephone follow-up.
- Mechanisms to gather and appropriately share information across sites of care.
- Engagement of patients and family caregivers in planning and executing the plan of care.
- Coordinated services during and following the hospitalization by a health care professional with special preparation in the care of chronically ill people, preferably a master's-prepared nurse.

Hospital Discharge Redesign

Randomized trials have demonstrated the benefits of redesigned hospital discharge processes to strengthen timeliness of primary care visits and/or reduce hospital readmissions or emergency room use (Balaban et al., 2008; Jack et al., 2009). The interventions included redesigned discharge forms or individualized information sent to primary care providers, medications with specific forms or having a clinical pharmacist call patients after discharge, and arranging patients' primary care visits and facilitating communication with the outpatient offices (i.e., sharing discharge forms). Redesigned discharge processes led to comparatively lower hospital use, especially for those with prior hospitalizations (Jack et al., 2009) and more patients following up with their primary care providers within 21 days (Balaban et al., 2008).

Other transition models that have been described in the literature include the following:

- Guided Care Model—Developed at Johns Hopkins University. It is described as an enhancement to primary care; it applies the Chronic Care Model (2011), including access to community resources and policies, and self-management (www.guidedcare.org/about-us.asp).
- The Bridge Model—Developed by the Illinois Transitional Care Consortium (ITCC). The model emphasizes addressing social determinants of health, biopsychosocial factors, community-specific focus, and hospital–community collaboration (www.transitionalcare.org/the-bridge-model).
- Better Outcomes for Older Adults through Safe Transitions (BOOST)—A project funded by a grant from the John A. Hartford Foundation that provides face-to-face training and a year of expert mentoring and coaching to customize and implement BOOST interventions based on the TCM and CTI (www.hospitalmedicine.org/Web/Quality___Innovation/Mentored_Implementation/Project_BOOST/Project_BOOST.aspx).
- Geriatric Resources for Assessment and Care of Elders (GRACE)—A model of primary care for low-income

seniors and their primary care physicians (PCPs) aimed to improve the quality of geriatric care, optimize health and functional status, decrease excess health care use, and prevent long-term nursing home placement (graceteamcare.indiana.edu/home.html).

- Project RED (Re-Engineered Discharge)—Supported by grants from the Agency for Healthcare Research and Quality (AHRQ) and the National Institutes of Health's (NIH) National Heart, Lung and Blood Institute (NHBLI), Project RED is a research group at Boston University Medical Center that develops and tests strategies to improve the hospital discharge process and reduce rehospitalization rates (www.bu.edu/fammed/projectred/index.html).
- Interventions to reduce acute care transfers (INTERACT)—This is a quality improvement program to improve early identification, assessment, documentation, and communication about changes in the status of residents in skilled nursing facilities (https://interact2.net).

Whichever model is adopted by the institution and stakeholders, staff training is of vital importance. Competency in cross-site collaboration is critical to the management of patients with complex acute and chronic illnesses.

Starting February 2012, the government established support of community-based transition programs under the PPACA with a $300 million budget. The CCTP, created by Section 3026 of the Affordable Care Act, tests models for improving care transitions from the hospital to other settings and reducing readmissions for high-risk Medicare beneficiaries. The law aims to dedicate transitional care services to patients with multiple chronic conditions or other risk factors associated with a hospital readmission or substandard transition into posthospitalization care. The law also provided funding for pilot projects with incentives for transitional care, including bundled payments to one entity for services by several providers (Health Affairs, 2012). The adaptation of these best practice models into legislation is a fine example of research translated into practice.

Initial evaluation of the federally funded CCTP (47 programs) for the first year of implementation did not show differences in 30-day unadjusted readmission rates between treatment and comparison hospitals. Only 9% of community-based organizations (CBO) achieved some reduction in 30-day readmission (Econometrica, 2014).

This evaluation demonstrates some of the challenges of implementing transitional care. Challenges included hiring qualified personnel and gaining access to hospitals' electronic records and case management data to identify those who are at risk. Critics of the report state that the statistical analysis lacked transparency and does not provide information about what works and what does not work to improve care transitions (Lynn, 2015).

CASE STUDY

Lin Kwon Ying is a 70-year-old widower who lives alone in an apartment in Chinatown. He was mostly independent up until 5 months ago when he started to develop shortness of breath, increasing fatigue, and cough. He has had three admissions for CHF exacerbation. His medical–surgical history includes hypertension (HTN), arthritis, peptic ulcer disease, and gastrointestinal (GI) bleeding. He is back in the hospital for another CHF exacerbation, a small left pleural effusion, and a left leg deep venous thrombosis (DVT). Although cognitively intact, Mr. Ying does not speak English and his family is very much involved in his care. A relative is present during most of the day and evening while he is in the hospital. Most of his relatives have poor English proficiency. Mr. Ying is scheduled for discharge home the next day after being in the hospital for 6 days. His current medications have been satisfactorily reconciled, with the addition of enoxaparin (low-molecular-weight heparin) injection for 7 days and to check with his primary care provider for possible oral anticoagulation. He is to continue taking prehospitalization medications: metoprolol, esomeprazole, multivitamins, and furosemide. The family reports that Mr. Ying uses Chinese liniment to ease his joint pains. He is described by his family as an obedient patient who will do whatever his doctor recommends although he has received little advice or "teachings" during his previous CHF admissions. He cannot recall being informed what lifestyle changes are required of him.

Factors, such as Mr. Ying's rehospitalization, a diagnosis of CHF, language barrier, family involvement, being cognitively intact, and a complex plan of care (i.e., self-injection of enoxaparin), indicate that he is an ideal candidate to receive dedicated transitional care services. If transition-care service were available in the current institution, he would have been referred for a consult on his admission. An assessment would have been made by an advanced practice TCN or "coach," preferably in the presence of the informal caregiver and a staff translator. From this transition-care evaluation, a multidisciplinary plan of care with emphasis on applying best practices, on family involvement, and patient

(continued)

CASE STUDY *(continued)*

teaching by the staff nurses would be drawn up. The handoff report would mention Mr. Ying's status as a transition-care patient and a disease-specific clinical pathway (in his case CHF) would be implemented and followed through during rounds and discharge planning.

To meet TJC standards, all his medication should have been reconciled within 24 hours of his admission and the record placed in a prominent location in his chart. The challenge is to create a medication reconciliation record written in Mr. Ying's own language (Mandarin) that he can take with him on discharge.

At the bedside level, the nurses (mostly bilingual Chinese) provided random or "ambush" teachings when they saw Mr. Ying consuming Chinese food brought from home that they considered high in sodium. No dedicated patient teachings were delivered and no printed materials in the patient's language were provided. How best to standardize patient teachings in acute care transitions is an ongoing challenge. Staff often report not having the time to teach patients and their families. Patient education must be held as an essential and independent nursing intervention. The facility must provide adequate training, not only for the licensed providers (nurses, APNs, physicians, and social workers), but also for the auxiliary staff such as patient-care technicians and other staff members with direct patient contact. Repetition and reinforcement with use of traditional printed media can easily be achieved. Numerous online patient teaching materials are now available. The institution could translate these materials into various languages based on local needs. In Mr. Ying's case, his ability to self-inject enoxaparin should be assessed, reinforced, and documented. During the handoff, the nurse would include the patient's teaching needs and the follow-up needed, focusing on health-promotion content, follow-up appointments, telephone numbers to call for questions, or to report changes in condition.

Depending on the TCM applied, Mr. Ying would receive a home visit from the nurse TCM coordinator or nurse "coach" within 24 hours postdischarge with an individualized and explicit plan of care, including following up on medications, availability of equipment, and self-report of any "red-flag" signs for CHF exacerbation or pulmonary embolism. On his first visit to his primary care provider, he would be accompanied by his transitional care coordinator/coach. In this visit and in future encounters with health care providers, Mr. Ying would be encouraged and provided with the skills necessary for self-advocacy and self-management of his condition. Success would depend on various factors such as patient readiness, literacy, and longitudinal follow-up. From the evidence-based models mentioned in this chapter, follow-up varies from day 1 of hospitalization to up to 3 months postdischarge. Patient follow-up must also address patients' and informal caregivers' satisfaction with the care received. Additionally, the postacute transition care nurse could also coordinate referrals to relevant, local community organizations to provide greater continuity and long-term social support.

SUMMARY

High-quality transitional care is especially important for older adults with multiple chronic conditions and complex therapeutic regimens, as well as for their family caregivers (Naylor & Keating, 2008). Nurses must recognize their critical role in safe transitions. Breakdown in communication is often cited as one of the major causes of poor-quality transitions that may lead to untimely rehospitalization, injury, and poor patient satisfaction. Clinicians and institutions must actively collaborate and communicate to ensure an appropriate exchange of information and coordination of care across health care settings among multiple providers (IOM, 2001).

The current evidence indicates that hospital discharge planning for frail older people can be improved if interventions address family inclusion and education, communication between health care workers and family, interprofessional communication, and ongoing support after discharge (Balaban et al., 2008; Bauer, Fitzgerald, Haesler, & Manfrin, 2009; Jack et al., 2009). In addition, evidence supports the need for close follow-up posthospitalization, including home visits, telephone calls, and timely primary care provider visits. This provides opportunities to reinforce previous patient and family education, especially medications, and monitoring of condition changes (Coleman et al., 2006; Naylor et al., 2004; Rich et al., 1995).

As more evidence on the value of transitional care programs in improving health outcomes emerges, we hope that nurse-sensitive quality indicators of transitional health care delivery will emerge as well as sustainable adaptation of these models. Full implementation and evaluation of the PPACA community-based transition programs is underway. Stakeholders in education, practice, research, and health policy will continue to assess the value of evidence-based transitional care interventions for the ever-growing older adult population.

NURSING STANDARD OF PRACTICE

Protocol 36.1: Transitional Care

I. GOAL

To facilitate the implementation of comprehensive and evidence-based transitional care services as patients transfer between different locations or different levels of care within the same location.

II. OVERVIEW

A. Evidence that both quality and patient safety are jeopardized for patients undergoing transitions across care settings continues to expand (Coleman, Mahoney, & Parry, 2005).
B. Care transitions are clinically dangerous times for older adults with complex health problems (Corbett et al., 2010).
C. Problems encountered with poor transition process can lead to unplanned readmission and ED visits (Jacob & Poletick, 2008).
D. Transitions are particularly vulnerable to breakdowns in care and, thus, have the greatest need for transitional care services (Coleman et al., 2006; Naylor & Keating, 2008).
E. Family caregivers play a major—and perhaps the most important—role in supporting older adults during hospitalization and especially after discharge (Naylor & Keating, 2008).

III. BACKGROUND AND STATEMENT OF PROBLEM

A. Definition

Transitional care: The American Geriatrics Society (2003) defines transitional care as "a set of actions designed to ensure the coordination and continuity of health care as patients transfer between different locations or different levels of care within the same location. Representative locations include (but are not limited to) hospitals, subacute and postacute nursing facilities, the patient's home, primary and specialty care offices, and long-term care facilities. Transitional care, which encompasses both the sending and the receiving aspects of the transfer, is based on a comprehensive plan of care and includes logistical arrangements, education of the patient and family, and coordination among the health professionals involved in the transition" (Coleman & Boult, 2003, p. 549).

Transitional care encompasses a broad range of services and environments designed to promote the safe and timely passage of patients between levels of health care and across care settings (Naylor & Keating, 2008).

B. Etiology and/or epidemiology
   1. Situations likely to result in failed transitions include poor social support, discharge during times when ancillary services are unavailable, uncertain medication reconciliation, depression, and patients' cognitive limitations (Cumbler, Carter, & Kutner, 2008).
   2. Medication errors related to medication reconciliation typically occur at the "interfaces of care"—when a patient is admitted to, transferred within, or discharged from a health care facility (TJC, 2012).
   3. Hospital discharge practices are placing an increasing burden of care on the family caregiver (Bauer et al., 2009).
   4. RCTs of transitional care interventions have been shown to reduce hospital readmissions and health care costs (Arbaje et al., 2010; Coleman et al., 2006; Naylor et al., 2004).
   5. APN interventions in transition care have consistently resulted in improved patient outcomes and reduced health care costs (Naylor, 2002).

IV. PARAMETERS OF ASSESSMENT

A. Patient population that is most likely to benefit from transitional care interventions are those who are diagnosed with one or more of the following diseases: CHF, cognitive impairment (dementia), chronic obstructive pulmonary disease, coronary artery disease, diabetes, stroke, medical and surgical back conditions (spinal stenosis), hip fracture, peripheral vascular disease, cardiac arrhythmias, DVT, and pulmonary embolism (Coleman, Smith, et al., 2004).

(continued)

Protocol 36.1: Transitional Care *(continued)*

B. On admission to an acute care setting, starting at the ED, patient evaluation must include referral of vulnerable older adults for transitional care services.
C. Compliance with TJC standards in medication reconciliation will be used as one of the quality indicators and predictors in overall patient safety.

V. NURSING CARE STRATEGIES

A. A synthesis of best practice guidelines based on existing transitional care models recommends the following key features of a fully developed transition care (TJC, 2012):
   1. Multidisciplinary communication, collaboration, and coordination, including patient/caregiver education, from admission through transition.
   2. Clinician involvement and shared accountability during all points of transition.
   3. Comprehensive planning and risk assessment throughout hospital stay.
   4. Standardized transition plans, procedures, and forms.
   5. Standardized training of every care provider involved.
   6. If a patient is readmitted within 30 days, gain an understanding of the factors associated with the admission.
   7. Evaluation of transitions of care measures
B. Successful and safe transitions demand active patient and informal caregiver involvement. To improve patient advocacy and safety, the nurse can:
   1. Promote the "Speak Up" initiative by the TJC (2015b). The brochure "Planning Your Follow-Up Care" lists patient-centered and safety-focused questions to be asked by the patients of their health care provider before they are discharged from the hospital.
   2. Encourage family involvement and direct them to the "Next Steps in Care" website (see Resources section).
   3. Provide the patient a complete and updated medication reconciliation record. The record should include medications the patient was taking before admission, medications prescribed during hospitalization, and medications to be continued on discharge (TJC, 2015a).
   4. Implement evidence-based interventions to reduce transition-related medication discrepancies (Corbett et al., 2010). Encourage the patients to carry a medication list (i.e., a copy of recent medication reconciliation from a recent hospital admission) and to share the list with any providers of care, including primary care and specialist physicians, nurses, pharmacists, and so forth (TJC, 2012).
C. Critical elements of successful transitions
   1. Team approach and preferably nurse led (APN or specialized nurse; Coleman et al., 2006; Naylor & Keating, 2008)
   2. Active and early family involvement across transitions (Almborg, Ulander, Thulin, & Berg, 2009; Bauer et al., 2009; Naylor & Keating, 2008)
   3. Proactive patient roles and self-advocacy (Coleman et al., 2006)
   4. High-quality and individualized patient and family discharge instructions (Clark et al., 2005)
   5. Apply interventions for improving comprehension among patients with low health literacy and impaired cognitive function (Chugh, Williams, Grigsby, & Coleman, 2009), such as the National Patient Safety Foundation's "Ask Me 3" campaign. Retrieved from www.npsf.org/askme3
   6. Patient and informal caregiver empowerment through education
   7. Commence interventions well before discharge (Bauer et al., 2009)
   8. Elements identified for effective and successful transitions (Coleman, 2003):
      a. Communication between the sending and receiving clinicians regarding a common plan of care
      b. A summary of care provided by the sending institution (to the next care interface providers).
      c. The patient's goals and preferences (including advance directives).
      d. An updated list of problems, baseline physical and cognitive functional status, medications, and allergies.
      e. Contact information for the patient's caregiver(s) and primary care practitioner.
      f. Preparation of the patient and caregiver for what to expect at the next site of care.

(continued)

Protocol 36.1: Transitional Care *(continued)*

g. Reconciliation of the patient's prescribed medications before the initial transfer with the current regimen and communicate changes to the patient and family.
h. A follow-up plan for how outstanding tests and follow-up appointments will be completed.
i. An explicit discussion with the patient and caregiver regarding warning symptoms or signs to monitor that may indicate that the condition has worsened and the name and phone number of who to contact if this occurs.

D. Barriers to successful transitions (Barriers to effective care transitions have been identified at three levels: the delivery system, the clinician, and the patient [Coleman, 2003].)
1. The delivery system barriers
a. The lack of formal relationships between care settings represents a barrier to cross-site communication and collaboration.
b. Lack of financial incentives promoting transitional care and accountability in fee-for-service Medicare; although such incentives exist in Medicare-managed care, most plans do not fully address care integration.
c. The different financing and contractual relationships that facilities have with various pharmaceutical companies impede effective transitions. As patients are transferred across settings, each facility has incentives to prescribe or substitute medications according to its own medication formulary. This constant changing of medications creates confusion for the patient, caregiver, and receiving clinicians.
d. Neither fee-for-service nor Medicare-managed care has implemented quality or performance indicators designed to assess the effectiveness of transitional care.
e. There is a lack of information systems designed to facilitate the timely transfer of essential information.
2. The clinician barriers
a. The growing reliance on designated institution-based physicians (i.e., hospitalists) and productivity pressures have made it difficult for primary care physicians to follow their patients when they require hospitalization or short-term rehabilitation.
b. Nursing staff shortages have forced an increasing number of acute care hospitals to divert patients to other facilities where a completely new set of clinicians, who often do not have timely access to the patients' prior medical records, manages them. SNF staff are also overwhelmed and do not have the time or initiative to request necessary information.
c. Clinicians do not verbally communicate patient information to one another across care settings.
3. The patient barriers
a. Lack of advocacy or outcry from patients for improving transitional care until they or a family member are confronted with the problem firsthand
b. Older patients and their caregivers often are not well prepared or equipped to optimize the care they will receive in the next setting.
c. Patients may have unrealistic expectations about the content or duration of the next phase of care and may not feel empowered to express their preferences or provide input for their care plan.
d. Patients may not feel comfortable expressing their concern that the primary factor that led to their disease exacerbation was not adequately addressed.

E. Evaluation/Expected outcomes
1. Clinician outcomes
a. Increase nurse involvement in leading transition care teams.
b. Enhance staff training of transitional care by a multidisciplinary team.
c. Include patient's transitional care needs during in-hospital handoff.
d. Improve medication reconciliation throughout all transition interfaces.
2. Patient outcomes
a. Improve patient satisfaction, increase involvement in their care during hospitalization and transitions across health care settings.
b. Increase feeling of empowerment in making health care decisions.

(continued)

Protocol 36.1: Transitional Care *(continued)*

c. Reduce rehospitalization and ED visits because of primary disease and comorbidities.
d. Increase timeliness of making follow-up appointments after hospital discharge.

3. Informal caregiver outcomes
   a. Improve informal caregiver satisfaction and exercise proactive roles during transitions across health care settings.
   b. Increase informal caregiver participation in all transition interfaces.
4. Institutional outcomes
   a. Adopt evidence-based TCMs and provide logistic support.
   b. Provide orientation and on-going education on transitional care strategies.
   c. Introduce transitional care content into nursing core curriculum, both at baccalaureate and graduate levels.
   d. Assess transition care interventions as part of hospital accreditation by TJC and CMS.

VI. FOLLOW-UP MONITORING

A. Institute comprehensive and multidisciplinary transition care planning as soon as the patient is admitted and sustain throughout hospitalization.
B. Identify transition care team members and perform periodic role reassessment, including roles of informal caregivers.
C. Incorporate continuous quality-improvement criteria into transition care programs such as monitoring for rehospitalization of targeted older adults, quality of discharge instruction, and medication reconciliation.
D. Develop ongoing transitional care educational programs for both formal and informal caregivers, using high-tech and traditional media.
E. Provide orientation and ongoing education on procedures for reconciling medications to all health care providers, including ongoing monitoring (TJC, 2012).
F. Periodic debriefing of high-risk discharges as a quality-improvement strategy.
G. Improve recognition of condition changes or adverse events caused by medications.
H. Increase patient and caregivers' knowledge concerning actions to take if condition worsens, including a contact information.
I. Consistently transmit hospital discharge summary with all the relevant information to primary care providers (Health Affairs, 2012).

VII. RELEVANT PRACTICE GUIDELINES

A. Ongoing chart and medical records review of patients being considered for discharge or awaiting transition should reflect the QI outlined in the ACOVE under the Continuity and Coordination of Care QI heading ("Assessing Care," 2007).
B. NPSG related to transitions of care include the following (TJC, 2015a): NPSG.03.06.01—Maintain and communicate accurate patient medication information. The elements of performance include the following (TJC, 2015a):
   1. Obtain information on the medications the patient is currently taking when he or she is admitted to the hospital or is seen in an outpatient setting. This information is documented in a list or other format that is useful to those who manage medications.
      a. Current medications include those taken at scheduled times and those taken on an as-needed basis.
      b. It is often difficult to obtain complete information on current medication from a patient. A good-faith effort to obtain this information from the patient and/or other sources will be considered as meeting the intent of the EP.
   2. Define the types of medication information to be collected in non–24-hour settings and different patient circumstances.
      a. Examples of non-24-hour settings include the ED, primary care, outpatient radiology, ambulatory surgery, and diagnostic settings.
      b. Examples of medication information that may be collected include name, dose, route, frequency, and purpose.

(continued)

Protocol 36.1: Transitional Care *(continued)*

3. Compare the medication information the patient brought to the hospital with the medications ordered for the patient by the hospital to identify and resolve discrepancies.
   a. Discrepancies include omissions, duplications, contraindications, unclear information, and changes. A qualified individual, identified by the hospital, does the comparison.
4. Provide the patient (or family as needed) with written information on the medications the patient should be taking when he or she is discharged from the hospital or at the end of an outpatient encounter (i.e., name, dose, route, frequency, and purpose).
   a. When the only additional medications prescribed are for a short duration, the medication information the hospital provides may include only those medications.
5. Explain the importance of managing medication information to the patient when he or she is discharged from the hospital or at the end of an outpatient encounter.
   a. Examples include instructing the patient to give a list to his or her primary care physician; to update the information when medications are discontinued, doses are changed, or new medications (including over-the-counter products) are added; and to carry medication information at all times in the event of emergency situations.

C. Project BOOST provides a toolkit for quality improvement based on best practices, provides technical support to hospitals implementing the toolkit, and provides mentoring to promote long-term sustainability of transitional care programs (Chugh et al., 2009).

D. Position Statement of the American Geriatrics Society Health Care Systems Committee on Improving the Quality of Transitional Care for Persons with complex care needs must be considered in developing practice guidelines (Coleman, 2003)

E. The NTOCC developed the guidebook *Improving on Transitions of Care: How to Implement and Evaluate a Plan* (http://www.ntocc.org/portals/0/pdf/resources/implementationplan.pdf). This book is intended for institutions ready to make changes in the processes their facilities use to send and receive patients. It includes an educational component about transitions of care, an implementation manual, and evaluation methodology that relates to nursing home to ED/hospital and vice versa. This implementation and evaluation plan aims to empower institutions to take the first step at measuring their own performance in transitions of care and identify areas for improvement (NTOCC, 2008). Guidelines on hospital-to-home and ED-to-home transitions are also available from the NTOCC website:
   www.ntocc.org/Portals/0/ImplementationPlan_HospitalToHome.pdf
   www.ntocc.org/Portals/0/ImplementationPlan_EDToHome.pdf

F. The PPACA addresses community-based transition programs under section 3026 of the law. The law provides incentives for hospital to establish and cultivate partnerships with CBOs to implement evidence-based transition care intervention. Proposals and programs must meet the criteria stipulated in the law. These criteria will lend themselves to evaluation of relevant practice guidelines (PPACA, 2010).

ABBREVIATIONS

ACOVE Assessing Care of Vulnerable Elders
APN Advanced practice nurse
BOOST Better Outcomes for Older Adults through Safe Transitions
CBO Community-based organization
CHF Congestive heart failure
CMS Centers for Medicare & Medicaid Services
DVT Deep venous thrombosis
ED Emergency department
EP Elements of performance
NPSG National Patient Safety Goals

(continued)

Protocol 36.1: Transitional Care *(continued)*

NTOCC	National Transitions of Care Coalition
PPACA	Patient Protection and Affordable Care Act
QI	Quality indicator
SNF	Skilled nursing facility
TCM	Transitional care model
TJC	The Joint Commission

ACKNOWLEDGMENT

We are grateful to Richard Hsu for his assistance in the literature search.

RESOURCES

Administration on Aging
http://www.aoa.gov

American Geriatrics Society. (2007). Assessing care of vulnerable elders-3 quality indicators. *Journal of the American Geriatrics Society, 55*(Suppl. 2), S464–S487. *Evidence Level VI.*

American Geriatrics Society Position Statement
http://www.caretransitions.org/documents/improving%20the%20quality%20-%20jags.pdf

Care Transitions Program: Eric Coleman. MD
http://www.caretransitions.org

Centers for Medicare & Medicaid Services: Patient Discharge Checklist
http://www.medicare.gov/Pubs/pdf/11376.pdf

Institute for Healthcare Improvement (IHI)
http://www.ihi.org/resources/Pages/Tools/HowtoGuideImproving-TransitionstoReduceAvoidableRehospitalizations.aspx

Meals on Wheels Association of America
http://www.mowaa.org

National Transitions of Care Coalition: Transition Care Advocacy Group
http://www.ntocc.org

Next Steps in Care: Family Caregivers and Health Professionals Working Together. United Hospital Fund
http://www.nextstepincare.org

NICHE—Transitional Care Models
http://www.nicheprogram.org/transitions

Partnership for Clear Health Communication and National Patient Safety Foundation "Ask Me 3" campaign
http://www.npsf.org/askme3

Robert Wood Johnson Foundation's (RWJF) Speaking Together Toolkit
The toolkit provides advice to hospitals on improving the quality and accessibility of their language services for limited-English-proficient populations.
http://www.rwjf.org/en/library/research.html?pn=Speaking+Together+Toolkit

The Joint Commission: "Speak Up" Initiative
http://www.jointcommission.org/topics/speakup_brochures.aspx

The Joint Commission—Transitions of Care: The Need for a More Effective Approach to Continuing Patient Care.
http://www.jointcommission.org/assets/1/18/Hot_Topics_Transitions_of_Care.pdf

Transition Care Model
http://www.transitionalcare.info/home

Visiting Nurse Associations of America
http://vnaa.org

REFERENCES

Albert, M., McCraig, L. F., & Ashman, J. J. (2013). *Emergency department visits by persons aged 65 and over: United States, 2009–2010.* Retrieved from http://www.cdc.gov/nchs/data/databriefs/db130.pdf. *Evidence Level V.*

Almborg, A. H., Ulander, K., Thulin, A., & Berg, S. (2009). Discharge planning of stroke patients: The relatives' perceptions of participation. *Journal of Clinical Nursing, 18*(6), 857–865. *Evidence Level IV.*

Arbaje, A. I., Maron, D. D., Yu, Q., Wendel, V. I., Tanner, E., Boult, C.,... Durso, S. C. (2010). The geriatric floating interdisciplinary transition team. *Journal of the American Geriatrics Society, 58*(2), 364–370. *Evidence Level II.*

Balaban, R. B., Weissman, J. S., Samuel, P. A., & Woolhandler, S. (2008). Redefining and redesigning hospital discharge to enhance patient care: A randomized controlled study. *Journal of General Internal Medicine, 23*(8), 1228–1233. doi:10.1007/s11606–008-0618–9. *Evidence Level II.*

Bauer, M., Fitzgerald, L., Haesler, E., & Manfrin, M. (2009). Hospital discharge planning for frail older people and their family: Are we delivering best practice? A review of the evidence. *Journal of Clinical Nursing, 18*(18), 2539–2546. *Evidence Level V.*

Bennett, H. D., Coleman, E. A., Parry, C., Bodenheimer, T., & Chen, E. H. (2010). Health coaching for patients with chronic illness. *Family Practice Management, 17*(5), 24–29. *Evidence Level IV.*

Bowles, K. H., Naylor, M. D., & Foust, J. B. (2002). Patient characteristics at hospital discharge and a comparison of home care referral decisions. *Journal of the American Geriatrics Society, 50*(2), 336–342. *Evidence Level III.*

Bradway, C., Trotta, R., Bixby, M. B., McPartland, E., Wollman, M. C., Kapustka H.,... Naylor, M. D. (2012). A qualitative analysis of an advanced practice nurse-directed transitional care model intervention. *The Gerontologist, 52*(3), 394–407. doi:10.1093/geront/gnr078. *Evidence Level IV.*

Care Transitions Program. (2014). *Encouraging patients and family caregivers to assert a more active role during care hand-offs: The care transitions intervention.* Retrieved from http://www.caretransitions.org/documents/Evidence_and_Adoptions_9_2014.pdf. *Evidence Level V.*

Centers for Medicare & Medicaid Services (CMS). (n.d.). *Community-based care transitions program.* Retrieved from http://innovation.cms.gov/initiatives/CCTP/. *Evidence Level VI.*

Choi, J. (2011). Literature review: Using pictographs in discharge instructions for older adults with low-literacy skills. *Journal of Clinical Nursing, 20*(21–22), 2984–2996. doi:10.1111/j.1365–2702.2011.03814.x. *Evidence Level V.*

Chugh, A., Williams, M. V., Grigsby, J., & Coleman, E. A. (2009). Better transitions: Improving comprehension of discharge instructions. *Frontiers of Health Services Management, 25*(3), 11–32. *Evidence Level V.*

Clark, P. A., Drain, M., Gesell, S. B., Mylod, D. M., Kaldenberg, D. O., & Hamilton, J. (2005). Patient perceptions of quality in discharge instruction. *Patient Education and Counseling, 59*(1), 56–68. *Evidence Level IV.*

Coleman, E. A. (2003). Falling through the cracks: Challenges and opportunities for improving transitional care for persons with continuous complex care needs. *Journal of the American Geriatrics Society, 51*(4), 549–555. *Evidence Level V.*

Coleman, E. A., & Boult, C. (2003). Improving the quality of transitional care for persons with complex care needs. *Journal of the American Geriatrics Society, 51*(4), 556–557. *Evidence Level VI.*

Coleman, E. A., Mahoney, E., & Parry, C. (2005). Assessing the quality of preparation for posthospital care from the patient's perspective: The care transitions measure. *Medical Care, 43*(3), 246–255. *Evidence Level IV.*

Coleman, E. A., Min, S. J., Chomiak, A., & Kramer, A. M. (2004). Posthospital care transitions: Patterns, complications, and risk identification. *Health Services Research, 39*(5), 1449–1465. *Evidence Level V.*

Coleman, E. A., Parry, C., Chalmers, S., & Min, S. J. (2006). The care transitions intervention: Results of a randomized controlled trial. *Archives of Internal Medicine, 166*(17), 1822–1828. *Evidence Level II.*

Coleman, E. A., Rosenbek, S., & Roman, S. P. (2013). Disseminating evidence-based care into practice. *Population Health Management, 16*(4), 227–234. doi:10.1089/pop.2012.0069. *Evidence Level IV.*

Coleman, E. A., Smith, J. D., Frank, J. C., Min, S. J., Parry, C., & Kramer, A. M. (2004). Preparing patients and caregivers to participate in care delivered across settings: The care transitions intervention. *Journal of the American Geriatrics Society, 52*(11), 1817–1825. *Evidence Level III.*

Corbett, C. F., Setter, S. M., Daratha, K. B., Neumiller, J. J., & Wood, L. D. (2010). Nurse identified hospital to home medication discrepancies: Implications for improving transitional care. *Geriatric Nursing, 3*(31), 188–196. *Evidence Level IV.*

Cumbler, E., Carter, J., & Kutner, J. (2008). Failure at the transition of care: Challenges in the discharge of the vulnerable elderly patient. *Journal of Hospital Medicine, 3*(4), 349–352. *Evidence Level V.*

Econometrica. (2014). *First annual report: Evaluation of community-based care transitions program.* Retrieved from http://innovation.cms.gov/Files/reports/CCTP-AnnualRpt1.pdf. *Evidence Level V.*

Forster, A. J., Murff, H. J., Peterson, J. F., Gandhi, T. K., & Bates, D. W. (2003). The incidence and severity of adverse events affecting patients after discharge from the hospital. *Annals of Internal Medicine, 138*(3), 161–167. *Evidence Level IV.*

Foust, J. B., Naylor, M. D., Bixby, M. B., & Ratcliffe, S. J. (2012). Medication problems occurring at hospital discharge among older adults with heart failure. *Research in Gerontological Nursing, 5*(1) 25–33. doi:10.3928/19404921–20111206-04. *Evidence Level IV.*

Foust, J. B., Vuckovic, N., & Henriquez, E. (2012). Hospital to home health care transition: Patient, caregiver, and clinician perspectives. *Western Journal of Nursing Research, 34*(2), 194–212. doi:10.1177/0193945911400448. *Evidence Level IV.*

Gardner, R., Li, Q., Baier, R. R., Butterfield, K., Coleman, E. A., & Gravenstein, S. (2014). Is Implementation of the care transitions intervention associated with cost avoidance after hospital discharge? *Journal of General Internal Medicine, 29*(6), 878–884. doi:10.1007/s11606–014-2814–0. *Evidence Level II.*

Health Affairs. (2012). *Improving care transitions.* Retrieved from http://www.healthaffairs.org/healthpolicybriefs/brief.php?brief_id=76. *Evidence Level VI.*

Horwitz, L., Moriarty, J. P., Chen, C., Fogerty, R. L., Brewster, U. C., Kanade, S.,... Krumholz, H. M. (2013). Quality of discharge practices and patient understanding at an academic medical center. *JAMA Internal Medicine, 173*(18), 1715–1722. *Evidence Level IV.*

Hu, S. H., Capezuti, E., Foust, J. B., Boltz, M. P., & Kim, H. (2012). Medication discrepancy and potentially inappropriate medication in older Chinese-American home-care patients after hospital discharge. *American Journal of Geriatric Pharmacotherapy, 10*(5), 284–295. doi:10.1016/j.amjopharm.2012.08.001. *Evidence Level IV.*

Hu, S. H., Foust, J. B., Boltz, M., & Capezuti, E. (2014). Subtypes of potentially inappropriate medications in older

Chinese-Americans during care transitions: cross sectional retrospective study. *International Journal of Nursing Studies, 51*(9), 1221–1229. doi:10.1016/j.ijnurstu.2014.01.014. *Evidence Level IV.*

Hung, D., & Leidig, R. C. (2015). Implementing a transitional care program to reduce hospital readmissions among older adults. *Journal of Nursing Care Quality, 30*(2) 121–129. doi:10.1097/NCQ.0000000000000091. *Evidence Level IV.*

Improving Chronic Illness Care. (2011). *The Chronic Care Model.* Retrieved from http://www.improvingchroniccare.org/index.php?p=The_Chronic_Care_Model&s=212. *Evidence Level V.*

Institute of Medicine (IOM). (2001). *Crossing the quality chasm: A new health system for the 21st century.* Washington, DC: National Academies Press. *Evidence Level VI.*

Jack, B. W., Chetty, V. K., Anthony, D., Greenwald, J. L., Sanchez, G. M., Johnson, A. E.,... Culpepper, L. (2009). A reengineered hospital discharge program to decrease rehospitalization: A randomized trial. *Annals of Internal Medicine, 150*(3), 178–187. *Evidence Level II.*

Jacob, L., & Poletick, E. B. (2008). Systematic review: Predictors of successful transition to community-based care for adults with chronic care needs. *Care Management Journals, 9*(4), 154–165. *Evidence Level I.*

Jencks, S. F., Williams, M. V., & Coleman, E. A. (2009). Rehospitalizations among patients in the Medicare fee-for-service program. *New England Journal of Medicine, 360*(14), 1418–1428. *Evidence Level V.*

Kanaan, A. O., Donovan, J. L., Duchin, N. P., Field, T. S., Tjia, J., Cutrona, S. L.,... Gurwitz, J. H. (2013). Adverse drug events after hospital discharge in older adults: Types, severity, and involvement of Beers Criteria Medications. *Journal of the American Geriatrics Society, 61*(11), 1894–1899. doi:10.1111/jgs.12504. *Evidence Level IV.*

Kessler, C., Williams, M. C., Moustoukas, J. N., & Pappas, C. (2013). Transitions of care for the geriatric patient in the emergency department. *Clinical Geriatric Medicine, 29*(1) 49–69. doi:10.1016/j.cger.2012.10.005. *Evidence Level IV.*

Kripalani, S., LeFevre, F., Phillips, C. O., Williams. M. V., Basaviah, P., & Baker, D. W (2007). Deficits in communication and information transfer between hospital-based and primary care physicians: Implications for patient safety and continuity of care. *Journal of the American Medical Association, 297*(8), 831–841. *Evidence Level IV.*

Levine, C., Halper, D., Peist, A., & Gould, D. A. (2010). Bridging troubled waters: Family caregivers, transitions, and long-term care. *Health Affairs (Project Hope), 29*(1), 116–124. *Evidence Level VI.*

Lynn, J. (2015). *Initial CMS evaluations of readmissions have serious flaws.* Retrieved from http://medicaring.org/2015/01/26/evaluation-flaws. *Evidence Level VI.*

Miller, J. F., Piacentine, L. B., & Weiss, M. (2008). Coping difficulties after hospitalization. *Clinical Nursing Research, 17*(4), 278–296. *Evidence Level IV.*

Moore, B., Levit, B. A., & Elixhauser, A. (2014). *Costs for hospital stays in the United States 2012.* Retrieved from http://www.hcup-us.ahrq.gov/reports/statbriefs/sb181-Hospital-Costs-United-States-2012.pdf. *Evidence Level V.*

National Center for Health Statistics. (2013). *Health, United States, 2013: With special feature on prescription drugs.* Retrieved from http://www.cdc.gov/nchs/data/hus/hus13.pdf#001. *Evidence Level V.*

National Transitions of Care Coalition (NTOCC). (2008). *Improving on transitions of care: How to implement and evaluate a plan.* Retrieved from http://www.ntocc.org/Portals/0/ImplementationPlan.pdf. *Evidence Level VI.*

Naylor, M. D. (2002). Transitional care of older adults. *Annual Review of Nursing Research, 20,* 127–147. *Evidence Level I.*

Naylor, M. D., Bowles, K. H., McCauley, K. M., Maccoy, M. C., Maislin, G., Pauly, M. V., & Krakauer R. (2013). High-value transitional care: translation of research into practice. *Journal of Evaluation in Clinical Practice, 19*(5), 727–733. doi:10.1111/j.1365-2753.2011.01659.x. *Evidence Level III.*

Naylor, M. D., Brooten, D. A., Campbell, R. L., Maislin, G., McCauley, K. M., & Schwartz, J. S. (2004). Transitional care of older adults hospitalized with heart failure: A randomized, controlled trial. *Journal of the American Geriatrics Society, 52*(5), 675–684. *Evidence Level II.*

Naylor, M. D., Feldman, P. H., Keating, S., Koren, M. J., Kurtzman, E. T., Maccoy, M. C., & Krakauer, R. (2009). Translating research into practice: Transitional care for older adults. *Journal of Evaluation in Clinical Practice, 15*(6), 1164–1170. *Evidence Level IV.*

Naylor, M. D., Hirschman, K. B., Hanlon, A. L., Bowles, K. H., Bradway, C.,... Pauly, M. V. (2014). Comparison of evidence-based interventions on outcomes of hospitalized, cognitively impaired older adults. *Journal of Comparative Effectiveness Research, 3*(3), 245–257. doi:10.2217/cer.14.14. *Evidence Level II.*

Naylor, M. D., & Keating, S. A. (2008). Transitional care. *American Journal of Nursing, 108*(Suppl.9), 58–63; quiz 63. *Evidence Level V.*

Naylor, M. D., & Sochalski, J. A. (2010). *Scaling up: Bringing the transitional care model into the mainstream.* The Commonwealth Fund. Retrieved from http://www.commonwealthfund.org/Content/Publications/IssueBriefs/2010/Nov/Scaling-Up-Transitional-Care.aspx. *Evidence Level V.*

Parrish, M. M., O'Malley, K., Adams, R. I., Adams, S. R., & Coleman, E. A. (2009). Implementation of the care transitions intervention: Sustainability and lessons learned. *Professional Case Management, 14*(6), 282–295. doi:10.1097/NCM.0b013e3181c3d380. *Evidence Level IV.*

Parry, C., Kramer, H., & Coleman, E. A. (2006). A qualitative exploration of a patient-centered coaching intervention to improve care transitions in chronically ill older adults. *Home Health Care Services Quarterly, 25*(3–4), 39–53. *Evidence Level IV.*

Parry, C., Min, S. J., Chugh, A., Chalmers, S., & Coleman, E. A. (2009). Further application of the care transitions intervention: Results of a randomized controlled trial conducted in a fee-for-service setting. *Home Health Care Service Quarterly, 28*(2–3), 84–99. doi:10.1080/01621420903155924. *Evidence Level II.*

Patient Protection and Affordable Care Act, 42 U.S.C. § 18001 *et seq.* (2010). Retrieved from http://docs.house.gov/energycommerce/ppacacon.pdf. *Evidence Level VI.*

Rich, M. W., Beckham, V., Wittenberg, C., Leven, C. L., Freedland, K. E., & Carney, R. M. (1995). A multidisciplinary intervention to prevent the readmission of elderly patients with congestive heart failure. *New England Journal of Medicine, 333*(18), 1190–1195. *Evidence Level II.*

The Joint Commission (TJC). (2012). *Transitions of care: The need for a more effective approach to continuing patient care.* Retrieved from http://www.jointcommission.org/assets/1/18/Hot_Topics_Transitions_of_Care.pdf. *Evidence Level VI.*

The Joint Commission. (2015a). *National Patient Safety Goals 2015.* Retrieved from http://www.jointcommission.org/assets/1/6/2015_HAP_NPSG_ER.pdf. *Evidence Level VI.*

The Joint Commission. (2015b). *Speak up initiatives.* Retrieved from http://www.jointcommission.org/speakup.aspx. *Evidence Level VI.*

Unroe, K. T., Pfeiffenberger, T., Riegelhaupt, S., Jastrzembski, J., Lokhnygina, Y., & Colón-Emeric, C. (2010). Inpatient medication reconciliation at admission and discharge: A retrospective cohort study of age and other risk factors for medication discrepancies. *American Journal of Geriatric Pharmacotherapy, 8*(2), 115–26. doi:10.1016/j.amjopharm.2010.04.002. *Evidence Level III.*

U.S. Department of Health and Human Services. (2012). *National hospital discharge survey 2010.* Retrieved from http://www.cdc.gov/nchs/data/nhds/1general/2010gen1_agesexalos.pdf. *Evidence Level V.*

Weiss, A. J., & Elixhauser, A. (2012). *Overview of hospital stays in the United States 2012.* Retrieved from http://www.hcup-us.ahrq.gov/reports/statbriefs/sb180-Hospitalizations-United-States-2012.pdf. *Evidence Level V.*

Weiss, A. J., Wier, L. M., Stocks, C., & Blanchard, L. (2014). *Overview of emergency department visits in the United States, 2011.* Retrieved from http://www.hcup-us.ahrq.gov/reports/statbriefs/sb174-Emergency-Department-Visits-Overview.pdf. *Evidence Level V.*

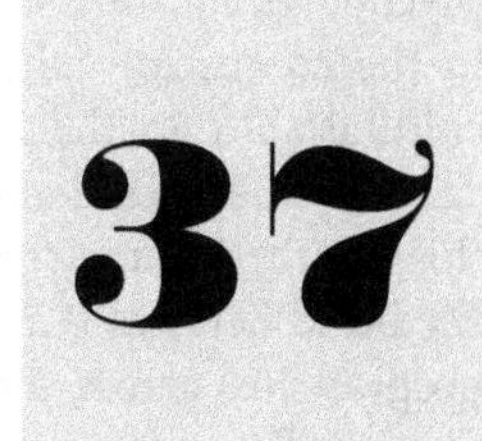

Palliative Care Models

Constance Dahlin

EDUCATIONAL OBJECTIVES

On completion of this chapter, the reader should be able to:

1. Define palliative care and how it differs from hospice
2. Describe how palliative care promotes quality care
3. Discuss the metrics that support the role of palliative care in health care costs
4. Delineate models of palliative care in the United States based on venue

OVERVIEW

The U.S. federal government defines *palliative care* as

> patient and family-centered care that optimizes quality of life by anticipating, preventing, and treating suffering. Palliative care throughout the continuum of illness involves addressing physical, intellectual, emotional, social, and spiritual needs and to facilitate patient autonomy, access to information, and choice. (Centers for Medicare & Medicaid Services, 2008, p. 1; National Quality Forum, 2006, p. 8).

There are specific characteristics that underpin palliative care: (a) care provision and care coordination are interdisciplinary; (b) the circle of care includes patients, families, palliative and non-palliative health providers who collaborate and communicate about care needs; (c) services are available concurrently either with or independent of curative or life-prolonging therapies; (d) patient and family hopes for peace and dignity are supported throughout the course of illness, during the dying process, and after death (National Consensus Project for Quality Palliative Care, 2013).

Palliative care is especially synergistic with nursing (Lynch, Dahlin, Hultman, & Coakley, 2011). The aims of nursing actions are to protect, promote, and optimize health; prevent illness and injury; and alleviate suffering (American Nurses Association, 2010). Nurses have been in the forefront of efforts to improve quality of life for patients and families throughout the experience of illness (Benoliel, 2010). Indeed, the establishment of palliative care in the United States occurred during the late 1970s. Dr. Florence Wald, the dean of Yale School of Nursing, visited Dame Cicely Saunders, founder of the modern hospice movement in England (Dahlin & Mazenec, 2011; Yale Bulletin and Calendar, 2001). Dr. Wald stated that, "hospice care was the epitome of good nursing care, as it enables the patient to get through the end of life on their own terms. It is a holistic approach, looking at the patient as an individual, a human being. The spiritual role nurses play in the end of life process is essential to both patients and families" (Yale Bulletin and Calendar, 2001). On return to Yale University, Dr. Wald developed a comprehensive nursing curriculum of the essential nursing skills necessary in the care of dying patients, including communication, as well as pain and symptom management (Adams, 2010).

This stimulated national interest in hospice care. The comprehensive care model, inclusive of physical,

For a description of evidence levels cited in this chapter, see Chapter 1, "Developing and Evaluating Clinical Practice Guidelines: A Systematic Approach."

psychological, spiritual, and emotional aspects of care in the context of culturally appropriate care, involved a cultural shift to the more technological type of health care in which death and dying were ignored. Reaction to this resulted in the creation of a Centers for Medicare & Medicaid Services (CMS) demonstration project of eight hospice sites across the country. In 1982, the Medicare Hospice Benefit was enacted as part of health care, offering benefits to patients with a terminal illness. At the time, the payment structure was progressive as its fee structure was a capitated rate of a specific rate per day. It became the gold standard by which to measure care of patients with life-limiting illnesses.

To promote consistency and quality, the hospice conditions of participation (CoPs) were created, which specified required services, and characteristics for hospice development and care delivery (CMS, 2008). Eligibility for hospice is determined by meeting three criteria: a life-limiting diagnosis, a prognosis of 6 months or less, and the desire to forgo curative treatment. Four categories of hospice care are available: home care, continuous care, inpatient care, and respite care. Patients and families receive a range of services: medications, equipment, and interdisciplinary care. In programs across the United States, the majority of hospice care centers on care delivery by nurses visiting the patient's home. These nurses represent all levels of practice from nursing assistant, licensed practical or vocational nurse, registered nurse, and advanced practice registered nurse. Patients receive care during benefit period in which attestations are made to the patient's continued eligibility.

CURRENT STATE OF PALLIATIVE CARE

Forty years later, the basic structure of the Medicare Hospice Benefit remains relatively intact. Eligibility criteria are unchanged, but are more tightly monitored. However, benefit periods have been redefined and recertification processes have been added. Revisions have occurred in reimbursement rates, and in the broader expansion of provider roles. Finally, the Affordable Care Act brought the Medicare Hospice Benefit care into the fold of quality-measurement reporting, similar to all other health care delivery providers (Patient Protection and Affordable Care Act [PPACA], 2010).

Hospice remains a wonderful model of care for patients with end-stage illness and who want to forgo curative treatment. The challenge became what to do for patients diagnosed with life-limiting illnesses who either: do not qualify for hospice; want to pursue curative therapies; or for whom hospice means "giving up" (Casarett & Quill, 2007). The answer is palliative care. Palliative care developed for patients diagnosed with serious illness for whom cure is not possible. However, the illness could have a trajectory of years to days.

Palliative care focuses on quality of life and can be provided concurrently with life-sustaining therapies. In the 1990s, a Canadian physician, Balfour Mount, coined the term *palliative care* when he brought hospice concepts of caring for patients with life-limiting illness into the academic hospital setting. The focus was on care for patients with serious illness at diagnosis with the potential for care to occur over longer periods. In the United States, this meant more time than possible under the hospice benefit. More specifically, care was moved upstream to diagnosis to provide care that was consistent with patients' values, preferences, and belief throughout the disease trajectory. Figure 37.1 provides a comparison of hospice and palliative care.

This focus on patient wishes was mandated by the *Study to Understand Prognoses and Preferences for Outcomes and Risks of Treatment* (SUPPORT), the 1995 landmark study that demonstrated a failure to honor patients' preferences (SUPPORT Principal Investigators, 1995). It revealed continued lack of communication between patients and their health care providers about end of life; high levels of pain reported by the seriously ill and dying; and that in spite of expressed patient preferences that suggested otherwise, aggressive care continued (SUPPORT Principal Investigators, 1995).

Other important documents about dying in America spoke to the demand for palliative care. In 1997, the Institute of Medicine published, *Approaching Death*, which set the groundwork for subsequent review and analysis (Institute of Medicine, 1997). This report recommended specialty palliative care, endorsed appropriate utilization of medications for pain and symptom management, supported financial investment in palliative care, and called for health care provider education with the inclusion of palliative care principles and practice in both training programs and curriculum textbooks (Institute of Medicine, 1997). The 2001 Institute of Medicine published *When Children Die* and *Crossing the Quality Chasm*, which called for significant changes in care of dying children and quality in health care (Institute of Medicine, 2001, 2002). These commentaries focused on the need for better care of dying children similar to adults and for better quality measurement in health care. In 2002, Last Acts—a Robert Wood Johnson Foundation supported entity—published a state-by-state report card of end-of-life care in America, which captured a fairly bleak picture of palliative care in the United States (Last Acts, 2002). Clearly, there was work to be done.

A monograph by the National Hospice Work Group (NHWG) and the Hastings Center, in association with

FIGURE 37.1

Comparison of hospice and palliative care.

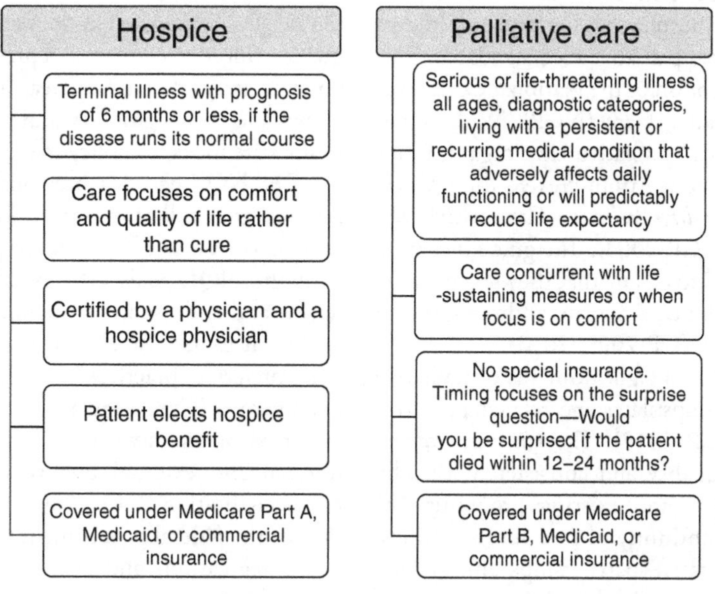

the National Hospice and Palliative Care Organization (NHPCO), titled *Access to Hospice Care: Expanding Boundaries, Overcoming Barriers,* argued for significant changes in access to palliative care, including all ages, all health settings, and all progressive chronic or serious life-threatening illness and injuries (Jennings, Ryndes, D'Onofrio, & Baily, 2003).

In 2013, the Institute of Medicine issued *Delivering High-Quality Cancer Care: Charting a New Course for a System in Crisis* (Institute of Medicine, 2013). There were two palliative care-specific recommendations. The first was that the cancer care team should provide patients and their families with understandable information on cancer prognosis, treatment benefits and harms, palliative care, psychosocial support, and estimates of the total and out-of-pocket costs of cancer care. The second was that in the setting of advanced cancer, the cancer care team should provide patients with end-of-life care consistent with their needs, values, and preferences.

Most recent, the Institute of Medicine released its 2014 report, *Dying in America—Improving Quality and Honoring Individual Preferences Near End of Life* (Institute of Medicine, 2014). The report provided five areas for quality palliative care in achieving health care improvement and moving care upstream to patients with serious illness, rather than focusing on end of life: (a) delivery of person-centered and family-focused palliative care; (b) clinician–patient communication and advance care planning; (c) professional education in palliative care; (d) policies and payment for palliative care; and (e) public education and engagement in palliative care (Institute of Medicine, 2014). Over the years, the field of palliative care has matured and is now available at diagnosis of a serious illness across all settings, populations, and ages.

QUALITY AND PALLIATIVE CARE

Quality is and has been an essential component of palliative care. Within hospice, there are guidelines and standards for care. From the outset of the hospice benefit, CMS created the CoPs, as previously described. Most recently updated in 2011, the CoPs articulate essential components of hospice care such as the eligibility criteria, core services, hospice care planning, benefit periods, and coverage. The NHPCO created 10 quality and practice standards: (a) patient- and family-centered care, (b) ethical behavior and consumer rights, (c) clinical excellence and safety, (d) inclusion and access, (e) organizational excellence, (f) workforce excellence, (g) standards, (h) compliance with laws and regulations, (i) stewardship and accountability, and (j) performance measurement (NHPCO, 2011).

Although hospice had standards of care, palliative care did not. This need for quality, consistency, and access was the backdrop to a national discussion regarding national guidelines for palliative care. In 2001, an interdisciplinary meeting of palliative, hospice, and end-of-life leaders convened to create national palliative care standards. This meeting served as the inception of the National Consensus Project for Quality Palliative Care (NCP). With representation from the national palliative care organizations in the United States, this consortium created the *Clinical Practice Guidelines for Quality Palliative Care*, which was first published in 2004 (NCP, 2004). The guidelines were updated in 2009 and 2013 to ensure that they reflected the maturity of the field, health care reform, and the growing literature within the field (NCP, 2009, 2013).

The document delineates eight domains of palliative care (Table 37.1) and encapsulates the related palliative care-related research (NCP, 2013). The *Clinical Practice Guidelines* (a) promote quality and consistency, thereby reducing variation in new and existing programs; (b) develop and encourage continuity of care across settings; and (c) facilitate collaborative partnerships among palliative care programs, community hospices, as well as a wide range of other health care delivery settings (NCP, 2013). Rather than set minimally acceptable practices, ideal practices and goals for quality palliative care service delivery are offered. The *Clinical Practice Guidelines* offer a framework for the future of palliative care in serving as a manual or blueprint to create new programs, guide developing programs, and set high expectations for excellence for existing programs.

In 2006, the National Quality Forum (NQF) adopted the *Clinical Practice Guidelines for Quality Palliative Care* within the document *A National Framework and Preferred Practice for Palliative and Hospice Care Quality* (NQF, 2006). The NQF is a private, nonprofit, membership organization created to develop and implement a national strategy for health care quality improvement. Its mission is to improve American health care through the endorsement of consensus-based national standards for measurement and public reporting of health care performance data. Because the NQF is recognized as the national leader in health care quality improvement and representative of the broadest possible array of practice areas and topics, it offered palliative care both legitimacy and recognition within a broad health care focus, to policy makers and payers.

The NQF had not previously addressed the topic of hospice and palliative care. Given the consensus-based process of the guideline development, it was consistent with the NQF goals. The NCP requested the NQF to review and endorse the guidelines. The NQF appointed a Technical Expert Panel to review the guidelines and propose preferred practices. The result was the *Framework* document, which formulated palliative care standards and preferred practices with implications for reimbursement, internal and external quality measurement, regulation, and accreditation (NQF, 2006). With important recognition of the federal government as the basis for reimbursement, regulation, and accreditation, the significance of this endorsement cannot be overstated. See Appendix 37.1 for the correspondence between the NCP *Clinical Practice Guidelines* and the NQF Preferred Practices.

The NQF has continued to recognize the importance of quality palliative care. In 2008, the National Priorities Partnership (NPP)—a consortium of U.S. health care organizations working with NQF, identified palliative care as one of six top priorities for improving the U.S. health system (NPP, 2008). They developed a National Priority Partners Palliative and End-of-Life Work Group to consider next steps. NPP released the report, *National Priorities & Goals—Aligning Our Efforts to Transform America's Healthcare*. It identified palliative care and end-of-life care as one of the six national priorities that, if addressed, would significantly improve the quality of care delivered to Americans (NPP, 2008). In 2010, the NPP convened a palliative and end-of-life meeting to develop strategies to promote palliative care, including quality-improvement stakeholders, insurers, consumer groups, certification groups, professional groups, and education institutions (NPP, 2010).

Within the federal reporting structures of health care reporting, palliative measure development remains a priority. In 2011, as required by the Affordable Care Act, NQF established the Measure Applications Partnership (MAP), as a public–private partnership entity that reports directly to the U.S. Department of Health and Human Services secretary and advises on quality measures for public reporting across all health care settings and performance-based payment programs (National Quality Forum, 2013). They evaluate

TABLE 37.1

Eight Domains of Palliative Care

Domain 1: Structure and Processes of Care
Domain 2: Physical Aspects of Care
Domain 3: Psychological and Psychiatric Aspects of Care
Domain 4: Social Aspects of Care
Domain 5: Spiritual, Religious, and Existential Aspects of Care
Domain 6: Cultural Aspects of Care
Domain 7: Care of the Patient at the End of Life (changed from Care of Imminently Dying Patient)
Domain 8: Ethical and Legal Aspects of Care

Source: National Consensus Project for Quality Palliative Care (2013).

measures for CMS for public reporting and reimbursement. There is palliative representation on all of these groups, which promotes and supports palliative-related measures.

A Palliative Care and End-of-Life Care Endorsement Maintenance Measures Project was established in 2011. Over the course of a year, it evaluated 22 measures that addressed assessment and management of conditions and symptoms in patients, including pain, dyspnea, weight loss, weakness, nausea, serious bowel problems, delirium, and depression; patient- and family-centered palliative and hospice care focused on psychosocial needs and care transitions; and patient, caregiver, and family experiences of care (NQF, 2012b). In February 2012, the NQF endorsed 14 quality measures for palliative and hospice care (NQF, 2012a, 2012b). The goal of these measures is to ensure the provision of high-quality palliative care and end-of-life care. The measures, some of which are applicable to all clinical settings and provider types, will help hospice and palliative care providers to improve quality of care and generate ideas for future research.

One of the MAP workgroups, the Post-Acute/Long Term Care (PAC/LTC) workgroup, is responsible for reviewing and advising on hospice and palliative care measures. However, there are measures that occur within the Clinician Workgroup and the Hospital Workgroup. The June 2012 MAP Final Report on Performance Measurement Coordination Strategy for Hospice and Palliative Care states that, "while measurement in this area is new, MAP suggests a phased approach that emphasizes clinically-focused measures at first, but quickly expands to more measures that follow the patient and their full set of experiences rather than the setting or fragments of a patient's care (often referred to in this report as 'cross-cutting')" (NQF, 2012a, p. 3). The MAP report also addresses quality reporting in palliative care, by stating "while there is not a formal quality reporting program for palliative care, settings in which palliative care is provided (e.g., hospitals, home health) are required to participate in federal quality initiatives" (NQF, 2012a, p. 4).

Another project on quality is the joint program between the American Academy of Hospice and Palliative Medicine and the Hospice and Palliative Nurses Association, *Measuring What Matters* (Dy et al., 2015). As the population ages and the demand for this type of care grows, the ability to assess quality throughout the country and across care settings is increasingly important. This project promotes the use of validated indicators in order to ensure consistent quality measures that can ultimately be used for benchmarking, comparison, and quality improvement (Dy et al., 2015). They have identified 10 measures that range from a complete assessment (including physical, psychological, social, spiritual, and functional needs) to a plan for managing pain and shortness of breath to having patients' treatment preferences followed. There is planning to promote further measurement as the field develops.

Finally, in terms of quality, palliative certification for both health care programs and providers demonstrates specialty practice. Speciality certification is now possible in each of the core services—chaplaincy, medicine, nursing, and social work; as well as hospital-based programs (AAHPM, 2015; Board of Chaplaincy Inc. [BCCI], 2015; Hospice and Palliative Credentialing Center [HPCC], 2015; National Association of Social Workers [NASW], 2015). Different discipline-specific organizations are responsible for certification, which occurs either by examination or meeting standards of practice. See Table 37.2 for a list of disciplines with the association responsible and the eligibility for certification.

In 2011, The Joint Commission (TJC) created voluntary advanced certification in palliative care for inpatient palliative care teams (TJC, 2011). This certification is based on the NCP guidelines. There are currently some 90 hospitals that are certified and information can be found on TJC website. However, currently both TJC and the Community Health Accreditation Partner (CHAP) are working on certification for community-based programs. Both TJC and CHAP are planning to create these from the NCP guidelines: TJC will continue to provide voluntary certification and CHAP will oversee accreditation.

OUTCOMES

Over the past 10 years, research has demonstrated the quality of palliative care. For years, many hospice and palliative providers have intuitively known that they promoted quality of life. However, there were no studies to support these claims. Several studies have now demonstrated better quality of life and survival in patients with the involvement of palliative care (Bakitas et al., 2009; Temel et al., 2010). Other studies in patients with non-cancer diagnoses in outpatient settings have also demonstrated more comprehensive care, higher satisfaction rates, and deaths at home (Brumley et al., 2007; Rabow, Hauser, & Adams, 2004; Rabow, Schanche, Petersen, Dibble, & McPhee, 2003).

In 2012, the American Society of Clinical Oncology (ASCO) released a statement stating that palliative care should be offered to patients with advanced stages of lung cancer as well as for metastatic disease (Smith et al., 2012). At the same time, the American College of Surgeons in collaboration with the Commission on Cancer issued a statement that palliative services should be offered to all patients across the cancer trajectory (American College of Surgeons, 2012). In cardiovascular care, there is a new emphasis on palliative care. In 2014, the American Heart Association

TABLE 37.2
Health Disciplines With Palliative Care Specialty Certification

Discipline	Organization	Certification Process	Credential	Eligibility
Chaplaincy	Association of Professional Chaplaincy	Application	BCCPC	3 years of clinical experience in hospice/palliative care 10-page essay documenting hospice and pallaitive care chaplain competencies 15 hours of CE in hospice and palliative care
Medicine	American Academy of Hospice and Palliative Medicine	Examination		1-year fellowship
Nursing	Hospice and Palliative Credentialling Center	Examination	CHPLN	LPN /LVN 500 hours in 1 year or 1,000 hours in 2 years of specialty palliative nursing practice
			CHPN	RN 500 hours in 1 year or 1,000 hours in 2 years of specialty palliative nursing practice
			ACHPN	APRN 500 hours in 1 year or 1,000 hours in 2 years of specialty palliative nursing practice
Social Work	National Association of Social Work and the National Hospice and Palliative Care Organization	Application	CHP-SW	BSW—A bachelor's degree in social work from an accredited university 3 years of practice 20 CEUs in hospice or palliative care
			ACHP-SW	MSW—master's degree in social work from an accredited college or university program is required 3,000 hours of post MSW practice 20 CEUs in H&P care Reference review of advanced SW palliative competencies

ACHPN, advanced certified hospice and palliative nurse; ACHP-SW, advanced certified hospice and palliative social worker; APRN, advanced practice registered nurse; BCC-HPCC, board certified chaplain-hospice/palliative care certified; CE, continuing education; CEU, continuing-education units; CHPLN, certified hospice and palliative licensed practical/vocational nurse; CHPN, certified hospice and palliative nurse; CHP-SW, certified hospice and palliative social worker; H&P, hospice and palliative; LPN/LVN, licensed practical nurse/licensed vocational nurse; RN, registered nurse; SW, social work.

and the American Stroke Association issued joint guidelines for palliative care in heart disease and stroke (Holloway et al., 2014). It recognized that palliative care should begin with the onset of such an event. In particular, this includes advance care planning, goal setting, and family support, especially for surrogate decision makers. As more research demonstrates the value and benefit of palliative care, it is expected that more professional organizations will release guidelines specific to integrating palliative care.

MODELS ACROSS HEALTH CARE VENUES

As the definition of palliative care has broadened to patients with serious illness, the potential to affect a range of populations is apparent. The NCP *Clinical Practice Guidelines* describe how a serious or life-threatening illness is assumed to encompass populations of patients at all ages within the broad range of diagnostic categories, living with a persistent or recurring medical condition that adversely affects their daily functioning or will predictably reduce life expectancy.

Therefore, palliative care covers a broad spectrum of care. It is "operationalized through effective management of pain and other distressing symptoms, while incorporating psychosocial and spiritual care with consideration of patient/family needs, preferences, values, beliefs, and culture. Evaluation and treatment should be comprehensive and patient-centered with a focus on the central role of the family unit in decision making. Palliative care affirms life by supporting the patient and family's goals for the future, including their hopes for cure or life-prolongation, as well as their hopes for peace and dignity throughout the course of illness, the dying process, and death" (NCP, 2013, p. 9).

As a model, palliative care has several tenets set forth by the NCP (Table 37.3). Both clinical model and service

TABLE 37.3
Tenets of Palliative Care

1. Palliative care is patient- and family-centered care.
2. There is comprehensive palliative care with continuity across health settings.
3. Early introduction of palliative care concepts should begin at diagnosis of a serious or life-threatening illness by the primary team. Specialist consultation may be offered as well.
4. Palliative care may be offered concurrent with or independent of curative or life-prolonging care. Patient and family hopes for peace and dignity are supported throughout the course of illness, during the dying process, and after death.
5. Palliative care is interdisciplinary and collaborative. Patients, families, palliative care specialists, and other health care providers collaborate and communicate about care needs.
6. Palliative care team members have clinical and communication expertise.
7. The goal of palliative care is the relief of physical, psychological, emotional, and spiritual suffering of patients and families.
8. Palliative care should focus on quality care.
9. There should be equitable access to palliative care services.

Adapted from the National Consensus Project (2013).

delivery models have been identified (Luckett et al., 2014). Clinically, they range from case management, to liaison, integrated care, and consultative models. Service delivery ranges from clinical networks, managed care networks, and collaboration among community providers (Luckett et al., 2014). Service delivery models have complex considerations and financial implications and are beyond the scope of this chapter. Clinical models range from models in the hospital, home, office, and long-term care setting and are discussed as follows.

Every palliative model provides comprehensive assessment in all domains (physical, spiritual, emotional, and social) related to quality of life. There is simultaneous evaluation and reevaluation of initiation of interventions to manage any of these aspects of care (Partridge et al., 2014). Specifically, palliative care addresses pain and symptoms, psychosocial distress, quality of life, and care preferences. This may look different depending on the diagnosis. The National Comprehensive Cancer Network suggests the following criteria for palliative care: (a) uncontrolled symptoms, (b) moderate to severe distress related to diagnosis and treatment, (c) serious comorbid physical and psychosocial conditions, (d) life expectancy less than 6 months, and (e) patient concerns about the course of disease and/or their treatment options, including when these are expressed by the family (Levy et al., 2014; National Comprehensive Cancer Network, 2012).

Palliative care is an essential aspect of health care, it occurs across a variety of settings. The venue will determine the model of care and the financial aspects of program development. Venues can be based on a health system, a hospital, an office, a long-term care setting, a hospice organization, a home health agency, and in the community. With all the models, there is the overarching principle of giving the right care to the right patients in the right settings.

Although hospice is considered the gold standard of care, it is a subset of palliative care. First of all, it focuses on end-of-life care as a result of the eligibility requirements of a prognosis of 6 months or less without curative measures. Patients must sign onto the benefit. Patients can receive care in the home, nursing home, hospice unit, or residential setting with different levels of intensity depending on the pain and symptom management. Palliative care programs can vary because there are no restrictions of prognosis, treatment direction, election of benefit, or necessity of specific interventions (Table 37.4).

There are positive and negative aspects to various hospice and palliative care models (Wiencek & Coyne, 2014). Hospital-based models are the most defined. Indeed, over the past 15 years, the focus has been on inpatient palliative care. These are inpatient consultative services that consist of an interdisciplinary team. They vary in resources and acuity by academic medical center, community hospital, rural hospital, and essential access hospital. These programs must have interdisciplinary teams; in particular, a team for each of the core service disciplines. These programs may be led by any one of the team members, but are often led by physicians or advanced practice registered nurses.

There can be a range of clinical responsibilities after consultation. This includes consultation only in which recommendations of pharmacological and nonpharmacological interventions are offered; comanagement of a specific pain or symptom in which the team writes orders and prescriptions; assuming the role of a primary care provider responsible for all the care, not just the serious diagnosis; or a mix of all clinical responsibilities. The financial structure is based on billing and reimbursement through Medicare, Medicaid, and other commercial payers, as well as hospital support. The palliative care team may see a range of patients all over a hospital or have specific beds or even a unit.

Hospital-based palliative care models are often the easiest to implement as they usually build off of current hospital structures. They are, by nature, crisis oriented and demand close to 24/7 access. They demand, however, the collaboration of an interdisciplinary team, which may or may not be under the auspices of a palliative care department. The benefits may be lower costs, earlier discharge, higher satisfaction, and better pain management (Casarett et al., 2008).

Office-based palliative care may offer more continuity to longer term issues. Models include outpatient or ambulatory

TABLE 37.4
Palliative Care Models

Model	Payment Structure	Clinical Responsibility	Team Composition	Referral/Duration/Limitation
Hospital-based palliative care				
Hospital based (academic medical center, community hospital, rural hospital, critical or essential access hospital)	Medicare B Medicaid Commercial	Consultative, comanagement, or primary care role	Medicine, nursing, social work, and chaplaincy	■ By referral of primary attending (APRN, DO, MD, PA), other disciplines, or self-referral ■ Length of hospital stay ■ May not cross to other settings
Community-based palliative care				
Office based (independent clinic, outpatient clinic, ambulatory clinic)	Medicare B Medicaid Commercial	Consultative, comanagement, or primary care role	Medicine, nursing, social work, and chaplaincy	■ By referral of primary attending provider (APRN, DO, MD, PA), other disciplines, or self-referral ■ Duration of disease/condition ■ May move easily cross settings
Home based (home, rest home, group home, senior housing, shelter)	Medicare B Medicaid Commercial	Comanagement or primary care role	Medicine and nursing	■ By referral of primary attending (APRN, DO, MD, PA), other disciplines, service organizations, or self-referral ■ Duration of disease/condition ■ Center of care coordination
Palliative care in long-term care settings				
Skilled nursing facility (skilled facility, long-term acute care, nursing home)	Medicare B Medicaid Commercial	Consultative comanagement	Medicine and nursing	■ By referral of primary attending (APRN, DO, MD, PA), other disciplines, service organizations, or self-referral ■ Duration of disease/condition ■ Center of care coordination
Assisted living	Medicare B Medicaid Commercial	Comanagement and/or primary care role	Medicine and nursing	■ By referral of primary attending (APRN, DO, MD, PA), other disciplines, service organizations, or self-referral ■ Duration of disease/condition ■ Center of care coordination

APRN, advanced practice registered nurse; DO, doctor of osteopathy; MD, medical doctor; PA, physician assistant.

care clinics as well as independent clinics in the community or clinics run by a hospice. These clinics may be imbedded in another specialty clinic such as oncology, heart failure, amyotrophic lateral sclerosis, liver failure, kidney failure, or gerontology. There are also stand-alone or free-standing palliative care clinics. These programs include either interdisciplinary or multidisciplinary teams depending on the structure. Often, however, they lack the full scope of an interdisciplinary team. The nature of these programs is care over a longer period of time with care coordination. The focus is on continuity and relationship building to promote and avoid both emergency visits and hospitalizations. Clinical responsibility of the palliative care team is most often comanagement of pain and symptoms as well as assuming primary care roles or a mix of comanagement and primary care.

Many office-based programs developed from hospital teams. However, many are growing in the community separate from hospital teams. Office-based models necessitate different resources depending on the type of practice and ownership—outpatient clinic as part of a hospital, ambulatory clinic as part of a health system, or independent clinic as part of a hospice or palliative care provider. Resources depend on the financial structure of the clinic, in particular whether it is hospital or system owned, independent, or supported philanthropically. Often, the primary providers are physicians and advanced practice providers because their visits are reimbursable under Medicare, Medicaid, and commercial insurance. The benefits are reduction in emergency room admissions, hospital admissions, and better patient satisfaction.

Home-based palliative care models are growing. The focus is coordinating care from service agencies and delivering clinical care in the home. These programs work well for geriatric patients who have avoided the clinic or hospital for any care, but also patients who are too sick to travel to

TABLE 37.5

Current Palliative Care Delivery Under Medicare and Medicaid Hospice and Home Health Benefits

Hospice	Medicare A—Hospice Benefit Medicaid Hospice Benefit varies by state	Mostly primary care role	Mandated by conditions of participation Medicine, nursing, social work, and chaplaincy	Limited by 6-month eligibility
Hospice benefit–based palliative care	Medicare A—limited palliative care under the Hospice Benefit Medicaid–may be included in Hospice Benefit	Consultative or comanagement	Physician and or APRN	Medicare hospice benefit allows three visits
Home health benefit–based palliative care	Medicare B–under home care Medicaid–may be included in Home Health Benefit	Consultative or comanagement	Nurse	Must be homebound

APRN, advanced practice registered nurse.

appointments. It is essential for these programs to coordinate with service agencies such as Councils on Aging, Meals on Wheels, Parish Nurses, and so on. Some programs have clinicians who visit patients whom they have seen in the hospital. Other program enroll patients from the community who lack primary care providers. Clinical responsibility is most often held by primary providers, although there may be comanagement of pain and symptoms as well. These teams are multidisciplinary in nature, depending on workforce availability and financial structure. Reimbursement occurs through Medicare, Medicaid, and commercial payers.

There is wide variability in home-based models differentiated by structure and services. Their benefit is keeping people in their homes and community. However, because of reimbursement and revenue streams, home-based models may not encompass a full interdisciplinary team. In addition, depending on the geography of the area covered, there may be issues in the number of patients seen or financial implications of transportation. However, there is research to suggest that home-based palliative care decreases health care costs, reduces 30-day hospital readmission rates, and increases patient satisfaction (Brumley et al., 2007; Enguidanos, Vesper, & Korenz, 2012; Kerr & Cassel, 2014).

Palliative care in the long-term care setting is less developed and not well delineated (Ersek & Carpenter, 2013). Broadly, it includes consultation to patients in the skilled nursing facility, assisted living, nursing home, and chronic and acute rehabilitation settings. Although there is research about pain and symptom management for this population as well as advance care planning, there are few commentaries on models (Ersek & Carpenter, 2013). It has been suggested that outside of hospice, there are two models—external consultative teams and internal consultative teams (Ersek & Stevenson, 2013). Either model includes a variety of interdisciplinary team members to provide consultation to these complex populations. However, palliative care initiatives in nursing homes are beset with the challenges of high staff turnover, staff shortages of qualified individuals, regulatory requirements, reimbursement, and various health policies (Strumpf, Tuch, Stillman, Parrish, & Morrison, 2008).

Within a health system, such as an accountable care organization (ACO) or Patient-Centered Medical Home (PCMH), care is focused on keeping the patient out of the hospital. This palliative care model focuses on primary palliative care in which there is a strong communication and care coordination across the system. In particular, there is a major presence of nurse case management with a focus on advance care planning. There is constant assessment of the needs of the patient and the right services. Here, quality care for patients with serious illness may include both hospital-, office-, and home-based palliative care. However, the model for palliative care will emanate from primary care practices.

Finally, there are palliative care models that occur broadly under Medicare programs such as under the Hospice or Home Health Benefit (Table 37.5). However, there are limitations because of Medicare regulations. First, under the Medicare Hospice or Home Health Benefit, palliative care may lack interdisciplinary care because nurses most often provide the care alone. Palliative care under the Medicare Hospice Benefit is time limited to only a few consultation visits. Palliative care under Home Health is limited by the necessity that the patient qualify for homebound status. Moreover, hospices and home health agencies must attend to antitrust issues. Therefore, palliative care programs under Hospice and Home Health Benefits are restricted in their breadth and scope.

CASE STUDY

Sally Martin, APRN-BC, ACHPN, is a palliative nurse practitioner who works in a health care system. She performs palliative care consultations for patients with serious illness in a community palliative care clinic 3 days a week. She then sees patients in the home 2 days a week. She receives referrals from all eligible licensed professionals. She provides consultation documentation for new patients as well as follow-ups. As part of her evaluation, she performs the Edmonton Symptom Assessment System to determine symptoms and distress. She orders diagnostics as necessary. In order to implement a care plan, she collaborates with the primary care providers. She writes orders and prescriptions for pain and symptom management when she makes recommendations and develops a palliative care plan. Her clinical responsibilites include both a consultative role in the clinic and a primary care role in the home. She offers 24/7 coverage during the week. On the weekends, the covering provider for primary care covers both her clinic patients and her home patients. She bills for her services under Medicare Part B professional billing for a palliative care encounter, as well as symptoms, and a primary diagnosis. There are occasions in which she visits a hospitalized patient to provide continuity in terms of goals of care. The health system tracks her visits and her patient satisfaction scores are high and her symptom assessment data demonstrate that patients symptoms are managed within 48 hours on average. The patient satisfaction scores demonstrate better quality of life and better communication with her care plan. She is able to recoup 40% of her salary in billing and reimbursement. However, her care offers the hospital cost savings of around $400,000 by preventing 30-day readmission hospitalizations and emergency visits.

SUMMARY

Palliative care is an important model of care. It promotes quality patient- and family-centered care that incorporates patient and family values and preferences of care in the settings where patients and families prefer to receive care. Nurses have a prominent role in all palliative care models as direct providers of care. Moreover, nursing is founded on the principles of palliative care. As health care reform continues, palliative care will be essential in promoting patient-centered, family-focused care in accordance with patient preferences. Palliative care promotes the notion of the right care at the right time in the right place. It has been demonstrated that palliative care increases patient quality of life, satisfaction, improves pain and symptom management, and reduces cost of care. Although no one model of palliative care fits every setting, palliative care is established in hospitals, offices, and the home. More work is needed to better understand palliative care in the long-term care setting.

RESOURCES

Certification

Community Health Accreditation Partner (CHAP)
Specialty certification/accreditation-Community-based programs
http://www.chapinc.org

Hospice and Palliative Credentialing Center
Specialty certification in hospice and palliative nursing—Nursing assistant, licensed practical/vocational nurse, registered nurse, advanced practice registered nurse, pediatrics
Non-Nursing—Hospice and palliative care administrator, perinatal loss
hpcc.advancingexpertcare.org/

The Joint Commission (TJC)
Specialty certification in palliative care
1. Hospital-based programs
2. Hospices and home health agencies

http://www.jointcommission.org/certification/palliative_care.aspx

Continuing Education

End of Life Nursing Education consortium (ELNEC)
Curriculum offerings—Core, pediatrics, geriatrics, veterans, critical care, APRN, international *products*—articles about ELNEC and nursing education, *15th Anniversary Report*
www.aacn.nche.edu/elnec

Palliative Care Communication
Curriculum—COMFORT Communication
Products—Online communication curriculum, *Communication in Palliative Nursing, Textbook of Palliative Care Communication*
http://pccinstitute.com/home/about-us/

Palliative Care Standards

National Consensus Project for Quality Palliative Care (NCP)
Clinical practice guidelines for quality palliative care, 3rd ed., 2013
1. Defines the domains and characteristics for quality palliative care across all settings in the United States.
2. Serves as the basis for standard development by *The Joint Commission* (TJC) and Community Health Accreditation Partner (CHAP).

http://www.nationalconsensusproject.org

National Quality Forum (NQF)
A National Framework and Preferred Practices for Care and Hospice Care—A Consensus Report 2006
Develops palliative care preferred practices based on the *NCP Clinical Practice Guidelines.*
National Priorities Partnership
National Priorities & Goals—Aligning Our Efforts to Transform America's Healthcare
Palliative Care and End-of-Life Convening Meeting Synthesis Report
Measure Applications Partnership—Performance Measurement Coordination Strategies for Hospice and Palliative Care Final Report
Palliative Care and End-of-Life Care—A Consensus Report
https://www.qualityforum.org

Professional Organizations—Non-Nursing

American Academy of Hospice and Palliative Medicine (AAHPM)—individual membership necessary
Online education—E-Learning
Conferences—Annual Assembly*Journals*
1. *Journal of Palliative Medicine*
2. *Journal of Pain and Symptom Management*

Products—Palliative care content—UNIPAC, position statements, AAHPM smart brief on current research and current events, primer of palliative care
www.aahpm.org

American Society of Clinical Oncology (ASCO)—individual membership necessary
Online Education—ASCO Learning
Conference—Palliative Care in Oncology Symposium
Journals
1. *Journal of Clinical Oncology*
2. *Journal of Oncology Practice*

www.asco.org

California Health Care Foundation—no membership necessary
Free products
1. *Snapshots of Palliative Care Practices*
2. *Up Close: A Field Guide to Community-Based Palliative Care in California*
3. *Innovative Models in Palliative Care Fact Sheet*
4. *Weaving Palliative Care Into Primary Care: A Guide for Community Health Centers*

http://www.chcf.org/topics/end-of-life-and-palliative

Center to Advance Palliative Care (CAPC)—organizational membership necessary
Online education—Clinical and technical assistance courses for palliative care delivery and program development.
Conferences—CAPC seminar, webinars, virtual office hours
Free products—Palliative Care Fast Facts (previously at University of Wisconsin EPERC site), Team Wellness Monograph, State-by-State Report Card
www.capc.org

NHPCO—organizational membership necessary
Online education—E-Learning
Conferences—Clinical Team and Pediatric Conference, Management and Leadership Conference

Networking
Products—Newsbriefs, position statements, technical assistance
www.nhpco.org

Professional Organizations—Nursing

American Association of Critical Care Nurses—individual membership necessary
Online education—Self-Assessment: Palliative and End-of-Life Care
Conferences—National Training Institute (NTI)
Journals
1. *Critical Care Nurse*
2. *American Journal of Critical Care*

Products—Acute and Critical Care Choices Guide to Advance Directives
AACN Protocols for Practice: Palliative Care and End-of-Life Issues in Critical Care
Repository for the Robert Wood Johnson Foundation Promoting Excellence in End of Life Care—Palliative Care in the Intensive Care Unit.
http://www.aacn.org

American Nurses Association (ANA)
General Resources and Individual Membership
Online education—E-Learning
Journal—American Nurse Today
Professional issues panel—Palliative and Hospice Nursing
Products—Nursing Scope and Standards, Code of Ethics for Nursing, Palliative Nursing Scope and Standards (ANA and HPNA)
Position statements
1. *Registered Nurses' Roles and Responsibilities in Providing Expert Care and Counseling at End of Life, Nursing*
2. *Nursing Care and Do Not Resuscitate (DNR) and Allow Natural Death (AND) Decisions*
3. *Euthanasia, Assisted Suicide, and Aid in Dying*

www.nursingworld.org

Hospice and Palliative Nurses Association (HPNA) —individual membership necessary
The specialty palliative nursing organization for all levels of nursing—the nursing assistant, the licensed practical/vocational nurse, the registered nurse, and the advanced practice registered nurse.
Online education—E-Learning
Conferences—Annual Assembly, Clinical Practice Forum
Journals
1. *Journal of Hospice and Palliative Nursing,*
2. *Journal of Palliative Medicine*

Networking—Special interest groups—APN, pediatrics, bioethics, research, heart failure, and intensive care
Products—Palliative Nursing Scope and Standards (ANA and HPNA), Compendiums of Non-Cancer Diagnoses, Core Curriculum for the Hospice and Palliative RN and APRN, Primer on APRN Reimbursement, Palliative Nursing Manuals, and Patient Teaching Sheets
www.gohpna.org

Oncology Nursing Society (ONS)—individual membership necessary

Online education—E-Learning

Conferences—Congress, Fall Institute

Journals

1. *Oncology Nursing Forum*
2. *Clinical Journal of Oncology Nursing*

Networking—special interest groups

Products—core curriculum, core competencies, position statements

www.ons.org

Additional Resources

National Comprehensive Cancer Network
Guidelines for palliative care
Guidelines for psychosocial distress
http://www.nccn.org

Oxford University Press

Nursing-specific references—Oxford Textbook of Palliative Nursing, 4th ed., 2015. B. Ferrell, N. Coyle, & J. Paice (Eds).

Advanced Practice Palliative Nursing 2016. C. Dahlin, P. Coyne, & B. Ferrell (Eds).

Palliative Nursing Manuals with HPNA based on the eight domains of the National Consensus Project for Quality Palliative Care

https://global.oup.com/academic/category/medicine-and-health/nursing

REFERENCES

Adams, C. (2010). Dying with dignity in America: The transformational leadership of Florence Wald. *Journal of Professional Nursing, 26*(2), 125–132. doi:10.1016/j.profnurs.2009.12.009. *Evidence Level VI.*

American Academy of Hospice and Palliative Medicine. (2015). *ABMS and AOA subspecialty certification in hospice and palliative medicine.* Retrieved from http://aahpm.org/certification/subspecialty-certification. *Evidence Level VI.*

American College of Surgeons. (2012). In Commission on Cancer (Ed.), *Cancer program standards 2012: Ensuring patient centered care. Standard 2.4 Palliative Care Services* (pp. 70–72). Retrieved from www.facs.org/cancer/coc/programstandards2012.pdf. *Evidence Level VI.*

American Nurses Association. (2010). *Nursing scope and standards of practice* (2nd ed.). Silver Spring, MD: Author. *Evidence Level VI.*

Bakitas, M., Lyons, K. D., Hegel, M. T., Balan, S., Brokaw, F. C., Seville, J., . . . Ahles, T. A. (2009). Effects of a palliative care intervention on clinical outcomes in patients with advanced cancer: The Project ENABLE II randomized controlled trial. *Journal of the American Medical Association, 302*(7), 741–749. *Evidence Level II.*

Benoliel, J. (2010). Foreword. In B. R. Ferrel & N. Coyle (Eds.), *Textbook of palliative nursing* (3rd ed., p. vii). New York, NY: Oxford University Press. *Evidence Level VI.*

Board of Chaplaincy Inc. (BCCI). (2015). *Hospice & palliative care specialty certification.* Retrieved from http://bcci.professionalchaplains.org/palliative. *Evidence Level VI.*

Brumley, R., Enguidanos, S., Jamison, P., Seitz, R., Morgenstern, N., Saito, S., . . . Gonzalez, J. (2007). Increased satisfaction with care and lower costs: Results of a randomized trial of in-home palliative care. *Journal of the American Geriatrics Society, 55*, 993. *Evidence Level II.*

Casarett, D., Pickard, A., Bailey, F. A., Ritchie, C., Furman, C., Rosenfeld, K., . . . Shea, J. A. (2008). Do palliative care consultations improve outcomes? *Journal of the American Geriatrics Society, 56*, 593–599. *Evidence Level II.*

Casarett, D. J., & Quill, T. E. (2007). "I'm not ready for hospice": Strategies for timely and effective hospice discussions. *Annals of Internal Medicine, 146*(6), 443–449. *Evidence Level V.*

Centers for Medicare & Medicaid Services. (2008). *Medicare and Medicaid programs: Hospice conditions of participation; final rule.* Washington, DC. Retrieved from www.gpo.gov/fdsys/pkg/FR-2008-06-05/pdf/08-1305.pdf. *Evidence Level VI.*

Dahlin, C., & Mazenec, P. (2011). Building from our past: Celebrating 25 years of clinical practice in hospice and palliative nursing. *Journal of Hospice and Palliative Nursing, 13*(6S), S20–S28. *Evidence Level VI.*

Dy, S., Kiley, K., Ast, K., Lupu, D., Norton, S., McMillan, S., . . . Casarett, D. (2015). Measuring what matters: Top-ranked quality indicators for hospice and palliative care from the American Academy of Hospice and Palliative Medicine and Hospice and Palliative Nurses Association. *Journal of Pain and Symptom Management, 49*(4), 773–778. *Evidence Level I.*

Enguidanos, S., Vesper, E., & Lorenz, K. (2012). 30-Day re-admissions among seriously ill adults. *Journal of Palliative Medicine, 15*, 1356–1361. *Evidence Level IV.*

Ersek, M., & Carpenter, J. (2013). Geriatric palliative care in long-term care settings with a focus on nursing homes. *Journal of Palliative Medicine, 16*(10). *Evidence Level V.*

Ersek, M., & Stevenson, D. (2013). Integrating palliative care into nursing homes: Challenges and opportunities. *Health Affairs Blog.* Retrieved from http://healthaffairs.org/blog/2013/12/02/integrating-palliative-care-into-nursing-homes-challenges-and-opportunities. *Evidence Level VI.*

Holloway, R., Arnold, R., Cruetzfeldt, C., Lewis, E., Lutz, B., McCann, R., . . . Zorowitz, R. (2014). Palliative care and end of life care in stroke: A statement for health professionals from the American Heart Association/American Stroke Association. *Stroke, 45. Evidence Level VI.*

Hospice and Palliative Credentialing Center. (2015). *Why certification?* Retrieved from http://hpcc.advancingexpertcare.org/competence/why-certification. *Evidence Level VI.*

Institute of Medicine. (1997). *Approaching death: Improving care at the end of life.* In M. Field & C. Cassel (Eds.). Washington, DC: National Academies Press. Retrieved from http://www.nap.edu/catalog/5801/approaching-death-improving-care-at-the-end-of-life. *Evidence Level VI.*

Institute of Medicine. (2001). *Crossing the quality chasm: A new health system for the 21st century.* Washington, DC: National Academies Press. *Evidence Level VI.*

Institute of Medicine. (2002). *When children die: Improving palliative and end-of-life care for children and their families.* Washington, DC: National Academies Press. Retrieved from http://iom.nationalacademies.org/Reports/2002/When-Children-Die-Improving-Palliative-and-end-of-life-care-for-children-and-their-families.aspx. *Evidence Level VI.*

Institute of Medicine. (2013). *Delivering high-quality cancer care: Charting a new course for a system in crisis.* Washington, DC: National Academies Press. Retrieved from http://iom.nationalacademies.org/Reports/2013/Delivering-High-Quality-Cancer-Care-Charting-a-New-Course-for-a-System-in-Crisis.aspx. *Evidence Level VI.*

Institute of Medicine. (2014). *Dying in America—Improving quality and honoring individual preferences near end of life.* Washington, DC: National Academies Press. Retrieved from http://iom.nationalacademies.org/Reports/2014/Dying-In-America-Improving-Quality-and-Honoring-Individual-Preferences-Near-the-End-of-Life.aspx. *Evidence Level VI.*

Jennings, B., Ryndes, T., D'Onofrio, C., & Baily, M. A. (2003). Access to hospice care: Expanding boundaries, overcoming barriers. *Hastings Center Report* (Supp.), *33*(2), S1–S59. *Evidence Level V.*

Kerr, K., & Cassel, J. B. (2014). *Quality and fiscal incentive alignment for community-based palliative care.* Retrieved from http://coalitionccc.org/documents/CBPC_biz_case_Aug_2013.pdf. Evidence *Level V.*

Last Acts. (2002). *Means to a better end: A report on dying in America Today.* Washington, DC: Author. *Evidence Level V.*

Levy , M., Smith, T., Alvarez-Perez, A., Back, A., Baker, J. N., Block, S., . . . National Comprehensive Cancer Network. (2014). Palliative care, Version 1.2014. Featured updates to the NCCN Guidelines. *Journal of the National Comprehensive Cancer Network, 12*(1379). *Evidence Level VI.*

Luckett, T., Phillips, J., Agar, M., Virdun, C., Green, A., & Davidson, P. (2014). Elements of effective palliative care models: A rapid review. *BMC Health Services Research, 14,* 136. *Evidence Level I.*

Lynch, M., Dahlin, C., Hultman, T., & Coakley, E. (2011). Palliative care nursing—Defining the discipline? *Journal of Hospice and Palliative Nursing, 13*(2), 106–111. *Evidence Level VI.*

National Association of Social Workers. (2015). The certified hospice and palliative social worker (CHP-SW). Retrieved from http://www.naswdc.org/credentials/credentials/chpsw.asp. *Evidence Level VI.*

National Comprehensive Cancer Network (NCCN). (2012). *NCCN clinical practice guidelines in oncology (NCCN Guidelines c), distress management; chaplaincy services.* Retrieved from http://www.nccn.org/professionals/. *Evidence Level VI.*

National Consensus Project for Quality Palliative Care (NCP). (2004). *Clinical practice guidelines for quality palliative care.* Pittsburgh, PA: Author. *Evidence Level VI.*

National Consensus Project for Quality Palliative Care (NCP). (2009). *Clinical practice guidelines for quality palliative care* (2nd ed.). Pittsburgh, PA: Author. *Evidence Level VI.*

National Consensus Project for Quality Palliative Care (NCP). (2013). *Clinical practice guidelines for quality palliative care* (3rd ed.). Pittsburgh, PA: Author. *Evidence Level VI.*

National Hospice and Palliative Care Organization. (2011). *Essential guide to hospice management.* Alexandria, VA: Author. *Evidence Level VI.*

National Priorities Partnership (NPP). (2008). *National priorities & goals—Aligning our efforts to transform America's healthcare.* Retrieved from http://psnet.ahrq.gov/resource.aspx?resourceID=8745. *Evidence Level VI.*

National Priorities Partnership (NPP). (2010). *Palliative care and end-of-life convening meeting synthesis report.* Paper presented at the Palliative Care and End-of-Life Convening Meeting, November 2010, Washington, DC. Retrieved from file:///C:/Users/connied/Downloads/ATTACHMENT%2014%20-%20PallEol_Report_FINAL_DMPaperExtracted.pdf. *Evidence Level VI.*

National Quality Forum (NQF). (2006). *A national framework and preferred practices for palliative and hospice care quality: A consensus report.* Washington, DC: Author. Retrieved from https://www.qualityforum.org/Publications/2006/12/A_National_Framework_and_Preferred_Practices_for_Palliative_and_Hospice_Care_Quality.aspx. *Evidence Level VI.*

National Quality Forum (NQF). (2012a). Measure applications partnership—Performance measurement coordination strategies for hospice and palliative care final report. June 2012. In National Quality Forum (Ed.). Washington, DC: Author. Retrieved from file:///C:/Users/connied/Downloads/MAPHospiceandPalliativeCareFinalReport.pdf. *Evidence Level IV.*

National Quality Forum (NQF). (2012b). *Palliative care and end-of-life care—A consensus report.* Retrieved from http://www.qualityforum.org/Publications/2012/04/Palliative_Care_and_End-of-Life_Care%e2%80%94A_Consensus_Report.aspx. *Evidence Level VI.*

National Quality Forum (NQF). (2013). *Mission and vision.* Retrieved from http://www.qualityforum.org/About_NQF/Mission_and_Vision.aspx

Partridge, A., Seah, D., King, T., Leighl, N., Hauke, R., Wollins, D., & Von Roenn, J. (2014). Developing a service model that integrates palliative care throughout cancer care: The time is now. *Journal of Clinical Oncology, 32*(29), 3330–3336. *Evidence Level V.*

Patient Protection and Affordable Care Act. (2010). Title III (B) (III) Section 3140,124. Retrieved from https://www.gpo.gov/fdsys/pkg/BILLS-111hr3590enr/pdf/BILLS-111hr3590enr.pdf. *Evidence Level VI.*

Rabow, M., Hauser, J., & Adams, J. (2004). Supporting family caregivers at the end of life—"They don't know what they don't know." *Journal of the American Medical Association, 291*(4), 483–489. *Evidence Level V.*

Rabow, M. W., Schanche, K., Petersen, J., Dibble, S. L., & McPhee, S. J. (2003). Patient perceptions of an outpatient palliative care intervention: "It had been on my mind before, but I did not know how to start talking about death." *Journal of Pain and Symptom Management, 25,* 1010. *Evidence Level V.*

Smith, T., Temin, S., Alesi, E., Abernathy, A., Balboni, T., Basch, E.,...Von Roenn, J. H. (2012). American Society of Clinical Oncology provisional clinical opinion: The integration of palliative care into standard oncology care. *Journal of Clinical Oncology, 30*(5), 880–887. *Evidence Level VI.*

Strumpf, N., Tuch, H., Stillman, D., Parrish, P., & Morrison, N. (2008). Implementing palliative care in the nursing home. *Annals of Long Term Care—Clinical Care and Aging, 17*, 54. *Evidence Level V.*

SUPPORT Principal Investigators. (1995). A controlled trial to improve care for the seriously ill hospitalized patients: The study to understand prognoses and preferences for outcomes and risks of treatment (SUPPORT). *Journal of the American Medical Association, 274*(20), 1591–1598. *Evidence Level II.*

Temel, J., Greer, J., Muzikansky, A., Gallagher, E., Admane, S., Jackson, V.,...Lynch, T. (2010). Early palliative care for patients with metastatic non-small cell lung cancer. *New England Journal of Medicine, 363*, 733–742. *Evidence Level II.*

The Joint Commission (TJC). (2011). *Advanced certification in palliative care.* Retrieved from http://www.jointcommission.org/certification/palliative_care.aspx. *Evidence Level VI.*

Wiencek, C., & Coyne, P. (2014). Palliative care delivery models. *Seminars in Oncology Nursing, 30*(5), 227–233. *Evidence Level VI.*

Yale Bulletin and Calendar. (2001). *American Academy honors three from YSN.* Retrieved from http://www.yale.edu/opa/arc-ybc/v30.n11/story9.html

APPENDIX 37.1

Mapping the National Consensus Project Domains and the National Quality Forum Preferred Practices

2013 NCP Domains	2006 NQF Preferred Practices
Domain 1—Structure and Processes of Care	
Guideline 1.1. General structure of care	Preferred practice 1 ■ Provide palliative and hospice care by an *interdisciplinary team* of skilled palliative care professionals, including, for example, physicians, nurses, social workers, pharmacists, spiritual care counselors, and others who collaborate with primary health care professional(s) Preferred practice 2 ■ Provide access to palliative and hospice care that is responsive to the patient and family *24 hours a day, 7 days a week.* Preferred practice 3 ■ Provide *continuing education* to all health care professionals on the domains of palliative care and hospice care. Preferred practice 4 ■ Provide *adequate training and clinical support* to assure that professional staff are confident in their ability to provide palliative care for patients. Preferred practice 5 ■ Hospice care and specialized palliative care professionals should be *appropriately trained, credentialed, and/or certified* in their area of expertise.
Guideline 1.2. General processes of care	Preferred practice 6 ■ Formulate, utilize, and regularly review a *timely care plan* based on a comprehensive interdisciplinary assessment of the values, preferences, goals, and needs of the patient and family and, to the extent that existing privacy laws permit, ensure that the plan is broadly disseminated, both internally and externally, to all professionals involved in the patient's care. Preferred practice 7 ■ Ensure that on *transfer between health care settings, there is timely and thorough communication* of the patient's goals, preferences, values, and clinical information so that continuity of care and seamless follow-up are assured. Preferred practice 8 ■ Health care professionals should *present hospice as an option to all patients* and families when death within a year would not be surprising, and reintroduce the hospice option as the patient declines. Preferred practice 9 ■ Patients and caregivers should be asked by palliative and hospice care programs to *assess physicians'/health care professionals' ability* to discuss hospice as an option.

(*continued*)

APPENDIX 37.1

Mapping the National Consensus Project Domains and the National Quality Forum Preferred Practices (*continued*)

2013 NCP Domains	2006 NQF Preferred Practices
	Preferred practice 10 ■ Enable patients to make *informed decisions* about their care by educating them on the process of their disease, prognosis, and the benefits and burdens of potential interventions. Preferred practice 11 ■ Provide *education and support to families* and unlicensed caregivers based on the patient's individualized care plan to assure safe and appropriate care for the patient.
Domain 2—Physical Aspects of Care	
Guideline 1	Preferred practice 12 ■ *Measure and document* pain, dyspnea, constipation, and other symptoms using available standardized scales.
Guideline 2	Preferred practice 13 ■ *Assess and manage symptoms* and side effects in a timely, safe, and effective manner to a level acceptable to the patient and family.
Domain 3—Psychological and Psychiatric Aspects of Care	
Guideline 1	Preferred practice 14 ■ *Measure and document* anxiety, depression, delirium, behavioral disturbances, and other common psychological symptoms using available standardized scales. Preferred practice 16 ■ *Assess and manage psychological reactions* of patients and families to address emotional and functional impairment and loss, (including stress, anticipatory grief and coping), in a regular ongoing fashion. Preferred practice 15 ■ *Manage* anxiety, depression, delirium, behavioral disturbances, and other common psychological symptoms in a *timely, safe, and effective* manner to a level acceptable to the patient and family.
Guideline 2	Preferred practice 17 ■ *Develop and offer a grief and bereavement care plan* to provide services to patients and families before and for at least 13 months after the death of the patient.
Domain 4—Social Aspects of Care	
Guideline 1	Preferred practice 18 ■ Conduct *regular patient and family care conferences* with physicians and other appropriate members of the interdisciplinary team to provide information, discuss goals of care, disease prognosis, and advance care planning, and offer support.
Guideline 2	Preferred practice 19 ■ *Develop and implement a comprehensive social care plan*, which addresses the social, practical, and legal needs of the patient and caregivers, including but not limited to relationships, communication, existing social and cultural networks, decision making, work and school settings, finances, sexuality/intimacy, caregiver availability/stress, and access to medicines and equipment.
Domain 5—Spiritual, Religious, and Existential Aspects of Care	
Guideline 1	Preferred practice 20 ■ Develop and document a plan based on *assessment of religious, spiritual, and existential concerns* using a structured instrument and integrate the information obtained from the assessment into the palliative care plan. Preferred practice 21 ■ Provide information about the availability of spiritual care services and make *spiritual care available* either through organizational spiritual counseling or through the patient's own clergy relationships. Preferred practice 22 ■ Specialized palliative and hospice care teams should include *spiritual care professionals appropriately trained and certified* in palliative care.

(*continued*)

APPENDIX 37.1

Mapping the National Consensus Project Domains and the National Quality Forum Preferred Practices (*continued*)

2013 NCP Domains	2006 NQF Preferred Practices
Guideline 2	Preferred practice 23 ■ Specialized palliative and hospice spiritual care professionals should build *partnerships* with community clergy, and provide education and counseling related to end-of-life care.
Domain 6—Cultural Aspects of Care	
Guideline 1	Preferred practice 24 ■ Incorporate *cultural assessment* as a component of comprehensive palliative and hospice care assessment, including, but not limited to, locus of decision making, preferences regarding disclosure of information, truth telling and decision making, dietary preferences, language, family communication, desire for support measures such as palliative therapies and complementary and alternative medicine, perspectives on death, suffering and grieving, and funeral/burial rituals. Preferred practice 25 ■ Provide professional interpreter services and culturally sensitive materials in the *patient's and family's preferred language*.
Domain 7—Care of Patient at End of Life	
Guideline 1	Preferred practice 26 ■ *Recognize and document* the transition to the active dying phase and *communicate* to the patient, family, and staff the expectation of imminent death. Preferred practice 27 ■ The *family is educated* on a timely basis regarding signs and symptoms of imminent death in a developmentally, age-, and culturally appropriate manner.
Guideline 2	Preferred practice 28 ■ As part of the ongoing care-planning process, routinely ascertain and *document patient and family wishes* about the care setting for site of death, and fulfill patient and family preferences when possible. Preferred practice 29 ■ Provide *adequate dosage of analgesics* and sedatives as appropriate to achieve patient comfort during the active dying phase and address concerns and fears about using narcotics and using analgesics to hasten death.
Guideline 3	Preferred practice 30 ■ *After death, treat the body with respect* according to the cultural and religious practices of the family and in accordance with local law.
Guideline 4	Preferred practice 31 ■ *Facilitate effective grieving* by implementing a bereavement care plan in a timely manner after the patient's death when the family remains the focus of care.
Domain 8—Ethical and Legal Aspects of Care	
Guideline 1	Preferred practice 32 ■ *Document the designated surrogate/decision maker* in accordance with state law for every patient in primary, acute, and long-term care and in palliative and hospice care. Preferred practice 33 ■ *Document the patient/surrogate preferences* for goals of care, treatment options, and setting of care at first assessment and at frequent intervals as conditions change. Preferred practice 34 ■ Convert the patient treatment goals into medical orders and ensure that the information is transferable and applicable across care settings, including long-term care, emergency medical services, and hospitals, such as the Physician Orders for Life-Sustaining Treatments (*POLST*) Program. Preferred practice 35 ■ Make *advance directives and surrogacy designations available* across care settings, while protecting patient privacy and adherence to Health Insurance Portability and Accountability Act (HIPAA) regulations, for example, by Internet-based registries or electronic personal health records.

(*continued*)

APPENDIX 37.1

Mapping the National Consensus Project Domains and the National Quality Forum Preferred Practices (*continued*)

2013 NCP Domains	2006 NQF Preferred Practices
	Preferred practice 36 ■ Develop health care and *community collaborations to promote advance care planning* and completion of advance directives for all individuals, for example, Respecting Choices, Community Conversations on Compassionate Care.
Guideline 2	Preferred practice 37 ■ *Establish or have access to ethics committees* or ethics consultation across care settings to address ethical conflicts at the end of life. Preferred practice 38 ■ For minors with decision-making capacity, *document the child's views and preferences for medical care*, including assent for treatment, and give appropriate weight in decision making. Make appropriate professional staff members available to both the child and the adult decision maker for consultation and intervention when the child's wishes differ from those of the adult decision maker.

Adapted from the National Consensus Project for Quality Palliative Care (NCP, 2013); the National Quality Forum (NQF, 2006).

38

Care of the Older Adult in the Emergency Department

Marie Boltz and Amala Sooklal

EDUCATIONAL OBJECTIVES

On completion of this chapter, the reader should be able to:

1. Identify evidence-based approaches and tools to assess the older adult in the emergency department (ED)
2. Describe interventions to prevent and manage geriatric syndromes in the ED
3. Discuss approaches to support effective transitions from the ED

OVERVIEW

Older adults aged 65 years and older use more ED services than any other age group, comprising approximately 21% to 40% of all consumers who use the ED (Niska, Bhuiya, & Xu, 2010). One in five patients aged 65 to 74 years and one in four patients aged 75 years and older visit the ED each year; the percentage of ED visits made by nursing home (NH) residents, patients arriving by ambulance, and patients admitted to the hospital increases with age (Albert, McCaig, Jill, & Ashman, 2013). Approximately 42% of ED visits of patients 65 years and older result in hospitalization.

The ED plays a critical role in the health care system for older adults. Most common, it is the point of entry for hospitalization. The higher prevalence of chronic disease and exacerbations of these conditions is one reason for high utilization (Salvi et al., 2007; Samaras, Chevalley, Samaras, & Gold, 2010). In other cases, older adults transition from the ED to other settings such as long-term care or mental health facilities. Finally, others receive care for crises such as mistreatment or displacement. The ED may be used for the performance of complex diagnostic workups, overflow, and off-hours medical care; for some older adults, the ED is the only source of health care evaluation and treatment (Gonzalez Morganti et al., 2013; Samaras et al., 2010). This chapter describes evidence-based approaches to assessing the older adult presenting to the ED, as well as interventions to prevent and manage common geriatric syndromes that occur before or during the ED admission. Transitions from the ED and organizational approaches to senior-friendly ED care are also discussed.

BACKGROUND AND STATEMENT OF PROBLEM

Older adults present to the ED with serious complaints, such as injury, dyspnea, chest pain, and abdominal pain, as well as nonspecific complaints, including weakness, fatigue, and dizziness, which may indicate serious disease (Wilber & Gerson, 2009). As compared to younger people, older adults have more diagnostic tests, longer stays in the ED, and are more likely to be admitted to the hospital (Banerjee, Dehnadi, & Mbamalu, 2011). Those older adults who are discharged from the ED are more likely to be readmitted; they also risk functional loss and higher rates of mortality (McCusker et al., 2007; Niska et al., 2010; Sklar et al., 2007).

For a description of evidence levels cited in this chapter, see Chapter 1, "Developing and Evaluating Clinical Practice Guidelines: A Systematic Approach."

Although they represent a cohort of frequent ED users, it has been argued that older adults typically do not receive specialized care. As compared to younger persons, older adults are more likely to experience missed or incorrect diagnoses (Salvi et al., 2007), inadequate pain management (Hwang, Richardson, Harris, & Morrison, 2010; Iyer, 2011), and less information (Baillie, 2005; George, Jell, & Todd, 2006). There is international consensus that care of older adults in the ED warrants close attention and systemic approaches that support uptake of evidence-based care (Gruneir, Silver, & Rochon, 2011; Parke & McCusker, 2008).

ASSESSMENT OF THE OLDER ADULT IN THE ED

The complex presentation of disease and illness in older adults, along with complicated polypharmacy, functional impairments (Schnitker, Martin-Khan, Beattie, & Gray, 2011; Wilber, Blanda, & Gerson, 2006), communication problems, and cognitive impairment (Press et al., 2009; Salvi et al., 2007), presents a challenge to the ED nurse. Therefore, assessment of older adults encompasses a comprehensive evaluation to detect critical health issues hidden within a complex clinical and social presentation. Whenever possible, and with the permission of the older adult, the emergency nurse should include the patient's significant other, family, and support person in the assessment process (Boltz, Parke, Shuluk, Capezuti, & Galvin, 2013). The three major components of assessment include triage, risk assessment to prevent adverse outcomes, and general assessment.

Triage/Primary Assessment

Accurate triage of elder patients is a key component of providing effective emergency care for this vulnerable population. The large number of ED visits by elders, the growing problem of ED crowding, and the longer time it takes to evaluate older adults often result in delays at the point of triage (Platts-Mills et al., 2010; Salvi et al., 2007). Delays in triage are associated with increased waiting time, anxiety, and discomfort for older adults (Miró et al., 1999). Moreover, the resulting delay in treatment increases the risk of mortality, especially in older trauma patients (Perdue, Watts, Kaufmann, & Trask, 1998). Thus, there is a need for triage that promotes timely treatment.

The Canadian Triage and Acuity Scale (CTAS) is widely used as an emergency patient triage tool. The CTAS has demonstrated high validity for older adults and it is an especially useful tool for categorizing severity and for recognizing older adults who require immediate life-saving intervention (Bullard, Unger, Spence, & Grafstein, 2008; Lee et al., 2011). See Table 38.1 for the CTAS levels and associated descriptions, examples of conditions, and recommended time to be seen by a physician in an ED. Another tool, the Emergency Severity Index (ESI), includes a comprehensive algorithm that describes symptoms, and physiological indicators as well as the resources anticipated to be used (Gilboy, Tanabe, Travers, & Rosenau, 2012). However, there has been reported under-triage in older adults when the ESI guidelines are not precisely followed (Platts-Mills et al., 2010).

Airway–Breathing–Circulation

The goal of the primary assessment is to identify and immediately treat the patient for all life-threatening conditions, incorporating prearrival information from emergency medical services. During the assessment of *airway* patency, the emergency clinician considers the physiological changes with age that may alter patency of the airway. Dentures can occlude the airway if dislodged; additionally, dentures can cause difficulty with bag-valve mask ventilation of the airway. Kyphosis and other spinal alignment changes may cause changes in positioning of a cervical collar or spinal backboard, which may inhibit appropriate airway patency. Cervical rigidity may present challenges to establishing of a definitive airway (Aresco & Stein, 2010). The quality of *breathing* and ventilation is evaluated. While assessing the volume of lung expansion and effectiveness of breathing, it is important to consider that pulmonary vascular tissue and parenchyma tissue may become stiff and cause decreased compliance as well as an increase in pulmonary vascular resistance. Lung capacity is diminished by alveolar changes in depth and width. Older adults are at risk to have decreased respiratory reserve and arterial blood oxygenation, which can lead to decompensation sooner than their younger counterparts (Blumenthal, Plummer, & Gambert, 2010). Assessment of *circulation* may also be affected by physiological changes with increased age. Patients with cardiac history may be consuming antihypertensive medications or rate-control medications that may inhibit or alter the physiological responses. Additionally, hypertension in the patient may mask the signs of a lowered blood pressure caused by hypovolemic shock (Criddle, 2013).

Patients older than age 65 years are more likely to present with dysrhythmias. During the assessment phase, other causes of abnormal cardiac function should be evaluated, such as electrolyte imbalances, hypoxia, cardiac injury, or hypovolemia (McQuillan, Makic, & Whalen, 2009). Vague and, in some cases, nondramatic presentations

TABLE 38.1

Canadian Triage and Acuity Scale (CTAS) Used in an ED

Evidence Level	Description: Conditions That	Examples	Time to Be Seen by a Physician
1. Resuscitation	Pose threats to life or limb (or imminent risk of deterioration) requiring immediate aggressive interventions	Cardiac/respiratory arrest, major trauma, shock states, unconscious patients, severe respiratory distress, severe dehydration	Immediately 98% of the time
2. Emergent	Pose potential threat to life, limb, or function; requiring rapid medical intervention or delegated acts	Altered mental states, head injury, severe trauma, MI, overdose, and CVA	Less than or equal to 15 minutes 95% of the time
3. Urgent	Could potentially progress to a serious problem requiring emergency intervention. May be associated with significant discomfort or affect ability to function at work or activities of daily living.	Moderate trauma, asthma, GI bleeds, acute psychosis and/or suicidal thoughts, and acute pain	Less than or equal to 30 minutes 90% of the time
4. Less urgent/ semi-urgent	Are related to patient age, distress, or potential for deterioration or complications that would benefit from intervention or reassurance within 1 to 2 hours	Headache, corneal foreign body, and chronic back pain	Less than or equal to 1 hour 85% of the time
5. Nonurgent	May be acute but nonurgent as well as conditions that may be part of a chronic problem with or without evidence of deterioration	Sore throat, URI, mild abdominal pain (chronic or recurring), with normal vital signs, vomiting alone, and diarrhoea alone	120 minutes 80% of the time

CVA, cerebrovascular accident; ED, emergency department; GI, gastrointestinal; MI, myocardial infarction; URI, upper respiratory infection.

indicate serious, life-threatening problems in older adults. Table 38.2 shows the common atypical presentation of geriatric emergencies. Additionally, "red flags" during triage that should be evaluated closely include acute change in mental status and/or physical function, dyspnea, fatigue, self-neglect, apathy, and falls (Fletcher, 2004).

TABLE 38.2

Atypical Presentation of Common Geriatric Emergencies

- Acute abdomen with constipation and decreased appetite, rather than severe pain
- Pneumonia with vague chest pain and dry cough, rather than fever
- Depression with agitation, rather than dysphoria
- Infection with falls, rather than fever or elevated white count
- Sepsis with functional decline and generalized weakness, rather than fever
- Myocardial infarction with dyspnea and confusion, rather than chest pain
- Heart failure with fatigue, rather than dyspnea

Adapted from Fletcher, (2004).

Screening for Risk of Adverse Outcomes

Two commonly used tools, the Identification of Seniors at Risk (ISAR) and the Triage Risk Screening Tool (TRST), evaluate the presence/absence of risk factors for adverse outcomes. These tools are useful in guiding a plan to preventing avoidable complications during the ED stay, if admitted during hospitalization, and after an ED visit, when transitioning to home or another setting. The TRST (Table 38.3) is considered positive when an older adult has cognitive impairment or has two or more of the remaining risk factors and the screening has been found to be predictive of subsequent ED use, hospitalization, and NH admission (Meldon et al., 2003). The ISAR tool (Table 38.4) is positive when the score is greater than or equal to 2 and is a predictor of increased risk of death, institutionalization, functional decline, and both repeat ED visit and hospital admission in the following 6 months after an ED visit (McCusker et al., 1999). ISAR or TRST is administered by a nurse just after triage, to identify high-risk patients more likely to benefit from a comprehensive geriatric evaluation and follow-up, a longer observation time (or access to observation units), and appropriate referrals (primary physician, geriatric evaluation and management unit, and social service). Furthermore, all patients noted to

TABLE 38.3
Triage Risk Screening Tool (TRST)

- History or evidence of cognitive impairment (poor recall or not oriented)
- Difficulty walking/transferring or recent fall(s)
- Five or more medications
- ED use in previous 30 days or hospitalization in previous 90 days
- RN professional recommendation[a]

[a]Emergency department (ED) nurse (RN) concern for elder abuse/neglect, substance abuse, medication noncompliance, problems meeting instrumental activities of daily living, or other.
Adapted from Meldon et al. (2003).

TABLE 38.4
Identification of Seniors At Risk Tool

- Before the injury or illness, did you need someone to help you on a regular basis?
- Since the injury or illness, have you needed more help than usual?
- Have you been hospitalized for one or more nights in the past 6 months?
- In general, do you see well?
- In general, do you have serious problems with your memory?
- Do you take more than three medications daily?

Adapted from McCusker et al. (1999).

be at risk who are admitted to the hospital are referred to case management; those who are discharged from the hospital can be followed up the following day, either through a home visit or telephone consultation (Salvi et al., 2012).

General Assessment

At a minimum, the social history should address the person's living situation, marital status, work status, and advance directives. A social assessment also focuses on supports within the family and in the community. A way to assess this is to ask, "If something bad happened, who would you call?" Stressors related to loss, grief, relationship changes, and environmental factors are often antecedents to acute onset or exacerbation of illness, and should be ascertained (Graf, Zekry, Giannelli, Michel, & Chevalley, 2011). In addition to the past medical/surgical history, medication use, and allergies, weight loss/changes in oral intake, and details of recent changes in diagnosis or medication regimes are standard data. When evaluating the reason for coming to the ED, the nurse should elicit a comparison between the older adult's condition before the acute illness and new or exacerbated symptoms. Information about baseline cognition, mood, and physical function is essential as changes within these dimensions can be early and sensitive indicators of physiological dysfunction (Ellis, Marshall, & Ritchie, 2014; Hare, Wynaden, McGowan, & Speed, 2008).

Cognition and Mood

It is estimated that one fourth of all older adults who present to the ED show impaired mental status associated with delirium, dementia, or both (Hustey & Meldon, 2002; Hustey, Meldon, Smith, & Lex, 2003). Although common in older ED patients, cognitive impairment is often undetected (Hustey & Meldon, 2002; Lewis et al., 1995). The Geriatric Emergency Medicine Task Force recommends a mental status evaluation for all older adults presenting to the ED (Wilber, Lofgren, et al., 2005). The Six-Item Screener (immediate recall of three words; orientation to year, month, day of the week; recall of three words) is short and easy to use and detects cognitive impairment with a sensitivity of 94% and a specificity of 86% in the ED setting (Callahan, Unverzagt, Hui, Perkins, & Hendrie, 2006). If cognitive impairment is detected, the family or formal caregiver should be questioned as to the baseline cognition; abrupt onset suggests delirium.

The Geriatric Emergency Department Guidelines Task Force (2014), developed by the Emergency Nurses Association, American College of Emergency Physicians, American Geriatrics Society, and Society for Academic Emergency Medicine, includes a two-step process to assess for delirium. Step 1 (Figure 38.1) is the highly sensitive delirium triage screen (DTS). Step 2 is the highly specific Brief Confusion Assessment Method (bCAM; Han et al., 2013).

The DTS is comprised of two parts: (a) level of consciousness as measured by the Richmond Agitation Sedation Scale (RASS); and (b) inattention by spelling the word "LUNCH" backwards. If the patient has an RASS other than 0 (0 = alert and calm; Ely et al., 2003) or makes more than one error on the "LUNCH" backward spelling test, then the DTS is considered positive. The bCAM is then used to rule in delirium.

A variety of ED-appropriate dementia and mild cognitive impairment screening instruments have been validated; they are useful to reduce the probability of nondelirium cognitive impairment (dementia or mild cognitive impairment) rather than to rule-in the diagnosis (Geriatric Emergency Department Guidelines Task Force, 2014). On the diagnosis of delirium, attention is paid to identifying the underlying cause, which can be infection, medications, dehydration, electrolyte imbalance, alcohol/drug use or withdrawal, depression, stroke or other neurological problems (Elie, Cole, Primeau, & Bellavance, 1998) Additionally, the following

FIGURE 38.1

(A) Step 1: Delirium triage screen. (B) Brief Confusion Assessment Method.

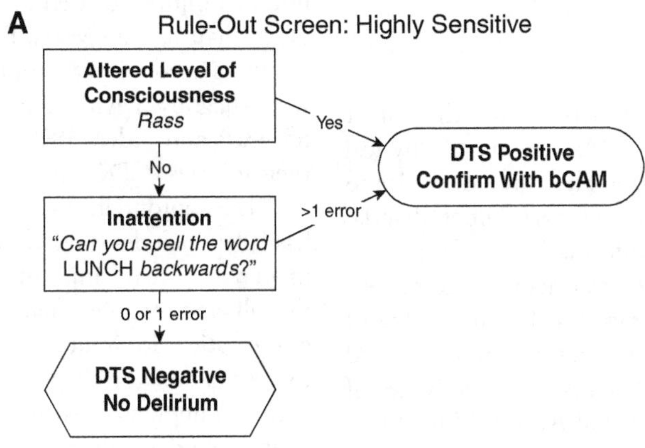

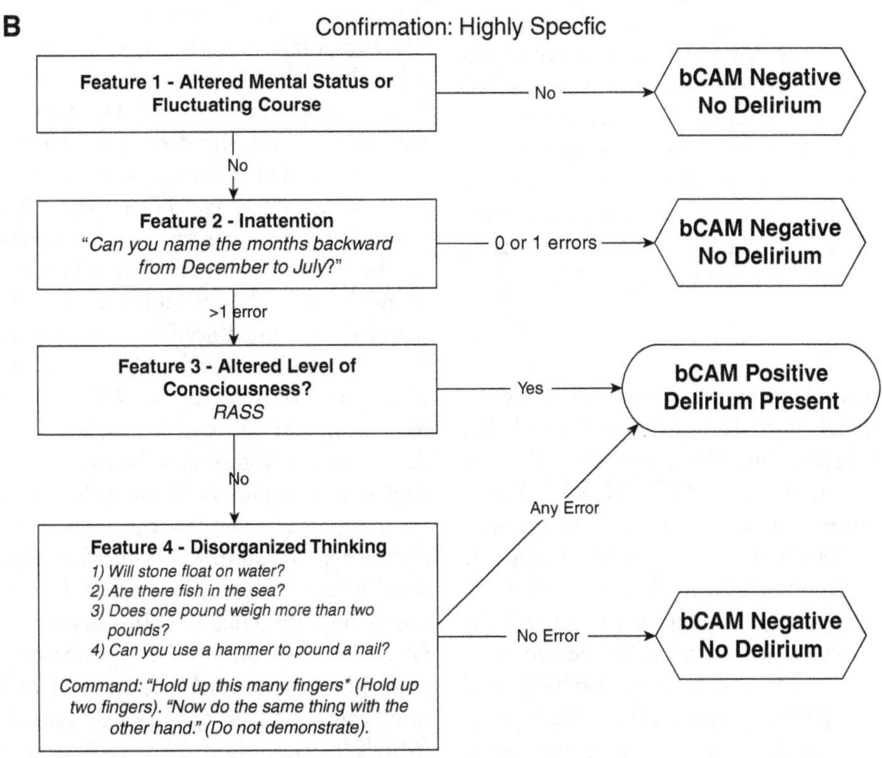

bCAM, Brief Confusion Assessment Method; DTS, delirium triage screen; RASS, Richmond Agitation Sedation Scale.

should be evaluated as risk factors for the development of delirium: decreased vision or hearing, decreased cognitive ability, severe illness, or dehydration/prerenal azotemia (Geriatric Emergency Department Guidelines Task Force, 2014).

Depression may interfere with the clinical presentation of acute medical disorders and results in a larger number of ED visits (Fabacher, Raccio-Robak, McErlean, Milano, & Verdile, 2002). Approximately one third of older ED patients present with depression (Meldon et al., 2003; Sanders, 2001). The Emergency Department Depression Screening Instrument (ED-DSI) is appropriate for the detection of depression in the ED; it is brief, consisting of three questions

(Do you often feel (a) sad and depressed? (b) helpless? (c) downhearted and blue?). The ED-DSI has a sensitivity of 79% and a specificity of 66% as compared with the longer Geriatric Depression Scale (Fabacher et al., 2002).

Physical Function

Physical function is an important metric of health in older adults, as described in Chapter 7, "Assessment of Physical Function." A recent loss of function often precedes a visit to the ED and can signify underlying illness (Wilber, Blanda, & Gerson, 2006). Additional, information on function is used to benchmark response to treatment as the patient transitions among various settings. Finally, the degree of services, including rehabilitation therapy, is largely guided by an assessment of functional status. Basic activities of daily living (ADL) and instrumental ADL (IADL) function should be assessed for each patient, including capacity for dressing, eating, transferring, toileting, hygiene, ambulation, and medication adherence. Measurement needs to capture baseline function (before the acute admitting problem, typically 2 weeks before admission) as well as current functional performance. Physical function is appraised using a valid measure of basic function such as the Katz ADL Index (Katz, Ford, Moskowitz, Jackson, & Jaffe, 1963) or Barthel Index (Mahoney & Barthel, 1965) and instrumental activities of daily living (IADL) using the Lawton IADL Scale (Lawton & Brody, 1969).

Medication Evaluation

A national surveillance study of adverse drug events (ADE) and a national outpatient survey estimated that Americans aged 65 years or older have more than 175,000 ED visits for ADE yearly. One third of ADE-related visits were attributed to three commonly prescribed drugs: warfarin, insulin, and digoxin (Budnitz, Shehab, Kegler, & Richards, 2007). Furthermore, older adults who are more frequent ED users have a greater number of potentially inappropriate medications (PIMs); they also tend to experience significant delay between hospital discharge and primary care follow-up (Wong, Marr, Kwan, Meiyappan, & Adcock, 2014). In addition to following established medication reconciliation processes, the emergency nurse has a pivotal role in facilitating systematic screening for polypharmacy and use of PIMs as well as detecting ADE in the ED (Samaras et al., 2010). For those patients who demonstrate polypharmacy, PIMs, and/or ADEs, and are admitted, a referral to the pharmacist and interdisciplinary team will enable collaborating with the attending physician to correct the medication problem (Geriatric Emergency Department Guidelines Task Force, 2014).

Fall Assessment

According to the Centers for Disease Control and Prevention (CDC, 2015a), falls are the number one cause of nonfatal injuries treated in hospital emergencies in people older than age 65 years. Furthermore, almost one third of adults aged 65 years and older who fell in a bathroom were diagnosed with a fracture and among adults aged 85 years and older, 38% were hospitalized as a result of their injuries (CDC, 2015).

The appropriate ED evaluation of an older adult who has fallen includes three components: (a) a thorough assessment for traumatic injuries, (b) an assessment of the cause of the fall, and (c) an estimation of future fall risk. Evaluation of the patient for injury should include a complete head-to-toe evaluation for all patients, including those presenting with seemingly isolated injuries. An EKG; complete blood count; standard electrolyte panel; evaluation of medications, including measurable levels; and appropriate imaging should be secured. For those older adults who present to the ED after a fall, traumatic injuries may be occult, presenting without classic signs or symptoms (Geriatric Emergency Department Guidelines Task Force, 2014). High-risk injuries, such as blunt head trauma, spinal fractures, and hip fractures, warrant a higher degree of suspicion and extensive workups (Sterling, O'Connor, & Bonadies, 2001). For example, hip fractures can present as isolated knee pain and can be underdetected on x-ray (Dominguez, Liu, Roberts, Mandell, & Richman, 2005; Guss, 1997). Older adults who have sustained head trauma, even when perceived by the patient to be slight, require neurological assessment and observation (Rathlev et al., 2006). Altered mental state, focal neurologic deficits, headache, and falls may indicate the presence of a chronic subdural hematoma (Adhiyaman, Asghar, Ganeshram, & Bhowmick, 2002).

A targeted interview with the patient and the family member should address previous falls as well as the location, activity, potential environmental factors, and symptoms proceeding the actual fall. This description helps identify a fall as a result of an underlying pathology or general frailty. Falls may be the chief symptom of orthostatic hypotension, cardiovascular syncope, or carotid sinus syndrome (Mitchell, Richardson, Davies, Bexton, & Kenny, 2002). Other responsible pathologies may include acute myocardial infarction, infection, medications (side effects, interactions, and toxicity), metabolic disturbances, neurological event or conditions (e.g., seizure and transient ischemic attack), acute abdominal pathology, or elder abuse (Sanders, 1999). Finally, environmental factors, including physical hazards and unfamiliar surroundings, are common culprits.

A recent systematic review revealed the paucity of evidence in the literature regarding ED-based screening for risk of future falls among older adults (Carpenter et al., 2014). Six fall predictors were identified in more than one study (past falls, living alone, use of walking aid, depression, cognitive deficit, and more than six medications), with a self-report of depression associated with the highest likelihood of falling. Additionally, the assessment of the etiology of a fall will help determine whether a patient will continue to be at risk for a fall at the time of discharge and the potential risk factors (Carpenter, Scheatzle, D'Antonio, Ricci, & Coben, 2009). This may include involving home health services (nursing, physical, or occupational therapies) to schedule a home safety evaluation. A home evaluation typically involves an assessment to determine whether home modifications/hazard removal is needed as well as whether use of assistive devices and proper footwear, medication management, and so forth, will decrease fall risk. Depending on hospital protocol, a physical therapy evaluation in the ED should be considered to ensure a safe discharge home, and is indicated for all patients admitted to the hospital after a fall (Aschkenasy & Rothenhaus, 2006). Communicating the details of the fall event and evaluation is critical during handoff to ensure mobilization of fall-prevention measures (see Chapter 19, "Preventing Falls in Acute Care").

Substance Misuse

The ED may be the portal to treatment for older adults dealing with substance misuse. Alcohol is the drug that is most commonly misused by older adults, followed by tobacco and psychoactive prescription drugs, with trends indicating an increase in the numbers of older individuals using marijuana (Moore et al., 2009). *Misuse* is defined as the use of a drug for purposes other than that for which it was intended. Alcohol abuse is present in 6% to 11% of older persons admitted to the hospital and 14% of older adults presenting to the ED have diagnosable alcoholism (Ferreira & Weems, 2008). Validated screening instruments for older adults, including the Alcohol Use Screening and Assessment for Older Adults, have shown to have good to excellent sensitivity and specificity (Ong-Flaherty, 2012). Other simple questions can also uncover a substance abuse problem. For example, the CAGE questionnaire, originally developed for alcohol (Ewing, 1984), has been modified to ascertain drug use and has been tested in older adults with some success. CAGE is an acronym for the four basic questions:

1. Have you felt you ought to *cut* down on your drinking or drug use?
2. Have people *annoyed* you by criticizing your drinking or drug use?
3. Have you felt bad or *guilty* about your drinking or drug use?
4. Have you ever had a drink or used drugs first thing in the morning to steady your nerves, get rid of a hangover, or get the day started (as an *eye-opener*)?

A complete social evaluation is vital given that social risk factors play a role in substance misuse. It is important to evaluate the patient's social network and identify which members are supportive of treatment and which are potentially hazardous to the patient. Harmful network members include active substance abusers; those who "enable" the patient's misuse; and those who abuse the patient physically, sexually, or emotionally. In addition, the evaluation should make sure the patient has adequate housing and access to food, adequate transportation, and medical care. The patient's mood, cognition, sleep patterns, and mental health history, including past treatment, should also be ascertained (Ross, 2005).

When there is evidence of substance misuse, nursing interventions focus on (a) monitoring for withdrawal; (b) providing an environment that is safe from potential harm to patient; and (c) collaborating with the patient, family, physician, and social worker to secure a mental health evaluation and program directed to the substance abuse needs and support. If the patient is admitted to the hospital, careful handoff should include the communication of the patient's history and clinical findings as well as safety issues, including fall risk and the presence of delirium (Center for Substance Abuse Treatment, 1998).

Elder Mistreatment

EDs are often the first point of contact for elder mistreatment (EM) victims (Fulmer, Paveza, Abraham, & Fairchild, 2000). EM includes physical, verbal, sexual, and psychological abuse, as well as abandonment, exploitation, and neglect (Acierno et al., 2010). The ED nurse needs to be vigilant to recognize the clinical features of EM, and to know their organization's policies for reporting suspected EM, as required by the Joint Commission on Accreditation and state mandatory reporting requirements (Dong, 2012; Falk, Baigis, & Kopac, 2012). The clinician should look for red flags of mistreatment—delays in seeking treatment, signs of withholding or giving too much medication, missed appointments, use of several hospitals, driving to a hospital farther away from home, description of an event that does not fit the injury sustained, and repetitive injuries (Heath & Phair, 2009). Signs of caregiver indifference, berating or threatening comments, hypervigilant/possessive behavior, or excessive concerns over finances warrant suspicion of EM (Bond & Butler, 2013; Stiegel, Klem, & Turner, 2007).

When EM is suspected, it is recommended to separate the older adult from the caregiver and obtain a detailed history and physical assessment; interviewing the patient about his or her feelings of safety is important (Bond & Butler, 2013). Care needs to be taken by clinicians to secure a careful medical history, including baseline conditions, and conduct a comprehensive physical examination. Physical examination cues may include poor hydration; poor hygiene; suspicious injuries in unusual locations and bruises in various stages of healing; unexplained abrasions and/or markings on skin, including human bite marks, skin tears, pressure ulcers, or genital complaints, including infections or injury (Stiegel et al., 2007).

NURSING INTERVENTIONS

Delirium and Dementia

In addition to collaborating with the physician to detect cognitive impairment, including delirium or delirium superimposed on dementia, the nurse provides key interventions to prevent delirium and promote comfort and safety. Strategies include controlling the environment: (a) supporting the family/familiar person (or volunteer) present with the patient; (b) providing sensory aides (glasses and hearing aids and offering hearing amplifiers and magnifiers as indicated); (c) controlling noise; (d) avoiding excessively bright lights when possible; and (e) providing comfort measures, including fluids and a warm blanket. Additional nursing interventions include promoting mobility and addressing need for pain management, toileting, rest/sleep, and fluid/hydration (Hshieh et al., 2015; Rivosecchi, Smithburger, Svec, Campbell, & Kane-Gill, 2015). Invasive procedures should be avoided as much as possible. Alternatives to physical restraints should be employed such as camouflaging dressings and securing intravenous and other lines to promote comfort. Adapting communication to cognitive loss through the use of verbal and physical cues, brief and clear instructions and inclusion of family in the sharing of information and decision making will promote a sense of security for the patient and promote effective collaboration with family (Boltz, Chippendale, Resnick, & Galvin, 2015; Boltz, Resnick, Chippendale, & Galvin, 2014).

When delirium is detected, interventions are aimed at reversing the cause (which may include the use of supplemental oxygen, hydration, etc.) while continuing to provide supportive preventive measures. The use of physical and chemical restraints should be avoided (American Association of Critical-Care Nurses, 2011). Education about the etiology of delirium and planned interventions will reassure anxious family members and help enlist their involvement in promoting safety and comfort for the patient (Boltz et al., 2014, 2015).

Prevention of Falls and Related Injuries

The aforementioned interventions will also mitigate the risk for falls and injuries. In addition to addressing modifiable fall risk factors, such as offending medications or dehydration, attention to the patient's safety is paramount. Patients often fall when trying to get out of bed unsupervised or unassisted; bedrails do not reduce the amount of falls and may increase the severity of the fall (Capezuti, Maislin, Strumpf, & Evans, 2002). For the person who is at risk of injury as a result of cognitive impairment, weakness, and low mobility, and who is nonambulatory and at risk of leaving the bed unsafely, low beds should be considered with bedside mats. Close oversight is essential (Capezuti et al., 2002). Encouraging physical activity (e.g., range of motion) and helping the older adult to walk to the bathroom when possible or use of a commode is helpful to prevent early deconditioning and thereby to mitigate fall risk (Alexander, Kinsley, & Waszinski, 2013; Capezuti et al., 2002).

Prevention of Pressure Ulcers

The use of pressure-redistributing foam mattresses has shown to be a cost-effective approach to prevent ED-acquired pressure ulcers (Pham et al., 2011). The use of reclining chairs in the ED instead of ED gurney beds has been shown to reduce pain and improve patient satisfaction (Wilber, Burger, Gerson, & Blanda, 2005). Evidence-based guidelines to prevent and manage pressure ulcers (as described in Chapter 24, "Preventing Pressure Ulcers and Skin Tears") should be followed, including skin assessment, pressure relief/off-loading, prevention/treatment of infection, pain control, and nutritional evaluation and management (Ayello, 2011; Reddy, Gill, & Rochon, 2006).

Prevention of Catheter-Associated Urinary Tract Infection

A catheter-associated urinary tract infection (CAUTI) is a urinary tract infection (UTI) that occurs while a patient has an intrauterine catheter (IUC) or within 48 hours of its removal. The use of preventive practices is associated with a lower incidence of CAUTIs. These practices include avoiding unnecessary urinary catheter use, removal prompts and nurse-initiated urinary catheter discontinuation protocols, alternatives to indwelling urinary catheterization, portable bladder ultrasound monitoring, and insertion care and maintenance (Oman et al., 2012; Saint et al., 2013).

In the ED, the identification of appropriate patients for urinary catheter insertion is an essential component of a protocol to prevent CAUTIs. According to the Infectious Disease Society of America and other expert opinion (Apisarnthanarak et al., 2007; Fink et al., 2012; Saint et al., 2013), these indications are as follows: (a) urinary retention/obstruction; (b) need for very close monitoring of urine output and patient unable to use urinal or bedpan; (c) open wound in sacral or perineal area with urinary incontinence; (d) patient too ill, fatigued, or incapacitated to use alternative urine collection method; (e) patient status postrecent surgery, hip fracture, emergency pelvic ultrasound, neurogenic bladder, and other urologic problems; and (f) hospice/palliative care. After receiving a physician order with the appropriate indications documented, the nurse should insert the indwelling catheter as per protocol, using the smallest size catheter and sterile technique (Fink et al., 2012; Hooton et al., 2010). There should be a plan for the earliest removal, which is communicated during the handoff to the nurse on the transferred unit. Daily catheter rounds guide decision making for continued use or removal of indwelling catheters (Wald & Kramer, 2011).

TRANSITIONS FROM THE ED

In a 12-state survey study of a combined 65.5 million ED visits from 2006 to 2007, carried out with patients older than 65 years, approximately 40% had medication errors after a hospital discharge, and 18% of Medicare patients discharged from a hospital were readmitted within 30 days (Steiner, Barrett, & Hunter, 2010). Older ED patients have identified misinformation, a factor associated with ED readmissions, as a primary source of dissatisfaction with ED care. Factors associated with misinformation include underrecognition of cognitive dysfunction, lower health literacy, and financial impediments for prescriptions and recommended outpatient follow-up (Baraff et al., 1992; Carpenter et al., 2009; Han et al., 2011).

ED-based interventions that emphasize patient education and care coordination have demonstrated mixed results on the rate of ED readmissions and the prevention of complications (Basic & Conforti, 2005; Corbett, Lim, Davis, & Elkins, 2005; Hegney et al., 2006). Experts agree, however, that the transition from the ED to other settings includes three systematic processes: discharge planning, patient/family education, handoff, and follow-up (Geriatric Emergency Department Guidelines Task Force, 2014).

Discharge Planning

Discharge planning from the ED is a multidisciplinary process that includes the family or significant others. The process is tailored to the individual needs of the older adult patient according to his or her discharge diagnosis and the destination setting. Components of discharge planning include (a) evaluation of the clinical status related to the admitting problem, (b) assessment of physical and psychosocial functional status (including fall/safety risk), (c) risk assessment for subsequent functional decline (e.g., ISAR or TRST), (d) assessment of caregiver availability and ability, (e) an appraisal of the patient/family readiness and ability to learn, (f) medication review, (g) review of advance directives, and (h) referrals with follow-up arrangements (Agency for Healthcare Research and Quality [AHRQ], 2009; Centers for Medicare & Medicaid Services [CMS], 2014). If the assessment by the nurse, physician, and other relevant disciplines determines that post-ED care is indicated, active engagement of patients and families and offering a range of options will support the patient's preferences and goals (Popejoy, 2011). The CMS (2014) recommends that the EDs maintain a complete and accurate file of appropriate community-based services, supports, and facilities to which the patient can be referred.

Patient/Family Education

ED patients frequently do not understand their discharge instructions (Crane, 1997; Jolly, Scott, Feied, & Sanford, 1993; Zavala & Shaffer, 2011). In a recent study of patient and caregiver understanding of discharge instructions, the investigators assessed patient and caregiver understanding of discharge instruction in four domains: (a) diagnosis and cause, (b) ED care, (c) post-ED care, and (d) return instructions. Seventy-eight percent of participants demonstrated deficient comprehension in at least one domain. Greater than one third of the deficiencies involved understanding of post-ED care (Engel et al., 2009). Within the emergency medicine literature, commonly cited challenges to patient/caregiver understanding are limited literacy and numeracy (Ginde, Clark, Goldstein, & Camargo, 2008; Ginde, Weiner, Pallin, & Camargo, 2008). Adding to the problem, print discharge instructions are not written at appropriate reading levels (Jolly et al., 1993; Williams, Counselman, & Caggiano, 1996).

To address these challenges, written instructions should be at the sixth-grade level (established using a literacy calculator). Nurses use plain language, focusing on "need to know" information, limiting the documents to essential content in order to avoid information overload (McCarthy et al., 2012). Also, information and educational material should be provided in large font suitable for older adults. The use of the teach-back method has demonstrated a positive impact on recall of discharge instructions in the

ED regardless of age and education (Slater, Dalawari, & Huang, 2013). This teaching method assesses the effectiveness of teaching by having the person explain and/or demonstrate back to the nurse what he or she has just been taught, ensuring that the patient is actively involved in the teaching process (Schillinger et al., 2003).

The nurse may use a standardized tool that assesses older adults' ability to self-administer their medication such as the Drug Regimen Unassisted Grading Scale (DRUGS), which takes approximately 5 minutes to complete. This tool requires subjects to perform the following four tasks with each of their medications: (a) identify the appropriate medication, (b) open the container, (c) select the correct dose, and (d) report the appropriate timing of doses (Edelberg, Shallenberger, Hausdorff, & Wei, 2000; Kripalani et al., 2006).

Handoff

Communication with primary care providers regarding an ED visit is considered to be a necessary process, particularly for vulnerable elders (ACOVE-3 Investigators, 2007). In an effort to improve continuity of care between the ED and other settings, the Geriatric Emergency Department Guidelines Task Force (2014) recommends standardized information be provided to the patient/family and outpatient care providers, including NHs and primary care providers (Table 38.5). Structured focus group interviews with NH staff, ED staff, and a county-wide emergency medical service (EMS) system identified the following additional approaches to support handoffs between EDs and NHs: (a) a verbal report from ED nurses provided to the NH as well as written documentation, (b) an emergency form in NH residents' charts that contains predocumented information with an area to write in the reason for transfer, and (c) brief NH-to-ED and ED-to-NH transfer forms that are accepted and used by local NHs and EDs (Terrell & Miller, 2006).

TABLE 38.5
Standardized Discharge Information

- Presenting complaints
- Test results and interpretation
- ED therapy and clinical response
- Consultation notes (in person or via telephone) in ED
- Working discharge diagnosis
- ED physician note, or copy of dictation
- Patient condition (including fall risk, functional and cognitive status)
- New prescriptions and alterations with long-term medications
- Discharge recommendations: physical activity, diet, resources/services
- Support systems
- Advance directives
- Follow-up plan

ED, emergency department.
Adapted from Geriatric Emergency Department Guidelines Task Force (2014).

Follow-Up

Telephone follow-up is recommended for patients discharged from the ED; home visits are ideally provided to high-risk individuals. Telemedicine alternatives hold promise for effective follow-up and should be considered, especially in rural areas (Kessler, Williams, Moustoukas, & Pappas, 2013).

CASE STUDY

EMS transported an 86-year-old woman to the ED from a nearby assisted living facility (ALF). She was evaluated 3 days ago in the ED for UTI presenting with increased lethargy and a fall without injury. She was started on antibiotic therapy and returned to the ALF. Forty-eight hours later a nurse from the ALF contacted the on-call physician to report continued confusion, poor oral intake, and declining functional status. She was sent back to the ED; her daughter is alarmed by her confusion and inability to respond to questions coherently, stating, "She is normally as clear as a bell." Transfer records indicate new-onset urinary and fecal incontinence in addition to the mental status changes. Because the triage nurse identifies the emergent nature of the patient's condition because of the change in mental status, she is evaluated by the physician within 15 minutes of arrival. Before this, the ED nurse determines her past medical history (positive for hypertension, depression, and gastroesophageal reflux disease [GERD]), baseline cognition of being oriented three times with no apparent problems with recall and managing her daily routine at the ALF, and requiring assistance getting in and out of the bathtub. The Six-Item Screener indicates impaired recall and orientation and the Brief Confusion Assessment Method is positive for delirium.

The patient's medications include verapamil SR = 360 mg daily, donezepil = 10 mg daily, levafloxacin = 500 mg daily, ranitidine = 150 mg daily,

(continued)

CASE STUDY *(continued)*

hydrochlorothiazide (HTCZ) = 12.5 mg daily, and paroxetine 20 = mg daily. The labs are remarkable for a blood urea nitrogen (BUN) of 42 and creatinine of 2.6, and urinalysis with 15 to 20 red blood cells (RBCs) per high-power field, 0 to 2 white blood cells (WBCs) per high-power field, + 1 protein, and +2 leukocyte esterase.

The ED nurse ascertains that a UTI is a likely cause of delirium. Additionally, the patient's medications may be contributing to her altered cognition. Ranitidine and paroxetine (unlike most other selective serotonin reuptake inhibitors [SSRIs]) exhibit anticholinergic activity and sedation as a side effect. Verapamil can cause constipation, which can contribute to UTI and delirium. Quinolone antibiotics cause delirium in a small percentage of older adults. A medication review is conducted with the physician and pharmacist to eliminate offending agents.

Important nursing interventions focus on safety, comfort, and preventing complications. The nurse encourages the daughter to stay with the patient, and advises her let to the staff know when she needs to leave, in which case a volunteer will cover. The patient is located in a quiet area, with gentle lighting and warming blankets. A pressure-relieving mattress and repositioning are provided to prevent ED-acquired pressure ulcers. The intravenous line is camouflaged and secured to minimize discomfort, as an alternative to a physical restraint. The nurse provides education to the daughter about delirium and its approaches, in addition to correcting the underlying problems, to support comfort and recovery (including familiar presence, calm approach, early mobility, and adequate food/fluids). The case manager covering the ED and the receiving nurse on the medical floor are notified of the patient's risk of functional decline, NH placement, and subsequent readmission, based on her TRST findings (cognitive impairment, use of five or more medications, recent fall, recent ED admission, and need for ADL support). During the handoff to the medical floor, the following are communicated: the patient's health and social history; details of ED admission, including findings; baseline and current cognitive status; fall and pressure ulcer risk; and daughter's involvement in her care. The daughter is present during the handoff.

SUMMARY

The nurse has the opportunity to positively influence the experience and outcomes of the older adult admitted to the ED. Careful assessment and planning, as well as considering age-related changes and the interaction of the acute illness with comorbid conditions are critical to prevent complications and promote resolution of the admitting problem. Clear and comprehensive communication during transitions and engaging family in care delivery and decision making support effectiveness and patient comfort.

NURSING STANDARD OF PRACTICE

Protocol 38.1: Care of the Older Adult in the Emergency Department

I. GOALS

To ensure nurses in acute care are able to

A. Identify evidence-based approaches and tools to assess the older adult in the ED
B. Describe interventions to prevent and manage geriatric syndromes in the ED
C. Discuss approaches to support effective transitions from the ED

II. OVERVIEW

A. One in five patients aged 65 to 74 years and one in four patients aged 75 years and older visit the ED each year (Albert et al., 2013).
B. The ED is:
   1. The portal to other settings, including the hospital, long-term care, and mental health facilities (Samaras et al., 2010)
   2. Used for the performance of complex diagnostic workups, overflow, and off-hour medical care

(continued)

Protocol 38.1: Care of the Older Adult in the Emergency Department *(continued)*

3. For some older adults, the only source of health care evaluation and treatment (Gonzalez Morganti et al., 2013; Samaras et al., 2010)

III. BACKGROUND AND STATEMENT OF THE PROBLEM

A. As compared to younger people, older adults:
   1. Have more diagnostic tests, longer stays in the ED, and are more likely to be admitted to the hospital (Banerjee et al., 2011)
   2. Are more likely to be readmitted on discharge from the ED; they also risk functional loss and higher rates of mortality (McCusker et al., 2007; Niska et al., 2010; Sklar et al., 2007)
   3. Are more likely to experience missed or incorrect diagnoses (Salvi et al., 2007), inadequate pain management (Hwang et al., 2010; Iyer, 2011), and less information (Baillie, 2005; George et al., 2006)

IV. ASSESSMENT OF THE OLDER ADULT IN THE ED

A. Triage/primary assessment
   1. Delays in triage for older adults are associated with increased waiting time, anxiety, and discomfort (Miró et al., 1999), and increased risk of mortality (Perdue et al., 1998).
   2. Tools
      a. The CTAS demonstrated high validity for older adults, especially useful for categorizing severity and for recognizing older adults who require immediate life-saving intervention (Bullard et al., 2008; Lee et al., 2011).
      b. The ESI includes a comprehensive algorithm that describes symptoms and physiological indicators as well as the resources anticipated to be used (Gilboy et al., 2012). There are reports of under-triage using this tool when guidelines are not precisely followed (Platts-Mills et al., 2010).
   3. A–B–C: identify and treat life-threatening conditions
      a. Airway: Challenges to establishing an airway include the presence of dentures, kyphosis, and cervical rigidity (Aresco & Stein, 2010).
      b. Breathing and ventilation: Consider age-related changes, including decreased pulmonary compliance, respiratory reserve, and arterial oxygenation (Blumenthal et al., 2010).
      c. Circulation: Use of antihypertensive medication may inhibit physiological response and/or mask signs of hypovolemic shock (Criddle, 2013).
   4. Consider atypical presentation and "red flags" (acute change on mental status and/or physical function, dyspnea, fatigue, self-neglect, apathy, and falls; Fletcher, 2004).

B. Screen for risk of adverse outcomes: useful in guiding a plan to prevent avoidable complications during the ED stay, if admitted during hospitalization, and after an ED visit when transitioning to home or another setting.
   1. TRST: Is predictive of subsequent ED use, hospitalization and NH admission (Meldon et al., 2003)
   2. ISAR: Is predictive of increased risk of death, institutionalization, functional decline and both repeat ED visit and hospital admission in the following 6 months after an ED visit (McCusker et al., 1999)

C. General assessment
   1. History
      a. Social history: living situation, marital status, work status, advance directives, supports within family and community, and stressors (Graf et al., 2011)
      b. Past medical/surgical history, medication use, allergies, weight loss/changes in oral intake, recent changes in diagnosis or medication regimens
      c. Baseline cognition, mood, and physical function: early and sensitive indicators of physiological dysfunction (Ellis et al., 2014; Hare et al., 2008)
   2. Cognition and mood
      a. Cognitive impairment: Geriatric Emergency Medicine Task Force recommends a mental status examination for older adults presenting to ED (Wilber, Lofgren, et al., 2005).
         i. Six-Item Screener (Callahan et al., 2006)

(continued)

Protocol 38.1: Care of the Older Adult in the Emergency Department *(continued)*

b. Delirium: suggested by abrupt onset of cognitive impairment
   i. Two-step process included in the Geriatric Emergency Department Guidelines Task Force (2014): Delirium triage screen followed by the Brief Confusion Assessment Method (Han et al., 2013)
c. Depression: May interfere with clinical presentation and may be associated with greater number of ED visits (Meldon et al., 2003; Sanders, 2001).
   i. ED-DSI: Three-question screener (Fabacher et al., 2002)

3. Physical function: Recent loss often precedes the visit to the ED and can signify underlying illness (Wilber et al., 2007).
   a. Basic ADL: Katz ADL Index (Katz et al., 1963) or Barthel Index (Mahoney & Barthel, 1965)
   b. IADL: Lawton IADL Scale (Lawton & Brody, 1969)
4. Medications:
   a. ADEs: One third are related to one of the following: warfarin, insulin, and digoxin (Budnitz et al., 2007)
   b. PIMs: Greater number is associated with frequent ED use (Wong et al., 2014).
   c. Geriatric Emergency Department Guidelines Task Force (2014) recommendations:
      i. Medication reconciliation
      ii. Screening for polypharmacy, PIMs, ADEs; collaborate with pharmacist, interdisciplinary team as indicated, and attending physician to correct.
5. Falls: Number one cause of nonfatal injuries treated in hospital emergencies in people older than 65 years (CDC, 2015b).
   a. ED evaluation
      i. Assess for injury (consider occult presentation): complete physical examination; EKG; complete blood count; electrolytes; medication evaluation, including measurable levels; and appropriate imaging (Adhiyaman et al., 2002; Dominguez et al., 2005; Rathlev et al., 2006; Sterling et al., 2001).
      ii. Assess the cause of the fall (Mitchell et al., 2002; Sanders, 1999).
         a) Targeted interview with patient and family: previous falls, location, activity, potential environmental factors, and symptoms preceding the fall
         b) Comprehensive history and physical examination
      iii. Estimation of future fall risk: guided largely by determination of reasons for past falls (Carpenter et al., 2009)
6. Substance misuse
   a. Misuse defined: use of a drug for purposes other than that for which it was intended
   b. Alcohol abuse: present in 14% of older adults presenting to the ED
      i. Screening tool: Alcohol Use Screen and Assessment in Older Adult has been shown to have good to excellent sensitivity and specificity (Ong-Flaherty, 2012).
   c. Evaluation (Center for Substance Abuse Treatment, 1998)
      i. Patient's social network; Identify which members are supportive of treatment and which are potentially hazardous to the patient. Harmful network members include active substance abusers; those who "enable" the patient's misuse; and those who abuse the patient physically, sexually, or emotionally.
      ii. Patient's mood, cognition, sleep patterns, and mental health history, including past treatment, should also be ascertained.
      iii. It should also be verified that the patient has adequate housing and access to food, adequate transportation, and medical care (Ross, 2005).
      iv. When there is evidence of substance misuse, nursing interventions focus on (a) monitoring for withdrawal; (b) providing an environment that is safe from potential harms to patient; (c) collaborating with the patient, family, physician, and social worker to secure a mental health evaluation and program directed to the substance abuse needs and support.
      v. Careful handoff should include the communication of the patient's history and clinical findings as well as safety issues, including fall risk and the presence of delirium.

(continued)

Protocol 38.1: Care of the Older Adult in the Emergency Department *(continued)*

7. EM
   a. Definition: physical, verbal, sexual, and psychological abuse, as well as abandonment, exploitation, and neglect (Acierno et al., 2010)
   b. Nurse is expected to know the organization's policies for reporting suspected EM, as required by The Joint Commission on Accreditation and state mandatory reporting requirements (Dong, 2012; Falk et al., 2012).
   c. Red flags of EM: delays in seeking treatment; signs of withholding or giving too much medication; missed appointments; use of several hospitals; driving to a hospital farther away from home; description of an event that does not fit the injury sustained; repetitive injuries (Heath & Phair, 2009); and signs of caregiver indifference, berating or threatening comments, hypervigilant/possessive behavior, or excessive concerns over finances warrant suspicion of EM (Bond & Butler, 2013; Stiegel et al., 2007).
   d. When EM is suspected:
      i. Separate the older adult from the caregiver and obtain a detailed history and physical assessment; interview the patient about his or her feelings of safety is an important screening question (Bond & Butler, 2013).
      ii. Conduct a careful medical history, including baseline conditions, and a comprehensive physical examination.
         a) Physical examination cues may include poor hydration; poor hygiene; suspicious injuries in unusual locations and bruises in various stages of healing; unexplained abrasions and/or markings on skin, including human bite marks, skin tears, pressure ulcers, or genital complaints, including infections or injury (Stiegel et al., 2007).
         b) Follow mandatory reporting procedures.

V. NURSING CARE STRATEGIES

A. Delirium and dementia
   1. Preventing delirium
      a. Control the environment:
         i. Support the family/familiar person (or volunteer) present with the patient
         ii. Provide sensory aides (glasses and hearing aids and offering hearing amplifiers and magnifiers as indicated)
         iii. Control noise
         iv. Avoid excessively bright lights when possible and
         v. Provide comfort measures, including fluids and a warm blanket
      b. Additional nursing interventions include promoting mobility and addressing need for pain management, toileting, rest/sleep and fluid/hydration (Hshieh et al., 2015; Rivosecchi et al., 2015).
   2. Managing delirium: in addition to interventions aimed at reversing the cause:
      a. Continue to provide aforementioned supportive measures
      b. Avoid physical and chemical restraints (American Association of Critical-Care Nurses, 2011)
      c. Educate patient/family about the etiology of delirium and interventions
      d. Involve family in promoting safety and comfort for the patient (Boltz et al., 2014, 2015)
B. Prevention of falls and related injuries
   1. Collaborate with the interdisciplinary team to modify fall risk (e.g., correct orthostasis, remove offending medications, etc.; Alexander et al., 2013)
   2. Provide close oversight (Capezuti et al., 2002)
   3. Encourage physical activity (e.g., range of motion)
   4. Pay attention to toileting (Alexander et al., 2013; Capezuti et al., 2002)
   5. For the person who is at risk for injury caused by cognitive impairment, weakness, and low mobility, provide low beds with bedside mats (Capezuti et al., 2002)
C. Prevention of pressure ulcers
   1. The use of pressure-redistributing foam mattresses has shown to be a cost-effective approach to prevent ED-acquired pressure ulcers (Pham et al., 2011)

(continued)

Protocol 38.1: Care of the Older Adult in the Emergency Department *(continued)*

2. The use of reclining chairs in the ED instead of ED gurney beds has been shown to reduce pain and improve patient satisfaction (Wilber, Burger, et al., 2005)
3. Evidence-based guidelines to prevent and manage pressure ulcers should be followed, including skin assessment, pressure relief/off-loading, prevention/treatment of infection, pain control, and nutritional evaluation and management (Ayello, 2011; Reddy et al., 2006)

D. Prevention of CAUTI
1. Definition: a UTI that occurs while a patient has an IUC or within 48 hours of its removal
2. Preventive practices
   a. Avoid unnecessary urinary catheter use (Apisarnthanarak et al., 2007; Fink et al., 2012; Hooton et al., 2010; Saint et al., 2013)
   b. Consider removal prompts and nurse-initiated urinary catheter discontinuation protocols (Fink et al., 2012)
   c. Use an aseptic technique and sterile products during catheter insertion; maintain cleanliness (Oman et al., 2012; Saint et al., 2013)
   d. Handoff: Communicate plan/need for surveillance and for the earliest removal (Wald & Kramer, 2011)

VI. TRANSITIONS FROM THE ED

A. Problem: misinformation (Steiner et al., 2010)
1. Primary source of older adults' dissatisfaction with ED care
2. Contributes to readmission

B. Factors associated with misinformation include underrecognition of cognitive dysfunction, lower health literacy, and financial impediments for prescriptions and recommended outpatient follow-up (Baraff et al., 1992; Carpenter et al., 2011; Han et al., 2011).
1. Three systematic processes to ensure appropriate transfer of information to patient/family and providers: (Geriatric Emergency Department Guidelines Task Force, 2014).
   a. Discharge planning
      i. Components: (a) evaluation of the clinical status related to the admitting problem, (b) assessment of physical and psychosocial functional status (including fall/safety risk), (c) risk assessment for subsequent functional decline (e.g., ISAR or TRST), (d) assessment of caregiver availability and ability, (e) an appraisal of the patient/family readiness and ability to learn, (f) medication review, (g) review of advance directives, and (h) referrals with follow-up arrangements (AHRQ, 2009; CMS, 2014)
      ii. Patients and families prefer active engagement and a range of options will support the patient's preferences and goals (Popejoy, 2011)
      iii. CMS (2014) recommends that EDs maintain a file of appropriate community-based services, supports, and facilities to which the patient can be referred
   b. Patient/family education
      i. Challenges to patient/caregiver understanding are limited literacy and numeracy (Ginde, Clark, et al., 2008; Ginde, Weiner, et al., 2008)
      ii. Print discharge instructions are often not written at appropriate reading levels (Williams et al., 1996; Jolly et al., 1993)
      iii. To address challenges (Geriatric Emergency Department Guidelines Task Force, 2014):
         a) Written instructions should be at the approriate grade level (established using a literacy calculator)
         b) Use plain language, focusing on "need to know" information, limiting the documents to essential content in order to avoid information overload (McCarthy et al., 2012)
         c) Information and educational material provided in large font suitable for older adults.
         d) Use the teach-back method (Schillinger et al., 2003; Slater et al., 2013)
         e) A standardized tool that assesses older adults' ability to self-administer medication such as the DRUGS. This tool requires subjects to perform the following four tasks with each of their medica-

(continued)

Protocol 38.1: Care of the Older Adult in the Emergency Department *(continued)*

tions: (a) identify the appropriate medication, (b) open the container, (c) select the correct dose, and (d) report the appropriate timing of doses (Edelberg et al., 2000; Kripalani et al., 2006)

c. Handoff
   i. Recommended standardized information (Geriatric Emergency Department Guidelines Task Force, 2014) to provide cross-settings:
      a) Presenting complaints
      b) Test results and interpretation
      c) ED therapy and clinical response
      d) Consultation notes (in person or via telephone) in ED
      e) Working discharge diagnosis
      f) ED physician note, or copy of dictation
      g) Patient condition (including fall risk, functional and cognitive status)
      h) New prescriptions and alterations with long-term medications
      i) Discharge recommendations: physical activity, diet, resources/services
      j) Support systems
      k) Advance directives
      l) Follow-up plan
   ii. Additional approaches: (a) a verbal report from ED nurses provided to the NH as well as written documentation; (b) an emergency form in NH residents' charts that contains predocumented information with an area to write in the reason for transfer, and (c) brief NH-to-ED and ED-to-NH transfer forms that are accepted and used by local NHs and EDs (Terrell & Miller, 2006)

d. Follow-up (Kessler et al., 2013)
   i. Telephone follow-up for patients discharged from the ED
   ii. Home visits provided to high-risk individuals
   iii. Telemedicine alternatives when indicated, especially in rural areas

VII. EVALUATION AND EXPECTED OUTCOME(S) FOR CARE OF OLDER ADULTS IN ED

A. Improved patient/family satisfaction and experience
B. Processes:
   1. Adherence to evidence-based practice and guidelines
   2. Throughput and waiting times
C. Better clinical outcomes: fewer falls, pressure ulcers, hospital-acquired infections, and improved diagnostic accuracy
D. Improved organizational outcomes: readmission rates (ED and hospital) and cost
E. Enhanced staff competencies and satisfaction

ABBREVIATIONS

A–B–C	Airway–breathing–circulation
ADE	Adverse drug events
ADL	Activities of daily living
CAUTI	Catheter-associated urinary tract infection
CMS	Centers for Medicare & Medicaid Services
CTAS	Canadian Triage and Acuity Scale
DRUGS	Drug Regimen Unassisted Grading Scale
ED	Emergency department
EM	Elder mistreatment
ESI	Emergency Severity Index
IADL	Instrumental activities of daily living
ISAR	Identification of Seniors at Risk

(continued)

Protocol 38.1: Care of the Older Adult in the Emergency Department *(continued)*

IUC	Indwelling urinary catheter
NH	Nursing home
PIMs	Potentially inappropriate medications
TRST	Triage Risk Screening Tool
UTI	Urinary tract infection

RESOURCES

*C*ollaboration for *H*omecare *A*dvances in *M*anagement and *P*ractice (CHAMP) website
http://www.champ-program.org/page/55/about-champ

Department of Health and Human Services Centers for Medicare & Medicaid Services Discharge Planning Guide
http://www.cms.gov/Outreach-and-Education/Medicare-Learning-Network-MLN/MLNProducts/Downloads/Discharge-Planning-Booklet-ICN908184.pdf

Emergency Nurses Association
www.ena.org

Geriatric Emergency Department Guidelines
http://www.acep.org/geriEDguidelines

Geriatric Emergency Nursing Education (GENE) Course
http://www.ena.org/education/education/GENE/Pages/Default.aspx

National Center on Elder Abuse Administration on Aging
http://www.ncea.aoa.gov/index.aspx

Portal of Geriatrics Online Education
www.pogoe.org

REFERENCES

Acierno, R., Hernandez, M. A., Amstadter, A. B., Resnick, H. S., Steve, K., Muzzy, W., & Kilpatrick, D. G. (2010). Prevalence and correlates of emotional, physical, sexual, and financial abuse and potential neglect in the United States: The National Elder Mistreatment Study. *American Journal of Public Health, 100*(2), 292–297. *Evidence Level IV.*

ACOVE-3 Investigators. (2007). Assessing Care of Vulnerable Elders-3 Quality Indicators. *Journal of the American Geriatrics Society, 55*(Suppl. 2), S464–S487. *Evidence Level VI.*

Adhiyaman, V., Asghar, M., Ganeshram, K. N., & Bhowmick, B. K. (2002). Chronic subdural haematoma in the elderly. *Postgraduate Medical Journal, 78*(916), 71–75. *Evidence Level V.*

Agency for Healthcare Research and Quality (AHRQ). (2009). *Discharge process reduces hospital use in the 30 days following discharge.* Retrieved from http://www.ahrq.gov/research/jun09/0609ra29.htm. *Evidence Level V.*

Albert, M., McCaig, L. F., Jill J., & Ashman, J. J. (2013). *Emergency department visits by persons aged 65 and over: United States, 2009–2010.* Statistical Brief #130. Retrieved from http://www.cdc.gov/nchs/data/databriefs/db130.htm. *Evidence Level V.*

Alexander, D., Kinsley, T. L., & Waszinski, C. (2013). Journey to a safe environment: Fall prevention in an emergency department at a level I trauma center. *Journal of Emergency Nursing, 39*(4), 346–352. *Evidence Level V.*

American Association of Critical Care Nurses. (2011). *AACN practice alert: Delirium assessment and management.* Retrieved from http://www.aacn.org/wd/practice/content/practicealerts/delirium-practice-alert.pcms?menu=practice. *Evidence Level VI.*

Apisarnthanarak, A., Rutjanawech, S., Wichansawakun, S., Ratanabunjerdkul, H., Patthranitima, P., Thongphubeth, K., . . . Fraser, V. J. (2007). Initial inappropriate urinary catheters use in a tertiary-care center: Incidence, risk factors, and outcomes. *American Journal of Infection Control, 35*(9), 594–599. *Evidence Level IV.*

Aresco, C., & Stein, D. (2010). Cervical spine injuries in the geriatric patient. *Clinical Geriatrics, 18*(2), 30–35. *Evidence Level V.*

Aschkenasy, M. T., & Rothenhaus, T. C. (2006). Trauma and falls in the elderly. *Emergency Medicine Clinics of North America, 24*(2), 413–32, vii. *Evidence Level V.*

Ayello, E. A. (2011). Changing systems, changing cultures: Reducing pressure ulcers in hospitals. *Joint Commission Journal on Quality and Patient Safety/Joint Commission Resources, 37*(3), 120–122. *Evidence Level VI.*

Baillie, L. (2005). An exploration of nurse-patient relationships in accident and emergency. *Accident and Emergency Nursing, 13*(1), 9–14. *Evidence Level V.*

Banerjee, A., Dehnadi, H., & Mbamalu, D. (2011). The impact of very old patients in the ED. *British Journal of Healthcare Management, 17,* 72–74. *Evidence Level V.*

Baraff, L. J., Bernstein, E., Bradley, K., Franken, C., Gerson, L. W., Hannegan, S. R., . . . Wolfson, A. B. (1992). Perceptions of emergency care by the elderly: Results of multicenter focus group interviews. *Annals of Emergency Medicine, 21*(7), 814–818. *Evidence Level V.*

Basic, D., & Conforti, D. A. (2005). A prospective, randomised controlled trial of an aged care nurse intervention within the emergency department. *Australian Health Review, 29*(1), 51–59. *Evidence Level II.*

Blumenthal, J., Plummer, E., & Gambert, S. (2010). Trauma in the elderly: Causes and prevention. *Clinical Geriatrics, 18*(1), 21–24. *Evidence Level V.*

Boltz, M., Chippendale, T., Resnick, B., & Galvin, J. E. (2015). Testing family-centered, function-focused care in hospitalized persons with dementia. *Neurodegenerative Disease Management, 5*(3), 203–215. *Evidence Level III.*

Boltz, M., Parke, B., Shuluk, J., Capezuti, E., & Galvin, J. E. (2013). Care of the older adult in the emergency department: Nurses views of the pressing issues. *The Gerontologist, 53*(3), 441–453. *Evidence Level IV.*

Boltz, M., Resnick, B., Chippendale, T., & Galvin, J. (2014). Testing a family-centered intervention to promote functional and cognitive recovery in hospitalized older adults. *Journal of the American Geriatrics Society, 62*(12), 2398–2407. *Evidence Level III.*

Bond, M. C., & Butler, K. H. (2013). Elder abuse and neglect: Definitions, epidemiology, and approaches to emergency department screening. *Clinics in Geriatric Medicine, 29*(1), 257–273. *Evidence Level V.*

Budnitz, D. S., Shehab, N., Kegler, S. R., & Richards, C. L. (2007). Medication use leading to emergency department visits for adverse drug events in older adults. *Annals of Internal Medicine, 147*(11), 755–765. *Evidence Level V.*

Bullard, M. J., Unger, B., Spence, J., & Grafstein, E.; CTAS National Working Group. (2008). Revisions to the Canadian Emergency Department Triage and Acuity Scale (CTAS) adult guidelines. *Canadian Journal of Emergency Medicine, 10*(2), 136–151. *Evidence Level IV.*

Callahan, C. M., Unverzagt, F. W., Hui, S. L., Perkins, A. J., & Hendrie, H. C. (2002). Six-item screener to identify cognitive impairment among potential subjects for clinical research. *Medical Care, 40*(9), 771–781. *Evidence Level IV.*

Capezuti, E., Maislin, G., Strumpf, N., & Evans, L. K. (2002). Side rail use and bed-related fall outcomes among nursing home residents. *Journal of the American Geriatrics Society, 50*(1), 90–96. *Evidence Level III.*

Carpenter, C. R., Avidan, M. S., Wildes, T., Stark, S., Fowler, S. A., & Lo, A. X. (2014). Predicting geriatric falls following an episode of emergency department care: A systematic review. *Academic Emergency Medicine, 21*(10), 1069–1082. *Evidence Level I.*

Carpenter, C. R., Scheatzle, M. D., D'Antonio, J. A., Ricci, P. T., & Coben, J. H. (2009). Identification of fall risk factors in older adult emergency department patients. *Academic Emergency Medicine, 16*(3), 211–219. *Evidence Level IV.*

Centers for Medicare & Medicaid Services (CMS). (2014). *Department of Health and Human Services discharge planning.* Retrieved from http://www.cms.gov/Outreach-and-Education/Medicare-Learning-Network-MLN/MLNProducts/Downloads/Discharge-Planning-Booklet-ICN908184.pdf. *Evidence Level VI.*

Center for Substance Abuse Treatment. (1998). Identification, screening, and assessment. In *Substance abuse among older adults.* (Treatment Improvement Protocol [TIP] Series, No. 26). Rockville, MD: Substance Abuse and Mental Health Services Administration (US) (Treatment Improvement Protocol [TIP] Series, No. 26). Retrieved from http://www.ncbi.nlm.nih.gov/books/NBK64420/. *Evidence Level VI.*

Corbett, H. M., Lim, W. K., Davis, S. J., & Elkins, A. M. (2005). Care coordination in the Emergency Department: Improving outcomes for older patients. *Australian Health Review, 29*(1), 43–50. *Evidence Level III.*

Crane, J. A. (1997). Patient comprehension of doctor–patient communication on discharge from the emergency department. *Journal of Emergency Medicine, 15*(1), 1–7. *Evidence Level IV.*

Criddle, L. M. (2013). *Geriatric trauma, in Sheehy's manual of emergency care* (7th ed.). St. Louis, MO: Saunders Elsevier. *Evidence Level V.*

Dominguez, S., Liu, P., Roberts, C., Mandell, M., & Richman, P. B. (2005). Prevalence of traumatic hip and pelvic fractures in patients with suspected hip fracture and negative initial standard radiographs—A study of emergency department patients. *Academic Emergency Medicine, 12*(4), 366–369. *Evidence Level IV.*

Dong, X. (2012). Advancing the field of elder abuse: Future directions and policy implications. *Journal of the American Geriatrics Society, 60*(11), 2151–2156. *Evidence Level VI.*

Edelberg, H. K., Shallenberger, E., Hausdorff, J. M., & Wei, J. Y. (2000). One-year follow-up of medication management capacity in highly functioning older adults. *Journals of Gerontology. Series A, Biological Sciences and Medical Sciences, 55*(10), M550–M553. *Evidence Level IV.*

Elie, M., Cole, M. G., Primeau, F. J., & Bellavance, F. (1998). Delirium risk factors in elderly hospitalized patients. *Journal of General Internal Medicine, 13*(3), 204–212. *Evidence Level I.*

Ellis, G., Marshall, T., & Ritchie, C. (2014). Comprehensive geriatric assessment in the emergency department. *Clinical Interventions in Aging, 9*, 2033–2043. *Evidence Level V.*

Ely, E. W., Truman, B., Shintani, A., Thomason, J. W., Wheeler, A. P., Gordon, S., . . . Bernard, G. R. (2003). Monitoring sedation status over time in ICU patients: reliability and validity of the Richmond Agitation-Sedation Scale (RASS). *Journal of the American Medical Association, 289*(22), 2983–2991. *Evidence Level IV.*

Engel, K. G., Heisler, M., Smith, D. M., Robinson, C. H., Forman, J. H., & Ubel, P. A. (2009). Patient comprehension of emergency department care and instructions: Are patients aware of when they do not understand? *Annals of Emergency Medicine, 53*(4), 454–461.e15. *Evidence Level IV.*

Ewing, J. A. (1984). Detecting alcoholism: The CAGE Questionnaire. *Journal of the American Medical Association, 252*, 1905–1907. *Evidence Level IV.*

Fabacher, D. A., Raccio-Robak, N., McErlean, M. A., Milano, P. M., & Verdile, V. P. (2002). Validation of a brief screening tool to detect depression in elderly ED patients. *American Journal of Emergency Medicine, 20*(2), 99–102. *Evidence Level IV.*

Falk, N. L., Baigis, J., & Kopac, C. (2012). Elder mistreatment and the Elder Justice Act. *Online Journal of Issues in Nursing, 17*(3), 7. *Evidence Level V.*

Ferreira, M. P., & Weems, M. K. (2008). Alcohol consumption by aging adults in the United States: Health benefits and detriments. *Journal of the American Dietetic Association, 108*(10), 1668–1676. *Evidence Level V.*

Fink, R., Gilmartin, H., Richard, A., Capezuti, E., Boltz, M., & Wald, H. (2012). Indwelling urinary catheter management and catheter-associated urinary tract infection prevention practices in Nurses Improving Care for Healthsystem Elders hospitals. *American Journal of Infection Control, 40*(8), 715–720. *Evidence Level IV.*

Fletcher, K. (2004). Geriatric emergencies part 1: Vulnerability and primary prevention. *Topics in Advanced Practice Nursing, 4*(2), 1–3. *Evidence Level V.*

Fulmer, T., Paveza, G., Abraham, I., & Fairchild, S. (2000). Elder neglect assessment in the emergency department. *Journal of Emergency Nursing, 26*(5), 436–443. *Evidence Level IV.*

George, G., Jell, C., & Todd, B. S. (2006). Effect of population ageing on emergency department speed and efficiency: A historical perspective from a district general hospital in the UK. *Emergency Medicine Journal, 23*(5), 379–383. *Evidence Level VI.*

Geriatric Emergency Department Guidelines Task Force. (2014). The geriatric emergency department guidelines. *Annals of Emergency Medicine, 63*(5), e7–25. *Evidence Level VI.*

Gilboy, N., Tanabe, T., Travers, D., & Rosenau, A. M. (2012). *Emergency Severity Index (ESI): A triage tool for emergency department care, Version 4.* Implementation Handbook 2012 Edition (AHRQ Publication No. 12–0014). Rockville, MD: Agency for Healthcare Research and Quality. *Evidence Level VI.*

Ginde, A. A., Clark, S., Goldstein, J. N., & Camargo, C. A. (2008). Demographic disparities in numeracy among emergency department patients: Evidence from two multicenter studies. *Patient Education and Counseling, 72*(2), 350–356. *Evidence Level IV.*

Ginde, A. A., Weiner, S. G., Pallin, D. J., & Camargo, C. A. (2008). Multicenter study of limited health literacy in emergency department patients. *Academic Emergency Medicine, 15*(6), 577–580. *Evidence Level IV.*

Gonzalez Morganti, K., Bauhoff, S., Blanchard, J. C., Abir, M., Iyer, N., Smith, A. C., . . . Kellermann, A. L. (2013). The evolving role of emergency departments in the United States. RAND Report. Retrieved from http://www.rand.org/content/dam/rand/pubs/research_reports/RR200/RR280/RAND_RR280.pdf. *Evidence Level V.*

Graf, C. E., Zekry, D., Giannelli, S., Michel, J. P., & Chevalley, T. (2011). Efficiency and applicability of comprehensive geriatric assessment in the emergency department: A systematic review. *Aging Clinical and Experimental Research, 23*(4), 244–254. *Evidence Level I.*

Gruneir, A., Silver, M. J., & Rochon, P. A. (2011). Emergency department use by older adults: A literature review on trends, appropriateness, and consequences of unmet health care needs. *Medical Care Research and Review, 68*(2), 131–155. *Evidence Level V.*

Guss, D. A. (1997). Hip fracture presenting as isolated knee pain. *Annals of Emergency Medicine, 29*(3), 418–420. *Evidence Level V.*

Han, J. H., Bryce, S. N., Ely, E. W., Kripalani, S., Morandi, A., Shintani, A., . . . Schnelle, J. (2011). The effect of cognitive impairment on the accuracy of the presenting complaint and discharge instruction comprehension in older emergency department patients. *Annals of Emergency Medicine, 57*(6), 662–671.e2. *Evidence Level IV.*

Han, J. H., Wilson, A., Vasilevskis, E. E., Shintani, A., Schnelle, J. F., Dittus, R. S., . . . Ely, E. W. (2013). Diagnosing delirium in older emergency department patients: Validity and reliability of the delirium triage screen and the brief confusion assessment method. *Annals of Emergency Medicine, 62*(5), 457–465. *Evidence Level IV.*

Hare, M., Wynaden, D., McGowan, S., & Speed, G. (2008). Assessing cognition in elderly patients presenting to the emergency department. *International Emergency Nursing, 16*(2), 73–79. *Evidence Level V.*

Heath, H., & Phair, L. (2009). The concept of frailty and its significance in the consequences of care or neglect for older people: An analysis. *International Journal of Older People Nursing, 4*(2), 120–131. *Evidence Level V.*

Hegney, D., Buikstra, E., Chamberlain, C., March, J., McKay, M., Cope, G., & Fallon, T. (2006). Nurse discharge planning in the emergency department: A Toowoomba, Australia, study. *Journal of Clinical Nursing, 15*(8), 1033–1044. *Evidence Level IV.*

Hooton, T. M., Bradley, S. F., Cardenas, D. D., Colgan, R., Geerlings, S. E., Rice, J. C., . . . Nicolle, L. E.; Infectious Diseases Society of America. (2010). Diagnosis, prevention, and treatment of catheter-associated urinary tract infection in adults: 2009 International Clinical Practice Guidelines from the Infectious Diseases Society of America. *Clinical Infectious Diseases, 50*(5), 625–663. *Evidence Level VI.*

Hshieh, T. T., Yue, J., Oh, E., Puelle, M., Dowal, S., Travison, T., & Inouye, S. K. (2015). Effectiveness of multicomponent nonpharmacological delirium interventions: A meta-analysis. *JAMA Internal Medicine, 175*(4), 512–520. *Evidence Level I.*

Hustey, F. M., & Meldon, S. W. (2002). The prevalence and documentation of impaired mental status in elderly emergency department patients. *Annals of Emergency Medicine, 39*(3), 248–253. *Evidence Level IV.*

Hustey, F. M., Meldon, S. W., Smith, M. D., & Lex, C. K. (2003). The effect of mental status screening on the care of elderly emergency department patients. *Annals of Emergency Medicine, 41*(5), 678–684. *Evidence Level IV.*

Hwang, U., Richardson, L. D., Harris, B., & Morrison, R. S. (2010). The quality of emergency department pain care for older adult patients. *Journal of the American Geriatrics Society, 58*(11), 2122–2128. *Evidence Level IV.*

Iyer, R. G. (2011). Pain documentation and predictors of analgesic prescribing for elderly patients during emergency department visits. *Journal of Pain and Symptom Management, 41*(2), 367–373. *Evidence Level IV.*

Jolly, B. T., Scott, J. L., Feied, C. F., & Sanford, S. M. (1993). Functional illiteracy among emergency department patients: A preliminary study. *Annals of Emergency Medicine, 22*(3), 573–578. *Evidence Level IV.*

Katz, S., Ford, A. B., Moskowitz, R. W., Jackson, B. A., & Jaffe, M. W. (1963). Studies of illness and the aged. The index of ADL: A standardized measure of biological and psychosocial function. *Journal of the American Medical Association, 185*, 914–919. *Evidence Level IV.*

Kessler, C., Williams, M. C., Moustoukas, J. N., & Pappas, C. (2013). Transitions of care for the geriatric patient in the emergency department. *Clinics in Geriatric Medicine, 29*(1), 49–69. *Evidence Level VI.*

Kripalani, S., Henderson, L. E., Chiu, E. Y., Robertson, R., Kolm, P., & Jacobson, T. A. (2006). Predictors of medication self-management skill in a low-literacy population. *Journal of General Internal Medicine, 21*(8), 852–856. *Evidence Level IV.*

Lawton, M. P., & Brody, E. M. (1969). Assessment of older people: Self-maintaining and instrumental activities of daily living. *The Gerontologist, 9*(3), 179–186. *Evidence Level IV.*

Lee, J. Y., Oh, S. H., Peck, E. H., Lee, J. M., Park, K. N., Kim, S. H., & Youn, C. S. (2011). The validity of the Canadian Triage and Acuity Scale in predicting resource utilization and the need for immediate life-saving interventions in elderly emergency department patients. *Scandinavian Journal of Trauma, Resuscitation and Emergency Medicine, 19*, 68. *Evidence Level IV.*

Lewis, L. M., Miller, D. K., Morley, J. E., Nork, M. J., & Lasater, L. C. (1995). Unrecognized delirium in ED geriatric patients. *American Journal of Emergency Medicine, 13*(2), 142–145. *Evidence Level IV.*

Mahoney, F. I., & Barthel, D. W. (1965). Functional evaluation: The Barthel Index. *Maryland State Medical Journal, 14*, 61–65. *Evidence Level IV.*

McCarthy, D. M., Engel, K. G., Buckley, B. A., Forth, V. E., Schmidt, M. J., Adams, J. G., & Baker, D. W. (2012). Emergency department discharge instructions: Lessons learned through developing new patient education materials. *Emergency Medicine International, 2012*, 306859. *Evidence Level V.*

McCusker, J., Bellavance, F., Cardin, S., Trépanier, S., Verdon, J., & Ardman, O. (1999). Detection of older people at increased risk of adverse health outcomes after an emergency visit: The ISAR screening tool. *Journal of the American Geriatrics Society, 47*(10), 1229–1237. *Evidence Level IV.*

McCusker, J., Ionescu-Ittu, R., Ciampi, A., Vadeboncoeur, A., Roberge, D., Larouche, D., . . . Pineault, R. (2007). Hospital characteristics and emergency department care of older patients are associated with return visits. *Academic Emergency Medicine, 14*(5), 426–433. *Evidence Level IV.*

McQuillan, K., Makic, M., & Whalen, E. (2009). *Trauma nursing: From resuscitation through rehabilitation* (4th ed.). St. Louis, MO: Saunders Elsevier. *Evidence Level VI.*

Meldon, S. W., Emerman, C. L., Schubert, D. S., Moffa, D. A., & Etheart, R. G. (1997). Depression in geriatric ED patients: Prevalence and recognition. *Annals of Emergency Medicine, 30*(2), 141–145. *Evidence Level IV.*

Meldon, S. W., Mion, L. C., Palmer, R. M., Drew, B. L., Connor, J. T., Lewicki, L. J., . . . Emerman, C. L. (2003). A brief risk-stratification tool to predict repeat emergency department visits and hospitalizations in older patients discharged from the emergency department. *Academic Emergency Medicine, 10*(3), 224–232. *Evidence Level IV.*

Miró, O., Antonio, M. T., Jiménez, S., De Dios, A., Sánchez, M., Borrás, A., & Millá, J. (1999). Decreased health care quality associated with emergency department overcrowding. *European Journal of Emergency Medicine, 6*(2), 105–107. *Evidence Level IV.*

Mitchell, L. E., Richardson, D. A., Davies, A. J., Bexton, R. S., & Kenny, R. A. (2002). Prevalence of hypotensive disorders in older patients with a pacemaker in situ who attend the Accident and Emergency Department because of falls or syncope. *Europace, 4*(2), 143–147. *Evidence Level IV.*

Moore, A. A., Karno, M. P., Grella, C. E., Lin, J. C., Warda, U., Liao, D. H., & Hu, P. (2009). Alcohol, tobacco, and nonmedical drug use in older U.S. Adults: Data from the 2001/02 national epidemiologic survey of alcohol and related conditions. *Journal of the American Geriatrics Society, 57*(12), 2275–2281. *Evidence Level V.*

Niska, R., Bhuiya, F., & Xu, J. (2010). National Hospital Ambulatory Medical Care Survey: 2007 emergency department summary. *National Health Statistics Reports*, (26), 1–31. *Evidence Level V.*

Oman, K. O., Makic, M. F.-M., Fink, R., Hulett, T., Keech, T., Schraeder, N., & Wald, H. L. (2012). Nurse-directed interventions to reduce catheter-associated urinary tract infections. *American Journal of Infection Control, 40*(6), 548–553. *Evidence Level III.*

Ong-Flaherty, C. (2012). Screening, brief intervention, and referral to treatment: A nursing perspective. *Journal of Emergency Nursing, 38*(1), 54–56. *Evidence Level VI.*

Parke, B., & McCusker, J. (2008). Consensus-based policy recommendations for geriatric emergency care. *International Journal of Health Care Quality Assurance, 21*(4), 385–395. *Evidence Level VI.*

Perdue, P. W., Watts, D. D., Kaufmann, C. R., & Trask, A. L. (1998). Differences in mortality between elderly and younger adult trauma patients: Geriatric status increases risk of delayed death. *Journal of Trauma, 45*(4), 805–810. *Evidence Level IV.*

Pham, B., Teague, L., Mahoney, J., Goodman, L., Paulden, M., Poss, J., . . . Krahn, M. (2011). Early prevention of pressure ulcers among elderly patients admitted through emergency departments: A cost-effectiveness analysis. *Annals of Emergency Medicine, 58*(5), 468–78.e3. *Evidence Level IV.*

Platts-Mills, T. F., Travers, D., Biese, K., McCall, B., Kizer, S., LaMantia, M., . . . Cairns, C. B. (2010). Accuracy of the Emergency Severity Index triage instrument for identifying elder emergency department patients receiving an immediate lifesaving intervention. *Academic Emergency Medicine, 17*(3), 238–243. *Evidence Level IV.*

Popejoy, L. (2011). Participation of elder persons, families, and health care teams in hospital discharge destination decisions. *Applied Nursing Research, 24*(4), 256–262. *Evidence Level IV.*

Press, Y., Margulin, T., Grinshpun, Y., Kagan, E., Snir, Y., Berzak, A., & Clarfield, A. M. (2009). The diagnosis of delirium among elderly patients presenting to the emergency department of an acute hospital. *Archives of Gerontology and Geriatrics, 48*(2), 201–204. *Evidence Level IV.*

Rathlev, N. K., Medzon, R., Lowery, D., Pollack, C., Bracken, M., Barest, G., . . . Mower, W. R. (2006). Intracranial pathology in elders with blunt head trauma. *Academic Emergency Medicine, 13*(3), 302–307. *Evidence Level V.*

Ross, S. (2005). Alcohol use disorders in the elderly. *Primary Psychiatry, 12*(1), 32–40. *Evidence Level VI.*

Reddy, M., Gill, S. S., & Rochon, P. A. (2006). Preventing pressure ulcers: A systematic review. *Journal of the American Medical Association, 296*(8), 974–984. *Evidence Level I.*

Rivosecchi, R. M., Smithburger, P. L., Svec, S., Campbell, S., & Kane-Gill, S. L. (2015). Nonpharmacological interventions to prevent delirium: An evidence-based systematic review. *Critical Care Nurse, 35*(1), 39–50; quiz 51. *Evidence Level I.*

Saint, S., Greene, M. T., Kowalski, C. P., Watson, S. R., Hofer, T. P., & Krein, S. L. (2013). Preventing catheter-associated urinary tract infection in the United States: A national comparative study. *Journal of the American Medical Association Internal Medicine, 173*(10), 874–879. *Evidence Level IV.*

Salvi, F., Morichi, V., Grilli, A., Giorgi, R., De Tommaso, G., & Dessì-Fulgheri, P. (2007). The elderly in the emergency department: A critical review of problems and solutions. *Internal and Emergency Medicine, 2*(4), 292–301. *Evidence Level V.*

Salvi, F., Morichi, V., Grilli, A., Lancioni, L., Spazzafumo, L., Polonara, S., . . . Lattanzio, F. (2012). Screening for frailty in elderly emergency department patients by using the Identification of Seniors At Risk (ISAR). *Journal of Nutrition, Health & Aging, 16*(4), 313–318. *Evidence Level III.*

Samaras, N., Chevalley, T., Samaras, D., & Gold, G. (2010). Older patients in the emergency department: A review. *Annals of Emergency Medicine, 56*(3), 261–269. *Evidence Level V.*

Sanders, A. B. (1999). Changing clinical practice in geriatric emergency medicine. *Academic Emergency Medicine, 6*(12), 1189–1193. *Evidence Level V.*

Sanders, A. B. (2001). Older persons in the emergency medical care system. *Journal of the American Geriatrics Society, 49*(10), 1390–1392. *Evidence Level V.*

Schillinger, D., Piette, J., Grumbach, K., Wang, F., Wilson, C., Daher, C., . . . Bindman, A. B. (2003). Closing the loop: Physician communication with diabetic patients who have low health literacy. *Archives of Internal Medicine, 163*(1), 83–90. *Evidence Level IV.*

Schnitker, L., Martin-Khan, M., Beattie, E., & Gray, L. (2011). Negative health outcomes and adverse events in older people attending emergency departments: A systematic review. *Australasian Emergency Nursing Journal, 14*, 141–162. *Evidence Level I.*

Sklar, D. P., Crandall, C. S., Loeliger, E., Edmunds, K., Paul, I., & Helitzer, D. L. (2007). Unanticipated death after discharge home from the emergency department. *Annals of Emergency Medicine, 49*(6), 735–745. *Evidence Level IV.*

Slater, B., Dalawari, P., & Huang, Y. (2013). Does the teach-back method increase patient recall of discharge instructions in the emergency department? *Annals of Emergency Medicine, 62*(4 Suppl. 2). *Evidence Level III.*

Steiner, C., Barrett, M., & Hunter, K. (2010). *Hospital readmissions and multiple emergency department visits, in selected states, 2006–2007. Statistical Brief #90.* Retrieved from http://www.hcup-us.ahrq.gov/reports/statbriefs/sb90.jsp *Evidence Level IV.*

Sterling, D. A., O'Connor, J. A., & Bonadies, J. (2001). Geriatric falls: Injury severity is high and disproportionate to mechanism. *Journal of Trauma, 50*(1), 116–119. *Evidence Level IV.*

Stiegel, L., Klem, E., & Turner, J. (2007). *Neglect of older persons: An introduction to legal issues related to caregiver duty and liability.* Retrieved from http://www.ncea.aoa.gov/Resources/Publication/docs/NeglectOfOlderPersons.pdf. *Evidence Level V.*

Terrell, K. M., & Miller, D. K. (2006). Challenges in transitional care between nursing homes and emergency departments. *Journal of the American Medical Directors Association, 7*(8), 499–505. *Evidence Level IV.*

Wald, H. L., & Kramer, A. M. (2011). Feasibility of audit and feedback to reduce postoperative urinary catheter duration. *Journal of Hospital Medicine, 6*(4), 183–189. *Evidence Level III.*

Wilber, S. T., Blanda, M., & Gerson, L. W. (2006). Does functional decline prompt emergency department visits and admission in older patients? *Academic Emergency Medicine, 13*(6), 680–682. *Evidence Level IV.*

Wilber, S. T., Burger, B., Gerson, L. W., & Blanda, M. (2005). Reclining chairs reduce pain from gurneys in older emergency department patients: A randomized controlled trial. *Academic Emergency Medicine, 12*(2), 119–123. *Evidence Level II.*

Wilber, S. T., & Gerson, L. W. (2009). *Emergency department care. Hazzard's geriatric medicine and gerontology* (6th ed.). Columbus, OH: McGraw-Hill Professional. *Evidence Level V.*

Wilber, S. T., Lofgren, S. D., Mager, T. G., Blanda, M., & Gerson, L. W. (2005). An evaluation of two screening tools for cognitive impairment in older emergency department patients. *Academic Emergency Medicine, 12*(7), 612–616. *Evidence Level III.*

Williams, D. M., Counselman, F. L., & Caggiano, C. D. (1996). Emergency department discharge instructions and patient literacy: A problem of disparity. *American Journal of Emergency Medicine, 14*(1), 19–22. *Evidence Level IV.*

Wong, J., Marr, P., Kwan, D., Meiyappan, S., & Adcock, L. (2014). Identification of inappropriate medication use in elderly patients with frequent emergency department visits. *Canadian Pharmacists Journal, 147*(4), 248–256. *Evidence Level IV.*

Zavala, S., & Shaffer, C. (2011). Do patients understand discharge instructions? *Journal of Emergency Nursing, 37*(2), 138–140. *Evidence Level IV.*

39

Advance Care Planning

Linda Farber Post and Marie Boltz

EDUCATIONAL OBJECTIVES

On completion of this chapter, the reader should be able to:

1. Distinguish instruction directives and appointment directives in terms of their strengths and weaknesses
2. Describe assessment parameters that would ensure that older adults receive advance directive information
3. Identify strategies to ensure good communication about advance directives among patients, families, and health care professionals
4. Guide a discussion of the benefits and burdens of various treatment options to assist proxy treatment decision making
5. Describe measurable outcomes to be expected from implementation of this practice protocol

OVERVIEW

As discussed in Chapter 4, one of the most important yet difficult situations health care professionals face is decision making about care for those who can no longer communicate their health goals, values, and treatment preferences. Surrogate decision making has particular relevance in the geriatric setting because the decisional capacity of older adults may be diminished, fluctuating, or lapsed. Precisely because individuals may lack the capacity to participate in discussions when decisions about treatment are required, advance care planning (ACP) has become an increasingly important priority. ACP enables individuals with decisional capacity to prospectively articulate their health goals, values, and treatment preferences so that they can be communicated and honored when the ability to make and communicate decisions has lapsed. It must be emphasized, however, that ACP is not about death, dying, or aging. It is how responsible adults control their future and should be an integral part of routine health care for every age at every stage of health.

One indispensable ACP tool is the advance directive, a simple and effective mechanism for the clear and legally enforceable documentation of these important decisions; all capable adults are empowered to complete such a document. Although health care professionals agree that all decisionally capacitated individuals should be encouraged to execute advance directives, the right *not* to do so must also be respected. When patients and residents are engaged in discussion about ACP, they should be informed and reassured that neither their providers nor the facilities in which they receive treatment will condition care or make assumptions about their care preferences if they do not have an advance directive.

For a description of evidence levels cited in this chapter, see Chapter 1, "Developing and Evaluating Clinical Practice Guidelines: A Systematic Approach."

BACKGROUND

Advance directives are legal instruments intended to secure an individual's ability to set out prospective instructions regarding health care. Conceived during the 1970s, they responded to the concern that patients who had lost the ability to make health care decisions might be subjected to medical interventions they would not have chosen, especially at the end of life. The 1990 federal Patient Self-Determination Act (PSDA) codified the right to conduct ACP by requiring all health care facilities that receive federal funds to offer patients or residents the opportunity to execute advance directives and assistance in doing so.

Although all 50 states and the District of Columbia have statutory and/or case law governing advance directives and all states honor them, their standards and restrictions differ (Olick, 2012; see also advance directives by state link in the Resources section). Although advance directives are useful whenever substitute decision making is required, they are most often invoked in the geriatric and critical care settings, as disease trajectory declines and the end-of-life approaches.

TYPES OF ADVANCE DIRECTIVES

Advance directives commonly come in two varieties—instruction directives, also known as living wills, and appointment directives, also known as health care proxies or durable powers of attorney for health care. In different ways, they provide direct access to patient preferences, enabling caregivers and families to rely on the most immediate and authentic of the decision-making standards. The first advance directive was the instruction directive or living will, a written set of value-neutral instructions about specified medical, surgical, or diagnostic interventions the individual *would* or *would not* want under particular circumstances, usually at the end of life. The structure of the document typically has a trigger phrase, such as, "If I am ever in an irreversible coma..." or "If I am ever terminally ill...," followed by instructions related to treatment in the specified circumstances.

Because the living will presents explicit articulation of the patient's previously expressed preferences, it is assumed to provide helpful guidance to family and caregivers about what she or he would choose in current circumstances. As became apparent, however, this type of directive is significantly limited by the fact that it is a static document that requires an individual to anticipate, often years in advance, some future medical condition(s) and determine the preferred treatment(s). Quality-of-life assessments and care preferences evolve over time, however, and it is not unusual for patients to change their minds about medical interventions that they thought they would or would never be able to tolerate.

Moreover, these documents do not always mean what they say. A living will that states, "I don't ever want to be on dialysis" probably does not mean, "I don't want three dialysis treatments if they will return me to baseline kidney function." What the individual probably means is, "I don't want to be on dialysis for the rest of my life." But living wills typically do not provide that kind of nuanced interpretation. Finally, this type of directive usually refers only to end-of-life care. The result is a set of instructions that reflect what the patient *believed* and *tried to communicate* at a *particular time* about what she *thought she would want under different circumstances* at a *later time*. Because of their significant limitations, living wills are most appropriate for someone without trusted friends or family to make surrogate decisions in the event of her or his incapacity.

The preferred advance directive is the appointment directive, also known as a health care proxy or a durable power of attorney for health care (DPOAHC). This document enables a capacitated individual to legally appoint another person to make medical decisions on her or his behalf after capacity has been lost. Depending on the type of appointment directive and the jurisdiction, the designated person may be known as a *health care agent, proxy, representative,* or *power of attorney (POA)*. For purposes of this discussion, the term *health care agent* will be used to represent any person legally appointed to make surrogate health care decisions. Appointment of an *alternate agent* is also recommended as a backup in the event the agent is unavailable or unable to make decisions on the patient's behalf.

The appointment directive is preferred over the instruction directive because it authorizes decision making in the event of *temporary* or *permanent* incapacity and enables greater flexibility in responding to unanticipated or rapidly changing medical conditions. Although the agent is generally required to honor the patient's previously expressed care preferences, if those instructions do not apply to or are inconsistent with the patient's current health needs, the agent is empowered to exercise judgment and use his knowledge of the patient's health goals, values, preferences, and decision history to make choices that promote the patient's best interest. Because the agent and alternate agent have the same decisional authority as the patient once the powers are activated, he or she may make any and all care decisions the patient could make if capable. Moreover, the authority of the agent and alternate supersedes that of anyone else (except a court-appointed guardian), including next of kin. This scope of authority presupposes a patient–agent relationship characterized by trust; familiarity with the patient's goals, values, and preferences; and the agent's willingness to exercise judgment and make often difficult decisions in the patient's interest.

As noted in Chapter 4, appointing a health care agent requires a lower level of capacity than that needed to make the often complex decisions the agent will make. All the individual must be able to do is understand that, at some future time, another person will be needed to make care decisions on her or his behalf and consistently designate the same person. Assessing this level of capacity can be as simple as asking, "If you couldn't make decisions about your care, who would you trust to do it?" Return in 30 minutes, ask the same question and, if the same person is named, that is sufficient. The importance of this provision, especially in the geriatric setting, is that even patients with diminished or fluctuating capacity who are unable to make complex medical decisions may still be able to appoint an agent and an alternate to assume this responsibility.

As noted previously, one type of appointment directive is the DPOAHC, but the term POA, when applied to advance health care planning, can cause confusion. Powers of attorney are delegations of legal authority for specified tasks. Often, a well-meaning person will show up in the clinical setting, clutching a document, and saying, "I'm the POA so I'm responsible for making decisions." Encourage staff to read the document. Very often, it will be a POA for banking or real estate or some other nonmedical responsibilities. Unless the document includes "health care decisions" or similar language, the document should be returned to the person with the explanation that the delegated powers do not include health care decision making (Post & Blustein, 2015).

A key presumption of the appointment directive is that the individual and the appointed agent(s) have engaged in candid and comprehensive discussions about the individual's goals, values, and treatment preferences (Span, 2015). The literature reveals that older adults with a DPOAHC or other advance directive are less likely to die in a hospital or receive unwanted or nonbeneficial care in comparison with those without an advance directive that provides insight into treatment preferences and guidance in making decisions about care (Silveira, Kim, & Langa, 2010). Some states require the agent's signature on the advance directive as confirmation that he is aware of the appointment and has accepted the decision-making responsibilities that are entailed. In states without that requirement, however, health care agents may first learn of their appointment when they are called from an emergency department.

Although an instruction directive, such as a living will, typically addresses treatment decisions at the end of life, the appointment directive becomes activated any time the individual has a *temporary* or *permanent* loss of decisional capacity, such as might be associated with trauma, illness, states of diminished awareness or impaired cognition (e.g., dementia, stroke, and delirium), alcohol or other substance use or abuse, elective or emergency surgery, or any other condition that impairs decisional capacity. In these situations, a health care agent has the legal authority to infer or interpret the patient's treatment preferences in real time, based on current medical circumstances and likely prognosis, as well as knowledge of the patient's goals, values, and preferences. These decisions address a wide range of clinical issues and are not restricted to decisions about forgoing life-sustaining measures as death nears. In essence, the agent is able to say, "If Mama had known then what we know now about her condition and prognosis, this is what she would have decided."

As discussed in Chapter 4, in the absence of an advance directive, the care team typically turns to informal surrogates, usually family, for guidance and consent in care planning. *Family consent laws* are state-specific statutes that set out the state-approved decision-making hierarchy—the order in which persons are authorized to make decisions on behalf of a patient who lacks decisional capacity and has not appointed a health care agent by means of an advance directive or DPOAHC.

Variations in Advance Directives

Some states have a combined directive that provides for the appointment of a health care agent and an alternate agent, as well as optional instructions regarding treatment specifics. A section on organ donation ("anatomical gift") has been added to the advance directives in some states, enabling the expression of preferences about organ donation. Some states limit the authority of the appointed agent or alternate to activate these preferences, unless this person is also the identified decision maker(s) for organ donation, a distinct statutory authority that is separate from the agent's rights and responsibilities to make decisions about the patient's treatment.

Instructional/medical directives have been suggested to address specific clinical situations and interventions. Individuals must decide prospectively which interventions they would want in the context of four scenarios: coma with virtually no chance of recovery; coma with a small chance of recovery but restored to an impaired physical and mental state; advanced dementia and a terminal illness; and advanced dementia. Among the interventions are cardiopulmonary resuscitation (CPR), artificial nutrition and hydration (ANH), dialysis, invasive diagnostic tests, antibiotics, and blood transfusion. This type of directive shares and even exacerbates the problems with living wills by requiring individuals to anticipate hypothetical clinical conditions and make choices about interventions she or he may or may not understand. In addition, the instructional/medical directive does not address the patient's desired goals of care, willingness to allow a short-term intervention, or treatment choices associated with stage of chronic illness or exacerbation.

Five Wishes is a hybrid directive that provides the opportunity to communicate decisions about (a) the person I want to make care decisions for me when I can't, (b) the kind of medical treatment I do or don't want, (c) how comfortable I want to be, (d) how I want people to treat me, and (e) what I want my loved ones to know. For many people, this is an accessible and nonthreatening way to frame the issues. Five Wishes is currently recognized in 42 states and is available in 26 languages (Five Wishes, Aging with Dignity, www.aginwithdignity.org/catalog/productsinfo.php?productsid=28). The "values statements" embedded in the Five Wishes document generally does not explore or express the patient's understanding of the benefits and burdens of various treatments, sometimes making it difficult to act on the patient's wishes and preferences (Lo & Steinbrook, 2004).

ADVANCE DIRECTIVES AND DECISION MAKING

The literature reveals that quality-of-life concerns, family influence, and pragmatism inform most adults' decisions to create an advance directive (Crisp, 2007). Older adults who execute advance directives tend to believe that their physicians know their wishes and do not feel that the directive would constrain their care. Those who do not create an advance directive tend to prefer that their families make decisions for them and may not appreciate the decision-making flexibility provided by an advance directive (Beck, Brown, Boles, & Barrett, 2002). Among participants of the original Framingham Heart Study, almost 70% discussed their end-of-life care preferences and advance directives with someone, but not necessarily a physician or other health care provider. More than half had a health care proxy or living will; slightly less than half had both types of directive. Most respondents wanted a comfort care plan at the end of life, but few agreed to forgo life-sustaining treatment interventions (e.g., ventilator and feeding tube) and said they would endure a burdensome health status (e.g., intense pain, confusion, and forgetfulness) in order to prolong life (McCarthy et al., 2008).

The literature also reveals the relationship between ACP and the degree to which individuals' care preferences are known, understood, and followed. Surrogate decision makers for hospice patients who talked with their surrogates about their end-of-life treatment wishes demonstrated greater understanding of the patients' preferences than the surrogates of patients who did not have these discussions (Engelberg, Patrick, & Curtis, 2005). Although surrogate decision making by families demonstrated greater accuracy than primary physicians in predicting older patients' preferences for life-sustaining treatments in hypothetical scenarios, having an advance directive did not necessarily improve congruence between patients' wishes and decisions made for them by others (Coppola, Ditto, Danks, & Smucker, 2001).

Studies have revealed that surrogate decision makers do not necessarily make treatment choices that reflect patients' preferences (Ditto et al., 2001; Mitchell, Berkowitz, Lawson, & Lipsitz, 2000). Although a small study found that communication between patients and their agents improved the accuracy of agent representations of patient preferences (Barrio-Cantalejo et al., 2009), a meta-analysis of surrogate decision making did not find that prior discussion between patient and agent improved agent accuracy in representing patient preferences (Shalowitz, Garrett-Mayer, & Wendler, 2006). Lack of concordance between patients' stated wishes and physicians' orders, however, was not shown to be simply a denial of patient rights; rather, physicians may have been relying on additional information to guide their treatment decisions (HardinHardin & Yusufaly, 2004).

Advance directives and high-quality end-of-life care have been associated with patients dying in their preferred location (e.g., at home or in hospice rather than in an acute care hospital), less likelihood of being burdened with an unwanted respirator or feeding tube, fewer concerns about family/significant others being informed about what to expect, and good physician communication (Bakitas et al., 2008; Detering, Hancock, Reade, & Silvester, 2010; Teno, Gruneir, Schwartz, Nanda, & Wetle, 2007). Patients with advanced illness requiring end-of-life care who were randomized to an Advanced Illness Coordinated Care Program reported increased satisfaction with care and communication, completed more advance directives, and their surrogates reported fewer support problems than patients receiving standard care (Engelhardt et al., 2006). As reported in a similar study (Teno et al., 2007), no difference was found in survival rates between the experimental and control groups. Unmet needs were reported, however, for adequate pain management and emotional support for patient and family (Teno et al., 2007).

Factors considered important by older patients with regard to their medical decision making and ACP included their religious beliefs, dignity, physical comfort, dependency, and finances (Hawkins, Ditto, Danks, & Smucker, 2005). Few patients indicated a desire to document their specific medical treatment preferences, but they highly valued verbal communication about these matters. Spouse surrogates were less likely than child surrogates to believe that prospective documentation of treatment preferences was necessary and more likely than child surrogates to consider financial issues important. Most patients accorded their surrogate considerable leeway in decision making. Patients indicated greater confidence in their child surrogates' understanding of their wishes than in the understanding of their spouse surrogates. An association between recent hospitalization and reduced desire to receive life-sustaining interventions (e.g., CPR, artificial nutrition, and hydration) was noted during an interview conducted just after recovery, but returned to baseline several months after hospitalization. These results challenge assumptions about the stability of treatment preferences and the temporal context during which treatment decisions are made (Ditto, Jacobson, Smucker, Danks, & Fagerlin, 2006; Hawkins et al., 2005).

Surrogate decision making has traditionally been grounded in the notion that an individual's characteristic preferences, long-held values, and cherished convictions provide the touchstone for decisions made on her or his behalf when capacity has lapsed. ACP in general, and advance directives in particular, have been held to be reliable guides for surrogate decision making because they authentically reflect the choices and principles that have given the individual's life meaning.

Mrs. B is an 82-year-old nursing home resident. Except for increasing dementia and an irregular heartbeat that requires a pacemaker, she is in good health and appears to have a very pleasant and comfortable life. She enjoys music, walking in the garden, and visits from her grandchildren, even though she is not entirely sure who they are. She has been admitted to the hospital to have her pacemaker changed, an intervention her two devoted daughters have refused. When asked their reason for refusing, they replied, "Our mother was an elegant, fastidious woman who always said that, if she were ever in diapers, she wouldn't want to live. If she could see herself now, she would be humiliated" (Post & Blustein, 2015).

A thought-provoking debate within the bioethics community challenges the justification for adhering to previously articulated preferences that may not adequately meet the markedly different needs of a now-incapacitated individual. Commentators have argued that persons with advanced dementia are, in effect, different people in terms of their health status and interests, for whom care decisions should be based on their current needs and preferences rather than their prior instructions (Blustein, 1999; Dresser, 1995; Post & Blustein, 2015). Ultimately, the ethical analysis would seem to rest on the imperative to preserve the dignity of the individual before us, as well as that of the individual she was.

Research Advance Directives

The notion of a research advance directive has been suggested because of the ethical implications of including in research studies participants with dementia who cannot provide informed consent (National Bioethics Advisory Commission, 1998). A research advance directive must be executed while the individual still has decisional capacity and must contain a detailed description and confirmation that the individual understands the purpose of research, including the concepts of risk, benefit, and burden. At the time of recruitment for a research study, the appointed surrogate decision maker must determine whether the individual's previously articulated intention to participate in research is congruent with the proposed research.

A study involving individuals with moderate dementia and their family surrogate sought to learn whether the patients wanted to retain decision-making control of their participation in future research or allow their surrogates to make the decision at the time of recruitment. Although many but not all individuals authorized their surrogates to make future decisions about research participation, surrogates did not always want to make these decisions (Stocking et al., 2006).

Psychiatric Advance Directives

Psychiatric advance directives are written by decisionally capable individuals who want to articulate their preferences about psychiatric treatment so that these preferences may be communicated and honored during periods when decisional capacity has lapsed. Research has shown that, given the opportunity to meet with a trained facilitator, adults with psychiatric disorders demonstrated sufficient capacity to make and document treatment decisions (Elbogen et al., 2007). Psychiatric outpatients have demonstrated a desire for assistance in creating an advance directive. This population tends to be female; non-White; with limited autonomy; a history of self-harm, arrest, and perceived pressure to take psychiatric medications (Swanson, Swartz, Ferron, Elbogen, & Van Dorn, 2006). Patients who complete a psychiatric advance directive typically exhibit good insight and reliably keep their outpatient mental health treatment appointments (Swanson et al., 2006).

Psychiatric advance directives in which patients identified their preferred psychiatric medications predicted not only that the medications were likely to be prescribed but also that medication adherence persisted over time (Wilder, Elbogen, Moser, Swanson, & Swartz, 2010). Most psychiatrists, psychologists, and social workers agreed that psychiatric advance directives would be helpful for patients with severe mental illness who are capable of creating them. The positive attitude of these mental health professionals is also supported by their knowledge that their respective state laws do not require them to follow a directive that contains a patient's refusal of appropriate mental health treatment or a request for treatment that is not clinically indicated (Elbogen et al., 2006).

Verbal Advance Directives

Although courts tend to prefer written advance directives, oral directives are typically respected, especially in emergency situations, and can be persuasive in a judicial decision about withholding life-sustaining treatment. Some states permit patients to verbally designate a health care agent in discussion with their physicians, rather than executing a written directive (Lo & Steinbrook, 2004). In determining the validity of a verbal advance directive, courts seek information about whether the statement was made by a mature person who understood the underlying issues, in a deliberate rather than casual or emergency context, was consistent with characteristic values and statements exhibited in other aspects of the individual's life, including religious or philosophical convictions, and addressed the specific medical condition necessitating a decision (Lo & Steinbrook, 2004). What might seem like an off-hand comment made by a patient in a practitioner's office or at the bedside should be recorded for just such an occasion, when clear and convincing evidence of the individual's wishes may be required.

OTHER TYPES OF ACP

In addition to advance directives, other mechanisms enable prospective medical decision making in specific circumstances.

Do-Not-Resuscitate Orders

Almost all diagnostic and therapeutic interventions require the informed consent of a decisionally capable patient or an authorized surrogate on behalf of a patient lacking decisional capacity. The few exceptions include emergency treatment that, if delayed, would result in significant harm or death, interventions to manage pain and other symptoms, and CPR. In the event of cardiopulmonary arrest, consent to resuscitation is presumed unless a physician enters a do-not-resuscitate (DNR) order, which is a specific order to refrain from performing CPR. Because of their life-and-death implications, most jurisdictions require DNR orders to have explicit informed consent, with few carved-out exceptions. Absent a DNR order, the patient's code status is presumed to be "full code" and, in the event of cardiopulmonary arrest, CPR must be performed.

Determining, communicating, and honoring a patient's code status often causes moral distress for caregivers, especially nurses. Care professionals are often conflicted and believe that CPR should not be instituted when it is considered medically futile, will not provide clinical benefit to the patient, or when death is inevitable and impending. Even in these situations, however, patients or surrogates often insist on CPR because of the misperception, fueled by television and film dramas, that it is always effective in restarting cardiac function. In the interest of clarity and accuracy, an increasing number of states have changed the name of the order from DNR to DNAR—do not *attempt* resuscitation.

Decisionally capable individuals or surrogates on behalf of incapacitated individuals have the right to *consent to or refuse* any proposed medical intervention. State-specific Natural Death Acts codify the right of capable patients to decline unwanted life-sustaining interventions, a right supported by the U.S. Supreme Court *(Cruzan v. Director*, 1990). Accordingly, capable patients and surrogates have the right to refuse CPR by consenting to a DNR order after they have been informed and demonstrate their understanding of the implications, including the relevant benefits, burdens, and risks. Because these are *medical orders* written by *physicians*, they are not considered advance directives, which are *patient*-generated statements of care preference.

Not uncommonly, conflict arises between and among patients, families, and care professionals regarding the necessity and appropriateness of DNR orders. For example, a physician may be unwilling to write a DNR order requested by a patient or surrogate because forgoing CPR would be considered clinically inappropriate. In this situation, the physician is required to notify the requestor that the order will not be entered and offer to transfer the patient's care to a physician willing to write the order.

The more typical scenario is a patient who has consented to a DNR order suffering a cardiopulmonary arrest and a hysterical family member imploring the care team, "You must save my loved one!" Too often, the patient is resuscitated and the code status is changed to full code with the reasoning, "When the patient can't make decisions, we always turn to the family." Reframing this dynamic is essential to the fundamental ethical obligation to respect patient autonomy. A medical order consented to by a capable patient is a compact between the patient and the care team. The patient's consent implicitly expresses confidence that his or her wishes will be honored and the care team implicitly promises, "When you are at your most vulnerable and cannot advocate for yourself, we will advocate for you." Accordingly, a DNR order consented to by a family member, health care agent, or other surrogate on behalf of an incapacitated patient may subsequently be modified or rescinded by an authorized surrogate. A DNR order consented to by a *decisionally capable patient*, however, *may be rescinded or modified only by the patient.* The rare exception is when *a health care agent appointed by the patient* determines that, in the context of *current changed clinical realities, the patient would have rescinded or modified the DNR order.*

Out-of-hospital DNR orders can protect individuals at home, in long-term care, rehab facilities, or other nonacute care settings from unwanted and clinically inappropriate CPR. Like in-hospital DNR orders, these are written by physicians based on clinical assessment and consented to by capable patients or surrogates. In one study, interest in and consent to DNR orders by patients on palliative home care programs were associated with sleep and incontinence problems, acceptance of their clinical condition and impending death, and their wish to die at home (Brink, Smith, & Kitson, 2008).

Artificial Nutrition and Hydration

Artificial nutrition and hydration (ANH) poses ethical, legal, and cultural challenges, primarily because of the traditional association between nourishing and nurturing. Before the PSDA became law, the U.S. Supreme Court ruled that capable patients have a constitutionally protected right to refuse unwanted medical treatment, a category in which the Court included ANH (*Cruzan v. Director*, 1990). Thus, ethical and legal reasoning that considers ANH the same as any other medical treatment recognizes no distinction between withholding and withdrawing life-sustaining measures, including ANH.

Powerful emotional and cultural influences persist, however, and are reflected in the varying state-specific legal evidentiary rules and procedures required to forgo or discontinue ANH. Some states hold that health care agents may not make decisions about forgoing ANH unless explicitly authorized to do so by the patient's advance directive. Some DPOAHC documents include a statement that the patient may check to verify that the POA is aware of the patient's wishes about ANH, without indicating the nature of those wishes. Living will statutes in some states regard ANH as a medical treatment, whereas other states consider it a comfort measure (Gillick, 2006). Given states' varying legislation, nurses need to be aware of the relevant laws of the state in which they practice and what those laws require, permit, and prohibit. They should also understand the extent to which patients and their surrogates are correctly informed about the clinical benefits and burdens of ANH at the end of life; the palliative alternatives; the cultural, religious, and language influences that may equate forgoing ANH with "starving" the patient to death; and strategies to address those concerns.

Orders for Life-Sustaining Treatment (POLST/MOLST)

An entirely different type of ACP is a consolidated set of medical orders for life-sustaining interventions. Originated in Oregon in 1995, this is a decision-making model that has been adopted by or is in development in approximately 40 states, which accounts for the variety of names (e.g., Physician or Practitioner or Pennsylvania Orders for Life-Sustaining Treatment [POLST], Medical Orders for Life-Sustaining Treatment [MOLST], Louisiana Physician Orders for Life-Sustaining Treatment [LaPOLST]; Span, 2015). In the interest of simplicity, the term *POLST* is used in this discussion to refer to all documents of this type.

Although POLST is a legal mechanism for ACP, it is fundamentally different from advance directives and, as noted in the following, distinguishing them is crucial to their proper implementation.

- Advance directives are *statements of patient intention, not medical orders.* Thus, an advance directive that stipulates, "If I am ever in one of the following three clinical conditions, I would not want cardiopulmonary resuscitation" is not a DNR order. That instruction may be translated into a DNR order by a physician if forgoing resuscitation is deemed clinically indicated. In contrast, POLST is a consolidated set of *medical orders* that are immediately actionable.
- *Every decisionally capable person 18 years of age or older* should have an advance directive, regardless of health status. POLST is intended for a subsection of the population, *individuals who have life-limiting illnesses and, typically, are expected to live 1 year or less.*
- Advance directives become *active only when the individual is determined to have lost decisional capacity.* POLST is *active from the moment it is signed.*

POLST is a comprehensive and specific product of discussion between a practitioner and a capacitated individual or the authorized surrogate for an incapacitated individual. It begins with a statement about the goals of care, which inform decisions about medical interventions, including CPR, airway management, ANH, hospitalization, and symptom management. Precisely because of the life-limiting nature of the individual's illness(s), POLST orders respond to current rather than anticipated or hypothetical clinical circumstances. The specificity of the POLST protocol provides guidance in honoring the individual's preferences, such as wishing to die at home or in a nursing facility, rather than a hospital; wanting to be alert, even if that means incomplete pain relief; and declining intubation in the event of respiratory compromise.

The literature reveals that, for appropriate individuals, POLST enables greater specificity and accuracy in communicating end-of-life care preferences in comparison with advance directives (Bomba & Vermilyea, 2006). Nursing home residents who have completed POLST are more likely to have documented their preference for limited life-sustaining measures and are less likely to be hospitalized if they have specified comfort measures only. There is no evidence of differences in symptom assessment or management between residents who have completed POLST and those who have not (Hickman et al., 2010).

DECISIONAL CAPACITY TO ENGAGE IN ACP

A threshold consideration is assessing the decisional capacity of individuals to engage in the various types of ACP. Chapter 4 includes an in-depth discussion of decisional capacity, its assessment, and its implications for health care decision making. The following section considers the role of capacity assessment in ACP.

As noted in Chapter 4, capacity is decision specific because different decisions require different levels of capacity. To suggest that, because an individual lacks sufficient capacity to make a complex treatment decision, he lacks the capacity to make other treatment decisions risks disenfranchising and disempowering him from any participation in planning his health care. To promote the exercise of patient autonomy to the fullest extent while protecting patients from the harms of deficient decision making, capacity assessment typically employs a sliding scale based on the notion of risk. The greater the risk attached to a decision, the higher the level of capacity required to honor the decision.

Chapter 4 explains that decisional capacity refers to an individual's ability to (a) understand and process information about diagnosis, prognosis, and proposed treatment options; (b) weigh the benefits, burdens, and risks of the options; (c) apply a set of values; (d) arrive at a decision that is consistent over time; and (e) communicate the decision. The sliding scale assessment strategy has particular application in the setting of ACP. An individual lacking the capacity to execute a living will or an instructional/medical directive may still have sufficient capacity to create a health care proxy or other type of appointment directive (Mezey, Leitman, Mitty, Bottrell, & Ramsey, 2000). The former task requires the individual to envision and make decisions about complex hypothetical clinical scenarios; the latter task requires only that the individual understand that someone else will make health care decisions on his behalf and consistently designate the same person.

Benefit–Burden–Risk Assessment

All health care decision making invokes an analysis that considers the intended and unintended consequences of a particular intervention; identifies the potential benefits, burdens, and risks; estimates the likelihood that they will occur; and weighs their importance to the patient. Based on this information, the analysis determines whether the likely benefits of the intervention will outweigh the burdens and risks. Not uncommonly, patients or surrogates are encouraged to consent to tests or treatments that are uncomfortable, burdensome, and even risky. The ethical justification is the conviction that the benefits, including clinical improvement, palliation, or improved function, will not only result but will outweigh the burdens and risks. Making the benefit–burden–risk assessment an integral part of care planning is a safeguard against performing tests and treatments because they are available rather than indicated.

Patients are not necessarily consistent in their treatment preferences, especially if the degree of burden or the chance to avoid death is unclear. Patients exhibit varying degrees of readiness for ACP, including communication with their families, other surrogates, and physicians about their health goals and the execution of an advance directive. Prior experience with health care decision making can influence a patient's perceptions of and readiness to engage in ACP (Fried, Bullock, Iannone, & O'Leary, 2009; Fried, O'Leary, Van Ness, & Fraenkel, 2007). An appointed agent can be helped to infer how the now-incapacitated patient would likely evaluate the benefits and burdens based on knowledge of the patient's values, preferences, and past behavior. Nurses can helpfully ask the agent, "If Mama could join this discussion, knowing what we know about her condition, prognosis, and treatment options, what would she say?" "Faced with similar situations in the past, how did she decide?" "What did she say when her brother was very ill?" Higher congruence between patient and agent regarding patients' end-of-life care preferences has been associated with a nurse-led discussion intervention: patients in the experimental group were more knowledgeable about life-sustaining measures, less willing to receive these interventions for a new, serious medical event, and less willing to live in a state of poor health (Schwartz et al., 2002).

The rationale for forgoing (either withholding or withdrawing) a treatment is eliminating a burdensome intervention that has neither produced nor is expected to produce the desired clinical result. Under these circumstances, analysis reveals that the burdens and risks significantly outweigh any compensating benefit. As discussed in Chapter 4, surrogate decision-making standards include *substituted judgment*, used when knowledge of the patient's goals, values, preferences, and decision-making history can be used to infer her or his likely decision about current clinical conditions, and the *best interest* standard, used when making decisions for a patient whose goals, values, and preferences are unformed or unknown. In guiding the process, nurses may helpfully ask, "What does this patient have to gain or lose as a result of this intervention?" "In what ways will this patient be better or worse off as a result of having or not having this treatment?"

CULTURAL PERSPECTIVES ON ACP

The notion of ACP and written directives is not universally accepted. In some cultures, the close-knit family may consider an advance directive intrusive, irrelevant, or a refusal, if not a legal denial, of care. Many in African American and other minority populations do not view an appointment directive as relevant, nor do they regard a DNR order as a summative value statement (Cox et al., 2006). Disinterest in creating an advance directive may reflect a present-day rather than a future orientation, and unwillingness to write about, speak of, or plan for death is a pervasive cultural influence on decisions not to engage in ACP. Likewise, deference to physician authority, the family's role in protecting the patient from the burdens of life and death decision making, and spiritual obligations or beliefs can exert a powerful influence on the willingness to address future health care.

Studies indicate different life-sustaining treatment preferences and decision-making contexts among racial and ethnic groups (Cox et al., 2006). Overall, Asian and Hispanic patients tend to prefer family-centered decision making, in contrast to White and African American patients' preference for patient-directed decision making (KwakKwak & Haley, 2005). Many studies have shown that White patients are more comfortable discussing treatment preferences, executing an advance directive, refusing certain life-sustaining treatments, and appointing health care agents than Black or Hispanic patients (Hopp & Duffy, 2000). Much of the reluctance of minority populations can be traced back to a regrettable history of exploitation in the clinical and research settings. Advance directive completion is more concentrated among White patients with higher education and income levels than among Black and Hispanic patients with low-income levels and less than a high school education (Mezey, Leitman, Mitty, Bottrell, & Ramsey, 2000). In comparison with White patients, Latino patients are less likely to complete an advance directive or communicate their preferences, even though there are no other differences between the groups with regard to advance directive preferences (Froman & Owen, 2005).

In contrast, African American patients have been shown more likely to want life-sustaining treatments to forestall death. The literature reveals that some African American patients perceive advance directives as a legal way to deny access to treatment and care, and tend to be more skeptical about the health care system than Mexican Americans and Euro-Americans (Perkins, Geppert, Gonzales, Cortez, & Hazuda, 2002). Among African American patients, spirituality and beliefs that conflict with palliative care goals, views of suffering, death and dying, and mistrust of the health care system discourage creation of advance directives (Bullock, 2006; Gerst & Burr, 2008; Johnson, Kuchibhatla, & Tulsky, 2008; Morrison, Zayas, Mulvihill, Baskan, & Meier, 1998). An intervention study using same-race peer mentors to discuss ACP with dialysis patients demonstrated a significant positive effect on Black patients but not on White patients. Positive outcomes included greater comfort in discussion, increased completion of advance directives, and enhanced feelings of well-being (Perry et al., 2005).

Cultural assimilation, as well as diversity, makes even basic assumptions about why people do and do not create advance directives very difficult. When patients and health care professionals are from different ethnic backgrounds, the value systems that inform ACP and decision making may conflict, often creating ethical and interpersonal tensions. Older Japanese American patients in the United States have been shown to prefer making their own decisions about forgoing life-sustaining measures, whereas older Japanese patients residing in Japan tend to defer decision making to their physicians and families (Matsui, Braun, & Karel, 2008). Subtle themes that resonate with elder

Japanese patients include feelings about being a burden to others, family obligations to support the dying person, and the overall utility of an advance directive as a means to reduce conflict without being intrusive (Bito et al., 2007). High religiosity, strong family decision-making history, and belief that the family should support the patient's wishes have been negatively correlated with advance directive creation in many cultural groups in the United States, including patients of Greek (MakridouMakridou, Efklides, Economidis, & Peonidis, 2006), Bosnian (Searight & Gafford, 2005), Asian Indian (Doorenbos, & Nies, 2003), and Malaysian heritage (Htut, Shahrul, & Poi, 2007). Predictors of advance directive completion for multi-ethnic urban seniors include what investigators called "modifiable factors," such as an established relationship with a primary care physician and their doctor's willingness to initiate the ACP discussion, being knowledgeable about ACP, recognizing the family role in decision making, and prior experience with decisions about mechanical ventilation (Morrison & Meier, 2004).

NURSES' ROLES IN ACP

All capable adult patients, regardless of their gender, religion, socioeconomic status, diagnosis, or prognosis, should be engaged in discussion about ACP and provided with information and assistance in creating advance directives. Rather than focusing on "The Conversation," these discussions should occur regularly as part of routine health care. Unlike interviews, they are most effective as patient-centered exchanges of information between patients and their care professionals.

Nurses have an essential role in assessing their patients' understanding of ACP and its importance at every age and stage of health. They can be crucial in reframing ACP as a way for responsible adults to control their health care future, rather than something reserved for the end of life. Providing accurate information about advance directives, the right to refuse as well as consent to treatment, palliative care, and hospice can counteract misinformation and apprehension about measures that permit rather than promote death. Oncology nurses tend to be more knowledgeable about advance directives than about the PSDA and the relevant laws in their respective states. They reported lacking confidence in their knowledge and ability to assist patients in creating advance directives (Jezewski et al., 2005). The ability to accurately distinguish treatment refusal and treatment withdrawal, assisted dying, and euthanasia was associated with being college educated, White, and having had prior experience as a health care agent for another person (Silveira, DiPiero, Gerrity, & Feudtner, 2000). They reported viewing their role as patient advocates, especially for adequate pain management at the end of life, despite knowing that it may hasten death.

Patients have reported that they complete advance directives to ease their family's financial and emotional burden and facilitate decision making. They want to discuss ACP, including end-of-life care, but they expect their health care professionals to initiate these discussions. Indeed, ACP discussions between patients and their primary care physicians were found to be a statistically significant predictor of patient satisfaction with their primary medical doctors (Tierney et al., 2001). Community-dwelling older patients receiving care in a general medical clinic were more likely to create an advance directive when they had received ACP information by mail before their appointments and their physicians had received a reminder to discuss ACP. Patients in the control group, whose physicians had received only a reminder to document having asked their patients whether they had advance directives, were less likely to create directives (Heiman, Bates, Fairchild, Shaykevich, & Lehmann, 2004).

When medical residents caring for hospitalized older adults were surveyed about their attitude, skills, and knowledge regarding ACP, they were found to have incomplete, often inaccurate, understanding of patients' decision-making processes, which influenced their willingness to have ACP discussions (Gorman, Ahern, Wiseman, & Skrobik, 2005). Not only did training in ACP improve the residents' knowledge of and comfort in discussing advance directives, it also positively influenced patients' interest in creating directives (Alderman, Nair, & Fox, 2008). Case managers reportedly vary in their knowledge about ACP, as well as their skills, response to family involvement and patient receptivity, and the ACP support they provide patients (Black & Fauske, 2007). Physicians have found advance directives that address hospitalization and emergency treatment to be most useful, but they also report that these directives are not always available, especially in emergency departments (Cohen-Mansfield & Lipson, 2008; Weinick, Wilcox, Park, Griffey, & Weissman, 2008).

A persistent myth, especially in minority populations, and one influenced by a history of abuse and denial of health care, is that an advance directive signals "do not treat," "withdraw life-sustaining measures" or, in some instances, "provide all interventions to keep me alive." Another pervasive belief is that, as soon as care professionals take possession of an advance directive, all its provisions, including discontinuing life-sustaining measures, will be implemented. This may explain why families will often acknowledge that the patient has an advance directive but not bring it to the care-providing facility until the end of life is near. Families, agents, and other surrogates should be helped to understand that the patient's preferences and instructions are applicable only in the indicated clinical circumstances.

Some patients erroneously believe that a lawyer is needed to execute an advance directive and that each state has only one specific advance directive document that must be used. In fact, state-approved directives may vary slightly and individuals need only ensure that their directives are consistent with the approved model in their respective states. Absent an appointed health care agent or alternate, the default surrogate decision maker is drawn from a state-approved hierarchy of family members authorized to serve as authorized health care surrogates. Typically, the list runs from those in closest relation to the individual to those more distantly related. This reflects the recognition in tradition and law that family plays a central role in making important decisions and the presumption that family is likely to know the individual's goals, values, and preferences. The reality in many cases is that families disagree or might be unaware of the patient's wishes. Nurses are in a position to identify potential family conflict and act to mitigate the effects of misinformed or delayed treatment decisions.

The language of some advance directives can be confounding, especially for those with limited literacy. Randomized to a standard advance directive form (12th-grade reading level) or one that had been modified to address literacy needs (fifth-grade reading level with graphics), most English- and Spanish-speaking patients preferred the modified form, resulting in a greater number of completed advance directives in the experimental group (Sudore et al., 2007). Most community-dwelling older adults were found to understand the purposes of various treatments, but understood less about potential outcomes, and vague terms, such as, "improvement" or "vegetable," were idiosyncratically interpreted (Porensky & Carpenter, 2008).

ACP INTERVENTIONS AND STRATEGIES

One way for nurses in the geriatric setting to begin discussion about ACP is by engaging the patient and/or health care agent in discussion about the quality of life valued by the patient, the importance of preserving or prolonging life, and how the patient's illness (and, ultimately, death) will affect others emotionally, financially, and in other significant ways. Some patients might want to focus on the quality of living, whereas others, nearing the end of life, may target the quality of their dying. Some might want to talk about where and from whom they prefer to receive care, including at the end of life. Some may fear their dependence on others, whereas some may find that inevitability more tolerable. Those considering hospice may specify a preference for receiving those services at home or an inpatient facility. Patients, families, agents, and others important to the patient might need encouragement and support in expressing what they each fear most and what will be important as death approaches.

Communication About ACP

Under state laws, Joint Commission standards, and patient bills of rights, patients have the right to have a qualified interpreter translate and transmit their discussions with their health care professionals. The interpreter may be the only person who recognizes subtleties in language, signaling that patients and their families may have a totally different understanding than the care team of words like "health," "illness," "improvement," and "decline;" what a treatment is expected to accomplish; and how dying and death are acknowledged clinically and culturally. If ACP or advance directives are associated with end of life, they are likely to be resisted as topics of conversation. If telling or contemplating "bad news" is culturally prohibited, it may be difficult to discuss end-of-life planning. Sensitive terms and concepts are not value neutral; nuance and syntax can make all the difference. Although a translator may provide literal word-for-word translation, an interpreter communicates fact and nuance, explanation and rationale.

Families should not be responsible for communicating between or among languages. Deliberately or inadvertently, facts may be omitted, shaded, or emphasized to protect or influence patient decisions. If it is difficult to translate medical terms and concepts from English to English, it is infinitely harder to do it while bridging language and cultural differences. Families should be reassured that their most important job is providing support and advice, which is why Joint Commission standards and hospital policies require trained interpreters when patients are more comfortable in another language.

CASE STUDY

Mrs. R is an 88-year-old woman, widowed for 22 years, with no next of kin, who lived alone before her admission to the nursing home 2 years ago. At that time, after consultation with her physician, she consented to an out-of-hospital DNR order. She had several comorbidities,

(continued)

CASE STUDY *(continued)*

including severe chronic obstructive pulmonary disease (COPD), chronic renal failure (blood urea nitrogen [BUN] = 58); mild to moderate dementia (Mini-Mental State Exam score of 20/30); mild depression (by Geriatric Depression Scale [GDS] score); and had lost 22 pounds, putting her below her ideal body weight (IBW).

Mrs. R now requires one-person assistance with all personal care needs and bruises easily. Her prognosis is poor and the goals of care are symptom management with a focus on comfort. She has had multiple hospitalizations for pneumonia, most recently 10 weeks ago, after which she had further weight loss and developed a grade II pressure ulcer on her right hip. She is receiving the standard meds for COPD, anxiety, sleeping problems, and appetite stimulation. Recent discussion about her quality of life by the interdisciplinary team noted that she no longer attends parties, Sabbath candle lighting, or discussion groups, all of which she used to enjoy. Beginning 6 months ago, Mrs. R has seemed unable to make decisions about her health care and her decisional capacity appears to fluctuate in relation to her O_2 saturation.

Five years ago, Mrs. R executed a living will that stipulated "aggressive comfort care, including ventilatory support" in the event she experienced respiratory distress, but no documentation addresses her preferences about being hospitalized if she has another COPD exacerbation, which is to be expected given the trajectory of the disease.

Two days ago, Mrs. R began to have stertorous breathing, a nonproductive cough, and episodes of diaphoresis. She appears exhausted, her solid food intake is minimal, and she becomes very dyspneic when taking small sips of fluid. A chest x-ray was equivocal and will be repeated today. Her current vital signs are: temperature: 100.8, pulse oximetry: 82%; pulse and blood pressure within normal limits. The nursing home has the resources to provide oxygen, intravenous (IV) fluids, and antibiotics.

Discussion

This case is complicated by the instructions in the living will, which illustrate the weaknesses of the instruction directive. These instructions were written before Mrs. R's disease trajectory had reached a terminal state; they may not be applicable to her clinical condition or in her best interest because nonaggressive, disease-directed measures are likely to be more burdensome than beneficial. How and by whom will the balance of benefits and burdens of hospitalization be assessed against remaining in the nursing home for palliative care? What was Mrs. R envisioning when she created her living will and what would she decide if she could do so now?

The nursing assistants, who have been very involved in Mrs. R's care, believe that she should be hospitalized, based on their knowledge of and affection for her. The professional staff argue from prognostications about the burdens and risks of ventilatory support, especially if it becomes permanent, as well as the likely multiple skin breakdowns that will occur if she is hospitalized. The standard of substituted judgment used by surrogates is not available because the living will is silent about her goals, values, and desired quality of life, and no close or trusted person is available to provide insight into what she would decide in the current situation. The best interest standard asks what a surrogate thinks would promote Mrs. R's well-being. At this point, the benefit–burden risk assessment becomes a critical part of the discussion.

However, Mrs. R's living will does not provide the necessary information or insight to confidently make decisions on her behalf. It stipulates "aggressive comfort care," without explaining what that meant to her. It mentions "ventilatory support" in the event of respiratory distress but does not specify whether she would find it tolerable as a long-term intervention or agree to it only as a temporary measure.

Mrs. R would have been much better served had she completed an appointment directive, authorizing a health care agent and alternate to make these decisions in real time after consultation with her physicians. Understanding her goals, values, and preferences, her agent would have been able to address the following questions: What is the potential for improvement or return to baseline? Would intubation prolong a life she would find acceptable or merely prolong her dying? Would intubation and hospitalization be responding to Mrs. R's needs or institutional anxiety? To what extent can the facility provide a quality of life with comfort and safety that might meet Mrs. R's interests at this time, even if this life quality were different from that which the staff previously enjoyed with her? In what way would hospitalization benefit Mrs. R and how might it harm her? What role might the administration of morphine play in relieving symptoms of air hunger, even though it risks shortening life? Mrs. R's agent would be authorized to make decisions that her instructions do not address or even depart from instructions that do not apply to her current medical condition.

(continued)

CASE STUDY *(continued)*

After discussion with an ethics consultant during an interdisciplinary meeting that included Mrs. R's involved family, the nursing home medical and nursing directors, the nurse assistants responsible for her care, and the director of social work who knows her well, a consensus decision was made not to hospitalize Mrs. R. The decision was guided by the clinical facts, the nursing home's ability to provide the necessary resources, Mrs. R's stated wishes for "aggressive comfort care," the likely downward trajectory of COPD, and reflection about Mrs. R's deteriorated condition after each hospitalization. Mechanical ventilation was determined likely to be more of a burden than a benefit at this point in her illness, one that would be inconsistent with a focus on comfort, which could be provided in familiar surroundings with judicious use of medication and intensive nursing care.

This case illustrates that ACP is not a static one-time event. Whether an individual's wishes and preferences are expressed in an advance directive or verbally, they must be documented and periodically reviewed whenever there is a change of clinical condition, life style, health care agent, goals, values, and/or preferences. The ability to reach consensus through discussion that addressed the concerns of all caring professionals while keeping the focus resident centered was key to arriving at a clinically and ethically principled, goal-driven plan of care.

SUMMARY

Discussions about ACP should occur over time, at every age and stage of health. Having such discussions shortly after hospitalization for an acute event can refocus on the goals of care and indicate where care can most effectively be provided (Happ et al., 2002). Rather than choosing specific interventions or technologies of life-sustaining treatment, nurses can help refocus the discussion with patients or residents, families, and agents on the health goals, values, and preferences; the characteristics of an acceptable quality of life, including comfort and function; and valued life activities. Among the things that nurses do better than anyone else is help individuals, their families, and other surrogates create a decision-making framework that enables care planning that most authentically and effectively meets patient/resident-centered needs and interests.

An environment conducive to meaningful ACP discussions requires appropriate time and location. An emergency admission is not an ideal time for thoughtful deliberation about these important matters. Distribution of advance directive forms without discussion, commonly done in hospital admission offices at the time of an elective admission, does not provide sufficient information or assistance in completing them, which is why nursing homes tend to wait 2 weeks before discussing advance directives with new residents. Many studies report that the most effective intervention for ACP is verbal information exchanged over several interactive sessions with health care professionals (Bravo, Dubois, & Wagneur, 2008; Tamayo-Velázquez et al., 2010), including the opportunity to ask questions (Jezewski, Meeker, Sessanna, & Finnell, 2007). Passive use of printed material and lack of opportunity to receive assistance in understanding directives do not promote their creation (Ramsaroop, Reid, & Adelman, 2007). Ultimately, however, the most effective way to encourage ACP is to reframe the perceptions of health care professionals and the lay public, disconnecting ACP from end of life and making it an integral part of routine health care throughout the entire therapeutic continuum.

NURSING STANDARD OF PRACTICE

Protocol 39.1: Advance Directives

I. GUIDING PRINCIPLES

1. All decisionally capable persons have the right to decide, in consultation with their health care providers, what will be done with their bodies.
2. All individuals are presumed to have decision-making capacity unless and until they are determined to lack this capacity.

(continued)

Protocol 39.1: Advance Directives *(continued)*

3. All adults who can participate in a conversation, either verbally or through alternate means of communication, should be offered the opportunity to engage in ACP and document their health care goals and preferences.
4. Health care professionals can promote enhanced quality of life for older patients and residents, including care at the end of life, by encouraging ACP and the creation of advance directives.

II. BACKGROUND

A. Education about ACP and advance directives
   1. Patients clearly indicate that they want information about advance directives.
   2. Patients indicate that they want nurses and physicians to engage them in discussions about ACP and advance directives.
   3. Despite indications of interest in ACP, only 19% to 36% of Americans have completed an advance directive.
   4. Documentation of treatment preferences is insufficient unless individuals discuss their health goals and values with their health care providers, families, and appointed health care agents.

B. Advance directives
   1. Enable capable individuals to designate and legally appoint trusted persons—a health care agent/representative/proxy/POA and one or more alternates—who will be authorized to make health care decisions on behalf of the individuals during any period of temporary or permanent decisional incapacity
   2. Are legal mechanisms that enable capable individuals to articulate and document their health goals and preferences regarding the kind of medical care they would or would not want in specified clinical circumstances if they lack the capacity to make or communicate their decisions
   3. Provide guidance for health care professionals, families, and surrogate decision makers about health care decisions that reflect an individual's goals, values, and preferences
   4. Provide immunity from civil and criminal liability for health care professionals, families, and appointed health care agents who follow in good faith the provisions of advance directives

C. Types of advance directives
   1. An *appointment directive* (also known as a health care proxy or DPOAHC) enables a decisionally capable individual to designate and legally appoint trusted persons—a health care agent/representative/proxy/POA and one or more alternates—who will be authorized to make health care decisions on behalf of the individual during any period of temporary or permanent decisional incapacity. An appointment directive enables the agent or alternate to confer with the care team in real time and respond to clinical conditions that are changing or were unanticipated by the now-incapacitated individual. Because the agent and alternate will have the same decisional authority as the individual to start, stop, or forgo treatment, the appointment directive is the preferred type of advance directive.
   2. An *instruction directive* (also known as a living will) enables a decisionally capable individual to provide instructions about medical treatment that would or would not be acceptable in specified clinical circumstances, typically at the end of life. The provisions of a living will are limited to what the individual *thought* that he or she *might want* in clinical circumstances that *have not yet occurred.*

D. An instructional or medical directive is intended to compensate for the weaknesses of living wills by posing hypothetical medical scenarios and asking the individual to indicate specific medical interventions that would or would not be acceptable. They suffer from the same limitations as living wills.

E. Verbal advance directives are honored in some states if there is clear and consistent evidence of the capable individual's preferences for care in current specific clinical circumstances. Legal rules governing oral advance directives vary by state.

III. ASSESSMENT PARAMETERS

A. All decisionally capable adults, regardless of age or health status, should be engaged in discussion about ACP and asked whether they have created advance directives. If they have an advance directive, a copy should be requested for the medical record. If they have not created an advance directive, information and assistance should be offered.

(continued)

Protocol 39.1: Advance Directives *(continued)*

B. Discussions about ACP and advance directives should be an integral part of routine health care throughout the arc of the health care continuum.
C. Discussions about advance directives should be conducted in the patient's preferred language to promote the exchange of information, questions, and answers.
D. Discussions should be conducted with sensitivity to the individual's health status, capacity to understand and process information, and degree of interest in participating in care planning.
E. Because capacity is decision specific rather than global, individuals who have been determined to lack the capacity to make specific decisions may still have the capacity to make less complex decisions or to designate an agent and alternate(s) to make health care decisions on their behalf.
F. When an advance directive has been completed:
   1. A copy of the document should be accessible in real time in the patient's current medical record.
   2. The primary care doctor should have a copy of the directive and be familiar with its provisions.
   3. The appointed health care agent and alternate agent(s) should have copies of the document and be familiar with its provisions.
   4. The directive should be reviewed periodically by the individual in consultation with the primary care doctor to determine whether it reflects the patient's current health status and preferences.

IV. CARE STRATEGIES

A. Nurses should assist patients/residents, appointed agents, and families in addressing ACP, including end-of-life care issues.
B. Patients should be encouraged to discuss their health goals, values, preferences, and concerns with their primary care physician, family, or other trusted surrogates.
C. In some instances, patients/residents may be more willing to discuss their health goals, values, preferences, and concerns with a nurse or clergy than a family member or other surrogate, and should be supported in doing so.
D. Patients should be assessed for their capacity to understand and process the provided information about their health status, prognosis, and treatment options.
E. Nurses must be mindful of and sensitive to the factors of race, culture, ethnicity, and religion that can influence the health care decision-making process. The fact that patients from non-Western cultures may not subscribe to Western notions of autonomy does not mean that these patients may not want to talk about their treatment preferences or concerns, or that they would not have conversations with their families about these matters.
F. Patients'/residents' decisions not to complete an advance directive must be respected, with the understanding that these decisions will be revisited at a later time. They should be reassured that they will not be abandoned or receive substandard care if they elect not to formulate an advance directive at this time.
G. Nurses should be aware of the institution's mechanisms for resolving conflicts between and among the patient/resident, family members, and the appointed health care agent or alternate, and assist the parties in using these resources to achieve resolution.
H. Nurses should be aware of the professional(s) responsible for managing introduction, explanation, assistance in creating, and storage of advance directives in their institution. These responsibilities may include checking with the patient/resident to ensure that a copy of the advance directive has been given to the primary health care provider(s), the appointed agent and alternate(s), and that the patient/resident is carrying a wallet-size card that includes advance directive and agent/alternate contact information.

V. EVALUATION OF EXPECTED OUTCOMES

To determine whether implementation of this protocol has influenced the type, as well as the number, of advance directives created, changes should be measurable and contribute to the facility's ongoing quality-improvement program. Special attention should be paid to the following:

A. Documentation in medical records of:
   1. Whether patients have been engaged in discussion about ACP and advance directives
   2. What was learned during the discussions about patients' health goals, values, preferences, and concerns

(continued)

Protocol 39.1: Advance Directives *(continued)*

3. Whether patients have completed advance directives

B. Presence of advance directives in patients' medical records, including
   1. Whether copies of patients' advance directives are in their medical records
   2. Whether the directives are easily accessible for reference by the care team

C. The use of trained or certified interpreters to assist staff in ACP discussions with patients whose primary language is not English

D. The number of requests by nurses for ethics committee consultation regarding questions, concerns, or conflicts related to advance directives

ABBREVIATIONS

ACP	Advance care planning
DPOAHC	Durable power of attorney for health care
DNR	Do not resuscitate
POA	Power of attorney

ACKNOWLEDGMENT

The author acknowledges the work of Ethel Mitty, PhD, RN, whose knowledge, wisdom, and collaboration enriched the previous iterations of this chapter. Her influence continues to touch and improve the lives of patients, students, and colleagues.

RESOURCES

Advance Directives by State
http://www.noah-health.org/en/rights/endoflife/adforms.html.
http://www.caringinfo/stateaddownloa

American Nurses Association (ANA)
ANA Center for Ethics and Human Rights
www.nursingworld.org
- Code for Nurses with Interpretive Statements
- Position statements on assisted suicide and active euthanasia, do-not-resuscitate, comfort and relief, Patient Self-Determination Act
- Selected bibliographies on ethical issues such as end-of-life decisions, foregoing artificial nutrition and hydration, nursing ethics committees, and assisted suicide and euthanasia

American Society for Bioethics + Humanities
www.asbh.org
- *International Journal of Nursing Ethics*

Caring Connections
A program of the National Hospice and Palliative Care Organization (NHPCO) includes Partnership for Caring, Inc. (formerly, Choice in Dying)
http://www.caringinfo.org
- Questions and answers: advance directives and end-of-life decisions; medical treatments and your advance directives; artificial nutrition and hydration and end-of-life decision making; do-not-resuscitate orders and end-of-life decisions
- Video: *Who's Death Is It, Anyway?* (PBS special)

End-of-Life Nursing Education Consortium (ELNEC)
American Association of Colleges of Nursing
www.aacn.nche.edu/elnec/curriculum.htm

Five Wishes AD
www.agingwithdignity.org/five-wishes.php
fivewishes@agingwithdignity.org

Physician Education Research Center
End of Life/Palliative Education Resource Center (EPERC)
www.eperc.mcw.edu/EPERC/FastFactsandConcepts

Physician's Orders for Life-Sustaining Treatment (POLST)
Washington State Medical Association
http://www.wsma.org/patient_resources/polst.cfm

REFERENCES

Alderman, J. S., Nair, B., & Fox, M. D. (2008). Residency training in advance care planning: Can it be done in the outpatient clinic? *American Journal of Hospice & Palliative Care, 25*(3), 190–194. *Evidence Level IV.*

Bakitas, M., Ahles, T. A., Skalla, K., Brokaw, F. C., Byock, I., Hanscom, B.,... Hegel, M. T. (2008). Proxy perspectives regarding end-of-life care for persons with cancer. *Cancer, 112*(8), 1854–1861. *Evidence Level IV.*

Barrio-Cantalejo, I. M., Molina-Ruiz, A., Simón-Lorda, P., Cámara-Medina, C., Toral López, I., del Mar Rodríguez del Aguila, M., & Bailon-Gómez, R. M. (2009). Advance directives and proxies' predictions about patients' treatment preferences. *Nursing Ethics, 16*(1), 93–109. *Evidence Level II.*

Beck, A., Brown, J., Boles, M., & Barrett, P. (2002). Completion of advance directives by older health maintenance organization members: The role of attitudes and beliefs regarding life-sustaining treatment. *Journal of the American Geriatrics Society, 50*(2), 300–306. *Evidence Level II.*

Bito, S., Matsumura, S., Singer, M. K., Meredith, L. S., Fukuhara, S., & Wenger, N. S. (2007). Acculturation and end-of-life decision making: Comparison of Japanese and Japanese-American focus groups. *Bioethics, 21*(5), 251–262. *Evidence Level IV.*

Black, K., & Fauske, J. (2007). Exploring influences on community-based case managers' advance care planning practices: Facilitators or barriers? *Home Health Care Services Quarterly, 26*(2), 41–58. *Evidence Level IV.*

Blustein, J. (1999). Choosing for others as a continuing life story: The problem of personal identity revisited. *Journal of Law, Medicine & Ethics, 27*, 20–31. *Evidence Level V.*

Bomba, P. A., & Vermilyea, D. (2006). Integrating POLST into palliative care guidelines: A paradigm shift in advance care planning in oncology. *Journal of the National Comprehensive Cancer Network, 4*(8), 819–829. *Evidence Level V.*

Bravo, G., Dubois, M. F., & Wagneur, B. (2008). Assessing the effectiveness of interventions to promote advance directives among older adults: A systematic review and multi-level analysis. *Social Science and Medicine, 67*(7), 1122–1132. *Evidence Level I.*

Brink, P., Smith, T. F., & Kitson, M. (2008). Determinants of do-not-resuscitate orders in palliative home care. *Journal of Palliative Medicine, 11*(2), 226–232. *Evidence Level IV.*

Bullock, K. (2006). Promoting advance directives among African Americans: A faith-based model. *Journal of Palliative Medicine, 9*(1), 183–195. *Evidence Level IV.*

Cohen-Mansfield, J., & Lipson, S. (2008). Which advance directive matters? An analysis of end-of life decisions made in nursing homes. *Research on Aging, 30*(1), 74–92. *Evidence Level IV.*

Coppola, K. M., Ditto, P., Danks, J. H., & Smucker, W. D. (2001). Accuracy of primary care and hospital-based physicians' predictions of elderly outpatients' treatment preferences with and without advance directives. *Archives of Internal Medicine, 161*(3), 431–440. *Evidence Level II.*

Cox, C. L., Cole, E., Reynolds, T., Wandrag, M., Breckenridge, S., & Dingle, M. (2006). Implications of cultural diversity in do not attempt resuscitation (DNAR) decision-making. *Journal of Multicultural Nursing & Health, 12*(1), 20–28. *Evidence Level V.*

Crisp, D. H. (2007). Healthy older adults' execution of advance directives: A qualitative study of decision making. *Journal of Nursing Law, 11*(4), 180–190. *Evidence Level IV.*

Cruzan v. Director, Missouri Department of Health, 497 U.S. 261 (1990).

Detering, K. M., Hancock, A. D., Reade, M. C., & Silvester, W. (2010). The impact of advance care planning on end of life care in elderly patients: Randomised controlled trial. *British Medical Journal, 340*, c1345. doi:10.1136/bmj.c1345. *Evidence Level II.*

Ditto, P. H., Danks, J. H., Smucker, W. D., Bookwala, J., Coppola, K. M., Dresser, R.,... Zyzanski, S. (2001). Advance directives as acts of communication: A randomized controlled trial. *Archives of Internal Medicine, 161*(3), 421–430. *Evidence Level II.*

Ditto, P. H., Jacobson, J. A., Smucker, W. D., Danks, J. H., & Fagerlin, A. (2006). Context changes choices: A prospective study of the effects of hospitalization on life-sustaining treatment preferences. *Medical Decision Making, 26*(4), 313–322. *Evidence Level IV.*

Doorenbos, A. Z., & Nies, M. A. (2003). The use of advance directives in a population of Asian Indian Hindus. *Journal of Transcultural Nursing, 14*(1), 17–24. *Evidence Level IV.*

Dresser, R. (1995). Dworkin on dementia: Elegant theory, questionable policy. *Hastings Center Report 25*(6), 32–38. *Evidence Level VI.*

Elbogen, E. B., Swanson, J. W., Appelbaum, P. S., Swartz, M. S., Ferron, J., Van Dorn, R. A., & Wagner, H. R. (2007). Competence to complete psychiatric advance directives: Effects of facilitated decision making. *Law and Human Behavior, 31*(3), 275–289. *Evidence Level II.*

Elbogen, E. B., Swartz, M. S., Van Dorn, R., Swanson, J. W., Kim, M., & Scheyett, A. (2006). Clinical decision making and views about psychiatric advance directives. *Psychiatric Services, 57*(3), 350–355. *Evidence Level IV.*

Engelberg, R. A., Patrick, D. L., & Curtis, J. R. (2005). Correspondence between patients' preferences and surrogates' understandings for dying and death. *Journal of Pain and Symptom Management, 30*(6), 498–509. *Evidence Level III.*

Engelhardt, J. B., McClive-Reed, K. P., Toseland, R. W., Smith, T. L., Larson, D. G., & Tobin, D. R. (2006). Effects of a program for coordinated care of advanced illness on patients, surrogates, and healthcare costs: A randomized trial. *American Journal of Managed Care, 12*(2), 93–100. *Evidence Level II.*

Fried, T. R., Bullock, K., Iannone, L., & O'Leary, J. R. (2009). Understanding advance care planning as a process of health behavior change. *Journal of the American Geriatrics Society, 57*(9), 1547–1555. *Evidence Level IV.*

Fried, T. R., O'Leary, J., Van Ness, P., & Fraenkel, L. (2007). Inconsistency over time in the preferences of older persons with advanced illness for life-sustaining treatment. *Journal of the American Geriatrics Society, 55*(7), 1007–1014. *Evidence Level IV.*

Froman, R. D., & Owen, S. V. (2005). Randomized study of stability and change in patients' advance directives. *Research in Nursing & Health, 28*(5), 398–407. *Evidence Level II.*

Gerst, K., & Burr, J. A. (2008). Planning for end-of-life care: Black–White differences in the completion of advance directives. *Research on Aging, 30*(4), 428–449. *Evidence Level IV.*

Gillick, M. R. (2006). The use of advance care planning to guide decisions about artificial nutrition and hydration. *Nutrition in Clinical Practice, 21*(2), 126–133. *Evidence Level V.*

Gorman, T. E., Ahern, S. P., Wiseman, J., & Skrobik, Y. (2005). Residents' end-of-life decision making with adult hospitalized patients: A review of the literature. *Academic Medicine: Journal of the Association of American Medical Colleges, 80*(7), 622–633. *Evidence Level V.*

Happ, M. B., Capezuti, E., Strumpf, N. E., Wagner, L., Cunningham, S., Evans, L., & Maislin, G. (2002). Advance care planning and end-of-life care for hospitalized nursing home residents. *Journal of the American Geriatrics Society, 50*(5), 829–835. *Evidence Level IV.*

HardinHardin, S. B., & Yusufaly, Y. A. (2004). Difficult end-of-life treatment decisions: Do other actors trump advance directives? *Archives of Internal Medicine, 164*(14), 1531–1533. *Evidence Level II.*

Hawkins, N. A., Ditto, P. H., Danks, J. H., & Smucker, W. D. (2005). Micromanaging death: Process, preferences, values, and goals in end-of-life medical decision making. *The Gerontologist, 45*(1), 107–117. *Evidence Level IV.*

Heiman, H., Bates, D. W., Fairchild, D., Shaykevich, S., & Lehmann, L. S. (2004). Improving completion of advance directives in the primary care setting: A randomized controlled trial. *American Journal of Medicine, 117*(5), 318–324. *Evidence Level II.*

Hickman, S. E., Nelson, C. A., Perrin, N. A., Moss, A. H., Hammes, B. J., & Tolle, S. W. (2010). A comparison of method to communicate treatment preferences in nursing facilities: Traditional practice versus the physician orders for life-sustaining treatment program. *Journal of the American Geriatrics Society, 58*(7), 1241–1248. *Evidence Level IV.*

Hopp, F. P., & Duffy, S. A. (2000). Racial variations in end-of-life care. *Journal of the American* Geriatrics *Society, 48*(6), 658–663. *Evidence Level IV.*

Htut, Y., Shahrul, K., & Poi, P. J. (2007). The views of older Malaysians on advanced directive and advanced care planning: A qualitative study. *Asia-Pacific Journal of Public Health, 19*(3), 58–67. *Evidence Level IV.*

Jezewski, M. A., Brown, J., Wu, Y. W., Meeker, M. A., Feng, J. Y., & Bu, X. (2005). Oncology nurses' knowledge, attitudes, and experiences regarding advance directives. *Oncology Nursing Forum, 32*(2), 319–327. *Evidence Level IV.*

Jezewski, M. A., Meeker, M. A., Sessanna, L., & Finnell, D. S. (2007). The effectiveness of interventions to increase advance directive completion rates. *Journal of Aging and Health, 19*(3), 519–536. *Evidence Level I.*

Johnson, K. S., Kuchibhatla, M., & Tulsky, J. A. (2008). What explains racial differences in the use of advance directives and attitudes toward hospice care? *Journal of the American Geriatrics Society, 56*(10), 1953–1958. *Evidence Level IV.*

KwakKwak, J., & Haley, W. E. (2005). Current research findings on end-of-life decision making among racially or ethnically diverse groups. *The Gerontologist, 45*(5), 634–641. *Evidence Level V.*

Lo, B., & Steinbrook, R. (2004). Resuscitating advance directives. *Archives of Internal Medicine, 164*(14), 1501–1506. *Evidence Level V.*

MakridouMakridou, S., Efklides, A., Economidis, D., & Peonidis, F. (2006). Advance directives: A study in Greek adults. *Hellenic Journal of Psychology, 3*(3), 227–258. *Evidence Level IV.*

Matsui, M., Braun, K. L., & Karel, H. (2008). Comparison of end-of-life preferences between Japanese elders in the United States and Japan. *Journal of Transcultural Nursing, 19*(2), 167–174. *Evidence Level IV.*

McCarthy, E. P., Pencina, M. J., Kelly-Hayes, M., Evans, J. C., Oberacker, E. J., D'Agostino, R. B., Sr., . . . Murabito, J. M. (2008). Advance care planning and health care preferences of community-dwelling elders: The Framingham Heart Study. *Journals of Gerontology. Series A, Biological Sciences and Medical Sciences, 63*(9), 951–959. *Evidence Level IV.*

Mezey, M. D., Leitman, R., Mitty, E. L., Bottrell, M. M., & Ramsey, G. C. (2000). Why hospital patients do and do not execute an advance directive. *Nursing Outlook, 48*(4), 165–171. *Evidence Level IV.*

Mitchell, S. L., Berkowitz, R. E., Lawson, F. M., & Lipsitz, L. A. (2000). A cross-national survey of tube-feeding decisions in cognitively impaired older persons. *Journal of the American Geriatrics Society, 48*(4), 391–397. *Evidence Level IV.*

Morrison, R. S., & Meier, D. E. (2004). High rates of advance care planning in New York City's elderly population. *Archives of Internal Medicine, 164*(22), 2421–2426. *Evidence Level IV.*

Morrison, R. S., Zayas, L. A., Mulvihill, M., Baskan, S. A., & Meier, D. E. (1998). Barriers to completion of health care proxies: An examination of ethnic differences. *Archives of Internal Medicine, 158*(22), 2493–2497. *Evidence Level IV.*

National Bioethics Advisory Commission. (1998). *Research involving persons with mental disorders that may affect decision making capacity* (Vol. 1). Rockville, MD: Author. *Evidence Level V.*

Olick, R. S. (2012). Defining features of advance directives in law and clinical practice. *Chest, 141*(1), 232–238. *Evidence Level V.*

Perkins, H. S., Geppert, C. M., Gonzales, A., Cortez, J. D., & Hazuda, H. P. (2002). Cross-cultural similarities and differences in attitudes about advance care planning. *Journal of General Internal Medicine, 17*(1), 48–57. *Evidence Level IV.*

Perry, E., Swartz, J., Brown, S., Smith, D., Kelly, G., & Swartz, R. (2005). Peer mentoring: A culturally sensitive approach to end-of-life planning for long-term dialysis patients. *American Journal of Kidney Diseases, 46*(1), 111–119. *Evidence Level II.*

Porensky, E. K., & Carpenter, B. D. (2008). Knowledge and perceptions in advance care planning. *Journal of Aging and Health, 20*(1), 89–106. *Evidence Level IV.*

Post, L. F., & Blustein, J. (2015). *Handbook for health care ethics committees* (2nd ed.). Baltimore, MD: Johns Hopkins University Press. *Evidence Level V.*

Ramsaroop, S. D., Reid, M. C., & Adelman, R. D. (2007). Completing an advance directive in the primary care setting: What do we need for success? *Journal of the American Geriatrics Society, 55*(2), 277–283. *Evidence Level V.*

Schwartz, C. E., Wheeler, H. B., Hammes, B., Basque, N., Edmunds, J., Reed, G., . . . Yanko, J. (2002). Early intervention in planning end-of-life care with ambulatory geriatric patients: Results of a pilot trial. *Archives of Internal Medicine, 162*(14), 1611–1618. *Evidence Level II.*

Searight, H. R., & Gafford, J. (2005). "It's like playing with your destiny": Bosnian immigrants' views of advance directives and end-of-life decision-making. *Journal of Immigrant Health, 7*(3), 195–203. *Evidence Level IV.*

Shalowitz, D. I., Garrett-Mayer, E., & Wendler, D. (2006). The accuracy of surrogate decision makers: A systematic review. *Archives of Internal Medicine, 166*(5), 493–497. *Evidence Level I.*

Silveira, M. J., DiPiero, A., Gerrity, M. S., & Feudtner, C. (2000). Patients' knowledge of options at the end of life: Ignorance in the face of death. *Journal of the American Medical Association, 284*(19), 2483–2488. *Evidence Level IV.*

Silveira, M. J., Kim, S. Y., & Langa, K. M. (2010). Advance directives and outcomes of surrogate decision making before death. *New England Journal of Medicine, 362*(13), 1211–1218. *Evidence Level IV.*

Span, P. (2015, March 13). The trouble with advance directives. *The New York Times.*

Stocking, C. B., Hougham, G. W., Danner, D. D., Patterson, M. B., Whitehouse, P. J., & Sachs, G. A. (2006). Speaking of research advance directives: Planning for future research participation. *Neurology, 66*(9), 1361–1366. *Evidence Level IV.*

Sudore, R. L., Landefeld, C. S., Barnes, D. E., Lindquist, K., Williams, B. A., Brody, R., & Schillinger, D. (2007). An advance directive redesigned to meet the literacy level of most adults: A randomized trial. *Patient Education and Counseling, 69*(1–3), 165–195. *Evidence Level II.*

Swanson, J., Swartz, M., Ferron, J., Elbogen, E., & Van Dorn, R. (2006). Psychiatric advance directives among public mental health consumers in five U.S. cities: Prevalence, demand, and correlates. *Journal of the American Academy of Psychiatry and the Law, 34*(1), 43–57. *Evidence Level IV.*

Tamayo-Velázquez, M. I., Simón-Lorda, P., Villegas-Portero, R., Higueras-Callejón, C., García-Gutiérrez, J. F., Martínez-Pecino, F., & Barrio-Cantalejo, I. M. (2010). Interventions to promote the use of advance directives: An overview of systematic reviews. *Patient Education and Counseling, 80*(1), 10–20. *Evidence Level I.*

Teno, J. M., Gruneir, A., Schwartz, Z., Nanda, A., & Wetle, T. (2007). Association between advance directives and quality of end-of-life care: A national study. *Journal of the American Geriatrics Society, 55*(2), 189–194. *Evidence Level IV.*

Tierney, W. M., Dexter, P. R., Gramelspacher, G. P., Perkins, A. J., Zhou, X. H., & Wolinsky, F. D. (2001). The effect of discussion about advance directives on patients' satisfaction with primary care. *Journal of General Internal Medicine, 16*(1), 32–40. *Evidence Level II.*

Weinick, R. M., Wilcox, S. R., Park, E. R., Griffey, R. T., & Weissman, J. S. (2008). Use of advance directives for nursing home residents in the emergency department. *American Journal of Hospice & Palliative Care, 25*(3), 179–183. *Evidence Level IV.*

Wilder, C. M., Elbogen, E. B., Moser, L. L., Swanson, J. W., & Swartz, M. S. (2010). Medication preferences and adherence among individuals with severe mental illness and psychiatric advance directives. *Psychiatric Services, 61*(4): 380–385. *Evidence Level II.*

Index

CPSIA information can be obtained
at www.ICGtesting.com
Printed in the USA
LVHW062139280120
645144LV00013B/68